AJN / MOSBY

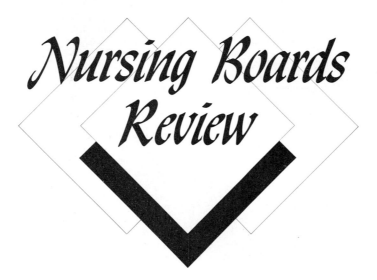

Nursing Boards Review

For the NCLEX-RN Examination

Managing Editor

Rose Mary Carroll-Johnson, MN, RN. *Nurse Editor, Valencia, California*

Coordinators for this Edition

Patricia E. Downing, MN, RN. *Formerly with University of California, San Francisco School of Nursing, San Francisco, California*

Susan Colvert Droske, MN, RN. *Assistant Professor, Texarkana College School of Nursing, Texarkana, Texas*

Alene Harrison, EdD, RN. *Associate Professor, Idaho State University Department of Nursing, Pocatello, Idaho*

Paulette D. Rollant, MSN, RN, CCRN. *President, Multi-Resources, Inc., Grantville, Georgia*

Marybeth Young, PhD, MSN, RNC. *Assistant Professor, Loyola University Niehoff School of Nursing, Chicago, Illinois*

Contributing Authors

Quilla D. Bell-Turner, PhD, RN. *Assistant Professor, University of Colorado Health Science Center, Denver, Colorado*

Karen S. Bernardy, MSN, RNC. *Atlanta, Georgia*

Suzette Cardin, MS, RN, CCRN. *Nurse Manager, Cardiac Care Unit/Cardiac Observation Unit, University of California, Los Angeles Medical Center, Los Angeles, California.*

Virginia L. Cassmeyer, PhD, RN. *Associate Professor, University of Kansas Medical Center School of Nursing, Kansas City, Kansas*

Robin Donohoe Dennison, MSN, RN, CCRN, CS. *Critical Care Clinical Nurse Specialist, Central Baptist Hospital, Lexington, Kentucky*

Gita L. Dhillon, CNM, MA, MS, MEd, RNC. *Certified Nurse Midwife, Memorial Medical Center, Las Cruces, New Mexico*

Deborah A. Ennis, MSN, RN, CCRN. *Associate Professor of Nursing, Harrisburg Area Community College, Harrisburg, Pennsylvania*

Alice Copp Franz, MA, RN. *Associate Professor, Maternal-Child Nursing, formerly with Indiana University-Purdue University at Fort Wayne, Fort Wayne, Indiana*

Peg Gray-Vickrey, MS, RNC. *Doctoral Student University at Buffalo School of Nursing, Buffalo, New York*

Sharon Golub, MN, RN. *Instructor of Nursing, Mount St. Mary's College, Los Angeles, California*

E. Ingvarda Hanson, MSN, RN

Kathleen Haubrich, MSN, RNC. *Assistant Professor, Miami University, Hamilton, Ohio*

Ann L. Jessop, MSN, RN. *Associate Chief, Nursing Service for Education, Veteran's Administration Medical Center, Marlin, Texas*

Roberta A. Kordish, MSN, RN. *Owner, Clinical Nurse Specialist, Professional Nurse Associate, Inc., Cleveland, Ohio*

Janet E. Bloomer Kristic, MSN, RN, CS. *Assistant Professor, Psychotherapist/Consultant. University of Oklahoma College of Nursing, Oklahoma City, Oklahoma*

Alma Joel Labunski, EdD, MS, RN. *Associate Professor, St. Xavier School of Nursing, Chicago, Illinois*

Judith K. Leavitt, MEd, RN, *Consultant, Ithaca, New York*

Mariann C. Lovell, MS, RN. *Doctoral Student, Ohio State University, Columbus, Ohio*

Michele A. Michael, PhD, RN. *Assistant Professor, University of Maryland School of Nursing, Baltimore, Maryland*

Maribeth L. Moran, MSN, RN. *Assistant Professor, University of Oklahoma College of Nursing, Oklahoma City, Oklahoma*

Judith K. Sands, EdD, RN. *Associate Professor, University of Virginia School of Nursing, Charlottesville, Virginia*

Marianne Scharbo-DeHaan, CNM, MN, RN. *Assistant Professor, Nurse-Midwifery, Emory University Nell Hodgson Woodruff School of Nursing, Atlanta, Georgia*

Bernadette Mazurek Vulcan, MSN, RNC, PNP. *Doctoral Candidate and Senior Associate, University of Rochester School of Nursing, Rochester, New York*

Janet Sullivan Wilson, MEd, RN. *Assistant Professor and Clinical Consultant, University of Oklahoma College of Nursing, Oklahoma City, Oklahoma*

Contributors to Previous Editions

Ida M. Androwich, MS, RN
Janis P. Bellack, PhD, MN, RN
Kay Bensing, MA, RN
Cecily Lynn Betz, PhD, RN
Carolyn V. Billings, MSN, RN, CS
Phyllis Gorney Cooper, MSN, RN
Olivian DeSouza, MSN, RN
Cynthia Dunsmore, MSN, RN
Jackie Flaskerud, PhD, RN
Carolyn Vas Fore, MSN, RN
Elizabeth Anne Gomez, MSN, RN
Anne C. Holland, MSN, RN
Stephen Jones, MSN, RNC
Michele M. Kamradt, EdD, RN
Carol W. Kennedy, PhD, RN
Deborah Koniak, EdD, RN
Beverly Kopala, MS, RN
Karen Krejci, MSN, RN
Esther Matassarin-Jacobs, PhD, RN
Susan McCabe, MS, RN
Edwina A. McConnell, PhD, MS, RN
Jerry R. Myhan, MSN, RN
B. Patricia Nix, MSN, RN
Kathleen Deska Pagana, PhD, RN
Tamra Parsons, MSN, RN
Joan Reighley, MN, RN
Constance M. Ritzman, MSN, RN
Mary Charles Santopietro, EdD, MS, EdM, RN, CS
Ann M. Schofield, MS, RN
Victoria Schoolcraft, MSN, RN
Diane S. Smith, MSN, RN, CS
Diane M. Taylor Snow, MSN, RN
Karen Stefaniak, MSN, RN
Deborah L. Ulrich, MA, RN
Francene Weatherby, MSN, RNC
Gail D. Wegner, MSN, RN

AJN/MOSBY

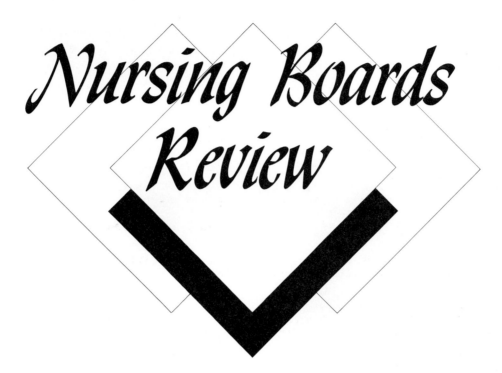

Nursing Boards Review

For the NCLEX-RN Examination

EIGHTH EDITION

with **61** illustrations

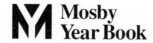 **Mosby**
Year Book

St. Louis Baltimore Boston Chicago London Philadelphia Sydney Toronto

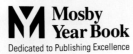

Mosby
Year Book
Dedicated to Publishing Excellence

Senior Editor: Nancy L. Coon
Managing Editor: Susan R. Epstein
Project Manager: Karen Edwards
Production Editor: James Russell
Production Assistant: Ginny Douglas
Book and Cover Design: Gail Morey Hudson

EIGHTH EDITION

Printed in the United States of America

Mosby–Year Book, Inc.
11830 Westline Industrial Drive
St. Louis, MO 63146

International Standard Book Number 0-8016-0019-7

GW/MV 9 8 7 6 5 4 3 2 1

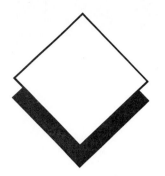

Introduction

Congratulations! You have passed a big milestone—completing your nursing program. A new and exciting career awaits you. Only one more challenge remains: passing the NCLEX-RN.

The *AJN/Mosby Nursing Boards Review* gives you a comprehensive review of the essential content you need to pass the NCLEX-RN. Your educational program laid the groundwork to take the boards, but review and study now are essential ingredients to guarantee success on the examination.

The NCLEX-RN examination focuses on two areas: the nursing process and client needs. It emphasizes the care of both healthy and ill clients. Content areas covered by the test include care of the adult, the child, the childbearing family, and the client with an emotional problem.

The *AJN/Mosby Nursing Boards Review* has three distinct components. The first, Section One, introduces you to the format of the NCLEX-RN test and its scoring method.

To augment your test-taking skills, this section reviews strategies to increase your competence and confidence. To help you on the day of the examination, it presents techniques to reduce stress. As you study, refer to this section frequently to reinforce principles you will need during the examination.

The second component, contained in Sections Two through Five, covers the four clinical areas. The nursing process provides a consistent framework for organizing client care. Assessment and implementation actions are listed in order of priority. Goals are client centered. Evaluation statements are measurable and reflect the goals. Nursing diagnoses reflect the latest list approved by the North American Nursing Diagnosis Association (NANDA).

The content in each section is supplemented by tables, summaries, and illustrations to clarify information and reinforce your knowledge of specific health problems, pharmacology, growth and development, and nutrition. Reprints of articles from the *American Journal of Nursing* and *MCN* are collected at the end of each section. These provide a convenient reference to supplement some content and may be especially useful if many months have separated one clinical rotation from your exam preparation.

Review one clinical area at a time. Start with the one you feel the most comfortable with; this will bolster your confidence to continue. Use a highlighter pen to underline areas you want to return to for more study. Make notes in the margins. Use your nursing texts to look up unfamiliar material or to broaden your knowledge base.

Section 6 contains a practice exam, simulating the actual NCLEX-RN exam. It consists of four integrated tests of approximately 94 questions each, to parallel the four parts of the NCLEX. You may want to use this exam as a pretest before you begin your review to identify your strengths and weaknesses. Take the exam again after you have completed your review to see how much you have improved your score. These tests will also help you learn to pace yourself for the NCLEX. Allow 90 minutes for each test.

Answers and rationales for both the correct and incorrect answers are provided for all test questions. The rationales can help clarify faulty thought processes, correct misinformation, and help you learn from your mistakes. Also included is a reference to the section and subsection of the book where relevant content may be found.

You may decide to take an *intensive review course,* such as the AJN/Mosby Nursing Boards Review. This five-day program gives you the opportunity to listen to specialists in clinical areas who are also experienced in the review process.

Your success with the NCLEX-RN sets you firmly on the road to a fulfilling and varied career that is full of opportunities. All those responsible for this volume—from the staffs at the American Journal of Nursing Company and Mosby–Year Book to the coordinators and contributing authors who prepared this material—join me in wishing you the best of luck on the exam and in your career as a professional nurse.

Rose Mary Carroll-Johnson, MN, RN
Managing Editor

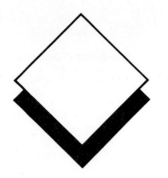

Contents

3   NURSING CARE OF THE ADULT, 111

Coordinators

Patricia E. Downing, MN, RN
Paulette D. Rollant, MSN, RN, CCRN

Contributors

Suzette Cardin, MS, RN, CCRN
Virginia L. Cassmeyer, PhD, RN
Robin Donohoe Dennison, MS, RN, CCRN, CS
Deborah A. Ennis, MSN, RN, CCRN
Peg Gray-Vickery, MS, RN, C
Alma J. Labunski, EdD, MS, RN
Judith K. Sands, EdD, RN

4 NURSING CARE OF THE CHILDBEARING FAMILY, 309

Coordinator

Marybeth Young, PhD, MSN, RNC

Contributors

Quilla D. Bell-Turner, PhD, RN
Gita Dhillon, MA, MS, MEd, RNC
Kathleen Haubrich, MSN, RNC
Roberta Kordish, MSN, RN
Marianne Scharbo-DeHaan, CNM, MN, RN

5 NURSING CARE OF THE CHILD, 427

Coordinator

Susan Colvert Droske, MN, RN

Contributors

Karen S. Bernardy, MSN, RNC
Alice Copp Franz, MA, RN
Judith K. Leavitt, MEd, RN
Mariann C. Lovell, MS, RN
Michele A. Michael, PhD, RN
Maribeth L. Moran, MSN, RN
Bernadette Mazurek Vulcan, MSN, RNC, PNP

The Healthy Child, 428

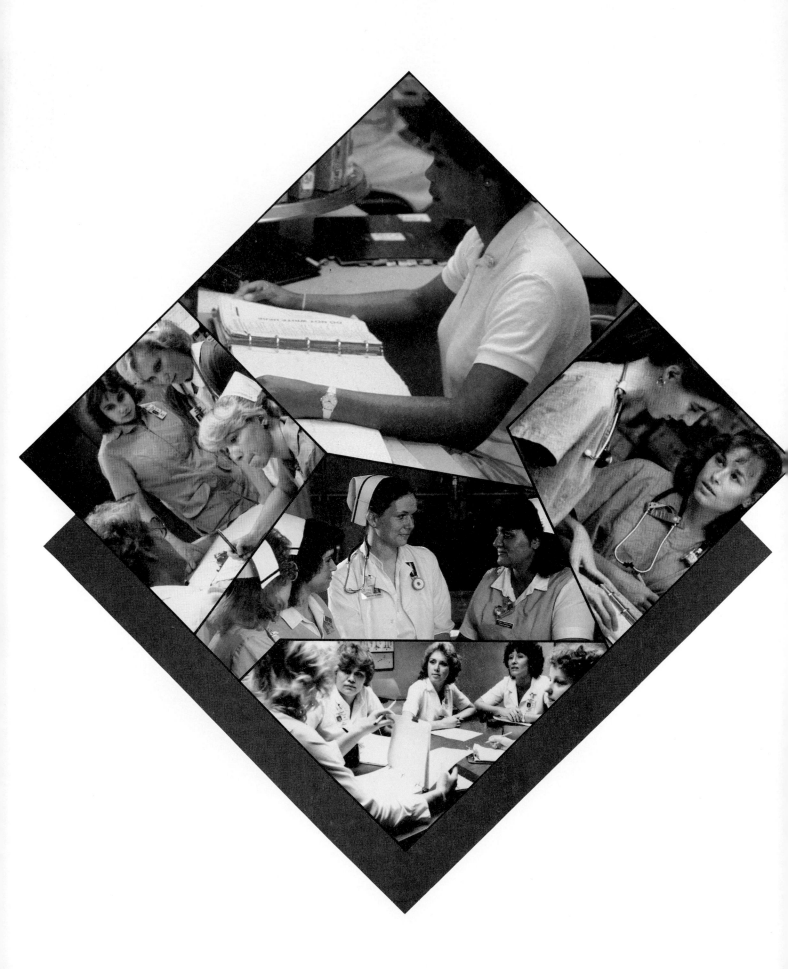

Preparing for the NCLEX-RN

Marybeth Young, PhD, MSN, RNC

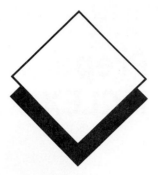

PRETEST

1. Test items on the NCLEX-RN are based on case studies
   a. describing actual or potential health problems.
   b. emphasizing knowledge of physiology and safe, effective care.
   c. focusing on situations encountered by entry-level nurses.
   d. All of the above choices are correct.
2. The examination requires that the graduate nurse select
   a. one single, correct response.
   b. answers from "multiple-multiple" options.
3. Time allotted for each of the approximately 93 items in each section is
   a. 20 seconds.
   b. 30 seconds.
   c. 45 seconds.
   d. 60 seconds.
4. The integrated nursing exam contains about the same number of questions measuring applied knowledge of
   a. pediatric, maternity, and medical-surgical nursing.
   b. assessment, analysis, planning, implementation, and evaluation.
   c. acute illnesses and chronic health problems.
   d. risk factors and measures to promote health.
5. Which of the following test-taking hints is *not* useful in taking the licensure examination?
   a. Try to narrow the possible answers to two choices.
   b. Focus on key words such as *initially* or *least effective*.
   c. *Do not guess* if you are unsure of an answer.
   d. Be careful when erasing responses and changing them.

After completing the above pretest, you may find that you want more accurate information about the licensure examination ahead. Reading the following information may contribute to your success.

KNOW THE TEST FORMAT

Just as the novice driver needs to know what to expect on the state driving test, each graduate nurse needs a clear idea of the professional licensure exam format. Knowing that you have some questions about the test itself or are unsure of your responses on the pretest, the following brief summary will provide answers.

Success on the national examination is required for entry into professional practice. The same multiple-choice test currently is administered throughout the United States twice each year. Computerized Adaptive Testing (CAT) currently is offered as a field test in selected sites across the nation. Eventually, this computer-interactive approach will eliminate some stress often experienced in a massive testing environment. If your state is involved in this testing approach or you participate in clinical simulation testing, information will be shared with you in advance. Until the test format changes in every state, which will take several years, the current paper-and-pencil test will be used to measure competence.

There are approximately 93 test items in each of four separate, integrated sections. (Some questions are "pilot items" and are not counted toward the pass/fail score. However, since these are not identified as such, respond to each item with equal attention.) Situations and questions represent a variety of client health problems and needs. One case study describing a plan for health promotion of a young family may be followed by another case study focusing on the safe care environment of an adolescent in an acute-care setting. Test items focus on critical requirements for competent practice rather than on separate specialty content, such as pediatric or surgical nursing.

The National Council of State Boards of Nursing organizes the licensure examination around a broad framework comprising the "Nursing Process" and "Categories of Human Needs." Each part of this plan is summarized briefly; implications for review are suggested.

Nursing Process

The nursing process provides organization for the test as it does for care planning in every clinical setting. Each nursing process phase is equally important in resolving health problems. This consistency is immediately evident to test takers who perceive this equal emphasis. These same graduates are quick to point out that the numbers of items testing maternity and psychiatric nursing are not equal; medical-surgical nursing is heavily emphasized. Table 1-1 suggests a possible test item focus for each phase of the nursing process.

Categories of Human Needs

Concepts that contribute to understanding human needs are another exam focus. Among these are basic human needs, the teaching-learning process, therapeutic communication, crisis intervention, and developmental theory. Knowledge of anatomy, physiology and pathophysiology, asepsis, nutrition, accountability, the group process, and mental health concepts is basic to the practice of nursing and also is incorporated into many test items. The organization of client needs based on these concepts is identified by the National Council of State Boards of Nursing as "Categories of Human Needs" and is part of the test format. These four categories flow from the ANA Nursing Social Policy Statement and current research on job analysis for beginning practitioners. The greatest NCLEX-RN exam emphasis is on the categories of physiological integrity (42%-48%) and safe care environment (25%-31%). Health promotion and maintenance (12%-18%) and psychosocial integrity (9%-15%) are also incorporated (see Tables 1-2 and 1-3).

Some overlap is evident as you look at the nursing process framework and the categories of client needs. For example, the nursing process phase of planning addresses both physiological and psychosocial needs. However, if an individual has a severe deficit in fluid volume related to dehydration, emotional needs are attended to *after* setting a goal to resolve life-threatening physiolog-

Table 1-1 Test item focus suggested by the nursing process

Phase	Possible item focus
Assessment	Identifying data base
	Selecting appropriate means to gather data
	Gathering information from client/family
	Noting significant observations/data
	Considering environmental factors
	Recognizing client/family strengths, limitations
Analysis	Prioritizing potential/actual problems
	Selecting an appropriate nursing diagnosis
	Interpreting meaning of test results
Planning	Setting measurable long/short-term goals
	Prioritizing goals
	Involving client/family in goal setting
	Examining/modifying existing plan
	Sharing plan with client/family/staff
Implementation	Carrying out nursing actions safely
	Understanding rationale for care
	Prioritizing care
	Assisting with self-care
	Calculating/administering medications safely
	Suggesting diet modifications
	Ensuring safety/comfort
	Preventing infection/injury
	Promoting mobility/independence
	Responding to emergencies
	Recording/sharing information
	Teaching to client's intellectual level
	Communicating appropriately with client/family/staff
	Supervising/delegating care
Evaluation	Comparing outcomes to goals
	Examining response to therapy
	Seeking more information
	Identifying learning outcomes
	Recognizing risks/problems of therapy
	Communicating outcomes to staff/family
	Reassessing/revising plan

Table 1-2 Categories of human needs

Categories	Nursing focus
Safe, effective care environment	Coordinating care
	Ensuring quality
	Setting goals
	Promoting safety
	Preparing client for treatments/procedures
	Implementing care
Physiological integrity	Promoting adaptation
	Identifying/reducing risks
	Fostering mobility
	Ensuring comfort
	Providing care
Psychosocial integrity	Promoting adaptation
	Facilitating coping
Health promotion/maintenance	Promoting growth and development
	Directing self-care
	Fostering support systems
	Prevention/early treatment of disease

Table 1-3 Test item focus suggested by categories of human needs

Human needs category	Possible test item focus
Safe, effective care environment	Understanding basic principles
	Using management skills
	Implementing protective measures
	Promoting safety
	Ensuring client/family rights
	Preventing spread of infection
Physiological integrity	Recognizing altered body function
	Using body mechanics
	Providing comfort measures
	Using equipment safely
	Understanding effects of immobility
	Recognizing untoward responses to therapy/medication/procedures
	Documenting emergency actions
Psychosocial integrity	Identifying mental health concepts
	Recognizing behavior changes
	Referring to resources
	Communicating appropriately
Health promotion/maintenance	Understanding family systems
	Teaching nutrition
	Promoting wellness
	Strengthening immune responses
	Recognizing adaptive changes to health alterations
	Considering cultural/religious impact on childbearing
	Supporting the dying/family

ical problems. Priority setting is critical to exam success, just as it is in clinical care giving.

Use your knowledge of the test format to help you identify and review concepts learned throughout your nursing education and to prepare thoughtfully for the examination. However, during the actual NCLEX-RN exam, do not attempt to identify whether safe, effective care or physiological integrity is tested in a particular item.

Applied knowledge, rather than mere recall of facts, is measured in most test questions. Detailed and sometimes lengthy case studies describe a client or family with emphasis on health needs, followed by several questions. In order to answer these, you will need to use knowledge gained from clinical experience and classroom learning to identify and resolve client problems. Expect to find test questions challenging and varying in difficulty. Application of knowledge may be subtle, such as selecting a toy appropriate for a hospitalized toddler

in traction, or suggesting emergency treatment for a neighbor who splashes cleaning solution in her eyes. Remember that standards for care are based on general principles. Although environmental factors may affect client needs, priorities for safe care are based on those general principles.

HOW THE TEST IS SCORED

The exam grading method differs significantly from standardized achievement or aptitude tests. For example, instructions given before college placement exams urge students to avoid guessing. Directions given to you before the nursing licensure exam stress that guessing is not penalized. An educated guess may thus contribute to success. If you can narrow the four options to two possibilities, the probability is 50% for making a correct choice. Completing all questions becomes a critical goal because the grading process results in a pass/fail score based on the number of correct responses. Although individuals who fail the exam are informed of the approximate number of items missed, there is no numerical score.

There is no separate answer sheet, and responses are marked by filling in circles at the left of each option. All stray pencil marks and underlining must be erased before turning in the test booklet so that the scanner does not pick them up during the grading process. A blank page is provided for mathematical calculations of medication doses and IV flow rates. This is also an ideal "scratch sheet" on which to note items you skip initially but plan to reexamine after completing the rest of the exam. This approach saves time and eliminates the need to scan the entire booklet to locate omitted responses.

Remember, the NCLEX-RN test plan has been developed to measure critical thinking and nursing competence. Knowing the framework of the exam should dispel some of your fears and help you to anticipate and prepare for the test. When the actual date arrives, do not think about the "test plan," but concentrate on the challenge of each case study and the related questions. Just as the driver attends the road test without wondering, "What is being tested now?" you need only address the problem-solving task.

WHERE SHOULD YOU BEGIN?

When you are familiar with this text and the test format, map out a personal plan for preparation and review. If independent study is planned, set realistic goals within the time available. Ideally, reviewing content over several months is preferable to "cramming" in a few weeks. Studying regularly, over time, helps to reinforce knowledge and improves your ability to apply that knowledge.

Begin your review plan by focusing on content that is less familiar to you or about which you feel insecure. Your results on standardized national tests, such as the AssessTest, could serve as a guide, or you may select

several case studies from Section 6 and answer the questions that follow after reviewing related content. After completing the test items, refer to the correct responses, rationale, and test format classification; then compare your problem-solving abilities to those of content experts. You may find it helpful to return to the review book outline, to a nursing specialty or fundamentals text, or to your class notes to resolve doubts or increase understanding. Look for patterns of test-taking difficulties as you review responses. Becoming aware of your strengths and weaknesses in test taking is an important phase of review and gives more meaningful feedback than counting correct and incorrect responses. By beginning with the greatest challenge and reinforcing understanding, your confidence is renewed as the date of the exam approaches.

COGNITIVE AND AFFECTIVE KEYS TO SUCCESS

There are three factors that are important in achieving success: *reading,* which affects both reviewing and test taking; *test wiseness,* which is defined as the ability to use a test situation to demonstrate learning; and the ability to *control tension* in a major examination, freeing the mind to concentrate on the written questions. Although these factors are interrelated, they are discussed separately. Suggestions and strategies are offered for use during your licensure exam experience (Table 1-4).

Cognitive Strategies to Promote Success

Reading with concentration is a learned skill that is critical for study, review, and successful examination performance. When preparing for the NCLEX-RN, select an environment that is well-lighted and suits your learning style. Avoid reading on a bed—its comfort may induce sleep rather than reinforce knowledge. Gather all materials in advance for the planned study session, including this review book, other appropriate texts, notes, and marker pens to highlight content needing subsequent review.

Skim the review text material, then read for understanding. Look up any unfamiliar terms. Make a note of further questions that come to mind as you review information. Use your knowledge of anatomy, physiology, and pathophysiology to visualize the impact of a specific health alteration. Review the disease process, preventive measures, restoration, and rehabilitation. Refresh your memory of procedures specifically used in treatment. Think about ways in which health might be improved.

While reading test items as practice or in a real situation, be especially observant of *key words*. Notice cues such as *age, risk factors,* and *coping mechanisms.* Clearly identify the question focus (e.g., the concerned parent, the ill child, or the caregiver). Use your knowledge of nursing to think through the question and consider

Table 1-4 Cognitive strategies for success

Prepare	for safe practice
Plan a review	to broaden knowledge
Read carefully	for understanding
Identify key words	to focus attention
Narrow options	by critical thinking
Use an educated guess	not random choice
Set priorities	based on health risk
Trust decisions	avoid many erasures

possible responses even before reading all possible options.

Be sure to control the time you spend considering each situation and question. During each 90-minute test section you will not have the luxury of time to thoughtfully *reread* and reflect. For this reason, it is wise to omit the very complex problems that may take several minutes to resolve. Return to those challenges after completing the less difficult items.

Although you must read carefully to understand the questions, avoid reading into the words more than is actually stated. Assume that the health care agency described is ideal and well staffed. If you think that the client's needs would be met by a midnight snack of milk and crackers, do not qualify this with ". . . but it may be impossible to provide this at night."

During the exam, you have no resource for defining vocabulary. Use the sentence context to deduce the meaning of unfamiliar words. Refer to the case study for insight and clarification, and remember to apply your understanding of pathophysiology throughout the exam.

One word of caution about rereading questions as you complete a test section. Occasionally, a series of items describes a client's progress over several days of treatment. Do not alter care priorities for the day of admission based on results of later diagnostic tests.

The following examples give you an opportunity to apply several testing strategies to varied questions typical of the NCLEX-RN. Priority setting can be a challenge on a written test. One approach is to view each option as a true/false statement. This is especially helpful if several nursing implementations are correct but you are asked to select a *best* or *initial* action. Ask yourself, "Will the client's health or recovery be affected if one action is *not* carried out initially?"

Consider this test item:

Ms. Travis, a 44-year-old kindergarten teacher, was admitted last evening with a medical diagnosis of endocarditis. History includes a cholecystectomy 2 years ago and childhood rheumatic fever. Two days ago her dentist extracted an infected molar after an unsuccessful root canal procedure. Although she usually takes prophylactic penicillin before dental treatment, she forgot to do so. Present temperature is 103° F. IV ampicillin is ordered every 6 hours. She seems uncom-

fortable and very anxious, asking repeatedly if her son has arrived from a distant state.

1. During the initial assessment of Ms. Travis, the nurse notes that 600 ml of 5% dextrose in 0.225% normal saline has infused in 2 hours. Since the physician ordered 1000 ml in 10 hours, the *initial action* should be to
   - ☐ 1. notify the attending physician.
   - ☐ 2. assess respirations and breath sounds.
   - ☐ 3. recalculate the infusion rate.
   - ☐ 4. report the problem to the supervisor.

Note that the case study is very detailed. As you would do in a clinical setting, review the assessment data and filter out the information that has less impact on the client's present condition. Identify the actual and potential problems; then read the question and consider each option thoughtfully. As fluid volume is altered, physiological integrity clearly dictates priority assessments and *immediate* interventions.

In this example say to yourself, "The priority action is to notify the physician. True or False?"; then proceed to the other options. Although responses 1, 2, and 3 are appropriate, the *priority action* is to detect signs of fluid volume excess related to very rapid infusion (option 2). Pulmonary edema could further complicate the client's condition. Option 4 is not an initial action, nor should the supervisor be notified until after consulting with the head nurse or unit manager.

2. After examining the client, the cardiologist orders the remaining 400 ml of IV fluids administered over 8 hours. The drop factor is 10/ml. The nurse would adjust the fluid rate to
   - ☐ 1. 4 drops per minute.
   - ☐ 2. 8 drops per minute.
   - ☐ 3. 12 drops per minute.
   - ☐ 4. 16 drops per minute.

Calculate the fluid rate using the standard equation. Be sure to label all values such as minutes and milliliters. The correct response for this question is option 2, 8 drops per minute. The client must be assessed very carefully during the next few hours. Lab data will be analyzed for further problems related to overhydration.

Other priority test items may focus on emergency nursing actions in varied health care settings. Problem solve thoughtfully and select an initial lifesaving action. Consider this item:

Mr. Kent had a bronchoscopic examination several hours ago. A topical anesthetic spray was used during the procedure. Since the physician ordered diet as tolerated and the client tolerated sips of water, he was given a general diet for lunch. As he begins to eat, his color turns gray; he appears to have difficulty breathing and then grasps his throat.

3. Select the correct priority action.
   - ☐ 1. Notify the anesthesiologist.
   - ☐ 2. Suction secretions from his oral pharynx.
   - ☐ 3. Perform a thrust maneuver.
   - ☐ 4. No action can be taken until further information is gathered.

The priority action is to ensure a patent airway, option 3. Further reflection may lead you to question if the client's swallowing and gag reflexes were assessed before the meal. In this example, as in many NCLEX-RN test items, one choice suggests the need for further information. Be very careful in selecting this response. Although it may be very helpful to have more assessment data, this case study provides sufficient data to direct quick and safe action.

Communication test items present a special challenge. As in actual practice, nonverbal cues and the environment affect the communication process. When reading case studies and questions focusing on nurse/client/family interactions, consider all information very carefully. Realize that a reference to an interaction or the presence of quotation marks does not automatically imply therapeutic

Table 1-5 Focus of communications test items

Type of interaction	Approach
Interview	Asking purposeful questions
	Identifying risk factors
	Using appropriate vocabulary
	Listening to responses
	Maintaining confidentiality
Information giving	Describing tests/procedures
	Clarifying data
	Explaining treatment to client/family
Teaching/learning	Assessing health, learning needs
	Using developmentally appropriate terms
	Giving instructions to promote safety
	Demonstrating self-care
	Reinforcing group learning
	Observing a return demonstration
	Involving family in basic care
	Evaluating learning outcome
Therapeutic use of self	Establishing trust
	Identifying own communication skills
	Developing goal direction
	Listening actively
	Clarifying, reflecting
	Sharing observations
	Anticipating needs
	Reinforcing positive coping styles
	Supporting in loss
	Referring for help

use of self. Refer to Table 1-5 for suggested ways in which communication test items might vary with *nurse-client* interactions. Apply basic principles and be aware of possible communication blocks. Base choices on sound rationale, rather than selecting a response that "sounds like" what you actually might say.

Consider the following case study and test items:

Ms. Fox, 57, visits the clinic for a Pap smear and describes occasional hot flashes and irregular menstrual periods. She plans to discuss estrogen replacement therapy with her gynecologist. In response to questions about life-style, she describes regular activity and rest patterns, and a well-balanced diet. A review of her history reveals that two sisters had breast cancer. When asked if she performs breast self-exams regularly, Ms. Fox appears upset. "I am so afraid of cancer! I'd rather not know if there is a problem! I could not cope with finding a mass."

4. Select an appropriate reply to the client:
   □ 1. "Fear is no reason to neglect your health."
   □ 2. "Your risk is very high because of family history."
   □ 3. "Tell me more about what you are feeling."
   □ 4. "You should not feel afraid; early detection is critical."

5. After further discussion, the client agrees to view videotapes on menopause and regular breast examination. Which of the following statements made by Ms. Fox indicates that further teaching is necessary?
   □ 1. "When my periods stop, I won't need to check my breasts."
   □ 2. "I understand that I should continue to take calcium."
   □ 3. "Even though my body is changing, I know I can get pregnant."
   □ 4. "If I take estrogen, I'll decrease fat intake and stop smoking."

Question 4 indicates an initial need for therapeutic communication. Although correct information should be conveyed, risk factors identified, and teaching emphasized, this client needs to express her feelings and concerns. Response 3 indicates the nurse's availability as a listener.

In question 5, the client verbalizes understanding of several elements of teaching and plans to take a more active role in health maintenance. All statements, except response 1, indicate learning has occurred. This lack of understanding about continuing breast self-exams even after menopause indicates a need for further teaching.

Some questions focusing on Human Needs Categories address potential problems within the environment. Consider the following test questions.

6. During a busy day in the outpatient clinic, the nurse suspects that a young child may have rubella. Of the following clients who were in contact with the child, which individual is at greatest risk?

□ 1. John Norris, HIV positive, recovering from tuberculosis
□ 2. Celia Moran, 8 months pregnant; rubella titer positive
□ 3. Lori Ruiz, 1 month old; breastfeeding
□ 4. Frances Long, chronic alcoholic with cirrhosis

7. As a nurse makes rounds on a pediatric unit, each of the following is observed. Which situation must be corrected immediately to ensure client well-being?

□ 1. A school-aged amputee leaves his wheelchair at the bedside.
□ 2. Several toddlers spread their toys on the playroom floor.
□ 3. The stereo volume in the adolescent lounge is quite loud.
□ 4. The newborn step-down ICU is 68° F.

Risk factors are very different in the above situations. In question 6, rubella exposure is particularly dangerous for any immunosuppressed client (option 1). Although insufficient information is given about the 1-month-old baby's nursing mother and there may be a risk to the client described in option 4, you are asked to identify the individual for whom exposure is *most dangerous*. That client is John Norris. In assessing environmental conditions that may affect physiological functioning and safety, the very low nursery temperature (option 4) is a serious problem and may lead to cold stress. Examine the other options for potential safety problems. The child with a disability should have access to his wheelchair. Although toys should not be left in an area where they create a hazard, risk is minimal in the playroom. The loud music may subsequently affect hearing, but this is typical for adolescents. Since the case study does not mention that other clients are disturbed, there is no need for immediate action.

Some test items ask you to consider potential or actual problems identified in several clients and then decide on an appropriate action. Consider this item:

8. Each of the following assessments is documented by a night nurse on an adult surgical unit. Which observation should be reported *immediately* to the physician?

□ 1. Jenny Bocci has a temperature of 100° F the night following surgery for a ruptured appendix.
□ 2. Karen Rosen's knee is hot and swollen 2 days after cartilage repair.
□ 3. William Clifford's dressing has purulent drainage shortly after the incision of an abscess.
□ 4. George Henderson has blood-tinged urine 12 hours after a transurethral prostatectomy.

In reviewing the data, visualize the operative procedure and expected recovery. Identify problems that may delay healing. The physician should be notified immediately about the orthopedic client's postoperative condition. Option 2 indicates a serious problem that may lead to subsequent bone or systemic infection. All other observations are expected during convalescence for the surgical procedures described.

Affective Strategies for Success

It is difficult to separate cognitive and emotional factors in test performance. There are, however, distinctly separate ways to prepare for the mental and emotional challenges of the examination.

Long-range goal setting must include realistic life plans. Anticipate the time that study and review demand; avoid a major life change that increases tension. While a wedding date may be difficult to reschedule, consider delaying other emotionally charged events, such as a three-week hiking trip through Europe just before the exam.

Realistically evaluate your personal responses to test challenges. Look at past successes and ways you maintain energy and confidence under stress. How have you reacted to past major examinations? What physiological or psychological responses to stress are common for you? Many graduates report that tension headaches or gastrointestinal distress occur during the two days of testing. Some suggest that lapses of concentration are frequent during a tiring day of problem solving. Expect that your thoughts may "drift" or that you may experience a "failure fantasy," as many other nurses have described. Expect some anger about a specific test item. You may feel that you could have written "better answers than those!"

In order to use your mind to its fullest and to demonstrate your competence as a nurse, you need to control the effects of anxiety. Several effective ways exist to reduce tension, including:

- relaxing and contracting muscles progressively from head to toe
- slow, deep breathing and deliberate calming
- guided imagery with focus on a peaceful scene
- meditation, prayer, positive thoughts
- focusing on a confident self

Select the method of stress reduction that has worked for you in the past, learn new approaches, and practice them during times of tension while studying. For example, to use imagery, see yourself in the setting that is most peaceful for you. Close your eyes and imagine the quiet, the scents, the scenery around you. Feel the warmth and energy. Relax and feel calm. Change the setting as you need to until it is the perfect relaxing pause. Recall these images during difficult moments in the exam when you need a brief recharge. You will feel your spirits lift and will experience clearer thinking.

Close to the test date, plan your travel to the exam site. If distance allows, visit the area in advance so that you know the best route and alternates. Consider seasonal problems that may affect travel time. It is critical to arrive at the testing site ahead of time, or you may be refused entry.

Table 1-6   Keys to success on the NCLEX-RN

Know the Test Format
   An integrated exam
   Pass/fail score
   Single-response, multiple-choice items
   Based on measurement of safe nursing behaviors for
     common health problems
Review Concepts
   Growth and development
   Pharmacology and pathophysiology
   Effects of culture and nutrition on health
   The nursing process
   Categories of human needs
Where Should You Begin?
   Consider your strengths and your learning style
How Should You Prepare?
   Review course notes and texts
   Consider a review program
   Use human resources and support services
Strategies to Promote Success
   Begin with self-evaluation
   Sharpen test-taking skills
   Learn methods to reduce stress
   Be self-confident
Just Before the Exam
   Get a good night's rest
   Avoid late cramming
   Eat breakfast
During the NCLEX-RN
   Be precise in marking answer spaces
   Use time wisely
   Be "test wise"
   Keep emotions under control

Used with permission © 1982, 1988. Young, M., & Kopala, B.

Anticipate that the massive test setting may be overwhelming. Plan ways that you can block out environmental distractions such as a noisy lobby, classmates who desire a last-minute review of content, or friends who wish to hold a lunch-hour postmortem on test items. Replace those stimuli with a walk during the noon break, a brief nap on the steps, or reminiscence about school experiences. This is one time in your professional life that *your* needs are a priority. Do what you must to remain calm and confident.

On the exam days, consider your own comfort and nutritional needs. Dress in nonconstricting and attractive clothing that helps you to feel good about yourself. It is wise to carry a jacket in anticipation of temperature changes within the testing room. Eat a high-protein breakfast, but avoid excessive caffeine and fluids so that repeated trips to the restroom can be avoided during the examination period. Carry fruit, a can of juice, and other quick-energy sources for breaks. This suggestion is especially helpful to prevent overwhelming fatigue during the final test section.

If you know that you often have a tension headache

during a long day of concentration, carry a remedy with you. Prepare for other problems by bringing cough drops or antacids. However, do not take medications that might cause drowsiness, since you need to remain alert and attentive during the 90-minute test periods.

Expect to encounter at least one unfamiliar health problem in the NCLEX-RN exam. Remain confident that you can use your knowledge of anatomy, physiology, pathophysiology, and nursing to solve the problem. Do not allow anger to destroy your concentration with thoughts such as "Why didn't we learn about that condition in school?" Rather, think to yourself, "I can try to answer these questions." Read cues that help you understand the nature of the health problem, or perhaps omit unfamiliar items and return to them later.

The keys to success are within you (see Table 1-6). Discover your strengths and potential by preparing thoroughly—mentally and emotionally. Study, review, practice test-taking strategies, and learn how to reduce personal tension. The rewards begin with your license to practice as a professional nurse. You are needed in the health care field of the 1990s, and you are welcomed as a caregiver and a colleague!

Answer Key for Pretest Questions, p. 2

1. d
2. a
3. d
4. b
5. c

REFERENCES

Kane, M., Kinsgsbury, C., Colton, D., & Estes, C. (1986). *A study of nursing practice, role delineation, and job analysis of entry-level performance for registered nurses*. Chicago: National Council of State Boards of Nursing, Inc.

National Council of State Boards of Nursing. (1987). *Test plan for the National Council licensure examination for registered nurses*. Chicago: National Council of State Boards of Nursing, Inc.

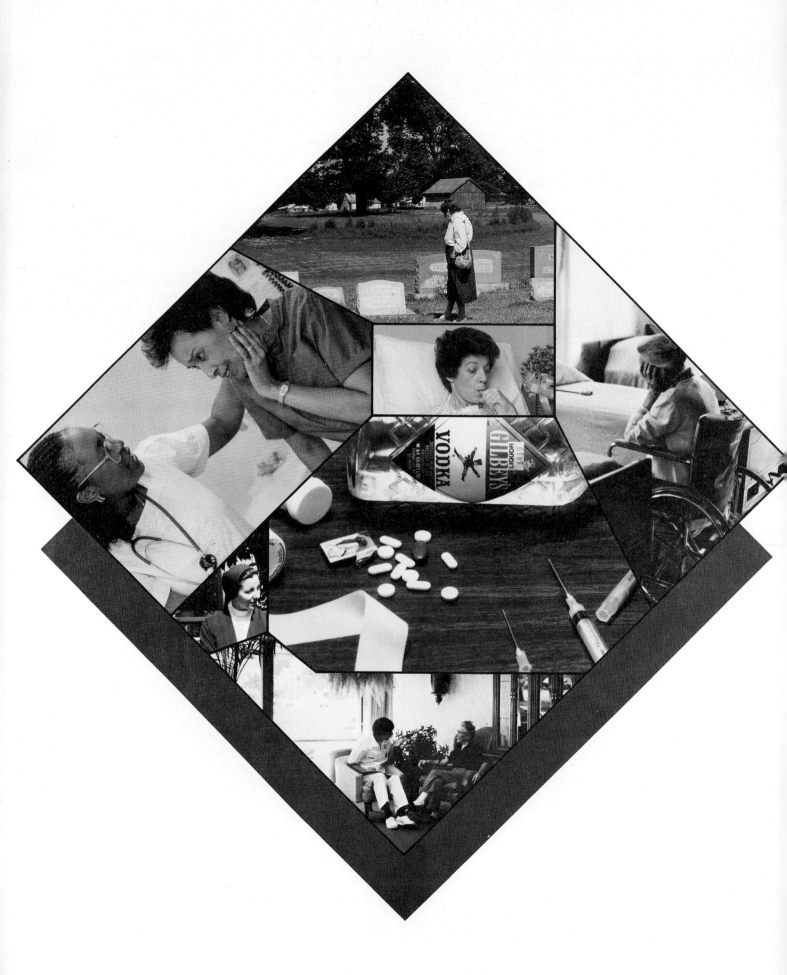

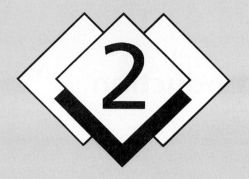

Nursing Care of the Client with Psychosocial and Mental Health Problems

Coordinator

Alene Harrison, EdD, RN

Contributors

Sharon Golub, MN, RN
E. Ingvarda Hanson, MSN, RN
Ann L. Jessop, MSN, RN
Janet Elizabeth Bloomer Kristic, MSN, RN
Janet Sullivan Wilson, MEd, RN

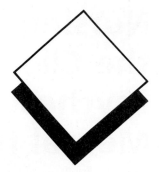

Introduction

OVERVIEW

1. This section reviews content that is general to all nursing—that is, communicating with clients and the nurse-client relationship—as well as content that is specific to psychiatric nursing. The NCLEX-RN examination will test your knowledge of communication and interpersonal relationships in *all* sections of the examination.

2. DSM-III-R: The sections in this book are organized in the format of client problem behaviors and the *Diagnostic and Statistical Manual of Mental Disorders,* 3rd ed.-revised (American Psychiatric Association: 1987). The DSM-III-R categorizes and codes psychiatric diagnoses. These categories and codes are used by physicians and other health care providers to make diagnoses, to compile statistics, to apply for grants, and to report for third-party payment (insurance). Each diagnosis includes a description of diagnostic criteria. NCLEX-RN will not ask you to diagnose the client's disorder.

SCOPE OF THE PROFESSION

1. Psychiatric nursing is a specialized area of nursing that utilizes both science and art to provide nursing care to individuals and groups in a wide variety of settings. The nurse-client relationship is the vehicle through which the nurse fulfills independent, interdependent, and dependent roles. Psychiatric/mental health nursing includes promoting mental health and preventing mental illness. It includes the care and rehabilitation of the psychiatrically ill and the mental health care of the physically ill.

2. Scientific focus: on human behavior
   a. To understand biopsychosocial principles underlying emotional problems
   b. To be aware of safe and effective treatment measures such as psychotherapy, medications, electroconvulsive therapy (ECT)

3. Purposeful use of self
   a. To apply principles of the nurse-client relationship to all interactions
   b. To be aware of oneself as a principal in the relationship and countertransference issues
   c. To recognize and use one's own feelings and reactions as a guide to increasing empathy and trust, and understanding the client
   d. To act as an appropriate behavioral/social role model

4. Dependent practice involves implementation and coordination of physician's orders
   a. Know important aspects of each client problem in order to assess, report, and document findings accurately
   b. Apply knowledge and use skills therapeutically in assessment and treatment
   c. Work collaboratively, sharing information about the client's progress

5. Independent practice involves use of the nursing process and development of individualized nursing care plans

6. Interdependent practice involves working with the interdisciplinary team in a variety of settings

INTERPERSONAL RELATIONSHIPS

1. Therapeutic relationships
   a. Relationship between nurse and individual client includes
      1. the initiation, development, and termination of a therapeutic relationship (objective, professional, empathic interactions)
      2. the nurse role-modeling appropriate behavior
      3. the nurse treating the client as a unique individual worthy of respect, focusing on the client's symptoms and strengths
      4. the nurse being consistent and reliable in increasing the client's trust and security and decreasing defensive acting-out behavior
   b. Group relationship includes
      1. working with clients concerning the here-and-now living problems they confront
      2. providing information and role modeling
      3. clients getting feedback from other group members

2. Collaboration with other professionals
  a. Coordinating and planning holistic health care
  b. Sharing implementation of the care plan according to skills needed (e.g., physical therapist, occupational therapist, rehabilitation counselor)
  c. Working interdependently with other health professionals

ROLES ASSUMED BY THE NURSE

Nurses are involved directly in the care of the client and may assume many different, overlapping roles.
1. Therapist
  a. Therapy may focus on problems of daily living
    1. on a one-to-one basis (nurse-client communication); focus is on problem solving
    2. in groups such as assertiveness groups, grooming groups, adolescent groups; focus is on dealing with specific problems, providing emotional support and reality orientation, and increasing social skills and social acceptance
  b. Individual psychotherapy
    1. therapist and client meet regularly; the client learns to identify own problems and practices new ways of handling them
    2. the client has the opportunity to develop a close relationship with another person (the therapist), to grow from that experience, and to direct new insights and behavior to other areas of life
  c. Group psychotherapy: nurse may be group leader or co-leader
  d. Family therapy
    1. the therapist meets with the client and the family in various combinations
    2. family dynamics are stressed, and scapegoating of the "identified client" is decreased
  e. Sociotherapy: within the community mental health movement, psychiatric nurses provide services aimed at preventing mental illness and reinforcing healthy adaptation; specifically, this is done by teaching, by developing therapeutic relationships, and by recognizing early indications of problems and intervening appropriately
2. Surrogate parent: the nurse is perceived in the role of nurturer, authority figure, parent as part of therapy with adults and children
3. Teacher: the nurse educates clients regarding biopsychosocial health needs, medications, nutrition, and constructive ways of interacting and coping with stress
4. Social agent: the nurse assists the client in using community agencies and social networks and helps people learn about mental health, mental illness, and the prevention of mental illness
5. Coordinator of client care
6. Client advocate

7. Researcher
8. Administrator
9. Supervisor
10. Expanded and advanced roles (e.g., clinical specialists, consultants, liaison nurses)

LOCATIONS OF PRACTICE

The role of the nurse is often dictated by the type of mental health facility.
1. In hospitals: the type of involvement the nurse has in client care varies with the theoretical model in use at the individual facility; the nurse may
  a. Work with psychiatrists
  b. Formulate care plans
  c. Observe, support, and listen to clients
  d. Assist clients in developing new behaviors
  e. Provide clients with an environment to try new behaviors
  f. Administer medicines and physical nursing care
  g. Facilitate individual/group counseling
2. In community mental health centers
  a. The nurse may
    1. provide outpatient care using a variety of therapies
    2. enhance primary prevention in the community through
      a. classes designed to fulfill community needs
      b. crisis intervention
  b. There is a blurring of roles
    1. psychiatrists, psychologists, social workers, psychiatric nurses, and community mental health care workers work together in counseling, home visits, record keeping
    2. psychiatrists prescribe drugs; nurses administer medications; both make physical and emotional assessments

LEGAL ASPECTS

The court protects the rights of psychiatric clients using civil and criminal legal procedures. Many individuals are referred to psychiatric services through the courts. Psychiatric expert testimony is used by the courts when a person uses insanity or inability to stand trial as a defense.
1. Civil admission procedures
  a. General information
    1. the Mental Health Systems Act (1980) provides states with a Recommended Bill of Rights for mentally ill clients
    2. each state has its own mental health code determined by the legislature; the code provides guidelines for admission procedures of the mentally ill to hospitals that treat mental illness
    3. state laws differ in legal commitment procedures
  b. Voluntary admission: any legal adult can apply for admission to an institution that treats mental illness

1. admission implies that the individual agrees to accept treatment and abide by hospital rules
2. many states require that the client give written notice to the hospital if requesting early discharge
3. if a physician believes this release to be dangerous to the client or others, involuntary admission will be arranged according to state laws
4. in most states a child under the age of 16 may be admitted if the parents sign the required application form
5. in some states the minor has the right to protest admission by parents and petition the court for dismissal
6. clients retain all rights with voluntary admission

c. Involuntary admission: application for admission is initiated by someone other than the client and presupposes lack of client consent; state codes have two types of involuntary admissions
   1. emergency involuntary admission
      a. person is an immediate danger to self or others
      b. can be initiated by any official or person
      c. client is held temporarily for evaluation and emergency care (usually 3-5 days; American Bar Association recommends a maximum of 72 hours for emergency involuntary admission)
      d. hearing usually occurs within 48 hours
   2. indefinite involuntary admission
      a. includes initial and indefinite commitments
      b. client is hospitalized for treatment if dangerous to self or others
      c. hearing required by court
      d. client cannot be committed without adequate proof of danger

d. Competency hearings: different and separate from admission hearings
   1. *admission to mental hospital does not mean a person is incompetent* to manage own affairs
   2. legally, *incompetency* indicates the person is no longer able to make responsible decisions for himself, his dependents, or his property
   3. person declared incompetent has legal status of a minor and cannot
      a. vote
      b. make contracts or wills
      c. manage personal property
      d. drive a car
      e. sue or be sued
      f. hold a professional license
   4. a guardian is appointed for the incompetent person and has the power of consent

5. procedure can be instituted by state or family admission

2. Criminal admission procedures
   a. *Insanity:* a legal, not psychiatric, term meaning that because of mental illness the accused did not realize the extent or consequences of his actions, did not know right from wrong, or had impaired ability to resist "wrong," and thus is *not criminally responsible* for the unlawful act
      1. sanity is determined by jury, based on psychiatric expert testimony
      2. the person accused of a crime will stand trial and plead not guilty by reason of insanity
         a. persons found guilty can be sentenced to prison
         b. persons found not guilty are committed to a mental hospital until judged sane by staff
         c. when released, a person who was found not guilty by reason of insanity usually is free and has no legal ruling against self
   b. *Inability to stand trial:* a person accused of committing a crime is not mentally responsible at time of trial
      1. the person is unfit to stand trial if at that time he cannot understand the charge against him, or is incapable of cooperating with his own defense
      2. if found unfit to stand trial, the person must be sent to a psychiatric unit until legally determined to be competent for trial
      3. once mentally fit, the person must stand trial and serve sentence if actually convicted

3. Client rights (recent judicial precedents)
   a. Give clients the right to treatment and active participation in treatment
   b. Require institutions to devise specific plans of treatment for their individual clients
   c. Require that plans of treatment be the least restrictive of client's liberty considering the individual's condition
   d. Protect civil rights
   e. Support confidentiality
   f. Give client right to refuse treatment
   g. Support informed consent

4. Role of the nurse
   a. Functions as advocate for client
   b. Gives care that reflects knowledge of client's legal rights as determined by the mental health code of the state in which the nurse practices
   c. Implements nursing care that meets ANA Standards of Psychiatric-Mental Health Nursing Practice
   d. Charts both legible and accurate *subjective* client data as well as *objective* observations and interventions in accordance with accepted nursing practice

e. Maintains confidentiality of client information
f. Consults a lawyer when legal clarification is needed
g. Knows difference between acts of omission and commission
   1. omission: failing to do what should have been done
   2. commission: doing what should not have been done
h. Ascertains client's understanding of consent to treatment
i. Provides necessary information at client's level of understanding
j. Monitors nursing actions relative to client protection to prevent assault or battery

1. assault: words or actions that produce genuine belief that action will occur without consent
2. battery: unconsented touching or restraining of a person without legitimate rationale

PSYCHOSOCIAL CHARACTERISTICS OF THE HEALTHY CLIENT

1. Infant through adolescent
   a. See Table 2-1 and *The Healthy Child*, p. 428
2. Young adult years (20-40)
   a. Cognitive development
      1. thinking and learning are problem centered
      2. thinks at an abstract level and compares ideas mentally or verbally with previous memories, knowledge, and experience

Table 2-1 Life-cycle stages

Common name/ age	Freud	Erikson	Sullivan	Tasks
Infancy Birth-18 months	Oral sexual gratification through mouth dependent drives pleasure of biting aggressive drives and body image develop differentiates self from mother	Trust vs Mistrust exchanges with parents lay basis for trust or mistrust of others in later life	Development of a self-system Others gratify needs and satisfy wishes	Dependent drives Aggressive drive Differentiation from mother/sense of self trust/security
Toddler 18 months-3 years	Anal excretory control learned concepts of cleanliness, punctuality, self-control, personal independence learned	Autonomy vs Shame and Doubt self-control personal independence and self-worth develop	Acculturation Delay gratification	Shame, disgust Control, cleanliness Punctuality Independence Self-worth
Preschool 3-6 years	Phallic/Oedipal pleasure through genitals attachment to parent of opposite sex competition with parent of same sex resolves by identifying with parent of same sex develops sexual identity, guilt	Initiative vs Guilt sharing, competing, self-motivation learns to control jealousy, rage, envy, guilt	Playmates: forms satisfactory relationships with peers	Guilt, values Establishment of masculine or feminine role Sharing, competing Self-motivation
School age 6-12 years	Latency limited sexual image socialization outside home intellectual and social growth friends control over aggressive, destructive impulses	Industry vs Inferiority skill mastery work and play in groups intellectual growth	Chums: relates to friend of same sex	Intellectual and social growth Mastery of skills Establishment of friendships Group work and play Control over aggressive, destructive impulses

Continued.

Table 2-1 Life-cycle stages—cont'd

Common name/age	Freud	Erikson	Sullivan	Tasks
Adolescence 12-20 years	Genital sexuality focuses on genitals establishes identity learns independence from parents, responsibility for self, intimacy with one of opposite sex	Identity vs Role Diffusion sense of self and identity apart from parents	Early: satisfactory relationships with members of opposite sex Late: intimate relationship with member of opposite sex	Independence from parents Responsibility for self Independent identity Acceptance of sexual and peer relationships
Young adult 20-40 years		Intimacy vs Isolation learns to establish relationship with partner, gratifying social relationships		Establish intimate relationship with partner Gratifying social relationships Work adjustment
Middle age 40-60 years		Generativity vs Stagnation productivity at home, work, community child rearing		Productivity at home, work, community Can include reproduction, child rearing
Older adult 60 years-death		Integrity vs Despair views past and remaining life as meaningful whole		Fulfillment Increased dependence Death of spouse, friends, self

3. learns formally and informally by emphasizing principles and concepts
4. objective, realistic
  b. Emotional development
    1. sexuality is a powerful determinant
    2. expected to be responsible, have good impulse control
    3. Erikson's task: intimacy vs self-isolation or self-absorption
  c. Moral/religious development
    1. challenges values, principles defined by parents and identifies those to be retained or modified
    2. values become individualized, integrated, and provide basis for future ethical decision making
  d. Body-image development
    1. body image is flexible, subject to constant revision, may not reflect actual body structure
    2. a social creation
    3. close interdependence between body image and personality, self-concept, and identity; may be altered by illness, injury, disability
  e. Life-style options
    1. separates from parents in 20s and develops peer relationships

2. makes decisions regarding types of relationships to form (marriage, child rearing, communal, homosexual)
3. settles into career
4. establishes leisure activities
  f. Developmental tasks
    1. accepts self: stabilizing self-concept and body image
    2. establishes independence
    3. establishes a vocation to make worthwhile contributions
    4. learns to appraise and express love responsibly
    5. establishes intimate bond with another
    6. establishes and manages residence
    7. finds congenial social group
    8. decides on option of a family
    9. formulates philosophy of life
    10. establishes role in community
3. Middle adult years (40-65)
  a. Cognitive development
    1. goal oriented
    2. enhanced by experiences, motivation
    3. decreased memory functioning
    4. less retained from oral information

5. continued learning emphasized
6. emphasis on realistic thinking
7. problem-centered thinking
8. attitudes may be less flexible
   b. Emotional development
   1. transitional, self-assessment period
   2. channels emotional drives without losing initiative and vigor
   3. masters environment
   4. controls emotional responses
   5. values age and life experiences
   6. Erikson's task: generativity vs self-absorption and stagnation
   c. Moral/religious development
   1. integrates new concepts from wider sources
   2. beliefs are less dogmatic
   3. personal philosophy offers comfort, happiness
   d. Body-image development
   1. adapts to climacteric; changes accepted as part of maturity
   2. reinforces positive self-concept
   3. prefers experiences, insights, values of current age
   e. Life-style options
   1. reflects work ethic
   2. increasing leisure time
   3. differentiates compulsive work and play from healthy work and play
   4. recognizes self-creativity
   5. increases preparation for retirement
   f. Developmental tasks
   1. develops new satisfaction as a mate; supportive to mate; develops sense of unity with mate
   2. helps offspring become happy, responsible adults
   3. takes pride in accomplishments of self and spouse
   4. balances work with other roles
   5. assists aging parents
   6. achieves social and civic responsibility
   7. maintains active organizational membership
   8. accepts physical changes of middle age
   9. makes an art of friendship
   10. balances leisure with service pursuits
   11. develops more depth of personal philosophy by reevaluating values and examining assets

4. Elderly (over 65)
   a. Cognitive development
   1. may decrease as a result of physiological deterioration
   2. environmental events may affect cognition
      a. loss of self-esteem
      b. isolation
   3. must deal with a will, financial status, and property

   b. Emotional development
   1. reflects on meaningfulness of life, puts success and failure into perspective
   2. sense of wisdom, knowledge, and self-reliance, of being able to cope with whatever comes along
   3. Erikson's task: integrity vs despair
   c. Moral/religious development
   1. may become more spiritually oriented
   2. value system changes from a material orientation to a more value-oriented outlook
   d. Body-image development
   1. must integrate continued physiological changes
   2. may see body as less dependable, therefore less desirable
   e. Life-style options
   1. may depend on finances, family situation, state of health
   2. increased leisure time upon retirement
   3. adjusting to fixed income
   4. developing new hobbies and friends
   f. Developmental tasks
   1. continued self-development (recognizing positive experience of aging)
   2. adapting to family responsibilities
   3. maintaining self-worth, pride, and usefulness
   4. dealing with multiple losses (e.g., spouse, friends; changes in life-style, body function; upcoming end to life)

5. Sexuality and cultural components related to the healthy client
   a. Sexuality
   1. an intrinsic part of each human
      a. biological, sociocultural, psychological, and ethical components
      b. significant part of Maslow's higher-order needs
      c. integral part of Erikson's task for early adulthood: intimacy vs isolation
   2. definitions
      a. *gender:* internal sense of masculinity or femininity
      b. *sexual role behavior:* all we do to disclose ourselves as male or female to others
      c. *self-concept/self-esteem:* the perceptions each individual has of self
      d. *body image:* a person's opinion of the appearance, function, and separateness of one's own body; a component of self-concept
   3. sexual role dissatisfaction can occur with a wide variety of problems/disease states
      a. common physical problems
         ◆ spinal cord injuries, neuromuscular disease
         ◆ cancer of reproductive organs, genitals

◆ diabetes mellitus
◆ hypertensive drug regimens
◆ cardiac problems (fear)
◆ advancing age, menopause
◆ colostomy
◆ obesity
◆ venereal diseases
◆ infertility
◆ endocrine disorders
◆ chronic illness
◆ rectal, prostate carcinoma
b. common biopsychosocial problems
◆ disturbances in body image, self-concept
◆ transvestitism, transexualism
◆ orgasmic or erectile dysfunction
◆ post-traumatic stress disorder
c. drugs that adversely affect sexuality
◆ alcohol
◆ antipsychotic tranquilizers, antidepressants, monoamine oxidase (MAO) inhibitors
◆ antihypertensives
◆ chemotherapeutic agents
◆ hormones and hormone antagonists
4. sexual functioning is multidimensional and influenced by a large number of variables; it is relative to each individual, the individual's life-style, culture, values, and choice of love object (e.g., heterosexuality, homosexuality, bisexuality)

5. a critical part of nursing care of the client with respect to sexuality is that the nurse understand his/her own thoughts, feelings, beliefs, and misconceptions about this sensitive area
6. psychosocial counseling with client and significant others includes
a. verbalizing feelings/concerns/fears
b. encouraging client to maximize unaltered sexual characteristics
c. realizing and verbalizing other characteristics that are part of client's individuality

b. Cultural variables
1. definition: culture is the organized system of behavior or way of life for an identified social group; it includes knowledge, art, beliefs, morals, laws, customs, and values that are transmitted from one generation to the next
2. psychosocial support for client and significant others includes
a. awareness of the components of a cultural orientation
◆ social institutions: family, religion, education, economics, politics
◆ communication systems
b. identifying client's specific, culturally related nursing care needs
c. tailoring interventions to be consistent with cultural practices of client
3. if culture is mentioned in an NCLEX-RN question, base answer on theory, not past experience

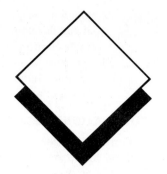

Therapeutic Use of Self

THEORETICAL KNOWLEDGE OF BASE

1. Theories of behavior: nursing interventions in the realm of human behavior are based on a variety of theories; see Table 2-2
2. Life-cycle stages (refer to Table 2-1)
   a. Freud: each stage must be negotiated successfully to avoid arrest at any one stage
   b. Erikson: focuses on psychosocial crises and developmental tasks; each crisis must be resolved successfully so the individual will be able to meet subsequent crises
   c. Sullivan: focuses on social and environmental factors; a healthy personality develops through meaningful, gratifying interpersonal experiences with others in the environment
3. Defense mechanisms (Freud)
   a. Psychological techniques the personality develops to manage anxiety, aggressive impulses, hostilities, resentments, frustrations, and conflicts between the id (pleasure-seeking impulses) and the superego (inhibiting)
   b. Used by both mentally healthy and mentally ill persons
   c. Measure of mental health is determined by the degree that defense mechanisms
      1. distort the personality
      2. dominate behavior
      3. disturb adjustment with others
   d. Specific defense mechanisms
      1. *suppression:* the conscious, deliberate forgetting of unacceptable or painful thoughts, impulses, feelings, or acts
      2. *repression:* unconscious, involuntary forgetting of unacceptable or painful thoughts, impulses, feelings, or acts
      3. *isolation:* separating thought and affect, allowing only the former to come to consciousness; it is a compromise mechanism
      4. *dissociation:* walling off certain areas of the personality from consciousness

5. *denial:* treating obvious reality factors as though they do not exist because they are consciously intolerable
6. *rationalization:* attempting to justify feelings, behavior, and motives that would otherwise be intolerable, by offering a socially acceptable, intellectual, and apparently logical explanation for an act or decision
7. *symbolization:* using an object or idea as a substitute or to represent some other object or idea
8. *idealization:* conscious or unconscious overestimation of another's attributes (e.g., hero worship)
9. *identification:* attaching to oneself certain qualities associated with others; it operates unconsciously and is a significant mechanism in superego development
10. *introjection:* incorporating the traits of others, internalizing feelings toward others
11. *conversion:* the unconscious expression of mental conflict by means of a physical symptom
12. *compensation:* putting forth extra effort to achieve in one area to offset real or imagined deficiencies in another area
13. *substitution:* unconsciously replacing an unobtainable or unacceptable goal with a goal that is more acceptable or obtainable; the process is more direct and less subtle than sublimation
14. *sublimation:* directing energy from unacceptable drives into socially acceptable behavior
15. *reaction formation:* expressing unacceptable wishes or behavior by opposite overt behavior
16. *undoing:* thinking or doing one thing for the purpose of neutralizing something objectionable that was thought or done before
17. *displacement:* transferring unacceptable feel-

ings aroused by one object or situation to a more acceptable substitute

18. *projection:* unconsciously attributing one's own unacceptable qualities and emotions to others

19. *ideas of reference:* believing that one is the object of special and ill-disposed attention by others

20. *fantasy:* satisfying needs by daydreaming

21. *regression:* going back to an earlier level of emotional development and organization

22. *fixation:* never advancing the level of emotional development beyond that in which one feels comfortable

23. *withdrawal:* separating oneself from interpersonal relationships in order to avoid emotional expression or responsiveness

NURSE-CLIENT RELATIONSHIP

1. Purpose: provide counseling, crisis intervention, individual therapy
2. Characteristics

Table 2-2 Theoretical models

Models/proponents	Assumptions	Treatment
Medical-Biological	Emotional disturbance is an illness or defect Illness is located in body or is biochemical Disease entities can be diagnosed, classified, and labeled	Physical/somatic: surgery, electroconvulsive therapy (ECT), chemotherapy Therapists: physicians, others treating under MD's orders
Psychoanalytical (Freud, Erikson)	Emotional disturbance stems from emotionally painful experiences Feelings are repressed Unresolved, unconscious conflicts remain in the mind Symptoms and defense mechanisms develop	Therapy uncovers roots of conflicts through interviews within long-term therapy Therapists: psychoanalysts, usually MDs
Interpersonal (Sullivan, Peplau)	Emotional disturbance results from problematic interpersonal interaction Client is seen as a subsystem of larger systems (e.g., family and community)	Client is approached in a holistic way Intervention includes health promotion/illness prevention and alteration of harmful environments Constructive interpersonal relationship is developed with therapist Therapists: physician or nurse
Behavioral-Cognitive (Pavlov, Skinner, Wolpe, Beck, Ellis)	Behavior can be modified by operant conditioning behavior that is reinforced tends to be repeated behavior that is ignored tends to be eliminated Client needs to eliminate faulty thought processes, self-defeating ideas	Treatment aims at eliminating unwanted behavior by ignoring it and reinforcing wanted behavior Response to behavior by therapists must be consistent Therapists: physicians, nurses, psychologists, trained assistants
Social	When stresses and supports are in balance, the individual is socially competent Emotional disturbance results from imbalance between stresses and supports (see Table 2-3) too much stress and not enough support leads to social disorientation and disintegration too much support and too little stress leads to social dependence, immobility, regression	Treatment is aimed at maintaining or restoring balance between stresses and supports Levels of prevention of mental illness *primary:* promotion of mental health and disease prevention (anticipatory guidance, education, community organization, crisis prevention) *secondary:* early treatment to prevent long-term illness (screening, early diagnosis, case finding, brief hospitalization, crisis intervention) *tertiary:* treatment of chronic, long-term problems (halfway houses, partial hospitalization, day hospitals) Therapists: physicians, nurses, social workers, psychologists, other trained mental health workers

    a. Mutually defined relationship
    b. Mutually collaborative
    c. Goal directed
    d. Interpersonal techniques facilitate communication
    e. Development of therapeutic relationship fostered
    f. Relationship differs from friendship
       1. specific boundaries established
       2. purpose, time, and place of interaction are specific
       3. professional demeanor and objectivity maintained
    g. Nurse assists client with problem resolution
    h. Successful relationship leads to mutual growth for client and nurse

3. Facts to remember
    a. It is not a friendship
    b. Its main benefit is to the client
    c. It presents an opportunity for the client to deal with the problems brought to treatment
    d. The nurse's approach to the relationship is crucial to the client's being able to express feelings
    e. Increased experience and education allow the nurse to have more discretion in relating to clients, but new practitioners should "go by the book"

4. Therapeutic communication
    a. Interpersonal techniques that facilitate communication
    b. Factors that influence the nurse's response
       1. client's stage of growth and development
       2. stage of the nurse-client relationship
       3. client's level of readiness
       4. goals of the interaction/priorities of care

Table 2-3   Social determinants of mental health and illness

Stress	Individual	Support
Social	Genetic information	Social
poverty	Constitutional traits	churches and
poor housing	Developmental	synagogues
unemploy-	traits	schools
ment	coping mecha-	social welfare
crowding	nisms	agencies
high rate of	ego strength	
mobility		
Personal		Personal
maturational		family net-
adolescence		work
aging		friends
role changes		clergy
situational		bartender
loss		hairdresser
divorce		
separation		
illness		

    c. General guidelines: the best responses focus on
       1. actual client behaviors and nursing observations rather than inferences
       2. the here-and-now rather than the past
       3. description rather than judging, to promote trust
       4. sharing information and exploring alternatives rather than giving advice/solutions
       5. how/what rather than why
       6. orientation and presentation of reality (particularly for confused, disoriented clients)
       7. maintenance of biological integrity
       8. nursing interventions rather than roles designated to other health team members
    d. See Table 2-4, Communication Skills in the Nurse-Client Relationship

5. Phases of the nurse-client relationship: correct response to NCLEX-RN questions may be based on initial phase of the relationship
    a. *Initiating or orientating phase:* establishes boundaries
       1. when, how long, how often nurse will meet with client
       2. focus of relationship defined with client
       3. usually time of anxiety for client and nurse
         a. client may come late to or miss meetings; test boundaries
         b. client may exhibit nervous mannerisms
         c. client may sit silently, hallucinate, or exhibit delusions
         d. nurse may be more likely to use responses that block communication because of own anxiety
       4. preparation for termination begins at this stage
    b. *Working phase:* exhibits reduction of anxiety in both client and nurse
       1. client accepts boundaries of relationship
       2. nurse uses interpersonal skills that foster communication
       3. client confronts problems and feelings
       4. client develops insights, learns methods of coping and problem solving
         a. begins to come to meetings on time
         b. uses the time with nurse as a "working" time
       5. nurse and client see each other as unique people
    c. *Terminating phase:* begins when work of relationship is over and builds on preparation made during orientation phase; focus on loss, separation anxiety
       1. client and nurse summarize and evaluate work of relationship
       2. both express thoughts and feelings about termination

Table 2-4 **Communication skills in the nurse-client relationship**

Therapeutic communication techniques

TECHNIQUE	EXAMPLE
Attending: indicating awareness of what is going on in interaction; includes giving feedback/recognition	Yes (nodding). You're wearing a different blouse.
Encouraging Verbalization: promoting continued client verbalization	Um-hmm. And then? Go on.
Verbalization Observations: commenting on what nurse has perceived	You sound frustrated. I notice that you're biting your nails.
Reflecting Feelings: verbalizing either stated or implied client feelings	You're feeling anxious. You feel that no one cares about you.
Paraphrasing: restating the content of the message	Client: The doctor said I could go home tomorrow but I'm still having a lot of trouble walking. Nurse: You're wondering if you're ready to go home.
Open Questioning: promotes freedom of response	What would you like to talk about today? What happens when you feel angry?
Closed Questioning: limits freedom of response to short answer or yes/no	Have you ever been hospitalized before? Did you eat breakfast?
Giving Information: providing factual data	My name is. . . . Lunch is at noon. Visiting hours are 2-8 PM
Clarifying: promotes understanding of what is unclear	I'm not sure I understand what you are saying.
Validating: checking perception of client verbalization	This is what I heard you say. . . . Let me know if this is how you see it.
Focusing: directing flow of interaction	You were saying. . . .
Requesting Description/Comparison: asking client to verbalize perceptions/similarities/differences	Describe how you are feeling now. Tell me when you feel angry. How does this compare with what happened when. . . . ? What other times have you felt this way?
Summarizing: pulling together the salient points of an interaction	Today we have discussed three alternatives for. . . . Last time we talked you were going to. . . .
Presenting Reality	I don't hear any voices except yours and mine **or** Today is Monday, September 24, and you're in the hospital
Seeking Consensual Validation: ensuring understanding of client verbalization	Tell me if I understand you correctly. . . .
Decoding or Desymbolizing: interpreting meaning of client verbalization	Client: I'm the son of God sent to take care of man. Nurse: Do you feel like you want someone to take care of you?
Suggesting Collaboration	Let's figure out together what makes you anxious.

BLOCK	EXAMPLE
False assurance	Everything will be all right. You don't need to worry. You're doing fine.
Giving advice	What you should do is. . . . Why don't you. . . . ?
Giving approval	That's the right attitude. That's the thing to do.
Requesting an explanation	Why are you upset? Why did you do that?
Agreeing with the client	I agree with you. You must be right.
Expressing disapproval	You should stop worrying like this. You shouldn't do that.
Belittling the client's feelings	I know just how you feel. Everyone gets depressed at times.
Disagreeing with the client	You're wrong. That's not true. No, it isn't.
Defending	Your doctor is quite capable. This hospital is well equipped. She's a very good nurse. **Or:** The doctor wouldn't have ordered this for you if it weren't for your own good.
Rejection	I don't think you should be talking about this. . . .
Clichés or stereotypical comments	Look on the bright side **or** Every dark cloud has a silver lining.
Literal responses	Client: The TV is controlling my mind. Nurse: You need to turn it off then.

NURSING PROCESS

Elicit client participation in each stage as appropriate.

1. Assessment: collecting and organizing data about the client by observation, interview, and examination; strengths and problem areas are identified
   a. Observation: note the ABCs (appearance, behavior, communication)
   b. Interview
      1. informal
      2. nursing history
   c. Examination
      1. psychosocial assessment
         a. general appearance and behavior: age, grooming, dress, posture, body movements, eye contact, speech, affect, mood, attitude during interview
         b. thought processes, sensation, perception: logical, circumstantial, perseveration, flight of ideas, delusions, hallucinations, illusions
         c. cognitive functions: orientation, memory, attention and concentration, intellect, judgment, insight, communication, abstract thinking
         d. social processes: self-concept, interpersonal relations (family, peers, community), activities of daily living (ADL), leisure activities
      2. physical: complete review of systems, growth and development history, diet, exercise, rest, tobacco/drug/alcohol use, body image
2. Analysis: evaluating information gathered during assessment and making nursing diagnoses
3. Planning: developing client goals and nursing interventions to meet them
   a. Develop long- and short-term goals with client
   b. Goals should be stated in behavioral terms
   c. Specify nursing interventions that will meet each goal
   d. Include nursing actions such as setting limits on unacceptable behavior without rejecting the client as a person, increasing or decreasing environmental stimuli, and providing individually appropriate activities
4. Implementation: carrying out the nursing care plan
   a. Carry out nursing interventions
   b. Establish a suitable environment for implementation (i.e., therapeutic milieu)
5. Evaluation: appraising client's response to nursing interventions and modifying the plan as necessary
   a. Appraise client response to nursing intervention based on the effect of the intervention on the client's behavior, concerns, and achievement of short-term goals
   b. Carried out by the individual nurse as well as by the total staff involved in the care
   c. Revise nursing care plan as necessary

INTERPERSONAL TREATMENT MODALITIES

1. Psychotherapy
   a. Definition: goal-oriented, corrective emotional experience with a therapist in order to effect behavioral change, including
      1. increased well-being
      2. improved psychological performance
      3. improved social performance
   b. Length of treatment
      1. may be long term, to allow client to gain insight and slowly take on new coping mechanisms
      2. may be short term, such as crisis intervention
2. Crisis intervention
   a. Definition: a time-limited (approximately 6 weeks), directive approach to help a client cope with a crisis
      1. person is in crisis when traditional methods of coping are not effective
      2. crises tend to resolve after several weeks; however, if the present one is ineffectively resolved, the person may have lost some ability to cope with future crises
   b. Therapy
      1. includes helping an individual or family cope with an immediate problem that is intolerable
      2. does not go into cause or require insight
      3. deals directly and briefly with the individual's present situation to return client to previous level of coping
         a. clarifies situation and identifies problem
         b. teaches client new coping skills
         c. identifies and mobilizes external and internal resources
      4. helps the client learn to problem solve, and thus client may grow because of the intervention
      5. may prevent maladaptation, development of more serious psychiatric symptoms
   c. The process of therapy includes
      1. establishing a nurse-client relationship
      2. being as active and directive as necessary to help client deal with crisis
      3. helping the client to establish therapeutic goals
      4. reinforcing that the relationship is time-limited, and therefore it is necessary to establish a termination date
      5. actively encouraging the client to express feelings and emotions regarding the crisis situation
      6. helping the client develop new and more effective coping mechanisms
      7. having the client take more responsibility in subsequent sessions (if there is more than one)
3. Behavior modification
   a. Definition: altering undesirable behavior by systematically changing its consequences
      1. operates on the principle that behavior is determined by consequences

2. changes in consequences result in change in behavior
3. does not deal with cause of behavior

b. Process of treatment
1. identify the behavior to be changed (e.g., child throws temper tantrum when told it is time for bed)
2. obtain baseline data regarding the behavior (e.g., frequency)
3. identify the conditions and reinforcers that promote the behavior (e.g., child allowed to stay up late [rewarded] to stop temper tantrum)
4. identify the conditions and reinforcers that will change or eliminate the behavior

c. Techniques: systematic desensitization, ignoring the behavior, time out, token economy, aversion

d. Positive reinforcers (rewards) are much preferable to aversion techniques

4. Therapeutic milieu
a. Uses all interaction to assist client in developing interpersonal and social skills in a conducive physical and emotional environment
b. Manipulates (increases or decreases) environmental stimuli to provide limits, protect client
c. Nurse's role
1. provide 24-hour milieu management
2. provide positive role model
3. plan/coordinate care
d. Activities
1. government: distributes power, promotes open communications; client-elected officers run meetings, negotiate with staff, run unit activities (e.g., cleanups, unit parties)
2. self-care: client required to maintain room, clothing, etc., to promote independence
3. occupational therapy: specific programs developed by occupational therapists to encourage client nonverbal expressions, increase self-esteem, and increase living skills
4. activity therapy: art, music, and recreation planned by nurses or activity therapists to increase social interactions and skills

5. Therapeutic groups: more closely resemble real-life situations than does one-to-one therapy
a. Leading these groups requires training beyond basic nursing education
b. Beginning nurse may co-lead a group
c. Group members provide feedback to each other
d. Variety of responses and reactions available for behavior displayed in group setting
e. Three stages of development
1. group orientation and development of identity
2. group interaction and observation of dynamics

3. resolution of dynamics and production of insights

f. Members may examine patterns of relating to each other and authority figures in supportive atmosphere

g. Group therapy more economical than one-to-one therapy; there are usually two therapists and 7-12 clients

h. The goals and purposes are essentially the same as in one-to-one therapy

6. Family therapy: focuses on the family rather than on the individual
a. Major problem: intolerance of differences
1. healthy family can tolerate differences
2. maladjusted family experiences differences as threats to individual identity and family unity; conflicts lead to splits, coalitions, scapegoating, alignments

b. Major objective: to reestablish rational communication between family members
1. family can reassess and recognize alliances
2. family can resolve to accept differences between members

c. Important difference between family therapy and group therapy
1. in family therapy, the participants enter therapy with a long-standing system of roles and interactions, which the nurse-therapist must learn
2. in group therapy, the relationship between participants begins with the first session; they have no history of a relationship

7. Self-help groups: use persons who have themselves surmounted problems. Nurses may serve as consultants/resource persons.
a. Recovery, Inc.
1. a consumer-funded group consisting of former mental clients and persons with emotional problems
2. focus is on the use of will power in avoiding deviant behavior

b. Other self-help groups
1. Parents Without Partners
2. groups for colostomy clients
3. parents whose children have terminal diseases
4. Overeaters Anonymous
5. Reach for Recovery
6. Alcoholics Anonymous (see p. 76)
7. Narcotics Anonymous
8. groups for child/wife abusers

8. Other therapies
a. Sex therapy
1. geared toward improving a person or couple's sexual functioning

2. treatment includes psychotherapy and pre-scribed experiential learning
3. Masters and Johnson treatment program has served as model for sex therapy treatment

b. Hypnotherapy
   1. may be used for specific symptoms such as anxiety, pain, high blood pressure, smoking, overeating, and phobias
   2. also may be used in conjunction with other therapies to decrease repression
   3. only done by trained professionals
   4. nurse's role is to support client in treatment; communicate with therapist

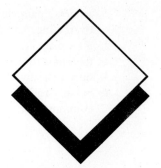

Loss and Death and Dying

GENERAL CONCEPTS
Overview

1. Every human being experiences several losses during a lifetime (e.g., loss of health, loss of a relationship or loved one, change in life-style); people deal with loss by grieving and integrating the subsequent changes into their life
   a. Responses to loss vary greatly depending upon the individual's personality, previous experience with losses, and value of the person or thing lost
   b. Behavior during normal grieving is similar to that seen in a depressed person (e.g., crying, fatigue, feelings of emptiness); unlike grief, depression is a chronic state characterized by low self-esteem
   c. People who are dying experience fear (e.g., pain, loneliness, meaninglessness)
2. Definitions
   a. *Loss:* the anticipated or actual removal of something or someone of value to a person
   b. *Grief:* the normal emotional responses to a loss, which subside after a reasonable time
   c. *Unresolved grief:* failure to complete the grieving process and cope successfully with the loss because of social and psychological factors; some circumstances that increase the likelihood of unresolved grief responses include
      1. socially unspeakable loss (e.g., suicide)
      2. uncertainty over loss (e.g., person missing in action)
      3. need to be strong and in control
      4. ambivalence over lost object or person
      5. multiple losses
      6. reawakening of an old, unresolved loss
   d. *Mourning:* the expression of sorrow with outward signs of grief as a result of a perceived or threatened loss
   e. *Grief and mourning process:* the process a person goes through in adapting to a loss; this process is triggered by an *actual* or a *threatened* loss

3. According to Kübler-Ross (the theorist most often associated with the study of death and dying), there are five stages in the grief and mourning process of the dying person (these stages can be applied in evaluating other losses)
   a. Denial: unconscious avoidance that varies from a very brief period to the remainder of life; allows a person to mobilize defenses to cope with death
      1. adaptive responses: crying, verbal denial
      2. maladaptive responses: absence of crying or verbal recognition of loss
   b. Anger: covert or overt expression of realization of loss
      1. adaptive responses: verbal expression of anger
      2. maladaptive responses: persistent guilt or low self-esteem, aggression, self-destructive ideation or behavior
   c. Bargaining: an attempt to change reality of loss, often done with God
      1. adaptive responses: bargains for treatment control, expresses wish to be alive for specific events in near future
      2. maladaptive responses: bargains for unrealistic activities or events in distant future
   d. Depression: sadness resulting from actual and anticipated losses
      1. adaptive responses: crying, withdrawing from interactions
      2. maladaptive responses: self-destructive actions, despair
   e. Acceptance: resolution of feelings about death resulting in feeling of peace
      1. adaptive behaviors: may wish to be alone, limit visitors, limit conversation, complete personal and family business
      2. may never reach this stage
4. A child's understanding and responses to death depend on
   a. Age

1. preschooler can't differentiate between death and absence
2. from 5–6 years old, they see death as something others experience, begin to accept death as a fact, believe death is reversible, not final
3. from 6–9 years old, children associate death with injury; personify death (someone bad carries them away), or death is "old people"
4. from 9–10 years old, they recognize everyone must die
5. early adolescents understand permanence of death; difficult to see self dying before having a chance to live; may experience resentment, withdrawal, see self as different from others; also concerned about possible different reaction of others (e.g., withdrawal of friends); fantasies of rebirth, reunion, and reincarnation result
6. all ages: underlying fear is of separation and pain, rather than fear of death itself

b. Previous experience with death: relatives, friends, pets, family responses to death
c. Knowledge of what is happening
d. Other influences
   1. whether child is hospitalized; staff behavior
   2. parents' anxieties
   3. reaction of other family members, siblings

Application of the Nursing Process to the Client Experiencing a Loss

Assessment
1. Current behavior
   a. Stage of grief and mourning
   b. Adaptive or maladaptive
2. Previous losses
3. Support system

Analysis
1. Safe, effective care environment
   a. High risk for violence: self-directed or directed at others
   b. Knowledge deficit
   c. Sensory—perceptual alteration (visual, auditory, kinesthetic, gustatory, tactile, olfactory)
2. Physiological integrity
   a. High risk for activity intolerance
   b. Pain
   c. Impaired verbal communication
3. Psychosocial integrity
   a. Body image disturbance, personal identity disturbance, self-esteem disturbance
   b. Anticipatory grieving
   c. Dysfunctional grieving
4. Health promotion/maintenance
   a. Altered family processes
   b. Altered growth and development
   c. Altered health maintenance

General Nursing Planning, Implementation, and Evaluation

> **Goal:** Client will move through the grief and mourning process within an acceptable time frame.

Implementation
1. Allow the client to use own method of coping as long as it is not physically destructive.
2. Reinforce adaptive behavior; remember that suicidal ideation is not adaptive in any stage.
3. Tell client that it is normal and expected to grieve over a loss.
4. Help client to express feelings ("You look sad. What are you feeling right now?"); listen attentively and with empathy.
5. Recognize impact of previous losses, help client resolve past and present losses.

Evaluation
Client talks about specific loss; asks questions about future; bargains verbally; expresses anger, sadness.

SELECTED HEALTH PROBLEMS
☐ Loss (Other than Death and Dying)
General Information
1. Types of loss
   a. Physical losses include loss of
      1. body part
      2. usual function of a body part (e.g., paralysis of a limb)
      3. a valued object (e.g., a house)
      4. economic status
      5. youth, beauty, health
      6. a significant other, either through loss of a relationship or through death
   b. Psychological losses include losses/changes in
      1. meaning in life, beliefs, and values
      2. status, recognition, prestige
      3. meaningful work, creative abilities
      4. self-esteem and self-worth
      5. nurturance and sense of belonging
      6. expected outcome (e.g., a stillborn infant)
      7. role identity, self-concept

Nursing Process
Assessment
1. Specific loss
2. Meaning of loss to client
3. Support system
Analysis (see p. 27)
Planning, Implementation, and Evaluation

> **Goal:** Client will respond adaptively to the loss.

Implementation

1. Allow client to cry, express anger, or exhibit other adaptive responses to the loss.
2. Provide support for adaptive behavior (e.g., "It must be very difficult for you right now.").
3. Help client to express feelings (e.g., "Other people in your situation often feel sad or angry. How do you feel?").
4. When client asks questions about living with loss, tell the client only what he or she wants to know at that time (in-depth teaching can be done later when client is ready).
5. Reinforce all adaptive behaviors.
6. Expect that client will alternate between behaviors of consecutive stages.

Evaluation

Client asks questions about adapting to the loss; cries, feels sad, plans for future.

☐ Death and Dying

General Information

1. Responses to the dying process are highly individualized and may be greatly influenced by the client's physical status and personality; the interaction of client and family will have a strong bearing on the client's healthy progression through the process
2. Nurse's responses
   a. In order to be effective in helping the dying person, the nurse must focus on own beliefs, feelings, and behaviors in regard to death
   b. The nurse who is unaware of own feelings, fears, and beliefs about death may unwittingly inhibit client's expression of feelings
   c. By looking at own beliefs about death and how people should respond to death, nurse can be aware of expecting others to respond in accordance with nurse's belief system
3. Establishing priorities
   a. Priorities may be determined by the client's psychological and physical status
      1. at some point, pain or fatigue may demand more attention than the psychological factors
      2. a client who cannot keep any food down or cannot feel relief from pain needs the nurse to respond to those factors immediately
   b. The next most important action is to assist the client in dealing with the manifestations of whatever stage client is in
   c. Help the family interact in healthy ways with client by healthy role modeling, discussing illness and death with the client and family
4. DSM-III-R classification: uncomplicated bereavement

Nursing Process: Adult

Assessment

1. Physical condition and relationship to psychological stimulus

2. Knowledge of and response to diagnosis; people respond to dying similarly to the way they have responded to other major crises
3. Stage in dying process: the stage can fluctuate, or client/family may exhibit behaviors of more than one stage at a time
   a. Current behavior
   b. Current affect and feelings expressed
4. Support from significant others
5. Expectations and resources
6. Feelings about treatment setting
7. Family assessment
   a. Perception of diagnosis and prognosis
   b. Stage of loss
   c. Feelings and their influence on client
   d. Communication patterns
   e. Needs and resources
   f. Response to dying person and impact on client

Analysis (see p. 27)

Planning, Implementation, and Evaluation

Goal 1: (Stage 1) Client will begin to cope with the impending death through denial.

Implementation

1. Plan several brief interactions with client each shift (client may try to protect others by being "brave" and perhaps not seek out help and support from others).
2. Teach client that some isolation and denial are normal responses.
3. Allow denial until client has mobilized other defenses to deal with the impact of diagnosis and prognosis.
4. Be honest when answering the client's questions about life, death, and treatment. Do not be too harsh in your honesty, but do not minimize client's concerns; allow client to maintain hope.
5. Do not reinforce or reject client's denial; accept need for denial (e.g., if client says, "I can't believe it! It's not happening," nurse might say, "It must seem a bit unreal to you").
6. Support client in dealing with denial expressed by family and friends.

Evaluation

Client initially denies and then begins to acknowledge the reality of the impending death.

Goal 2: (Stage 2) Client will verbalize anger about impending death.

Implementation

1. Permit and encourage the verbal expression of anger (often the anger is directed toward the nurse). Remember that fear underlies anger; do not take the anger as a personal attack and react defensively.
2. Allow expression of guilt (not seeking or following treatment), but help client move away from self-blame.

3. Listen to client's expressions of anger without offering any judgment; help client deal with anger arising from distancing behaviors of relatives and friends.
4. Discuss possible alternative treatment and lifestyle changes introduced by the client; offer clear, factual information about any alternatives to assist client in making choices.

Evaluation

Client verbalizes anger about impending death.

Goal 3: (Stage 3) Client will use bargaining in an attempt to prolong life.

Implementation

1. Permit client to cope by bargaining; client may say things like, "If only . . ." or "Maybe I could . . ."; know that this characteristic "magical thinking" allows client to feel some control.
2. Help client to make amends for past failures or grievances (perceived or real); help client to find meaning in life by reminiscing.
3. Discuss importance of what is being bargained for using a sensitive, accepting approach.
4. Allow client to make appropriate decisions (e.g., timing of, intervals between, or lack of interventions); explore risks and possible consequences, but allow client to make the decisions.

Evaluation

Client continues progress through the grief and mourning process by bargaining.

Goal 4: (Stage 4) Client will verbalize recognition of the inevitable and allow self to feel sadness and depression.

Implementation

1. Allow client to express sadness by crying, talking, or withdrawing into silence; avoid trying to "cheer" client.
2. Answer questions such as "Am I going to die?" with a response such as "Do you feel you are going to die?"; support and discuss client's responses.
3. Provide opportunities for client to express feelings about the impending loss of everything known and loved, and changes in body image and self-esteem; accept sadness as grieving behavior, not as self-pity.
4. Remind client that sadness is normal; explore the difference that coping with the impending death rather than giving up can make.
5. Help client to focus on the present and to make the most of each day.

Evaluation

Client verbalizes sad, depressed feelings; begins to talk about own death.

Goal 5: (Stage 5) Client will accept the inevitability of impending death.

Implementation

1. Help client take care of personal and family matters as desired.
2. Continue to allow discussion of the impending death but realize that full acceptance may not be achieved (rather, the client becomes resigned to the situation); do not try to force acceptance.
3. Allow client to continue to participate in making decisions about care as desired.
4. Allow client to decide when and if to spend some time alone; allow client to restrict visitors to short periods of time as desired.
5. Promote a peaceful conclusion of the dying process by offering comfort and security measures as necessary.
6. Know that the family may not be at the same level of coping as the client.
   a. Assess the potential disruption the death will have on the family.
   b. Use clear and factual terminology and information when speaking with them.
   c. Remain as calm and unreactive as possible so as not to further stress the family with your own emotions and needs.
   d. Use family rituals and customs whenever possible.
   e. Spend time with them discussing their feelings.
   f. Know that families respond to the dying member much as they handled other major crisis situations.
   g. Family's greatest needs may be competent physical care for the ill member and empathy for the difficulty of their situation.
   h. Help family with packing, arrange a comfortable place to sleep in the hospital, or allow family to call at any time to find out how their ill relative is.

Evaluation

Client moves through the fifth stage of loss at own rhythm to a comfortable and dignified death; expresses feelings and concerns about impending death; participates in decision making for own activities of daily living (ADL) for as long as possible; the family or significant other discuss feelings and concerns about death of loved one.

Nursing Process: Child

Assessment

1. Child's level of understanding and reaction/feelings about situation; ability to express self
2. Parents' level of understanding and reaction/feelings about situation; parents' strengths and needs; support systems
3. Child's physical condition (e.g., vital signs, pain, hydration), ability to perform ADL
4. Staff members' feelings and concerns, need for support
5. Siblings' level of understanding; their responses to

behavior of, health changes in, and separation from ill sibling

Analysis (see p. 27)

Planning, Implementation, and Evaluation

> **Goal 1:** Child/family will express feelings, fears, anxieties, guilt they may be experiencing; will verbalize their understanding of the physical health status and the terminal process.

Implementation

1. Determine what the child knows.
2. Work through own feelings with other staff members.
3. Allow and encourage the parents to express their feelings, and accept those expressions in a nonjudgmental manner.
4. Be available to client and family for frequent interactions.
5. Permit child to express anger and hostility, but at the same time do not be totally permissive regarding unacceptable behavior (child may perceive this permissiveness as total hopelessness and abandonment).
6. Encourage child to draw or play with toys to express feelings:
   a. Draw own body.
   b. Draw a feeling.
   c. Draw family.
   d. Play doctor/nurse and act out feelings, including angry feelings; let nurse be the client.
7. Acknowledge family responses, stages of grieving:
   a. Shock, denial, guilt, bodily distress, anxiety.
   b. Acceptance, belief in God.
8. Encourage interaction/involvement of ill child and siblings.
9. Help reduce marital stress by encouraging couple to spend an evening away from the hospital and to call when they feel concerned about their child.

10. Help siblings to express their feelings, use drawing, storytelling, play therapy.
    a. Help parents understand that siblings' perceptions/interpretations/reactions may not be as intense as parents'.
    b. "Favorite child" angers other siblings; stress is also on siblings who need a chance to discuss feelings; they, too, may feel they did something to cause sibling to become ill.
11. Refer family to self-help groups in community.

Evaluation

Child/family expresses some degree of awareness of the terminal process; verbalizes some feelings associated with grief and mourning.

> **Goal 2:** Child will maintain as much independence as possible in ADL; will have minimal pain and discomfort; will ingest adequate food and fluid to meet body needs.

Implementation

1. Encourage child's participation in ADL as long as energy levels are not depleted.
2. Ensure adequate fluid and food; use supplements when necessary and allow child choice of food if possible.
3. Preserve skin integrity by massage, lotions, sheepskin, water mattress.
4. Provide pain medication and comfort measures as needed (PRN).
5. Use passive and active range of motion (ROM).
6. Permit child to have toys, music, and special objects.
7. Allow parents to participate in care; explain procedures to parents/child.

Evaluation

Child maintains independence in ADL; has minimal pain and discomfort; ingests food and fluid to meet body needs.

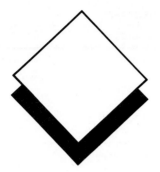

Anxious Behavior

GENERAL CONCEPTS
Overview

1. Anxiety can be a problem in and of itself, but it is also an aspect of other psychosocial problems. Anxiety is a persistent feeling of dread, apprehension, and impending disaster brought on by a nonspecific threat to self. In mild degrees, it is a normal experience that motivates a person to take constructive action in a situation. As anxiety becomes more severe, it can interfere with perception, judgment, and behavior, and it requires outside intervention to help the person to function constructively. Its prominence as a human occurrence makes it one of the most common concerns in psychosocial nursing. Recognition of anxious behaviors and the appropriate use of helping interventions are essential nursing skills in any health care setting (see Table 2-5).

2. Anticipatory anxiety, anxiety, and fear are all accepted official nursing diagnoses with established defining characteristics
   a. *Anticipatory anxiety:* an increased level of arousal associated with a perceived *future* threat to the self
   b. *Anxiety:* a generalized feeling of dread and apprehension, which is a subjectively painful warning of a threat to the self or to significant relationships
   c. *Fear:* a feeling of dread related to an *identifiable* source that is perceived as a threat or danger to the self or significant relationships
   d. *Anxious behavior:* a manifestation of a subjective feeling resulting from the experience of anxiety, conflict, fear, or stress; such response ranges from mild to severe and represents a usual human reaction to a sense of threat

3. General causes
   a. A threat to biological integrity
   b. A threat to security of self; anxiety is a warning signal stimulating the organism to act against the threat

   c. A person's own defenses/coping mechanisms are not working as well as they usually do
   d. An unconscious conflict brought on by a nonspecific threat to self (psychoanalytic theory)
   e. Genetic predisposition

4. Four levels of anxiety: on a continuum from mild to panic, which primarily involves sensory perception and level of functioning
   a. *Mild anxiety:* characteristics
      1. more alert than usual, increased questioning
      2. heightened capacity to deal with perception of impending danger
      3. focus of attention on immediate events
      4. person experiences mild discomfort, restlessness
      5. may be a useful motivating force (e.g., if a person experiences mild anxiety during NCLEX-RN, this may help to increase ability to answer questions)
   b. *Moderate anxiety:* characteristics
      1. narrowed perception
      2. reduced ability to listen, perceive, comprehend, and communicate
      3. selective inattention, focus on one specific thing; "tunnel vision" develops
      4. increased tension; increased discomfort; verbalization about expected danger
      5. decreased ability to function
      6. physical symptoms (e.g., pacing, hand tremors, diaphoresis, increased heart rate, sleep and/or eating disturbances)
   c. *Severe anxiety:* characteristics
      1. greatly reduced perception; difficulty attending to, understanding, and processing information
      2. sense of impending doom; dread, horror
      3. increased physical symptoms (e.g., diaphoresis, dizziness, increased muscle tension, pallor, nausea, trembling)
      4. survival response (fight or flight)

Table 2-5 **DSM-III-R classification of anxiety-related disorders**

Anxiety Disorders	Somatoform Disorders	Dissociative Disorders
Panic Disorder	Somatization Disorder	Depersonalization Disorder
General Anxiety Disorder	Hypochondriasis	Psychogenic Amnesia
Phobias	Somatoform Pain Disorder	Psychogenic Fugue
Obsessive-Compulsive Disorder	Conversion	Multiple Personality Disorder
Post-Traumatic Stress Disorder	Somatoform Disorder NOS*	Dissociative Disorder NOS*
Anxiety Disorder NOS*		

Psychological factors affecting physical condition	Disorders usually first evident in infancy, childhood, or adolescence
Physical condition specified	Eating disorders
	Anorexia nervosa
	Bulimia nervosa
	Pica
	Rumination disorder of infancy
	Eating disorder NOS*

The above disorders all have anxiety as the underlying dynamic. Multiple defenses are used, but they are repetitive and ineffective in lowering the anxiety.
*NOS = Not otherwise specified

  d. *Panic:* characteristics
    1. altered perception of and focus on reality
    2. helpless, fearful, panicky feelings
    3. physical symptoms (e.g., tachycardia, hyperventilation)
    4. extreme discomfort; extreme measures to decrease anxiety
    5. feeling of personal disintegration
    6. severe hyperactivity, loss of control
    7. inability to communicate or function
  5. Diagnosis of anxiety: inferred from three kinds of data: physiological changes, psychological changes (see Table 2-6), and use of coping or defense mechanisms
    a. Physiological changes
      1. involve primarily the autonomic nervous system
      2. physiological operations tend to be speeded up by mild and moderate anxieties
      3. functioning tends to be slowed down by severe panic; can result in complete functional paralysis and death (in prolonged panic)
      4. knowledge of physical manifestations allows the nurse to intervene prior to the panic stage
      5. during panic, when the physical symptoms are severe, immediate intervention is imperative
    b. Psychological changes
      1. psychological manifestations accelerate as anxiety level increases and can become extremely uncomfortable to the person
      2. maladaptive behaviors are mechanisms used to avoid accelerating anxiety to the panic state (e.g., rumination, rituals, compulsivity)
    c. Coping mechanisms: may be a defense mechanism

Table 2-6 **Manifestations of anxiety**

Physiological	Psychological
Tachycardia	Tension
Palpitations	Nervousness
Excessive perspiration	Apprehension
Dry mouth	Irritability
Cold, clammy, pale skin	Indecisiveness
Urinary frequency	Oversensitivity
Diarrhea	Tearfulness
Muscle tension	Agitation
Tremors	Dread
Narrowing of focus	Horror
	Panic

or any means used to resolve, or at least delay, the conflict
    1. constructive: client, alerted by warning signal that something is not going as expected, resolves the conflict
    2. destructive or disturbed: client tries to protect self from anxiety without resolving the conflict, which can be expressed in maladaptive or dysfunctional behavior

Application of the Nursing Process to the Client Exhibiting Anxious Behavior

NOTE: The same nursing process is used with all anxiety-related behaviors regardless of whether they are functional or dysfunctional.
Assessment
1. Level of anxiety (signs and behavior)
2. Physiological and psychological signs and symptoms
3. Cause, if known

4. Coping mechanisms (constructive and/or destructive)
5. Problem behavior (e.g., weekly episodes of gastritis indicating moderate anxiety related to work conflict)
6. Strengths
7. Support systems and their involvement with client
8. Insight

Analysis

1. Safe, effective care environment
   a. Impaired home maintenance management
   b. High risk for trauma
   c. Knowledge deficit
2. Physiological integrity
   a. Impaired verbal communication
   b. Altered nutrition: less/more than body requirements
   c. Sleep pattern disturbance
3. Psychosocial integrity
   a. Anxiety
   b. Ineffective individual coping
   c. Self-esteem/body image/personal identity disturbance
   d. Post-trauma response
4. Health promotion/maintenance
   a. Impaired adjustment
   b. Altered family processes
   c. Altered health maintenance
   d. Self-care deficit (specify)

General Nursing Planning, Implementation, and Evaluation

Goal 1: Client will develop an open, trusting relationship with the nurse.

Implementation

1. Approach client in unhurried way and actively listen to concerns and feelings.
2. Encourage client to express feelings and concerns about unmet needs or stressful situation.
3. Be aware of feelings and behavior and their impact upon client.

Evaluation

Client expresses concerns and unmet needs to the nurse (e.g., concern about failure or rejection).

Goal 2: Client will use anxiety as a motivation for change.

Implementation

1. Help client express feelings about stressful situations, unmet needs.
   a. Help client to acknowledge or name the feelings being experienced.
   b. Express genuine interest and concern.
2. Be nonjudgmental and offer unconditional acceptance.
3. Offer reassurance by giving appropriate information,

correcting misinformation; repeat the process if necessary as client may have reduced hearing perception; use short, concise statements.
4. Work with client to identify anxiety-causing situations that can be avoided.
5. Teach client to recognize how client is manifesting anxiety in behavior and body responses.
6. Help client identify situations that trigger anxiety.
7. Assist client in using stress-reduction techniques (e.g., biofeedback, visualization, talking it out) to cope with anxiety; refer to Table 2-7.
8. Be aware that client and nurse have reciprocal influence on each other.
   a. Anxiety is contagious.
   b. Find constructive ways to control own anxiety, frustration, or anger.
9. Prevent mild anxiety from escalating by intervening early, whenever possible.
10. Provide physical care as needed to severely anxious client.

Evaluation

Client expresses feelings; identifies situations that cause anxiety; incorporates at least one stress-reduction technique into daily routine; experiences no more than moderate anxiety.

Goal 3: Client will recognize own anxious behaviors and gain insight into cause of problems.

Implementation

1. Help client recognize anxiety by exploring the feelings that precede anxious behavior.
2. Help client distinguish between thoughts, feelings, and behaviors.
3. Use the nurse-client relationship to increase the client's ability to gain insight into the cause of problems.
4. Provide a new perspective on the situation (i.e., help client "redefine" the problem).
5. Use biofeedback learning to help client recognize own tensions.
6. Teach client to evaluate the threat, expectations, or unmet needs and to assess own capabilities realistically.

Evaluation

Client identifies own behaviors that are linked to current anxiety; tells nurse when feeling increasingly anxious; can state cause(s) of current anxiety.

Goal 4: Client will demonstrate alternative methods of coping with anxiety.

Implementation

1. Examine client's patterns of coping with anxiety.
2. Reinforce effective and constructive coping mechanisms.

Table 2-7   Stress management

Stress is a generalized, nonspecific response of the body to any demand, change, or perceived threat, whether positive or negative. *Stressors* are the circumstances or events that elicit this response and may be real or anticipated. *Distress* is damaging or unpleasant stress.

Signs of distress		
accident proneness	frequent urination	irritability
alcohol and drug abuse	grinding teeth	neck or back pain
chronic fatigue	headache	neurotic or psychotic behavior
decrease or increase of appetite	impulsive behavior	nightmares
diarrhea or constipation	inability to concentrate	sexual problems
emotional instability	increased smoking	stuttering
emotional tension	insomnia	sweating

GOAL

The client will maintain homeostasis or optimal adaptive coping by preventing, or recognizing promptly, excessive levels of stress; the client will use effective measures to manage stress by describing a plan to cope with stress in an adaptive way that includes exercise, relaxation, creative problem solving, and sharing feelings and concerns with a significant other.

Stress-reduction techniques	Nursing implications	Stress-reduction techniques	Nursing implications
Identify stressors (e.g., work, relationships, environment, health, age, finances, spiritual/emotional factors)	Have client examine own reaction to life occurrences (e.g., frustration, knot in stomach, loss of control). Discern between positive and negative stressors; explain that stress is unavoidable and can be used to motivate.	relaxation techniques progressive relaxation autogenic training guided imagery	Guide patient through a relaxation exercise to experience its usefulness. Begin relaxation with deep breathing. Use guided imagery to induce relaxation (e.g., "Take another deep breath and let all the tension release. With each breath you become more relaxed. Now, imagine yourself in a peaceful, quiet setting [garden, beach, etc."]).
Modify or eliminate stressors	Review possibilities for simple and major changes. Discuss alternatives, advantages, and disadvantages of reducing stressors.		Refer to cassettes, books, and classes on learning and practicing relaxation techniques.
Develop effective coping mechanisms daily exercise	Suggest methods to reduce stress through exercise (e.g., walking, running, dancing, swimming, gardening, participating in sports, body movement exercises, yoga). Assist in developing a plan of regular activity. Refer to community gyms, health clubs, and YMCAs. Advise consultation with personal physician for contraindications to exercise program.	diaphragmatic breathing; periodic deep breathing	Practice diaphragmatic breathing with client Sit or recline in a comfortable position with legs uncrossed. Place one hand on the chest and the other hand on the diaphragm, approximately 2 inches below the bottom center of the breastbone. Inhale so the diaphragm expands and the hand covering the diaphragm moves out while the other hand remains almost still.
develop alternative ways to relax (e.g., drawing, pottery, carpentry, writing, music, photography, reading, watching the sunset, taking a bubble bath).	Review with client activities enjoyed and suggest client devote at least an hour a day to an activity. Refer to recreation departments, adult education programs, community colleges.		As you exhale, the diaphragm relaxes and the hand covering it moves inward.

Table 2-7   Stress management—cont'd

Stress-reduction techniques	Nursing implications	Stress-reduction techniques	Nursing implications
positive affirmations creating positive, active, new beliefs about oneself and immersing them into the subconscious mind by repeating them frequently	Teach to write out the statements and place them on mirror, steering wheel, refrigerator, desk, etc. repeat the statements several times daily. be specific, positive, and brief (e.g., "I am relaxed," not "I am not tense."). use the present tense, "I am," not "I will." (e.g., "I am learning to express my feelings. I am expressing anger in a positive way. I am lovable.").	improve self-care	Discuss personal habits that contribute to distress. self-medication poor nutrition neglecting early warning signs of tension nonassertiveness drinking, smoking Demonstrate positive ways to express and become more aware of feelings. Teach creative problem solving; brainstorm for alternatives. Discuss importance of setting priorities, taking one thing at a time.
balance work and recreation	Teach importance of seeking work that one enjoys and is capable of doing or learning. learning to take relaxation breaks. taking regularly scheduled vacations. taking a "mental health" day away from work in lieu of a sick day.		

From Caine, R., & Bufalino, P. (1987). *Nursing care planning guides for adults.* Baltimore, Williams & Wilkins. Used with permission.

3. Teach client alternative methods of coping (e.g., visual imagery, relaxation, talking it out).
4. Know that the client with mild or moderate anxiety is generally not hospitalized for treatment depending upon:
   a. Severity of the symptoms.
   b. Incapacity of function.
   c. Threat to self or others.
   d. Nature of the home environment.
5. Observe physical status and intervene directly as necessary for client's well-being.

Evaluation

Client learns two new coping mechanisms (e.g., talking about feelings, guided imagery; experiences more control over anxiety).

> **Goal 5:** Client will be able to cope with severe to panic anxiety and reduce anxiety at least one level.

Implementation

1. Understand that a severely anxious client may neglect physical needs, exhaust self, or actually injure self. Give physical care and protection as indicated; maintain safe environment.
2. Remove client from other clients if anxiety is increasing, but do not leave a highly anxious client alone.
3. Anticipate mild disturbances and prevent them from developing into severe or panic stage by identifying early signs of disturbance with client.
4. Allow client to determine what stresses client can handle.
5. Know that coping mechanisms keep the anxiety within tolerable limits.
6. Remain calm in your approach to client.
7. Do not attempt to argue, ridicule, or reason with a client regarding defense mechanisms.
8. Help client to adopt and develop effective, positive coping mechanisms.
9. When tranquilizing agents are prescribed:
   a. Refer to Table 2-8.
   b. Administer as ordered to provide symptomatic relief of anxiety and to create stability so client may be more able to participate in process of therapy.

Table 2-8 Antianxiety agents (minor tranquilizers)

Drug	Action	Side effects	Nursing implications
BENZODIAZEPINE DERIVATIVES			
Chlordiazepoxide hydrochloride (Librium) 5-10 mg po 3-4 x/day (mild-moderate anxiety) 20-25 mg po 3-4 x/day (severe anxiety) 50-100 mg po for acute alcohol withdrawal Oxazepam (Serax) 10-15 mg po 3-4 x/day (mild, moderate anxiety) 15-30 mg po 3-4 x/day (severe anxiety) Chlorazepate dipotassium (Tranxene) 15-60 mg/day po in divided doses for maintenance Diazepam (Valium) 2-10 mg po 2-4 x/day 10 mg po 3-4 x first day for acute alcohol withdrawal Alprazolam (Xanax) 0.25-0.5 mg po tid Maximum dosage 4 mg/day in divided doses Lorazepam (Ativan) 2-3 mg po divided into 2-3 doses/day	Appears to act on limbic, thalamic, and hypothalamic levels of CNS; produces hypnotic, sedative, anxiolytic, skeletal muscle relaxant, and anticonvulsant effects. Range of CNS depression is from mild sedation to coma.	Hypotension, drowsiness, dizziness, ataxia, lethargy, headache, dry mouth, constipation, urinary retention, changes in libido, paradoxical excitement. Psychic and physical dependence.	Caution client to avoid potentially hazardous activities because of drowsiness. Warm client of danger of concurrent use of alcohol or other CNS depressants. Be aware that these drugs may potentiate suicidal tendencies. Monitor vital signs. Report paradoxical excitement. Avoid abrupt withdrawal (may produce reactions). Tolerance and psychological and physiological dependence may occur after prolonged use. Do not give antacids concurrently. In geriatric clients, doses are initiated at lower levels.
Meprobamate (Equanil, Miltown) 1.2-1.6 g daily in 3-4 divided doses Maximum dose 2.4 g	CNS depressant action is similar to barbiturates. Apparently acts on multiple CNS sites—hypothalamus, thalamus, limbic, and spinal cord.	Drowsiness, ataxia, dizziness, vertigo, slurred speech, headache, skin rash, weakness. Psychic and physical dependence.	Know that meprobamate is highly lethal in overdose; consider the possibility of suicide attempts and take precautions. Caution client regarding the concurrent use of alcohol or other CNS depressants. Avoid rapid withdrawal (convulsions and death can result). Caution client to avoid potentially hazardous activities because of drowsiness.
ANTIHISTAMINES			
Hydroxyzine hydrochloride (Vistaril) Hydroxyzine pamoate (Atarax) 50-100 mg po qid	Has central cholinergic effect and CNS properties; used for sedative effects as nighttime sleep aid.	Drowsiness, dry mouth, headache.	Caution client to avoid potentially hazardous activities because of drowsiness. Warm client of additive effects with alcohol and other drugs.

Table 2-8 Antianxiety agents (minor tranquilizers)—cont'd

Drug	Action	Side effects	Nursing implications
BARBITURATES			

The following are sedative doses (hypnotic doses are higher for sleep inducement and preop anxiety)
Amobarbital
    30-50 mg po bid or tid
Aprobarbital
    40 mg po tid
Butabarbital sodium
    15-30 mg tid or qid
Mephobarbital
    32-100 mg po tid or qid
Pentobarbital
    20-40 mg po bid or tid
Phenobarbital
    30-120 mg po od
Secobarbital sodium
    100-300 mg od in 3 divided doses (not usually used for sedation; used mostly as a hypnotic)
Talbutal
    30-60 mg po bid or tid
	Decreases the excitability of both presynaptic and postsynaptic membranes to produce sedative/hypnotic effect. Barbiturates are capable of producing all levels of CNS depression. Used for anxiety, insomnia, alcohol withdrawal syndrome, preoperative sedation, anticonvulsant (only phenobarbital, metharbital, and mephobarbital are effective as oral anticonvulsants).	Tolerance, psychological and physiological dependence may occur after prolonged use when used for insomnia; should not be used over 2 weeks; drowsiness.	Warn clients that barbiturates may impair the ability to perform tasks requiring mental alertness (e.g., driving, operating machinery)
			Warn clients not to consume alcohol while taking these drugs.
			Do not withdraw drug abruptly after prolonged use.
			May potentiate side effects of other CNS depressants.
			Dosage in elderly is reduced.
			Obtain BP, P&R before administration.
			Watch for paradoxical reactions (e.g., excitement, hyperactivity, confusion, depression).
			Watch for drug interactions (other CNS depressants, anticoagulants, corticosteroids, antidepressants, doxycycline).

MISCELLANEOUS			
Buspirone hydrochloride (BuSpar)	Anxiolytic; takes 3 weeks for therapeutic effect.		
Propranolol hydrochloride (Inderal)	Beta-adrenergic blocker used to relieve physical symptoms; attaches to sensors and blocks messages that arouse anxiety states	See Table 3-9.	See Table 3-9.
Imipramine hydrochloride (Tofranil)	Antidepressant; regulates brain's reaction to serotonin to prevent panic attacks.	See Table 2-10.	See Table 2-10.

c. Know that drugs have potential for addiction and should be prescribed for only short periods; drugs may also rob client of motivation for change.

d. Teach client that minor tranquilizers should not be taken with alcohol, since each affects the central nervous system (CNS) and enhances the effect of the other (potentiation).

e. Teach the client actions and side effects of drugs (a common side effect of tranquilizers is drowsiness; therefore persons taking these drugs should avoid driving or any potentially dangerous activity).

10. When client's anxiety has decreased, negotiate reasonable limits on anxious behavior.

11. Do not reinforce manifestations of anxiety by giving them undue attention.

12. Provide physical activity as appropriate to client's condition.

Evaluation

Client reduces anxiety to at least a moderate level; does not injure self or others; has a constructive, effective coping mechanism (e.g., talking about feelings, using relaxation techniques, punching bag).

SELECTED HEALTH PROBLEMS
☐ Obsessive-Compulsive Disorders
General Information

1. Definition: presence of obsession (uncontrollable, recurring thoughts) or compulsion (a ritualistic act done in an attempt to relieve the anxiety related to the thoughts or to make the thoughts go away); considered to be a psychological conversion reaction to anxiety

2. Ego defense mechanisms: displacement and undoing; the person attempts to displace unconscious, hostile, aggressive impulse with unrelated acts (e.g., hand washing); in so doing, the person attempts to undo or negate the unacceptable impulse

3. Signs and symptoms: may include ritualistic behaviors, (e.g., compulsive hand washing or cleanliness, or habitual responses such as extreme thrift, neatness, or insistence on same daily routine) with panic or bizarre behavior if usual routine is broken

4. Treatment: individual, family, or group psychotherapy; desensitization; behavior modification; antidepressants

5. DSM-III-R classification: subclassification of anxiety disorders, obsessive-compulsive disorder

Nursing Process
Assessment

1. Note patterns of compulsive behaviors, including preceding events, and client's reactions to specific situations and persons

2. Listen for description of obsessions

Analysis (see p. 33)

Planning, Implementation, and Evaluation

> **Goal:** Client will accept limits on repetitive acts and participate in alternative adaptive activities.

Implementation

1. Give client a schedule to follow so that ritualistic/repetitive behaviors are *limited,* but not prohibited.

2. Allow client to have choices in schedule and participate in decisions about use of time and energy.

3. Do not abruptly interrupt the repetitive act, since it is allaying anxiety; interruption allows the anxiety to break through and can cause panic.

4. Set reasonable limits on repetitive behavior; give the client adequate warning that at a certain time another activity will begin.

5. Engage in alternative activities with client; do not expect the client to proceed in another activity alone.

6. Provide physical protection from repetitive acts; some ritualistic behaviors can cause physical discomfort (e.g., compulsive hand washing).

7. As ritualistic/repetitive behaviors decrease, help client express feelings and concerns in socially acceptable ways.

Evaluation

Client washes hands (or other compulsive act) fewer times a day compared with admission; begins to participate in other activities.

☐ Anorexia Nervosa
General Information

1. Definition: a symptom complex with compulsive resistance to eating and maintaining body weight; intense fear of becoming obese, yet obsessed with food; loss of weight in excess of 15% of recommended body weight with no known physical illness to account for weight loss; body-image disturbance (feel fat when thin and emaciated); in females, absence of at least three consecutive menstrual periods

2. Onset: usually 12-18 years of age

3. Possible etiologies: primary hypothalamic disorder; atypical affective disorder; phobic avoidance of adulthood; control of one's identity; disturbance in family relationships, especially with mother; societal demands for perfection and control; ambivalence toward mother and independence

4. Prevalence reported in 12- to 18-year-old girls ranges from 1 in 100 to 1 in 800; 90%-95% are females

5. Prognosis: reports that up to 21% die from malnutrition, intercurrent infection, or other physical problems; 17%-77% recover

6. DSM-III-R classification: listed with other eating disorders of childhood and adolescence, such as bulimia and pica (craving unnatural foods such as plaster from walls, dirt, clay)

7. Complications: metabolic abnormalities, muscle

wasting, weakness, fatigue, bradycardia, orthostasis, decreased systolic BP, body temperature below 36° C.

8. Treatment: bed rest, hospitalization for intravenous or oral feedings to restore electrolyte and nutritional balance, psychotherapy, behavior modification, family therapy, pharmacotherapy (tricyclics, cyproheptadine [Periactin] with caution)

Nursing Process

Assessment

1. Weight and percentage of normal body weight lost
2. Eating patterns (time, amount and types of foods taken)
3. Vomiting after eating, or if food is forced
4. Anemia, hypotension
5. Amenorrhea
6. Physical activities
7. Sleep
8. Relationships and interactions with parents, friends, staff, other clients
9. Feelings about eating, body image, self
10. Positive coping mechanisms, strengths, interests
11. Family history of anorexia or bulimia
12. Fluid/electrolyte balance
13. Dental erosion, oral hygiene
14. Vital signs

Analysis (see p. 33)

Planning, Implementation, and Evaluation

> **Goal 1:** Client will regain/maintain fluid and electrolyte balance and have adequate nutrition for growth and development.

Implementation

1. Avoid threats, pleas, and health advice.
2. Keep accurate intake and output record (I&O); observe amounts and types of food eaten.
3. Observe for 2 hours after eating to prevent vomiting/regurgitation.
4. Administer tube feedings/intravenous feedings as ordered.
5. Provide positive reinforcement for weight gain rather than amount of food eaten.

Evaluation

Client regains/maintains fluid and electrolyte balance and has adequate nutrition for growth and development.

> **Goal 2:** Client will express feelings and concerns about self and treatment plan; will improve self-concept, will participate in treatment plan.

Implementation

1. Provide opportunities for decision making in treatment plan and ADL (e.g., time of meal, type of food to be eaten, hygiene, exercise, leisure activities).

2. Know that control issues are important dynamics; client needs to accept responsibility for self without guilt or ambivalence. Set and maintain firm limits; be clear about limits and consistent with treatment plan.
3. Provide opportunities for staff to meet to vent feelings about manipulative and self-destructive behavior.

Evaluation

Client expresses feelings and concerns about self/treatment plan; participates in treatment plan (e.g., makes decisions about schedule and activities).

☐ Bulimia

General Information

1. Definition: syndrome characterized by recurrent binge eating with lack of control (average of two binge episodes per week for 3 months), regular self-induced vomiting, use of laxatives or diuretics, dieting/fasting, vigorous exercise to prevent weight gain, overconcern with weight and body shape; usually maintains normal weight and appears healthy
2. Onset: adolescence or early adulthood (17-23 years of age)
3. Prevalence: reports of 1%-4.5% of women affected, 0.4% men
4. Etiology: same as anorexia
5. Prognosis: good if identified early; tends to be episodic with remissions and relapses
6. Complications (usually result of vomiting and laxative abuse): callus formation on back of hand due to trauma from teeth while stimulating gag reflex; dental erosions and cavities; Mallory-Weiss tears resulting in bloody vomitus and blood loss; acid-base changes, especially hypokalemia; ipecac toxicity; hyperactivity; depression/suicide attempts
7. Treatment: psychotherapy, family therapy, behavioral therapy, hospitalization, outpatient treatment, pharmacotherapy (tricyclic antidepressants and MAO inhibitors), diet therapy, restoration of normal fluid/electrolyte balance
8. DSM-III-R classification: listed with other eating disorders of childhood or adolescence

Nursing Process

See assessment, planning, implementation, and evaluation for "Anorexia," p. 38.

☐ Psychogenic Disorders

General Information

1. Definition: psychologically meaningful environmental stimuli are temporarily related to the initiation or exacerbation of a physical condition with demonstrable organic origin or known pathophysiological process
2. Psychogenic disorders are sometimes confused with hypochondriasis; the latter is an exaggerated concern

with one's physical health, and there is no associated organic, pathological condition

3. Reactions: include eczema (skin), migraine headaches (cardiovascular system), backaches (musculoskeletal system), gastrointestinal and respiratory disorders, and psychogenic pain
4. Ego defense mechanism used is repression: emotional tension is unconsciously channeled through organs
5. Occurrence: often seen in medical settings and becomes a psychiatric problem when anxiety escalates in spite of physical disorder
6. Possible secondary characteristics
   a. *Dependence:* a person may manifest abnormal dependency needs resulting from lack of confidence and poor living skills
      1. difficulty in making decisions
      2. extreme lack of confidence
      3. a need for more help in dealing with problems
   b. *Controlling behavior:* attempts to exercise a dominating influence over another person because of helpless feelings. Manipulative techniques include negativism, obstinancy, silence, avoidance, talkativeness, crying
   c. Self-centeredness (narcissism):
      1. excessive self-attention because of low self-esteem
      2. DSM-III-R: classified under "Psychological Factors Affecting Physical Condition" and the physical condition specified

Nursing Process

Assessment (see p. 32)
Analysis (see p. 33)
Planning, Implementation, and Evaluation

> **Goal:** Client will express feelings, perceptions, and concerns about symptom and treatment plan; client will participate in treatment plan.

Implementation

1. Verbally recognize and reinforce authentic communication of feelings, concerns, and perceptions.
2. Give appropriate information about medications and treatment.
3. Negotiate areas of self-care and independent activity.
4. Focus intervention on understanding and alleviation of primary symptoms.
5. Encourage joint exploration of the motivation for client's behavior.
6. Explore alternatives to the primary symptom for handling anxiety (e.g., talking directly about the concern, asking for help and support, setting limits with others, saying "no" appropriately).
7. Set limits on controlling/manipulative behaviors; state time limits; make expectations clear; do not impose unnecessary controls.
8. Permit the client to retain control when appropriate; avoid a battle of wills.
9. Be consistent and support other staff to be consistent.
10. When manipulative behaviors occur, provide opportunities for staff meetings to vent feelings and coordinate care.

Evaluation

Client accepts limits on controlling/manipulative behaviors; develops alternative coping mechanisms; participates in self-care.

☐ Post-Traumatic Stress Disorder
General Information

1. Definition: anxiety neurosis resulting from severe external stress that is beyond what is usual or tolerable for most people
2. Stressors: rape, military combat, natural disasters (e.g., earthquakes), physical accidents involving loss of life of another or loss of body part or its functions (e.g., permanent paralysis following an accident), accidental disasters caused by people (e.g., crashes,

---

Table 2-9 Additional anxiety disorders

Disorder	Characteristics	Additional nursing interventions
Phobia	Persistent, irrational, fearful reactions to objects or situation (e.g., social phobia, claustrophobia)	Promote behavior modification, relaxation, and desensitization.
Dissociative reactions	Splitting off of one portion of conscious mind that represents major, unresolvable conflict; psychogenic amnesia, multiple personality, etc.	Assess physical condition to help rule out organic causes. Assess reaction to milieu, persons, and events.
Somatiform disorders	Hysterical reactions manifest by dysfunction of organ with no pathophysiological basis for loss of function; symptoms do not follow motor-nerve paths; person shows little concern about incapacity	Assist with physical exam to rule out organic causes. Do not focus on physical symptoms.

fires), intentional disasters (e.g., bombing, torture), victims of criminal assaults (e.g., robbery)

3. Characteristics
   a. Reexperiencing trauma in at least one of the following ways
      1. recurrent/intrusive recollections of event
      2. recurrent dreams of event
      3. sudden acting out or feeling as if traumatic event were recurring, because of environmental or ideational stimulus
   b. Numbing of responsiveness to or decreased involvement with external world after the trauma
      1. markedly diminished interest in one or more significant activities
      2. feeling of detachment or estrangement from others
      3. constricted affect
   c. At least two of the following symptoms not present before the trauma
      1. hyperalertness or exaggerated startle response
      2. sleep disturbance
      3. guilt about surviving or about behavior required for survival
      4. memory impairment or trouble concentrating
      5. avoidance of activities that arouse recollection of traumatic event
      6. intensification of symptoms by exposure to events that symbolize or resemble traumatic event
4. Related factors
   a. Physical injury may be present because of the nature of the trauma
   b. Depression and anxiety are usually present
5. Dynamics: loss of self-esteem and loss of control in the traumatic situation have led to the behavior and feelings described above
6. DSM-III-R classification: Subclassification of anxiety disorders, posttraumatic stress disorder

Nursing Process

Assessment
1. Nature of the traumatic event
2. Duration of disorder
3. Degree of impairment
4. Preexistence of problems that may complicate situation (e.g., anxiety, depression)
5. Presence and degree of symptoms
6. Positive support system available

Analysis (see p. 33)

Planning, Implementation, and Evaluation

> **Goal 1:** Client will recount the traumatic event and cope with feelings related to it.

Implementation
1. Support client through process of recounting the event and venting feelings.
2. Acknowledge significance of the traumatic event and the appropriateness of client's feelings.
3. If there is a need to return to the scene of the trauma, help the client select supportive accompanying resources.
4. Review goals and plans for crisis intervention (p. 23), depression, rape, and loss (p. 27).
5. Involve client in a recovering group of people with similar problems (e.g., Victims for Victims).

Evaluation
Client describes the event and discusses feelings related to it (e.g., sadness, anger).

> **Goal 2:** Client will resume involvement in external world.

Implementation
1. Take measures to prevent the client from becoming isolated.
2. Gradually increase reinvolvement in pretrauma activities.
3. Discuss feelings about activities.
4. Reinforce client's involvement in activities.
5. Give information about social, financial, or health resources.

Evaluation
Client gradually resumes involvement in activities important to client.

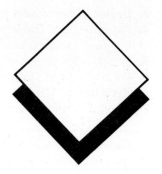

Confused Behavior

GENERAL CONCEPTS
Overview

Confusion can be related to physiological or psychological disturbances and can range from mild to severe in acute, temporary, or chronic forms. It is a biopsychosocial disorder involving the inability to comprehend and/or integrate words, relationships, or events.

Confusion can be a symptom of physical disturbances such as respiratory abnormalities, electrolyte imbalance, infection, biochemical or nutritional imbalances, cerebral disease or destruction, and physical or psychological trauma. It also may be seen in functional psychotic disorders, severe depression, acute psychological crises, and substance abuse.

Application of the Nursing Process to the Client Exhibiting Confused Behavior

Certain physiological and environmentally induced confused behaviors are short-lived and directly associated with factors that can be controlled, changed, or improved. When the causative factors create permanent or progressive changes, the confusion becomes chronic — the selected health problem outlined below.

SELECTED HEALTH PROBLEM
☐ Chronic Confusion
Definition

1. A mental dysfunction related to the response of the brain to disease, damage, or an aging process; a persistent clinical syndrome
2. Specific syndromes
   a. Alzheimer's disease: degeneration of the cortex and atrophy of cerebrum; usually begins in persons in their early 60s, death 1-10 years after onset
   b. Korsakoff's syndrome: associated with chronic alcoholism
   c. Trauma-induced confusion (e.g., stroke, residual problems related to neurosurgery)

3. Confusion of varying degree and influence is noted in chronic organic brain syndromes
4. DSM-III-R classification: organic mental syndromes: delirium and dementia, amnestic syndrome, organic mental syndrome not otherwise specified, primary degenerative dementia of the Alzheimer type, multi-infarct dementia, senile dementia not otherwise specified, presenile dementia not otherwise specified, dementia associated with alcoholism

Nursing Process
Assessment
1. Onset history
2. Orientation to person, time, and place
3. Problems with cognition; decreased attention, comprehension, abstract thinking, and calculation
4. Memory: impairment of recent or remote memory; may fabricate experiences or situations in plausible manner to cover memory loss (confabulation)
5. Judgment and decision making
6. Speech patterns
7. Paranoid ideation
8. Self-care abilities
9. Previous coping mechanisms
10. Personality and affectual changes
11. Social interaction
12. Feelings and concerns about treatment, impairment
13. Family involvement
14. Physiological problems: respiratory, skin, cardiac, nutrition, rest, and activity

Analysis
1. Safe, effective care environment
   a. High risk for trauma
   b. Sensory-perceptual alteration (specify)
   c. Knowledge deficit
2. Physiological integrity
   a. Activity intolerance
   b. Sleep pattern disturbance
   c. Altered nutrition: less than body requirements

3. Psychosocial integrity
   a. Altered role performance
   b. Social isolation
   c. Personal identity disturbance
4. Health promotion/maintenance
   a. Self-care deficit
   b. Ineffective family coping
   c. Impaired adjustment

Planning, Implementation, and Evaluation

> **Goal 1:** Client will maintain or improve self-care activities to maintain optimal physiological functioning.

Implementation
1. Arrange for client to have needed eyeglasses, hearing aid, false teeth, and other assisting devices for activities of daily living (ADL).
2. Plan ADL schedule based on client's established patterns; allow client to make schedule and activities decisions as appropriate.
3. Give client specific, simple directions for ADL. Provide assistance only if client cannot function alone; allow sufficient time for activities, and give advance notice.
4. Provide range-of-motion (ROM) exercises at least once daily; assist with ambulation as necessary.
5. Schedule rest periods during the day as needed.
6. Follow client's established bedtime routine; avoid use of sedatives, which may *increase* confusion.
7. Offer and encourage nutritionally balanced foods and fluids.
8. Keep skin clean, dry, and free from surface irritants or pressure that impedes circulation
9. Assist client in maintaining neat, appropriate, attractive appearance.
10. Supervise medication consumption (kind, time, and amount); know side effects of drugs given and carefully observe and record client responses to all medications and treatments.
11. Record vital signs and I&O daily.

Evaluation

Client performs ADL; attains and maintains ambulation; sleeps sufficient hours to obtain optimal rest; maintains adequate nutritional intake; maintains skin integrity; receives assistance only as required.

> **Goal 2:** Client will regain and maintain contact with reality.

Implementation
1. Establish routine; avoid changes in routine or environment.
2. Provide hourly orientation to time/place/person using clocks, calendars, signs, pictures, and written reminders.
3. Put client's picture and name (big letters) on room door and the bed.
4. Use concrete symbols, photographs of client's past to strengthen sense of continuity.
5. Answer questions as often as needed, using short, simple sentences; demonstrate acceptance nonverbally to reinforce verbal communications; build on the reality-based statements of the client to strengthen conversation; talk about familiar subjects; establish eye contact; and face directly when addressing client.
6. Help client to use previously successful coping mechanisms.
7. Provide adequate sensory stimulation, avoiding both sensory deprivation and overload.
8. Use touch: back rub, skin care; hold hands if nurse and client are comfortable doing so.
9. Respect client's privacy, space, time, and possessions.
10. Avoid physical restraints or environmental confinement, which increase helplessness; assign staff to wandering clients for short times.
11. Obtain necessary orders and administer appropriate symptomatic chemotherapy; observe and record behavioral changes.
12. Educate and relate to the family and friends, so they will not withdraw from the client.
    a. Discuss client's behavior, memory loss, and confusion; recognize and help them to work through their own feelings of helplessness, anger, depression, love, and guilt. Discuss importance of continued interaction for client and significant others.
    b. Help them prepare for client's continuing care by raising questions, exploring alternatives, and deciding on a goal and plan of action that meets their needs as well as the client's.
    c. Refer to Alzheimer's support group.

Evaluation

Client is oriented to person, time, and place; interacts with others appropriately; family and friends maintain interaction with client; client and family make reasonable plans for client's continuing care.

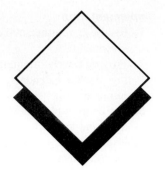

Elated-Depressive Behavior

GENERAL CONCEPTS
Overview

1. Affective disorders comprise a variety of states and syndromes; they include extremes in mood and affect such as depressive or manic behavior and unresolved grief (affect is the mood or emotion an individual shows in response to a given situation)
2. Affective states may be viewed as mood states or as full clinical syndromes; for example, the mood state of depression may occur in a normal person who feels sad, in a client with a major depression, or in a medical client who at intervals may be sad, irritable, anxious, or angry
3. Management modalities (treatments) depend on the severity of the symptoms and include psychotherapy, chemotherapy, convulsive therapy (electroshock), and milieu therapy in a hospital setting or on an ambulatory basis
   a. Chemotherapy consists of antidepressant drugs (see Table 2-10 and reprints)
   b. Psychotherapy focuses on developing insight into the underlying depression, acknowledging feelings of worthlessness, and increasing self-esteem
   c. Therapeutic milieu offers client safe emotional and physical environments by protecting client from self-injury and by providing problem-solving opportunities in a supportive environment
   d. Staff reaction to elated or depressed clients may be characterized by a feeling of ineffectiveness
      1. this can lead to avoiding the client or requesting an assignment change
      2. engenders further feelings of worthlessness in client, creating further withdrawal
      3. the feelings must be dealt with to ensure a therapeutic milieu
      4. staff must recognize potential for this rejection cycle and avoid it; the staff can support each other in treating client
      5. avoid becoming defensive with manic clients
         a. clients have uncanny sensitivity to others' weaknesses and inadequacies; they constantly point these out
         b. staff must tolerate criticisms without becoming defensive
         c. defensiveness fuels attack and is counterproductive
   e. Electroconvulsive therapy (ECT)
      1. only form of shock (convulsive) therapy still in use
      2. one of the chief benefits is that it often makes a client more accessible to psychotherapy
      3. electric shock is delivered to brain through electrodes on one or both temples
         a. produces immediate unconsciousness
         b. produces a cerebral seizure
         c. effective in remission of symptoms
      4. Usually given every other day, 3 times a week for a total of up to 20 in a series
      5. Candidates for ECT
         a. severely depressed elderly with chronic disease that precludes use of antidepressants
         b. severely depressed, suicidal clients who do not respond to antidepressants or psychotherapy
         c. in patients when tricyclic and tetracyclic antidepressants are contraindicated (e.g., clients with cardiac disease, pregnant women)
      6. side effects: temporary confusion, amnesia

Application of the Nursing Process to the Client with an Affective Disorder

Assessment

1. Affect
   a. Powerlessness, worthlessness
   b. Helplessness
   c. Fear and crying
   d. Anger, hostility (directed inwardly in depression, outward in elation)
   e. Elation, exaltation

f. Anxiety

g. Depression related to guilt and repressed hostility; leads to self-condemnation and punishment

2. Cognition

a. Narrowed perception and interests

b. Impaired concentration

c. Delusional thinking

d. Loquaciousness, flight of ideas in elated stage

3. Behavior

a. Decreased motor activity, agitation, or hyperactivity

b. Decreased or increased communications

c. Changes in social interactions

d. Inappropriate dress

4. Physical changes

a. Eating disorders (excessive or insufficient eating)

b. Sleep disturbances (too much or too little)

c. Interest in sex (increase or decrease)

d. Weakness, fatigue

e. Constipation/diarrhea

5. Strengths and capabilities

a. Usual coping strategies

b. Family and peer relationships

c. Hobbies and pastimes (often very limited in depression)

Analysis

1. Safe, effective care environment

a. Impaired home maintenance management

b. High risk for violence: self-directed

c. Knowledge deficit

2. Physiological integrity

a. Altered bowel elimination

b. Altered nutrition: less/more than body requirements

c. Sleep pattern disturbance

d. Sexual dysfunction

3. Psychosocial integrity

a. Hopelessness

b. Chronic/situational low self-esteem

c. Social isolation

4. Health promotion/maintenance

a. Impaired adjustment

b. Altered family processes

c. Altered health maintenance

d. Self-care deficit (specify)

General Nursing Planning, Implementation, and Evaluation

Goal 1: The elated or depressed client will demonstrate increased ability to cope with feelings by sharing feelings with others.

Implementation

1. Spend time with client at least twice daily; start with 5-10 minutes, and increase time as nurse and client can tolerate it; encourage client to identify and verbalize feelings, accept what is said; use silence when appropriate—the presence of a caring person is helpful when learning to cope with painful feelings; *avoid* false reassurance, overcheerfulness.

2. Focus on client's feelings; allow ventilation in ways that seem comfortable to the client; express to client that the only way to work through feelings is to stay with them and experience them.

3. Help client explore meaning of loss, somatic symptoms, and feeling tone. The client may say, "It seems like it just isn't worth it." Proper responses might include, "You've had a hard time lately, and you're learning to deal with your feelings," "You've lost someone you loved, and you're going through grief and mourning," or, "Sounds like you remember the good parts and the rough parts of this relationship, and you're beginning to be ready to risk again."

Evaluation

Client discusses feelings with nurse and others; shares feelings of sadness and wanting to cry.

Goal 2: The elated or depressed client will use acceptable expressions of anger.

Implementation

1. Help client identify angry feelings.

2. Explore sources of anger and help client to express anger verbally.

3. Avoid arguments or involvement in client's set of rules, and avoid discussions that involve moral values.

4. Prevent punishment that extends to self-mutilation (remove sharp objects, matches, and cigarettes).

5. Involve client in minimal tasks and activities.

6. Help client explore ways to cope with anger; talk about alternate ways to express anger (handball, racquetball, hitting a punching bag or mattress, shouting, singing, confronting with words, swearing, tearing up phone books, or throwing sponges or bean bags).

Evaluation

Client shoots baskets in the gym; tells staff "it feels good to let off steam."

Goal 3: The elated or depressed client will identify feelings of guilt.

Implementation

1. Acknowledge client's view of guilt but show that this is client's view, not nurse's.

2. Help client to express guilt: explore situation and persons with whom the client experiences guilt, "I feel guilty when I . . ."; have client try to replace the word "guilt" with "resentment"; explore feelings about this; most situations that involve guilt also involve feelings of anger and resentment; work on these feelings with client.

Table 2-10 Medications used to treat affective disorders

Name	Usual daily dose (mg)	Action	Side effects	Nursing implications
TRICYCLIC ANTIDEPRESSANTS				
Amitriptyline (Elavil)	100-300	Blocks reuptake of neurotransmitters at neuronal membrane; effects of norepinephrine and serotonin may be potentiated resulting in antidepressant effect; strong anticholinergic activity	Dizziness, nausea, excitement, blurred vision, constipation, dry mouth, anorexia, insomnia, drowsiness, excessive perspiration, gynecomastia, skin rash, hypotension	Assess suicide potential. Observe side effects and treat symptomatically. Do not give with or immediately following treatment with MAO inhibitors. Monitor blood pressure. Teach client avoid alcohol check with MD before taking over-the-counter medications ways to avoid problems with orthostatic hypotension importance of oral hygiene take with meals to avoid gastric irritation
Amoxapine (Asendin)	150-450			
Imipramine (Tofranil)	100-300			
Doxepin (Sinequan)	100-300			
Combination-Clordiazepoxide/Amitriptyline (Limbitrol)	100-300 100-300			
Desipramine (Norpramin)	100-200			
Maprotiline (Ludiomil)	50-150			
Nortriptyline (Pamelor)	15-60			
Protriptyline (Vivactil)	100-300			
Trimipramine (Surmontil)				
TETRACYCLIC ANTIDEPRESSANTS				
Maprotiline hydrochloride (Ludiomil)	75-150	Similar to the tricyclics but do not appear to influence reuptake of serotonin	Same as tricyclics	Institute seizure precautions.
Zimelidine (Zelmid)	100-300			
ATYPICAL ANTIDEPRESSANTS				
Fluoxetine hydrochloride (Prozac)	40-80	Inhibition of CNS neuronal uptake of serotonin	Rash, anxiety, nervousness, insomnia, drowsiness, fatigue or asthenia, tremor, sweating, anorexia, nausea, diarrhea, weight loss, dizziness, lightheadedness; may activate mania	Assess suicide potential. Observe for mania, side effects. Teach client avoid alcohol avoid driving car or operating heavy machinery until response is determined check with MD before taking other prescribed medications or over-the-counter medications notify MD if client becomes pregnant

Table 2-10 Medications used to treat affective disorders—cont'd

Name	Usual daily dose (mg)	Action	Side effects	Nursing implications
ATYPICAL ANTIDEPRESSANTS—cont'd				

Trazodone (Desyrel)	150-300	Blocks reuptake of serotonin at the presynaptic neuronal membrane	Dizziness, fainting, cardiac irritability, conduction defects, headache, nausea, priapism	Teach client
				  take with food
				  avoid alcohol, CNS depressants
				  notify MD if priapism occurs
				  do not drive

MONOAMINE OXIDASE (MAO) INHIBITORS				
Phenelzine (Nardil) Tranylcypromine (Parnate) Isocarboxazid (Marplan)	15-90 10-30 10-30	Inhibition of monoamine oxidase enzyme (mainly in nerve tissue, liver, and lungs) increases concentration of amines (epinephrine, norepinephrine, dopamine, serotonin), causing an antidepressant effect	Headache, dizziness, dry mouth, blurred vision, postural hypotension, increased appetite, dermatitis, hepatitis, euphoria; activates latent schizophrenia	Potentiates action of narcotics, barbiturates, sedatives, atropine derivatives. Avoid natural foods (e.g., aged cheese) and alcohol (may cause severe headaches, hypertension) Teach client food restrictions
LITHIUM				

Lithium carbonate (Eskalith, Lithane). Dosage determined by blood level and by behavior. Typically 900-1800 mg in divided daily doses.	Blood level: 0.8-1.5 mEq/L
	Maintenance level: 0.5-1.3 mEq/L (300 mg/day tid)
	Toxic level: 2.0 mEq/L or above
	Acute mania: 1-1.4 mEq/L (20-30 mg/kg/day in 2-3 doses)
		Monovalent action that competes with potassium, sodium, calcium, and magnesium at cellular sites; interferes with reuptake of central monoamine neurotransmitters	GI discomfort (nausea, vomiting, stomach, pain, diarrhea), thirst, dazed feeling, drowsiness, hand tremor, tinnitus, blurred vision	Remind client to take medications.
				Assess drug level every 3-4 days.
				Assess suicide potential.
				Monitor salt and fluid intake.
				Teach client
				  importance of administration and blood work schedule
				  to control salt and fluid intake
				  avoid caffeine
				  take with meals
				Wait 5-14 days for clinical effect

3. Give positive reinforcement to reality-oriented behavior and realistic expectations.

Evaluation

Client acknowledges guilty feelings; discusses reasonableness of feelings.

Goal 4: The elated or depressed client will improve interpersonal relationships.

Implementation

1. Explore the identity of persons in client's life with whom feelings can be shared; if there is no one, explore how this came about, feelings about this situation, and ways to change situations; use role playing or psychodrama to try alternative ways to begin sharing feelings.

2. Explore client's feelings about listening to others' feelings; often people who have problems tolerating their own feelings feel overwhelmed with others' feelings; practice sharing feelings and setting limits on listening to problems; practice reciprocal sharing of feelings in role playing; discuss how to set limits and keep relationship.

3. Discuss effect of irrational demands and negativity on relationships; support self-direction and decision making; role-play interpersonal relationships, decision making; use assertiveness training; explore needs met by dependency, helplessness; discuss what client would lose if behavior changed.

4. Explore expectations of self and others in relationships; discuss consequences of unrealistic expectations; realistically assess expectations, strengths in relationships.

Evaluation

Client reinstates relationships with family and friends; initiates contact with a significant person at least once a week; follows through with social engagements as feasible.

SELECTED HEALTH PROBLEMS
☐ Depression
General Information

1. Definitions
   a. A disorder of mood or affect characterized by feelings of dejection, sadness, and hopelessness
   b. Operational definition: gratification is received from a love object; loss of love object leads to frustration, anxiety, grief, guilt, and hostility; this results in loss of self-esteem and depression
2. Precipitating factors
   a. Loss of a loved one through separation or death is the most common precipitant; the loss must be significant to the person
   b. Threats to self-esteem: disruption in the interpersonal and intrapersonal input of love, respect, and approval results in decreased self-esteem

   c. Success: paradoxically, one may become depressed upon achieving success; this is due to the anticipation of loss of self-esteem if one does not live up to the expectations implied by the success
   d. Physical illness: depression is interrelated with many physical illnesses because of real or anticipated loss of function, independence, role of well person
   e. Self-image: changes in perception of self as a result of physical, emotional, or life-style changes including role changes, body changes
3. States of depression: depression may be felt to some degree by anyone; in terms of severity of disruption, there are five kinds of depression
   a. *Transitory depression*
      1. seldom seen as presenting problem
      2. may be related to environmental or physiological stress
      3. symptoms
         a. affect: quiet, unhappy, helpless or hopeless
         b. cognition: difficulty making decisions, self-deprecation, feelings of inadequacy, focus on personal problems
         c. behavior: decreased activity, restrained, inhibited
         d. physical changes: mild physical discomforts
      4. short-lived; person institutes own cure
   b. *Grieving*
      1. DSM-III-R classification: uncomplicated bereavement
      2. related to precipitating environmental or physiological stress or personal loss (e.g., death of someone close)
      3. responses follow stages of grief and mourning process (refer to Loss and Death and Dying, p. 26).
      4. symptoms
         a. affect: withdrawn, apathetic, angry
         b. cognition: personal derogation, suicidal thoughts, preoccupation with loss or stress
         c. behavior: serious impairment of activity, domestic disturbances
         d. physical changes: mild changes, weight loss or gain of less than 10 lb, feels worse as day progresses
      5. the crisis period takes about 6 weeks; complete resolution is usually achieved in 6-12 months; grief is normal reactive depression
   c. *Depressive neurosis*
      1. DSM-III-R classification: dysthymic disorder
      2. cognitive changes much greater and may be long-standing based on inability to get love from others and lack of supportive experiences
      3. symptoms
         a. affect: powerlessness, helplessness, anxiety, hostility, anger, fear, crying

b. cognition: cognitive triad present—negative self-image, negative view of world, negative expectations for future; indecisive, self-blame, decreased concentration and memory, suicidal ideation

c. behavior: psychomotor retardation, decreased grooming and self-care, constant repetition of a life experience or regret, decreased social interaction but maintains ability to work

d. physical changes: weakness, fatigue, somatic preoccupation, eating changes, sleep changes, decreased sexual interest

d. *Major depression*

1. DSM-III-R classification

a. major depressive episode with psychotic features including severe impairment of reality testing and physiological disturbances

b. manic episode with psychotic features

2. depression brought on by severe environmental blows to security; mobilization of extreme guilt; may have biochemical/genetic causes

3. symptoms

a. affect: despondent, little feeling tone, helplessness, worthlessness, emptiness

b. cognition: delusional thinking, cognitive triad present and marked; thought pattern more despondent in morning, lifts as day progresses

c. behavior: markedly depressed (vegetative) or agitated depending on type

◆ *agitated depression:* anxious, tense, extremely restless; pacing, hand wringing, skin picking, poor eating and sleeping

◆ *retarded depression:* general physical and cognitive slowness, sitting idly, hanging head, looking haggard; indecisive and uncooperative

◆ *bipolar depression (manic-depression):* episodes of well-defined, self-limiting mania or depression, usually in repeating cycles, with or without an interval of normalcy

• person usually recovers completely from both phases, but there is a tendency for recurrence

• may experience only the depressive phase, only the manic phase, or both at different times in life

d. physical changes

◆ vegetative signs: anorexia, weight loss of more than 10 lb, constipation, insomnia, amenorrhea/impotence

◆ insomnia, early morning awakening

◆ lack of self-care

e. *Seasonal affective disorder*

1. cyclical major depressive disorder that is affected by changes in day length occurring in the fall and winter months

2. symptoms (appear as the days shorten during winter months)

a. sadness, irritability, and anxiety during depressed periods

b. overeating

c. carbohydrate craving, weight gain

d. sleep duration increases

e. quality of sleep decreases

f. drowsiness during daytime, fatigue

g. difficulties at work, in interpersonal relationships

3. symptoms may be mediated by the secretion of melatonin, a hormone secreted by the pineal gland. It is thought to mediate seasonal behavior and to be affected by day-night rhythms

4. treatment: studies have shown good results with bright light application in the morning or evening hours every day (reverses the depressive changes by extending the photoperiod by 4-6 hours); clients respond to treatment after 2-4 days.

5. DSM-III-R classification: recurrent major depression, seasonal pattern

Nursing Process

Assessment

1. Signs and symptoms (refer to "States of Depression," p. 48)

a. Affect

b. Degree of cognitive change: cognitive triad (i.e., emotional, physical, and behavioral changes), unlike other symptoms, occurs only in depression; the more severe the cognitive triad, the more debilitating the depression

c. Behavior

d. Physical changes

2. Severity and level of depression (refer to "States of Depression," p. 48)

3. Priorities for care

a. Safety

b. Physical needs

c. Self-esteem

4. Suicide potential

a. Suicidal risk: persons at high risk for suicide include

1. adolescents and people over 50 years old

2. single males

3. black males

4. alcoholics, isolated and unhappy persons

5. police, physicians

6. depressed persons

7. hallucinating persons responding to voice commands

8. those with a history of family suicide
9. persons experiencing a maturational or situational crisis or a chronic or painful illness
10. previous attempters

b. Suicidal plan
1. method—assess degree of lethality (margin for error)
2. availability (the more available, the higher the risk)
3. specificity of plan

c. Change in behavior (e.g., calmness: may mean person has worked out a plan); as depression lifts, client may have energy to carry out plan

d. Giving away valued things: saying good-bye, making amends, asking medical questions

e. Ambivalent feelings
1. Coexistence of opposing emotions in client (e.g., wants to live/die, experiences love and hate toward deceased or absent person)
2. inability to express anger and hostility toward another person, turns hate and aggression inward toward self, leading to self-destructive thoughts or actions
3. feelings of ambivalence are common in severely depressed clients, particularly when the depression is related to the loss of a person important to them

f. Changes in activities of daily living
1. sleep patterns
2. work habits
3. eating patterns (refer also to reprints)

Analysis (see p. 45)

Planning, Implementation, and Evaluation

Goal 1: Client will be protected from suicidal gestures.

Implementation
1. Assume responsibility for safety of client; inspect unit for dangerous items such as sharp items (e.g., scissors, nail files, razor blades), pills; remove from client area.
2. Restrict client to observable areas; observe closely for suicidal ideation/gestures.
3. Use open questioning about suicidal plans and ideas.
4. Set limits on repetition of story of suicidal feelings or gesture.
5. Establish nurse-client relationship that shows nurse as respectful, knowledgeable, able to help solve problems; nurse's attitude should reflect firmness and confidence.
6. Allow client to express feelings.
7. Involve client in activities that ensure success (e.g., attaining small goals in activities of daily living [ADL], exercise).
8. Provide realistic reassurance; convey attitude that client will succeed.

9. Assess client's abilities realistically and provide only the help needed; irrational demands should be discussed openly and refused.
10. Stress client's capabilities/strengths.
11. Work with client to prepare list of problems and corresponding solutions; use all resources available, including family and community resources; give client sense that problems are manageable.
12. Know that suicidal client behavior may cause nurse to feel anger, guilt, or to experience rescue fantasies; staff needs to meet daily for mutual support, planning, and reality testing.
13. Do not withdraw when ambivalence is directed toward nursing staff; continue to offer listening and socialization.
14. Use emergency methods to counteract suicidal attempts (e.g., lavage, one-to-one observation).
15. If suicide attempt occurs, help client/family to share and work through feelings and concerns.
16. Acknowledge the coexistence of opposing (ambivalent) emotions in the client and family.

Evaluation

Client makes no gestures of physical harm; gives all potentially dangerous materials to staff; lists problems, solutions, resources.

Goal 2: Client will meet physical care needs independently.

Implementation

Food and Fluid Intake
1. Find acceptable eating pattern based on client's likes, dislikes, and usual eating habits. If client is anorexic and apathetic to food, provide frequent, small meals and snacks of easy foods to eat (leave a thermos of hot chocolate, oatmeal cookies, crackers and cheese, 7-Up, etc., at bedside for small snacks at night or during day). Monitor food and fluid intake.
2. Weigh weekly (continued loss of weight may indicate deepening depression; weight gain may indicate decreased depression).

Sleep/Rest
3. Help client follow usual bedtime routine. If client sleeps continuously during the day and does not rest at night, work with client to maintain schedule of activity and rest during daytime. Recognize that insomnia increases fatigue, and fatigue increases depression. Sedatives are generally ineffective; therefore, use other nursing measures (e.g., warm milk, snacks, back rub, warm bath).

Elimination
4. Maintain adequate fluid intake.
5. Provide adequate fiber in diet.
6. Monitor elimination.

Grooming and Hygiene
7. Help client establish routine and schedule for bath-

ing, care of hair, skin, nails, clothes. If client is unable to initiate self-care, approach in matter-of-fact manner (e.g., "It's time to bathe, Mr. Watkins"). Convey expectation that client can perform self-care. Give positive reinforcement to any self-care.

Activity

8. Consider personal preferences and needs; help client do things for self (many depressed clients become dependent on others, but activity usually helps them to feel better).

9. Assign daily responsibility for ward-maintenance to help renew sense of self-worth and purposefulness. Simple tasks (emptying ashtrays, straightening chairs, putting away cards, games, or crafts equipment) with supervision may be appropriate for deeply depressed clients; more difficult tasks can be gradually assigned as client tolerates. Assignments should not be demeaning or demanding.

10. Assess previous hobbies and pastimes. Assist with simple crafts that can be finished in one sitting to increase sense of accomplishment; encourage group singing, poetry reading, painting, working with clay, to help client become more comfortable in groups and to establish community and group socialization; client may need nurse's presence to tolerate group activities at first; simple exercises, walks, may progress to group sports; avoid competitive activities.

11. Plan activity schedule based on client's morning and evening mood variation; teach client about variation
    a. Reactive depression: plan group and other activities in morning and following afternoon rest period
    b. Endogenous: do not plan therapy sessions or demanding activities early in day.

Medications

12. Discuss rationale for medication as client can tolerate and assimilate teaching.

13. Teach side effects, administration (see Table 2-10).

Evaluation

Client ingests adequate food and fluids; achieves adequate sleep and activity patterns; has adequate elimination; dresses and grooms self daily; participates in activities.

Goal 3: Client receiving ECT will be free from preventable injury.

Implementation

1. Prep client as if going to OR.
2. Explain procedure thoroughly, and answer client questions and concerns.
3. Ensure consent form is in chart.
4. Arrange for spine x-ray, if required.
5. Keep client NPO.
6. Remove dentures, hairpins, etc.
7. Give medications as ordered: muscle relaxant (e.g., succinylcholine) to reduce tonic/clonic movements;

atropine sulfate to dry secretions and prevent bradycardia and asystole; short-acting barbiturate (e.g., pentothal) for sedation.

8. Sit with client before treatment to provide support, and assign staff member to stay with client.
9. After treatment, check client's pulse and respirations; observe reaction upon awakening.
10. Monitor vital signs every 15 minutes for the first hour and hourly for the next 4 hours.
11. Orient client to time and place and to the fact that treatment has been administered (temporary memory loss and confusion are the most distressing side effects following ECT).
12. Stay with client a minimum of 1 hour after ECT; check vital signs; monitor confusion; observe closely for 6-8 hours after treatment.

Evaluation

Client recovers from ECT safely; is oriented to time, place, and person.

Goal 4: Client will increase interactions with staff, other clients, and family.

Implementation

1. Help client identify, define, and solve difficult problems in social relationships (e.g., client who is hypercritical of self and others can discuss and practice a softer, more accepting approach).
2. Help client to look at situations where client may push others away out of fear of rejection (i.e., reject them before being rejected).
3. Practice social skills, use role playing.
4. Go with client to group activities, choosing short, simple group activities that client identifies as least threatening (exercise, sports, music).
5. Involve client in activity that provides chance for success (e.g., simple occupational therapy activities).
6. Refer to "Activity," p. 51.

Evaluation

Client spends more time with staff, other clients, and family; identifies problems in relationships; practices new social skills with staff and other clients.

Goal 5: Client will discuss feelings about self and situation (refer to General Nursing Goals 1, 2, and 3, p. 45).

Goal 6: Client will increase independent decision making.

Implementation

1. Assess areas in which client is making own decisions and give positive reinforcement to self-enhancing ones.
2. Assist with decision making when client is profoundly depressed.

3. Expect client to make own decisions, with support as depression lifts.

Evaluation

Client participates in planning own activities and schedule.

> **Goal 7:** Family members will maintain relationship with client.

Implementation

1. Provide family members with an opportunity to discuss their feelings of anger, guilt, inability to help client.
2. Help family understand client's anger, dependency, negativism.
3. Discuss ways family can respond to excessive demands and dependency.
4. Review expectations and goals for family and individual family members; explore alternatives for unrealistic expectations.

Evaluation

Family members discuss feelings, expectations, and goals with appropriate staff; interact with client by letter, phone, or visit; bring client home when appropriate and assist with recreation and socialization.

☐ Elation and Hyperactive Behavior

General Information

1. Definition: elation is a seemingly pleasurable affect that is characterized by an air of happiness and self-confidence as well as extreme motor activity
2. Precipitating factors
   a. Results from a real or threatened loss of self-esteem
   b. Massive denial of depression
   c. May develop from early childhood
      1. child first begins to be independent of mother
      2. mother is threatened by this; responds as if this independence is bad
      3. child fears loss of mother's love
      4. child attempts to meet expectations for compliance
3. Types
   a. *Mild:* euphoric state of mind, mild exhilaration
      1. happy, unconcerned, uninhibited, expansive, "life-of-the-party" mood
      2. mood can change rapidly to irritability and anger; irritability is expression of anxiety and hostile impulses
      3. very active, but activity is sometimes inappropriate for age and place
      4. relationships are superficial
      5. DSM-III-R classification: hypomanic episode
   b. *Acute:* moderate degree of mania called hypomania

   1. extreme emotional lability ranging from wild euphoria to fury; readily provoked by harmless remarks, seems to forgive and forget
   2. thought disorders: flight of ideas, delusions of grandeur, short attention span, pressure of speech
   3. little sleep, fatigue, very uninhibited, possibly sexually indiscreet
   4. psychomotor activity is extremely exaggerated
   5. often requires hospitalization
   6. DSM-III-R classification: manic episode, moderate or severe without psychotic features
   c. *Delirium* or *delirious mania:* maximum intensity of reaction
      1. disorganized, seriously delusional
      2. disoriented, incoherent, agitated
      3. prone to self-injury, burnout, and dehydration
      4. immediate intervention is necessary to meet physical needs
      5. DSM-III-R classification: manic episode, severe with psychotic features
   d. *May alternate* between *manic and depressive phases*
      1. usually hospitalized first for manic episode
      2. may have rapid cycling (manic and depressive) phases succeed each other without a period of remission; DSM-III-R classification: bipolar disorder, manic
      3. may have numerous hypomanic and mild depressive episodes; DSM-III-R classification: cyclothymia
4. Prognosis: good, even without treatment, provided that the person does not suffer from complete physical exhaustion in manic phase or commit suicide in depressed phase

Nursing Process

Assessment

1. Physical needs
   a. Nutrition: decreased appetite or unwillingness to stop activity to eat may lead to weight loss
   b. Hydration
   c. Sleep/rest: activity pattern and insomnia may lead to exhaustion
   d. Elimination: may be incontinent; constipation
   e. May ignore injuries or symptoms of physical illness
   f. Hygiene and grooming: inappropriate dress, excessive makeup; diaphoresis
2. Affect
   a. Degree of euphoria
   b. Lability: rapid mood change from happy to sad without apparent provocation
   c. Anger
   d. Anxiety

3. Cognition
   a. Feelings of worthlessness, loneliness are masked by elation
   b. Flight of ideas
   c. Delusions of grandeur and/or persecution
   d. Inadequacy, low self-esteem
   e. Short attention span
4. Behavior
   a. Degree and appropriateness of activity
   b. Aggression, manipulation, acting out
   c. Demanding, verbally hostile
   d. Pressured speech (loquaciousness)
   e. Impulsivity
   f. Decreased inhibitions leading to profanity, sexually indiscreet acts
   g. Pseudoindependence (false independence and confidence)
   h. Superficial relationships

Analysis (see p. 45)

Planning, Implementation, and Evaluation

Goal 1: Client will meet physical needs independently.

Implementation

Food and Fluid Intake

1. Nutrition: provide high-calorie finger foods that can be eaten on the run; note amount of food ingested; monitor weight.
2. Hydration: provide fluids at frequent intervals; fluid intake of 2000 ml/day.

Sleep/Rest

3. Provide medication to induce sleep and rest; provide opportunities for frequent short naps.
4. Reduce stimuli in environment to help calm client; use soft lighting, low noise level, simple room decorations; quiet room if necessary.

Elimination

5. Monitor elimination, maintain fluid intake, establish toileting schedule if necessary.

Hygiene and Grooming

6. Provide flexible schedule for showering and changing clothing; provide loose, comfortable clothing; limit access to clothing if necessary to maintain appropriate dress or decrease frequency of changes; assist with hygiene.

Safety

7. Watch for physical symptoms.

Medications

8. Administer lithium and other medications as ordered (see Table 2-10); observe for side and/or toxic effects, teach client and family about lithium therapy.

Evaluation

Client receives adequate sleep and rest; ingests appropriate amounts of food and fluids; maintains hygiene and grooming; remains free from injury and verbalizes knowledge of medication regimen.

Goal 2: Client will cope adaptively with hostility and aggression.

Implementation

1. Ignore or respond minimally to hostile behavior that is not destructive to avoid positive reinforcement.
2. Nurse or other staff should not react defensively to criticism or profanity from client.
3. Set limits on behavior: "I cannot allow you to hurt people. You'll have to go to the quiet room for half an hour." Be consistent in expectations and limits; collaborate with other staff members to set, enforce, and evaluate limits; enforce limits in a clear, firm manner.
4. After a hostile or aggressive episode, discuss feelings before, during, and after the episode. Explore effect of client's behavior on self and others; explore alternative behavior.
5. Reduce stimuli; use solitary time for hygiene, laundry, etc.
6. Develop behavioral contract.
7. Do not hurry manic clients; hurrying them will result in more anger and hostility.
8. Use measures to prevent overt aggression, (e.g., distraction, reduction of environmental stimuli); avoid competitive games; use large motor skill activities that are not highly structured or confining (e.g., walks, exercise, dance, painting).
9. Using quiet persuasion is most effective.

Evaluation

Client discusses feelings related to hostility and aggression; engages in appropriate physical activities to relieve tension.

Goal 3: Client will demonstrate realistic independence; will develop ability to problem solve, make requests appropriately, and negotiate.

Implementation

1. Do not discuss grandiose ideas/plans.
2. Assess client's abilities realistically.
3. Give help only when client is incapable.
4. Discuss capabilities calmly with client; reinforce client's self-esteem; convey expectation that client can function independently.
5. Involve client in planning ADL.
6. Inform client that staff will not comply with unreasonable demands while conveying acceptance of client.
7. Give client feedback about effects of dependency and demands: "I become annoyed when you repeatedly ask me to do things for you that we decided you would do."

8. Help client to identify feelings, needs, means of seeking gratification.
9. Assist client in developing decision-making skills; explore possible consequences of decisions/behavior.
10. Help client develop alternate behavior; teach client to use assertion, problem solving, negotiation.

Evaluation

Client makes decisions and takes actions independently, makes requests in a quiet voice, and sets limits on own demanding behavior.

Goal 4: Client will recognize and set limits on own manipulative, acting-out behaviors and impulsivity.

Implementation

1. Avoid impatience and anger if client is manipulative or acts out.
2. Inform client of behaviors expected in short, clear sentences.
3. Set firm, definite limits on client's behavior; consistently enforce limits.
4. Teach client that it is the manipulative behavior that is being rejected, not client.
5. Avoid arguments or displaying disapproval of vulgarity, profanity, or overt sexual behavior resulting from extreme euphoria.

6. Remove client from public places when this behavior could embarrass client or family.
7. Protect other clients from sexual overtures.
8. Use chemical or physical restraints as necessary to prevent leaving hospital or injuring self or others.

Evaluation

Client displays manipulative, acting-out behaviors and impulsivity less frequently than on admission.

Goal 5: Family will recognize indications that client needs treatment.

Implementation

1. Discuss expectations of family and client.
2. Explore need for and ways of setting limits.
3. Teach family criteria for seeking treatment:
   a. noncompliance with lithium regimen
   b. anorexia, weight loss, insomnia
   c. hyperactivity, excessive spending
   d. increased use of alcohol
   e. delusions of grandeur or persecution
   f. sexual impulsivity
   g. aggressive, demanding, acting-out behavior
   h. rapid mood changes

Evaluation

Family lists indications of need for treatment.

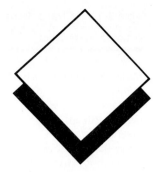

Socially Maladaptive Behavior

GENERAL CONCEPTS
Overview

Socially maladaptive or acting-out behavior includes many problem behaviors and conditions. All human beings live within a social system, and each social system has values and rules by which to live with other human beings. When an individual copes with tension and anxiety by acting out against the social system's values and rules, society considers the individual to be socially maladapted.

Societies use different ways to deal with socially maladaptive or acting-out behavior. Courts, jails, and prisons may be used if laws are broken. Psychotherapy may be used; it helps such persons reenter society and change maladaptive behaviors to adaptive, healthy behaviors.

A strong social structure minimizes stress, social disorder, and upheaval by promoting a healthy environment and providing services essential to physical and mental health. These services include health care, schools, religious institutions, the justice system, recreational facilities, and welfare.

When the structure and expectations of society are stable forces, the family and individual will decrease acting-out behavior. Social unrest, economic stress, health care inequities, moral decay, or dysfunctional families may precipitate or perpetuate stress and anger.

Application of the Nursing Process to the Client Exhibiting Socially Maladaptive Behavior

Assessment

1. Immediate events that precipitated socially maladaptive/acting-out behavior: characteristics and frequency
2. Physiological changes that accompany anger
3. Coping behavior that client uses to handle stress and anger: adaptive and maladaptive
4. Defense mechanisms used to cope with anger
5. DSM-III-R classification: three clusters
   a. Paranoid, schizoid, and schizotypal
   b. Antisocial, borderline, histrionic
   c. Avoidant, dependent, obsessive-compulsive, passive-aggressive

Analysis

1. Safe, effective care environment
   a. High risk for violence: self-directed or directed at others
   b. High risk for injury
2. Psychosocial integrity
   a. Ineffective individual coping
   b. Self-esteem disturbance, personal identity disturbance
   c. Impaired social interaction
   d. Rape trauma syndrome
   e. Altered patterns of sexuality
3. Health promotion/maintenance
   a. Noncompliance
   b. Ineffective, disabling family coping
   c. Altered family processes

General Nursing Planning, Implementation, and Evaluation

> **Goal:** The socially maladaptive client will decrease unacceptable behavior; will use assertive behaviors as a means of expressing independence and control.

Implementation

1. Provide structure and set limits on behavior that is physically destructive to others or the environment.
2. Consistently enforce limits (inconsistent limit setting increases the client's belief that manipulative behavior is productive).
3. Be aware of own nonverbal messages to client; avoid acting defensively or aggressively.
4. Stress to staff the importance of not chastising client or rejecting client's efforts to cope by using aggressive behavior.
5. Teach client the difference between assertiveness (asking for what one wants, standing up for rights)

and aggression (getting what one wants at the expense of others).

6. Recognize and point out manipulative behaviors in a nonjudgmental way; do not allow client to manipulate staff or other clients; discuss effect of manipulation on relationships.
7. Reinforce positive (assertive) approaches ("I would . . ." versus "Do this . . .").
8. Discuss consequences of impulsive actions; help client develop problem-solving skills.
9. Increase self-esteem by supporting strengths.
10. Teach stress-reduction techniques (e.g., imagery, relaxation).
11. Praise efforts of family and significant others as they assist the client in coping.

Evaluation

Client reduces frequency of unacceptable behavior; can describe the difference between assertion and aggression; can demonstrate at least one assertive behavior; uses positive coping mechanisms to handle stress (e.g., relaxation).

SELECTED HEALTH PROBLEMS
☐ Violence in the Family
General Information

1. Definitions
   a. Violence: aggressive drives expressed in a destructive manner
   b. A learned behavior, learned either through exposure and imitation or indirectly as seen when an individual is unable to channel aggressive impulses constructively.
2. Some violent persons feel guilty about their behavior, and others do not. Behaving violently, either with or without feeling guilty, can cause a mental health problem for the person or those dependent upon him.
3. Victims can include
   a. Children
   b. Spouse
   c. Elderly parents or other adults
   d. Children or adults in long-term care settings
4. Characteristics of victims and abusers: see Tables 2-11 and 2-12.
5. Multidisciplinary treatment
   a. Case finding: health care personnel are often the ones who have the opportunity to assess children and adults for possible abuse, especially when they are seen for injuries
      1. be alert for abuse cases, especially in emergency rooms, pediatrics, ambulatory clinics
      2. carefully document bruises, cuts, etc., as well as their size and location; also document interaction patterns of client and significant others; these may become evidence
      3. all suspected child abuse cases must be re-

Table 2-11 Characteristics of abuse

Victim characteristics	Abuser characteristics
Weaker than abuser	Stronger than victim
Emotionally dependent	Physically abused as child
Physically dependent	May or may not feel guilt/remorse
Low self-esteem; may feel need for punishment	Defensive about behavior with victim
Ashamed of being abused	Low self-esteem, self-acceptance
Fearful of retaliation from abuser	Hostility
	Impulsivity
	Experiences chronic anxiety
	Inadequate knowledge of growth and development
	Seductive behavior toward child
	Aloof, impersonal, dysfunctional attachment
	May have experienced recent crisis—separation; divorce; housing, financial, or personal crisis

ported and will be investigated by the state child welfare agency; in some states elder abuse is also reportable

4. medical personnel cannot be charged with defamation of character if they report an abuse that does not check out as such
5. help both abuser and abused receive emotional treatment if they are willing
   b. Community services: numerous branches of the health care system respond to client abuse situations
      1. treatment and intervention by child welfare agencies may include alternative living situations for the abused
      2. various community agencies provide classes on parenting, dealing with older parents, problem-solving skills, and appropriate expression of emotion (e.g., Parents Anonymous—a self-help group for actual or potential child abusers)

Nursing Process
Assessment
1. Assess characteristics of victim and abuser (see Table 2-11)
2. Assess victim for indicators of abuse (see Table 2-12)

Analysis (see p. 55)

Planning, Implementation, and Evaluation

Goal 1: The abuser will discuss feelings and needs related to violence openly and honestly with nurse.

Table 2-12   Indications of abuse

Multiple injuries
Injuries that do not fit description of accident
Old, healed fractures
Poor hygiene
Retarded growth or development with no pathological
   explanation
Child has not had immunizations
Child is not properly dressed for weather
Wary of caretaker
Does not seek comfort or affection from caregiver
Young child does not cry when parents leave
Grabbing behavior/lap hunger
Provocative behaviors
Delinquent or runaway behavior
Teenage pregnancy

Implementation

1. Acknowledge own feelings about abuser and abused; recognize the needs of both (nurse may feel angry with abuser and sympathetic with victim); be aware of impact of own feelings on client care.
2. Treat abuser with respect; know that the abuser may not view own actions as abusive, may be unable to stop the behavior, or may have low self-esteem and need assistance in developing positive self-regard.
3. Help abuser or caretakers to recognize importance of meeting own needs for affection, belonging, and self-esteem.
4. Discuss appropriate ways to express and meet need.
5. Discuss expectations for need fulfillment by those in abuser's care.
6. Explore expectations related to meeting abuser's needs and needs of those in abuser's care.
7. Help client identify events that trigger anger and violence.
8. Teach stress-reduction skills.

Evaluation

Abuser begins to talk about feelings, anxieties, and frustrations rather than acting out violently.

Goal 2: Victim will manage psychological and physical trauma related to violence.

Implementation

1. Encourage expression of feelings in both adult and child victims; provide child with drawing materials and dolls to act out feelings.
2. Discuss adult victim's strengths, coping abilities, ability to function independently.
3. Attend to physical needs caused by specific trauma (e.g., burns, fractures).
4. Provide physical and emotional comfort (e.g., analgesics, therapeutic use of touch: stroking, holding).
5. Refer to in-hospital support services and community

services (e.g., mental health center, crisis intervention hot-line, individual and group counseling).
6. Discuss use of support services if violence recurs.
7. If unsafe to return home, contact social service or child/adult protective services for placement.

Evaluation

Victim expresses feelings; has physical needs met; identifies available support services; verbalizes plan of escape if violence recurs.

Goal 3: Abuser will learn ways to relate to victim without the use of violent behavior.

Implementation

1. Practice open, direct communication that does not attack listener.
2. Help abuser to acknowledge emotional problems when they occur, explore childhood experiences with violence (some were abused as children and need to learn new ways of handling conflicts).
3. Explore alternative ways of expressing anger (e.g., physical activities, discussion, relaxation).
4. Teach effective problem-solving skills.
5. Teach parents normal growth and development, and realistic expectations of children at various ages; discuss appropriate methods of limit setting and discipline as opposed to physical use of force.
6. Reinforce positive parenting strategies.
7. Assist in incorporating older parent into family home and life-style while maintaining independence for all family members.
8. Identify resources in community to assist family in managing situation: day/home care agencies to provide partial relief from total care for elderly, Parents Anonymous to help discuss feelings and problems and share solutions, mental health center for counseling.

Evaluation

Abuser identifies appropriate alternatives to handle feelings, seeks referral for counseling; attends peer support groups.

☐ Hostile and Aggressive Behavior
General Information

1. Definitions
   a. Aggression: forceful, goal-directed action that may be verbal or physical; the motor counterpart of the affect of rage, anger, and hostility
      1. defensive response to anxiety and loss of self-esteem and power
      2. constructive when it is problem-solving and appropriate as a defense against realistic attack, expressed appropriately (e.g., assertiveness)
      3. pathological when it is unrealistic, self-destructive, not problem-solving, the outcome of unresolved emotional conflict and results in physical or emotional harm to others

b. *Passive-aggressive behavior:* resistance to demands for adequate performance in occupational or social functioning are met by timidity, sullenness, stubbornness, forgetfulness, and obstruction
   1. if the behavior is characteristic of the person, it may be considered a personality disorder (DSM-III-R classification)
   2. the person acts out anger in very indirect ways (e.g., always late, forgetting to do things that are important to another person); criticizes persons in authority
   3. the anger of the other person provides the passive-aggressive person with attention and release for anger
2. Dynamics
   a. Behavior is a response to a perceived threat
   b. Feelings of anxiety occur, accompanied by helplessness
   c. Judgment and reasoning decrease as anxiety increases
   d. Verbal or physical aggression occurs as an attempt to alleviate anxiety

Nursing Process

Assessment
1. Refer to assessment, p. 55
2. Aggressive behaviors
   a. Increase in motor agitation
   b. Verbal threat or abusive language
   c. Tense and angry affect
   d. Demanding
   e. Self-directed anger
   f. Manipulative
   g. Noncompliant
3. Level of control
   a. Ability to listen and follow directions
   b. Ability to identify source of anger and verbalize feelings appropriately
   c. Ability to explore alternative ways of expressing anger
4. Nurse's perception of impending violence

Analysis (see p. 55)

Planning, Implementation, and Evaluation

Goal 1: Client will increase control and decrease aggressive behavior.

Implementation
1. Refer to General Nursing Plan, p. 55.
2. Encourage verbal identification of source of angry feelings.
3. Explore alternative ways of dealing with anger.
4. Avoid power struggles:

   a. Allow flexibility in decision making as long as it is within safe parameters.
   b. If decision poses risks to self, other clients, or staff, explain why you cannot go along with it and do not give in.
   c. Set limits on disruptive behavior; apply limits consistently.
5. At signs of increased loss of control:
   a. Reduce stimuli; remove objects or persons that agitate client; move client to area with few people and minimal noise, light, or activity.
   b. Explain what is happening, that client will be safe; ask whether client has any questions; maintain calm, helpful approach.
   c. If client expresses fear of hurting self or others, initiate steps to avert it; remove weapons or objects that could be used destructively.
   d. Explain to client that the behavior can be controlled externally if client cannot regain self-control.
   e. Offer medication, explaining that client is unable to control the behavior voluntarily and will be restrained if medication is refused.

Evaluation
   Client decreases aggressive behavior, calms self, begins to verbalize feelings.

Goal 2: Client will be safely restrained to restore control and prevent injury to self and others.

Implementation
1. Be aware of state laws governing use of restraints and care of client in restraints.
2. Follow agency's policy and procedure in applying and documenting the subsequent care of client in restraints.
   a. Have sufficient number of staff members available to apply restraints.
   b. Give range-of-motion (ROM) exercises for each extremity, and check for full circulation at periodic intervals.
   c. Remove each restraint at specified intervals.
   d. Monitor client in restraints continually and document behavior and care at regular intervals.
   e. Never leave restrained client alone.
3. Remove physical restraints when medication takes effect.
4. Explain use of restraints to any other clients who observed episode; encourage discussing fears of loss of control and availability of help.
5. Explain that restraints were used to help client regain control and prevent injury to self and others.

Evaluation
   Client is free of restraint-related injury; staff applies restraints uneventfully.

☐ Sexual Acting Out
General Information
1. Definitions
   a. Includes sex acts with partners who are legally unable to consent, such as children (pedophilia), with persons who choose not to consent, sex acts accompanied by force or violence (rape), and invasion of another person's privacy without that person's knowledge (e.g., voyeurism)
   b. Voyeurism: the person observes other people's naked bodies without their knowledge or consent in order to obtain sexual gratification
   c. Exhibitionism: a person exposes sexual organs when it is socially inappropriate
   d. Sadomasochism: obtaining sexual pleasure from having pain inflicted upon oneself or others; may be part of a rape incident or may also be part of other sexual encounter
   e. Rape: legal definitions of rape vary from state to state, but most include sexual intercourse without the consent of the other person; statutory rape is the seduction of a minor, even though the minor consented; victims may be any age; the majority are female, but males can be raped (usually by other males)
2. Profile of a rapist
   a. Rape is an aggressive sexual act and a crime of violence and power
   b. Rapists act for the purposes of venting anger and hostility and exercising control and power
   c. Many rapes are planned
   d. The majority of rapists are male, and in the case of child victims, usually someone the child knows; acquaintance rape is also a possibility with an adult victim
3. Responses to rape
   a. Shame and embarrassment may lead to not reporting rape
   b. Common reactions of the victim are shame, guilt, embarrassment, self-blame, anger; fears of injury, mutilation, sexually transmitted diseases, and pregnancy; fear of how significant others will react to incident
   c. The victim's response varies from expressing feelings through talking or behavioral manifestations (e.g., crying, trembling, agitation) to controlled (outwardly quiet, exerting control over behavior to regain physical and emotional control)
   d. The significant others' reactions to the rape are similar to the victim's and also vary (e.g., anger, support, isolation)
   e. The psychological effect of rape may be long lasting, affecting interpersonal relationships with significant others, impairing sexual functioning, and creating feelings of helplessness, anxiety, and depression
   f. Self-awareness of one's own reaction to rape is imperative to deal therapeutically with the victim and significant others

Nursing Process
Assessment
1. Victim's perception of incident
2. Victim's coping ability
3. Anxiety level
4. Signs of physical trauma (e.g., bruises, scratches)
5. Availability of significant others, support network
6. Impact of rape incident on significant others
7. Victim's immediate concerns (e.g., emotional control, legal information or assistance, physical care, pregnancy, or venereal disease protection/information)

Analysis (see p. 55)
Planning, Implementation, and Evaluation

Goal 1: Victim will return to prerape level of functioning; immediate physical and psychological needs met by staff.

Implementation
1. Provide a private location for interview, examination, and crisis intervention.
2. Document client's perception of incident, physical trauma, psychological status, coping ability, and physical assessment findings; assist in collecting physical evidence.
3. Use empathetic, nonjudgmental approach; do not give advice; be sensitive to victim's feelings while gathering information and physical evidence; avoid asking for unnecessary repetition of events by client.
4. Encourage verbalization of rape incident; if client is unable to talk about incident, acknowledge difficulty of traumatizing experience; allow immediate use of denial; explain that anger, sadness may occur later.
5. Encourage client to ventilate present feelings about incident; do not dwell on actual sexual act unless client needs to discuss this; allow expression of anger (may be directed at staff).
6. Help client assess present coping ability.
7. Explain common behavior and feeling responses that may occur.
8. Encourage client to actively problem solve, prioritize concerns, and make decisions (e.g., who to tell, legal recourse, physical care, pregnancy prevention).
9. Explore feelings of guilt or self-blame; reinforce responsibility of rapist, not of victim, for the act; suggest that whatever client did (either fighting or submitting) was necessary for self-protection.
10. If victim is child:
    a. Use drawing, play to help child ventilate feelings.

   b. Use calm approach, be aware of own nonverbal communications that may convey anger to child.
   c. Reinforce that child has done nothing wrong and will not be punished.
   d. Explain all procedures thoroughly.
11. Give victim and significant others information about community resources (e.g., rape trauma group, legal aid, rape crisis center, counseling)
12. Refer for follow-up to crisis counseling, marital and sexual functioning counseling.

Evaluation
Victim verbalizes need for intervention, complies with intervention, and verbalizes willingness to seek referral.

Goal 2: Significant others will verbalize feelings and assist victim.

Implementation
1. Assess significant others' reactions (self-blame or victim blame are common) and present coping abilities.
2. Reinforce rapist's responsibility for act and necessity of victim's actions for self-preservation.
3. Teach about typical reaction of victim and significant others to rape trauma (increased anxiety and fear within 48 hours followed by adjustment; reappearance of anxiety later).
4. Explain how significant others can assist victim.
   a. Encourage victim to ventilate but do not force discussion of rape.
   b. Help victim to resume daily activities.
   c. Support victim's decision for follow-up care, litigation, etc.
   d. Do not withhold emotional and physical comfort (e.g., touching, holding, stroking).
   e. Avoid overprotection or isolation.
   f. Provide the safety and protection measures victim needs to feel safe (e.g., new locks, escort at night).
5. Talk with family away from victim; encourage verbalizing anger to nurse rather than to victim
6. If victim is child:
   a. Help parents recognize that victim is still child and has age-related needs for physical comfort, reassurance, and protection.
   b. Help family plan ways to return to usual family activities as soon as possible.
7. Provide referral to community resources for additional support and assistance.

Evaluation
Significant others discuss traumatic experience and give support to victim.

☐ Antisocial Behavior
General Information
1. Definition: disorder manifested by persistent pattern of violating the rights of others; pattern of lifelong maladaptive behaviors

2. DSM-III-R classification: personality disorder
3. Characteristics
   a. Dysfunctional interpersonal relationships
   b. Poor work history
   c. May engage in sexually deviant behavior
   d. Alcohol or drug dependency
   e. Articulate communication skills, average to superior intelligence
   f. Able to rationalize or justify behavior
   g. Charming, fabricates stories to impress listener
   h. Manipulative
   i. Lack of responsibility, unreliable
   j. Poor judgment, insight, impulse control, and frustration tolerance; does not learn from experience or punishment
   k. Does not experience guilt or remorse
   l. Prior to age 15: poor school performance, truancy, petty crimes, lack of satisfactory relationships with family, peers, and authorities
4. Treatment: apply external controls to limit the acting-out behavior
   a. These behavior patterns are difficult to change; respond poorly to treatment
   b. Long-term psychotherapy is of some success, but relatively few clients remain in psychotherapy because of expense, time involved, poor motivation, and lack of insight
   c. Self-help groups have had some success

Nursing Process
Assessment
1. Characteristics of personality disorders
2. Behavior: manipulation, impulsiveness, narcissism, seductiveness, demanding, histrionics, acting out, violence
Analysis (see p. 55)
Planning, Implementation, and Evaluation

Goal 1: Client will interact with peers and staff within socially accepted norms; will follow treatment program.

Implementation
1. Refer to General Nursing Plan, p. 55.
2. Set firm limits to be consistently applied by all staff.
3. Call staff conferences to discuss behavior and plans for setting limits and dealing with behavior; write limits on care plans so all staff can follow intervention.
4. Communicate verbally and give written information to client on unit's rules and routines; explain consequences if expectations are violated; give concrete information on rules or limits.
5. Be aware of manipulative behavior, such as setting up staff, playing one staff member against another, and using other clients.

6. Do not make agreements with client without checking what all other staff members have told the client.
7. Confront client in a matter-of-fact way when behavior is not acceptable.
8. Encourage development of positive goals for change.
9. Give positive feedback when client is conforming to socially accepted norms.
10. Explore social relationships and problem areas; role-play social situations; use group therapy to point out problem behaviors.

Evaluation

Client increasingly complies with rules of the treatment program; interacts acceptably with others.

☐ Borderline Personality Disorder

General Information

1. Definition: long-standing pattern of unstable self-image, interpersonal relationships, and moods
2. Dynamics: stems from the toddler's experience with identity development and separation from significant other
3. Onset: early adolescence
4. Characteristics
   a. Splitting: seeing people as "all good" or "all bad"; leads to idolizing or devaluing people; causes relationships to be intense while idolizing person and short-lived as a result of devaluing
   b. Often angry, with extreme and rapid shifts in mood
   c. Poor judgment
   d. Feelings of emptiness, loneliness, and boredom
   e. Underdeveloped self-concept, identity diffusion
   f. Impulsivity
   g. Physically assaultive
   h. Suicidal ideation and gestures
   i. Poor school and work histories

Nursing Process

Assessment

1. Use of splitting
2. Quality and consistency of relationships with staff, peers, and family
3. Mood
4. Acting-out behaviors
5. Risk of self-injury
6. Ability to accept and express caring
7. Self-concept
8. Judgment and decision making
9. Strengths

Analysis (see p. 55)
Planning, Implementation, and Evaluation

Goal 1: Client will increase socially acceptable behavior.

Implementation

1. Protect client from self-injury (see *Depression,* Goal 1, p. 50).
2. Establish consistent time and setting for interactions with client.
3. Limit impulsive, acting-out behavior in a nonpunitive manner.
4. Discuss meaning and pattern of acting-out behavior with client.
5. Encourage adaptive expression of feeling (e.g., verbalization, physical activity, relaxation exercises).
6. Develop a behavioral contract (will write down angry feelings rather than acting-out, then discuss feelings with nurse to gain privileges).
7. Role-play behavioral responses to social situations.

Evaluation

Client adheres to behavioral contract, expresses feelings verbally, and uses relaxation exercises.

Goal 2: Client will express improved self-identity.

Implementation

1. Provide opportunities for client to relate to staff and persons in positive manner.
2. Explore client's self-expectations, potential strengths, and goals; assist in developing realistic expectations and goals.
3. Assist client in developing solitary activities.
4. Reinforce positive behaviors, constructive use of solitary time.

Evaluation

Client discusses realistic self-expectations; lists own strengths; uses solitary time constructively.

Goal 3: Client will improve interpersonal relationships.

Implementation

1. Recognize idolizing or devaluing of staff as part of client's pathology; do not act on feelings of hostility or flattery.
2. Be consistent in approach to client; use multidisciplinary conferences to prevent problems of transference and countertransference.
3. Examine client's expectations of others.
4. Help client develop realistic expectations of others.
5. Help client identify communication problems in interpersonal situations.
6. Role-play social situations.
7. Provide social skills training.

Evaluation

Client establishes and maintains at least one relationship; verbalizes improved ability to evaluate faults and strengths of others.

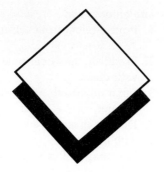

Suspicious Behavior

GENERAL CONCEPTS
Overview

Suspicious behavior occurs when a person is hypersensitive to, and preoccupied with, the behavior and motivations of others. In mild forms, such behavior may include taking normal protective precautions to avoid becoming the victim of a truly dangerous person. In severe forms, such behavior results from abnormal and unwarranted distrust of others and results in extreme, unwarranted, and inappropriate efforts to protect self.

Suspicious behavior may be part of an organic mental disorder or schizophrenic disorder, may be the predominant problem as in paranoid disorders or paranoid personality disorders of a nonpsychotic type, or may occur with substance abuse.

Application of the Nursing Process to the Client Exhibiting Suspicious Behavior

All adults have some level of sensitivity and preoccupation with the behavior and motivation of others. When this behavior becomes exaggerated, it is paranoia, the selected health problem discussed below.

SELECTED HEALTH PROBLEM
☐ Paranoia
General Information

1. Definition: behavior characterized by hostility, unwarranted suspiciousness, and mistrust of others resulting from grandiose and/or persecutory delusions
2. Types
   a. Paranoia: an insidious development of a permanent, well-organized, well-defined, unshakable delusional system that is contradicted by social reality; chronic; seen less frequently than paranoid schizophrenia
   b. Acute paranoid disorder: this is the sudden onset in individuals who have experienced drastic environmental changes (e.g., immigrants, boot camp recruits, POWs); rarely becomes chronic

3. Characteristics
   a. Suspiciousness
   b. Grandiose, persecutory, jealous, or erotic delusions
   c. Usually no hallucinations
   d. Haughty, superior manner
   e. Constant vigilance
   f. Tendency toward hostility, anger, and aggression; projected outward
   g. Usually no impairment of intellectual or occupational functioning; distrust may be in only one area of life, with others relatively untouched
   h. Often severe impairment of social and marital functioning with progressive estrangement from others as client "gathers evidence" to support delusion
   i. Duration of at least one week
   j. Rarely seeks help; client sees nothing unusual about delusions; brought in by associates or relatives for help
   k. Client tends to stimulate avoidance and dislike in others
4. Dynamics
   a. Lack of trust
   b. Low self-esteem
   c. Increased anxiety level
   d. Denial
   e. Projection resulting in delusions
   f. Decreased repression
   g. Poor reality testing in area related to delusions
5. DSM-III-R classification: paranoid disorder

Nursing Process
Assessment

1. Duration: at least 1 week; chronic if over 6 months; acute if less than 6 months
2. Delusions
3. Anxiety level
4. Problem behavior
   a. Superiority

    b. Expression of hostility, anger, or aggression

    c. Social and/or marital impairment

5. Self-esteem

Analysis

1. Safe, effective care environment

    a. High risk for violence: self-directed or directed at others

    b. Knowledge deficit

    c. Sensory-perceptual alteration (specify)

2. Physiological integrity

    a. Altered nutrition: less than body requirements

    b. Sleep pattern disturbance

3. Psychosocial integrity

    a. Anxiety

    b. Social isolation

    c. Altered thought processes

4. Health promotion/maintenance

    a. Noncompliance

    b. Self-care deficit (specify)

    c. Diversional activity deficit

Planning, Implementation, and Evaluation

Goal 1: Client will develop a trusting relationship with a staff member.

Implementation

1. Establish regular times and places for meetings; keep appointments or notify in advance of cancellation.

2. Be honest, accurate, and matter-of-fact in communication.

3. Make mutual expectations and promises clear, and abide by them.

4. Be accepting and nonjudgmental.

Evaluation

Client develops a trusting relationship with a staff member as evidenced by a willingness to cooperate with and confide in staff member.

Goal 2: Client will learn to define and test reality regarding the delusional system.

Implementation

1. Help client to recognize delusions as signs of anxiety and poor self-esteem.

2. Do not argue about content of delusions, but focus on reality (arguing results in client defending the delusions).

3. Limit discussion of delusions.

4. Acknowledge client's feelings and beliefs, but point out that these are not shared; appear quizzical and express some doubt about delusions.

5. Be honest and reliable.

6. Focus on the here and now.

Evaluation

Client gives up delusion; verbally expresses feelings of anxiety.

Goal 3: Client will demonstrate improved self-esteem.

Implementation

1. Identify strengths: encourage client to focus on them.

2. Assist client in developing a relationship with another client.

3. Assist client in gradually developing relationships within groups.

4. Assist client in gaining insight into underlying dynamics of behavior.

5. Intervene with problem behavior (e.g., superiority, hostility and anger, aggression; refer to those behaviors in *Socially Maladaptive Behavior*).

Evaluation

Client is able to begin an appropriate relationship with other clients and groups; controls problem behavior.

Goal 4: Client will improve social and marital functioning.

Implementation

1. Encourage client to discontinue behavior that disrupts social and marital relationships (e.g., spying, accusations, letter writing, threats).

2. Identify feelings that lead to problem behavior.

3. Encourage client to express anxiety, tension, anger, and fears verbally.

4. Find constructive outlets for the feelings (e.g., relaxation techniques, physical exercise, public service); avoid overly aggressive, competitive activities.

5. Help client to establish or reestablish trusting, supporting relationship with family members (e.g., promote open, direct communication and involvement in mutually agreed-upon activities).

6. Help family explore feelings about client's behavior; provide information about client's status; help family examine ways to respond to client.

Evaluation

Client improves social and marital relationships; communicates feelings, needs, and wants to family; family members state they feel comfortable around client.

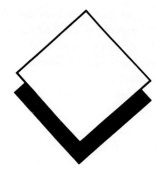

Withdrawn Behavior

GENERAL CONCEPTS
Overview

1. Definition: a retreat from interactions with people and environment; in extreme situations, the person retreats from reality
2. Behavioral continuum
   a. Healthy: temporary pulling back from a stressful situation and focusing psychic energy internally to think, plan, reflect, and regroup before acting — a healthy and sometimes necessary response
   b. Unhealthy: isolating onself from others and the world to the extent that relationships and the ability to function in society are seriously impaired
      1. may retreat to avoid facing important social situations; social skills are not learned and a cyclical pattern of withdrawal results
      2. examples of unhealthy uses of withdrawal include
         a. excessive fantasizing that keeps the person from having to deal with day-to-day problems of living
         b. excessive TV watching or involvement in only solitary activities to avoid social encounters
      3. schizophrenia is the most severe form of withdrawal; the person's thought patterns, communications, and relationships with others prevent functioning in a productive manner
3. Withdrawn behaviors: though withdrawn behaviors occur on a continuum, this section focuses primarily on the most severe form of withdrawal, schizophrenic disorder
   a. Etiological factors: no consensus about cause; various theories
      1. biological: physical defect or genetic potential
      2. psychological: internal dynamics related to difficulties in thought process, affect, and behavior
      3. sociological: family relationships and rigid so-

cial expectations; schizophrenic behavior is learned (i.e., communication patterns, response to double-bind communication are learned from parents)
   b. Dynamics: the person views the world as so threatening that withdrawal from interpersonal relationships, social situations, and reality are seen unconsciously as the only alternative
   c. Management: long-term management with continuing follow-up is frequently necessary
      1. medications: major tranquilizers (see Table 2-13)
         a. actions: modify intense anxiety, tension, and psychomotor excitement; alleviate delusions and hallucinations
         b. benefits: allow the client to participate in other forms of therapy
         c. side effects: not addictive but do have troublesome, sometimes irreversible, and occasionally dangerous side effects (see Table 2-14)
         d. nursing role
            ◆ administer the medications, observe client response, intervene to prevent complications related to drug side effects, and teach client and family about the drug (e.g., action, side effects, and need to take on long-term basis)
            ◆ record and report side effects or problems
      2. therapeutic milieu: used to increase independence, social skills; see p. 24
      3. nurse-client relationship
         a. purpose: helps the client to function as independently as possible and learn to deal with problems
         b. focuses on development of trust as model for healthy relationships with others
         c. DSM-III-R classification: schizophrenia

Table 2-13   Major tranquilizers (neuroleptics)

Generic name (trade name)	Dosage	Action	Nursing implications for all major tranquilizers
PHENOTHIAZINES			
Chlorpromazine (Thorazine)	100-1000 mg/day	Block dopamine-mediated transmission, depress lower levels of central nervous system, antipsychotic activity, decrease psychomotor activity; in combination with piperazine stimulate withdrawn client to increasing socialization and communication	Check BP prior to administration; observe for orthostatic hypotension; teach client to rise slowly from sitting or lying position; have client remain in lying position 30-60 minutes after IM dose.
Acetophenazine (Tindal)	6-120 mg/day		Monitor periodic liver function tests, blood counts.
Carphenazine (Proketazine)	75-400 mg/day		Notify physician of complaints of sore throat, nosebleed, rash, fever, or other infections.
Perphenazine (Trilafon)	6-64 mg/day		Observe for early signs of pseudoparkinsonism; if it occurs, explain to client and administer prescribed antiparkinsonian drug.
Trifluoperazine (Sterazine)	4-10 mg; may be slowly increased to 15-20 mg		Observe for warning signs of tardive dyskinesia (tonguelike movements) and report.
Fluphenazine hydrochloride, decanoate or enanthate (Prolixin, Permitil)	0.5-1.0 mg po daily, not to exceed 20 mg; 12.5-25 mg q2wk IM		
Thioridazine hydrochloride (Mellaril)	20-800 mg/day		
Mesoridazine (Serentil)	initial: 50 mg tid optimal: 100-400 mg/day		
Promazine (Sparine)	10-20 mg q4-6 hrs maximum: 1000 mg/day		
BUTYROPHENONES			
Haloperidol (Haldol)	1.5-6 mg/day; 6-15 mg, up to 100 mg to achieve control	Similar to the phenothiazines; more potent dopaminergic effects	Warn client that drowsiness may occur until tolerance is developed; avoid driving a car or operating machinery until tolerant.
THIOXANTHENES			Observe for dryness of mouth, visual or retinal changes, rash, gastric irritation, constipation. May be administered with food, water, or milk to reduce gastric irritation.
Chloroprothixene (Taractan)	100-600 mg		Maintain fluid intake to decrease mouth irritation and constipation.
Thiothixene (Navane)	6 mg daily, slowly increase to 20-30 mg; rarely exceeds 60 mg		
DIHYDROINDOLONES			
Molindone hydrochloride (Moban)	25-225 mg	As per phenothiazines; suppress aggressive behavior	Do not administer antacids within 1 hour of these medications given orally.
DIBENZOXAZEPINES			Teach client avoid alcohol
Loxapine hydrochloride (Loxitane C)	25-250 mg	Act on ascending reticular activating system; activate withdrawn client	consult MD before taking other medications
Loxapine Succinate (Loxitane)	25-250 mg		report sore throat in absence of other cold symptoms appropriate diet and exercise to avoid weight gain precautions to avoid skin damage from photosensitivity side effects high-fiber diet, fluids, exercise to prevent constipation

Table 2-14 Side effects of major tranquilizers

Parkinsonian-type
  pseudoparkinsonism
  dystonia (tonic muscle spasms, especially of eyes,
    tongue, jaw, and neck)
  akathisia (restlessness, inability to sit or lie quietly)
Hypotension
Photosensitivity
Anticholinergic effects (blurred vision, dry mouth, consti-
  pation, difficulty starting urination)
Agranulocytosis (rare)
Jaundice (rare)
Increased restlessness
Drowsiness
Weight gain
Skin rashes
Amenorrhea with false-positive pregnancy test, galactor-
  rhea
Ejaculation difficulties, gynecomastia
Decreased libido

Application of the Nursing Process to a Client Exhibiting Withdrawn Behavior

Assessment

1. Behavioral manifestations
   a. *Affect* (feeling tone or mood)
      1. a specific judgment criterion is the appropri-
         ateness of the affect; that is, the degree to
         which it is in keeping with the situation at hand,
         both quantitatively and qualitatively
      2. responses may be excessive, or they may be
         inappropriately minimal (flat). Flat affect is
         demonstrated by a blunt or dull emotional tone
         of expression; it is a generalized impoverish-
         ment of emotional reactivity
      3. inappropriate affect is that which is incon-
         gruent with the situation or the content of
         thought
   b. *Behavior disorganization*, in which the client
      reacts to stress in an unpredictable or bizarre man-
      ner (e.g., pacing, rigid posturing)
   c. *Disregard of hygiene and grooming* can range
      from looking unkempt to bizarre clothing and
      makeup or disregard for bodily care
   d. *Disregard of physical safety* includes not being
      concerned about placing self in dangerous situa-
      tions, such as walking in a busy street or causing
      self-inflicted wounds; these persons need close ob-
      servation
   e. *Nutrition deficits* because of poor eating habits
   f. *Regression*, in which the client returns to behavior
      patterns exhibited at an earlier stage of develop-
      ment (e.g., thumb sucking, baby talk, fetal po-
      sition)

1. main defense mechanism used in schizophrenia
2. allows the person to be dependent and return
   to the predictable behavior experienced in
   childhood
2. Psychological manifestations
   a. *Autism:* extreme withdrawal from real world and
      preoccupation with idiosyncratic thoughts and fan-
      tasies
      1. a common characteristic of schizophrenic be-
         havior
      2. this persistent tendency to withdraw from in-
         volvement with the external world and to be-
         come preoccupied with ideas and fantasies that
         are egocentric and illogical causes autistic
         clients to be unresponsive
      3. it is difficult to establish communication with
         them; they may be mute; their conversations
         may be irrelevant or lack coherence
   b. *Hallucinations:* a sensory perception that occurs
      without an external stimulus
      1. can be auditory, visual, or tactile, olfactory, or
         gustatory
      2. usually occurs in psychotic disorders but can
         occur in both chronic and acute organic brain
         disorders
      3. auditory hallucinations are the most common
         form occurring in clients with schizophrenia,
         although visual, tactile, olfactory, and gusta-
         tory hallucinations may be experienced; some
         clients describe the experience as very definite;
         others describe it with an element of vagueness
      4. auditory hallucinations are often threatening
         and aggressive; client's response to them may
         account for acts of violence
      5. hallucinations temporarily lessen anxiety be-
         cause they offer a substitute for interaction with
         real persons whom the client fears; such ex-
         periences are therefore counterproductive and
         conducive to further withdrawal from reality;
         when anxiety and loneliness increase, client
         becomes aware that others recognize that client
         is hallucinating and becomes ashamed and em-
         barrassed
   c. *Delusion:* a false belief or opinion that is unrea-
      sonable and causes distortion in judgment
      1. delusion of grandeur: false, grandiose, or ex-
         pansive belief that one is a very important or
         powerful person or entity (e.g., sees self as
         royalty or as Jesus)
      2. delusion of persecution: false belief that one is
         victim of others' hostility and aggressiveness
         (e.g., "The FBI is after me")
      3. although delusions represent a withdrawal
         from reality into fantasy, their function is to
         secure the client's identity; therefore delusional

systems are rigid and inaccessible to reason; any attempt to correct the client's beliefs makes the nurse seem like an enemy

    4. trying to reason the client out of false beliefs will make client work harder to improve the delusion, thus reinforcing it and making it more entrenched

  d. *Depersonalization:* feelings of unreality or strangeness concerning either the environment or the self, or both

    1. results from the client's poor self-concept

    2. client treats self as an object

    3. client seems to have resigned not only from the world of reality but also from self; this leads to extreme social isolation

  e. *Associative looseness:* one experience or idea reminds the client of a completely different experience, which is interpreted in an autistic manner

    1. the thought process loses its continuity so that thinking and expression become confused, bizarre, incorrect, and abrupt

    2. communication is disconnected, follows no logical sequence, and is confusing to the listener

  f. *Ambivalence*

    1. occurs normally, from time to time, in all persons and is popularly known as "mixed feelings"

    2. classic behavior in schizophrenia; characterizes the stormy, chaotic relationships the schizophrenic has with relatives, friends, and associates

    3. because of the ambivalence, minor difficulties can lead to disruption of relationships with significant others

3. Sociological manifestations

  a. Poor social skills: difficulty with conversation and even physical closeness

  b. Retreat from social situations

  c. Few or no friends: often has no friends, or relationships are considered to be friendships in spite of minimal contact

  d. Pathological family relationships: often severe communication problems

  e. Erratic employment history

  f. Difficulty maintaining an independent living situation: unable to care for self, will not pay rent regularly or take care of physical needs; some can do the caretaking tasks but tend to isolate themselves

4. Suicide potential

  a. Autistic thinking; aggressive/hostile voices; a confused, depressed mood, and low self-esteem increase suicide risk

  b. See "Elated-Depressive Behavior," p. 44

Analysis

1. Safe, effective care environment

  a. High risk for violence: self-directed or directed at others

  b. Sensory-perceptual alteration (visual, auditory)

  c. Impaired home maintenance management

2. Physiological integrity

  a. Impaired verbal communication

  b. Sleep pattern disturbance

  c. Altered nutrition: less than body requirements

3. Psychosocial integrity

  a. Ineffective individual coping

  b. Chronic low self-esteem

  c. Altered thought processes

  d. Impaired social interaction

4. Health promotion/maintenance

  a. Impaired adjustment

  b. Ineffective family coping: compromised

  c. Noncompliance

General Nursing Planning, Implementation, and Evaluation (see Table 2-15)

> **Goal 1:** Client will remain physically safe.

Implementation

1. Keep harmful objects away from clients.
2. Observe client at frequent intervals.
3. Observe for physical problems (e.g., infection, constipation) that may be outside client's awareness.
4. Observe for side effects of drugs.
5. Monitor rest and sleep; use comfort measures such as pillows, snacks, warm baths to induce sleep.

Evaluation

  Client does not injure self; experiences only minimal side effects of drugs; has adequate rest or sleep.

> **Goal 2:** Client will maintain adequate nutrition, and fluid and electrolyte balance.

Implementation

1. Observe for signs of dehydration (e.g., dry skin, lips); encourage fluids.
2. If client is not eating, assess the reasons (e.g., delusions about food being poisoned, too agitated to sit for meals, unaware of poor eating habits).
3. Help client find methods to ensure adequate food intake (e.g., permit food from home if client fears hospital food is poisoned; provide finger foods client can eat while walking).
4. Provide positive reinforcement for good eating habits.
5. Teach about nutrition as needed.

Table 2-15 Selected problem behaviors and interventions

Behavior	Interventions
Aggression	Prevention—early recognition of increased excitement. Encourage verbal expression of feelings surrounding behavior. Reduce stimuli. Avoid reinforcement (e.g., competitive games). Provide distraction. Set limits. Protect other clients.
Anger	Acknowledge or name feeling. Explore sources. Encourage to express verbally. Explore appropriate outlets. Avoid arguing.
Anxiousness	Acknowledge or name the behavior or feeling. Explore sources. Encourage appropriate expression. Give reassurance. Recognize that anxiety in nurse increases client's anxiety.
Associative looseness (thought disorder)	Relate in a concrete manner. Focus on immediate situation. Point out reality. Clarify verbalizations that are not understood.
Autism	Accept at stage client is in; do not push. Give ample time for responses. Do not reinforce dependency. Use silence appropriately.
Controlling behavior	Recognize means of controlling: negativism, obstruction, silence, avoidance, insults, yelling, increased chatter, or crying. Do not impose unnecessary controls. Allow client some control. Develop trust, security in giving up control.
Delusions	Avoid arguing. Avoid arousing suspicion. Be honest and reliable. Be consistent. Acknowledge client's feelings. Point out reality: client's beliefs are not shared.
Dependence	Assess abilities and capabilities. Provide only help needed. Encourage to solve problems and make decisions. Display attitude of firmness and confidence. Discourage reliance beyond actual need. Encourage successful participation.
Hallucinations	Help to recognize as manifestation of anxiety. Encourage to give up hallucinations. Help to relate with real persons. Do not give attention to content.
Hopelessness, helplessness	Structure small successes. Give encouragement. Exhibit expectation that client will succeed. Encourage identification of strengths.
Hostility	Avoid arguing with the client. Acknowledge and name feelings. Explore the source of hostility with client. Encourage to express hostility verbally rather than resort to physical aggression. Explore appropriate outlets for hostility (e.g., physical activities).
Low self-esteem, feeling worthless	Prevent isolation. Acknowledge client's view. Avoid system of shoulds and should nots and discussions regarding moral judgments. Avoid power struggles. Give minimal tasks, and grade them to manageable size. Prevent self-mutilation.
Manipulation/acting out	Spell out acceptable and unacceptable behavior. Set firm and definite limits. Consistently enforce limits. Avoid involvement in intellectualization (i.e., responsibility for behavior rests with client). Treat infractions with withdrawal of privileges. Ensure that staff is united, firm, and consistent. Maintain sense of authority.
Ritualistic behaviors	Do not interrupt repetitive act: could lead to panic. Set limits on repetitive behavior. Engage in alternative activities with client. Provide physical protection from repetitive acts.
Secondary gain	Understand unconscious motivation of the behavior and differentiate it from malingering. Understand and alleviate primary symptoms. Encourage client to explore the motivation of the behavior. Explore alternatives to the primary symptom for handling anxiety.
Somatic behaviors	Do not focus on physical symptoms. Give appropriate information regarding somatic complaints. Point out reality (i.e., correct misinformation).
Superiority	Suggest solitary activities for client. Put client in charge of things, not people. Give client activities at which client can succeed.

Evaluation

Client maintains adequate food and fluid intake; skin is hydrated.

Goal 3: Client will demonstrate improved hygiene and grooming.

Implementation

1. Identify specific client needs for assistance (e.g., with severe withdrawal, client may need nurse to provide care; client with poor reality orientation or attention span may need assistance; more self-sufficient client may only need encouragement).
2. Use gentle firmness and consistent interest in client's needs.
3. Provide matter-of-fact positive reinforcement for appropriate grooming and cleanliness.
4. Be sure equipment for physical care is available to client.

Evaluation

Client performs own hygienic care (hair, nails, clothing, bathing).

Goal 4: Client will develop a trusting relationship with staff member; will demonstrate increased ability in social interaction.

Implementation

1. Know that staff reactions can be the crucial element negating or facilitating attainment of the therapeutic goal for the client.
   a. Staff members may find themselves withdrawing from the client because the disorder is often chronic, the prognosis is pessimistic, and client's behavior provokes feelings of frustration, helplessness, and incompetence.
   b. Withdrawal on the part of the staff reinforces the client's past experiences of rejection and feelings of low self-esteem (mutual withdrawal).
   c. In own defense, the client will withdraw further into world of fantasy, negating progress toward the therapeutic goal planned.
   d. In addition, the client may test staff involvement by trying to push staff away.
   e. Offer support and encouragement to other staff members; meet regularly to provide support.
   f. Schizophrenics develop relationships slowly and use their ambivalence to push others away; therefore the orientation phase of the relationship is the most difficult.
2. Use consistent, predictable behavior with client.
3. Persevere even though client may be unreliable or rejecting.
4. Meet for short intervals at regularly scheduled times to increase trust.

5. Use silence; show willingness to spend time without talking if client so chooses.
6. Allow ample time for response if client is very regressed; use general comments that do not push client for answer.
7. Allow client to set the pace of the relationship.
8. Accept client's particular stage of illness; if communication is to be restored, the nurse must understand that client is frightened and both wants and fears contact from others, makes responses slowly, and needs ample time to trust nurse's sincerity and interest.
9. Listen in nonjudgmental way to client's thoughts and feelings.
10. Know that autistic clients are extremely sensitive to the feeling tones of others; they pick up negative cues from the nurse, who may be unaware of them.
11. Role-model socially appropriate behavior.
12. As client begins to accept the nurse, client may become very dependent; a therapeutic goal requires that the nurse maintain contact on a professional level and not reinforce the dependency.
13. Observe verbal and nonverbal behaviors that may indicate any interest in activities; give support to any expression of interest.

Evaluation

Client develops a relationship with one staff member; begins to interact with other clients.

Goal 5: Client will define and test reality; will dismiss internal voices, hallucinations, and delusions.

Implementation

1. Recognize disorientation as manifestation of severe withdrawal related to anxiety and frustration.
2. Be meticulously honest and reliable, especially with the suspicious client.
3. Do not give attention to content of hallucinations or delusions (gives them legitimacy): avoid arguing about content.
4. Acknowledge client's feelings and beliefs; point out that these are not shared.
5. Relate to client in a realistic and concrete manner, focusing on the immediate situation; it is helpful for the nurse to point out reality to the client by saying, "I don't understand," and asking for clarification as needed.
6. Help to recognize hallucinations or delusions as sign of anxiety.
7. Reassure that hallucinations and delusions do go away and can be dismissed as client focuses on real people and situations.
8. Help client relate to real persons.

9. Help client who has depersonalization to discuss feelings of estrangement with trusted individuals:
   a. First with a nurse with whom client has developed a trusting relationship.
   b. As client's condition permits, in group therapy sessions or similar groups involving other persons who may recount similar experiences.
10. Focus on reality of the client's body and environment during these discussions.

Evaluation

Client dismisses internal voice, hallucinations and delusions; increases ability to relate to real persons and situations.

Goal 6: Client will increase communication with family members.

Implementation

1. Accept client's feelings and thoughts, and help client do the same.
2. Explore present family patterns with client; family assessment and intervention during the client's hospitalization may be needed.

3. Help client identify feelings associated with family interactions.
4. Help client view self as unique person with values and beliefs that are sometimes different from family's.
5. Practice social skills to use with family members; use role playing, assertion techniques.
6. Provide opportunity for family members to talk about the client's illness and treatment to decrease hostility and withdrawal from client; help family explore social resources.

Evaluation

Client increases adaptive communication with family members.

Goal 7: Client will increase successful decision-making skills.

Implementation

1. Relate in a concrete manner; focus on the immediate situation.
2. Encourage decision making at level of client's ability; use therapeutic milieu as tolerated by client.
3. Increase complexity of decisions as tolerated.

Table 2-16 Types of withdrawn behavior (schizophrenia)

Type	Characteristics	Additional nursing care
Paranoid	Delusions of persecution/grandeur Hallucinations Ideas of reference Hostility/aggression Superiority	Interventions specific to delusions (see *Suspicious Behavior*, p. 62), hostility, superiority, and aggression (see *Socially Maladaptive Behavior*, p. 55)
Catatonic	Severe withdrawal, regression Catatonic stupor, waxy flexibility, muteness or Catatonic excitement, severe agitation, grimacing, bizarre gestures/posturing	Prevent complications of immobility: infection, skin breakdown, urinary and fecal incontinence, constipation
Undifferentiated	Mixed schizophrenic symptoms over long time	See General Nursing Plan, p. 67
Childhood	Onset in early childhood Withdrawal, impaired relationships, disturbed affect Ritualism Self-mutilation Increased or decreased sensitivity to sensory stimuli *No* hallucinations or delusions	Prevent self-mutilation Behavior modification

Other psychotic disorders
  schizophreniform disorders
  brief reactive psychosis
  schizoaffective disorder
  atypical psychosis
	Sudden onset
	Last less than 6 months
	No prior history of disturbed interpersonal relationships
	Minimal residual defects
		See General Nursing Plan, p. 67

4. Provide with tasks of increasing complexity.
5. Do not reinforce unneeded dependency.
Evaluation
Client increases ability to make decisions.

Goal 8: Client will demonstrate social skills in individual and group settings.

Implementation
1. Role-model appropriate social interaction.
2. Role-play social situation with client.
3. Help client develop a relationship with one other client.
4. Encourage client to relate to others during activities.
5. Do not push client beyond present abilities; may need encouragement to begin developing social skills.
6. Help client to relate to others in more complex situations, slowly as tolerated.

Evaluation
Client behaves appropriately in individual and group settings; interacts with other clients; demonstrates fewer problem behaviors.

Goal 9: Client will develop ability to be as self-supporting as possible.

Implementation
1. Support client in finding a healthy living situation; may be at home, a halfway house, or in own apartment depending on client's social skills and ability to be self-motivating.
2. Support client in finding employment as appropriate; employment history and assessment of skills in occupational therapy can help in developing employment plan.
3. Allow family to discuss feelings about plans for client's living and employment plans; help them evaluate their expectations and role in supporting client in living and employment settings.

Evaluation
Client finds healthy living situation; develops a plan to be self-supporting.

SELECTED HEALTH PROBLEM
☐ Specific Schizophrenic Disorders

Characterized by withdrawal, all are distinguished by other characteristic behaviors. General Nursing Plans and Evaluations, p. 67 (see also Table 2-15), are used in addition to care specific to the distinguishing characteristics; see Table 2-16.

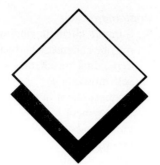# Substance Use Disorders

GENERAL CONCEPTS
Overview
1. Definitions
   a. Substance use disorder: behavioral changes associated with somewhat regular use of a substance that affects the central nervous system
   b. Polydrug abuse: mixing drugs and alcohol in varying degrees (particularly dangerous because of potentiating and toxic interactions of drugs and alcohol)
2. Etiology: not known, but thought to be an interplay of physiological, psychological, and sociocultural factors
3. Interaction variables
   a. The person
      1. no specific personality type identified
      2. most frequently, the person shows signs of immaturity, low tolerance for frustration, low self-esteem, environmental deprivation, conflicts over parental upbringing, and conflict between values and behavior
      3. it is not known if substance abuse fosters development of these characteristics or if the characteristics trigger the abuse
      4. major psychiatric disorders generally associated with substance abuse are antisocial personality and affective disorders
   b. The family: substance abuse may relate to overall anxiety level in family as well as in individual
   c. The environment: social aspects and peer pressure may lead the person into drug culture and antisocial acts
   d. The substance: which substance the person uses depends on the cultural group, availability, costs, and federal regulation of the item (alcohol and/or drug substances other than alcohol)
4. Three criteria distinguish substance *abuse* from substance *use*
   a. Pattern of pathological use: depending on the substance, client manifests inability to cut down or stop use despite physical problems; needs daily use for adequate functioning; intoxication through out the day; episodes of a complication of substance intoxication (e.g., alcoholic blackouts)
   b. Impairment of social or occupational functions: legal and economic difficulties because of cost, procurement, or complications of intoxication (e.g., auto accident)
   c. Duration of abuse: disturbance of at least a month
5. Substance dependence
   a. Definition: a more severe form of substance use disorder than substance abuse
   b. Manifestations
      1. a physiological need for a substance evidenced by withdrawal or tolerance
      2. almost always, a pathological use pattern occurs that causes impairment in social or occupational functioning
      3. rarely, manifestations are limited to physiological dependence
      4. alcohol or cannabis dependence requires evidence of occupational or social impairment; diagnosis of other substance-dependence categories requires only evidence of withdrawal or tolerance
   c. Length of dependence: regular maladaptive use for over 6 months qualifies as "continuous dependence"
   d. Social implications: although accessibility, chance, peer pressure, and curiosity play a part in who will ingest a drug and who will not, they do not account for the fact that one person becomes addicted and another does not
   e. Concepts
      1. physiological dependence: an altered physiological state produced by the repeated administration of the drug, which necessitates its continued administration to prevent a withdrawal syndrome
      2. addiction: the compulsive use of a chemical substance with physiological and psychological dependence

3. habituation: repeated use of a substance that results in psychological dependence
4. tolerance: markedly increased amounts of the substance are required to achieve the desired effect, or there is a markedly diminished effect with regular use of the same dose
5. withdrawal: a substance-specific syndrome following cessation or reduction of intake
6. lethality: the amount of a substance that constitutes a fatal dose
7. potentiation: two or more substances combined have a greater effect than simple summation (e.g., 1 + 1 = 3)

6. Substance use disorders among health professionals is a serious problem
   a. Narcotic addiction by physicians estimated at 1%-2%, or 30 times greater than in general population
   b. Estimated 40,000 alcoholic nurses in United States
   c. Problems with impaired health professionals' job performance compromise teamwork and result in danger to clients and the professionals themselves
   d. It is the responsibility of health professionals to report concerns about a colleague to supervisor, and for supervisor to take appropriate actions
   e. Professionals are helping, not harming, a substance-abusing colleague by bringing problems to the attention of someone qualified to help

Application of the Nursing Process to a Client with a Substance Use Disorder

Assessment

1. Substance use history (substance abusers are well-known for denying use or seriously understating extent of use; to increase likelihood of accurate history, ask questions in a logical and nonthreatening manner; family and friends may provide more accurate information or use denial)
   a. History of recent prescription and nonprescription drug use
   b. Drugs client has prescribed for self (e.g., nicotine, alcohol, cocaine, marijuana)
2. Work performance
   a. Excessive use of sick time
   b. Decreasing productivity or "job shrinkage"
   c. Decreasing ability to meet schedules and deadlines
   d. Sloppy or illogical work
   e. Frequent errors in judgment; in drug-addicted nurses, medication errors, incorrect controlled-drug wastage, or incorrect narcotic counts
3. Blood levels of suspected substance of abuse
4. Level of consciousness, reality orientation, mental status exam
5. Family history of substance abuse

Analysis

1. Safe, effective care environment
   a. High risk for injury
   b. Sensory-perceptual alteration: visual, auditory, kinesthetic, gustatory, tactile, olfactory
   c. High risk for violence: self-directed or directed at others
2. Physiological integrity
   a. Altered nutrition: less than body requirements
   b. Impaired physical mobility
   c. Sleep pattern disturbance
3. Psychosocial integrity
   a. Anxiety
   b. Ineffective individual coping
   c. Chronic low self-esteem
4. Health promotion/maintenance
   a. Ineffective family coping: compromised
   b. Altered family processes
   c. Noncompliance

General Nursing Planning, Implementation, and Evaluation

Goal 1: Client will withdraw from substance that is abused or creating dependency.

Implementation

1. It is important *not* to do any of the following:
   a. Scold, argue, moralize, blame, or threaten.
   b. Lose one's temper.
   c. Enable person to cover up consequences of actions.
   d. Be overly sympathetic.
   e. Put off facing problem.
2. Control symptoms with medication when required (PRN); take vital signs every 2 hours and report elevations to physician.
3. Assess risk of violence.
4. If client is agitated, confused, assaultive, or belligerent, stay with client; reassure that current symptoms are only the result of body's responding to the abused substance, and that they are temporary; reassure that client will regain control; use restraints only if necessary for safety (follow hospital policy carefully).
5. Deal with hallucinations by reinforcing reality; speak to client slowly in a calm voice; provide a quiet environment; stay with client until the frightening symptoms have decreased.
6. Provide physical care advocated for additional diseases/conditions that client may have.
7. Keep client ambulatory as much as possible; if necessary, walk with client several times a day.

Evaluation

Client withdraws from abused substance, free from complications.

Goal 2: Client will obtain treatment necessary to abstain from substance abuse or dependence.

Implementation

1. Sit and talk with client at least twice daily; your presence will say client is not being rejected; be aware of your own nonverbal distancing maneuvers; establish good eye contact.
2. Do not punish or reprimand client for failures or nonresponse to your suggestions and interventions (punishment serves only to give client fuel for continuing to deal with failure or rejection by drinking or taking drugs); ignore it, but do praise *any* positive responses.
3. Have client make decisions about daily care in hospital; involve in some type of occupational therapy, anything in which client can achieve some measure of success (helps increase self-confidence and self-esteem).
4. Provide opportunities to decrease social isolation and improve social skills (mealtimes, groups, recreation periods); calmly and gently point out unacceptable behavior such as manipulative acts; reinforce positive social behaviors (e.g., initiating friendly conversations); praise all efforts at participation in activities.

Evaluation

Client participates in prescribed treatment.

Goal 3: Client will develop a positive life-style that is free from substance use, abuse, or dependence.

Implementation

1. Help the client to gradually become aware of the denial by poking holes in denial process; encourage client's assessment of how denial serves client, including delineation of the self-defeating aspects.
2. Help client look at alternative coping methods and deal with abstinence one day (or one morning, one evening) at a time.
3. Work with client to develop sound discharge planning regarding employment counseling, ongoing support via outpatient counseling, or long-term inpatient treatment.
4. Provide information about other types of therapy available (e.g., stress-reduction programs, employee assistance, aftercare programs, and local mental health clinics or self-help groups).

Evaluation

Client's approach to daily living is positive and free from substance abuse or dependence.

Goal 4: Family will explore enabling behaviors.

Implementation

1. Arrange for client and family to attend group counseling sessions, if available in hospital, to discuss feelings, problems, changing behaviors, pressures, sources of support, etc.
2. Encourage family to allow time to take care of needs that may have been neglected during years of substance abuse.
3. Teach family new ways to manage frustrations; role-model assertion skills.
4. Discuss need for realistic expectations of client behaviors.

Evaluation

Family members participate in group counseling; discuss expectations of client.

SELECTED HEALTH PROBLEMS

☐ Alcohol

General Information

1. Definitions
   a. *Alcohol* is a mind- and mood-altering substance classified as a central nervous system depressant
   b. *Alcoholism (alcohol dependence)*
      1. no agreement on definition; clinical features: chronicity; preoccupation with drinking; loss of control over drinking; damage to health, relationships, and/or work; using alcohol as a solution to most problems
      2. the World Health Organization definition: a chronic disease or disorder of behavior characterized by alcohol consumption that exceeds customary use and interferes with the drinker's health, interpersonal relations, or economic functioning
2. Effects
   a. At low levels of consumption, there is little apparent effect on the drinker; moderate levels may produce euphoria; and in large amounts, alcohol acts as a sedative
   b. Alcohol depresses higher cortical functions, acts as a disinhibitor and tranquilizer, and serves to reduce anxiety rapidly (excessive drinking is often the way a person copes with anxiety)
3. Scope of alcohol abuse and dependence
   a. Estimates
      1. one third of general hospital clients, but these clients are rarely admitted with alcoholism diagnosis
      2. one out of 10 Americans who drink is an alcoholic
      3. 6.6 million adults in United States are alcoholic
      4. one in 10 alcoholics is diagnosed and treated
   b. Occurrence: alcoholism and related problems are widespread among
      1. city residents
      2. minorities
      3. poor men under 25 years of age
      4. persons who have experienced childhood disruptions (e.g., broken homes, alcoholic parents)

5. rural or small-town persons who have moved to urban areas

6. people of Swedish, Polish, Irish, northern French, and Russian origin

4. Characteristics common but not exclusive to alcoholics

   a. Low self-esteem

   b. Feelings of isolation, depression

   c. Emotional immaturity and excessive dependence

   d. Anger and hostility

   e. Highly anxious in interpersonal relationships

   f. Inability to express emotions adequately

   g. Ambivalence toward authority

   h. Grandiosity

   i. Compulsiveness, perfectionism

   j. Sexual-role confusion

   k. Excessive use of denial, projection, rationalization

5. Withdrawal from alcohol and detoxification

   a. Symptoms develop when there is a physiological dependence and the intake of alcohol is interrupted or decreased without substitution of other sedation

   b. Complete cessation of use of alcohol is not necessary for the development of withdrawal symptoms; the beginning of withdrawal can be a reflection of diminished use in those who have developed a marked tolerance and physical dependence

   c. Monitored detoxification for withdrawal is the top-priority need of the alcoholic client

   d. Withdrawal syndrome has four major manifestations: tremulousness, hallucinations, convulsive seizures, and delirium tremens; this is a progressive process and involves four stages

      1. *stage 1*, 8 hours plus after cessation: symptoms include mild tremors, nausea, nervousness, tachycardia, increased blood pressure, diaphoresis

      2. *stage 2*, symptoms include profound confusion, gross tremors, nervousness and hyperactivity, insomnia, anorexia, general weakness, disorientation, illusions, nightmares; auditory and visual hallucinations begin

      3. *stage 3*, 12-48 hours after cessation: symptoms include all those of stages 1 and 2, as well as severe hallucinations and grand mal seizures ("rum" fits)

      4. *stage 4*, occurs 3-5 days after cessation: symptoms include initial and continuing delirium tremens (DTs), which are characterized by confusion, severe psychomotor activity, agitation, sleeplessness, hallucinations, and at onset, uncontrolled and unexplained tachycardia; DTs are a medical emergency (fatality rate is 20% even with treatment)

6. Prognosis: motivation and recognition of the problem are necessary for eliminating alcohol use; the person experiences fluctuations of sobriety, during which acknowledging illness and moving toward a new way of life are punctuated by relapse, shock, and denial; alcoholics are considered as recovering, not cured

7. Treatment: approaches used in all alcohol treatment models

   a. General measures include vitamin and nutritional therapy, sedatives, tranquilizers, and/or disulfiram (Antabuse); avoid drugs containing alcohol (e.g., elixirs, cough syrups, mouthwashes)

   b. Detoxification: the acute phase of treatment

      1. involves close observation and safety measures to prevent severe reaction while withdrawing from alcohol

      2. magnesium sulfate 50% solution and high doses of chlordiazepoxide (Librium) are used to prevent seizures and hallucinations

      3. thiamine 50-100 mg intramuscularly (IM) to treat malnutrition

      4. education and group process are frequently used after detoxification when client is able to understand instructions

   c. Rehabilitation

      1. aim is to build treatment motivation and overcome denial in clients and significant others

      2. the alcoholic has to learn to give up alcohol forever

      3. the person is helped to learn new ways of problem solving and living a satisfying life without alcohol; this is enhanced by a therapeutic relationship that increases the alcoholic's self-confidence, feelings of self-worth, and attempts to become more independent

   d. Major models of treatment

      1. chronic disease model

         a. views alcoholism as a primary, physiological, incurable disease

         b. views psychosocial problems as result of drinking

         c. includes a maintenance program of recovery

         d. emphasis is on self-diagnosis by the alcoholic

      2. psychiatric model

         a. focus on unique needs as defined by psychiatric perspective

         b. varying psychotherapeutic treatment regimen depends on individual

      3. family systems model

         a. views family relationships as a contributing factor; chemical dependency is viewed as a family illness

         b. examines childhood development of alcoholic, such as drinking patterns of parents, ethnic attitudes, and socialization process regarding drinking behaviors

   c. looks at family roles, communication patterns, family rules, and power structure in the family

   d. identifies how present family relations re-create old patterns of avoidance or dependence

   e. uses family commitment and caring to promote recovery

   f. integrates recovering alcoholic into revised family structure

  e. Alcoholics Anonymous (AA) is a self-help group of recovering alcoholics

   1. a 12-step program to achieve sobriety, which members do at their own pace

   2. run entirely by sober alcoholics

   3. requires members to devote themselves completely to mutual help

   4. remarkable success with chronic alcoholism

   5. has member groups for families of alcoholics who themselves suffer from codependency (i.e., dependency on the alcoholic)

     a. Al-Anon is an organization of friends and families of alcoholics

     b. Alateen is an organization of teenagers affected by alcoholism

     c. AC-A is an Al-Anon organization for adult children of alcoholics

     d. the emphasis is on changing oneself to make the most of one's life, education, guidance in relating to the alcoholic family member, the sharing of problems and experiences, and support based on a 12-step program

  f. Long-term treatment also may take place in the controlled environment of a private or public facility and in an outpatient setting

   1. depending on the particular model used, emphasis varies among group process, education, psychotherapy, family therapy, and AA

   2. AA is the backbone to maintain sobriety; some clients attend daily

8. Preventive measures: include helping the client learn to

  a. Tolerate psychological stress

  b. Do advance planning for anticipated painful events (surgery, separation from a loved one)

  c. Reduce social isolation

  d. Communicate honestly

9. DSM-III-R classifications: Alcohol intoxication, uncomplicated alcohol withdrawal, alcohol withdrawal delirium, alcohol hallucinosis, alcohol dependence abuse

Nursing Process

Assessment

1. Physical assessment/history

  a. Skin: spider angiomas, jaundice, acne rosacea, multiple bruises, age of bruises (purple, yellow), mahogany finger stains, "dirty tan," flushed ruddy complexion

  b. Orthopedic system: vaguely explained fractures, moderate muscle wasting of proximal muscle groups of lower and upper extremities

  c. Cardiovascular system: a first episode of paroxysmal atrial tachycardia as adult, ventricular premature contractions, paroxysmal atrial fibrillation, erratic hypertensive course (alcohol elevates blood pressure)

  d. Gastrointestinal system: early tooth losses, esophagitis, gastritis, pancreatitis, palpable liver, peptic ulcer, epistaxis, anorexia, weight loss, jaundice, cirrhosis

  e. Neurological system: tremors that worsen with movement, vertigo and nystagmus that clear during the day, vaguely described memory lapses (blackouts), insomnia, seizures, peripheral neuropathy, hallucinations

  f. Genitourinary system: mild proteinuria, orgasmic/erectile dysfunction; prostatitis

  g. Indications of fluid and electrolyte imbalance

  h. Respiratory system: repeated upper respiratory infections

2. Psychological assessment

  a. Suicide potential

  b. Extent of cognitive disturbance

  c. Mental status exam

  d. Occurrence of signs and symptoms related to major psychiatric disorders

3. Other: although not diagnostic themselves, the following raise possibilities and should be explored further

  a. Numerous transient medical symptoms in various organ systems without mention of drinking

  b. Unwarranted complaints and signing out against medical advice (hospitalized clients)

  c. Functioning at lower job level than intelligence and education would indicate; changing jobs frequently

  d. Alcoholism in close relatives (parental alcoholism increases likelihood fivefold)

  e. Child or spouse abuse

4. Strengths and stressors, coping mechanisms

5. Beliefs, attitudes, feelings, concerns about alcohol consumption

6. Codependency behaviors in family and friends: enabling behaviors that perpetuate the drinking behaviors, dependence on alcoholic, superresponsibility in children, denial and poor coping, signs of chronic stress

7. Prescription- or street-drug use

Analysis (see p. 73)

Planning, Implementation, and Evaluation

> **Goal 1:** Client will withdraw from alcohol free of systemic complications.

Implementation

1. Observe for withdrawal symptoms (anxiety, anorexia, insomnia, tremor, disorientation leading to delirium, tachycardia, hallucinations) beginning shortly after last drink and lasting 5-7 days.
2. Monitor for delirium tremens (severe withdrawal behaviors) beginning 2-3 days after cessation of alcohol ingestion and lasting 48-72 hours.
3. Give antianxiety drugs as ordered.
4. Institute seizure precautions.
5. Monitor I&O, administer 2500 ml/day; avoid caffeinated drinks.
6. Weigh daily to monitor fluid retention.
7. Monitor electrolytes; report abnormalities.
8. Give vitamin/mineral supplements, especially B vitamins.

Evaluation

Client withdraws from alcohol without evidence of nutritional imbalance, seizures, fluid and electrolyte imbalances; remains safe during episodes of disorientation, hallucinations.

> **Goal 2:** Client will develop healthier coping mechanisms to deal with the stress of life.

Implementation

1. Express concern for client's situation and confidence in ability to recover.
2. Intervene to decrease denial and manipulative behavior.
3. Discuss your observations of client's behavior with client, being as frank as possible; help client relate this behavior to alcohol intake.
4. Deal with angry behavior resulting from confrontation; know that although the anger may be directed at staff, it may stem from emerging insight into the problems; direct anger into nondestructive outlets (e.g., exercise, art, or music).
5. Intervene in withdrawal behavior that may result from grieving process and result in relapse; express confidence in client's ability to recover.
6. Discuss drinking pattern with client to identify triggers, cues, "slippery places"; talk about what a lifestyle without alcohol would be like.
7. If receiving Antabuse therapy to control impulsive drinking; explain symptoms if alcohol is ingested (headache, severe GI distress, tachycardia, hypotension).
8. Discuss possibilities of continuing psychotherapy, a 12-step program (AA, Al-Anon, Alateen), or a transitional living program; arrange for a referral if client is receptive.
9. Initiate frequent staff conferences to share therapeutic insights and ideas, and vent responses to client's manipulative or angry behavior.
10. Develop a mutually agreed-upon "contract" for behavior change.

Evaluation

Client practices new coping behaviors; increases self-esteem, social skills; explores group support; initiates insight or behavioral therapy.

> **Goal 3:** Client and family will accept the support of concerned others; will establish a life-style without alcohol.

Implementation

1. Involve client in assertion therapy; involve in group therapy to help client recognize the impact of behavior on others.
2. Reinforce contacts with 12-step programs and psychotherapy.
3. Encourage new relationships that do not involve alcohol; be supportive during loss of old relationships.
4. Permit family to express anger regarding client's behavior; help them see their roles as enablers.
5. Help family and staff understand that relapse is a strong possibility but does not mean failure or futility.
6. Know that alcohol-dependent persons are susceptible to adopting other dependencies and developing "cross addictions."

Evaluation

Client and family attend therapy and support groups; client engages in and practices behaviors that decrease social isolation and strengthen new behaviors; family recognizes and decreases "enabling" behaviors.

☐ Drugs Other Than Alcohol
General Information

1. Opiates and opiate derivatives, synthetic opiates (e.g., morphine, Demerol, Dilaudid, codeine, heroin): chronic abuse results in tolerance, physical dependence, habituation, and addiction
   a. Psychologically, most opiate addicts show a similarity to alcoholics in some aspects of their personality; they are emotionally immature, dependent, hostile, and aggressive, and they take drugs to relieve inner tensions
   b. Opiate addicts sometimes differ from alcoholics in that they handle their feelings passively, by avoidance rather than by acting out; choosing drugs (opiates) seems to suppress these inner tensions
   c. Availability (abuse may begin following surgery or illness), curiosity, and peer pressure play roles

in the use of opiates; social factors, such as urban versus rural differences and social class, also play a role

  d. Cultural values regarding the use of opiates may play a role in the rates of addiction
    1. Asian countries in which opiate addiction has been tolerated have a high rate
    2. Western European countries, where opiate addiction is treated as a medical rather than a legal problem, have low rates
  e. May be in methadone maintenance program as part of treatment and continue to misuse drugs
2. Barbiturates and other sedative drugs (e.g., mepro-

bamate, glutethimide, chlordiazepoxide, ethchlorvynol, diazepam); if compulsively and chronically abused, cause tolerance, habituation, addiction, and physical dependence

  a. There is a general, depressant, withdrawal syndrome associated with all of these drugs
  b. Many users of the sedative drugs began with a physician's prescription; prescription drugs are considered socially acceptable in Western society for the relief of tension and insomnia
  c. Persons who become chronic and compulsive users of these drugs have a variety of underlying psychological difficulties; they may be

Table 2-17 Common drugs of abuse

Drug	Route	Use	Dependency	Overdose	Withdrawal
Sedatives/Depressants					
Glutethimide (Doriden) Methyprylon (Noludar) Ethchlorvynol (Placidyl) Ethinamate (Valmid) Benzodiazepines Barbiturates Chloral hydrate Methaqualone (Quaalude)	Oral Injection	Relaxation Euphoria	Psychological Physical	CNS: depression Respiratory: bradypnea CV: decreased BP, P GI: cramps	CNS: marked agitation, insomnia, convulsions, poor muscle coordination GI: nausea/vomiting Psychotic behavior CV: increased BP with postural hypotension
Stimulants					
Amphetamines Cocaine Phenmetrazine (Preludin)	Oral Smoking Injection	Rush/high Fatigue	Psychological Tolerance	CV: increased BP, P; dysrhythmias Respiratory: nasal abnormalities GI: anorexia, dry mouth, vomiting CNS: dilated pupils, hyperactivity, headache Impulsiveness Delusions/hallucinations Poor judgment	Depression Suicide potential Lethargy Somnolence Headache "Crash" paranoia
Cannabinoids					
Cannabis (marijuana, hashish) Dronabinol (Marinol)	Smoking Oral	"Dreamy" state Euphoria, hilarity, excitement To control nausea/ vomiting of chemotherapy As a bronchodilator	Psychological	"Drop out" syndrome Paranoia Confusion Delusions/hallucinations GU; impotence CNS: tremors, poor coordination Red eyes	No clinically significant effects
Inhalants					
Ether Cleaning fluids Gasoline/kerosene Glue vapor Ethylene oxide Aerosols	Inhalation	Intoxication Exhilaration	Tolerance	Extreme toxicity Airway obstruction Death through damage to liver, kidneys, bone marrow	No clinically significant effects

1. anxious or insecure
2. trying to relieve hostile and aggressive impulses
3. trying to escape tension through the drug's intoxicating effect

d. Withdrawal must be managed gradually because of danger of seizures

3. Amphetamines and cocaine (see also reprint, p. 106) have a stimulating effect upon the user
   a. When these drugs are chronically and compulsively abused, they result in tolerance and habituation
   b. When the drug is withdrawn, general fatigue and depression occur, along with changes in sleep EEG pattern; these symptoms are not considered a clinical withdrawal syndrome, and physical dependence is not associated with the abuse of these drugs
   c. Chronic use can result also in a toxic psychosis, characterized by vivid hallucinations and persecutory delusions
   d. Social, cultural, and psychological factors have all been cited as causative: family history of alcoholism and psychopathology, availability, peer pressure, curiosity, and physician prescription; the use of these drugs by persons who are overweight

Table 2-17   Common drugs of abuse—cont'd

Drug	Route	Use	Dependency	Overdose	Withdrawal
Psychedelics					
PCP LSD Mescaline Psilocybin	Oral Injection Smoking Inhalation	Euphoria Ecstasy but with anxiety	No evidence	Delusions/hallucinations Poor time/space perception Poor memory Multiple individualized effects Depersonalization GI: anorexia, dry mouth, nausea/vomiting CNS: dizziness, dilated pupils CV: increased BP, P, temperature; sweating, chills; dysrhythmias Chromosomal damage Flashbacks Accidents	No clinically significant effects
Opiate/Synthetics					
Heroin Oxymorphone (Numorphan) Morphine Meperidine (Demerol) Hydromorphone (Dilaudid) Opium alkaloids (Pantopon)	Injection Inhalation	"High" Ecstasy Relaxation Pleasurable feeling	Tolerance Physical	CV: decreased BP GI: anorexia, cramps CNS: grand mal seizures, pinpoint pupils, coma, death Respiratory: slow, shallow breathing GU: urinary retention	*Stage 1* Restlessness Anxiety Craving *Stage 2* Yawning Lacrimation Rhinorrhea Diaphoresis *Stage 3* Dilated pupils Gooseflesh Anorexia Muscle pain *Stage 4* Insomnia Marked agitation Nausea/vomiting Diarrhea

or depressed is more socially acceptable than by those who take them for thrills

   e. Many amphetamine or cocaine addicts are also compulsive users of barbiturates, alcohol, or morphine

4. Hallucinogens (e.g., lysergic acid diethylamide [LSD], mescaline, PCP [angel dust], STP) produce tolerance, and in some persons, habituation

   a. These agents do not produce physical dependence with its concomitant withdrawal syndrome or addiction

   b. May produce acute panic and anxiety states and toxic psychosis, characterized by hallucinations and persecutory delusions

   c. Historically, these drugs were used in connection with religious practices of American and Mexican Indians

   d. Recently they have been used by persons who wish to explore their feelings in altered states of drug-induced intoxication

   e. Persons who abuse these drugs are thought to be psychologically insecure, dependent, hostile, and immature

   f. Social class seems to be a factor in the use of hallucinogens, with those in the middle or upper class being more frequent users

5. DSM-III-R classification: drug intoxication, drug withdrawal, personality disorder, drug dependence abuse

Nursing Process

Assessment

1. Physiological problems: respiratory, circulatory, neurological problems associated with withdrawal (priority); see Table 2-17

2. After emergency treatment, assess for problems arising from

   a. Consequences of drugs
      1. nasal septum erosion (cocaine)
      2. potential seizures (cocaine, barbiturate withdrawal)
      3. tolerance

   b. Sepsis associated with drug injection
      1. abscesses of skin and subcutaneous fat deposits
      2. hepatitis
      3. septicemia

   c. Neglect of nutritional needs
      1. malnutrition
      2. loss of teeth, dental caries
      3. respiratory infections

3. Behavior problems
   a. Denial and/or underreporting of use
   b. Somatic complaints
   c. Blaming others
   d. Anger, hostility, self-pity, mistrust

   e. Family, social employment, and financial problems
   f. Low frustration tolerance
   g. Criminal or "antisocial" behavior
   h. Grandiosity
   i. High dependency needs
   j. Violence
   k. Suicidal attempts

4. Pattern of drug use, family problems

Analysis (see p. 73)

Planning, Implementation, and Evaluation

Goal 1: Client will withdraw from drug, free from respiratory failure, shock, toxic psychosis.

Implementation

1. Intervene in respiratory failure: maintain a patent airway, give oxygen, administer naloxone hydrochloride (Narcan).
2. Administer IV fluids for shock, as ordered.
3. Assess the level of coma or stupor.
4. Administer drugs as ordered to suppress withdrawal or to counter a toxic psychosis.
5. Give antibiotics as ordered.
6. Restrain client as necessary for safety.

Evaluation

Client withdraws from drug; has patent airway; is free from signs of shock or toxic psychosis.

Goal 2: Client will decrease purposeful drug-seeking, manipulative, and acting-out behaviors.

Implementation

1. Set firm and consistent limits.
2. Clearly define acceptable and unacceptable behavior.
3. Know that the client often will complain that a nurse who does not cooperate lacks trust.
4. Be aware that the client may plead, cry, ask for money, steal, stimulate drug withdrawal syndrome to obtain drugs.
5. Have entire staff adopt consistent approach to client's behavior.

Evaluation

Client decreases purposeful drug-seeking, manipulative, and acting-out behaviors; accepts limits of unit.

Goal 3: Client will decrease intellectualization; will focus on problem solving and activities of daily living (ADL).

Implementation

1. Know that client may exhibit dependency behaviors, blame parents, society, world conditions for drug-taking behaviors; be aware that client may try to in-

volve nurse in intellectual discussion about the above, but do not discuss these with client.

2. Keep focus on client's responsibility for own behavior; do not plead or exhort.

3. Focus on problems in ADL and possible solutions.

Evaluation

Client discusses living problems and develops some solutions.

Goal 4: Client decreases denial and superficiality; explores alternative coping mechanisms; verbalizes some awareness of consequences of own actions.

Implementation

1. Confront the client face-to-face with facts about self that client attempts to avoid; use only after foundation of trust and acceptance has been laid or when group relationship is cohesive.

2. Avoid discussions of "why" client abuses drugs.

3. Avoid nagging client to promise total rehabilitation; realistic approach to possibilities of success must be taken.

4. Know that 90% of drug abusers relapse.
   a. The most effective treatment to date has been that given by former abusers (e.g., Narcotics Anonymous); having been in the situation, these persons are familiar with the demanding behaviors, manipulations, rationalizations, intellectualizations, and denial of drug abusers, and are able to handle them with firmness and with supportive concern; clients are less likely to "put one over" on them.
   b. Do not make moral judgments.
   c. Be aware of own rescue, angry or hostile feelings toward drug abusers; try to control your reactivity in client's presence.

Evaluation

Client decreases use of denial; begins to explore alternative coping; visits postdischarge treatment facility; decreases number and frequency of drug-abuse incidents.

Goal 5: Family will recognize roles as codependents.

Implementation

1. Recognize that 50% of families in United States have problems with substance abuse.

2. Avoid collusion with client or family; focus on analyzing and restructuring relationships; teach how to avoid enabling behaviors.

3. Initiate education on substances and addictions.

4. Refer to self-help groups and 12-step programs as adjuncts to family therapy.

5. Explore ways to adjust life-style to decrease unhealthy behaviors.

6. Recognize the real possibility of relapse; be supportive while encouraging positive life-style changes during relapse.

7. Explore judicious use of confrontation strategies and therapeutic and supportive interventions.

Evaluation

Family discusses healthier life-style behavior; confronts client about unhealthy behaviors.

BIBLIOGRAPHY

General

Aromando, L. (1989). *Mental health psychiatric nursing*. Springhouse, PA: Springhouse.

Beck, C., Rawlins, M., & Williams, S. (1992). *Mental health-psychiatric nursing: A holistic life-cycle approach* (3rd ed.). St. Louis: Mosby–Year Book.

Burgess, A. (1990). *Psychiatric nursing in hospital and community*. Norwalk, CT: Appleton and Lange.

Carpenito, L. (1989). *Nursing diagnosis: Application to practice*. Philadelphia: Lippincott.

Colorado Society of Clinical Specialists in Psychiatric Nursing. (1990). Clients rights. *Journal of Psychosocial Nursing and Mental Health Services, 28*(2), 38-40.

Colorado Society of Clinical Specialists in Psychiatric Nursing. (1990). Ethical Guidelines for Confidentiality. *Journal of Psychosocial Nursing and Mental Health Services 28*(3), 43-44.

Doenges, M., Townsend, M., & Moorhouse, M. (1989). *Psychiatric care plans: Guidelines for client care*. Philadelphia: F.A. Davis.

Forchiek, C., et al. (1989). Establishing a nurse-client relationship. *Journal of Psychosocial Nursing and Mental Health Services 27*(2), 30-34.

Haber, J., Hoskins, P., Leach, A., & Sidelau, B. (1992). *Comprehensive psychiatric nursing* (4th ed.). St. Louis: Mosby–Year Book.

Johnson, B. (1990). *Psychiatric-mental health nursing: Adaptation and growth*, (2nd ed.). Philadelphia: Lippincott.

Rawlins, R., & Heacock, P. (1988). *Clinical manual of psychiatric nursing*. St. Louis: Mosby–Year Book.

Stuart, G., & Sundeen, S. (1990). *Principles and practice of psychiatric nursing* (4th ed.). St. Louis: Mosby–Year Book.

Varcolis, E. (1990). *Foundations of psychiatric nursing*. Philadelphia: Saunders.

Wilson, H., & Kneisl, C. (1988). *Psychiatric nursing* (3rd ed.). Menlo Park, CA: Addison-Wesley.

Loss and death and dying

*Gifford, B. (1990). Supporting the bereaved. *American Journal of Nursing, 90*(2), 48-53.

Stephany, T. (1990). A death in the family. *American Journal of Nursing, 90*(4), 54-56.

Anxious behavior

Beeber, L. (1989). Update on medications for the treatment of anxiety. *Journal of Psychosocial Nursing and Mental Health Services 27*(10), 42-43.

Breakwell, H. (1990). Are you stressed out? *American Journal of Nursing, 90*(8), 31-33.

Grainger, R. (1990). Dealing with feelings: Anxiety interrupters. *American Journal of Nursing 90*(2), 14-15.

---

*Reprint.

Hayes, G., Goodwin, T., & Miars, B. (1990). After disaster: A crisis support team at work. *American Journal of Nursing, 90*(2), 61-64.

Taylor, C. (1990). *Mereness' essentials of psychiatric nursing* (13th ed.). St. Louis: Mosby–Year Book.

Townsend, M. (1990). *Drug guide for psychiatric nursing.* St. Louis: Mosby–Year Book.

Confused behavior

Blakeslee, J. (1988). Untie the elderly. *American Journal of Nursing, 88,* 833-834.

Elated-depressive behavior

Brant, B., & Osgood, M. (1990). The suicidal patient in long-term care institutions. *Journal of Gerontological Nursing 90,* 1518

*Bydlon-Brown, B., & Billman, R. (1988). At risk for suicide. *American Journal of Nursing 88,* 1358-1361.

*Harris, E. (1988). The antidepressants. *American Journal of Nursing, 88,* 1512-1518.

Harris, E. (1989). Lithium. *American Journal of Nursing, 89,* 190-194.

McEnany, G. (1990). Managing mood disorders. *RN, 90,* 28-33.

Rankin, W. (1989). Teenage suicide. *Journal of Pediatric Nursing, 89,* 130-131.

Saunders, J., & Buckingham, S., (1988). Suicidal AIDS patients: When depression turns deadly. *Nursing88, 18,* 59-64.

Socially maladaptive behavior

Curry, L., Colvin, L., & Lancaster, F. (1988). Breaking the cycle of family abuse. *American Journal of Nursing, 88,* 1188-1190.

Freeman, S. (1988). Inpatient management of patient with borderline personality disorder: A case study. *Archives of Psychiatric Nursing, 2,* 360-365.

Substance use disorders

Bennett, E.G., & Woolf, D. (1991). *Substance abuse: pharmacologic, developmental and clinical perspectives* (2nd ed.). Albany, NY: Delmar Publishers.

Kinney, J. (1991). *Clinical manual of substance abuse.* St. Louis: Mosby–Year Book.

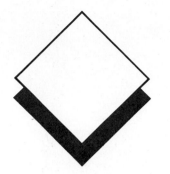

Reprints

Nursing Care of the Client with Psychosocial and Mental Health Problems

SUPPORTING
THE BEREAVED

By Bette J. Gifford/Beryl B. Cleary

The bereaved needs someone to listen—don't interrupt, don't tell your own story, don't change the subject, and don't offer platitudes.

My brother-in-law's telephone call sent shivers down my spine. He begged me to tell him how to comfort his brother, whose 21-year-old son had just been killed in an automobile accident. I thought of the other grieving people I'd tried to help recently—a young colleague whose husband had died and a patient with diabetes who'd lost her newborn. I realized that nurses are often called upon to support relatives, friends, coworkers, and patients who have lost a loved one. And we want to help, but many of us are quite unprepared to do so.

Probably the most basic truth about grief is that it lasts far longer than most people think. Grief is painful to witness, so many people, not knowing how to ease the sorrow, expect the bereaved to put their grief aside (easing everyone else's discomfort) and get right back to normal. Of course such sidestepping is not only impossible for the grieving person to do, it is also inappropriate because of the grief work needed before the loss is resolved.

The grim reality

The first task of grieving is accepting the reality of the loss: coming full face with the fact that the person is dead and will not return(1). The person who cannot accept that fact is manifesting denial and is stuck in the first task of grieving.

Most people deny a loss at least partially for a short while, but soon begin to realize that the loss has indeed occurred(2). Others deny the facts, the meaning, or the permanence of the loss for long periods. Some even continue arranging the environment as though the loss had not occurred(3). Such denial protects the person from the pain of acknowledging the loss.

Encourage the person to talk about the lost loved one.

To get the person to open up, say, "I'm so sorry about your loss. Would you like to tell me what happened?" or "Would you like to talk?"

If you don't know what to say or do, just give the person a hug or say, "I've been thinking about you." Cry if you feel like it. Showing the person you care might be all the encouragement he needs to talk. Don't worry that you'll "remind" the grieving person of the loss. You won't, because he hasn't forgotten—not for a moment. Encourage him to talk about memories of the loved one. Call the deceased by name and share a memory of your own. By doing so, you're telling the bereaved person that you feel comfortable sharing his grief.

Of course, if the bereaved does not want to talk, don't pursue the matter. Accept it and try again gently at a later date.

Listen.

Family members often ask the bereaved, "Why torture yourself by talking about it all the time?" But the bereaved needs someone to listen while he sorts out his complex emotional reactions to his new reality(4). Don't interrupt, don't tell your own story, don't change the subject, and don't offer meaningless platitudes such as "It's God's will" or "It's better this way." Such remarks don't help and can hurt. Simply *listen*.

Foster communication between family members.

They need to talk, too. Encourage them to set aside quiet times just for talking with each other. Explain to each the importance of listening to the others without criticizing or belittling them for their feelings. Once they start talking about the deceased, what they remember about him, and how they feel about his death, they begin to accept the unacceptable.

The cost of love

The second task is experiencing the pain of grief(1). As the meaning of the loss begins to register, the bereaved feels intense physical and emotional pain. Parkes describes that pain as "Just as much a part of life as the joy of love; it is perhaps the price we pay for love, the cost of commitment"(2).

To help with the second stage of grieving, **help the person express his feelings**. Many families encourage a stoic acceptance of death, so to avoid criticism, members often refuse

Bette J. Gifford, RN, MSN, is the director of the adolescent community services project for the Broome County Health Department, Binghamton, NY. Beryl B. Cleary, RN, MSEd, is an instructor of nursing at the Robert Packer Hospital School of Nursing, Sayre, PA. Both authors are bereaved parents; together they developed a program for nurses on supporting people through loss.

to cry or express emotions in front of the family(5). You can help by asking the bereaved, "How did that make you feel?" or "This must be a sad time for you." Be sure you have time to listen and steady yourself for the intense feelings that may rush out.

Many bereaved persons are confused about the **anger** they feel when a loved one dies. Anger is typically directed at the deceased for deserting the family; at nurses, physicians, clergy, funeral directors, or even God; and inward in the form of assuming some responsibility for the loved one's death(6).

Accepting anger as natural and encouraging its expression can help put it to rest. Open the door by saying, for example, "If my son died, I'd be angry," or "It must anger you to be left with so much responsibility since your husband died." Listen to the person's anger without taking any of it personally. Let the person know that, just as it's acceptable to thank God for the good times, it's reasonable to expect God to bear the brunt of our anger when a loved one dies. Suggest the person talk about his anger toward God with his religious counselor.

The "if only" element of grief (if only the bereaved had done something differently, the loved one might still be alive) can provoke overwhelming feelings of **guilt**. Guilt can virtually destroy a marriage if, for example, parents who cannot understand how their child could have died lash out at and blame each other for the death.

Help the bereaved identify the "if onlys" and put them into perspective. If the person says, "I didn't do enough" ask, "What did you do?" Keep exploring until he concludes that perhaps he did do all he could have under the circumstances.

The bereaved can also feel guilty as he recalls how he may have failed the deceased—with quarrels, disappointments, infidelities of thought or action, and negligence(3). Focusing on inconsequential "failings" may mask a more profound guilt over being the survivor(3).

Suggest to the bereaved that he

CONCRETE SUGGESTIONS THAT HELP

☐ Mark significant occasions on your calendar to remind yourself to send the bereaved a note or card.
☐ Help the person plan what he'll do on the first Christmas, the first birthday, the anniversary of the loss.
☐ Suggest that the person join special-interest groups or take college courses.
☐ Recall what the person likes to do—go out to dinner or see a play, for example. Plan such activities on a regular basis.
☐ Don't expect families to support each other. Each family member is struggling with his own personal grief. Encourage the bereaved to join a support group, such as Compassionate Friends, a self-help group for bereaved parents.

forgive himself. Say, "You're being awfully hard on yourself," "You seem to be blaming yourself for being human," or "I realize it's difficult for you, but try not to hurt yourself over something you could not have controlled." This conveys that others are willing to accept human failure.

Recognize normal responses to grief and offer reassurance.
After losing a loved one—especially a first loss—many people are so overwhelmed by their feelings that they think they are losing their minds. Let the bereaved know that their feelings are normal. One way to help is to make information about grief available to them and to their families and friends at the time of the loss. At some hospitals, information packets are available from the pastoral care department. Suggest one of the many books available for the bereaved (Harriet Schiff's *The Bereaved Parent,* for example, from Penguin Books).

Tell the bereaved that his feelings are temporary and necessary for getting the work of grieving done. Assure him that it is normal for painful periods of despair and helplessness to recur over many months, but that they'll alternate with periods of calmer, more normal functioning.

Stress individual differences.
Families are often upset when one member's grieving deviates from the behavior of the rest.

Explain that no two people in a family can be expected to go through the grief process in the same way.

**Suspect maladaptive grief when a person shows
no signs of grieving or displays intense grief
beyond the usual one- to two-year period.**

Encourage the family to accept and respect each person's unique style of grieving.

The missing person

The third task is adjusting to an environment that no longer includes the deceased(1). Someone who does not complete the third task promotes his own helplessness, refuses to develop new skills, and withdraws from the world. The person can remain in a state of suspended growth unless he redefines his goals(1).

Help the person adjust to the loss.

Immediately after the death, the bereaved feels distracted or "at loose ends." He's so stunned that he doesn't even know what he needs to do, let alone how others can help.

You can help the bereaved figure out what needs to be done and arrange the tasks in order of priority. Concrete interactions have more positive outcomes for the bereaved. For example, helping a widow collect insurance benefits or find a baby-sitter will mean more to her than general offers of help(7).

Loss of a spouse is extremely disruptive for an elderly partner, since family ties often weaken over the years and many peers have died. Elderly men have an especially difficult time when their wives die as they are often unfamiliar with domestic tasks and may have lost contact with co-workers and community members(8).

You can help an elderly widower by working with him to establish a structure for daily routines and by teaching him the basics of cooking

and laundering. Help him set specific and meaningful goals, such as reestablishing his peer network by eating three meals per week at the senior citizens center.

Loss typically disrupts appetite and sleep, so with this in mind, prepare food and bring it to a newly bereaved person, or invite him to dinner. Ask a widow to accompany you to the supermarket. Suggest techniques for getting to sleep, such as taking warm baths, avoiding caffeine, and getting up and doing something useful (reading or ironing, for example). Suggest regular exercise and explain that it can help relieve depression and improve appetite and sleep patterns. Invite the person to join you for after-dinner walks.

Don't discourage a bereaved person from cooking, cleaning, and returning to work. Relieving him of responsibility only thwarts his adjustment. Having to struggle with the pain of death, on the other hand, fosters feelings of strength and security.

Help the person make necessary changes.

The bereaved is often unaware of all the roles the deceased played until three months or so after the loss. Suddenly he or she has to come to terms with living alone, or raising children alone, or managing finances. That can be especially devastating for widows who had not previously built lives apart from their husbands(7).

Discuss with the person how he plans to develop new skills, leisure activities, interests, and social contacts. Explore what would pique his

interest, such as volunteer work or church activities that also promote self-esteem and a sense of belonging.

On the other hand, don't encourage major life changes, such as selling property, changing jobs, or adopting children too soon after a death. Few people can exercise their normal judgment while in acute grief.

That was then. . .

The fourth and final task of grieving is withdrawing emotional energy and reinvesting it in another relationship(1). The function of grief is to help survivors detach their memories and hopes from the deceased and begin to form new relationships(2,9). But many people think that doing so dishonors the memory of the deceased. Others fear that the new relationship might also end in a loss. However, a sign of final resolution of a loss is the person's ability to enjoy himself again and make new social contacts without feeling disloyal to the deceased(6).

Help the person withdraw his emotional attachment.

Begin by helping him dispose of the personal belongings of the deceased. Reluctance to do so is often a sign that the bereaved person fears losing his memories of the deceased. But if well-meaning family members do it for him, they are keeping the bereaved from accomplishing the last task of grief. Suggest, instead, that the bereaved and the family (including any children) find objects or mementos of the deceased that each wishes to keep.

Anticipate especially difficult times. Grieving is a process of cutting cords, and as such, it takes time. Many believe that four full seasons must pass before the bereaved can begin to think of the deceased without feeling intense emotional pain. Birthdays, anniversaries, and holidays trigger a variety of intense emotions, as do future life events that must be experienced without the deceased, such as weddings, births, and graduations. The bereaved needs extra support at those times and encouragement to reinvest his emotions back into life and in the living. Once the bereaved sees that he can get through various celebrations without the deceased, he begins to withdraw his emotional investment in the past(10).

Identify maladaptive grief reactions and refer accordingly. Some bereaved persons cannot get through all four tasks. They get stuck holding on to the past and refuse to move into the future. Watch for trouble and decide when the time is right for referring the person for grief therapy or psychotherapy. Generally, suspect maladaptive grieving when a person shows no signs of grieving at all or displays intense grief beyond the usual one- to two-year period.

Watch for the avoidance of grief—removing all reminders of the deceased or statements like, "I don't miss him." Radical changes in lifestyle, a tendency to shun people associated with the deceased, intense grief reactions triggered by minor events months after the loss, and preserving the environment exactly as the deceased left it, all indicate maladaptive grief that warrants professional counseling.

Unresolved grief leads to depression. Prolonged inactivity; despondency; feelings of helplessness and hopelessness; an inability to eat, sleep, or carry out usual activities; or prolonged withdrawal from social contacts are all signs of clinical depression.

The death of a loved one is a devastating emotional agony that takes a long time to subside. By maintaining contact with the bereaved over time, we can help turn the futility and despair of grief toward the direction of healthy recovery.

HELP FOR THE BEREAVED

☐ The Compassionate Friends, PO Box 3696, Oak Brook, IL 60522-3696.

☐ The Candlelighters Foundation, 2025 I St. NW, Washington, DC 20006.

☐ Survivors of Suicide (SOS): Directory of Survivor Groups, American Association of Suicidology, 2459 S. Ash St., Denver, CO 80222.

☐ Bereavement Outreach Network, 127 Arundel Rd., Pasadena, MD 21122.

☐ Growing Through Grief, PO Box 1664, Annapolis, MD 21404.

☐ Widow to Widow Program, 58 Fernwood Rd., Boston, MA 02115.

☐ The National SIDS Foundation, 8240 Professional Pl., Landover, MD 20785.

☐ Pregnancy and Infant Loss Center, 1415 E. Wayzata Blvd., Suite 22, Wayzata, MN 55391.

☐ SHARE, Sister Jane Marie, St. Johns Hospital, 800 E. Carpenter, Springfield, IL 62702.

☐ Widowed Persons Service, AARP, 1909 K St. NW, Washington, DC 20049.

REFERENCES

1. Worden, W. J. *Grief Counseling and Grief Therapy.* New York, Springer Publishing Co., 1982, pp. 11–19.
2. Parkes, C. M. *Bereavement: Studies of Grief in Adult Life.* New York, International Universities Press, 1972, pp. 3–7, 173.
3. Peretz, D. Development, object-relationships, and loss. IN *Loss and Grief: Psychological Management in Medical Practice,* ed. by B. Schoenberg and others. New York, Columbia University Press, 1970, pp. 15–28.
4. Attig, T. Death education and life-enhancing grief. IN *New Directions in Death Education and Counseling,* ed. by R. A. Pacholski and C. A. Corr. Decatur, IL, Association for Death Education and Counseling, 1981, p. 59.
5. Hampe, S. D. Needs of the grieving spouse in a hospital setting. *Nurs.Res.* 24:113–119, Mar.–Apr. 1975.
6. Speck, P. W. The experience of loss and normal grief. IN *Loss and Grief in Medicine,* ed. by P. W. Speck. London, Bailliere Tindall Publishers, 1978, pp. 11–12.
7. Lopata, H. Z. On widowhood: grief work and identity reconstruction. *J.Geriatr.Psychiatry* 8:1–55, Jan. 1975.
8. Barrineau, J. Sex differences in death and death-related concerns across the life span: old age. IN *New Directions in Death Education and Counseling,* ed. by R. A. Pacholski and C. A. Corr. Decatur, IL, Association for Death Education and Counseling, 1981, pp. 153–154.
9. Lindemann, E. Symptomatology and the management of acute grief. *Am.J.Psychiatry* 101:143, Sept. 1944.
10. Corr, C. A. Bereavement as a relative experience. IN *Loss and Grief in Medicine,* ed. by P. W. Speck. London, Bailliere Tindall Publishers, 1978, p. 6.

RELAXA

Six techniques you can teach to patients, incorporate into your care, and use yourself— even when you just have ten seconds to spare.

Relaxation, an effective adjunct to the treatment of a variety of ailments, can be achieved through simple techniques that can easily be taught to patients. Patients requiring minor invasive procedures—such as the drawing of blood, or insertion of intravenous catheters—can reduce their anxiety levels by following any one of a number of routes to relaxation. Those with asthma can learn to use these techniques when they anticipate attacks. Relaxation can relieve headaches and menstrual cramps and reduce both acute and chronic pain by alleviating tension in rigidly held muscles surrounding painful areas.

Several characteristics are common to all relaxation methods:

Rhythmic breathing. Most relaxation techniques start with slow deep breathing. As a person becomes relaxed, he consumes less oxygen; so breathing becomes slower and shallower. Although the rate and depth of breathing changes, the rhythm becomes constant. Thus, rhythmicity itself characterizes relaxation. (See chart, next page, for other physiologic changes brought about by relaxation.)

Reduced muscle tension. Some people relax so thoroughly that they can't move their arms or legs. Whether or not such profound relaxation is

Jean Wouters DiMotto, RN, MSN, is a psychophysiologist and educator. She is currently completing law school at Marquette Univerity, Milwaukee, WI.

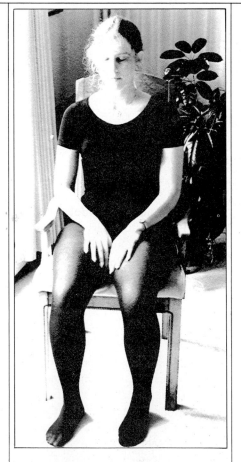

attained, almost any relaxation method will significantly ease muscle tension.

An altered state of consciousness. Your state of consciousness corresponds to your brain waves. The waking, alert state is called beta. During relaxation, you move to a level of consciousness called alpha[1]. In the alpha state, which falls between full consciousness and unconsciousness, thought processes become less logical and more associative and creative. Your sense of time and body may be distorted: A 15-minute relaxation exercise may seem to last two minutes or two hours; your body might feel very large or very small; you might feel a heavy, or a light, floating feeling; or, you might experience your body as boundless, at one with the surrounding environment[2].

You have a heightened ability to focus on one idea or image. Focus may be on breathing, sensory experiences, or tension[3]. Or, you might concentrate on a particular image, thought, or problem. Alpha state and focused mental activity are the major reasons why mental imagery is so effectively paired with relaxation. Although clients are seldom aware of moving from the beta to the alpha state, when relaxation is finished and they return to the beta level of consciousness they are aware of feeling more alert.

Clinical experience suggests there are individual differences in people's experiences of relaxation. Not everyone will demonstrate all characteristics of a relaxed psychophysiologic state.

RELAXATION TECHNIQUES

Full-body relaxation. A common type of relaxation, this 15-minute method—involves paying attention to different parts of your body, noting any ten-

ATION

BY JEAN WOUTERS DiMOTTO

Reprinted from American Journal of Nursing, June 1984

sion, and replacing it with warmth and relaxation.

If the patient is willing, this is a good relaxation technique to use while giving a bed bath. While preparing the patient for her bath, give the breathing instructions (see chart, p. 758). As you wash each part of her body, ask her to notice any tension in that part. For example, you could say, "As I wash your arm, notice any tightness or tension in it." As you rinse her arm say, "Breathe in warmth and relaxation to this arm and exhale the tension." Dry her arm with slower motions than you used to wash or rinse, saying, "Notice the warmth and relaxation you now feel in

this arm." Repeat these instructions as you wash each body part, dealing with her hands independently of her arms, her arms separately from her shoulders, her neck from her face, and her feet from her calves. The bath is likely to take about 20 to 30 minutes, so keep the water warm; cold water inhibits relaxation.

As is true of most relaxation exercises, it is fairly easy for patients to do the exercise themselves once you have done it with them a few times.

Modified autogenic relaxation. This method can be useful in the treatment of asthma, hyperventilation, high blood pressure, cold hands or feet, head-

ache, and ulcers(4). Relaxation is attained through a series of statements—or autosuggestions—about various bodily functions. After assuming a relaxing position, breathe in slowly and deeply, then slowly exhale, repeating to yourself the phrases shown in the chart on p. 0000. Inhale as you identify the parts of your body and exhale as you describe how relaxed you feel.

People enjoy this method and use it because the calming results are so obvious. After a while, subsequent use relaxes them more thoroughly and quickly. For some, just thinking the first statement produces relaxation.

Sensory pacing. While your uncon-

WHAT HAPPENS WHEN WE RELAX?

Physiologic manifestations	Cognitive manifestations	Behavioral manifestations
decreased pulse	altered state of consciousness, usually alpha level	lack of attention to and concern for environmental stimuli
decreased blood pressure	heightened concentration on single mental image or idea	no verbal interaction
decreased respirations	receptivity to positive suggestion	no voluntary change of position
decreased oxygen consumption		passive movement easy
decreased carbon dioxide production and elimination		
decreased muscle tension		
decreased metabolic rate		
pupil constriction		
peripheral vasodilation		
increased peripheral temperature		

Adapted from: Graves, H.H., & Thompson, E.A., "Anxiety: A Mental Health Vital Sign." In: Longo, D.C. and Williams, R.A. (Eds.), Clinical Practice in Psychosocial Nursing: Assessment and Intervention, N.Y., Appleton-Century-Crofts, 1978.

BODY POSTURES FOR RELAXATION

Sitting, reclining, or lying down are all postures conducive to relaxing. In each of these positions, the body should be well supported by a chair, bed, or couch. It is important that your primary position be balanced. Crossing your legs, dropping your head to one side, or leaning your upper body over a table will strain the affected muscles after ten to twenty minutes. Not only will these muscles remain tense, the discomfort will interfere with your attaining or remaining in alpha-level consciousness(5).

Sitting. Sit all the way back resting against the entire back of the chair. Place your feet flat on the floor. (If you're wearing high heels, remove your shoes.) Separate your legs so they're not touching each other. You can hang your arms by your sides or rest them on chair arms. Or, you can place each of your hands flat on each of your thighs. A fourth possibility is to rest your palms on your thighs, letting your fingers hang loosely between your legs.

Align your head with your spine. You can hold it comfortably straight, tilt it slightly forward, or rest your chin on your upper chest. If you choose to hold your head straight, you may unknowingly drop it forward as you relax. This is fine, since your head remains aligned with your spine.

You are now in a balanced, sitting position. Complete your preparation by loosening any tight clothing and making sure you are moderately warm.

Reclining and lying down. Many of the positioning principles for sitting apply. Separate your legs and point your toes slightly outward. Rest your arms at your sides without touching your sides. Keep your head aligned with your spine. You can lie flat or place a small, thin pillow under your head. Thick, large pillows will cause neck and back strain.

You will be able to maintain these postures for as long as you choose, without straining any muscle group. The only problem with reclining or lying down is that it's easy to fall asleep in these positions. In a recent study showing that relaxation training produces prolonged reduction of blood pressure, the author noted that the individual needs to remain awake to obtain maximum benefit from relaxation training(6). If, on the other hand, your purpose for relaxing is to induce sleep, then of course, reclining or lying down are the preferred positions.

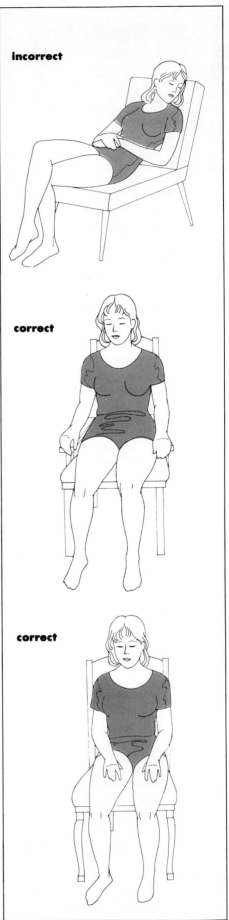

incorrect

correct

correct

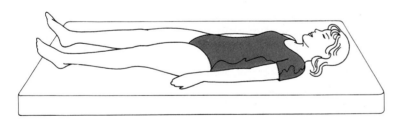

correct

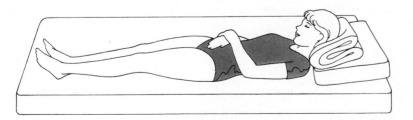

incorrect

scious mind constantly takes in information from all five senses, your conscious mind is seldom aware of input from more than one or two senses at any moment. By consciously calling attention to the sensory experience you are having at a particular instant, you synchronize, or pace, your conscious and unconscious minds. If your body is motionless in one of the relaxed postures and you continue pacing for two to four minutes, you will attain relaxation (see chart, next page).

The method is simple and effective, particularly for patients in units where there are a lot of environmental stimuli, such as critical care units and outpatient departments. It is also good for people who have trouble concentrating on different parts of their bodies.

If a patient is having difficulty with the exercise, repeat the first part of each sentence (as listed in the chart) and have the patient finish the sentence with what he is aware of at that moment. If at the end the patient doesn't feel relaxed, repeat the pacing.

Color exchange. This method uses two senses—kinesthetic and visual. Sensations of tension or pain are converted to colors, then exhaled. The exhaled color is replaced with white light that is inhaled (see chart, next page). The concept of white light— healing, peaceful energy—has been used by Eastern people for centuries.

Color exchange is especially effective in the late afternoon and early evening, a time when people who have worked all day feel fatigued, and when patients who spend most of their day in bed feel restless and uncomfortable. Using this method will reduce the day's tension, replenish energy, and relieve pain. It is also a good way to end a back rub.

Music. Any restful music is appropriate, but classical music is most conducive to relaxation because its rhythms and harmonic structures are often perceived as soothing. As people listen to classical music, they tend to let their thoughts wander, either away from their present concerns to more pleasant topics, or to creative perspectives on problems with which they are struggling.

A number of classical selections can be used. Pachelbel's Canon in D Major, Mozart's Piano Concerto No. 21 in C Major, and much of Vivaldi's and Bach's music are apt. Particularly, good selections from Vivaldi include *The Four*

Seasons, the concerti for mandolin, the baroque guitar concerti, and the six flute concerti (Opus 10). Relaxing selections from Bach include the *Goldberg Variations,* and the six concerti after Vivaldi.

The adagio, larghetto, and largo movements of Vivaldi and Bach have rhythms similar to the human heartbeat. When they listen to these movements, people's pulse rates and other biological rhythms tend to synchronize themselves with the beat of the music. This is particularly true with the largo movement's slow, stately, restful rhythm. The result is deeper, more efficient relaxation[7].

Another excellent choice is Halpern's *Soundscapes.* These are meditative col-

> # Postop patients who use relaxing techniques feel less pain and tension, and use fewer narcotics.

lections of sounds without any familiar rhythm that are designed to relax, balance, and attune the listener[8]. Similar selections include Horn's *Inside* albums, Andrew's *Kuthumi* and *The Violet Flame,* and Scott's and Yuize's *Music for Zen Meditations.*

Music can also serve as background accompaniment while using other relaxation methods. Recordings or tapes of environmental sounds (i.e., streams of water, soft rain, wind) are particularly helpful. You can create relaxation tapes for yourself or your patients.

Ten-second relaxation techniques. Even a short exercise can lower pulse and respiration rates, although using stimulants such as caffeine shortly before relaxing interferes with a person's ability to slow physiologic processes.

Two relaxation techniques take only 10 seconds. Both are useful when, for example, postoperative patients begin to feel incisional pain and become tense, as when ambulating or changing positions.

You yourself can use these tech-

niques during a busy day when there is no opportunity to take a break. While walking to a patient's room, taking an elevator, using the restroom, or sitting down to chart, you can lower your tension level with a 10-second exercise: Eyes open, let your lower jaw drop as if you were starting to yawn. Rest your tongue on the bottom of your mouth behind your lower teeth. Breathe slowly and rhythmically through your mouth: inhale, exhale, then rest. Do not form or even think words.

Research on patients who used this technique showed they felt significantly less incisional pain and bodily tension than those who didn't use the technique, and that they used fewer narcotics in the first 24 hours after surgery[9].

The second technique is done while sitting or standing. Close your eyes. Focus on a tiny imaginary star one inch in front of the tip of your nose. Take four deep breaths slowly through your mouth while continuing to focus on the star. This brief exercise requires intense concentration, and is especially helpful when you want to clear your mind as well as relax.

Ending relaxation techniques. The simplest and most comfortable way to end an exercise is to gradually open your eyes and stretch as though you were coming out of a deep sleep. Stretching helps move you from the alpha level of consciousness to the beta level of alert wakefulness. Although some people advocate jerking or contracting an arm or leg, it is more abrupt and less comfortable than stretching. After stretching, get up and move about a bit to become fully alert, especially if you are going to drive or operate medical machinery.

The more often you relax, the easier and faster you relax; relaxation becomes a conditioned response. Simply slowing your breathing, or performing a 10-second relaxation technique, or thinking of a phrase such as "relax," or "down you go," will trigger relaxation.

Relaxing regularly does not necessarily mean relaxing daily. Once a week is probably enough to establish a conditioned response. It is not necessary to use the same relaxation method each time in order to condition yourself; which relaxation method you choose is a matter of personal preference. Patients will also have preferences, so it is usually a good idea to teach them at least two methods.

USING RELAXATION TECHNIQUES

Relaxation by Sensory Pacing

Assume a relaxing position and slowly repeat and finish each of the following sentences, either in a low voice or to yourself.

Now I am aware of seeing . . .
Now I am aware of feeling . . .
Now I am aware of hearing . . .

Start with your eyes open, allowing them to close when they feel heavy. Begin by repeating and finishing each sentence four times. Then repeat and finish each sentence three times, then two times, then one time. Once your eyes are closed, what you see will be in your mind's eye.

Reference: Carter, P. and Gilligan, S. Personal Communication, 1980.

Full Body Relaxation

Assume a relaxing position. Note your breathing. Is it fast, slow, even or uneven, deep or shallow? Now, change your breathing to slow, abdominal breathing, breathing all the way in, down to your navel. Count to 4, inhaling on 1 and 2, exhaling on 3 and 4. Continue this.

Become aware of your face, your jaws, and your neck. Notice any tightness or tension in these parts. Breathe in warmth and relaxation. Exhale the tension.

Become aware of your shoulders, your arms, your hands and fingers. Notice any tightness or tension. Again, breathe in warmth and relaxation. Exhale the tension.

Become aware of your back—from your shoulders to your tailbone. Notice tightness or tension anywhere in your back. Breathe in, relaxing your back. Exhale the tension.

If you're feeling warm, you're relaxing.

Move to your chest and abdomen. Relax your abdominal muscles. Notice any tightness or tension. Breathe in warmth and relaxation. Exhale the tension.

You may notice that some parts of your body are tingling. It means you're relaxing.

Now move to your pelvic area and buttocks. Notice any tightness or tension in these parts. Breathe in warmth and relaxation to these areas and exhale the tension.

You may feel very heavy, as though you could sink deeply into your chair or bed. Or, you may feel light enough to float on a cloud or sit on a flower. Either way is fine. It means you're relaxing.

Move to your thighs. Notice any tightness or tension in those muscles. Breathe in warmth and exhale tension.

Move to your knees, then your calves, ankles, and feet. Notice any tightness or tension. Breathe in, relaxing all the way down to the tips of your toes. Exhale the tension.

Take time now to enjoy the peace you feel. When you're ready to end the relaxation period, count to ten, slowly open your eyes, wriggle your fingers and toes, and stretch as if you are just waking up.

Modified Autogenic Relaxation

Assume a relaxing position.

Slowly take in a very deep breath. Exhale very slowly.

Repeat each of the following phrases to yourself four times. Say the first part of the phrase as you breathe in for 2 to 3 seconds. Hold your breath in for 2 to 3 seconds. Then say the last part of the phrase as you breathe out for 2 to 3 seconds. Hold your breath out for 2 to 3 seconds.

Breathe in	Breathe out
1. I am	relaxed.
2. My arms and legs	are heavy and warm.
3. My heartbeat	is calm and regular.
4. My breathing	is free and easy.
5. My abdomen	is loose and warm.
6. My forehead	is cool.
7. My mind	is quiet and still.

References: Bauman, Edward, and others. The Holistic Health Handbook. Berkeley, And/Or Press, 1978.
Pelletier, Kenneth R. Mind as Healer, Mind as Slayer. New York, Dell, 1977.

Relaxation by Color Exchange

Assume a relaxing position. Concentrate on your breathing as you slowly take four deep breaths.

Notice any body tension, tightness, aches, or pains. Give the tension or discomfort a color, the first color you think of.

Now breathe in pure white light from the universe. Send the light to the tight or painful place in your body. Surround the color of your discomfort with the white light.

Exhale the color of your discomfort and inhale white light to take its place. Continue breathing in white light and exhaling the color of your discomfort.

Now, continue breathing in white light until your entire body is filled with the light and you have a sense of peace, well being, and energy.

Reference: Radtke, Dawn, D. Personal communication, 1980.

You may find that the more often you teach relaxation techniques to patients, the faster and more deeply you relax when you do an exercise yourself—one way the caregiver benefits directly from the care given.

For years, women preparing for childbirth have learned various breathing patterns and relaxation techniques in order to give birth without tranquilizers or analgesics. New mothers breastfeeding their babies can relax before feeding to increase the flow of milk. They are also more likely to feel at ease and to enjoy the experience.

Relaxation is useful preoperatively not only to help people sleep but to reduce their anxiety about upcoming surgery. Postoperatively, relaxation can be used to relieve pain. And, people can use relaxation to reduce the stress in their lives and to achieve even better health. In whatever nursing setting you choose to practice, there will be numerous indications for teaching relaxation to your patients.

REFERENCES

1. Wallace, R. K., and others. A wakeful hypometabolic physiologic state. *Am.J.Physiol.* 221:795-799, Sept. 1971.
2. Trygstad, Louise. Simple new ways to help anxious patients. *RN* 43:28-32, Dec. 1980.
3. McCaffery, Margo. *Nursing Management of the Patient with Pain.* 2nd ed. Philadelphia, J.B. Lippincott Co., 1979.
4. Davis, Martha, and others. *The Relaxation and Stress Reduction Workbook.* 2nd ed. Richmond, CA, New Harbinger, 1982.
5. Guyton, A. C. *Textbook of Medical Physiology.* 5th ed. Philadelphia, W.B. Saunders Co., 1976.
6. Agras, W.S. Relaxation therapy in hypertension. *Hosp. Prac.* May 1983, p. 134.
7. Ostrander, Sheila, and others. *Superlearning.* New York, Delacorte Press, 1979.
8. Halpern, Steven. *Tuning the Human Instrument.* Belmont, CA, Spectrum Research Institute, 1978.
9. Flaherty, G. G., and Fitzpatrick, J. J. Relaxation technique to increase comfort level of postoperative patients: a preliminary study. *Nurs.Res.* 27:352-355, Nov.-Dec. 1978.

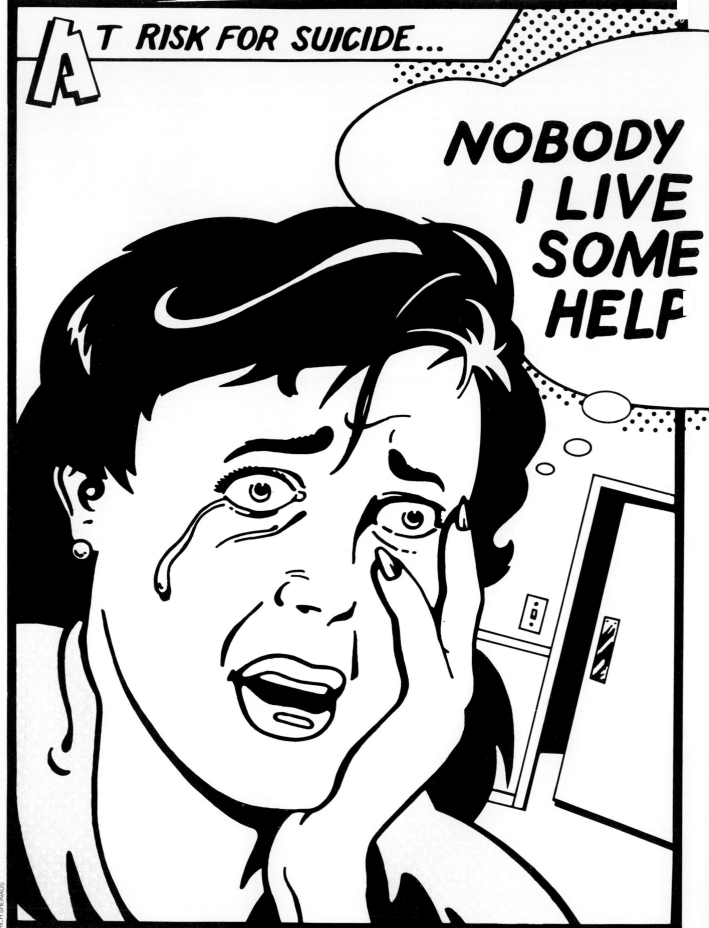

BY BARBARA BYDLON-BROWN/ROBERT R. BILLMAN

Reprinted from American Journal of Nursing, October, 1988.

CARES IF OR DIE! WILL ONE PLEASE ME?

Will you help me? I'm going to kill myself!" This frequent chant of 65-year-old Ms. C, a patient on our closed, acute-care psychiatric unit, was familiar to staff. Diagnosed as a chronic, agitated depressive person, Ms. C was being treated with electroconvulsive therapy and a PRN antianxiety agent.

Besides her constant refrain, Ms. C had a pattern of inappropriate behavior. She rarely communicated with staff, which made us anxious. She sometimes lay on the floor in the middle of the hall. Mood swings from cheerfulness to anger, sometimes accompanied by aggressive behavior, were becoming frequent.

One night her chants were louder than usual. Then Ms. C went to bed and appeared to sleep. The night shift reported that when she awoke she was calm and in good spirits. But things were not as they appeared. Shortly thereafter, the

Barbara Bydlon-Brown, RN, is a staff nurse, and Robert R. Billman, RN, certified in psychiatric/mental health nursing, is assistant head nurse, St. Marys Hospital, Rochester, MN.

nurse caring for Ms. C found a cloth restraint hidden in her room. Ms. C confided to the nurse, "I'm going to kill myself."

Nurses on units similar to our 29-bed psychiatric unit frequently face such situations(1). We use primary nursing to provide continuity of care, and we use routine suicide supervision levels. Every shift we also check rooms for sharp items such as nail files and razors(2). But what, we asked ourselves, are *appropriate* levels of supervision for the suicidal patient?

Are 5- to 10-minute checks adequate? Is one-on-one observation enough? Is there a correlation between patient behaviors and the intensity of nursing supervision?

To explore these issues, we formed a suicide assessment committee and observed nursing care given to suicidal patients. We found that many factors can interfere with suicide assessment, among them patient and staff transference; biased attitudes toward the diagnosis; reliance on intuition; and inconsistency because of differences in experience, expertise, education, and patient contact(3).

To begin to enhance our assessment technique, we realized we needed to standardize the way we

took psychosocial histories on suicidal patients. Our subjective (gut-level) responses to patients were *based* on objective data. However, we were not integrating our subjective feelings with our objective observations.

We also recognized that countertransference with specific patients had a major impact on which suicide supervision levels were used. In turn, these supervision levels affected patients' self-esteem. Observing a patient more closely to assure optimum safety may be perceived by the patient as mistrust. Consequently, he may become angry, feel he has lost control, and believe his condition is deteriorating(2).

However, to be less restrictive while attempting to maintain optimum patient safety places nurses in a difficult position. We realized we needed to balance risk factors and supervision levels with patients' rights and all the other factors influencing nurses' judgments. One way to achieve our goal was to develop a framework to assure assessment consistency.

The suicide assessment tool (on p. 1361) is based on subjective and objective data. When used in conjunction with nursing judgment, it helps determine the supervision level needed for suicidal or impulsive patients. The tool relies on the nurse's judgment of the way a patient is behaving.

WHAT TO WATCH FOR

Suicidal ideation is the thought of wanting to end one's life. When discussing such ideation with a patient it is important for the nurse to establish the patient's intent(4). If the intent (often called a suicide threat) is there, the patient is at greater risk of attempting the act. The act of planning a way to commit suicide (even if it is not a lethal plan) indicates the patient is prone to act on the thought.

Once the assessment is made, the nurse may make a contract with the patient(5). The patient agrees *not* to act on his suicidal thoughts until he first contacts the nurse, or he agrees to delay carrying out his threat for a specific time. If the patient cannot or will not agree to such a contract, the risk of his attempting suicide is greater.

Rapport, the ability of the patient to speak about his feelings to the nurse, eventually results in mutual trust. The less rapport there is, the freer the patient is to act on his thoughts(2).

How closely does the patient follow a **treatment plan?** Does he take medicines as prescribed? Does he attend assigned group therapy? If he does these things, he probably feels more hopeful about his ability to change and less helpless about his illness. The patient who does not, or cannot, comply with treatment is at greater risk of attempting suicide.

Socialization is another key issue. The patient who isolates himself may act on suicidal thoughts(1). Some minimally withdrawn patients will respond when spoken to but have little desire to make social contact. They will participate in social interaction if urged by the nurse. The highly withdrawn patient, even with constant encouragement, will not or cannot interact with staff and others. Thus, he should be considered at more risk of acting on suicidal thoughts, since he is not communicating his need for support. There is also less information on which to assess him.

What is the patient's **activity level?** The more anxious and hyperactive the patient, the higher the risk of attempting suicide.

Be alert to sudden changes in activity level: Note the highly withdrawn patient who becomes very agitated or the highly agitated patient who suddenly becomes calm(4). Either change may herald a patient's decision to kill himself. Close observation is needed.

What is the patient's **mood?** Does it change often, or is he constantly angry or frustrated? If the latter, he is at greater risk(6).

SUPERVISION STAGES

Once the nursing judgments are made, the behaviors are circled on the assessment form. The team leader or charge nurse will validate the data with the primary nurse. Then both nurses decide the supervision level for the patient.

For example, if many behaviors are marked in one column of the form, the patient may need to be supervised at the higher level of frequency. If the patient's behaviors range over several columns, the nurse considers how the lower-risk behaviors affect the higher-risk behaviors. (Higher-risk items appear at the bottom of the supervision columns.)

NEW CONFIDENCE

We were pleased with the results of using the assessment tool on our unit. Staff members exhibited increased confidence in making assessments. They also became more aware of the complex issues surrounding suicide intervention, leading to a heightened professionalism.

As a result of this new understanding, recently employed staff benefited from the close collaboration with experienced staff. At the same time, experienced staff were relieved that their judgments were no longer considered primarily subjective in nature but were based on a structured, systematic assessment.

A CASE IN POINT

Our unit's nurses were well acquainted with Mr. W, a manipulative and attention-seeking 30-year-old. He had been admitted to our unit several times over the last five years. Diagnosed with a bipolar illness, he was treated with an ECT series because his symptoms worsened after medication had failed. We checked him every 30 minutes.

One day, Julie, a staff nurse, approached the charge nurse with a concerned look on her face. "What's wrong?" asked the charge nurse. "Well, it's Mr. W," replied Julie. "I have him sitting in the lounge where I can observe him, but I don't know what to do. He says he has a plan to kill himself, and he is willing to come and get me before he acts on his plan. He's been withdrawn, anxious, and his thoughts are disorganized. I have a strange feeling about it. I don't want to overreact to his behavior by paying too much attention to his threats. At the same time, I'm afraid he might actually do something."

"Let's use the assessment checklist and see what it tells us," suggested the charge nurse.

After reviewing Mr. W's history and Julie's interactions with him that day, together they filled out the suicide assessment tool (at right) and were struck by the number of behaviors circled at the bottom of the third column.

"Even though manipulative, he is at risk and needs more observation," said the charge nurse.

"Yes, you're right," replied Julie. "Now that I see all the parts together, it's obvious that Mr. W needs to be checked every 5 to 10 minutes."

REFERENCES

1. Webster, M. Assessing suicide potential. IN *American Handbook of Psychiatric Nursing,* ed. by Suzanne Lego. Philadelphia, J. B. Lippincott Co., 1984, p. 29.
2. Barile, L. The client who is suicidal. IN *American Handbook of Psychiatric Nursing,* ed. by Suzanne Lego. Philadelphia, J. B. Lippincott Co., 1984, p. 40, 400–402.
3. Clunn, P. A., and Payne, D. B. *Psychiatric Mental Health Nursing.* 3d ed. New Hyde Park, NY, Medical Examination Publishing Co., 1982.
4. Carmack, B. J. Suspect a suicide? Don't be afraid to act. *RN* 46:43–45, 90, Apr. 1983.
5. Reubin, R. Spotting and stopping the suicide patient. *Nursing* 9:82–85, Apr. 1979.
6. Hatton, C., and others. *Suicide: Assessment and Intervention.* 2d ed. Norwalk, CT, Appleton & Lange, 1983, p. 76.

GUIDELINES FOR ASSESSING SUICIDE RISK

Current checks ___ Q 30 min ___
Any gestures in past 24 hours ___ No ___
Number of days of hospitalization ___ 35 days ___
Medications available ___ No ___

OFF CHECKS	OBSERVATION EVERY 30 MINUTES	OBSERVATION EVERY 15 MINUTES	CLOSE OBSERVATION EVERY 5–10 MINUTES	1:1 RESTRICTION	RESTRAINT OR SECLUSION
Verbalizes no suicidal ideation	Verbalizes suicidal ideation	(Verbalizes suicidal ideation with plan and/or intent)	Sudden change in activity level—i.e., becomes hyperactive—not chronic anxiety	Concealing equipment that could be used to harm self with available specific plan	Attempt made to kill self in front of staff, i.e., even 1:1 cannot resist impulse to kill self
Congruence shown in verbal and behavioral information	Verbalizes no plan	(No perception of support)	Unable to agree not to suicide	Attempt made while hospitalized to kill self	
100% compliance with treatment plan	Verbalizes no intention	Little compliance with treatment plan	Makes suicidal gesture currently		
	(Cooperative with treatment plan)	Subjective or objective frustration			
Has perception of support in community	(Withdrawn low)	Anger			
		Labile affect or mood			
	Multiple previous attempts	Mute or decreased amount of verbalization			
Verbalizes concerns on a feeling level to present nurse	(Verbalizes superficially to present nurse)	Avoidance of staff and others			
		Withdrawn high			
		Intoxicated			
		(Impaired reality testing)			
		(Hyperactive)			
		(Demonstrates limited problem-solving ability)			

SIGNIFICANT CONTRIBUTING DATA

Lives with parents.
Mother & father unable to visit — exhausted by pt's illness.
Previous attempt 3 yr. ago by carbon monoxide.
Paternal grandfather schizophrenic; suicide 10 yr. ago by carbon monoxide.
Tenth-grade education.
Oriented to person, place, and time.
Slight short-term memory loss.

PSYCH DRUGS

THE ANTI-DEPRESSANTS

BY ELIZABETH HARRIS

Reprinted from American Journal of Nursing, November, 1988.

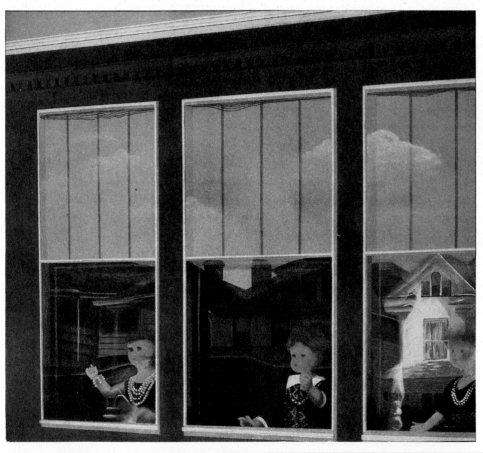

Art by Robin Price

Obviously, antidepressants are used to treat depression. More and more, though, some of these drugs are proving effective for a wide variety of other psychiatric and nonpsychiatric disorders, including panic attacks, bulimia, hyperactivity and enuresis in children, and chronic pain.

Antidepressant drugs fall into three major categories, each with its own unique effects and precautions: the tricyclics, the atypical antidepressants, and the monoamine oxidase inhibitors (MAOIs).

THE TRICYCLIC ANTIDEPRESSANTS

The tricyclic group is the gold standard of antidepressant drugs. In use longer and thus better understood than the atypicals, yet free of the dietary restrictions the MAOIs impose, the tricyclics are the drugs of choice for patients with major depression. Their long track record makes them likely candidates for some experimental uses as well (for hyperactivity, enuresis, and chronic pain syndromes, for example).

How they work. How the drugs lift depression is not quite clear. One time-honored theory is that depression is caused by the underactivity of certain amines in the parts of the brain responsible for

THE MOST COMMON SIDE EFFECTS OF TRICYCLIC AND OTHER NON-MAOI ANTIDEPRESSANTS

Anticholinergic side effects:

Dry mouth. *Management*: Assure the patient that this effect is usually temporary. Frequent sips of water help most. (Gum and candy may cause dental caries or monilial infections; sugarless products can trigger GI distress, especially when used excessively.) Oral hygiene *is* essential, since reduced salivation promotes caries. Cholinergic mouthwash may also help.

Blurred near vision. *Management:* Assure the patient that this is usually temporary. Recommend large-print reading materials. If vision does not clear within three weeks, the patient may need new eyeglasses. Cholinergic eyedrops may help.

Difficulty voiding, especially in starting the stream. *Management*: If conservative measures (such as running the water in the bathroom during urination attempts) do not help, reducing the dose of antidepressant or adding an oral cholinergic agonist such as bethanechol (Urecholine) may be nec-

essary. Catheterization may provide relief until other measures take effect.

Constipation. *Management:* Advise the patient to take several more glasses of fluid a day than usual, add fiber to his diet, and exercise regularly. If these measures fail, a bulking agent (such as Metamucil), a stool softener, or a laxative may help. Oral cholinergic agonists such as bethanechol are sometimes recommended. Unrelieved constipation can lead to severe obstipation and paralytic ileus, especially in elderly patients.

Sweating. *Management:* If the patient is plagued by persistent sweating, he probably needs to change to an antidepressant with less anticholinergic activity. Imipramine is the worst offender.

Erection/orgasm difficulty. *Management:* A lower dose or a less anticholinergic antidepressant may help.

Precipitation of glaucoma. *Management:* For chronic wide angle glau-

coma give cholinomimetic eyedrops (such as pilocarpine) while the patient is on antidepressant therapy. Recommend an ophthalmological consultation. Acute, narrow angle glaucoma is an emergency, requiring immediate treatment.

Anticholinergic delirium reveals itself with agitation, confusion, disorientation, dysarthria, hallucinations, dry, flushed skin, tachycardia, dilated pupils, reduced bowel motility, urinary retention, and fever. These symptoms are especially likely in a patient who takes an anticholinergic antidepressant along with other anticholinergic drugs (such as antipsychotics or antidyskinetics). *Management:* Stop all anticholinergic drugs. IV or IM physostigmine is sometimes given. Amitriptyline has the most anticholinergic activity followed by protriptyline, then trimipramine, and then doxepin. The antidepressant with the least anticholinergic activity is trazodone, then amoxapine, then maprotiline, desipramine, and fluoxetine.

Other side effects:

Cardiac effects, such as palpitations, mild tachycardia, cardiac conduction blocks, arrhythmia (although imipramine and some other tricyclics have a quinidine-like antiarrhythmic effect), or congestive heart failure. *Management:* Cardiac toxicity, other than mild palpitations or tachycardia, is rare in patients with no prior history of cardiovascular disease. For patients with a history of heart disease or for elderly patients at risk for stroke or MI, give antidepressants in smaller, divided doses, monitoring changes by serial ECGs.

Avoid antidepressants entirely in patients with known cardiac conduction defects or history of recent MI. Electroconvulsive therapy may be the best alternative for these patients. Nortriptyline and desipramine have the weakest cardiac effects; amitriptyline, imipramine, and trimipramine have the strongest cardiac effects.

Orthostatic hypotension may be the cause of lightheadedness, palpitations and/or nausea. *Management:* Usually temporary, it *may* abate with a reduced dose, with smaller divided doses, or by dramatically lowering the dose then raising it more gradually.

Adding triidothyronine, methylphenidate, dextroamphetamine, salt tablets, or fludrocortisone may help. Advise the patient to rise slowly from a sitting or lying position. When symptoms are present, take lying and standing blood pressures several times a day as long as this side effect is a problem. The least offensive agents are nortriptyline and fluoxetine; the most offensive agent is imipramine.

Sedation. *Management:* This effect is usually temporary and resolves within about two weeks. Warn the patient not to drive or operate other dangerous machinery until the sedation passes. The least sedative antidepressants are nortriptyline, desipramine, and protriptyline; the most, amitriptyline, trazodone, amoxapine, and doxepin.

Tremors. *Management:* If severe, give diazepam (Valium) or propranolol (Inderal). Advise the patient to avoid caffeinic beverages.

Grand mal seizures. *Management:* Since all antidepressants lower the seizure threshold somewhat, known epileptics may need more anticonvulsant. Seizures are especially likely with maprotiline, and even more so when the

patient's daily dose exceeds 200 mg or when the dose is escalated rapidly. The antidepressant least likely to provoke seizures is fluoxetine.

Nightmares or disturbed sleep. *Management:* Large doses at bedtime contribute to this effect; giving smaller, more frequent doses during the day may resolve it.

Weight gain. *Management:* Combining moderate calorie restriction and regular exercise seems to work best. Fluoxetine (which can produce weight *loss*) and trazodone are least likely to cause weight gain; amitriptyline and doxepin are most likely to do so.

Agitation, psychosis, or mania. *Management:* For psychosis, add an antipsychotic. For agitation, give an antipsychotic or sedative hypnotic. For a manic state, give lithium or stop the antidepressant.

Extrapyramidal side effects, including tardive dyskinesia, dystonia, akathisia, and others. *Management:* These occur almost exclusively with amoxapine. Adding an antidyskinetic drug, or for tardive dyskinesia, stopping amoxapine will help.

DRUGS

controlling mood and emotion. The tricyclics boost the activity of those amines—specifically norepinephrine and serotonin—by inhibiting their reuptake at the presynaptic junction.

More amine at the presynaptic junction means more amine activity at the synaptic cleft. It's not the whole story, though, since the tricyclics' chemical effect takes place instantly while their antidepressant effect takes a week or more to get underway.

We do know that taken orally (as most antidepressants are), the tricyclics are rapidly absorbed. They are fairly lipophilic and strongly bound to plasma protein and tissue. They are metabolized primarily by enzymes in the liver.

Selecting the right drug. The tricyclics and the atypicals are all about equally effective against depression. First, find out whether the patient has responded well to a specific antidepressant in the past. Since antidepressant response seems to "run in families," it can be helpful to find out if a close family member has had any experience with antidepressants(1).

Next, check the side effect profile of each antidepressant under consideration. Try to match the patient's symptoms and medical history with the drug's track record. (See chart.) For example, a patient with a history of disturbed sleep is likely to do well taking a sedating antidepressant at bed-

HOW ANTIDEPRESSANTS INTER

Tricyclic and other non-MAOI antidepressants plus:	Effect
cimetidine (Tagamet) methylphenidate (Ritalin) other stimulants acetaminophen (Tylenol, Anacin-3) thyroid hormones and TSH oral contraceptives chloramphenicol (Chloromycetin) MAOIs	inhibit metabolism, thus raising blood levels of the antidepressant
guanethidine (Ismelin Sulfate, Esimil) debrisoquine bethanidine	reduce the antihypertensive or antidepressant effect
quinidine (Quinaglute) procainamide (Pronestyl, Procan)	prolong cardiac conduction
coumarin anticoagulants	augment the anticoagulant effect
alcohol antihistamines phenytoin (Dilantin) barbiturates nicotine barbiturate hypnotics dichloralphenazone (Isocom) rifampin (Rifadin) doxycycline (Vibramycin) griseofulvin (Fulvicin) carbamazepine (Tegretol) phenylbutazone (Butazolidin)	induce hepatic metabolism, reducing the blood level and clinical effects of the antidepressant
epinephrine local anesthetics dissolved in epinephrine	augment hypotension, increase bleeding in nasal surgery
alcohol antihistamines barbiturates benzodiazepines other sedatives	increase CNS sedation, confusion
anticonvulsants	control seizures less effectively
anticholinergic agents	increase anticholinergic effects
MAOIs	may cause hypertensive crisis
clonidine (Catapres)	eliminate hypotensive action
beta-blockers	may antagonize hypotensive effects, augment cardiac depressant effects of the antidepressant, or cause blood levels of both drugs to rise

ACT WITH OTHER DRUGS

MAOI antidepressants plus:	Effect

amphetamines
ephedrine (Broncholate, Tedral)
methylphenidate (Ritalin)
phenylephrine (Neo-Synephrine)
pseudoephedrine (Chlorafed)
norephedrine
l-dopa
oxymetazoline
tranylcypromine (Parnate)
dopamine
epinephrine or other vaso-
   constrictors added to
   procaine
	may cause hypertensive crisis, ex-
	cess CNS stimulation, or intoxication

other antidepressants, including other MAOIs	may enhance clinical effects, or may cause hypertensive crisis or hypoten- sion; may induce catastrophic CNS excitation, seizures, or hyperpyrexia
general anesthetics alcohol antihistamines barbiturates benzodiazepines other sedatives antipsychotics anticonvulsants narcotics	potentiate the antidepressant, caus- ing excessive CNS depression; may reduce the blood level and effective- ness of the MAOI
meperidine (Demerol)	may cause hyperpyrexia, seizures, coma
anticholinergic agents	may intensify anticholinergic effects
levodopa	potentiate the MAOI; may cause CNS excitation, intoxication, or unpredict- able changes in BP
reserpine (Hydromox, Diupres) alpha-methyl-dopa guanethidine (Esimil)	may cause acute paradoxical hyper- tension or CNS excitation
clonidine (Catapres)	may potentiate the MAOI
hydralazine (Apresoline)	potentiate the MAOI
salt-depleting diuretics	lower BP
insulin oral hypoglycemics	potentiate the MAOI

time. And a patient with heart disease would best avoid strongly anticholinergic antidepressants.

Getting started. Keeping in mind patient-to-patient variability in metabolizing most drugs, start with a low dose—50 mg imipramine (Tofranil) per day or its equivalent. For an elderly patient, the clinician may prescribe an even lower starting dose. Every few days, the clinician adds another 25 or 50 mg until the patient's total daily dose is at the high end of the usual range, or until side effects become unpleasant or intolerable. Once the patient tolerates a dose that falls within the usual effective range, he continues on that dose for four to six weeks while waiting for an antidepressant response. He may improve in only a week, but resolving depression usually takes several weeks.

If you see no improvement in four to six weeks, check the patient's blood level of the drug. He may be metabolizing it too rapidly or absorbing it poorly. If so, the clinician may raise the dose, or select another antidepressant drug or a drug combination.

If a second or third drug fails and the patient's depression is too severe to continue drug trials, electroconvulsive therapy or some of the less conventional therapies (phototherapy, stimulant therapy, altering sleep-wake cycles) may be the next step.

Maintenance. Once the patient is stable, the clinician is likely to reduce his acute-phase dose by as much as 25 to 50 percent(2). At that point, one daily dose at bedtime is usually enough to control the patient's depression. If the patient's maintenance dose is over 150 mg of imipramine (Tofranil)

DRUGS

or its equivalent, or if troublesome side effects persist, the patient may be more comfortable continuing with divided doses.

When the patient is ready to stop the drug altogether, the clinician tapers the dose gradually over several weeks to avoid symptoms of withdrawal—restlessness, anxiety, malaise, chills, coryza, nausea, sweating, headache, and muscle aches(3). If tapering triggers symptoms of depression, the dose is brought back to maintenance levels.

Rarely is more than a one-week supply of antidepressants prescribed to an outpatient because of these drugs' potential lethality in the event of overdose.

ATYPICAL ANTIDEPRESSANTS

At the moment, only two drugs remain in this category—trazodone (Desyrel) and fluoxetine (Prozac). Bupropion (Wellbutrin) and nomifensine (Merital) were recently removed from the market—at least temporarily—because of unacceptably high rates of severe side effects(4).

Chemically different from other antidepressants but just as efficient, the atypicals have their own distinct side effects. Trazodone (Desyrel) may cause dizziness, fainting, cardiac irritability, conduction defects, headache, or nausea (especially when taken on an empty stomach) and (rarely) priapism, a painful condition that warrants immediate treatment or surgical intervention to avoid permanent loss of erectile ability. Fluoxetine (Prozac) may cause nausea, tremors, drowsiness, sweating, headache, insomnia, dry mouth, weight loss, and anxiety.

A QUICK LOOK AT THE ANTIDEPRESSANTS

Tricyclic Antidepressants	Usual Daily Dose (mg)
amitriptyline (Elavil, others)	100–300
amoxapine (Asendin)	150–450
desipramine (Norpramin)	100–300
doxepin (Sinequan, others)	100–300
imipramine (Tofranil, others)	100–300
maprotiline (Ludiomil)	100–200
nortriptyline (Pamelor, others)	50–150
protriptyline (Vivactil)	15–60
trimipramine (Surmontil)	100–300
Atypical Antidepressants	
trazodone (Desyrel, others)	150–300
fluoxetine (Prozac)	40–80
MAOI Antidepressants	
phenelzine (Nardil)	15–90
tranylcypromine (Parnate)	10–30
isocarboxazid (Marplan)	10–30

FOODS TO AVOID WHILE TAKING MAOI ANTIDEPRESSANTS

dairy foods	pizza, sour cream, cheese (except cottage, cream cheese), yogurt (more than 8 oz. per day)
meat/protein	beef and chicken liver, unrefrigerated fermented sausage, summer sausage, bologna, salami, pepperoni, pickled fish, pickled herring, smoked fish (such as lox), caviar, dried salted herring
vegetables	broad bean pods, fava beans, Italian green beans, snow pea pods, sauerkraut
fruits	banana peel, avocado
sweets	cakes, cookies, ice cream, pudding, or candy flavored with chocolate
alcohol	Chianti wine, sherry, red wine, burgundy, ale, beer, vermouth, Sauterne, Reisling, liqueurs
fats	avocado, salad dressings containing cheese or monosodium glutamate (MSG)
miscellaneous	food containing brewer's yeast or yeast extract (some soups, sauces, relishes, gravies), MSG, meat tenderizers, yeast vitamin supplements, hydrolyzed protein extracts (used as a base for soup, gravy, or sauce), soy sauce (more than one tablespoon per day)

MAOI ANTIDEPRESSANTS

This group seems to be regaining popularity despite the stringent dietary precautions associated with it (p. 1516) and the serious consequences of violations of those precautions. Effectiveness of MAOIs has never been an issue; they may even exceed the success of tricyclics with atypical depressions (those characterized by anxiety, reactivity of mood, fatigue, hyperphagia, hypersomnia). MAOIs also help bulimics and patients prone to panic attacks.

How MAOIs work. Like tricyclics, MAOIs also promote norepinephrine and serotonin activity, but they do so by inhibiting monoamine oxidase, an enzyme that breaks down the two amines in question. The end result is the same, though: More amine activity at the synapse lifts the patient's depression.

Dosing. Wait at least two weeks between a patient's last dose of any

CHECK BLOOD LEVELS

Obtain blood for a plasma level about 12 hours after the patient took his last dose of antidepressant (usually just before his morning dose).

Plasma levels of amitriptyline (Elavil) and imipramine (Tofranil) plus their active metabolites should fall between 100 and 300 nanograms (ng)/ml(3). The closer to 300, the more likely the antidepressant response. Levels above 300 usually indicate toxicity.

The therapeutic range for desipramine (Norpramin) is approximately 100 to 250 ng/ml; for nortriptyline (Pamelor), 50 to 150 ng/ml(3). Because levels *above* and *below* nortriptyline's therapeutic range are associated with a lack of response, that drug is said to have a "therapeutic window"(3).

other antidepressant and his first dose of the MAOI. Start with a low dose—30 mg of phenelzine (Nardil) is typical—and expect to see a therapeutic result in one to four

weeks. Tranylcypromine (Parnate) is an exception. Its amphetamine-like qualities put it to work after only a few days. Finding the therapeutic range and progressing to maintenance proceed much as with the tricyclics.

Blood levels of MAOIs are not used clinically, but some clinicians guide MAOI therapy by assays of the inhibition of platelet monoamine oxidase (MAO) activity. Inhibition over 85 percent is highly predictive of antidepressant effect.

The dietary connection. Why must patients taking MAOIs avoid the foods listed on page 1516? They all contain tyramine, a sympathomimetic pressor amine, which is normally broken down by the enzyme monoamine oxidase. Because this group of antidepressant drugs inhibits MAO, patients who take MAOIs without limiting their intake of tyramine can rapidly develop hypertensive crisis.

DRUGS

Tyramine restriction begins the day the patient takes his first dose of the MAOI and continues for two weeks after his last dose. Because tyramine content in food may vary (especially when the food is aged, overripe, or poorly refrigerated), teach the patient to watch for signs of hypertensive crisis—throbbing occipital headache, stiff neck, chills, nausea, flushing, retroorbital pain, apprehension, pallor, sweating, chest pain, and palpitations. Without immediate treatment, intracranial hemorrhage, collapse, and death may follow. Slow IV injection of an alpha-adrenergic blocker such as phento-

lamine (Regitine), or at least PO or IM chlorpromazine (Thorazine), may abort the crisis.

Patients unlikely to adhere to the dietary restrictions are obviously poor candidates for MAOI drug therapy. MAOIs are also inappropriate for patients who have pheochromocytoma or carcinoid syndrome; excess production of serotonin without enough monoamine oxidase to break it down can be deadly.

On the side. As with other antidepressants, the more benign side effects can usually be managed with dose reduction, re-dividing doses, adding another drug to control the symptom, or switching to another antidepressant. Orthostatic hypotension, sedation, weight gain (except with tranylcypromine), agitation, psychosis, and anticholinergic effects (with

phenelzine only) are the usual problems. Insomnia can be a particularly stubborn effect of tranylcypromine (Parnate). Taking the entire daily dose in the morning or early afternoon helps some patients; others need to take a benzodiazepine hypnotic such as lorazepam (Ativan) or temazepam (Restoril) along with the MAOI.

REFERENCES

1. Klein, D. F., and others. *Diagnosis and Drug Treatment of Psychiatric Disorders: Adults and Children.* 2d ed. Baltimore, Williams and Wilkins, 1980.
2. Schatzberg, A. F., and Cole, J. O. *A Manual of Clinical Psychopharmacology.* Washington, D.C., American Psychiatric Press, 1986.
3. Baldessarini, R. J. *Chemotherapy in Psychiatry: Principles and Practice.* Cambridge, MA, Harvard University Press, 1985.
4. Cole, J. O. Where are those new antidepressants we were promised? *Arch.Gen.Psychiatry* 45:193-194, Feb. 1988.

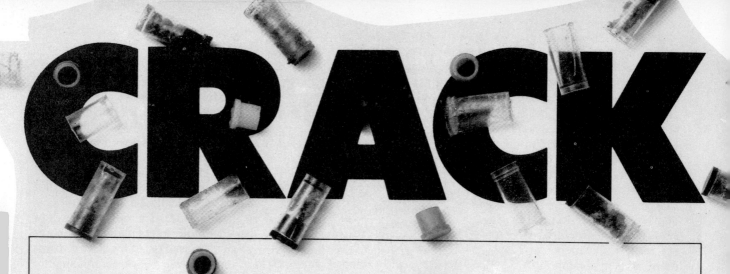

CRACK

These potent cocaine crystals cause explosive highs and easy addiction. This detox program helps to break the cycle.

Reprinted from American Journal of Nursing, June, 1987.

BY ANNA M. ACEE/DOROTHY SMITH

"Once you start using crack, you can't stop," observe those familiar with people trapped in the addiction.

Crack, a purified, free-base form of cocaine hydrochloride, acquired its name because of the sound made by crystals popping when it is heated. It is also called rock because of its appearance(1).

Crack differs from traditional cocaine powders—cocaine hydrochloride, cocaine sulfate, and cocaine base—in more than appearance. The powder is "snorted"—inhaled through the nose—or dissolved and taken intravenously. Unlike crack crystals, the powder is not smoked; in fact, smoking actually destroys powdered cocaine. Cocaine is somewhat self-limiting when it is inhaled. The inherent vasoconstrictive properties of cocaine actually diminish absorption through the nasal vasculature as the user continues to inhale the drug(2).

Anna M. Acee, RN, MA, is clinical specialist, psychiatric day treatment program, and Dorothy Smith, RN, MA, is assistant supervisor and clinical specialist, both at Bernstein Institute, Beth Israel Medical Center, New York, NY. Ms. Acee is also an adjunct clinical instructor, Lienhard School of Nursing, Pace University.

Crack, on the other hand, is always smoked: flakes are placed in a pipe or sprinkled on a tobacco or marijuana cigarette. The self-limiting property of inhaled cocaine is lost when crack is smoked because the drug is directly absorbed into the lungs. Moreover, crack reaches the brain in a more concentrated form(1).

Crack also differs from other street cocaine by its purity. Cocaine is usually 15 to 25 percent pure. But crack may be as much as 90 percent pure(1). The danger of overdose and severe toxicity is therefore heightened. And the cocaine-induced psychological symptoms—psychosis, paranoia, hallucinations, and violence—are intensified when crack is used(3).

Why is crack so popular? The sense of superiority, power, and exhilaration that cocaine brings undoubtedly makes it seductive. Crack is still associated with glamour—the way inhaled cocaine and heroin were in the 1960s and 1970s.

Crack's short, intense high is produced in four to six seconds with the euphoria lasting five to seven minutes. In contrast, when cocaine is snorted, its effects occur in one to three minutes and last up to half an hour. Crack's fleeting high is followed by a period of deep depression that strongly reinforces addictive behavior patterns and guarantees almost continuous use of the drug(1).

Crack users describe five stages as they come down from the drug's high: worries about where they can get more crack, deep depression, loss of energy and appetite, difficulty sleeping, and feelings of revulsion about themselves. Heavy crack smokers can go through all five stages after a single binge, which can last as long as the user can afford the habit(1).

The administration route also contributes to the drug's popularity. Many people perceive smoking as being less dangerous and less invasive than other routes. It does not destroy the nasal membranes the way inhaling cocaine does, nor is there the threat of infectious disease associated with IV use(1).

GETTING OFF CRACK

Widespread cocaine abuse has changed the way we think about treating drug addiction. Today, we think in terms of the broad concept of chemical dependency: the pathological relationship of a person to a mind-altering chemical(4).

The pathological relationship is

CRACK

Abnormal vital signs may indicate anxiety or infection. Cocaine-induced skin lesions may cause a negative self-image that influences interaction with staff and peers.

Cocaine abusers commonly complain of anxiety, impaired memory, and depression. Sometimes anxiety and depression are related to patients' concerns about their situations and their feelings of powerlessness to effect appropriate changes. Symptoms may also be due to psychosis that existed before their drug abuse.

To help patients whose memories are impaired, we give each patient written schedules of unit activities and we post daily schedules on the bulletin board.

An important assessment goal is to determine how drug abuse has eroded not only physical health (see box), but also familial, educational, social, and employment activities.

In both group sessions and individual counseling we encourage patients to discuss their feelings to help them gain perspective. Knowing that others experience similar feelings of guilt, doubt, or isolation can alleviate these feelings. Reality-testing can make such feelings less overwhelming.

Observing interactions among patients and between patients and staff is the primary way we assess motivation.

Surreptitious behavior suggests an attempt to obtain contraband drugs. For example, a patient may make frequent phone calls, then seek an excuse to leave the locked unit. To deter drug-seeking, we keep the unit locked and do not allow visitors. Of course, family members do come in to plan subsequent care together with the patient and counselor.

PHYSICAL EFFECTS OF COCAINE USE

While the exact physical effects of long-term crack use are unknown, long-term cocaine users lose weight, develop skin problems (such as facial dermatitis and perioral dryness and peeling), experience convulsions, have difficulty breathing, and spit up black phlegm. The source of the black phlegm is uncertain. Because crack is inhaled directly into the lungs, long-term crack users can also develop intermittent abnormal pulmonary gas exchange that subsides without treatment(2).

Cocaine slows digestion, masks hunger, stimulates the central nervous system, and induces agitation, restlessness, apprehensiveness, and sexual arousal. Cocaine also elevates blood pressure, temperature, pulse, and blood sugar. Cardiovascular problems, such as hypertension, tachyarrhythmias, myocardial infarction, cerebral hemorrhage, and even death, can result. IV users frequently develop cellulitis from using contaminated needles and syringes. Dental problems are common due to neglect and poor nutrition(2,6,7).

When we observe surreptitious behavior, we confront the person and point out how his actions inhibit his attaining or maintaining sobriety. Frequently, however, patients are very supportive with one another, extending encouragement and sympathy to someone experiencing discomfort. In fact, peer support is a key part of many rehabilitation programs: recovered users become mentors.

A daily meeting gives our multidisciplinary staff a chance to validate observations and correct possible misconceptions. It also allows us to examine a problem from each other's perspectives—sometimes perspectives that have not yet been considered regarding a given client.

Daily staff discussions also counter manipulative behavior that can promote staff dissension. A client may, for example, seek sympathy from one staff member by complaining about another. Another tactic is to misquote staff members so that it appears they are contradicting, or even demeaning, each other.

Motivations for treatment. A crack addict, like other chemically dependent people, uses both denial and compliance as major defense mechanisms.

We often see career addicts with dual addictions. Their motivation for treatment frequently centers on staying out of jail, obtaining welfare benefits, or retaining custody of their children.

For example, a 25-year-old woman had been attending a methadone maintenance treatment program for six years. She had been a model patient until she began snorting cocaine and smoking free-base five months before admission. She admitted that she came in to detoxify so that she could get a letter from her counselor to get her children back. They had been taken to a temporary shelter when she left them alone overnight while she was at a "crack house."

A crack user may experience severe difficulty sooner than users of other drugs. But since his relationship with the drug is not so long-standing, the seriousness of the crack addiction can be masked by the patient's denial. One 22-year-old man, for instance, maintained that he came in to detoxify only to satisfy his mother who, he said, overreacted when she found a marijuana cigarette in his room.

At first we were inclined to discharge this first-time client and

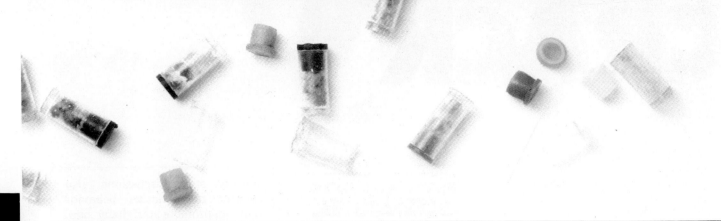

characterized by the addict's life revolving around obtaining the drug, by his inability to refuse the drug when it is offered, and by his continued use of the drug despite the hazards he experiences. The immediate goal of detoxification is to break the pattern of drug use.

Recreational users follow a different pattern: their involvement with a drug usually includes friends and is easily limited to when the drug is readily available. They can usually begin outpatient rehabilitation without the help of a detoxification unit.

Detoxification is only the first step in a substance abuser's rehabilitation. To be eligible for admission to our detox unit, patients must have used cocaine for at least four months. We also require referral from a long-term treatment facility, an employee assistance program, or a methadone maintenance program. The patient must demonstrate motivation toward making the essential long-term commitment for rehabilitation and recovery and follow-up care after discharge.

For those who cannot afford a 28-day inpatient rehabilitation program, whether due to financial or time constraints, the 7- to 10-day detoxification program serves as an orientation and preparation for outpatient rehabilitation programs.

When a patient is admitted, we note any signs and symptoms of withdrawal, oversedation, or acute intoxication (see box). Because of crack's short-lived effect, however, we rarely see intoxication symptoms when patients come to the detoxification unit.

In the first 12 hours, patients are often restless. Hypersomnia and overeating are also frequent. The paranoia and depression experienced when coming down from crack and other forms of cocaine are relatively short-lived and abate during the first 72 hours after the last drug dose.

We avoid antidepressants and anxiolytic agents. Instead we support clients through this period by assuring them that they will experience relief shortly. Meanwhile, we never minimize their discomfort.

SUBSTANCE HIGHS AND LOWS

	INTOXICATION	WITHDRAWAL
COCAINE	Elevated blood pressure, tachycardia, diaphoresis, tremors, pressured speech, euphoria, increased energy, alertness, insomnia, dilated pupils.	Lack of energy, depression, oversleeping, overeating, inability to concentrate, irritability, restlessness.
HEROIN	Respiratory depression, constricted pupils, lethargy, drowsiness, confusion, euphoria.	*Mild:* Lacrimation, rhinorrhea, gooseflesh, sneezing, sniffling, yawning. *Severe:* Extreme agitation, generalized body aches, nausea, vomiting.
BARBITURATES	Respiratory depression, slowed mental and physical activity, relaxation, drowsiness, slurred speech, ataxia. Loss of impulse control, resulting in mood swings, release of sexual and aggressive impulses; occasionally, combativeness.	Tremulousness, weakness, insomnia, diaphoresis, nausea, vomiting, loss of appetite, headache, malaise. Can progress to include suicidal thinking, grand mal seizures and status epilepticus, hallucinations, delirium, even death.
ALCOHOL	Basically the same as with barbiturate abuse. Smell of alcohol on breath.	Same as with barbiturates.

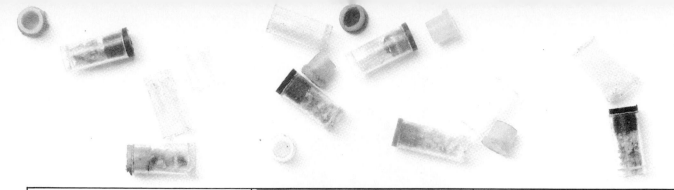

recommend outpatient treatment. When he then reassured his mother, "See, I don't have a drug problem," she called and told us that she and her husband had become alarmed when they had begun to miss sums of money and jewelry from their home. They had given their son an ultimatum to seek help or to move out of the house.

When we reviewed the conflicting stories at the staff meeting, we realized that, although he had appeared to comply with the unit's program, he had been simply going through the motions.

In fact, he was not acknowledging the extent of his addiction. He had been using crack for about a year. Already he was spending up to $1,500 a week on the drug—not only stealing but selling drugs to continue the habit.

He had experienced a seizure a month before admission during one of his heavier binges. During his last week's binge, which ended about three days before admission, he had lost at least 20 pounds.

Interactions with staff that focus on somatic complaints are another form of denial. We respond by helping the patient see how his physical problems are linked to his drug use.

The detoxification process provides an atmosphere that enables the patient to recognize the need for long-term treatment. To accomplish this, we use health teaching with peer-support and counseling groups to explain the nature of chemical dependency. Attendance at group sessions is mandatory: failure to comply is grounds for administrative discharge.

Despite emphasis on the group milieu, one-to-one staff–patient interaction is equally important. Individual counseling provides the

WHO USES CRACK?

A random survey of 458 people who called the 1-800-COCAINE national hotline during May 1986 found that 33 percent used crack. The majority of crack users were males (72%), 20 to 29 years old (94%), earned more than $16,000 a year (57%), and spent more than $100 a week on the drug (75%)(3,8).

Eighty-one percent had switched to crack from occasionally snorting cocaine powder. Eighty-two percent reported a compulsion to use the drug again as soon as the brief high wore off; 78 percent reported the onset of compulsive use and significant drug-related problems within two months of first use.

Drug-related physical complaints reported by the callers included chest congestion (64%), chronic cough (40%), and convulsions with loss of consciousness (7%). Psychiatric complaints included severe depression (85%), loss of sexual desire (58%), memory lapses (40%), violent behavior (31%), and suicide attempts (18%)(8).

chance to reflect on personal life direction and to synthesize the information that has been presented. We expect that the patients will understand:

☐ Chemical dependency is a progressively deteriorating disease if left unchecked.

☐ Individuals are not responsible for their disease, but they are responsible for their recovery.

☐ They cannot blame people, places, or things for their dependency. They must face their problems and their feelings.

☐ Rehabilitation and recovery are lifelong enterprises that begin with a commitment to a long-term treatment effort.

The value of detoxification by itself is limited. We now recognize that successful long-term treatment must address more than the psychodynamics related to addic-

tive behavior. The focus must be on the entrenched cycle of euphoria, abstinence, dysphoria, and continued abuse that gives detoxification its revolving door(5).

Rehabilitation must center on abstinence. Our program emphasizes self-help, supported through groups such as Cocaine Anonymous. Like Alcoholics Anonymous, the chemically dependent help each other in these groups without medical, political, or religious supervision. The career addict will need a more structured discharge plan, perhaps including escorted transportation to a halfway house or residential treatment facility.

During detoxification, we help patients take the first step: to admit they have become powerless in relation to the drug. For the chemically dependent, taking this first step—recognizing that the drug has made life unmanageable—is a step toward survival.

REFERENCES

1. New York State Division of Substance Abuse Services. *Report on Crack.* Albany, The Division, 1986, p. 2.
2. New York Department of Health, Poison Control Center, City Health Information. *Crack: Cocaine Repackaged.* The Department, New York City, 1986, Vol. 5, No. 10.
3. Gold, M. S. *800-COCAINE* New York: Bantam Books, 1984.
4. Peterson, R. M. *Hooked on a Line.* Palm Beach, FL, Palm Beach Institute Foundation, 1983.
5. Drakis, C. Brain mechanisms and pharmacologic treatment of cocaine abuse. Presented at *Cocaine: The Clinical Challenge* the first national conference on cocaine, sponsored by U.S. Journal Training, Inc., Nov. 17-19, 1985.
6. Mittelman, H. S., and others. Cocaine. *Am.J.Nurs.* 84:1092-1095, Sept. 1984.
7. Cregler, L. L., and Mark, H. Medical complications of cocaine abuse. *N.Engl.J.Med.* 315:1495-1500, Dec. 4, 1986.
8. Washton, A. M., and others. Survey of 500 callers to a national cocaine helpline. *Psychosomatics* 25:771-775, Oct. 1984.

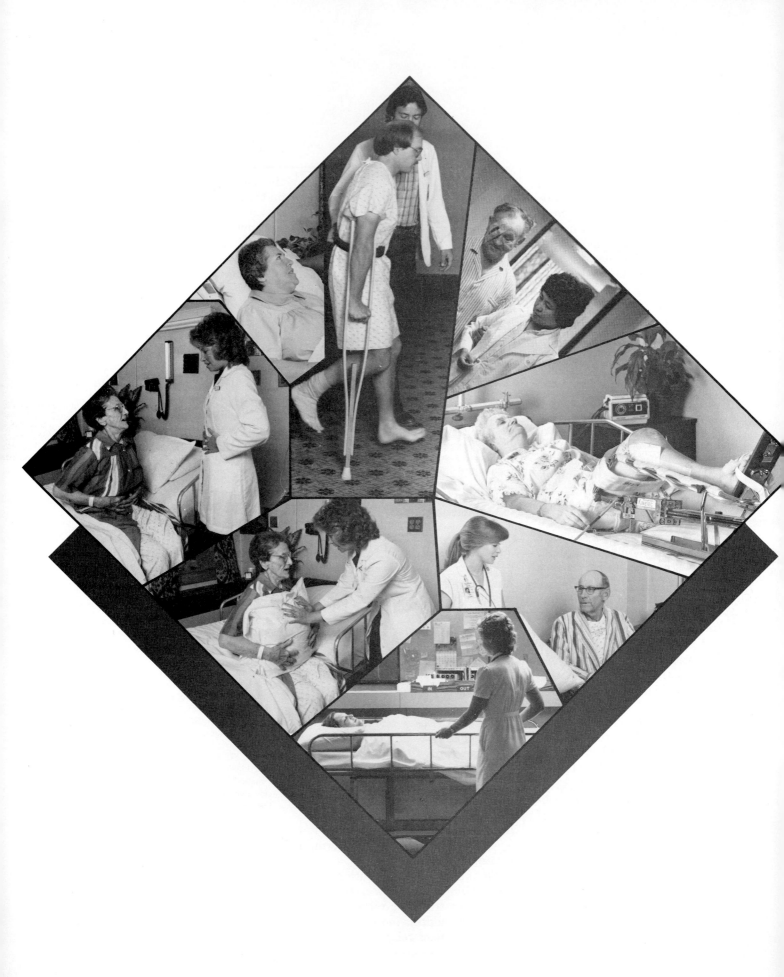

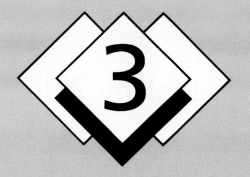

Nursing Care of the Adult

Coordinators

Patricia E. Downing, MN, RN
Paulette D. Rollant, MSN, RN, CCRN

Contributors

Suzette Cardin, MS, RN, CCRN
Virginia L. Cassmeyer, PhD, RN
Robin Donohoe Dennison, MSN, RN,
  CCRN, CS
Deborah A. Ennis, MS, RN, CCRN
Peg Gray-Vickery, MS, RN, C
Alma J. Labunski, EdD, MS, RN
Judith K. Sands, EdD, RN

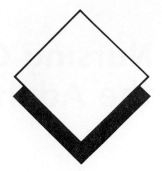

The Healthy Adult

HEALTH

1. Definition
   a. No universally accepted definition
   b. Defined by the World Health Organization (WHO) in 1946 as "state of complete physical, mental, and social well-being and not just absence of disease or infirmity . . . fundamental right of every human being"
   c. Defined by the American Nurses Association (ANA) in 1980 as "a dynamic state of being in which the developmental and behavorial potential of an individual is realized to the fullest extent possible. Each human being possesses various strengths and limitations, resulting from the interaction of hereditary and environmental factors. The relative dominance of the strengths and limitations determines an individual's place on the health continuum; it determines the person's biological and behavioral integrity, his wholeness."

2. Characteristics
   a. Dynamic state, dependent upon individual's ability to adapt continually to changing internal and external environments
   b. Continuous spectrum, extending from obvious disease through absence of discernible disease to state of optimal functioning
   c. Involves physical and psychosocial aspects
   d. Norms change with age

3. Duration of life
   a. Life span
      1. constant, genetically determined
      2. average appears fixed at 85 years, with maximum of 115 years
   b. Life expectancy (United States)
      1. changes with advances in disease control and treatment
      2. born in 1900: 47 years; born in 1989: 75 years

4. Levels of health promotion
   a. Primary: promotion of health and prevention of disease
   b. Secondary: early diagnosis, prompt treatment, and limitation of disability
   c. Tertiary: restoration and rehabilitation

Characteristics of the Healthy Young and Middle-Aged Adult (20-65 years)

1. Physiological characteristics
   a. General
      1. growth and development appropriate for age
      2. symmetrical body
      3. no pain
      4. balanced sleep pattern
   b. Integument
      1. skin
         a. clean, intact, smooth, warm, dry
         b. normal turgor and texture
         c. odorless
         d. no lesions
         e. normal color (e.g., no jaundice, cyanosis)
      2. mucous membranes
         a. pink, intact, hydrated
         b. no lesions
      3. hair
         a. normal distribution and amount
         b. normal texture
         c. no dandruff, scales
      4. nails
         a. pink nail beds
         b. rapid capillary filling of nail beds after compression
         c. no clubbing of fingers
   c. Neck
      1. trachea in midline
      2. no masses
   d. Eyes
      1. symmetrical placement
      2. white sclera
      3. pink conjunctiva
      4. normal lacrimation
      5. pupils equal, round, react to light and accommodation (PERRLA)
      6. eye movements coordinated and parallel
      7. visual acuity 20/20 without or with correction
   e. Ears
      1. symmetrical placement
      2. auditory acuity (hearing) normal (i.e., can distinguish softly whispered words at 1-2 feet)

3. no drainage from external auditory canal

4. equilibrium maintained (no vertigo)

f. Thorax and lungs
1. open, unobstructed airway
2. respirations (eupneic)
   a. effortless, noiseless, odorless
   b. rhythmical, normal depth
   c. rate: 12-20/min at rest
3. diaphragmatic breathing, bilateral equal excursion
4. thorax: symmetrical, normal anteroposterior (AP) diameter (i.e., AP diameter less than lateral-to-lateral diameter)
5. normal breath sounds: tracheobronchial, bronchovesicular, vesicular (no adventitious sounds)
6. resonant (no dullness) when percussion performed
7. no cough or sputum

g. Cardiovascular
1. normal sinus rhythm (NSR)
2. rate: 60-80/min at rest
3. normal heart sounds, no extra sounds or murmurs
4. blood pressure approximately 120/80 at rest
5. no chest pain
6. no palpitations
7. normal palpable arterial pulses in the extremities (radial, brachial, femoral, popliteal, tibial, dorsalis pedis)
8. normal skin color and temperature (e.g., no cyanosis or pigmentation)
9. no peripheral edema
10. no varicosities or ulcerations of extremities

h. Abdomen
1. soft, nontender
2. flat, no distension
3. normal, active bowel sounds
4. no palpable organomegaly, masses, or hernias

i. Gastrointestinal/nutrition
1. normal weight for height
2. normal appetite
3. balanced, adequate diet; see Tables 3-1 and 3-2 (see also Table 4-8)
4. normal digestion (e.g., no food intolerance or indigestion)
5. well nourished
6. teeth present, in good repair
7. normal mastication (i.e., no difficulty or pain with chewing)
8. no difficulty swallowing
9. regular bowel habits, stools brown and formed

j. Musculoskeletal
1. good posture and body alignment
2. body movements coordinated (no tremors or involuntary movements)
3. muscles firm, symmetrical, strong, normal tone (no spasms, contractures, weakness, atrophy, or paralysis)
4. normal gain (foot strikes heel to toe, normal base of support, arms swing in coordination with leg movements)
5. joints
   a. full, unimpaired range of motion
   b. no deformities
   c. nontender, nonswollen, no crepitation

k. Neurological
1. mental status and cognitive functioning

Table 3-1   The basic four food groups

MILK GROUP	FRUIT/VEGETABLE GROUP
Calcium	Vitamins A and C
Protein	Carbohydrates
Riboflavin	Daily servings: 4 or more
Daily servings (glasses)	Sources: dark green or yellow vegetables; citrus fruit or tomatoes; other fruits and vegetables
3 or more (children)	
4 or more (teens)	
2 or more (adults)	
Sources: milk, cheese, and other milk products	
MEAT GROUP	**GRAIN GROUP**
Protein	Carbohydrates
Niacin	Thiamin
Thiamin	Riboflavin
Iron	Iron
Riboflavin	Niacin
Daily servings: 2 or more	Daily servings: 4 or more
Sources: meat, fish, poultry, eggs or cheese; dry beans, peas, or nuts as alternates	Sources: whole-grain or enriched breads, cereals, pastas, and rice

From U.S. Department of Agriculture.

Table 3-2   U.S. recommended daily nutrition for an average healthy adult (23-50 years)

	Women	Men
	120 lb (55 kg)	154 lb (70 kg)
	64 in (163 cm)	70 in (178 cm)
Calories	2000 kcal	2700 kcal
Protein*	44 g	56 g
	(176 kcal)	(224 kcal)
Fat†	66 g	90 g
	(594 kcal)	(810 kcal)
Carbohy-drate‡	285 g	383 g
	(1140 kcal)	(1532 kcal)
Cholesterol	300 mg	300 mg
Sodium	1100-3300 mg	1100-3300 mg
Calcium	800 mg	800 mg
Iron	18 mg	10 mg
Fluids	1500 ml	1500 ml

From *Recommended Daily Allowances* (RDA), National Research Council. Daily Goals for the United States, U.S. Senate Select Committee on Nutrition & Human Needs. American Heart Association.
*8%-12% of total calories; 0.8 g/kg.
†30% of total calories (10% saturated fat and 20% from polysaturated or monosaturated fat).
‡58% of total calories (48% complex carbohydrate, 10% simple sugar).

    a. oriented to person, place, time
    b. alert, conscious
    c. responds appropriately to visual, auditory, tactile, and painful stimuli
    d. short- and long-term memory intact
    e. capable of abstract thinking
    f. articulates without difficulty
    g. appropriate dress, behavior and mood (no excessive aggression, violence, withdrawal, or depression)
  2. sensory
    a. pain perception intact
    b. light touch, pressure, and vibration perception intact
    c. temperature perception intact
    d. sight, hearing, taste, and smell perception intact
  3. motor (see also Musculoskeletal, p. 113)
    a. coordinated, balanced movement
    b. normal gait
    c. no tremors or involuntary movements
    d. no atrophy, weakness, or paralysis of muscles
    e. reflexes intact and normal (including deep tendon reflexes)
    f. proprioception (awareness of body position)
l. Genitourinary
  1. normal sexual function for age and sex

  2. genitals
    a. good hygiene
    b. normal pubic hair distribution
    c. normal appearance/structure
    d. no lesions or abnormal discharge
  3. breasts
    a. symmetrical size and placement
    b. no masses
    c. no abnormal discharge from nipples
  4. micturition (urination)
    a. nonpainful
    b. voluntary control
    c. no difficulty controlling stream
    d. no frequency or urgency
    e. bladder empty after voiding
    f. approximately 300 ml/voiding and 1000-1500 ml/day
    g. urine: amber, clear, specific gravity 1.001-1.025, pH 4.8-8.0; no RBCs, WBCs, protein, glucose, or bacteria
2. Psychosocial characteristics (see "Psychosocial Characteristics of the Healthy Client," p. 15)

Characteristics of the Elderly Healthy Adult (Over 65 Years)

1. Aging
  a. A normal progressive process, not a disease
  b. Norms: normal physiological changes (vs. abnormal pathological changes) have not been completely identified.
2. Physiological characteristics
  a. General changes
    1. general tissue desiccation and slowed cell division
    2. slowed, weakened speed of response to stimuli
    3. slowed rate of tissue repair
    4. decreased metabolism
    5. mechanisms of homeostasis less rapid and less efficient
    6. rate of change is individual, influenced by factors such as heredity and stress
    7. high incidence of health problems (e.g., congestive heart failure [CHF], osteoporosis, cataracts)
  b. Integument
    1. skin
      a. dry, wrinkled, loss of elasticity
      b. decreased perspiration and sebum
      c. fragile, easily injured
      d. decreased subcutaneous tissue
      e. decreased skin turgor
      f. increased sensitivity to cold
    2. hair
      a. decreased number of hair follicles, generalized loss
      b. scant, fine, greying

c. hirsutism (female)

d. possible hereditary baldness

3. nails

  a. dry

  b. thick

  c. brittle

c. Eyes

1. slowed accommodation to light

2. decreased visual acuity

  a. farsightedness due to slow lens accommodation (presbyopia)

  b. narrowed field of vision (tunnel vision)

d. Ears

1. decreased auditory acuity

2. sensorineural hearing deficit (presbycusis): gradual loss of ability to discriminate high-frequency tones

e. Thorax and lungs

1. decreased lung capacity

2. decreased elasticity of tissue

3. increased AP diameter of thorax

f. Cardiovascular

1. decreased vascular elasticity

2. increased systolic and diastolic BP

3. decreased cardiac output

4. less tolerance to position change

g. Gastrointestinal/nutrition

1. slowed digestion; increased food intolerances

2. decreased metabolism: caloric requirement of approximately 1000 calories/day

3. redistribution of body fat: increased fat in trunk, especially in the abdomen

4. teeth and gum problems common

5. atonia constipation common

h. Musculoskeletal

1. tire easily, less stamina

2. symmetrical decrease in muscle bulk

3. decreased muscle strength and tone

4. impaired range of motion resulting from stiff joints

5. generalized loss of 6-10 cm in stature because of

  a. flexion of knee and hip joints

  b. narrowing of intervertebral disks

6. body takes on bony, angular appearance

7. osteoporosis common (especially in vertebral bodies and neck of femur)

8. osteoarthritis common

i. Neurological

1. general

  a. slowed speed of impulse transmission

  b. progressive decrease in number of functioning neurons in CNS and sense organs

  c. normal neurological functioning possible because of tremendous reserve of numbers of neurons

2. mental and cognitive function

  a. altered capacity to retain new information and learn new tasks

  b. some impaired memory and mental endurance

3. sensory

  a. some impaired sensory perception (hearing, smell, sight, taste, touch, temperature, pain)

  b. gradual decrease of visual and auditory acuity

4. motor

  a. slowed reaction to stimuli; lengthening of reaction time

  b. decreased coordination and balance

j. Genitourinary

1. genital

  a. ability to function sexually may continue well into older years

  b. female: menopause secondary to decreased estrogen (see *Nursing Care of the Childbearing Family,* p. 309)

  c. male: decreased testosterone, spermatogenesis, and size of testes; increase in size of prostate

2. urinary

  a. decreased renal plasma flow (RPF), glomerular filtration rate (GFR), and tubular function

  b. decreased renal capacity to concentrate urine at night, resulting in nocturia

k. Immunity

1. diminished immune response with slower, less efficient response to infections

3. increased susceptibility to infections (e.g., pneumonia, influenza)

3. Psychosocial characteristics (see "Psychosocial Characteristics of the Elderly Healthy Client," p. 17)

Application of the Nursing Process to the Healthy Adult

Assessment

1. Health history

  a. Usual health status

  b. Present health status

  c. Family history (e.g., familial cancer, heart disease)

  d. Previous illness

  e. Immunization status

  f. Allergies

  g. Psychosocial

    1. age, sex, race, marital status

    2. role in family

    3. cultural heritage

    4. language

    5. education

6. economic status
7. occupation
8. housing
9. religious practices
10. recreational/social activities
11. personal habits (e.g., tobacco, alcohol)
   h. Physical
   1. personal hygiene habits/practices
   2. eating habits/patterns
   3. dental history
   4. bowel and bladder habits
   5. sleep and rest habits
   6. activity level
   7. work habits
   8. sexual habits
2. Physical exam
   a. Methods
   1. inspection: looking, observing
   2. auscultation: listening
   3. palpation: feeling, touching, pressing
   4. percussion: tapping
   b. Head-to-toe appraisal
   (see physiological characteristics of the young, middle-aged, and elderly adult, pp. 112-115)

Analysis
1. Safe, effective care environment
   a. Knowledge deficit
   b. High risk for injury
   c. Sensory or perceptual alteration (specify)
2. Physiological integrity
   a. Altered growth and development
   b. Altered nutrition: more/less than body requirements
   c. High risk for activity intolerance
3. Psychosocial integrity
   a. Self-esteem disturbance
   b. Spiritual distress
   c. Altered patterns of sexuality
4. Health promotion/maintenance
   a. Knowledge deficit
   b. Health-seeking behaviors
   c. Altered health maintenance

General Nursing Planning, Implementation, and Evaluation

Goal 1: Adult individual will use health practices that promote optimal health.

Implementation
1. Teach, support and act as role model as necessary to help individual to
   a. Maintain personal hygiene.
   b. Maintain good nutrition:
   1. eat nutritionally adequate, well-balanced diet (see Tables 3-1, 3-2, and 4-8).
   2. eat a variety of foods.
   3. avoid foods high in saturated fat, cholesterol, and simple sugars.
   4. eat adequate fiber and complex carbohydrates.
   5. limit alcohol use.
   6. limit use of salt and salty foods.
   c. Maintain proper body weight.
   d. Exercise regularly.
   e. Obtain adequate rest and sleep.
   f. Avoid tobacco use.
   g. Avoid prolonged sun exposure.

Evaluation
Individual maintains normal weight for height.

Goal 2: Adult individual will experience safe environment; will be free from accidental injury.

Implementation
1. Teach as necessary to ensure that individual
   a. Has safe home (e.g., fire alarms, ample lighting).
   b. Has safe working conditions (e.g., safety devices, no toxic material).
   c. Travels safely (e.g., automobile seat belts).
   d. Recreates safely (e.g., no diving in shallow water).

Evaluation
Individual is free from serious accidents.

Goal 3: Adult individual will undergo routine health exams.

Implementation
1. Recommend and help schedule as necessary
   a. Annual physical exam.
   b. Routine dentist or dental hygienist visits.
   c. Attendance at screening clinics (e.g., hypertension, glaucoma, diabetes).
2. Teach guidelines for early detection of cancer: see *Cellular Aberration*, general nursing goal 1, p. 270.

Evaluation
Individual has dental exam every 6 months and physical exam every year.

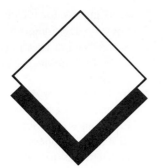

The Adult Client Undergoing Surgery

The nursing care presented in this unit concerns problems in the care of clients undergoing surgery.

GENERAL CONCEPTS
Overview/Physiology

1. Surgery is a stressful event
2. Close monitoring of cardiovascular, respiratory, and renal systems is needed particularly throughout the perioperative period
3. The most common problems during the immediate postanesthetic phase are obstruction of airway, hypoventilation, hypotension, cardiac dysrhythmias, and pain
4. The most common types of complications in the postoperative period
   a. Respiratory
      1. atelectasis (air blockage of portion of lung by mucus plugs, leading to lung collapse)
      2. hypostatic pneumonia
   b. Circulatory
      1. thrombophlebitis and phlebothrombosis (refer to "Circulatory Problems," p. 141)
      2. shock; volume depletion (refer to "Shock," p. 128)
   c. Wound
      1. hemorrhage
      2. infection
      3. dehiscence (separation of wound edges)
      4. evisceration (separation of wound edges with protrusion of viscera through incision)
   d. Urinary
      1. retention
      2. oliguria
   e. Gastrointestinal
      1. paralytic ileus (neurogenic disruption of intestine often related to hypokalemia or decreased autonomic innervation)
      2. singultus (hiccoughs)
   f. Negative nitrogen balance: greater nitrogen excretion than amount ingested

5. Factors affecting client's response to surgery and development of complications
   a. Age: very old and very young are less able to tolerate stress of surgery
   b. Nutritional status
      1. malnutrition: increases risk of infection and poor wound healing
      2. obesity: increases risk of poor wound healing, infection, respiratory complications, and thrombophlebitis
   c. Presence of other chronic illnesses
      1. chronic obstructive pulmonary disease (COPD) increases risk of pulmonary problems
      2. cardiovascular disease decreases ability to deal with stress of surgery
      3. renal disease increases risk of fluid and electrolyte problems, particularly hyperkalemia and fluid overload
      4. diabetes mellitus increases risk of poor wound healing
      5. chronic glucocorticoid therapy increases risk of fluid and electrolyte problems, poor wound healing
   d. Prolonged immobility after surgery increases risk of thrombophlebitis, abdominal distension, urinary retention, and pulmonary complications
   e. Type of operation: some operations are more frequently associated with complications (e.g., atelectasis after gallbladder surgery)
6. Each institution has basic admission, preoperative, intraoperative, and postoperative routines. The following content emphasizes general principles of care that apply to all situations.

PERIOPERATIVE PERIOD
General Information

1. Preoperative care may need to be completed within 1 or 2 hours in an emergency or day surgery situation, or it may be given over a longer period for elective surgery

117

2. Postoperative care may be given in recovery room, ICU, or on general floor
3. Adequate physiological and psychological preparation and care are extremely important to the client's successful recovery
4. For day surgery clients: Many procedures are now performed in ambulatory surgery or day surgery settings. These persons need the same care as that required by inpatients. Diagnostic tests are usually done on an outpatient basis during the week before surgery. The client may see the anesthesiologist, sign consents, and receive some preoperative teaching at this time. Postoperatively, a time and place must be provided to instruct the client and family about diet, fluids, activity, care of wounds, medications, and what to expect regarding comfort, nausea and vomiting, and returning to work. Clients need someone to help them get to and from the hospital if they receive a general anesthetic.

Nursing Process

Assessment

1. Total health status of the client and activities of daily living (ADL) preoperatively
2. General physical exam preoperatively as described for the healthy adult (if time is limited, focus on cardiovascular, pulmonary, neurologic, and renal exams)
3. Psychological readiness: anxiety, fears
4. Learning needs and expectations of surgery
5. For day surgery clients: ability to get home, do care at home
6. Diagnostic tests (preoperative)
   a. Every client
      1. CBC
      2. Electrolytes
      3. Urinalysis
      4. ECG
   b. Special considerations
      1. type and crossmatch blood (as necessary)
      2. prothrombin time, partial thromboplastin time (PTT), bleeding time and/or clotting time
         a. underlying bleeding or coagulation problem
         b. receiving anticoagulants or to receive anticoagulants during surgery
         c. liver problems or presence of jaundice
      3. blood gases and pulmonary function tests (if pulmonary problem is present or pulmonary-cardiovascular surgery is planned)
7. Diagnostic tests (postoperative) will vary with type of surgery
8. Postoperative assessment focuses on systems affected by surgery and by potential complications

Analysis

1. Safe, effective care environment
   a. Knowledge deficit (preoperative)
   b. High risk for injury (intraoperative)
   c. High risk for infection (postoperative)
2. Physiological integrity
   a. Ineffective breathing pattern, high risk for ineffective airway clearance (intraoperative, postoperative)
   b. High risk for decreased cardiac output (intraoperative, postoperative)
   c. Urinary retention (postoperative)
   d. Pain (postoperative)
   e. High risk for altered nutrition: less than body requirements (postoperative)
3. Psychosocial integrity
   a. Anxiety (preoperative)
   b. Fear (preoperative)
   c. Body image disturbance (postoperative)
4. Health promotion/maintenance
   a. Self-care deficit (specify) (postoperative)
   b. Knowledge deficit (postoperative)
   c. Altered health maintenance (postoperative)

Planning, Implementation, and Evaluation

Goal 1: Client and significant others will be prepared for surgery.

Implementation

Day before or immediately prior to surgery (for emergency or day surgery clients)

1. Explain surgical procedure.
2. Clarify expectations of surgery.
3. Explain preoperative procedures, postoperative routine to client and significant others.
4. Ensure that diagnostic tests are completed.
5. Evaluate nutritional status.
6. Prep bowel if required.
7. Ensure that client receives adequate rest the night before surgery; sedate prn.

Day of surgery

8. Monitor vital signs and report immediately if different from admission vital signs.
9. Have client shower.
10. Remove hairpins, jewelry, and medals to avoid loss or injury.
11. Remove prosthetic devices (i.e., dentures, artificial body parts).
12. Apply antiembolic stockings as ordered.
13. Have client void immediately before administering premedications.
14. Premedicate as ordered (not used as frequently as in the past).
15. Put side rails up following premedication.
16. Provide quiet environment.

Evaluation

Client and significant others explain surgery and postoperative routine correctly; client demonstrates coughing, rests well before surgery; diagnostic tests are completed.

Goal 2: Client will experience a safe environment in the operating room.

Implementation

1. Prepare skin as appropriate.
2. Maintain sterility of equipment and operating team.
3. Prevent static electricity by proper attire, safety of electrical equipment, proper grounding.
4. Position client appropriately.
5. Maintain contact with client during induction of general anesthesia (see Table 3-3).

Table 3-3 Stages of general anesthesia

Stage	Duration	Manifestations
I	Beginning of induction to loss of consciousness	Loss of judgment Hearing acute
II	Loss of consciousness to loss of eyelid reflex	Cerebral or voluntary control lost Hypersensitive to incoming impulses Hearing acute
III	Extends from loss of eyelid reflex to cessation of respiratory effort; surgery performed in this stage; reflexes absent and muscles relaxed	Functions of medulla retained
IV		Respiratory paralysis Cardiac failure Death

6. Assist in monitoring for potential complications of anesthetic agents (see Table 3-4).
7. Attend to client during intubation and extubation; be prepared to assist as necessary.
8. Promote hemostasis and have appropriate equipment, supplies available (hemostats, ligatures, electrocoagulation, bone wax, styptics, gelatin sponges, cryoprobe, laser beam, saline packs).
9. Monitor sponge usage; weigh sponges for blood loss as indicated.
10. Measure content of suction bottles; subtract irrigation fluid to approximate blood loss.
11. Estimate amount of blood on drapes and clothes of surgical team.

Evaluation

Client experiences no injuries from improper positioning; client's BP, pulse, rhythm, and oxygenation are maintained at normal levels during the induction of anesthesia and during surgery; client is free from signs of shock or cardiac dysrhythmias during surgery.

Goal 3: Postoperatively, client's respiratory, circulatory, fluid and electrolyte, and neurological status will be optimal.

Implementation

1. Monitor respiratory rate and character, vital signs, I&O, IV infusion, electrolytes, drainage tubes, neurological status, and surgical wound dressing.
2. Report changes to physician.
3. Begin turning, coughing, and deep-breathing exercises qh after airway tube is removed.
4. Suction nasopharyngeal secretions as needed.
5. Administer respiratory-assistance drugs as ordered.
6. Use inspiratory spirometer as indicated.

Table 3-4 General points regarding anesthetic agents

Type	Definition	Major complications
General inhalation	Gases and vapors administered through mask or endotracheal (ET) tube; block pathways to brain and render client unconscious; used for major operations of thorax, abdomen, head, and neck.	Cardiac dysfunction (dysrhythmias, arrest) Respiratory dysfunction (bronchospasms and laryngospasms, aspiration, failure) Cardiovascular dysfunction (shock, hypotension) Neurological complications (convulsions, cerebrovascular accident [CVA]) Others (renal and liver problems, malignant hyperthermia)
Intravenous	Drugs given directly into vein; used for induction and as adjuncts to inhalation agents; do not abolish all pain reflexes.	Respiratory dysfunction (arrest, bronchospasm and laryngospasms) Cardiac and cardiovascular dysfunction (hypotension, depression) Neurological dysfunction (convulsions)
Regional	Drugs injected into nerve track/endings to block selected fibers; may be given topically or locally (spinal, epidural, etc.); do not decrease anxiety, fear; must have a cooperative client.	Hypotension, anaphylactic shock Respiratory paralysis can occur with spinal anesthesia Headache

Table 3-5 Calculating IV rates

$$\frac{\text{amount of IV fluid (ml)}}{\text{time to infuse (min)}} \times \text{drip factor (gtt/ml)} = \text{IV rate (gtt/min)}$$

Example: The order is for 1000 ml D$_5$W to run for 10 hours. The drip factor is 15 gtt/ml.

$$\frac{1000 \text{ ml}}{\underset{(60 \times 10)}{600 \text{ min}}} \times \frac{15 \text{ gtt}}{1 \text{ ml}} = \text{IV rate of 25 gtt/min}$$

Table 3-6 Postoperative diet modifications

Diet	Foods Allowed	Comments
Clear liquids	Tea, Jell-O, broth, strained juices	Provide liquids, but inadequate calories and nutrients
Full liquids	Soups, milk, unstrained juices, ice cream, custards, pudding	Provides more calories and nutrients; if selected carefully, can meet many nutritional needs.

Table 3-7 Classes of analgesics

Morphine-like agonists
  codeine
  morphine
  hydromorphone (Dilaudid)
  methadone (Dolophine)
  levorphanol (Levo-Dromoran)
  oxycodone
  oxymorphone (Numorphan)
  meperidine (Demerol)
Partial agonist
  buprenorphine (Buprenex)
Mixed agonist-antagonists
  pentazocine (Talwin)
  nalbuphine (Nubain)
  butorphanol (Stadol)
Nonnarcotics
  aspirin
  acetaminophen
  ibuprofen (Motrin)
  fenoprofen (Nalfon)
  diflunisal (Dolobid)
  naproxen (Naprosyn)

7. Give IV therapy and drugs as ordered (see Table 3-5 for calculating IV rates).
8. Use voiding-inducement techniques as necessary.
9. Start oral fluids and food when appropriate (see Table 3-6).
10. Keep bed's side rails up until client's neurological status is normal.
11. Use restraints as necessary.
12. Care for surgical wound using aseptic technique.

Evaluation

Client's breath sounds are clear; client coughs well; BP remains stable; skin is warm and dry; nail beds blanch briskly; I&O is in balance; IV is infusing appropriately; client responds appropriately to commands; has dry and intact surgical dressing.

Goal 4: Client will be free from discomfort during the postoperative period.

Implementation
1. Position comfortably; turn q2h; begin ROM exercise as appropriate; ambulate to prevent abdominal distension and other complications of immobility as appropriate.
2. Assess pain
   a. Source of discomfort
   b. Location, character, intensity, and duration of pain
   c. Level of anxiety
   d. Factors that intensify or decrease discomfort
   e. Type of anesthetic administered
   f. Vital signs before and after administering medication
3. Give analgesics as appropriate (see Table 3-7 for common analgesics).

4. Use comfort measures, relaxation, and distraction.
5. Observe and document client's response to pain-relief measures (e.g., amount, onset, duration of relief).
6. Prevent nausea and vomiting
   a. Assess rationale for occurrence (e.g., type of anesthesia or surgery)
   b. Give antiemetics as ordered
   c. Give frequent oral hygiene

Evaluation

Client's pain is relieved; offers no complaints of nausea.

DISCHARGE
General Information

1. Discharge planning starts at admission

Nursing Process

Assessment

1. Client's ability to perform self-care at home

2. Significant others available to help
3. Home situation

Analysis (see p. 118)

Planning, Implementation, and Evaluation

> **Goal:** Client and significant others are prepared for client's discharge.

Implementation

1. Determine discharge date by consulting with physician.
2. Teach client and significant others appropriate information about medications, return appointments, treatments, activity, diet, and dressings.
3. Refer to appropriate community health agency.

Evaluation

Client states time of return appointment; lists medicines to take and how, activity allowed, and how to do treatments.

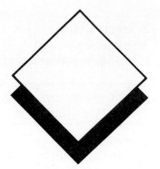

Oxygenation

The nursing care presented in this unit concerns selected health problems related to disturbances in the cardiovascular and respiratory systems.

GENERAL CONCEPTS
Overview/Physiology

1. The cardinal purpose of the cardiovascular and respiratory systems is to provide adequate oxygenation to the entire body
   a. Respiratory system: responsible for the intake of oxygen (O_2) and elimination of carbon dioxide (CO_2); plays a major role in maintaining acid-base balance
   b. Cardiovascular system: responsible for the transport of O_2, CO_2, nutrients, and waste products
2. The heart is a high-energy pump that forcefully ejects blood with enough pressure to perfuse the pulmonary and systemic circulatory system
3. Flow of blood through the heart: inferior and superior vena cava → right atrium → tricuspid valve → right ventricle → pulmonic valve → pulmonary arteries → lungs → pulmonary veins → left atrium → bicuspid (mitral) valve → left ventricle → aortic valve → aorta → systemic circulation (see Fig. 3-1)
4. Blood returning to the right side of the heart is unoxygenated, venous blood; blood ejected from the left side of the heart into the systemic circulation is oxygenated, arterial blood
5. The heart is surrounded by a sac of fibrous tissue known as the pericardium; between the pericardium and epicardium there is a small space that contains a few drops of fluid that lubricate the heart surface
6. The heart itself is composed of three layers
   a. Epicardium: outer layer; coronary arteries lie on this surface
   b. Myocardium: middle layer; cardiac muscle activity originates here
   c. Endocardium: inner layer; lines the valves, chordae tendineae, and papillary muscles
7. The cardiac impulse originates automatically in the sinoatrial (SA) node, travels to the right and left atria; atria contract. Then the impulse reaches the atrioventricular (AV) node, accelerates through the bundle of His, bundle branches, and Purkinje's fibers, and is distributed rapidly and evenly over the ventricles; ventricles contract. The conduction process is regulated by the autonomic nervous system
   a. Sympathetic stimulation increases the heart rate
   b. Parasympathetic or vagal stimulation decreases the heart rate
8. Mean arterial pressure = cardiac output × total peripheral resistance; cardiac output = stroke volume (amount of blood ejected/beat) × heart rate. Arterial pressure can be increased by increasing cardiac output (either stroke volume, heart rate, or both), or by increasing total peripheral resistance. Both cardiac output and total peripheral resistance are influenced by a variety of factors, particularly the autonomic nervous system. Stimulation of the sympathetic nervous system increases heart rate, stroke volume, and total peripheral resistance.
9. Blood pressure varies throughout circulation: greatest in the arterial system; lowest in the venous portion. Central venous pressure (CVP) is the pressure within the right atrium; normal = 4-10 cm H_2O (2-7 mm Hg).
10. The respiratory system is composed of upper and lower airway structures
    a. Upper airway: nose and nasopharynx, mouth, oropharynx, and larynx
    b. Lower airway: trachea, main stem of bronchi, bronchioles, alveolar ducts, and alveoli
    c. Airways filter, warm, and humidify inspired air
11. The lungs lie in and are protected by the thoracic cavity. This bony cage is composed of the sternum and ribs anteriorly and the ribs, scapulae, and vertebral column posteriorly. The thoracic cavity is lined with a serous membrane, the pleura; one surface of the pleura lines the inside of the rib cage (parietal pleura), and the other covers the lungs (visceral pleura). The pleural space (really a potential space) exists between the surfaces of the two pleurae. Subatmospheric pressure in the pleural space is responsible for the continued expansion of the lungs.

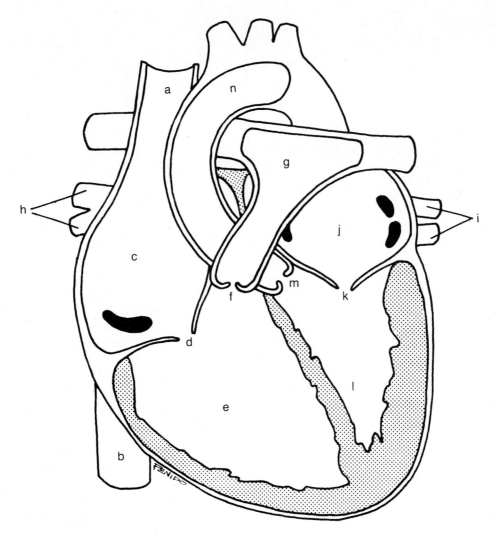

Fig. 3-1   The normal heart. *a,* Superior vena cava; *b,* inferior vena cava; *c,* right atrium; *d,* tricuspid valve; *e,* right ventricle; *f,* pulmonic valve; *g,* pulmonary artery; *h,* right pulmonary veins; *i,* left pulmonary veins; *j,* left atrium; *k,* bicuspid (mitral) valve; *l,* left ventricle; *m,* aortic valve; *n,* aorta.

12. The basic gas-exchange unit of the respiratory system is the alveolus. Pulmonary capillaries lie adjacent to each alveolus; O_2 and CO_2 are exchanged across the alveolar-capillary membrane by the process of diffusion.

13. The neural control of respirations is located in the medulla. Under normal conditions, this center is stimulated directly or reflexly by the concentration of CO_2 in the blood (P_{CO_2}). Chemoreceptors located in the carotid arteries and aortic arch also stimulate the respiratory center of the medulla and respond primarily to hypoxia in the blood (reduced P_{O_2}).

14. The rhythmic breathing pattern is dependent on the cyclical excitation of the respiratory muscles by the phrenic nerve (to the diaphragm) and the intercostal nerves (to the intercostal muscles)

15. Blood is the fluid that circulates through the cardiovascular system

    a. Composition
      1. cells: RBCs, WBCs, platelets
      2. plasma: water, protein, electrolytes, and various organic constituents
    b. Functions
      1. RBC (hemoglobin): carry O_2 from the lungs to tissue and CO_2 from tissue to lungs
      2. WBC: defense against microbial invasion
      3. platelets: hemostasis
    c. Volume: approximately 5000 ml

16. The major steps of clot formation are thromboplastin → prothrombin → thrombin → fibrinogen → fibrin (clot)

Application of the Nursing Process to the Client with Oxygenation Problems

Assessment
1. Health history

a. Dyspnea or chest pain/discomfort
   1. when (e.g., rest, activity)
   2. relieved by what
b. Cough
   1. when
   2. productive or nonproductive; character and amount of sputum, if productive
c. Smoking
   1. type, pack/years (number of packs per day × number of years)
   2. when stopped, duration
d. Allergies
   1. to what?
   2. symptoms
   3. relieved by what
e. Orthopnea or paroxysmal nocturnal dyspnea (PND)
   1. when
   2. relieved by what (e.g., number of pillows, rest)
f. Edema, syncope, dizziness, or headache
   1. when
   2. relieved by what
g. Fatigue or weakness
   1. when
   2. relieved by what
   3. compare with client's normal level of exercise
h. Changes in life-style
   1. ADL
   2. work
   3. leisure
i. Diet (have the client describe previous 24-hour intake)
   1. restrictions (e.g., sodium, cholesterol)
   2. difficulties complying with prescribed diet
   3. alcohol intake
   4. food preferences and intolerances
   5. who shops and prepares meals
j. Medications (prescription and nonprescription)
   1. dose
   2. side effects
   3. effectiveness
k. Personal or family history
   1. pulmonary problems (e.g., tuberculosis, pneumonia, asthma)
   2. cardiac problems (e.g., angina, myocardial infarction, hypertension)

2. Physical examination
  a. Vital signs
    1. blood pressure: lying, sitting, or standing, and in both arms
    2. pulse: rate and rhythm
    3. respirations: rate, depth, and effort
    4. temperature
  b. Inspection of chest
    1. use of accessory muscles
    2. presence of retraction

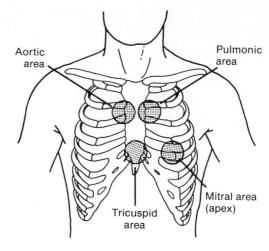

Fig. 3-2   Areas of auscultation of heart valves.

    3. degree of excursion
    4. chest deformity
  c. Palpation of chest
    1. areas of pain or tenderness
    2. presence of carotid thrills, atypical pulsation
    3. change in tactile fremitus
    4. point of maximal impulse (PMI): slight pulsation palpable at apex area (see Fig. 3-2)
  d. Percussion of chest
    1. resonance = normal air
    2. hyperresonance = trapped air
    3. dullness = fluid or consolidation
  e. Auscultation of the lungs
    1. normal breath sounds
     a. vesicular: heard over most of lungs
     b. bronchovesicular: heard over main stem of bronchi
     c. bronchial: heard over trachea and main stem of bronchi
    2. adventitious breath sounds
     a. rales or crackles
      ◆ high-pitched crackling
      ◆ predominantly inspiratory
      ◆ caused by air passing through abnormal secretions in alveoli
     b. rhonchi or gurgles
      ◆ loud, coarse gurgling
      ◆ predominantly expiratory
      ◆ caused by air passing through abnormal secretions in bronchi
     c. wheezing
      ◆ high-pitched whistling
      ◆ caused by air passing through narrowed bronchi
     d. bronchial (tubular) breath sounds audible over peripheral lung
      ◆ expiratory and inspiratory
      ◆ indicates consolidation (e.g., pneumonia)

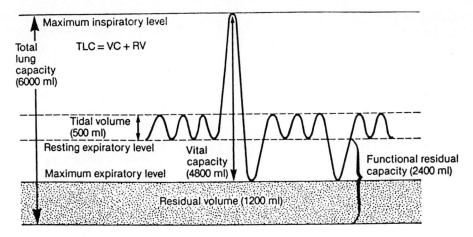

Fig. 3-3 Pulmonary volumes and capacities of an adult; values vary with age, sex, weight, and height. (From Kersten, L. [1989]. *Comprehensive respiratory nursing: A decision making approach.* Philadelphia: W.B. Saunders. Used with permission.)

f. Auscultation of the heart
1. anatomical landmarks: aortic, pulmonic, tricuspid, and mitral area correspond to where valve closing is the loudest (see Fig. 3-2)
   a. aortic: second intercostal space to the right of the sternum
   b. pulmonic: second intercostal space to the left of the sternum
   c. tricuspid: fourth and fifth intercostal space slightly left of the sternum
   d. mitral: at the apex of the heart in the fifth intercostal space in the midclavicular line
2. apical pulse (see Fig. 3-2)
   a. rate and rhythm
   b. pulse deficit = apical minus radial pulse (NOTE: the two pulses must be taken at the same time by *two* practitioners)
3. normal heart sounds
   a. S_1 (lub)
      ◆ closing of mitral and tricuspid valves
      ◆ at onset of ventricular systole
   b. S_2 (dub)
      ◆ closing of aortic and pulmonary valves
      ◆ at onset of ventricular diastole
4. extra heart sounds
   a. S_3, S_4
      ◆ abnormal in adults
      ◆ sometimes normal in children and young adults
   b. murmurs: caused by turbulent blood flow
g. Skin and extremities
1. skin color (e.g., pallor, cyanosis, rubor)
2. skin temperature
3. edema
4. peripheral pulses: presence, strength, equality
3. Diagnostic tests
a. Pulmonary function tests: the direct or indirect measurement of various lung volumes; done to assess lung function; see Fig. 3-3
1. *tidal volume* (TV): volume of gas inspired and expired with a quiet normal breath (500 ml)
2. *inspiratory reserve volume* (IRV): maximal volume that can be inspired at the end of a normal inspiration (3100 ml)
3. *expiratory reserve volume* (ERV): maximal volume that can be forcefully exhaled after a normal expiration (1200 ml)
4. *residual volume* (RV): volume of gas left in lung after maximal expiration (1200 ml)
5. *minute volume* (MV): volume of gas inspired and expired in 1 minute of normal breathing (6 liters/min)
6. *vital capacity* (VC): maximal amount of air that can be expired after a maximal inspiration (TV + IRV + ERV) (4800 ml)
b. Sputum specimens
1. examinations
   a. culture and sensitivity
   b. cytology
2. nursing care
   a. collect specimen in morning
   b. collect sterile specimen
   c. collect sputum, not saliva
c. Chest x-rays or tomograms
d. Lung scan: following injection of radioactive material, lung is scanned for presence of obstruction or areas that are poorly perfused
e. Bronchoscopy
1. insertion of a rigid or flexible fiberoptic bronchoscope through the oral cavity into the bronchus in order to view the area; bronchial brushing, biopsy, or bronchogram may be done during the procedure
2. nursing care: preparation

   a. explain procedure
   b. NPO 6-12 hours
   c. oral hygiene
   d. remove dentures
   e. premedicate
3. nursing care: postprocedure
   a. NPO until gag reflex returns
   b. observe respirations
   c. observe hoarseness, dysphagia
   d. observe for subcutaneous emphysema (crackling under the skin when pressed, caused by air from perforated airway)
   e. bloody sputum normal after biopsy
f. ECG
   1. monitor (see Fig. 3-4)
   2. resting 12-lead
   3. exercise (stress test)
      a. treadmill or bicycle
      b. ECG may show signs of ischemia during exercise
g. Myocardial scan: following injection of radioactive thallium, heart is scanned to detect areas of poorly perfused myocardium
h. Echocardiography: cardiac wall motion is viewed by ultrasound
i. Cardiac catheterization or angiography (see also Table 5-19, p. 480)

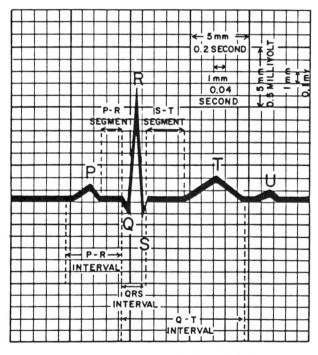

Fig. 3-4   Components of a normal electrocardiogram. The P wave represents atrial depolarization; the P-R segment, atrial depolarization and transmission of the cardiac impulse through the AV node. The QRS complex represents ventricular depolarization; the ST segment, the refractory period of the ventricular muscle. The T wave represents ventricular repolarization. The U wave may not be present.

1. under local anesthesia and fluoroscopy, a catheter is inserted into the femoral or brachial artery (left heart catheterization) or an antecubital vein (right heart catheterization). The injection of radiopaque dye permits viewing the heart vessels, chambers, and valves and measuring pressures and oxygen concentrations
2. preparation
   a. explain procedure
   b. NPO 6-12 hours
   c. take and record pulses and temperature of all extremities
   d. check for allergy to iodine
3. nursing care: after procedure
   a. monitor vital signs
   b. monitor pulse and temperature in area distal to arterial puncture site (spasms or emboli can cause these to diminish or disappear); emboli formation requires immediate intervention
   c. prevent stress on incision line (e.g., no bending of affected limb, no ambulation for 12-24 hours if femoral site)
   d. use pressure dressing at puncture site
j. Hematologic studies (normal values will vary slightly from laboratory to laboratory)
   1. arterial blood gases (ABG)
      a. test of arterial blood to assess oxygenation, ventilation, and acid-base status
      b. normal values
         ◆ pH: 7.35-7.45
         ◆ P_{O_2}: 80-100 mm Hg
         ◆ P_{CO_2}: 35-45 mm Hg
         ◆ % O_2 saturation: 95%-100%
   2. CBC
      a. WBC: 5000-10,000/mm³
      b. RBC: 4.7-6.1 million/mm³
      c. Hgb
         ◆ men: 14-18 g/dl
         ◆ women: 12-16 g/dl
      d. hematocrit (HCT)
         ◆ men: 42%-52%
         ◆ women: 37%-47%
      e. platelets: 150,000-400,000/mm³
   3. electrolytes
      a. sodium: 136-145 mEq/L
      b. potassium: 3.5-5.0 mEq/L
      c. chlorides: 90-110 mEq/L
   4. lipids
      a. cholesterol: 150-250 mg/dl
      b. triglycerides: 40-150 mg/dl

Analysis

1. Safe, effective care environment
   a. High risk for injury
   b. Knowledge deficit
   c. High risk for infection

2. Physiological integrity
   a. Decreased cardiac output
   b. Impaired gas exchange
   c. Activity intolerance
3. Psychosocial integrity
   a. Ineffective individual coping
   b. Anxiety
   c. Body image disturbance
4. Health promotion/maintenance
   a. Impaired adjustment
   b. Health-seeking behaviors
   c. Noncompliance

General Nursing Planning, Implementation, and Evaluation

Goal 1: Client will maintain patent airway and adequate oxygenation.

Implementation
1. Monitor respiratory status (e.g., vital signs, breath sounds, skin color).
2. Reduce anxiety.
3. Limit or space activities to decrease O_2 need.
4. Turn frequently if on bed rest.
5. Place in Fowler's position to increase air exchange.
6. Humidify air.
7. Administer O_2 as needed.
8. Cough and deep-breathe frequently.
9. Avoid sedatives that depress respirations and cough reflex (e.g., narcotics).
10. Force fluids to liquefy bronchial secretions.
11. Suction as needed; provide hyperoxygenation before and after suctioning to decrease chances of hypoxia.
12. Carry out postural drainage if needed.
    a. Give humidified air or bronchodilators 10-15 minutes before.
    b. No longer than 15 minutes at one time
    c. Clapping or vibrating can be done with postural drainage.
    d. Avoid clapping or vibrating over sternum, breast tissue, below ribs
    e. Folllow with coughing to be effective; do not allow client to cough in head-down position

Evaluation
Client is well oxygenated (PO_2 greater than 60 mm Hg).

Goal 2: Client's cardiac work load will be decreased.

Implementation
1. Monitor cardiovascular status (e.g., vital signs, pulse deficit, skin color).
2. Limit activity to decrease O_2 need.
3. Promote rest.
4. Administer O_2 as needed.

5. Monitor I&O of fluids to prevent circulatory overload.
6. Give diuretics as ordered to reduce circulating blood volume (see Table 3-16).
7. Prevent constipation (e.g., use stool softeners).
8. Reduce anxiety.

Evaluation
Client's cardiac work load is decreased; pulse decreases from 100 to 84.

Goal 3: Client will remain free from the hazards of immobility.

Implementation
1. Turn frequently.
2. Deep-breathe and cough as needed.
3. Provide passive ROM exercises as needed.
4. Teach client ankle flexion exercises.
5. Give good back care.
6. Apply antiembolic hose.
7. Give anticoagulants if ordered (see Table 3-11).

Evaluation
Client remains free from thrombophlebitis, decubitus ulcers, pulmonary consolidation.

SELECTED HEALTH PROBLEMS RESULTING IN INTERFERENCE WITH CARDIAC FUNCTION

☐ Cardiopulmonary Arrest

General Information
1. Definition: complete failure of the heart to perfuse adequately and the lungs to ventilate adequately
2. Classification: medical emergency

Nursing Process
Assessment
1. *A*-airway
   a. Determine unresponsiveness
   b. Determine airway patency
2. *B*-breathing
   a. Determine breathlessness
   b. Look for chest to rise and fall
   c. Feel for flow of air
3. *C*-circulation
   a. Determine pulselessness
   b. Check carotid pulse

Analysis (see p. 126)

Planning, Implementation, and Evaluation

Goal 1: Client will have an open airway and receive adequate ventilation.

Implementation
1. Place client in supine position on a flat, firm surface.
2. Assume rescuer position: kneel at level of client's shoulders.
3. Clear airway of foreign matter if present.
4. Open airway by head tilt–chin lift maneuver.

5. Watch for breathing.
6. Ventilate mouth-to-mouth if no breathing.
7. Give two full breaths of 1-1½ seconds each.
8. Use Heimlich's maneuver (subdiaphragmatic abdominal thrust) to clean airway if unable to ventilate.
9. Watch for breathing.
10. Continue mouth-to-mouth ventilation, if no breathing but pulse is present, at a rate of 12/min (once every 5 seconds).
11. If available
    a. Use airway and Ambu-bag.
    b. Administer 100% O_2.

Evaluation

Client is well ventilated (e.g., chest rises and falls with rescue breathing).

Goal 2: Client will circulate adequately oxygenated blood.

Implementation

1. Check carotid pulse.
2. Begin external chest compression after initial two breaths if carotid pulse absent.
   a. Assume rescuer position: arms straight, elbows locked, shoulders directly over hands.
   b. Locate proper hand position: hands one over other, long axis of heel over long axis of *lower half* of sternum, fingers *off* chest.
3. Depress lower half of sternum 1½-2 inches at a rate of 80-100/min.
4. One rescuer: give 15 compressions/2 ventilations.
5. Two rescuers: give 5 compressions/1 ventilation with a pause for ventilation (1-1½ seconds).
6. Continue CPR until spontaneous respirations and pulse return.

7. If available
   a. Monitor ECG.
   b. Defibrillate as soon as possible for ventricular fibrillation.

Evaluation

Client has carotid pulsation with each compression; maintains BP of 100 systolic.

Goal 3: Client will receive appropriate emergency drugs.

Implementation

1. Obtain cart with emergency drugs.
2. Start IV for drug administration.
3. Administer emergency drugs as needed (see Table 3-8).
4. Record accurately all drugs given.

Evaluation

Client receives appropriate doses of ordered drugs; client's heart resumes normal sinus rhythm.

☐ Shock
General Information

1. Definition: a syndrome associated with abnormal cellular metabolism; the pathology common to all shock is inadequate tissue perfusion
2. Etiological classification
   a. Hypovolemic (decreased volume)
   b. Cardiogenic (inadequate pump)
   c. Neurogenic (pooling due to vasodilation)
   d. Septic (caused by bacterial endotoxins; characterized by fever, early vasodilation, increased capillary permeability, and shift of fluid to interstitial space)

Table 3-8   Emergency drugs*

Name	Indications
Atropine sulfate	Bradycardia
Bretylium tosylate (Bretylol)	Ventricular dysrhythmias unresponsive to lidocaine
Calcium chloride	Not recommended for cardiac arrest except when hyperkalemia, hypocalcemia, or calcium channel block toxicity is present
Dobutamine hydrochloride (Dobutrex)	To increase cardiac contractility
Dopamine hydrochloride (Intropin)	To increase BP and cardiac contractility; in small doses improves renal perfusion
Epinephrine	Asystole and ventricular fibrillation; to increase heart rate, cardiac output, and BP
Lidocaine hydrochloride (Xylocaine)	Ventricular dysrhythmias
Procainamide hydrochloride (Pronestyl)	Ventricular dysrhythmias when lidocaine is not effective
Sodium bicarbonate	*Not recommended* routinely for metabolic acidosis during cardiac arrest; may be given in response to arterial blood gases
Verapamil (Calan)	Paroxysmal supraventricular tachydysrhythmias

*Drugs that should be readily available for all cardiac emergencies; recommended by American Heart Association.

e. Anaphylactic (massive capillary vasodilation due to release of histamine and related substances)
3. Precipitating factors
   a. Allergic reactions
   b. Infections, particularly gram negative
   c. Spinal anesthesia
   d. Spinal cord trauma
   e. Myocardial infarction
   f. Pulmonary emboli
   g. Dysrhythmias
   h. Hemorrhage
   i. Burns
   j. GI loss of fluid and electrolytes
4. Body's response to shock
   a. Stimulation of the adrenal medulla by the sympathetic nervous system
      1. tachycardia
      2. tachypnea
      3. vasoconstriction
      4. redistribution of blood
      5. cool, clammy skin; oliguria; decreased bowel sounds
   b. Stimulation of renin-angiotensin-aldosterone system and antidiuretic hormone (ADH)
      1. thirst
      2. decreased urine volume
      3. increased concentration of urine
   c. Stimulation of cortisol and growth hormone secretion
      1. increased glucose metabolism
      2. increased fat mobilization

Nursing Process

Assessment
1. Identify high-risk client
2. Vital signs: tachycardia, tachypnea; early BP may be normal because of compensatory mechanisms but will decrease later
3. Mental status: restless, early increased alertness, but as hypoxia occurs, alertness decreases, followed by lethargy, coma
4. Skin changes
   a. Pale, cool, clammy skin (hypovolemic and cardiogenic shock)
   b. Flushed, cool if vasodilation present (neurogenic shock)
   c. Flushed and warm early, then cool and clammy (septic shock)
5. Fluid status: check skin turgor, I&O, urine specific gravity, central venous pressure (CVP)
   a. CVP increased in cardiogenic shock
   b. CVP decreased in hypovolemic and vasogenic shocks
Analysis (see p. 126)
Planning, Implementation, and Evaluation

Goal 1: Client will remain free from any undetected change in cellular perfusion.

Implementation (high-risk client)
1. Assess vital signs q4h, more frequently if unstable.
2. Measure I&O at least q8h, qh if unstable.
3. Note skin turgor, temperature, and color q8h.
4. Monitor ECG if dysrhythmias are present.
5. Obtain blood work as appropriate (CBC, electrolytes, blood urea nitrogen [BUN], creatinine, blood gases).
Evaluation
Client maintains stable vital signs, fluid balance; has no signs of impending shock.

Goal 2: Client will have adequate perfusion.

Implementation
1. Monitor blood pressure (mean should be at least 80), pulse, and respiration.
2. Note and report dysrhythmias.
3. Monitor CVP (normal = 4-10 cm H_2O); measure the same way each time.
4. Maintain urine output of at least 30 ml/hr and equal to intake.
5. Monitor mental status.
6. Monitor GI function.
7. Administer fluids as ordered: blood, colloid fluids, or electrolyte solutions as necessary (until CVP = 6-10 cm H_2O).
8. Administer drugs only after circulating volume has returned to normal (see Table 3-8).
   a. Adrenergic stimulants (epinephrine, dopamine, dobutamine, norepinephrine [Levophed], isoproterenol [Isuprel]) cause increase in contractility and heart rate to increase cardiac output; some may also cause vasoconstriction.
      1. administer with a controlled-volume regulator.
      2. monitor BP q15min continually.
      3. wean off drugs as soon as possible.
      4. know that some of these drugs cause severe vasoconstriction and can worsen organ damage (renal failure, hepatic failure).
      5. watch for extravasation of vasopressors (if norepinephrine or dopamine extravasates, infiltrate around area with phentolamine [Regitine]).
      6. titrate drug infusion to keep BP at a mean of 80, or as ordered.
   b. Vasodilators (nitroprusside, hydralazine) may be used to decrease cardiac work in cardiogenic shock load
   c. When using adrenergic stimulants and vasodilators together
      1. if BP drops, decrease vasodilator first; then increase adrenergic stimulant.

2. if BP increases, decrease adrenergic stimulant and then increase vasodilator.
   d. Administer other drugs as ordered (e.g., cardiac glycosides to enhance cardiac contractility); see Table 3-15.
9. Place in modified Trendelenburg's position (feet up 45° and head flat).

Evaluation

Client's BP is maintained at a mean of 80 mm Hg.

> **Goal 3:** Client will have adequate O_2 and CO_2 levels.

Implementation

1. See General Nursing Goals 1 and 2, p. 127.
2. Provide comfort measures (NOTE: If giving pain medications, do not use IM or subcutaneous route since medications may accumulate and not be absorbed; when perfusion improves, client may get overdose).
3. Keep client warm, not hot or cold (heat causes sweating; cold causes shivering).

Evaluation

Client is well oxygenated (PO_2 greater than 60 mm Hg; no air hunger or cyanosis).

> **Goal 4:** Client will be protected from injury and complications.

Implementation

1. Keep bed's side rails up; if client is confused, watch carefully and avoid restraints.
2. Apply antiembolic stockings to prevent venous stasis.
3. Turn frequently to preven decubitus ulcers, pulmonary problems.
4. Use sterile technique with all procedures (e.g., changing IVs) since client has decreased resistance to infection.

Evaluation

Client is free from preventable complications (e.g., falls, infections).

☐ Angina Pectoris

General Information

1. Definitions
   a. Atherosclerosis: fatty plaque deposited in the intima of the artery
   b. Arteriosclerosis: calcium deposits in the media of the artery
   c. Angina pectoris: chest pain caused by temporary ischemia of the myocardium; usually caused by atherosclerosis, arteriosclerosis, thrombus, or coronary artery spasm
2. Risk factors (coronary artery disease)
   a. Risk factors that cannot be controlled
      1. age
      2. gender
      3. family history
   b. Risk factors that can be controlled with medical supervision
      1. hypertension
      2. hyperlipidemia
      3. diabetes
   c. Risk factors that can be controlled by the person at risk
      1. smoking
      2. high stress
      3. sedentary life-style
      4. obesity
3. Precipitating factors (immediate)
   a. Five "E"s
      1. *exercise*
      2. *exertion*: arteries are able to provide blood to myocardium at rest, but an increased demand on coronary circulation cannot be met temporarily
      3. *emotions*: stimulation of sympathetic nervous system leads to increased demand on heart
      4. *eating* a heavy meal: increased perfusion of the gastrointestinal tract for digestion; pressure from full stomach against diaphragm
      5. *exposure* to cold
   b. Smoking

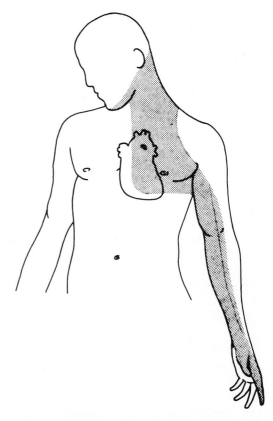

Fig. 3-5 Distribution of typical angina pain.

Nursing Process

Assessment

1. Precipitating factor(s)
2. Pain
   a. Pattern varies with each individual, but is usually the same for a specific person
   b. Usually retrosternal
   c. Tends to radiate into neck, jaw, shoulder, and down inner aspect of left arm (see Fig. 3-5).
   d. Short duration (1-3 minutes)
   e. Usually relieved by rest and nitroglycerin
3. ECG changes (if any) are not permanent

Analysis (see p. 126)

Planning, Implementation, and Evaluation

> **Goal 1:** Client will have improved perfusion of the myocardium.

Implementation

1. Give vasodilating and beta-blocking drugs (see Table 3-9).
2. Know action and side effects of these drugs.

Evaluation

Client performs daily activities without pain by spacing activities or by taking a nitroglycerin tablet before bathing, eating, or taking daily walks.

> **Goal 2:** Client will learn methods to prevent attacks.

Implementation

1. Teach client
   a. To recognize symptoms.
   b. To take medications and cope with side effects.
   c. When to take medications (e.g., before activity).
   d. To avoid precipitating factors if possible.

Table 3-9 Angina pectoris drugs

Name	Action	Side effects	Nursing implications
NITRATES			
Nitroglycerin (Nitro-Bid)	Generalized vasodilation Oxygen consumption and demand on myocardium are decreased	Pounding headache, flushing, tachycardia, dizziness, orthostatic hypotension	Usually taken sublingually. Take at pain onset; repeat in 5 min × 2; if no pain relief, go to nearest ER. Also taken prophylactically before pain onset.
Nitroglycerin ointment (Nitrol) Nitroglycerin disc (Transderm-Nitro)	Absorbed through skin; long-acting vasodilation	Relatively safe (same as nitroglycerin sublingual)	Applied to intact, hairless skin. Rotate sites. Use dermal patches intermittently (tolerance develops with use).
Erythrityl tetranitrate (Cardilate) Isosorbide dinitrate (Isordil, Sorbitrate) Pentaerythritol tetranitrate (Peritrate, Pentafin, and Pentritol)	Long-acting vasodilation	Less acute vasodilation effect due to slower absorption; can cause gastric irritation, nausea, vomiting	
CALCIUM CHANNEL BLOCKERS			
Nifedipine (Procardia) Diltiazem (Cardizem) Verapamil (Calan)	Coronary artery spasm is inhibited Oxygen consumption of myocardium is decreased	Fatigue, headache, transient hypotension, nausea, constipation	
BETA-ADRENERGIC BLOCKERS			
Propranolol (Inderal)	Heart rate, cardiac contractility, cardiac output, and BP are reduced; oxygen consumption of myocardium is decreased	Fatigue, bradycardia, postural hypotension, nausea, vomiting, diarrhea, bronchospasm	Heart rate must be 50 or more before the drug is administered.

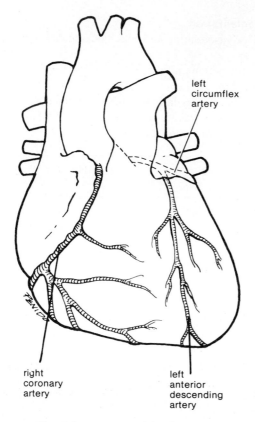

Fig. 3-6   Coronary blood supply.

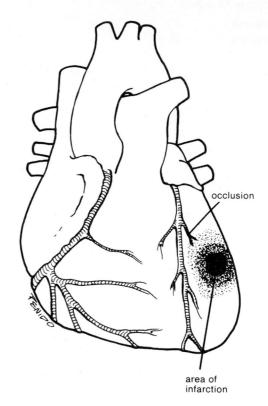

Fig. 3-7   Myocardial infarction.

e. To decrease risk factors (e.g., quit smoking, control hypertension).

f. To reduce dietary cholesterol and saturated fat to prevent further atherosclerosis (see Table 3-13).

2. Define activity level: space activities and eliminate those that might precipitate angina (e.g., mowing grass, shoveling snow).

Evaluation

Client is able to correctly explain medications, dosage, time schedule, side effects; has a balanced schedule of rest and activities.

> **Goal 3:** Client will be able to state what to do if symptoms change.

Implementation

1. Teach client to identify own pain pattern and to recognize change in pain.

2. Instruct client to notify physician of change.

Evaluation

Client explains ways of dealing with a change in anginal pain.

☐ Myocardial Infarction

General Information

1. Definition: occlusion of one or more coronary arteries causing death of a portion of the myocardial tissue (infarct); see Figs. 3-6 and 3-7

2. Incidence

a. Leading cause of death in the United States

b. More common in men; rate in women rises after menopause

3. Risk factors (see risk factors for coronary artery disease, p. 130)

Nursing Process

Assessment

1. Chest pain

a. Intense, crushing, substernal

b. Not relieved by rest or nitroglycerin

2. ECG changes: elevation or depression of ST segment; T wave inversion; pathological Q waves

3. Serum enzymes (see Table 3-10)

Analysis (see p. 126)

Planning, Implementation, and Evaluation

> **Goal 1:** Client's chest pain will be controlled.

Implementation

1. Give analgesics (e.g., morphine sulfate IV) until pain is relieved.

2. Administer O_2 (4-6 L/min).

3. Administer nitroglycerin IV drip as ordered.

4. Give sedatives prn to promote rest.

Evaluation

Client states pain was relieved.

Table 3-10   Cardiac enzyme changes after myocardial infarction

Enzyme	Normal value	Begins to rise (within x hours)	Peaks	Returns to normal
CPK	5-75 mU/ml	6	18 hr	2-3 days
CPK-MB	<5% total	3-6	12-24 hr	12-48 hr
AST (SGOT)	5-40 U/l	6-10	12-48 hr	3-4 days
LDH	90-200 ImU/l	24-72	3-4 days	14 days

From Pagana, K., & Pagana, T. (1990). *Diagnostic testing and nursing implications* (3rd ed.). St. Louis: Mosby-Year Book.

Goal 2: Client's coronary blood flow will be increased or reestablished.

Implementation
1. Administer thrombolytic drugs as ordered (see Table 3-11).
2. Monitor cardiac rhythm for reperfusion dysrhythmias.
3. Provide postprocedure care after percutaneous transluminal coronary angioplasty.
   a. Monitor arterial puncture site.
   b. Keep head of bed elevated less than 30° for 12 hours.
   c. Monitor pulses distal to puncture site.

Evaluation
Following angioplasty, client reports decreased chest pain; is free from dysrhythmias.

Goal 3: Client's cardiac work load will be decreased.

Implementation
1. See General Nursing Goal 2, p. 127.
2. Teach client to avoid Valsalva's maneuver (increases intrathoracic pressure and causes sudden temporary increase in work load).

Evaluation
Client's heart rate is decreased (e.g., from 88 to 72).

Goal 4: Client will remain free from new blood vessel occlusions.

Implementation
1. Administer anticoagulants as ordered (see Table 3-11).
2. Know action, side effects, and antidotes of anticoagulants.
3. Apply antiembolic hose.
4. Teach client ankle flexion and extension exercises.

Evaluation
Client's condition remains stable; has no signs of further occlusions.

Goal 5: Client will remain free from complications.

Implementation
1. Monitor ECG for dysrhythmias.
2. Monitor lab reports (enzymes and electrolytes); see Table 3-10.
3. Monitor for symptoms of cardiogenic shock (see p. 129).
4. Monitor for symptoms of congestive heart failure (see p. 136).
5. Monitor for symptoms of thrombophlebitis (see Fig. 3-11).

Evaluation
Client gradually improves without complications.

Goal 6: Client and significant others will be able to explain care during acute and recovery phase, and care that will follow discharge.

Implementation
1. Teach
   a. Level of activity
   b. Diet
      1. calories reduced if client is obese
      2. sodium restricted (see Table 3-12)
      3. cholesterol and saturated fat restricted (see Table 3-13)
      4. potassium increased if necessary (see Table 3-17)
   c. Medications
      1. administration
      2. schedule
      3. side effects
   d. Sexual activity: may resume sexual intercourse in 6-8 weeks following an *uncomplicated* MI
   e. Fluid retention

Evaluation
Client explains own activity; plans menu for a sodium-restricted diet; knows what symptoms to report to physician immediately.

☐ **Pacemaker**
General Information

1. Definition: An electronic device that delivers an electrical stimulus to the heart through electrodes placed directly on the epicardium or placed in contact with the endocardium; may be temporary or permanent

Table 3-11   Anticoagulant and thrombolytic drugs

Name	Action	Side effects	Nursing implications
ANTICOAGULANT AGENTS			
Heparin sodium	Prolongs clotting. Prevents formation of thrombin from pro-thrombin. Onset almost immediate. Lasts 4 hours. No effects on existing thrombi.	Hemorrhage epistaxis, he-maturia, melena, ecchy-mosis, bleeding gums, transient alopecia.	Parenteral: IV or subcutaneous. Monitor partial thromboplastin time (PTT). PTT maintained at 1½-2 times nor-mal (normal = 30-40 seconds). Discontinue heparin if there is evi-dence of bleeding or if the PTT is overly prolonged. ANTIDOTE: Protamine sulfate. Use bleeding precautions (e.g., soft toothbrush, electric razor).
Bishydroxycoumarin (Dicumarol)	Prolongs clotting. Inhibits synthesis of pro-thrombin and other vi-tamin K–dependent clotting factors. Slow onset (2-3 days). Lasts up to 9 days after last dose. No effect on existing thrombi.	Hemorrhage epistaxis, he-maturia, melena, ecchy-mosis, bleeding gums. GI disturbances: diar-rhea, vomiting, anorexia. INTERACTION: Salicylates *in-crease* anticoagulant ef-fect.	Oral. Monitor prothrombin time (PT). PT maintained at 1½-2 times nor-mal (normal = 12-15 seconds). Discontinue Dicumarol or Coumadin if the PT is overly prolonged or if bleeding occurs. No aspirin. ANTIDOTE: Vitamin K (Aqua-MEPHYTON). Use bleeding precautions as above. Wear ID stating anticoagulants are being taken.
Warfarin sodium (Coumadin)	Same as Dicumarol. Onset occurs within 18-24 hours. Cumulative effect lasts up to 7 days.	Same as Dicumarol.	Same as Dicumarol.
THROMBOLYTIC AGENTS			
Streptokinase (Streptase)	Activates plasminogen and converts it to plas-min, which degrades fibrin clots. Immediate onset; residual effects last up to 12 hours after infusion.	Hemorrhage, oozing at site of puncture, incision, or cut; fever, allergic reac-tion, reperfusion dys-rhythmias.	Parenteral: IV. Monitor PT, PTT, and thrombin time. Monitor for hemorrhage. Maintain bleeding precautions. Start heparin before streptokinase is discontinued. Solu-Cortef frequently given before infusion to prevent allergic reac-tion. Administer all drugs through preex-isting IV lines, by mouth, or by NG tube while streptokinase is in-fusing. Monitor cardiac rhythm for reperfu-sion dysrhythmias. No true antidote.
Tissue Plasminogen Activator (t-PA) (Activase)	Converts plasminogen to plasmin at fibrin sur-face; is more clot-spe-cific than streptokinase. Immediate onset; action lasts approximately 10 minutes.	Hemorrhage, oozing at site of puncture, incision, or cut; reperfusion dys-rhythmias.	Parenteral: IV bolus followed by 3-4 hour infusion. Monitor PT, PTT, and thrombin time. Monitor for hemorrhage. Maintain bleeding precautions. Start heparin before t-PA is discon-tinued. Administer all drugs through preex-isting IV lines, by mouth, or by NG tube while streptokinase is in-fusing. Monitor cardiac rhythm for reperfu-sion dysrhythmias.

Table 3-12 Approximate sodium content in selected food items*

Food items	Portion	Sodium content (mg)
BREADS AND CEREALS		
White bread	1 slice	200
Regular corn flakes	1 oz	260
DAIRY PRODUCTS		
Milk	8 oz	130
American cheese	1 slice	238
Cottage cheese, low fat	4 oz	435
FISH AND SHELLFISH		
Flounder, broiled filet	2 oz	355
Scallops	3½ oz	265
FRUITS AND VEGETABLES		
Tomato juice	6 oz	275
Peas, canned	5¼ oz	349
MEATS AND POULTRY		
Chicken, roasted	2 pieces	57
Bacon	1 slice	101
Bologna	1 slice	226
Beef	3 oz	381
MISCELLANEOUS FOOD ITEMS		
Olives	1	130
Catsup	1 tbsp	154
Peanut butter	1 tbsp	167
Potato chips	14 chips	191
Italian salad dressing	1 tbsp	315
Chocolate pudding, instant	½ cup	404
Dill pickle	1 large	1,137
Beef broth	1 cube	1,152
Salt	1 tsp	2,400

*Exact amount of sodium varies with brands of food items.

TEACHING GUIDELINES FOR SODIUM-RESTRICTED DIETS

1. Discuss salt and other sodium-containing compounds.
2. Explain relationship of sodium to high blood pressure, rationale for eliminating sodium from diet.
3. Stress avoiding foods and medications that contain multiple sodium compounds; read labels carefully.
4. Eat three well-balanced meals a day with foods naturally low in sodium.
5. Add no salt while preparing food and add no salt at table.
6. *If sodium intake is limited to only 2 g, food can be salted lightly during preparation, but no additional salt added at table.*
7. Season food with non-sodium flavorings.
8. Seek advice from physician concerning salt substitutes.

Table 3-13 Cholesterol and saturated fat content in selected items*

Food items	Serving	Cholesterol (mg)	Saturated fat (g)
DAIRY PRODUCTS			
Milk, skin	8 oz	0	0
Yogurt, low fat	8 oz	11	1.8
American cheese	1 oz	27	5.6
Butter	1 tbs	31	7.1
Milk, whole	8 oz	33	5.1
Ice cream	8 oz	59	8.9
FISH AND SHELLFISH			
Clams	3 oz	50	0.4
Fish, lean	3 oz	59	0.3
Shrimp	3 oz	126	0.5
MEATS AND POULTRY			
Beef liver	3 oz	372	2.5
Egg	1 whole	213	1.7
Beef, lean	3 oz	56	2.4
Chicken breast	3 oz	63	1.3
FRUITS AND VEGETABLES			
All fruits	No cholesterol and generally no satu-		
All vegetables	rated fats (vegetable oils in italics below are two exceptions)		
VEGETABLE OILS			
Coconut oil	1 tbs	0	11.8
Palm oil	1 tbs	0	6.7
Olive oil	1 tbs	0	1.8
Corn oil	1 tbs	0	1.7
Safflower oil	1 tbs	0	1.2

*Exact amount of cholesterol and saturated fat varies with brands of food items.

a. Fixed rate: continuously fires at preset rate
b. Demand rate: fires only if heart rate drops below given rate

Nursing Process

Assessment
1. Rate, rhythm, and quality of all pulses
2. ECG: alterations in P wave, PR interval, QRS complex, and T waves
3. Laboratory tests: electrolytes, serum digoxin levels

Analysis (see p. 126)
Planning, Implementation, and Evaluation

> **Goal:** Client will undergo pacemaker implantation free from preventable complications.

Implementation
1. Postprocedure
   a. Monitor for changes in pulse rate and rhythm.
   b. Keep insertion site clean; inspect for signs of infection.
   c. Monitor for temperature elevation.
   d. Support extremity on which pacemaker attached (external pacemaker).
2. Teach client with permanent pacemaker
   a. Level of activity.
   b. Take own pulse daily.
   c. Symptoms of pacemaker failure: vertigo, syncope, palpitations, hiccoughs, bradycardia.
   d. Avoid improperly grounded electrical appliances (e.g., some power tools).
   e. Avoid sources of high-frequency signals (e.g., radio towers).
   f. Avoid magnetic resonance imaging (MRI) procedures.
   g. Schedule for battery replacement.
   h. Carry identification card.
   i. Importance of follow-up care.

Evaluation
   Client maintains a regular, normal heart rate after pacemaker implantation.

☐ Congestive Heart Failure (CHF)
General Information
1. Definition: state in which cardiac output is inadequate to meet the metabolic needs of the body; characterized by circulatory congestion.
2. Etiology: one or more of the following
   a. Inflow of blood to heart greatly increased (e.g., excessive IV fluids or sodium and water retention)
   b. Outflow of blood from heart obstructed (e.g., damaged valves, narrowed arteries)
   c. Functional capacity of myocardium decreased; (e.g., myocardial infarction, dysrhythmias)
   d. Metabolic needs of body accelerated (e.g., fever, pregnancy)
3. Cardiac compensation
   a. Mechanisms
      1. *tachycardia:* increases cardiac output
      2. *ventricular dilation:* increases volume of chambers
      3. *myocardial hypertrophy:* fibers of nyocardium increase in length and diameter; heart contracts more forcibly
   b. Terminology
      1. *compensated CHF:* compensatory changes maintain adequate cardiac output
      2. *decompensated CHF:* compensatory changes unable to maintain adequate cardiac output; CHF becomes symptomatic
4. Left-sided congestive heart failure: left ventricle cannot accept all blood from pulmonary bed
   a. Etiology
      1. hypertension
      2. mitral and/or aortic valvular disease
      3. ischemic heart disease: damage or infarction of the left ventricle
   b. Pathophysiology: blood backs up in the *pulmonary bed* (see Table 3-14 for signs and symptoms)
5. Right-sided congestive heart failure: right ventricle cannot eject all blood from right atrium; therefore right atrium cannot accept all blood from systemic circulation
   a. Etiology
      1. left-sided CHF
      2. pulmonary disease
      3. tricuspid and pulmonic valvular disease
      4. ischemic heart disease: damage or infarction of the myocardium of the right ventricle
   b. Pathophysiology: blood backs up in systemic circulation (see Table 3-14 for signs and symptoms)

Table 3-14   Congestive heart failure

Results	Signs and symptoms
PATHOPHYSIOLOGY OF LEFT SIDE OF HEART: Blood backs up from left ventricle to *pulmonary* bed.	
Pulmonary congestion	Dyspnea, orthopnea, rales, paroxysmal nocturnal dyspnea
Pulmonary edema	(PND), decreased vital capacity, cyanosis
Cerebral anoxia	Irritability, restlessness, confusion
Decreased O_2 to cells	Extreme weakness, fatigue, oliguria
PATHOPHYSIOLOGY OF RIGHT SIDE OF HEART: Blood backs up from right ventricle to *systemic* circulation.	
Increased hydrostatic pressure in systemic circulation	Peripheral pitting edema, dependent edema: sacrum, ankles
Elevated venous pressure	Distended neck veins
Congestion in kidneys, retention of sodium	Oliguria
Venous congestion in extremities	Cool and cyanotic legs
Congestion in GI tract	Anorexia, nausea, bloating

Nursing Process

Assessment

1. Left-sided CHF
   a. Dyspnea
   b. Abnormal breath sounds (i.e., rales)
   c. Abnormal heart sounds (i.e., S_3)
   d. Arterial blood gas studies showing decreased Po^2 (i.e., less than 80mm Hg)
2. Right-sided CHF
   a. Elevated central venous pressure
   b. Distended neck veins
   c. Hepatomegaly (enlargement of the liver)
   d. Abnormal liver function (hepatic congestion)
   e. Peripheral pitting edema
3. Both right- and left-sided congestive heart failure (CHF)
   a. Cardiomegaly; displacement of point of maximal impulse (PMI)
   b. Oliguria
   c. Weight gain
   d. Tachycardia

Analysis (see p. 126)

Planning, Implementation, and Evaluation

Goal 1: Client will experience increased force and strength of contraction of the ventricles.

Implementation
1. Administer cardiac glycosides as ordered (see Table 3-15).
2. Monitor vital signs closely.

Evaluation
Client's heart rate is stable within normal range (e.g., 80 beats/min).

Goal 2: Client will eliminate excess fluid.

Implementation
1. Give diuretics as ordered (see Tables 3-16 and 3-42)
2. Keep accurate I&O.
3. Weigh daily.
4. Restrict sodium intake.

Evaluation
Client's weight decreases to preCHF level.

Goal 3: See General Nursing Goal 2, p. 127.

Goal 4: See General Nursing Goal 3, p. 127.

Goal 5: Client will remain free from pulmonary edema.

Implementation
1. Monitor closely for symptoms
   a. Severe dyspnea
   b. Audible rales
   c. Frothy, blood-tinged sputum
   d. Extreme anxiety
2. Institute therapy *immediately* if pulmonary edema develops.
   a. Place in Fowler's position.
   b. Give O_2 by positive pressure if available (increases O_2 and helps to push fluid from alveolar space).
   c. Apply rotating tourniquets (see Fig. 3-8) to reduce circulating blood volume by obstructing *venous* flow in three extremities.
      1. rotate one tourniquet every 15 minutes in *one* direction.
      2. remove one at a time when edema is controlled.
   d. Give morphine sulfate IV (relieves anxiety and dilates pulmonary vascular bed).
   e. Administer cardiac glycosides (see Table 3-15 as ordered.
   f. Give diuretic as ordered (e.g., furosemide); see Tables 3-16 and 3-42.
   g. Give aminophylline IV (see Table 3-18).

Evaluation
Client has normal respiratory rate (e.g., 16/min); client's lung fields are clear on auscultation.

Goal 6: Client and significant others will be able to explain need for care after discharge.

Implementation
1. Teach
   a. Level of activity, balance between activity and rest.

Table 3-15 Cardiac glycoside drugs

Name	Action	Side effects	Nursing implications
Digitalis leaf Digitoxin (Crystodigin, Purodigin) Digoxin (Lanoxin) Lanatoside C injection (Cedilanid)	Increases strength of myocardial contraction. Cardiac output is increased. Decreases heart rate. Promotes diuresis.	GI upset, visual disturbances, dysrhythmias, heart block. Hypokalemia potentiates digitalis action.	Take pulse before administration: if above 120 or below 60, hold medication and notify MD. Monitor serum K. High-potassium diet as needed.

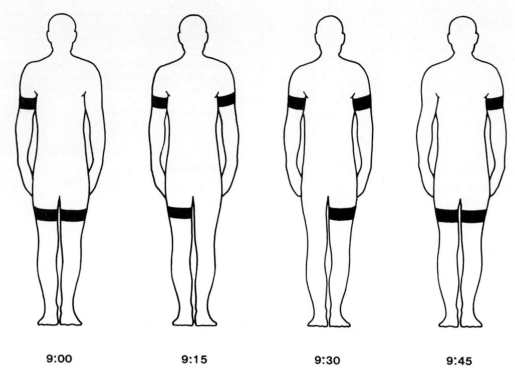

| 9:00 | 9:15 | 9:30 | 9:45 |

Fig. 3-8   Pattern for rotating tourniquets. Rotate one tourniquet every 15 minutes in the same direction.

Table 3-16   Antihypertensive drugs

Name	Action	Side effects	Nursing implications
DIURETIC AGENTS			
Thiazide diuretics Benzthiazide (Exna) Chlorothiazide (Diuril) Hydrochlorothiazide (Oretic, HydroDIURIL, Esidrix) **Potent, rapid-acting diuretics** Ethacrynic acid (Edecrin) Furosemide (Lasix)	Increases sodium and chloride excretion by inhibiting renal reabsorption. Enhances potassium excretion. Relaxes peripheral arteriolar smooth muscles. Increases sodium and chloride excretion by inhibiting renal reabsorption. Enhances potassium excretion.	*Hypokalemia:* weakness, paresthesias, muscle cramps, nausea, paralytic ileus, cardiac disturbances *Hyponatremia:* thirst, diminished sweating, fever, weakness, confusion *Hyperuricemia:* usually asymptomatic; can cause gouty arthritis *Hyperglycemia:* usually asymptomatic; can cause nausea, vomiting, polydipsia, polyphagia, weight loss, dehydration; sensitivity reactions, GI disturbances	Monitor I&O, BP, weight, serum electrolytes. Modify dietary sodium and potassium as needed.
Potassium-conserving diuretics Spironolactone (Aldactone)	Increases sodium and chloride excretion, and decreases potassium excretion by blocking aldosterone (adrenal cortex mineralocorticoid).	*Hyperkalemia:* weakness, paresthesias, cardiac disturbances *Hyponatremia:* GI disturbances, sensitivity reactions	

Table 3-16 Antihypertensive drugs—cont'd

Name	Action	Side effects	Nursing implications
SYMPATHETIC INHIBITING AGENTS			
Reserpine (Serpasil, Reserpoid, Sandril, Rau-Sed)	Acts by various complex mechanisms to inhibit synthesis, storage, and/or transport of norepinephrine, thereby depressing sympathetic nerve activity—as a result, cardiac output and/or peripheral vascular resistance are decreased. Reserpine and methyldopa also have central depressant effects.	Depression, nightmares, suicidal ideas, drowsiness, bradycardia, GI disturbances, dry mouth, increased appetite, excessive gastric secretion, nasal congestion	Monitor BP, P, weight. Teach importance of compliance. Advise hard candy for dry mouth. Instruct to rise and change position slowly.
Methyldopa (Aldomet)		Depression (less than reserpine), drowsiness (tends to subside with continued use), decreased mental acuity, GI disturbances, sodium and water retention, and loss of libido, sexual impotence and postural hypotension; less than guanethidine	
Guanethidine (Ismelin)		Postural hypotension, generalized muscle weakness especially on arising, diarrhea and other GI disturbances, sodium and fluid retention, failure to ejaculate, sensitivity to sympathomimetics found in some cold remedies (can result in hypertensive crisis)	
Propranolol (Inderal)	See Table 3-9		
VASODILATING AGENT			
Hydralazine (Apresoline) Nitroprusside (Nipride) injection	Acts directly on vascular smooth muscle to decrease peripheral resistance—relaxant effect more marked on arterioles than veins. Increases cardiac output, renal blood flow, and plasma renin activity.	Headache, flushing, tachycardia, palpitation, angina, GI disturbances, lupuslike syndrome (especially long-term administration with high doses), sodium and fluid retention	Monitor BP, P, weight. Teach importance of compliance. Instruct to rise and change position slowly.
ANGIOTENSIN-CONVERTING ENZYME (ACE) INHIBITORS			
Captopril (Capoten) Enalapril (Vasotec) Lisinopril (Prinivil, Zestril)	Inhibit conversion of angiotensin I to angiotensin II; prevent vasoconstriction and decrease aldosterone secretion; decrease vascular resistance and venous return.	Anorexia, tachycardia, hypotension, loss of taste, proteinuria, nephrotic syndrome, leukopenia, agranulocytosis, rash, dizziness	Monitor BP, heart rate. Caution elderly clients, clients with renal insufficiency or lupus, or clients taking other drugs that may affect WBC or immune response. Monitor WBC and differential. Check for proteinuria. Frequently used with a thiazide diuretic. Administer 1 hour before meals.
CALCIUM CHANNEL BLOCKERS			
Nifedipine (Procardia) Diltiazem (Cardizem) Verapamil (Calan)	See Table 3-9.		

Table 3-17 Foods high in potassium

Food	Portion	Potassium (mEq)
Whole milk	1 cup	9.0
Broiled meat	3 oz	9.6
Apricots (canned)	4 halves	7.9
Banana	1 small	9.5
Honeydew melon	⅛ medium	9.6
Fresh orange	1 medium	9.5
Dried prunes	4 large	12.0
Watermelon	½ slice (1 in. thick)	15.3
Baked potato	1 medium	12.9
Dried lima beans	½ cup cooked	14.5
Soybeans	½ cup cooked	13.8
Winter squash	½ cup cooked	10.0
Dried white beans	½ cup cooked	10.6

    b. Sodium-restricted diet (see Table 3-12), high-potassium diet as necessary (see Table 3-17).
    c. Medication administration, schedule, side effects.
    d. Application of antiembolic hose.
2. Instruct client to weigh daily to monitor fluid balance.

Evaluation

    Client correctly describes care needs for home (e.g., drug therapy, how to take own pulse).

☐ Hypertension

General Information

1. Definition: a chronic elevation of systemic arterial BP in which the systolic pressure is *consistently* over 140 mm Hg and the diastolic is 90 mm Hg or higher
2. Incidence
    a. Affects all age groups
    b. Prevalence increases with age
    c. One of the major causes of illness and death in the United States
3. Blood pressure physiology
    a. Determinants
        1. cardiac output
        2. total peripheral resistance
    b. Regulation
        1. neural stimulation: autonomic nervous system
        2. humoral stimulation (e.g., catecholamines, aldosterone, angiotensin)
4. Pathophysiology
    a. No obvious early pathological changes in blood vessels and organs
    b. Large vessels (aorta, coronary arteries, basilar artery to brain, peripheral vessels in limbs) eventually become sclerosed and tortuous
    c. Lumens narrow, resulting in decreased blood flow to heart, brain, and lower extremities
    d. Vessels become completely occluded, or rupture resulting in hemorrhage

    e. Damage to the intima of small vessels causes local edema and intravascular clotting
    f. Decreased blood supply to tissues of heart, brain, kidneys, and eyes causes dysfunction of these organs
5. Types
    a. *Primary* (essential): approximately 90% of all cases: etiology unknown; types include
        1. *benign:* slowly progressive
        2. *malignant:* rapidly accelerating
    b. *Secondary:* approximately 10%-15% of all cases; caused by an identifiable primary disease (e.g., pheochromocytoma, kidney disease)
6. Predisposing factors
    a. Stress
    b. Familial history
    c. Obesity

Nursing Process

Assessment
1. BP elevated on at least three different occasions
2. Headache
3. Change in vision (hemorrhages in retina, blurred vision)
4. Epistaxis
5. Personality change: forgetful and irritable
Analysis (see p. 126)
Planning, Implementation, and Evaluation

> **Goal 1:** Client's BP will decrease to safe level and permanent damage will be prevented.

Implementation
1. Monitor BP.
2. Modify life-style to reduce stress.
3. Modify diet.
    a. Calories reduced if client is obese.
    b. Sodium restricted (see Table 3-12).
    c. High potassium if needed (see Table 3-17).
4. Exercise in a regular, planned program.
5. Avoid smoking.
6. Administer antihypertensive medications as ordered (see Table 3-16).

Evaluation

    Client's elevated blood pressure is reduced to 140/90.

> **Goal 2:** Client will carry out self-care activities after discharge.

Implementation
1. Teach client to:
    a. Take own BP.
    b. Modify life-style.
    c. Institute exercise program.
    d. Manage diet (sodium-restricted and low-calorie, high-potassium as necessary) (see Tables 3-12 and 3-17).

e. Understand medications (see Table 3-16).
1. administration
2. schedule
3. side effects
4. importance of compliance
f. Stop smoking.
g. Remember importance of follow-up care.

Evaluation

Client lists all components of therapeutic regimen; keeps an appointment for return visit.

☐ Circulatory Problems

General Information

1. Definition: problems caused by changes in arterial and venous blood vessels peripheral to the heart
2. Types of arterial problems
   a. *Arteriosclerosis obliterans:* atherosclerotic plaque formation that involves arteries of lower extremities; occurs in men aged 50-70 and women after menopause
   b. *Raynaud's disease:* intermittent constricting spasms of arterioles of digits and extremities, resulting in pain and cyanosis
   c. *Buerger's disease* (thromboangiitis obliterans): disease characterized by diffuse, inflammatory, proliferative changes in arteries and veins of extremities
3. Types of venous problems
   a. *Varicose veins:* dilated, tortuous superficial veins; incompetent valves cause dilation; increased pressure causes tortuosity; increased capillary pressure causes edema
   b. *Varicose ulcers:* ulcers resulting from circulatory insufficiency
   c. *Thrombophlebitis:* inflammation of vessel with thrombus formation
   d. *Phlebothrombosis:* thrombus formation in a vein without inflammation

Nursing Process: Arterial Problems

Assessment

Signs or symptoms of impaired peripheral arterial circulation (see Fig. 3-9)

Analysis (see p. 126)

Planning, Implementation, and Evaluation

> **Goal 1:** Client will have adequate arterial blood flow to extremities.

Implementation

1. Teach client to eliminate or avoid
   a. Tobacco.
   b. Exposure to temperature extremes.
   c. Trauma
   1. tissue injury and infections
   2. maintain good foot care
   d. Excessive exercise

e. Vasospastic drugs (e.g., epinephrine)
f. Constrictive clothing
2. Walk to tolerance to promote collateral circulation.
3. Modify diet
   a. Low cholesterol
   b. Moderate fat
   c. Reduced calories if client is obese
4. Give thrombolytics or anticoagulants as ordered (see Table 3-11).

Evaluation

Client's extremities are warm; peripheral pulses are strong.

> **Goal 2:** Client will have minimal discomfort.

Implementation

1. Have client rest when pain occurs.
2. Administer vasodilator adrenergic medications as ordered (e.g., isoxsuprine [Vasodilan]).

Evaluation

Client develops schedule of activities that keeps pain under control.

> **Goal 3:** Client will be able to explain when surgery might be used; will be free from preventable complications.

Implementation

1. Know that bypass surgery may be used if client has localized occlusion with arteriosclerosis obliterans; that infrequently sympathectomy may be used to treat Buerger's disease; that amputation is the treatment for gangrene.
2. Provide postoperative care: avoid strain on incision (do not bend joint over which graft passes), monitor for hemorrhage resulting from disruption of graft or occlusion of graft, administer anticoagulants as ordered (see Table 3-11).
3. See "Amputation," p. 261.

Evaluation

Client explains the type of surgery that he may receive; is free from complications postoperatively (e.g., split incision, frank hemorrhage).

Nursing Process: Venous Problems

Assessment

Signs and symptoms of impaired venous circulation (see Fig. 3-9)

Analysis (see p. 126)

Planning, Implementation, and Evaluation

> **Goal 1:** Client will have adequate venous blood flow from extremities.

Implementation

1. Teach client to eliminate or avoid
   a. Tobacco

**Chronic Venous Insufficiency
(Advanced)**

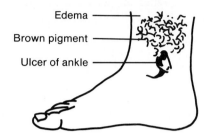

Edema ——
Brown pigment ——
Ulcer of ankle ——

**Chronic Arterial Insufficiency
(Advanced)**

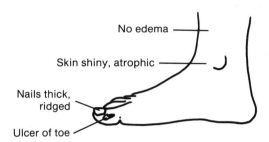

No edema ——
Skin shiny, atrophic ——
Nails thick,
ridged ——
Ulcer of toe ——

	Venous Conditions	Arterial Conditions
Pathophysiology	Impaired/occluded peripheral *venous* circulation	Impaired/occluded peripheral *arterial* circulation
Involved areas	Lower extremities	Upper and lower extremities
Signs and symptoms		
Pain	None or aching tiredness plus Homan's sign (thrombophlebitis)	Severe ischemic (e.g., intermittent claudication) Late: pain on rest
Edema	Pronounced	Usually none
Peripheral pulses	Present, difficult to palpate with edema	Diminished or absent
Skin	Thickened Stasis dermatitis	Trophic changes: shiny, hairless, tightly drawn, dry, and scaly skin; thick ridged nails
Color	Brawny pigmentation of ankle and lower leg Cyanosis with dependency	Pallor/cyanosis Rubor with dependency
Temperature	Warm	Cool or cold
Ulcers	May develop; nonpainful	May develop; painful
Gangrene	Not present	Present with occlusion
Effect of position		
Elevation	Improves symptoms	Aggravates symptoms
Dependency	Aggravates symptoms	Improves symptoms
Common conditions	Varicose veins Varicose ulcers Thrombophlebitis	Arteriosclerosis obliterans Raynaud's disease Buerger's disease

Fig. 3-9   Common manifestations of chronic arterial and venous peripheral vascular disease.

b. Injury and infections
c. Constrictive clothing (e.g., garters)
d. Standing or sitting for long periods
e. Crossing legs at knee
f. Oral contraceptives
2. Teach client to
    a. Wear antiembolic hose
    b. Elevate legs
    c. Do ankle push-ups when standing (promotes venous return)

Evaluation

Client's lower extremities are warm and free from edema.

Goal 2: Client with thrombophlebitis will be protected from dislodgement of thrombus.

Implementation
1. Maintain bed rest 7-10 days.
2. Prevent Valsalva maneuver.
3. Elevate legs.
4. Apply antiembolic hose.
5. Apply warm, moist packs to involved site (prevent burns).
6. Do not rub legs.
7. Give anticoagulant therapy as ordered (see Table 3-11).

Evaluation

Client is free from any signs or symptoms of pulmonary embolism.

Goal 3: Client's leg ulcers will heal.

Implementation
1. Maintain bed rest with leg elevated when ulcer is acute.
2. Monitor for signs of cellulitis and report immediately.
3. Give antibiotics as ordered if infected.
4. Know and inform client that skin grafting may be necessary.
5. Explain the long-term nature of treatment to client.

Evaluation

Client's ulcer remains clean, uninfected; heals well.

SELECTED HEALTH PROBLEMS RESULTING IN INTERFERENCE WITH PULMONARY FUNCTION

☐ Chronic Obstructive Pulmonary Disease (COPD) or Chronic Obstructive Lung Disease (COLD)

General Information

1. Definition: chronic respiratory disorders that involve a persistent obstruction of bronchial airflow
2. Incidence
    a. Fastest growing cause of death in the United States
    b. Occurs in adults and children

3. Predisposing factors
    a. Smoking
    b. Environmental factors: smoke, coal, hay, asbestos, air pollution
    c. Allergic factors
    d. Chronic, recurrent respiratory infections
    e. Genetic factors (possibly)
4. Pathophysiology
    a. Thoracic excursion is reduced because of bronchial obstruction, air trapping, and thoracic overdistension; possible inflammatory reaction in airways causes bronchial spasm and increased secretions
    b. Tidal volume, vital capacity, and inspiratory reserve necessary for effective coughing are decreased
    c. Person employs accessory muscles of respiration to facilitate breathing; purses lips to maintain open bronchioles with expiration
    d. Bronchial obstruction and air trapping lead to destruction of lung, permanently reduced alveolar ventilation, and CO_2 retention
    e. Decreased resistance increases susceptibility to respiratory infections (e.g., pneumonia)
    f. Respiratory acidosis (compensated) commonly occurs secondary to chronic CO_2 retention
5. Hypoxemia
    a. Definition: deficient oxygenation of the blood
    b. Frequently chronic, possibly acute
    c. Characterized by
        1. subtle changes in mentation such as restlessness, agitation, headache, drowsiness, and confusion (because of less O_2 to the brain and stimulation of the sympathetic nervous system)
        2. tachycardia, hyperventilation will be seen early in hypoxia; possibly followed by bradycardia and hypoventilation
        3. hypertension because of sympathetic nervous system stimulation may be present early with hypoxia
        4. decreased Po_2 (less than 80 mm Hg)
        5. late: cyanosis
6. Hypercapnia
    a. Definition: excess of CO_2 in blood
    b. Can occur with hypoxemia; may be chronic or acute
    c. Characterized by
        1. CNS depression: drowsiness, inability to concentrate, progressive loss of consciousness
        2. early behavioral changes: irritability; inability to get along with others; discontentment with food, care, etc; inability to sleep
        3. headache
        4. rubor
        5. tremors, dizziness, cardiac dysrhythmias
        6. increased Pco_2 (greater than 45 mm Hg)
7. Common examples of COPD

a. *Bronchial asthma:* a chronic disease characterized by episodic attacks of respiratory distress resulting from constriction of the bronchi and bronchioles (refer to *Nursing Care of the Child*, p. 427)

b. *Chronic bronchitis*

1. definition: chronic inflammation of the bronchi with production of large amount of sputum that causes bronchial obstruction

2. etiology and pathophysiology: air pollution or smoking cause inflammation of bronchial mucosa with resulting edema and copious production of mucus; also, person is predisposed to recurrent respiratory infections by reduced ciliary motility in the bronchi

c. *Emphysema*

1. definition: chronic lung condition characterized by abnormal enlargement of alveoli and alveolar ducts with destruction of alveolar walls

2. eitology: exact cause not identified

3. pathophysiology: air trapped behind partially obstructed bronchioles produces overdistention and destruction of alveoli; loss of elastic recoil of lungs reduces respiratory flow; barrel chest develops

Nursing Process

Assessment

1. Respiratory distress (dyspnea on exertion progressing to dyspnea at rest)
2. Apprehension
3. Cough (productive)
4. Lethargy (results from hypoxemia)
5. Use of accessory muscles
6. Abnormal breath sounds (rales, rhonchi, wheezing, decreased breath sounds)
7. Weight loss
8. Skin color
   a. flushed (hypercapnia)
   b. Cyanosis (hypoxemia)
9. Abnormal pulmonary function tests (e.g., decreased expiratory and inspiratory volumes, increased residual volume)
10. Blood gases
    a. PO_2 decreased only with activity at first, then decreased continuously
    b. PCO_2 increases as disease worsens
11. Respiratory acidosis, compensated (from chronic CO_2 retention)

Table 3-18   Bronchodilator drugs*

Name	Action	Side effects	Nursing implications
ADRENERGIC AGENTS			
Epinephrine (Adrenalin) Ephedrine	Stimulates alpha- and beta-adrenergic receptors of sympathetic nervous system. alpha: peripheral vasoconstriction, increased BP. beta: bronchodilation, increased cardiac irritability, increased heart rate.	Nervousness, tremors, headache, palpitation, tachycardia, dysrhythmias	Monitor BP, pulse. Use cautiously for clients with hypertension and coronary insufficiency.
Isoproterenol (Isuprel)	Stimulates beta-adrenergic receptors of sympathetic nervous system: relaxes bronchioles, stimulates heart.	Similar to epinephrine	
Terbutaline (Brethine) Albuterol (Proventil, Ventolin) Metaproterenol (Alupent)	Selective beta-2 agonists.	Similar to epinephrine and Isuprel with fewer cardiovascular effects.	
XANTHINE COMPOUNDS			
Aminophylline Theophylline	Relaxes smooth muscle of bronchial airway and blood vessels. Also has diuretic effect. Acts synergistically with adrenergic bronchodilators.	Dizziness, hypotension, restlessness, dysrhythmias, GI irritation (oral), cardiac stimulation	Monitor BP; observe for hypotension. Give oral preparations with food.

*See also Table 5-18.

12. Frequent respiratory infections (decreased resistance)

Analysis (see p. 126)

Planning, Implementation, and Evaluation

> **Goal 1:** Client will maintain a PO_2 of at least 60 mm Hg; airway will be clear, sputum will be thin and clear.

Implementation

1. See General Nursing Goal 1, p. 127.
2. Administer bronchodilators as ordered (see Table 3-18).
3. Administer expectorants (see Table 3-19) as ordered.
4. Administer nebulizer as ordered.
   a. Bronchodilators (see Table 3-18)
   b. Mucolytics (see Table 3-19)
5. Teach relaxation techniques and breathing exercises (e.g., pursed-lip breathing).
6. Administer low concentrations of humidified O_2 (1-2 L/min); CAUTION: high O_2 flow may precipitate respiratory failure in presence of hypercapnia and hypoxia.
7. Encourage activity to tolerance.
8. If client must be confined to bed for any period (usually infection or asthma attack)
   a. Use semi-Fowler's or Fowler's position.
   b. Turn frequently.
   c. Encourage to take frequent deep breaths and to breathe out slowly and completely.
   d. Perform active ROM exercises (passive if client too weak to do active exercises).
   e. Employ diversional activites to avoid napping during the day so as to prevent insomnia and nocturnal restlessness.
      NOTE: *avoid bed rest if at all possible to prevent hypoventilation, stasis of secretions, weakened ventilatory muscles, weakness of other muscles, and decreased cough reflex.*
9. Give diet as tolerated (e.g., small amounts of soft food 4-5 times/day); increase fluids unless contraindicated.

Evaluation

Client's PO_2 remains greater than 60 mm Hg; pH remains between 7.35 and 7.45; sputum is clear and thin.

> **Goal 2:** Client will be protected from any injuries.

Implementation

1. Know that with hypoxia, hypercapnia, or uncompensated respiratory acidosis, client may be lethargic, confused, or comatose.
2. Use bed's side rails, pad if necessary.
3. Keep bed low to floor.
4. Avoid restraints, sedatives, or tranquilizers.
5. If client is confused, have someone stay with client.
6. Maintain quiet environment.
7. Speak in low, calm, soothing tone.

Evaluation

Client is free from injury.

> **Goal 3:** Client will be protected from CO_2 narcosis.

Implementation

1. Know that uncontrolled O_2 delivery will eliminate hypoxic drive of respirations.
2. Administer O_2 at *low* concentrations (1-2 L/min).
3. Observe for symptoms of narcosis with O_2 therapy.
   a. Decreased respiratory rate and depth
   b. Headache
   c. Skin changes (flushing)
   d. Behavioral changes: confusion progressing to coma
   e. Blood gases
      1. increased PCO_2
      2. *increased* PO_2
   f. Respiratory failure

Table 3-19   Cough medications*

Name	Action	Side effects	Nursing implications
EXPECTORANTS			
Ammonium chloride Guaifenesin (Robitussin) Potassium iodide (SSKI)	Increases bronchial mucus secretion. Facilitates the expulsion of viscid, tenacious sputum.	Nausea, vomiting Drowsiness Gastric irritation	Force fluids: 6-8 glasses/day. Water alone may be the most effective expectorant.
MUCOLYTIC			
Acetylcysteine (Mucomyst, Airbron)	Inhalant; liquefies respiratory mucus.	Bronchospasm (especially asthmatics); nausea, vomiting, rhinitis, stomatitis	Use cautiously for clients with asthma.

*See also Table 5-18.

Table 3-20   Antibiotic drugs

Name	Action	Side effects	Nursing implications
			All antibiotics: take culture if ordered *before* starting antibiotic. instruct client to take *entire* prescription.
PENICILLIN			
Penicillin G: crystalline (Cryspen) IV or IM procaine (Wycillin) IM only benzathine (Bicillin) IM only **Penicillin V:** (Pen-Vee K) oral	Bactericidal (interferes with cell-wall synthesis); effective against numerous gram-positive cocci, spirochetes, actinomycetes, and some gram-negative organisms.	Hypersensitivity (rash, urticaria, anaphylaxis); GI disturbance (oral); superinfection	Check allergy history before giving. Observe for hypersensitivity.
Penicillin-resistant penicillin: oxacillin (Prostaphlin) methicillin (Staphcillin) nafcillin (Unipen)	Semisynthetic penicillin; effective against penicillin-resistant organisms such as *S. aureus.*	Same as Penicillin G and V	Same as Penicillin G and V.
Broad-spectrum penicillin: ampicillin (Polycillin) amoxicillin (Amoxil)	Semisynthetic penicillin; effective against many gram-positive and gram-negative organisms.	Same as Penicillin G and V	Same as Penicillin G and V.
CEPHALOSPORINS Cephalothin (Keflin) Cephalexin (Keflex)	Bactericidal (inhibits cell-wall synthesis); effective against most gram-positive cocci and many strains of gram-negative bacilli (similar to penicillin).	GI disturbance, hypersensitivity (rash), nephrotoxicity, cross-sensitivity to penicillin (but anaphylaxis rare)	Monitor renal function. Check for history of allergy to penicillin.
TETRACYCLINES Tetracycline* (Achromycin) Minocycline (Minocin)	Bacteriostatic (inhibits protein synthesis); effective against wide variety of gram-positive and gram-negative organisms, rickettsiae, chlamydia, trophozoite forms of amebae, and actinomycetes.	GI disturbance; hypersensitivity (rash, urticaria); photosensitivity; superinfection; permanent discoloration during tooth development	Do not give with milk, food, or antacids. Avoid sun exposure. Do not administer to pregnant women or children under 8 years.
AMINOGLYCOSIDES Neomycin* Gentamicin (Garamycin) Kanamycin (Kantrex) Streptomycin†	Bactericidal (inhibits protein synthesis); effective against a wide range of gram-positive and gram-negative organisms and mycobacteria.	Ototoxicity Nephrotoxicity	Monitor hearing function. Monitor renal function.

*See also Table 3-58.
†See also Table 3-21.

Table 3-20 Antibiotic drugs—cont'd

Name	Action	Side effects	Nursing implications
POLYPEPTIDES			
Bacitracin*	Bactericidal (hinders cell-wall synthesis); effective against most gram-positive organisms.	Nephrotoxicity	Used primarily as topical agent because of its nephrotoxicity.
Polymyxins*: Polymyxin B (Aerosporin) Colistin (Coly-Mycin)	Bactericidal (hinders cell-wall synthesis); effective against nearly all gram-negative organisms, except the *Proteus* group.	Nephrotoxicity Neuromuscular blockade	Used topically. Use parenterally with caution. Parenteral: monitor renal function; use cautiously for clients with respiratory insufficiency.

4. Help with ventilation when needed.

Evaluation

Client maintains spontaneous respirations.

Goal 4: Client will live as actively as possible within the limitations of the disease.

Implementation

1. Teach client
   a. Level of activity: balance of activity and rest
   b. Breathing and relaxation exercises
   c. Effective coughing
   d. Postural drainage
   e. Diet
      1. small, frequent, high-calorie meals
      2. adequate fluids
   f. Medications
      1. administration
      2. schedule
      3. side effects
   g. Use of O_2 equipment
   h. Preventive health habits
      1. stop smoking
      2. avoid respiratory infections
      3. seek *early* treatment for respiratory infections
      4. avoid factors that precipitate bronchospasms (e.g., pollens, air pollutants)
      5. take flu and pneumococcal vaccines

Evaluation

Client develops a schedule that allows activities of daily living, work obligations, and social activities.

☐ Pneumonia

General Information

1. Definition: acute inflammation of the alveolar spaces of the lung
2. Etiology
   a. Microorganisms
      1. bacteria
      2. viruses
      3. fungi
   b. Chemicals
      1. inhalation (e.g., smoke)
      2. aspiration (e.g., vomitus)
3. Predisposing factors
   a. Decreased immunity (e.g., COPD)
   b. Debility (e.g., malnutrition)
   c. Immobility (e.g., after surgery)
4. Pathophysiology
   a. Causative agent is inhaled
   b. Alveoli becomes inflamed and edematous
   c. Alveolar spaces fill with exudate
   d. Diffusion of O_2 and CO_2 is obstructed
   e. Involved lung tissue becomes consolidated

Nursing Process

Assessment

1. Chills, fever, and malaise
2. Chest pain (limits chest excursion)
3. Respirations: rapid, shallow, dyspneic; pain with pleuritic involvement
4. Tachycardia
5. Productive cough
6. Sputum
   a. Viscid, tenacious
   b. Color ranging from rusty to yellow
   c. Culture positive for causative microorganism
7. Breath sounds (diminished over involved areas, rales, and pleural friction rub)
8. Percussion dullness
9. Dehydration (if fever unchecked)
10. Leukocytosis
11. Abnormal chest x-ray
12. Cyanosis with advanced hypoxia

Analysis (see p. 126)

Planning, Implementation, and Evaluation

> **Goal 1:** Client's pulmonary ventilation will improve.

Implementation
1. See General Nursing Goal, p. 127.
2. Administer organism-specific antibiotics (see Table 3-20).
3. Administer expectorants prn (see Table 3-19).
4. Discourage antitussives.
5. Care for tracheostomy if present (see tracheostomy care, p. 155).
6. Administer analgesics for chest pain.
7. Provide good oral hygiene.

Evaluation
Client has decreased dyspnea.

> **Goal 2:** Client will remain free from atelectasis.

Implementation
1. Assess client status q2-4h for atelectasis (area of lung that is collapsed and airless).
2. Position client on unaffected side.
3. Check pulse rate.
4. See General Nursing Goal 1, p. 127.

Evaluation
Client has clear lungs on auscultation; breathes easily.

> **Goal 3:** Client will be able to care for self after discharge.

Implementation
1. Teach
   a. Activity level
   b. Avoid overfatigue
   c. Medications
      1. administration
      2. schedule
      3. side effects
   d. Breathing exercises
2. Prevent recurrence in high-risk clients: pneumococcal vaccine.

Evaluation
Client develops a realistic plan for balanced rest and activity; knows actions and side effects of all prescribed medications.

☐ Tuberculosis

General Information
1. Definition: a reportable, communicable disease usually affecting the respiratory system; opportunistic infection
2. Incidence: 9.3 cases/100,000 U.S. population; higher in nonwhites
3. Etiology: *Mycobacterium tuberculosis*, an acid-fast bacillus
4. Predisposing factors
   a. Lowered resistance caused by
      1. overcrowding
      2. poor sanitation
      3. poor nutrition
      4. poorly ventilated living conditions
      5. debilitating diseases
      6. immunosuppressive conditions
   b. Virulence of organism
   c. Length of exposure
5. Pathophysiology: tuberculosis bacillus is usually inhaled; transmitted by droplet produced by individual with active disease
   a. Most common site of implantation is on alveolar surface of lung parenchyma
   b. Induces hypersensitivity reaction in host
   c. Inflammation occurs, then acute pneumonia develops
   d. Caseous nodule (tubercle) is formed around organism
   e. Organism never completely disappears but is walled off in lungs
   f. May remain quiescent for long time, but physical and emotional stress can cause organism to become active and multiply (reactivation process)
   g. Inflammation can occur and tuberculous process begins again
   h. Disease may also spread through lymphatics and vascular system (miliary tuberculosis)
   i. If medical therapy fails, surgical resection of one or more lobes may be advised

Nursing Process
Assessment
1. Dyspnea
2. Pleuritic pain
3. Rales
4. Fatigue
5. Night sweats
6. Low-grade fever in afternoon
7. Weight loss
8. Anorexia
9. Hemoptysis (late symptom)
10. Positive skin testing
    a. OT (old tuberculin)
    b. PPD (purified protein derivative) is most reliable
       1. *Intradermal* injection on inner aspect of forearm
       2. Negative reaction: absence of erythema and/or induration after 48 hours
       3. Positive reaction: greater than 10 mm area of *induration* in 48 hours
          a. indicates contact with tuberculosis bacillus but not necessarily an active infection

b. do chest x-ray and sputum cultures if positive

c. do not repeat skin testing in future (screen with a chest x-ray)

d. prophylactic drug therapy may be indicated

11. Abnormal chest x-ray

12. Sputum culture positive for *Mycobacterium tuberculosis* (NOTE: May take 3-12 weeks to obtain positive result)

Analysis (see p. 126)

Planning, Implementation, and Evaluation

> **Goal 1:** Client's active tuberculosis will be arrested.

Implementation

1. Administer antituberculosis drugs as ordered (see Table 3-21).
   a. First-line drugs
   b. Second-line drugs

2. Provide adequate rest (*not* bed rest).
3. Institute nutritionally adequate diet.

Evaluation

Client's sputum culture converts to negative after 2 weeks of medications.

> **Goal 2:** Staff, client's family, and others will be protected from infection with tuberculosis.

Implementation

1. Maintain appropriate isolation.
   a. Necessary while client has positive sputum smear and culture or is coughing
   b. Discontinue after signs and symptoms disappear (often within 2 weeks after start of treatment)
2. Prevent the transmission of droplets.
   a. Cover mouth and nose when coughing, sneezing, or laughing
   b. Burn contaminated tissues
   c. Carefully wash hands when handling sputum

Table 3-21   Antituberculosis drugs

Name	Action	Side effects	Nursing implications
			All antituberculosis drugs: stress the importance of compliance.

FIRST-LINE DRUGS: Drugs used for primary therapy; often used in combination to potentiate effect (e.g., INH, rifampin, and ethambutol).

Name	Action	Side effects	Nursing implications
Isoniazid (INH)	Bactericidal (interferes with synthesis of cell wall)	Peripheral neuritis, pyridoxine deficiency (vitamin B_6); hepatotoxicity, glossitis, GI disturbance, hypersensitivity; fever	Give pyridoxine. Monitor liver function.
Rifampin (Rifadin)	Bactericidal (inhibits RNA synthesis)	Hepatotoxicity, GI disturbance, hypersensitivity; rash. May color urine and tears orange.	Instruct to expect orange body fluids.
Ethambutol (Myambutol)	Bacteriostatic (inhibits protein synthesis)	Optic neuritis: decreased acuity and loss of color discrimination; gout	Test vision frequently. Monitor serum uric acid.
Streptomycin	Bacteriostatic and bactericidal (inhibits protein synthesis)	Ototoxicity (eighth cranial nerve). Nephrotoxicity	Monitor ear and kidney function.

SECOND-LINE DRUGS: Therapy used when primary therapy cannot be used or has failed.

Pyrazinamide
Capreomycin (Capastat)
Cycloserine (Seromycin)
Ethionamide (Trecator-SC)
Kanamycin (Kantrex)
Paraaminosalicylic acid (PAS)

d. Adequately circulate air (air changes will dilute number of bacilli in air of isolated client's room)

e. Bacilli are killed by direct sunlight in 1-2 hours; boiling temperature of water kills bacilli in 5 minutes

3. Emphasize the importance of continuing prescribed medication.

4. Report to public health department for case finding.

Evaluation

Client's family does not contract tuberculosis.

Goal 3: Client will be able to cope with disease.

Implementation

1. Know there is a social stigma associated with tuberculosis.

2. Encourage expression of fears, concerns, or questions.

3. Spend time talking with client (see Table 2-4, p. 22)

Evaluation

Client verbalizes a desire to practice safe health measures.

Goal 4: Client will care for self at home and will practice health habits that prevent reactivation of infection.

Implementation

1. Teach

a. Medication administration, schedule, side effects, and importance of compliance.

b. Importance of activity.

c. Nutritious diet.

d. Isolation technique if necessary.

e. Not to swallow sputum.

f. Importance of follow-up care.

2. Arrange public health follow-up.

Evaluation

Client complies with medication regimen.

☐ Pulmonary Embolus
General Information

1. Definition: Obstruction of the pulmonary vascular bed; typically caused by a dislodged thrombus

2. Etiology: thrombus

3. Predisposing factors

a. Hypercoagulability (e.g., oral contraceptives, dehydration, aging)

b. Alterations in integrity of blood vessel (e.g., recent surgery, trauma to vessel wall, vasculitis)

c. Venous stasis (e.g., immobility, obesity, pregnancy, thrombus formation in heart, CHF)

4. Pathophysiology

a. Most emboli arise as detached portions of venous thrombi formed in the right side of the heart or in the deep veins of the legs or pelvic area

b. Dislodgment of thrombi is influenced by intravascular pressure changes, natural mechanism of clot dissolution

c. Acute pulmonary artery obstruction causes

1. increased alveolar dead space, loss of surfactant, alveolar collapse, regional atelectasis

2. increased resistance to pulmonary blood flow

3. acute right ventricular failure

Nursing Process
Assessment

1. Respirations: rapid, shallow, dyspneic

2. Tachycardia

3. Pleuritic chest pain

4. Cough, possibly hemoptysis

5. Anxiety, restlessness

6. Abnormal heart sounds (e.g., S_3, S_4)

7. Abnormal breath sounds (e.g., rales, pleural friction rub)

8. Fever, elevated WBC

9. Abnormal arterial blood gases; decreased P_{CO_2}, P_{O_2}

10. Abnormal chest x-ray and lung scan

11. Massive pulmonary embolism: sudden shock, cyanosis, tachypnea and respiratory distress, mental clouding and anxiety, feeling of impending doom

Analysis (see p. 126)
Planning, Implementation, and Evaluation

Goal 1: Client will be protected from development and dislodgment of thrombus.

Implementation

1. Encourage ambulation unless contraindicated.

2. Perform active and passive range of motion.

3. Apply antiembolic stockings.

4. Maintain adequate hydration, steady IV rates.

5. Avoid strain, Valsalva maneuver.

6. Turn, cough, deep-breathe every 2 hours.

7. Administer low-dose heparin as ordered.

Evaluation

Client is free from signs and symptoms of respiratory difficulty.

Goal 2: Client's pulmonary perfusion and ventilation will improve.

Implementation

1. Observe for signs and symptoms of hypoxia.

2. Monitor respiratory rate and rhythm.

3. Turn every 2 hours.

4. Administer O_2 at prescribed concentrations.

5. Administer thrombolytics or anticoagulants as ordered (see Table 3-11).

Evaluation

Client exhibits no respiratory distress; has pink nailbeds, normal skin and mucous membrane color.

Goal 3: Client will maintain adequate cardiac output.

Implementation

1. Monitor for signs and symptoms of acute right-ventricular heart failure.
2. Measure CVP as ordered.
3. Auscultate heart sounds.
4. Monitor cardiac rhythm.
5. Monitor I&O.
6. Administer pulmonary vasodilators (e.g., aminophylline) as ordered (see Table 3-18).
7. Administer diuretics (e.g., furosemide) (see Tables 3-16 and 3-42).

Evaluation

Client has normal heart rate and rhythm; BP, urine output within normal limits.

Goal 4: Client will experience reduced apprehension, fear, and anxiety.

Implementation

1. Administer sedation as ordered.
2. Provide a quiet, nonstimulating environment.
3. Provide calm reassurance.
4. Explain all procedures thoroughly.
5. Stay with client during episode of severe dyspnea or chest pain.

Evaluation

Client appears calm; verbalizes reduction in anxiety.

Goal 5: Client will remain free from recurrence of thrombus formation of pulmonary embolus.

Implementation

1. Teach
   a. Methods to prevent venous stasis
   b. Anticoagulant medication doses and side effects (see Table 3-11)

Evaluation

Client wears antiembolic stockings, avoids sitting or remaining in bed for long periods of time; takes anticoagulant drugs correctly.

☐ Chest Tubes and Chest Surgery
General Information

1. Clients who experience open-chest injuries or surgery require similar care because of the opening of the thoracic cavity and the subsequent use of chest tubes
2. Lung expansion: supported by
   a. Visceral and parietal pleura
   b. Pressure in pleural space
   c. Sucking effect on lung
3. Causes of disruption of airtight thoracic cavity
   a. Spontaneous pneumothorax

b. Stab wound
c. Bullet wound
d. Thoracotomy
e. Tear of pleura by fractured ribs

4. Tension pneumothorax
   a. Cause: closed chest wound; air is unable to escape on expiration; lung collapses and mediastinal contents shift to unaffected side of thorax as intrathoracic tension increases
   b. Emergency treatment: chest tube if available; otherwise, insert a needle to allow air to escape
5. Chest tube drainage
   a. Chest tube to open drainage bottle will not function: if atmospheric pressure is greater than intrathoracic pressure, lung will collapse
   b. Purpose of water seal: to seal off the end of chest tube so it acts as a one-way valve (air and fluid travel down the tube but atmospheric air cannot travel up the tube)
   c. 1-, 2-, or 3-bottle system of Pleur-Evac (see Figs. 3-10 and 3-11)
   d. Two chest tubes are used for client with lobectomy, segmental resection, or hemothorax; one chest tube is used with pneumothorax or cardiac surgery
      1. purpose
         a. to remove air and/or drainage from pleural space
         b. to help reexpand remaining lung tissue
         c. to prevent tension pneumothorax
      2. placement
         a. anterior, upper thoracic area for air removal
         b. second tube, if required, in posterior, lower thoracic area for drainage (drainage is heavier than air)
   e. No chest tubes used for client with pneumonectomy
      1. no lung left to reexpand
      2. increased danger of mediastinal shift
   f. Application of suction
      1. controlled suction: intermittent positive pressure is used to facilitate removal of secretions and aid in lung expansion
      2. uncontrolled suction: suction control bottle controls the amount of suction

Nursing Process
Assessment

1. Client: breathing (rate, regularity, depth, ease, breath sounds), anxiety, chest discomfort, level of understanding
2. Entry site: dressing, drainage, subcutaneous emphysema
3. Tubing: tight, taped connections; no kinks, compressions, dependent loops
4. Bottles (see Fig. 3-10)

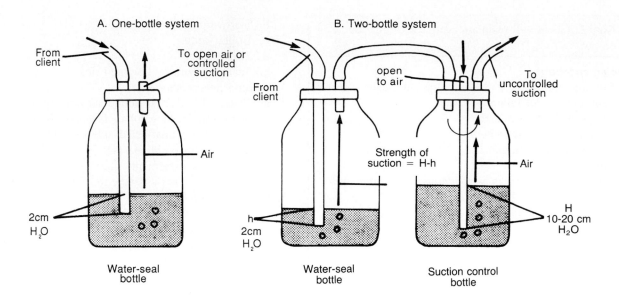

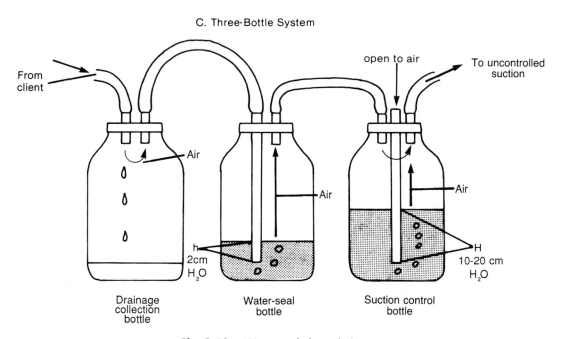

Fig. 3-10 Water-seal chest drainage.

a. *Water-seal bottle:* tube submerged and chamber filled to prescribed level (usually 2 cm); fluctuations with respirations; excessive bubbling indicates air leak; open vent to air if client not on suction

b. *Drainage collection bottle:* volume, type, rate of drainage; bottle below chest level

c. *Suction control bottle:* tube open to air with end submerged and chamber filled to ordered depth (usually 20 cm); gentle, continuous bubbling

5. Suction source
   a. No control bottle: suction set at ordered level
   b. Control bottle: suction set so that gentle, continuous bubbling occurs

Analysis (see p. 126)

Planning, Implementation, and Evaluation

Goal 1: Client will experience well-functioning water-seal system.

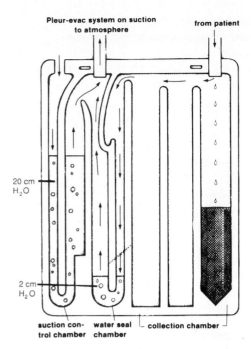

Fig. 3-11 Pleur-Evac system. A Pleur-Evac unit consists of three chambers comparable to a three-bottle water-seal drainage system. The suction control chamber is equivalent to bottle no. 3—the suction control bottle. The water-seal chamber is equivalent to bottle no. 2—the water-seal bottle. The collection chamber corresponds to bottle no. 1—the drainage collection bottle.

Implementation
1. Check functioning of system.
2. Check that tube(s) is submerged at appropriate level or that water level(s) in Pleur-Evac is correct.
3. Tape all connectors.
4. Know what to do if system breaks: have tube clamps at bedside and use clamps appropriately.

Evaluation
Client's water-seal drainage remains intact; client remains free from respiratory distress.

> **Goal 2:** Client will have tube patency maintained.

Implementation
1. Position tubes correctly; ensure that they are not kinked.
2. Attach tube to bed linens to prevent it from falling over side and pulling at insertion site.
3. Check for fluctuation of fluid in tube of water-seal bottle.

Evaluation
Client has adequate air and fluid drainage through patent tubes.

> **Goal 3:** Client will experience adequate lung reexpansion.

Implementation
1. Help with daily chest x-ray.
2. Measure amount of drainage by marking bottle with tape and time of measurement (usual blood loss; 50-100 ml/hr for the first few postoperative hours; then decreases to 10-20 ml/hr).
3. Monitor for respiratory distress.
4. Cough and deep-breathe q2h as needed.
5. Provide comfort measures as needed; pain medications as ordered (see Table 3-7).
6. Position the client to ensure optimal lung expansion
   a. Pneumonectomy: lie either on *affected* side or on back
   b. All other thoracotomies: lie on *unaffected* side or back
7. Help with removal of tube
   a. Equipment needed: gauze sponges, tape, and scissors to cut suture holding the tube
   b. Instruct client to exhale or inhale and hold breath
   c. Apply tight dressing of 4 × 4s over a piece of petrolatum gauze

Evaluation
Client has adequate lung reexpansion; breathes easily, has normal skin color.

☐ Cancer of the Lung
General Information
1. Incidence
   a. Leading cause of cancer death in men and women; peaks in middle age
   b. Increasing in frequency, especially among women
2. Mortality rate is 20 times higher for those who smoke two or more packs of cigarettes daily

Nursing Process
Assessment
1. No early signs
2. Cough: chronic, persistent
3. Abnormal chest x-ray
4. Positive findings from sputum cytology
5. Positive biopsy results
6. Hemoptysis, weakness, anorexia, weight loss, dyspnea, chest pain: symptoms of advanced disease
7. Pleural effusion (peripheral tumors)
Analysis (see p. 126)
Planning, Implementation, and Evaluation

> **Goal 1:** Client and significant others will be able to explain diagnostic tests and postprocedure care.

Implementation
1. Assess level of knowledge of client and significant others.
2. Explain procedures (e.g., bronchoscopy, sputum exams, p. 125).

Evaluation
Client and significant others describe what to expect during and after procedures.

Goal 2: Client and significant others will be able to explain planned medical treatment.

Implementation
1. Know that radiation therapy and chemotherapy are often given if surgery is not possible, or preoperatively in conjunction with surgery.
2. Prepare client and significant others for radiation and chemotherapy (see *Cellular Aberration,* p. 267).

Evaluation
Client describes expected actions and side effects of planned medical therapy.

Goal 3: Client and significant others will be able to explain preoperative care, postoperative needs, OR-RR-SICU environment, and purpose of chest tubes.

Implementation
1. Refer to "Perioperative Period," p. 117; *Cellular Aberration,* General Nursing Goal 2, p. 270; and chest tube care, p. 152.
2. Tour ICU.

Evaluation
Client demonstrates adequate coughing and deep-breathing; correctly describes ICU environment.

Goal 4: Postoperatively, client will have adequate respiratory function, stable cardiac function, and adequate pain control.

Implementation
1. Refer to "Perioperative Period," p. 117.
2. Monitor chest tubes; position appropriately for lung expansion (see chest tube care, p. 153).

Evaluation
Client remains free from postoperative complications (breathes easily, has adequate I&O, experiences good pain control).

Goal 5: Client and significant others will discuss fears and concerns.

Implementation
1. Assess level of anxiety.
2. Give emotional support and help relieve anxiety (see Table 2-4, p. 22).

3. Maintain hope.
4. Refer to appropriate support groups.

Evaluation
Client and significant others discuss fears and ask questions concerning diagnosis.

Goal 6: Client and significant others will be prepared for discharge.

Implementation
1. Teach
   a. Levels of activity and rest.
   b. How to prevent respiratory infections (e.g., avoid crowds).
2. Encourage client to stop smoking.
3. Arrange follow-up appointment.

Evaluation
Client knows date for return appointment with physician; states a willingness to comply with restrictions.

☐ Cancer of the Larynx
General Information

1. Incidence: most common malignancy of upper respiratory tract
2. Risk factors
   a. Irritants to mucous membranes (e.g., chemicals, allergens)
   b. Smoking
   c. Excessive alcohol intake
   d. Familial predisposition
   e. Chronic laryngitis
   f. Voice abuse
3. Medical treatment
   a. Surgical intervention
      1. laryngectomy
      2. laryngectomy with modified, radical neck dissection
   b. Medical intervention
      1. radiation therapy
      2. chemotherapy *not* used

Nursing Process
Assessment
1. Persistent hoarseness (early symptom)
2. Dysphagia, burning with hot liquids
3. Persistent sore throat
4. Pain in laryngeal prominence
5. Feeling that something is in throat
6. Swelling of the neck
7. Diagnostic tests: abnormal results of laryngoscopy and biopsy

Analysis (see p. 126)
Planning, Implementation, and Evaluation

Goal 1: Client and significant others will be able to explain planned medical treatment.

Implementation

1. Know that radiation is often used as adjuvant therapy to surgery.
2. Prepare client and significant others for radiation (see *Cellular Aberration*, p. 267).

Evaluation

Client describes expected actions and side effects of radiation therapy.

> **Goal 2:** Client and significant others will be able to explain preoperative care, postoperative needs, and the OR-RR environment.

Implementation

1. Refer to "Perioperative Period," p. 117, and *Cellular Aberration*, General Nursing Goal 2, p. 270.
2. Give frequent oral care.
3. Advise no smoking or drinking alcohol.
4. Teach about postoperative procedures.
   a. Presence of drains and HemoVac
   b. Tracheostomy care and suctioning
   c. Breathing through tracheostomy tube and inhalation treatments
   d. Possible IVs or tube feedings
5. Discuss communication problems that will result.
6. Determine methods of postoperative communication (e.g., writing pad, picture board, call bell, magic slate, hand signals).

Evaluation

Client explains tracheostomy care; client, significant others, and nurse have plan for postoperative communication.

> **Goal 3:** Postoperatively, client will have adequate respiratory function.

Implementation

1. Refer to "Perioperative Period," p. 117.
2. Assess frequently
   a. Patency of airway
   b. Breath sounds, respiratory rate and depth
3. Elevate head of bed 30°-45° (promotes drainage and facilitates respirations).
4. Support head and neck.
5. Administer humidified oxygen.
6. Suction tracheostomy frequently.
   a. Sterile suction setup
   b. Prepare equipment
   c. Hyperoxygenate client (suctioning can lower PO_2 10-30 mm Hg)
   d. Lubricate catheter (with H_2O-soluble lubricant) and insert catheter with suction turned off until obstruction is met
   e. Withdraw catheter 1 cm (away from mucosa)
   f. Withdraw catheter while rotating and applying suction
   g. Limit suctioning to 10-15 seconds at a time
   h. Hyperoxygenate client
   i. Repeat procedure, allowing client to rest and be hyperoxygenated between suctionings
   j. Observe cardiac monitor if in use; if bradycardia or dysrhythmias occur, terminate suctioning immediately and hyperoxygenate client
   k. If client has inflated endotracheal or tracheostomy tube in place and cuff must be deflated, use the following procedure
      1. suction trachea secretions through tube as outlined above
      2. suction oropharynx and nasopharynx
      3. open new sterile setup and then deflate cuff and apply suction through tube immediately
      4. reinflate cuff just until air can no longer be heard, being careful not to overinflate cuff
7. Give laryngeal-tube care; clean tube at least q8h.
8. Suction nasopharyngeal secretions and tracheostomy using separate sterile catheters (or apply suction to tracheostomy first and nasopharynx second with same catheter).
9. Give frequent oral hygiene.
10. Check neck drains and HemoVac for drainage.

Evaluation

Client remains free from respiratory distress; has stable vital signs; rests comfortably.

> **Goal 4:** Client will have satisfactory communication with staff and significant others postoperatively.

Implementation

1. Use communication measures decided upon preoperatively.
2. Stay with client as often as possible.
3. Explain to client how to summon nurse; respond promptly when called.
4. Have significant others remain with client.

Evaluation

Client communicates needs effectively.

> **Goal 5:** Client will receive adequate nutrition postoperatively.

Implementation

1. Give IV therapy as ordered.
2. Give NG tube feedings as ordered.
3. Give vitamin supplements as ordered.
4. Supervise first oral intake; know that aspiration is not possible unless a fistula has formed.
5. Check skin turgor to monitor adequate hydration of tissues.
6. Monitor I&O.

Evaluation

Client's weight remains stable; fluid output approximates intake.

Goal 6: Client will cope with change in body image.

Implementation
1. See *Loss and Death and Dying*, p. 26.
2. Enlist help of role models such as rehabilitated laryngectomy clients.

Evaluation
Client's grooming and attitude demonstrate a positive self-concept.

Goal 7: Client and significant others will be prepared for discharge.

Implementation
1. Teach importance of
   a. Tube care
   b. Stoma care
   c. Proper clothing
   d. Diet
   e. Activity and recreation
   f. Bathing
   g. Oral hygiene
   h. Medic Alert bracelet (neck breather)
2. Refer to community health agency (e.g., Laryngectomee Club of American Cancer Society).
3. Make referral to speech therapist.
4. Arrange follow-up appointment.

Evaluation
Client correctly explains care of tube and stoma.

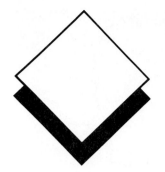

Nutrition and Metabolism

The nursing care presented in this unit concerns selected health problems related to disturbances in the digestive tract and the endocrine system.

The Digestive Tract

GENERAL CONCEPTS

Overview/Physiology

1. Function: to transfer food and water from the external to the internal environment of the body and transform these substances into a form suitable for distribution to the cells by way of the circulatory system
2. Anatomy (see Fig. 3-12)
   a. Upper gastrointestinal tract
      1. mouth, teeth, and salivary glands
      2. esophagus
      3. stomach
   b. Lower gastrointestinal tract
      1. small bowel
      2. large bowel
      3. rectum
      4. anus
   c. Accessory organs of digestion
      1. liver
      2. gallbladder
      3. pancreas
3. Processes
   a. Digestion: the process of breaking down proteins, polysaccharides, and fat; accomplished by the action of acid and enzymes secreted into the GI tract
   b. Secretion: the process of elaborating a specific product as a result of glandular activity (see Table 3-22)
      1. saliva (mouth): contains salivary amylase (hydrolyzes starch into maltase)
      2. gastric secretions
         a. mucus: lubricates stomach lining and content
         b. hydrochloric acid (HCl): essential to provide the acid medium necessary for the function of pepsin

c. pepsin: breaks down proteins to polypeptides, proteoses, and peptones
         d. lipase (small amounts): digests butterfat
         e. gastrin: involved in stimulation and release of HCl
      3. small bowel secretions
         a. peptidases: split polypeptides into amino acids
         b. sucrase, maltase, isomaltase, and lactase: split disaccharides into monosaccharides
         c. intestinal lipase splits fats into glycerol and fatty acids
         d. secretin and cholecystokinin-pancreozymin stimulate the pancreas and gallbladder
      4. pancreatic secretions
         a. trypsin, chymotrypsin, nucleases, carboxypeptidase, pancreatic lipase, and pancreatic amylase break down protein, fats, and carbohydrates
         b. bicarbonate-rich isosmotic electrolyte solution
      5. gallbladder secretes bile
   c. Absorption: the process by which the small molecules that are the result of digestion cross cell membranes of the intestine and enter the blood and lymph
      1. carbohydrates and proteins are absorbed by active transport along with sodium
      2. fatty acids are absorbed by diffusion
      3. water and electrolytes are absorbed in the small and large intestines
      4. synthesis and absorption of vitamin K, thiamin, riboflavin, vitamin B_{12}, folic acid, biotin, and nicotinic acid take place in the large intestine as a result of bacterial activity, primarily *E. coli*
   d. Motility: the process by which contractions of the smooth muscle lining the walls of the GI tract produce movement of substances through the GI tract while digestion and absorption occur
      1. GI tract contains an intrinsic nerve supply that controls tone and peristaltic action

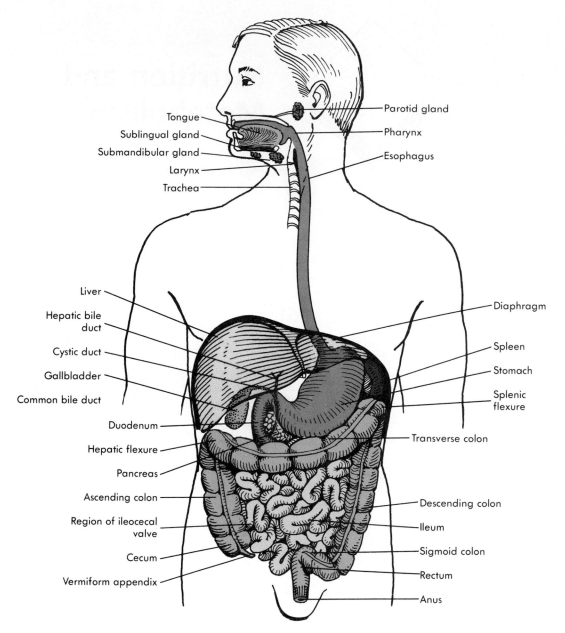

Fig. 3-12 The primary and accessory organs of digestion. (From Long, B.C., & Phipps, W.J. [1989]. *Medical-surgical nursing: A nursing process approach* [2nd ed.]. St. Louis: Mosby—Year Book.)

2. nerve fibers from both the sympathetic and parasympathetic branches of the autonomic nervous system supply the intestinal tract and interact with intrinsic nerve supply
3. the vagus nerve (the major autonomic nerve supplying the GI tract) is composed of motor parasympathetic fibers and many sensory fibers; parasympathetic stimulation *increases* motility and secretion; sympathetic stimulation *decreases* motility and secretion

e. Metabolism
1. all of the changes or body processes that take place in order to sustain life; the chemical changes that occur allow chemical energy to be changed to other forms of energy so that cellular functions can be maintained
2. intermediary metabolism includes all the cellular functions in the body's internal environment; this phase of metabolism begins after the ingestion and digestion of foodstuff from the external environment
3. two-part process
   a. anabolism: the process of synthesis of smaller molecules to larger molecules; energy is saved
      ◆ building process: proteins from amino

Table 3-22   Digestive enzymes

Enzymes that digest	Source	Selected action and products
CARBOHYDRATES		
Amylase	Parotid and submaxillary glands	Hydrolyzes starch to maltose.
Sucrase, maltase, isomaltase, lactase	Intestinal fluids	Split disaccharides into monosaccharides.
Pancreatic amylase	Pancreas	Splits starches into maltose and isomaltose.
FATS		
Gastric lipase	Gastric mucosa	Digests butterfat.
Intestinal lipase	Intestinal fluids	Splits fats into glycerol and fatty acids.
PROTEIN		
Pepsin	Gastric mucosa	Breaks down dietary protein into proteoses, peptones, and polypeptides.
Peptidases	Intestinal glands	Splits polypeptides into amino acids.
Trypsin	Pancreas	Splits proteins into peptide and amino acids.
Chymotrypsin	Pancreas	Splits proteins into polypeptides.
Carboxypeptidase	Pancreas	Splits polypeptides into smaller peptides.
OTHER		
Enterokinase	Duodenal mucosa	Activates trypsin.
Nucleases	Pancreas	Splits nucleic acids.

acids, fats from fatty acids, and polysaccharides from monosaccharides
   ◆ increased during growth, pregnancy, recovery states, or times of increased intake
   b. catabolism: the breaking down of larger molecules into smaller molecules
   ◆ protein, fats, and carbohydrates are broken down into units that can be used by the cells
   ◆ excesses in catabolism are seen in starvation, illness, and trauma
   ◆ breakdown involves the release of CO_2, water, and urea with amino acid metabolism
4. adenosine triphosphate (ATP) is the high-energy phosphate that is the major source of energy for cellular function
5. adenosine diphosphate (ADP) is one of the end products released when energy is used and ATP is broken down
6. metabolic balance remains unless a change in the internal or external environment produces imbalances (for the balance to be maintained, the rate of catabolism must equal anabolism)
7. variances in metabolic rate occur with differences in sex, age, hormonal environment, seasonal and environmental temperature changes, culture, activity levels, and ingestion of drugs (e.g., caffeine, nicotine, epinephrine)

8. materials needed for metabolism
   a. nutrients to supply energy and build tissue: glucose, glycerol, fatty acids, and amino acids
   b. minerals, electrolytes
   c. materials (primarily proteins) to promote synthesis of enzymes and hormones
   d. vitamins that function as coenzymes
   e. enzymes and hormones to function as organic cellular catalysts
9. metabolism governs the activities of muscle contraction, nerve impulse transmission, glandular secretion, absorption, and elimination

Application of the Nursing Process to the Client with Digestive Tract Problems

Assessment
1. Health history
   a. Normal dietary pattern: changes in appetite
   b. Normal weight: changes in weight (how much, time period, planned vs. unplanned)
   c. Change in energy level: weakness, fatigue, and general malaise
   d. Stool: changes in frequency, color, character
   e. Urine: dark, orange or clear color, frequency
   f. Indigestion or heartburn: pattern, frequency, drugs used, effectiveness
   g. Difficulty in swallowing: dysphagia with onset by solids or liquids
   h. Eructation or regurgitation

i. Difficulty tolerating certain foods: allergies

j. Vomiting or nausea: character of vomitus; pattern of nausea; relationship to intake, other events

k. Abdominal pain: presence, location, character, or pattern

l. Abdominal distension, flatus

m. History of abdominal surgery or trauma

n. Bleeding: onset, duration, and extent

o. Alcohol habits

2. Physical examination

  a. Inspection

   1. oral assessment: gums, tongue, teeth, and mucous membranes

   2. skin characteristics: turgor, scars, striae, engorged veins, spider angiomas, bruising, and jaundice

   3. abdominal structure: visible peristalsis, pulsations, or masses

   4. abdominal contour: rounded, protuberant, concave, or asymmetrical

  b. Auscultation: listen to all four quadrants of abdomen

   1. bowel sounds: location, frequency (normally 8-20/min in each quadrant), characteristics

    a. normal: succession of clicks and gurgles

    b. abnormal

     ◆ hyperperistalsis: prolonged, loud, multiple gurgles

     ◆ paralytic ileus: absent or infrequent sounds

     ◆ intestinal obstruction: loud clicks and gurgles, high-pitched tinkling sounds; late in the obstructive process bowel sounds are hypoactive as the intestine becomes fatigued

  c. Percussion

   1. stomach (tympany normal)

   2. liver size (liver area is normally dull to percussion)

   3. large intestinal areas: check for gaseous distension

  d. Palpation (Note: done first to avoid stimulating bowel sounds)

   1. pain, tenderness

   2. masses, especially liver enlargement

3. Diagnostic tests

  a. Hematological studies: normal values will vary slightly from laboratory to laboratory

   1. general function

    a. electrolytes

     ◆ sodium: 136-145 mEq/L

     ◆ potassium: 3.5-5.0 mEq/L

     ◆ chloride: 90-110 mEq/L

    b. CBC

     ◆ WBC: 5000-10,000/mm^3

     ◆ RBC: 4.2-6.1 million/mm^3

     ◆ Hgb
      • men: 14-18 g/dl
      • women: 12-16 g/dl

     ◆ HCT
      • men: 42%-54%
      • women: 37%-47%

   2. liver function

    a. aspartate aminotransferase (AST) (formerly SGOT): 5-40 units/L

    b. alanine aminotransferase (ALT) (formerly SGPT): 5-35 units/L

    c. alkaline phosphatase (ALP): 30-85 ImU/L

    d. ammonia: 15-110 g/dl

    e. albumin: 3.2-4.5 g/dl

    f. globulin: 2.3-3.5 g/dl

    g. total bilirubin: 0.1-1 mg/dl

    h. cholesterol: 150-250 mg/dl

    i. prothrombin time: 11-12.5 seconds

   3. GI function: gastrin—40-150 pg/ml

   4. pancreatic function

    a. glucose levels

     ◆ glucose: 70-115 mg/dl

     ◆ postprandial: less than 140 mg/dl

     ◆ glucose tolerance: peak of less than 200 mg/dl

    b. lipase: up to 1.5 units/ml

    c. amylase: 56-190 IU/L

  b. Urine tests

   1. glucose, acetone

   2. urobilinogen

  c. Stool tests

   1. ova and parasites (stool must be warm)

   2. occult blood (guaiac)

   3. fecal fat (after a 72-hour collection)

   4. culture

  d. Radiographic studies

   1. flat plate of abdomen

   2. GI series (barium swallow)

    a. definition: x-ray of esophagus, stomach, and duodenum following oral intake of 16-20 oz of contrast medium (barium)

    b. nursing care pretest: keep NPO for 8 hours before test

    c. nursing care posttest

     ◆ give laxatives, force fluids to remove barium

     ◆ encourage mobility to stimulate peristalsis

   3. cholecystography

    a. definition: x-ray visualization of gallbladder and biliary tract following oral ingestion of iodine dye (isopanoic acid tablets)

    b. nursing care pretest

     ◆ check for iodine allergies

     ◆ administer tablets (usually 6 with specified amount of water) one at a time at

5-minute intervals 12 hours before test
- assess for side effects of tablets: diarrhea, nausea, vomiting, or abdominal cramps; report to physician or radiologist
- give low-fat evening meal the day before in order to avoid contraction of the gallbladder
- keep NPO for 8 hours before test
- if serum bilirubin level is less than 1.8 mg/dl, report to physician since adequate visualization is unlikely

4. IV cholangiography
   a. definition: x-ray visualization of gallbladder and biliary tract following injection of iodine dye
      NOTE: test may also be performed via T-tube or during surgery
   b. nursing care pretest
      - check for iodine allergies
      - keep NPO for 8 hours before test
      - ensure signed consent is on chart if needed
      - give laxative as ordered on the day before exam
      - give cleansing enema if ordered
   c. nursing care posttest: force fluids (dye acts as diuretic)

5. abdominal CAT scan: with or without contrast medium

6. percutaneous transhepatic cholangiography (PTHC):
   a. definition: passing a needle through the liver into a dilated intrahepatic bile duct and directly injecting iodinated dye; used with clients who have elevated bilirubin and jaundice
   b. nursing care pretest: refer to IV cholangiography
   c. nursing care posttest
      - assess for signs and symptoms of peritonitis, bleeding, sepsis
      - keep client NPO and on bed rest as ordered
      - assess vital signs according to postprocedure routine

e. Endoscopy
   1. definition: direct visualization of a part or parts of the GI tract through a lighted scope; may be a treatment modality as well (e.g., polypectomy, removal of foreign objects, cauterization of GI bleeding sites)
   2. types
      a. esophagogastroduodenoscopy
      b. peritoneoscopy (liver, gallbladder, and mesentery)
      c. endoscopic retrograde cholangiopancreatography (ERCP) (pancreas and biliary tree)
      d. colonoscopy (entire colon)
      e. proctoscopy (rectosigmoid) sigmoidoscopy
   3. nursing care pretest
      a. keep NPO for 8 hours before test
      b. administer bowel prep for lower GI endoscopy
      c. ensure a signed consent is on the chart
      d. give pretest sedation as ordered
   4. nursing care posttest
      a. check vital signs frequently the first 24 hours
      b. feed when gag reflex returns after upper GI endoscopy
      c. observe for bleeding (indicated by frequent swallowing and bloody emesis following exam of the upper GI system or bloody stools following exam of lower GI system), sharp pain (indicates perforation)
      d. force fluids as needed

f. Ultrasound (sonogram)
   1. definition: use of high-frequency sound waves to evaluate organ size, shape, and structure; painless, safe procedure
   2. nursing care pretest
      a. if client has had prior barium contrast studies, laxatives and cathartics may be given the evening before
      b. gallbladder: keep NPO for 8 hours before test
      c. pelvic: have client drink 6-8 glasses of water just before test and not void until test is over, or clamp Foley catheter (full bladder acts as a landmark)
      d. all other organs: no food or fluid restrictions
   3. nursing care posttest: no special concerns

g. Analytical studies
   1. gastric analysis
      a. definition: to determine amount of gastric secretion with and without stimulation; may be done with NG insertion or administration of Diagnex blue tablets by mouth
      b. nursing care (with NG tube)
         - keep NPO for 8 hours
         - insert NG tube
         - collect fasting specimen and a specimen following stimulation by food or drugs
      c. nursing care (without NG tube)
         - keep NPO for 8 hours
         - have client empty bladder, discard urine
         - give Diagnex blue tablet
         - collect urine after 2 hours and check color (if gastric secretion has a pH of 3 or less, the dye will have been excreted)
   2. Schilling test

a. definition: to identify the reason for vitamin B_{12} deficits—either a lack of intrinsic factor (pernicious anemia) or a defect in absorption

b. nursing care
   - ◆ keep NPO 8-12 hours before exam
   - ◆ following administration of radioactive oral vitamin B_{12} by nuclear medicine personnel, administer vitamin B_{12} IM as directed (usually 1-2 hours after oral dose)
   - ◆ start 24-hour urine specimen collection after IM injection to assess levels of radioactive B_{12} excreted (normal = 8%-40% excretion of injected activity within 24 hours)
   - ◆ allow client to resume eating after IM injection

h. Biopsies
   1. excisional
      a. rectal (done at time of sigmoidoscopy)
      b. gastric (done at time of gastroscopy)
   2. needle (percutaneous liver biopsy)
      a. definition: a blind needle biopsy of liver tissue to establish a microscopic picture of the liver
      b. nursing care pretest
         - ◆ ensure informed consent is on chart
         - ◆ check prothrombin time (if less than 40%, test will not be done)
         - ◆ check platelet count (test may not be done if count is less than 100,000)
         - ◆ instruct client to hold breath for 1-2 seconds while biopsy is being done and not to move during procedure
      c. nursing care posttest
         - ◆ have client lie on right side with pillow or sandbag over the insertion point under costal margin
         - ◆ take frequent vital signs the first 24 hours
         - ◆ assess for pain or respiratory difficulty (pneumothorax or hemothorax)

Analysis
1. Safe, effective care environment
   a. Knowledge deficit
   b. High risk for infection
2. Physiological integrity
   a. Pain
   b. Constipation or diarrhea
   c. Altered nutrition: less than body requirements
3. Psychosocial integrity
   a. Ineffective individual coping
   b. Self-esteem disturbance
4. Health promotion/maintenance

a. Health-seeking behaviors
b. Noncompliance

General Nursing Planning, Implementation, and Evaluation

Goal 1: Client will ingest a diet that conforms to prescribed restrictions yet contains all needed nutrients.

Implementation
1. Increase or decrease dietary nutrients as ordered.
2. Teach client the rationale for dietary restrictions.
3. Help client identify factors in life-style that may interfere with compliance.
4. Provide needed support and encouragement; involve family if possible.

Evaluation
Client selects appropriate diet from sample menus; verbalizes rationale for restrictions; expresses positive attitude toward diet alteration.

Goal 2: Client will be as comfortable and as pain-free as possible.

Implementation
1. Administer pain medications as appropriate.
2. Use noninvasive pain-relieving techniques such as positioning, massage, and distraction.
3. Teach client and significant others about measures that will minimize pain when client is discharged (e.g., dietary regimen, medications).

Evaluation
Client states that pain is either minimal or nonexistent; verbalizes measures to control pain after discharge.

Goal 3: Client's fluid and electrolyte balance will return to normal.

Implementation
1. Institute replacement therapy or restrictions as ordered.
2. Keep accurate I&O.
3. Monitor daily weight.

Evaluation
Client's fluid and electrolyte levels are within normal limits.

Goal 4: Client will be knowledgeable about disease process, medications, and the prevention of complications.

Implementation
1. Explain disease process.
2. Discuss rationale for ordered treatment regimen.
3. Provide information regarding the administration and side effects of all medications.

4. Help client and significant others to identify factors that might trigger complications of the disease.

Evaluation

Client lists medications and describes the prevention of complications.

SELECTED HEALTH PROBLEMS RESULTING IN PROBLEMS WITH DIGESTION

☐ **Gastroesophageal Reflux**
☐ **Hiatal Hernia**
☐ **Acute Gastritis**

Refer to General Nursing Planning, Implementation, and Evaluation, p. 162. Additional nursing care can be found in Table 3-23.

☐ Peptic Ulcer Disease

General Information

1. Definition: sharply defined break in mucosa, which may involve the submucosa and muscular layers of the esophagus, stomach, and duodenum
2. Incidence: estimated that 25% of men and 17% of women have peptic ulcer disease but only 5%-10%
become symptomatic; incidence varies widely by age, sex, and site
   a. Duodenal: most common form, peak occurrence at age 40
   b. Gastric: risk higher in elderly, peak occurrence after age 50
3. Predisposing factors (see Table 3-24)
4. Pathophysiology (see Table 3-24)
5. Diagnostic aids
   a. Fiberoptic endoscopy (essential to rule out malignancy)
   b. Barium swallow
   c. Stool exams (occult blood)
6. Complications
   a. Bleeding: occurs in 15%-20%; may involve coffee-ground emesis, tarry stools (melena) with slower rates of bleeding, or the passage of bright-red blood rectally (hematochezia) with profuse upper GI tract hemorrhage
   b. Hemorrhage: occurs when ulcer erodes a blood vessel; treatment of shock and emergency surgery may be necessary
   c. Perforation: ulcer penetrates entire stomach or du-

Table 3-23 Related problems of ingestion and digestion

Disorders	Description	Medical management	Nursing management
Gastroesophageal reflux	Reflux of stomach and duodenal contents into esophagus causing heartburn and regurgitation; in severe cases it may progress to painful or difficult swallowing, ulceration, or stricture	PRN use of antacids; bethanechol (Urecholine) or metoclopramide (Reglan) to increase lower esophageal sphincter (LES) pressure; avoid anticholinergic agents	Diet—smaller, more frequent meals; high-protein, low-fat diet; avoid caffeine, alcohol, and chocolate Position—remain upright after eating; elevate head of bed 6-12 inches Activity—avoid activity that increases intraabdominal pressure (e.g., lifting, tight clothes, bending over)
Hiatal hernia	Herniation of a portion of stomach or other abdominal organ through enlarged esophageal opening in diaphragm; common problem that is usually asymptomatic but may be accompanied by reflux	(See above regimen) If reflux is severe, surgical repair (fundoplication of stomach around esophagus) may be performed	(See above regimen) Surgical care involves meticulous respiratory management; small feedings due to reduced stomach capacity
Acute gastritis	Transient inflammation of the gastric mucosa, mucosal hemorrhage and erosion; associated with aspirin ingestion, extreme physical stress, alcohol abuse, smoking, infection, and food or substance poisoning; symptoms vary with severity but may include nausea, vomiting, pain, and eructation	Condition is usually self-limited; treatment may necessitate fluids, antiemetics, antacids, or antibiotics; vitamin B_{12} may be needed in chronic cases	NPO status or liquids; comfort measures; monitor I&O and electrolyte status; NG lavage

Table 3-24   A comparison of gastric and duodenal ulcers

	Predisposing factors	Pathophysiology	Clinical manifestations
Gastric ulcers	Excessive use of salicylates, non-steroidal antiinflammatory drugs (NSAIDs) Cigarette smoking Dietary indiscretion Genetic predisposition Severe physiological stress	Mechanism remains unclear. Acid secretion rate is below normal. Theorized that ulcer results from failure of mucous barrier of stomach allowing back diffusion of H^+ ions into cells. Role of *Campylobacter pylori* bacteria under investigation.	Epigastric pain—often severe. Not related to food intake and may not respond to antacids. Anorexia, nausea and vomiting, bloating and weight loss. Hemorrhage is common.
Duodenal ulcers	Heterogenous group of disorders, 40% of which are a result of actual acid oversecretion related to: excess parietal cell mass increased postprandial gastrin release increased gastrin sensitivity	Gastrin stimulates acid secretion, which overwhelms the mucosal integrity. Gastric emptying also may be accelerated, causing acid load to exceed the buffering capacity.	Similar pain to gastric but episodic and rhythmic—relieved by food or antacid. Nighttime pain is common. Bleeding is more likely to be chronic, and perforation is more common.

odenal wall, releasing stomach contents, which results in a chemical burn and peritonitis; more common in long-term disease states

   d. Obstruction: repeated cycles of ulceration and healing in the pyloric region may cause scar tissue buildup

7. Medical treatment

   a. Drugs (see Table 3-25)

      1. histamine receptor antagonists

      2. antacids and mucosal healing agents

      3. anticholinergics

   b. Diet pattern modification

   c. Rest

   d. Surgical intervention (required in 10%-15% of clients)

      1. Billroth I: removal of part of stomach, anastomosis of remaining portion to duodenum

      2. Billroth II: resection of distal two thirds of the stomach; anastomosis of jejunal loop to remaining portion with remaining duodenal stump sutured shut

      3. vagotomy: severing of vagus nerve to eliminate acid-secreting stimulus to gastric cells

      4. pyloroplasty: revision of passage between pyloric region and duodenum to enhance emptying in gastric atony associated with vagotomy

Nursing Process

Assessment

1. Pain: type; severity; location; and duration; response to food, liquid, or antacid; may by asymptomatic

2. Anorexia, nausea, or vomiting

3. Weight loss

4. Alcohol and smoking histories

5. Melena or occult blood in stool

6. Hematemesis

7. Complications of peptic ulcers

   a. Perforation or peritonitis

      1. sudden onset of severe abdominal pain

      2. diffuse abdominal tenderness

      3. diminished bowel sounds

      4. boardlike abdomen with diffuse distension

   b. Obstruction

      1. fullness, nausea

      2. profuse vomiting of undigested food

Analysis (see p. 162)

Planning, Implementation, and Evaluation

Goal 1: Client will be free from pain.

Implementation

1. Give 30 ml antacid drugs 1-3 hours after meals, at bedtime, and PRN but not within 30 minutes of sucralfate ingestion.

2. Give histamine receptor antagonists as ordered with meals and at bedtime.

3. Teach client to eliminate foods from diet that cause increased pain.

   a. Try small, frequent meals; avoid eating at bedtime.

   b. Avoid common stimulants of gastric acid secretion (e.g., caffeine, alcohol, and spicy foods).

4. Provide for increased rest; ensure a calm, peaceful environment.

5. Teach client to stop smoking, if possible.

Evaluation

   Client can tolerate diet without discomfort; states or institutes measures that decrease or prevent pain.

Table 3-25 Drug therapy for peptic ulcer disease

Generic name (trade name)	Action	Use	Side effects
ANTACIDS			
Aluminum hydroxide (AlternaGEL, Amphojel) Dried form (Alu-Cap)	Nonsystemic; works by neutralization	To treat gastric and duodenal ulcers; and manage phosphate stone formation	Constipation, phosphorus deficiency, intestinal obstruction
Basic aluminum carbonate (Basaljel)	As with Amphojel	As with Amphojel	Constipation
Calcium carbonate (Alka-2, Tums)	Rapid onset; high neutralizing capacity	Peptic ulcers	Constipation, hypercalcemia, rebound hyperactivity
Magaldrate (Riopan)	Combination of aluminum and magnesium hydroxide; nonsystemic neutralizing substance	Antacid	Mild constipation or diarrhea Hypermagnesemia in renal failure
Magnesium hydroxide (Milk of Magnesia)	Neutralizes HCl; demulcent effect	Antacid Laxative	Diarrhea, abdominal pain, nausea
Sodium bicarbonate	Systemic and local alkalizer	Antacid	Acid rebound, systemic alkalosis
ANTIFLATULENT			
Simethicone (Mylicon)	Decreases surface tension of gas bubbles, prevents formation of mucus-surrounded gas bubbles	Antiflatulent	None
COMBINATION OF MIXTURES			
Aluminum and magnesium hydroxide (Maalox; Maalox 1, 2, and Concentrate)	As above	Antacid	As above
Aluminum and magnesium hydroxide and simethicone (Mylanta, Mylanta II, Maalox Plus)	As above	Antacid Antiflatulent	
HISTAMINE RECEPTOR BLOCKING AGENT			
Cimetidine (Tagamet)	Inhibits release of HCl by occupying histamine receptors in gastric mucosa	Duodenal ulcers; gastric hypersecretory states; prevent recurrent ulcers	Mild diarrhea, mental confusion, dizziness, gynecomastia
Ranitidine (Zantac)	As above; greater reduction of acid secretion, longer duration of action		As above, but side effects are fewer; no gynecomastia or confusion
MUCOSAL HEALING AGENTS			
Sucralfate (Carafate)	Action unclear; may stimulate release of gastric prostaglandins or adhere to protein in ulcer base	Duodenal ulcers	Constipation; do not take with antacids
ANTICHOLINERGICS			
Propantheline (Pro-Banthine)	Decreases quantity of GI secretions by inhibiting action of acetylcholine	Adjunct to ulcer treatment	Dry mouth, constipation, drowsiness

Goal 2: Client will identify activities to prevent ulcer recurrence.

Implementation

1. Teach client to avoid factors that tend to activate ulcer.
2. Help client plan to balance work, play, and rest.
3. Clarify dietary modifications.
4. Encourage reduction or elimination of smoking, alcohol, caffeine intake.
5. Encourage follow-up health care.
6. Teach regarding medications, side effects; time and method of administration; medications that irritate ulcer (e.g., ASA, NSAIDs, steroids).

Evaluation

Client states measures that will reduce the chances of recurrence; follows prescribed diet; takes medication correctly; has a balanced activity schedule; stops or decreases smoking or alcohol ingestion.

Goal 3: Client will recover from GI hemorrhage or ulcer perforation with minimal complications.

Implementation

1. Monitor vital signs q5-15 minutes; record I&O.
2. Establish large-bore IV line for fluid replacement.
3. Institute measures to control bleeding as ordered.
   a. Insert gastric lavage tube; irrigate stomach with tap water or saline until clear; connect to suction. (NOTE: controversy exists as to irrigant temperature [iced vs. cool] and type [saline vs. tap water])
   b. Give antacids or cimetidine (Tagamet) after acute bleeding has stopped.
   c. Administer IV fluids; type and crossmatch client's blood in order to replace blood loss as ordered.
   d. Offer emotional support.
4. Minimize consequences of perforation.
   a. Give antibiotics as ordered.
   b. Keep client in Fowler's position to localize gastric contents to one area of peritoneum.

Evaluation

Client experiences control of gastric bleeding; maintains vital signs within normal limits.

Goal 4: Client undergoing gastric surgery will recover free from complications.

Implementation

1. Provide standard postoperative care; refer to "Perioperative Period," p. 117.
2. Keep client NPO for 5-7 days to allow incision to heal; monitor for return of peristalsis; progress to clear liquids and diet as tolerated.
3. Keep client in semi-Fowler's position.
4. Maintain NG tube to suction.

   a. Do not irrigate or reposition unless ordered.
   b. Record all NG drainage as output.
   c. Observe color of drainage: should progress from bloody drainage to old blood to gastric secretions (greenish) within 24 hours.

Evaluation

Client recovers from surgery free from respiratory complications, infection or hemorrhage.

Goal 5: Client will recover from gastric surgery with minimal anemia.

Implementation

1. Know that 20%-50% of clients will experience anemia 1-2 years after resection.
   a. Vitamin B_{12} deficiency (pernicious anemia) if parietal cells of the stomach were removed
   b. Iron deficiency from blood loss
2. Give dietary supplements as ordered.

Evaluation

Client recovers, is free from anemia; if anemic, accepts follow-up care.

Goal 6: Client will understand dumping syndrome and ways to control it.

1. Teach client
   a. Symptoms of dumping syndrome (following subtotal or total gastrectomy: food enters duodenum rapidly; hyperosmolarity of intestinal contents pulls H_2O from vascular bed and stimulates a neuroendocrine response)
      1. reaction occurs within *30 minutes* after eating
      2. client feels dizzy, weak, and nauseated
      3. tachycardia, diaphoresis, orthostatic hypotension
      4. skin cool, clammy
   b. Prevention techniques
      1. eat six small meals that are dry and contain moderate protein and fat and reduced carbohydrate (avoid refined sugars)
      2. drink liquids between meals only
      3. rest or lie down on left side for 30 minutes after meals if possible to slow gastric emptying
   c. Blood glucose levels can rise rapidly after a meal containing simple sugars, triggering a reactive hypoglycemia several hours after the meal
   d. Control of diarrhea if present
      1. eliminate lactose and fluids during meals, limit glutens
      2. use antidiarrheal medications as needed
      3. report incidence of steatorrhea and weight loss

4. supplement vitamins and minerals as needed
5. decreases in severity in first year

2. Know that if the above does not relieve the problem, surgical intervention may be necessary to narrow the opening between stomach and intestine.
3. Know that for some clients, dumping syndrome and subsequent malabsorption become chronic, unrelieved problems.

Evaluation

Client states symptoms of and methods to prevent dumping syndrome; selects appropriate foods from diet list.

☐ Cholecystitis with Cholelithiasis
General Information

1. Definition: inflammation of the gallbladder usually caused by presence of stones (composed of cholesterol, bile pigment, or calcium)
2. Incidence: higher in white women over age 40
3. Predisposing factors
   a. Four times more common in women
   b. Obesity
   c. Middle age
   d. Multiparity, use of birth control pills, pregnancy
   e. Diabetes
4. Medical treatment
   a. Medical intervention
      1. low-fat diet (see Table 3-26)
      2. weight reduction
      3. dissolution therapy (chenodeoxycholic acid [CDCA])
      4. lithotripsy
   b. Surgical intervention
      1. cholecystectomy (removal of gallbladder and cystic duct): Jackson-Pratt or Penrose drain in gallbladder bed
      2. removal of stones from common bile duct usually necessitates placement of T-tube (see Fig. 3-13) to maintain duct patency during healing

Nursing Process

Assessment

1. Abdominal pain, usually in the right upper quadrant; may radiate to back
2. Fullness, eructation, dyspepsia following fat ingestion
3. Nausea and vomiting (distension of bile duct initiates stimulation of vomiting center)
4. Low-grade fever
5. Abnormal ultrasound or cholecystogram
6. Signs of obstructed bile flow
   a. Jaundice, pruritus
   b. Clay-colored stools, dark amber urine

Analysis (see p. 162)
Planning, Implementation, and Evaluation

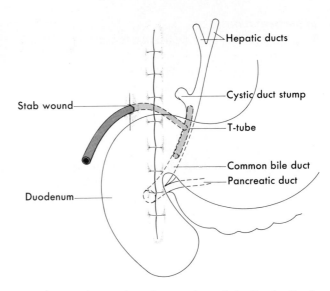

Fig. 3-13 The T-tube. The crossbar of the T-tube lies in the common bile duct. The long end is brought out through a stab wound in the abdomen and connected to gravity drainage. (From Beare P., & Myers, J. [1990]. *Principles and practice of adult health nursing.* St. Louis: Mosby–Year Book.)

Goal 1: Client with an acute attack will be comfortable and relieved of symptoms.

Implementation

1. Relieve pain with analgesics as ordered; meperidine (Demerol) is usually ordered since morphine causes spasms of bile ducts.
2. Relieve reflex spasms with antispasmodic drugs PRN as ordered.
3. Relieve vomiting and decrease gastric stimulation with NG tube to suction.
4. Give broad-spectrum antibiotics as ordered (ampicillin, tetracycline, and cephalosporins are frequently used).

Evaluation

Client is pain free without nausea or vomiting.

Goal 2: Client will recover from surgery without complications (refer to General Nursing Plans, p. 162.)

Table 3-26   Principles of a low-fat diet

Trim all visible fat from foods.
Use only lean meats; remove skin from poultry.
Restrict use of eggs.
Do not use fat for food preparation; no frying.
Use skim milk, and low-fat cottage cheese.
Avoid use of sauces, gravies, and rich desserts.
Increase use of fish and seafood.

Implementation
1. Provide liberal pain medication (postoperative pain is severe).
2. Place in low to semi-Fowler's position; encourage frequent coughing and deep breathing to prevent atelectasis.
3. Change dressings as needed (bile with a pH of 7.6-7.8 is very irritating to skin).
4. Care for T-tube if present.
   a. Avoid tension and obstruction of tubing.
   b. Measure amount of drainage carefully; record as output (drainage will be 200-1000 ml/day for first several days; continuing large amounts indicate obstruction).
   c. Clamp as ordered in 3-4 days before meals to allow bile to drain into duodenum; assess tolerance.
   d. Usually removed 10-12 days postoperatively following T-tube cholangiogram to determine status of duct.
5. Advance from clear liquids to low-fat diet as tolerated when ordered.

Evaluation
Client recovers from surgery free from skin irritation, diet intolerance, and biliary tract complications; ambulates without difficulty.

☐ Pancreatitis
General Information
1. Definition: acute or chronic inflammation of the pancreas
2. Pathophysiology: stimulation of the pancreas triggers digestive enzyme release; movement is blocked by edema or stones in the duct resulting in
   a. Duct rupture and enzyme escape
   b. Autodigestion within the pancreas
   c. Interstitial hemorrhage, tissue necrosis, or development of pseudocysts
   d. Chronic pancreatitis: precipitated protein blocks the duct, causing dilation, acinar tissue destruction, and fibrosis
3. Risk factors
   a. Alcohol abuse
   b. Gallbladder disease
   c. Abdominal trauma or surgery
   d. Infections (especially viral)
   e. Peptic ulcer disease
   f. Idiopathic causes
4. Medical treatment: generally conservative: control pain, rest pancreas, support nutrition and hydration

Nursing Process
Assessment
1. Extreme abdominal pain usually epigastric or left upper quadrant
2. Vomiting

3. Abdominal distension and tenderness
4. Elevated serum amylase and lipase
5. Elevated urinary amylase
6. Low-grade fever
7. Shock (kinin is a vasodilator activated by trypsin secretion)
8. Chronic steatorrhea
9. Hyperglycemia

Analysis (see p. 162)
Planning, Implementation, and Evaluation

> **Goal 1:** Client will be free from or have minimal pain.

Implementation
1. Keep NPO until inflammation subsides.
2. Know that meperidine (Demerol) is narcotic of choice; morphine may cause spasm of the sphincter of Oddi.

Table 3-27   Total parenteral nutrition (TPN)

DEFINITION

TPN is a method for nutritionally sustaining clients who cannot or should not ingest, digest, or absorb nutrients. TPN solutions consist of an individually calculated combination of amino acids, glucose, minerals, vitamins, and trace elements. Lipid emulsions are frequently added to make the feedings complete.

ADMINISTRATION

TPN may be delivered through either a peripheral or central vein. Peripheral delivery necessitates excellent venous access, and glucose concentrations are restricted to 10%-15%. Solutions of 25%-35% glucose may be administered centrally. TPN is associated with significant potential risks of infection and metabolic imbalance and necessitates careful monitoring.

NURSING INTERVENTIONS

Monitor insertion site; provide site care and dressing changes according to institution policy.
Administer TPN solutions through inline filters (lipids do not require filters).
Weigh client daily and maintain records.
Monitor laboratory values daily.
Avoid drawing blood or administering other fluids and medications through TPN catheter.
Monitor blood glucose levels throughout therapy; provide sliding-scale insulin coverage as needed.
Encourage active exercise as tolerated to support the production of muscle rather than fat cells.
Monitor respiratory rate (excess carbohydrates increase CO_2 production and may cause tachypnea).
Instruct client to use Valsalva maneuver and clamp tube during tubing changes to prevent air emboli.

3. Give anticholinergics such as propantheline (Pro-Banthine) as ordered to decrease secretions and relax the sphincter.
4. Administer antacids frequently in mild cases.
Evaluation
Client states pain is subsiding.

Goal 2: Client will be free from shock in the acute phase (refer to "Shock," p. 128)

Goal 3: Client will maintain adequate nutrition.

Implementation
1. Maintain NPO during. acute phase; NG suctioning may be used. Carry out specific mouth care orders.
2. Administer total parenteral nutrition (TPN) (see Table 3-27) as ordered if inflammation persists; gradually progress to a low-fat, bland diet after inflammation subsides.
3. Teach to avoid stimulants, alcohol.
4. Monitor blood glucose, urine glucose, and acetone levels (PRN insulin may be necessary).
5. Know that pancreatic enzymes may be given to aid fat digestion in chronic pancreatitis if damage is severe.
Evaluation
Client is free from nutritional deficiencies and digestive problems; ingests and tolerates prescribed diet; has no weight loss; chooses bland foods from diet menu.

Goal 4: Client will institute measures to prevent chronic pancreatitis.

Implementation
1. Discuss with client ways to eliminate the underlying cause when possible.
2. Avoid alcohol and caffeine.
3. Suggest alcohol rehabilitation programs if indicated.
Evaluation
Client has no recurrences; joins and consistently attends Alcoholics Anonymous.

☐ **Hepatitis**
General Information
1. Definition: acute inflammatory disease of the liver caused by virus (most common), bacteria, or toxic or chemical injury.
2. Types (see Table 3-28)
3. Pathophysiology
   a. Virus invades portal tracts and lobules of liver, causing inflammation and destruction of parenchymal cells
   b. Hyperplasia of Kupffer cells
   c. Damaged cells are gradually phagocytized and cell regeneration occurs
4. Medical treatment
   a. Rest, symptomatic support
   b. Interventions to minimize transmission

Nursing Process
Assessment
Preicteric
1. Flulike symptoms (malaise, fever, and chills)
2. Dull pain and tenderness in right upper quadrant (RUQ) of abdomen; liver enlargement
3. Nausea and vomiting
Icteric (2-6 weeks)
4. Jaundice
5. Clay-colored stools, dark-amber urine
6. Pruritus
7. Continued fatigue, anorexia, abdominal tenderness
8. Abnormal liver function tests (bilirubin, AST, and ALT)
Posticteric (2-6 months)
9. Resolving jaundice
10. Gradual return of appetite and energy
Analysis (see p. 162)
Planning, Implementation, and Evaluation

Goal 1: Significant others and staff will be protected from the client's infection.

Implementation
1. Follow guidelines for universal precautions.

Table 3-28 Major forms of hepatitis

Factor	Hepatitis A	Hepatitis B	Non A–non B hepatitis
Primary route of infection	Oral, fecal, parenteral	Parenteral, direct and sexual contact, secretions and breast milk	Parenteral, sexual contact
Primary sources of infection	Contaminated food and water	Contaminated blood, blood products, and instruments	Contaminated blood, instruments, and dialysis
Incubation	15-50 days	50-150 days	14-182 days
Age group primarily affected	Children and young girls	Any age	Any age
Severity	Usually mild	Severe	
Vaccine	Not available	Available	Not available

2. Reinforce importance of scrupulous personal hygiene and good hand-washing.

Hepatitis A

3. Use disposable eating utensils and dishes.

4. Follow hospital protocol for handling linens.

5. Provide gamma globulin to close household and sexual contacts.

Hepatitis B, non A–non B

6. Provide hepatitis B immune globulin to exposed persons.

7. Suggest hepatitis B vaccine for high-risk persons (e.g., dialysis workers, critical care health workers, and medical and dental staff); repeat every 3-5 years.

Evaluation

Staff members and client's significant others remain free from disease.

Goal 2: Client will have reduced metabolic demand on liver.

Implemenation

1. Place on bed rest; explain reason to client
  a. Limit activities until symptoms have subsided
  b. Provide environment for adequate rest
  c. Provide diversionary activities as needed

2. Monitor liver function tests throughout care.

3. Avoid administering drugs toxic to the liver; use sedatives and opiates with caution.

4. Provide general comfort measures and interventions to control pruritus (refer to "Cholecystitis" Goal 1, p. 167).

Evaluation

Client rests most of the day; sleeps throughout the night.

Goal 3: Client will have adequate nutrition.

Implementation

1. Encourage well-balanced diet with adequate nutrients and calories; restrict fats if poorly tolerated; encourage fluids.

2. Use mild antiemetics if needed before meals; offer small, frequent meals.

3. Know that good nutrition is hard to maintain because of anorexia and nausea.

4. Have food available at client's bedside (e.g., hard candy).

Evaluation

Client's nutritional status appears adequate (no weight loss, intake equals output, normal energy level).

Goal 4: Client will remain free from reinfection.

Implementation

1. Provide health teaching and information about preventive measures

  a. Encourage optimal sanitation and hygiene
  b. Instruct not to share personal care items
  c. Instruct to wash clothing separately in hot water
  d. Avoid sexual activity until blood values normalize
  e. Refrain from alcohol use
  f. Instruct not to donate blood

Evaluation

Client states methods to prevent transmission and recurrence.

☐ Cirrhosis
General Information

1. Definition: chronic degenerative disease of the liver causing inflammation, destruction, fibrotic regeneration, and hepatic insufficiency

2. Incidence: twice as common in men as in women, higher in people 40-60 years old

3. Predisposing/precipitating factors
  a. Malnutrition
  b. Effects of alcohol abuse
  c. Chronic impairment of bile excretion
  d. Necrosis from hepatotoxins or viral hepatitis
  e. Chronic congestive heart failure

4. Pathophysiology
  a. Liver cell damage results in inflammation and hepatomegaly
  b. Attempts at regeneration eventually result in fibrosis and a small nodular liver
  c. Hepatic function is slowly impaired
  d. Obstruction of venous and sinusoid channels blocks hepatic blood flow and causes portal hypertension

5. Medical treatment
  a. Eliminate or relieve causative factors
  b. Rest, nutritional and fluid support
  c. Prevent further liver damage

Nursing Process

Assessment

1. Early signs
  a. History of failing health
  b. Anorexia, nausea, indigestion
  c. Aching or heaviness in right upper quadrant
  d. Weakness, fatigue

2. Later signs
  a. Abnormal liver function tests: elevated bilirubin, AST, ALT, alkaline phosphatase
  b. Intermittent jaundice and pruritus
  c. Edema and ascites, prominent abdominal wall veins, decreased serum albumin
  d. Bleeding tendencies, prolonged prothrombin time, decreased platelet count
  e. Anemia: folic acid deficiency, decreased RBC production, increased RBC destruction in spleen
  f. Frequent infections, decreased WBC
  g. Hormonal abnormalities, elevated estrogen levels

1. palmar erythema, vascular spiders
2. testicular atrophy, gynecomastia, amenorrhea, or impotence

Analysis (see p. 162)

Planning, Implementation, and Evaluation

> **Goal 1:** Client will have reduced metabolic demands on liver.

Implementation

1. Provide bed rest during periods of acute malfunction.
2. Have client rest before and between activities if anemia becomes worse.
3. Eliminate ingestion of all substances toxic to liver: sedatives and opiates, alcohol, acetaminophen.

Evaluation

Client rests quietly most of the day; keeps activities to a minimum; sleeps through the night.

> **Goal 2:** Client will have adequate nutrition and hydration.

Implementation

1. Give a high-protein, high-carbohydrate, high-calorie (over 2000), sodium-restricted diet.
2. Plan small, frequent meals.
3. Administer multiple-vitamin therapy as ordered (higher doses of thiamin and fat-soluble vitamins if there is deficient fat absorption).
4. Restrict fluids and sodium intake if there is edema and/or ascites.
5. Provide mouth care before meals (foul taste may be present).
6. Monitor I&O and daily weights.

Evaluation

Client eats prescribed diet; is adequately hydrated; maintains weight.

> **Goal 3:** Client will be free from infection.

Implementation

1. Encourage scrupulous personal hygiene.
2. Know that reverse isolation may be necessary with extreme leukopenia.
3. Assess for signs of urinary or respiratory infection.
4. Encourage frequent deep-breathing and position changes.

Evaluation

Client has normal temperature; remains free from skin abrasions or inflammation.

> **Goal 4:** Client will be protected from bleeding.

Implementation

1. Monitor urine, stool, gums, and skin for signs of bleeding or bruising.
2. Avoid injections; apply pressure to venipuncture sites for at least 5 minutes.
3. Monitor prothrombin time and PTT.
4. Teach client to use soft toothbrush for oral care.
5. Handle client gently and prevent scratching from pruritus.
6. Administer vitamin K as ordered.

Evaluation

Client remains free of bleeding.

☐ Complications of Liver Disease: Esophageal Varices, Ascites, Hepatic Encephalopathy
General Information: Esophageal Varices

1. Definition: dilation of collateral veins that bypass a scarred liver to carry portal blood to vena cava; may occur in esophagus and stomach
2. Pathophysiology
   a. As liver becomes increasingly cirrhotic, portal hypertension increases
   b. Collateral circulation in the esophagus develops in vessels that are weaker than normal vessels
   c. As pressure in collateral vessels increases, vessels become overdistended and can rupture and bleed
3. Usually asymptomatic until the varices rupture
4. Mortality rate associated with hemorrhage is high
5. Treatment
   a. Medical intervention: Sengstaken-Blakemore tube; vasopressin infusion
   b. Endoscopic sclerotherapy
   c. Surgical intervention: portacaval shunt (anastomosis between the portal vein and inferior vena cava [has a high mortality rate])

Nursing Process: Esophageal Varices
Assessment

1. Abrupt, active bleeding following
   a. Increased abdominal pressure (physical exertion, Valsalva maneuver, coughing)
   b. Mechanical trauma (abrasions from swallowing poorly chewed food)
   c. Esophageal irritation by HCl, pepsin
2. Hematemesis

Analysis (see p. 162)

Planning, Implementation, and Evaluation

> **Goal:** Client will have esophageal bleeding effectively controlled.

Implementation

1. Assist with insertion of Sengstaken-Blakemore tube (see Fig. 3-14).
   a. Ensure balloon patency and accurate labeling of all ports before insertion.
   b. Monitor balloon pressure frequently (at least qh);

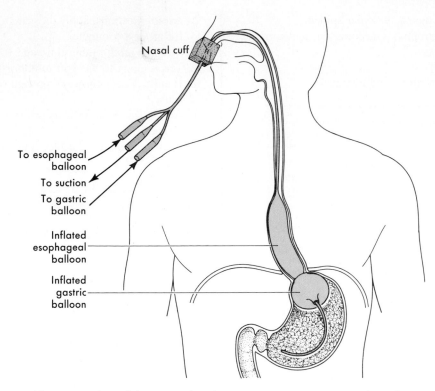

Nasal cuff

To esophageal balloon

To suction

To gastric balloon

Inflated esophageal balloon

Inflated gastric balloon

Fig. 3-14 The Sengstaken-Blakemore tube. (From Beare, P., & Myers, J. [1990]. *Principles and practice of adult health nursing.* St. Louis: Mosby—Year Book.)

deflate balloons to relieve tissue pressure as ordered.

c. Help client expectorate secretions or gently suction secretions from oral cavity (client cannot swallow around tube).

d. Monitor airway (danger of airway obstruction if tube moves); elevate head of bed 30°-45°.

e. Provide comfort measures such as mouth and nasal care and positioning (esophageal balloon may be left inflated for up to 48 hours).

f. Administer antacids as ordered.

2. Monitor and treat client for shock as needed (see "Shock," p. 128).

a. Establish adequate venous access.

b. Administer blood transfusions as ordered.

c. Administer vitamin K to correct clotting problems.

3. Administer gastric lavage, saline cathartics, lactulose, and enemas as ordered to reduce ammonia formation and possibility of hepatic coma.

4. Give intestinal antimicrobials (e.g., neomycin) as ordered to decrease intestinal bacterial action.

Evaluation

Client's esophageal bleeding is promptly identified and controlled; condition remains stable.

General Information: Ascites

1. Definition: an abnormal intraperitoneal accumulation of watery fluid containing small amounts of protein

2. Pathophysiology: results from a complex series of factors

a. Decreased colloid osmotic pressure from decreased liver albumin production

b. Increased capillary hydrostatic pressure from portal hypertension

c. Hypovolemia-related renin, angiotensin, aldosterone, and ADH secretion resulting in sodium and water retention

3. Medical treatment (dependent on severity of ascites)

a. Sodium (200-1000 mg) and fluid restriction (500-1000 ml)

b. Diuretic therapy: spironolactone (Aldactone) is often first drug used; a thiazide diuretic may be added

c. Salt-poor albumin to restore plasma volume

d. Placement of LeVeen shunt (catheter to move ascites from peritoneum to vena cava)

e. Paracentesis

1. used only for diagnosis or when fluid volume compromises comfort and breathing

2. fluid tends to reaccumulate rapidly

Nursing Process: Ascites

Assessment

1. Enlarged abdominal girth

2. Increased weight

3. Fatigue

4. Fluid status, dehydration
5. Abdominal discomfort, respiratory difficulty
Analysis (see p. 162)
Planning, Implementation, and Evaluation

> **Goal:** Client will experience a reduction of ascites and an increase in comfort.

Implementation
1. Maintain bed rest or restricted activity.
2. Give fluid- and sodium-restricted diet.
3. Monitor fluid and electrolyte balance and I&O.
4. Monitor daily weights.
5. Measure abdominal girth at least every shift.
6. Maintain high-Fowler's position for maximum respiratory effectiveness and comfort.
7. Support abdomen with pillows.
8. Administer diuretics as ordered.
9. Administer salt-poor albumin IV as ordered; monitor carefully for signs of CHF, pulmonary edema, dehydration, and electrolyte imbalance.
10. Assist with paracentesis if performed.
    a. Get a permit signed if appropriate.
    b. Have client void before the procedure.
    c. Prepare the client for a dangling or high-Fowler's position during the procedure.
    d. Monitor client during and after the procedure for hypovolemia and electrolyte imbalance.
    e. Observe puncture wound for leakage, signs of infection.

Evaluation
Client is comfortable; undergoes paracentesis without complications; has ascites reduced; experiences a reduction in abdominal girth and respiratory distress.

General Information: Hepatic Encephalopathy

1. Definition: cerebral dysfunction associated with severe liver disease
2. Pathophysiology: inability of the liver to metabolize substances that can be toxic to the brain such as ammonia, which is produced by the breakdown of protein in the intestinal tract
3. Medical treatment (depends on severity)
    a. Restriction or elimination of dietary protein
    b. Lactulose or neomycin to inhibit protein breakdown, decrease bacterial ammonia production, cleanse bowel of bacteria and protein

Nursing Process: Hepatic Encephalopathy
Assessment
1. Mental status, level of consiousness: lethargy progressing to coma
    a. Dullness, slurred speech
    b. Behavioral changes, lack of interest in grooming or appearance

2. Neurological exam: twitching, muscular incoordination, asterixis (a flapping tremor)
3. Elevated serum ammonia level
Analysis (see p. 162)
Planning, Implementation, and Evaluation

> **Goal 1:** Client will have decreased ammonia production.

Implementation
1. Reduce dietary protein to 20-40 g/day (see Table 3-43); maintain adequate calories.
2. Decrease ammonia formation in the intestine
    a. Give laxatives, enemas as ordered.
    b. Administer lactulose (Cephulac) and neomycin (oral or rectal) as ordered.

Evaluation
Client's serum ammonia level returns to normal limits; client tolerates a low-protein diet.

> **Goal 2:** Client will remain free from injury.

Implementation
1. Perform general nursing measures for the unconscious client (refer to *Sensation and Perception,* p. 228).
2. Assess mental status frequently.

Evaluation
Client regains consciousness free from injury.

> **Goal 3:** Client and significant others will learn to prevent future episodes of encephalopathy.

Implementation
1. Counsel client regarding low-protein diet and prescribed medications.
2. Ensure that client and family understand how to avoid and treat constipation.
3. Teach family early signs of encephalopathy (restlessness, slurred speech, decreased attention span).

Evaluation
Client states measures to ensure proper bowel functioning; states principles of a low-protein diet and planned rest periods.

The Endocrine System
GENERAL CONCEPTS
Overview/Physiology

1. The endocrine system is a chemical communication system that functions together with the nervous system as the body's communication network
    a. Endocrine glands synthesize and secrete chemical substances (hormones) that control and integrate body functions (see Table 3-29)
        1. secreted in minute amounts
        2. circulated in the blood

Table 3-29   Hormones

Gland	Hormone	Action
Hypothalamus	Releasing hormones	Stimulates release of hormones from pituitary gland.
	Inhibiting hormones	Inhibits release of hormones from pituitary gland.
	Antidiuretic hormone (ADH)	See Pituitary, posterior lobe.
Pituitary, anterior lobe	Growth hormone (GH)	Acts directly on bones and other tissues to stimulate growth.
	Prolactin (LTH)	Stimulates development of mammary tissue and lactation.
	Thryotropic hormone (TSH)	Stimulates thyroid gland.
	Adrenocorticotropic hormone (ACTH)	Stimulates adrenal cortex.
	Melanocyte-stimulating hormone (MSH)	Stimulates darkening of the skin.
	Luteinizing hormone (LH)	Initiates ovulation and formation of corpus luteum.
	Follicle-stimulating hormone (FSH)	*Women:* stimulates ovarian development of graafian follicle. *Men:* maintains spermatogenesis.
Pituitary, posterior lobe	Antidiuretic hormone (ADH): produced in hypothalamus and stored in pituitary	Facilitates reabsorption of H_2O in the kidneys, vasoconstriction in arterioles.
	Oxytocin	Initiates expression of breast milk; stimulates uterine contractions at delivery.
Thyroid	Triiodothyronine (T_3) Thyroxine (T_4)	Control body metabolism and influence physical and mental growth; nervous system activity; protein, fat, carbohydrate metabolism; reproduction.
	Calcitonin	Lowers serum calcium levels, inhibits bone resorption.
Parathyroid	Parathormone (PTH)	
Pancreas	*Endocrine function*	Regulates calcium and phosphorus metabolism.
	Insulin	Enables glucose to freely enter cells; helps muscle and tissue oxidation of glucose; promotes storage of glycogen.
	Glucagon	Increases gluconeogenesis in liver.
	Exocrine function (digestive enzymes)	
	Amylase	Aids carbohydrate digestion.
	Trypsin	Aids protein digestion.
	Lipase	Aids fat digestion.
Adrenal cortex	Glucocorticoids: cortisone, cortisol	Decrease protein synthesis; regulate serum glucose by increasing rate of gluconeogenesis; suppress the inflammatory and immune response; increase fat mobilization; support adaptation during stressful situations.
	Mineralocorticoids: aldosterone	Facilitate reabsorption of NA^+ and elimination of K^+.
	Sex hormones: primarily androgens	Responsible for development of secondary sex characteristics.
Adrenal medulla	Epinephrine	Initiates stress response.
	Norepinephrine	Causes vasoconstriction.
Ovaries	Estrogen	Responsible for secondary sex characteristics, mammary duct system, growth of graafian follicle in women.
	Progesterone	Prepares corpus luteum; maintains pregnancy.
Testes	Testosterone	Responsible for secondary sex characteristics, normal reproductive function in men.

3. regulated by
   a. negative feedback systems
   b. changes in the plasma concentration of specific substances
   c. direct autonomic nervous system activity
   d. circadian rhythms
4. action alters specific physiological responses
   a. growth and development
   b. reproduction
   c. metabolism
   d. responses to stress and injury

b. Health problems involving the endocrine system result from hormone imbalances
   1. primary problems: involvement of the target gland of the hormone
   2. secondary problems: involvement of the primary gland of secretion (i.e., pituitary or hypothalamus)

2. Glands

a. Pituitary

1. anatomy

a. lies in the sella turcica above the sphenoid at the base of the brain

b. consists of two lobes connected by the hypothalamus

2. functions (see Table 3-29)

a. anterior lobe (adenohypophysis) secretes ACTH, MSH, TSH, FSH, GH, and prolactin

b. posterior lobe (neurohypophysis) secretes ADH (vasopressin) and oxytocin

c. regulates the function of the other endocrine glands through the stimulation of target organs

d. controlled through the action of releasing and inhibiting factors from the hypothalamus

b. Thyroid gland

1. anatomy

a. located at or below the cricoid cartilage in the neck, anterior to the trachea

b. consists of two highly vascular lobes

2. functions (see Table 3-29)

a. controls the rate of body metabolism through the production of thyroxine (T_4) and triiodothyronine (T_3)

b. produces calcitonin

c. Parathyroid glands

1. anatomy: four small glands located near or imbedded in the thyroid gland

2. functions: secrete parathyroid hormone (PTH) and control calcium and phosphorus metabolism in the body

d. Adrenal glands

1. anatomy: two small glands lying in the retroperitoneal region, capping each kidney

2. functions (see Table 3-29)

a. adrenal cortex (outer capsule)

◆ secretes the adrenocortical steroids (cortisol, cortisone, corticosterone)

◆ secretes the mineralocorticoids (aldosterone)

◆ secretes the adrenal sex hormones (androgen, estrogen, progesterone)

b. adrenal medulla (inner parenchyma of gland)

◆ stimulated by the sympathetic nervous system

◆ secretes catecholamines (epinephrine and norepinephrine)

e. Pancreas

1. anatomy

a. long, soft gland that lies retroperitoneally

b. head of the gland is in the duodenal cavity and the tail lies against the spleen

2. functions

a. exocrine function to produce digestive enzymes

b. endocrine function to control carbohydrate metabolism

◆ glucagon secreted by alpha cells

◆ insulin secreted by beta cells

Application of the Nursing Process to the Client with Endocrine System Problems

Assessment

Hormones have very diverse systemic effects. Hypofunction or hyperfunction can result in dysfunction in a wide variety of organs and organ systems.

1. Health history

a. Current symptoms

1. change in client's energy level or stamina

2. change in personal appearance

a. size of head, hands, or feet

b. weight, skin, or hair

c. secondary sex characteristics

3. increased sympathetic nervous system activity

4. change in alertness or personality

5. change in sexual functioning

b. Past or family history

1. abnormal progression in growth and development

2. family history of diabetes, hypertension, infertility, mental illness

2. Physical exam

a. Inspection: subtle or dramatic deviations from normal in body size, muscle tone, skin, hair, voice, and sexual characteristics

b. Palpation: limited to the thyroid gland

3. Diagnostic tests (multiple tests available for each gland)

a. Measurement of the amounts of hormones present in serum or urine

b. Fluctuations in daily pattern of hormone secretion causes random specimens to have limited value

4. Medical treatment

a. Medical intervention: hormone replacement therapy, diet adjustment

b. Surgical intervention: partial or total gland removal

Analysis

1. Safe, effective care environment

a. Knowledge deficit

b. High risk for injury

2. Physiological integrity

a. Activity intolerance

b. High risk for fluid volume deficit

c. Altered nutrition: more or less than body requirements

3. Psychosocial integrity

a. Anxiety

b. Ineffective individual coping

c. Body image disturbance
4. Health promotion/maintenance
   a. Impaired adjustment
   b. Noncompliance
   c. Health-seeking behaviors

General Nursing Planning, Implementation, and Evaluation (refer to General Nursing Goals 1, 3, and 4 for Digestive Tract Problems, p. 162)

> **Goal:** Client will adapt to changes in body image.

Implementation
1. Assess client's perceptions of body.

2. Encourage client to verbalize concerns.
3. Provide client with correct information about the degree of symptom reversibility.

Evaluation
Client expresses self-acceptance and engages in usual social activities.

SELECTED HEALTH PROBLEMS
☐ Disorders of the Pituitary Gland
General Information (see Table 3-30)
Nursing Process: Hyperfunction
Assessment (see Table 3-30)
Analysis (see p. 175)

Table 3-30   Pituitary disorders

Disorder	Description	Symptoms	Medical management
HYPERPITUITARISM			
Anterior pituitary (acromegaly or gigantism)	Excess growth hormone secretion results in gigantism in childhood and acromegaly after puberty. Usually caused by a benign adenoma or ectopic stimulation. More common in women.	Coarse facial features; protruding, enlarged jaw and nose; enlarged hands and feet. Voice changes, fatigue and lethargy. Headache.	Options include a) transsphenoidal hypophysectomy b) radiotherapy c) drugs to suppress growth hormone Hypopituitarism is a risk with all treatments.
Posterior pituitary (syndrome of inappropriate secretion of ADH [SIADH])	Disorder is characterized by the inappropriate continued release of ADH, which can result in water intoxication, water excess, and hyponatremia. Disorder may be triggered by neoplasms, trauma, surgery, and drugs.	Depend on severity and rapidity of development. Weight gain, falling urine output, anorexia and nausea, confusion and lethargy. Seizures and coma may accompany very low sodium levels.	Fluid restriction to 500 ml will usually reverse the disorder. Drug therapy may inhibit renal ADH response; 3%-5% IV saline administration may be needed.
HYPOPITUITARISM			
Anterior pituitary	Rare disorder that usually involves partial or complete deficiency of hormone secretion and results in multiple deficiencies. May be triggered by neoplasms, infection, or hereditary conditions.	Symptoms are variable and depend upon the specific deficiencies. Most result from hypogonadism. They include menstrual irregularities, impotence, lethargy and fatigue, decreased stress response.	Options include hormone replacement (corticosteroids, levothyroxine, estrogen or testosterone), transsphenoidal surgery, or radiotherapy.
Posterior pituitary (diabetes insipidus)	Condition of impaired renal water conservation resulting from a deficiency in ADH. It may develop idiopathically or result from trauma, surgery, tumors, infections, or in response to drugs.	The syndrome causes abrupt onset of extreme thirst, polyuria, and polydipsia. Urine volume may reach 4-20 L/day with frequent urination. Dehydration may develop rapidly.	Treatment involves fluid replacement and drug therapy, usually with intranasal or injectable vasopressin.

Planning, Implementation, and Evaluation

> **Goal 1:** Client who has been treated by trans-sphenoidal hypophysectomy will be free from postoperative complications.

Implementation
1. Refer to "Intracranial Surgery," p. 236.
2. Note any nasal leakage of cerebrospinal fluid.
3. Prevent increased intracranial pressure (ICP).
4. Monitor signs of diabetes insipidus or adrenal crisis.

Evaluation
Client remains free from postoperative infection or alteration in mental status; maintains stable vital signs and fluid balance.

> **Goal 2:** Client treated by hypophysectomy will be prepared for knowledgeable self-care (see General Nursing Goals 2 and 4, p. 162.

Implementation
1. Provide information about the importance of lifelong replacement therapy with regular medical supervision.

Evaluation
Client follows prescribed medication regimen, experiences minimal fluctuations in hormone levels, expresses self-acceptance.

> **Goal 3:** Client with SIADH will reestablish normal fluid and electrolyte balance.

Implementation
1. Restrict fluid intake as ordered (less than 1000 ml/ day).
2. Maintain accurate I&O and daily weight records.
3. Monitor for symptoms of sodium or potassium imbalance.
4. Assess for signs of cerebral edema (refer to *Sensation and Perception*, p. 228).

Evaluation
Client's weight is stable; urinary output is within acceptable limits.

Nursing Process: Hypofunction

Assessment (see Table 3-30)
Analysis (see p. 175)
Planning, Implementation, and Evaluation

> **Goal 1:** Client's hormone levels will be restored and maintained in the normal range.

Implementation
1. Provide information about medications (i.e., name, dosage, side effects) and the importance of lifelong replacement with ongoing medical supervision.

2. Teach client the effects of physical and psychological stress on hormone needs.

Evaluation
Client follows prescribed medication regimen; adjusts life-style to maintain hormone balance.

> **Goal 2:** Client with diabetes insipidus will reestablish and maintain normal fluid and electrolyte balance.

Implementation
1. Administer replacement fluids as ordered.
2. Keep accurate I&O; monitor daily weight, urine specific gravity.
3. Monitor for signs of hypovolemic shock (refer to "Shock," p. 128).
4. Administer vasopressin nasal spray or vasopressin (Pitressin) IM as ordered (usually every 36-72 hours).
5. Teach client safe administration of nasal preparation.
6. Teach signs and symptoms of fluid volume excess.

Evaluation
Client's fluid balance is within normal limits; client self-administers replacement medications safely.

☐ Hyperthyroidism
General Information

1. Definition: oversecretion of the thyroid gland; second to diabetes in incidence; also called thyrotoxicosis
   a. A recurrent syndrome; may appear after emotional shock, stress, or infection
   b. Occurs primarily in women 30-50 years of age
   c. A variety of causes have been identified including adenoma, goiter, viral inflammation, and autoimmune glandular stimulation; Graves' disease is most common cause
2. Diagnosis
   a. Classic clinical picture
   b. Elevated T_3, T_4, protein-bound iodine (PBI), ^{131}I uptake values
   c. Abnormal findings from thyroid scan
3. Complications
   a. Cardiovascular disease (hypertension, angina, CHF)
   b. Exophthalmos caused by abnormal deposits of fat and fluid in the retroocular tissue
   c. Thyroid storm or crisis: life-threatening hypermetabolism and excessive adrenergic response
4. Medical treatment
   a. Medications
      1. propylthiouracil (PTU): antithyroid drug that depresses the synthesis of thyroid hormone; takes about three months to be completely effective
      2. propranolol (Inderal) or other adrenergic blockers: adrenergic antagonist that relieves the adrenergic effects of excess thyroid hormone

(e.g., sweating, tachycardia, tremors)

   3. iodine preparations (SSKI): decrease the size and vascularity of the gland (short-term use)

  b. Radioactive iodine: limits the secretion of hormone by damaging or destroying thyroid tissue; treatment of choice for most adults

  c. Surgical intervention (only performed when client is in a euthyroid state)

   1. subtotal thyroidectomy (for large goiters)

   2. total thyroidectomy (if carcinoma present)

Nursing Process

Assessment

1. Cardiovascular: elevated BP, bounding pulse, tachycardia, palpitations
2. Nutrition: weight loss, increased appetite, frequent stools
3. Integument: flushed, moist skin; heat intolerance
4. Musculoskeletal: fatigue, muscle weakness and wasting, fine tremors
5. Psychological: anxiety, insomnia, mood swings, personality changes
6. Other: menstrual irregularities, change in libido
7. Exophthalmos

Analysis (see p. 175)

Planning, Implementation, and Evaluation

Goal 1: Client will return to and remain in euthyroid state.

Implementation

1. Provide calm, restful physical environment with low levels of sensory stimulation.
   a. Ensure physical comfort; cool environmental temperature.
   b. Provide adequate rest, avoid muscle fatigue.
2. Provide adequate nutrients.
   a. High-calorie (4000-5000), balanced diet.
   b. Increased fluid intake.
   c. Small, frequent meals if hypermotility is present.
3. Provide eye care if exophthalmos present.
   a. Eye drops, dark glasses, patch eyes if necessary.
   b. Elevate head of bed for sleep.
   c. Assess adequacy of lid closure.
   d. Restrict dietary sodium.

Evaluation

Client enjoys restful sleep; verbalizes decreased discomfort and fatigue; maintains or increases body weight; is free from corneal damage.

Goal 2: Client undergoing thyroidectomy will be free from postoperative complications.

Implementation

1. Prepare client's room before return from OR with O_2, suction, tracheostomy set, and calcium gluconate at bedside.

2. Monitor for signs of bleeding or excessive edema.
   a. Elevate head of bed 30°; support head and neck
   b. Check dressings frequently, assess for constriction
   c. Check behind the neck for bleeding
3. Assess for signs of respiratory distress, hoarseness (laryngeal damage is possible, but worsening hoarseness is usually the result of edema).
4. Be alert for the possibility of
   a. Tetany (owing to hypocalcemia caused by accidental removal of parathyroid glands): assess for numbness, tingling, or muscle twitching.
   b. Thyroid storm: markedly increased temperature and pulse with increasing restlessness and agitation.
5. Administer food and fluid with care (dysphagia is common).
6. Encourage client to gradually increase range of motion of neck.

Evaluation

Client maintains normal vital signs; experiences no excessive bleeding or respiratory distress; supports head and neck during movement.

Goal 3: Client will maintain normal levels of thyroid hormone.

Implementation

1. Provide client with information about prescribed medications (i.e., name, dosage, side effects) and the importance of ongoing medical supervision.
   a. Total thyroidectomy necessitates lifelong replacement medication
   b. Subtotal thyroidectomy necessitates careful monitoring of the return of thyroid function
2. Teach client receiving radioactive iodine treatment symptoms of thyroid deficiency (hypothyroidism is common within 2-5 years).

Evaluation

Client follows prescribed medication regimen; is euthyroid.

☐ Hypothyroidism
General Information

1. Definitions: underactive state of the thyroid gland resulting in diminished secretion of thyroid hormone
   a. Creates a diffuse clinical syndrome
   b. Most common in women in their middle years
   c. Effects may be overt or extremely subtle
2. Diagnosis
   a. Decreased T_3 and T_4
   b. Elevated TSH and cholesterol
3. Complications
   a. Cretinism: severe physical and mental retardation resulting from severe deficiency in infancy or childhood
   b. Myxedema: rare syndrome that may occur from prolonged severe disease

1. accelerated development of coronary artery disease
2. organic psychosis
3. myxedema coma: rapid development of impaired consciousness and suppression of vital functions

4. Medical treatment: thyroid replacement
   a. Levothyroxine (Synthroid) is the drug of choice, if client does not have disabling cardiac involvement
   b. Liothyronine (Cytomel) is useful in clients who experience allergic responses to other preparations

Nursing Process

Assessment

1. Fatigue, weight gain, constipation
2. Dry skin, cold intolerance
3. Coarse, thinning hair
4. Mental sluggishness
5. Thick tongue, swollen lips
6. Menstrual irregularities, infertility
7. Extreme sensitivity to narcotics, barbiturates, anesthetics

Analysis (see p. 175)

Planning, Implementation, and Evaluation

> **Goal:** Client will return to and remain in euthyroid state.

Implementation

1. Provide a warm environment conducive to rest.
2. Avoid use of all sedatives.
3. Assist client in choosing low-calorie diet.

4. Increase intake of fluid and roughage to relieve constipation.
5. Increase physical activity and sensory stimulation gradually as condition improves.
6. Monitor cardiovascular response to increased hormone levels carefully.
7. Provide information about prescribed medication (i.e., name, dosage, side effects) and the importance of lifelong medical supervision.

Evaluation

Client follows prescribed medication regimen; loses weight; experiences increased activity tolerance and alertness.

☐ Disorders of the Parathyroid Gland

General Information (see Table 3-31)

Nursing Process: Hyperfunction

Assessment (see Table 3-31)

Analysis (see p. 175)

Planning, Implementation, and Evaluation

> **Goal:** Client undergoing parathyroidectomy will be free from complications.

Implementation

1. Provide low-calcium diet preoperatively; avoid milk and milk products.
2. Encourage high fluid intake preoperatively (at least 3000 ml/day).
3. Perform general postoperative care as for thyroidectomy, and in addition
   a. Observe carefully for tetany.
   b. Institute *high*-calcium diet.

Table 3-31 Parathyroid gland disorders

Disorder	Description	Symptoms	Medical management
Hyperparathyroidism	Disorder of calcium, phosphate, and bone metabolism characterized by hypersecretion of parathyroid hormone (PTH) from increased gland mass. May be caused by benign adenomas or secondary responses to hypocalcemic states. Incidence rises sharply after age 50.	Usually detected on routine chemistry profiles since most clients are asymptomatic. If present, symptoms are related to excess calcium and include hypertension, renal stones, muscle weakness, GI distress, constipation, and bone pain.	Surgical removal of affected gland; low-calcium diet, fluids, and calcium-blocking agents.
Hypoparathyroidism	May be produced by a variety of disease states associated with impaired secretion of parathyroid hormone (PTH). Rare disorders and autoimmune involvement is likely.	Symptoms are variable and primarily related to the severity and rapidity of the deficiency. Calcium deficiency is primary aspect with muscle tetany, abdominal cramping. Cardiac depression and seizures may occur.	Medications to replace calcium and vitamin D and control phosphate levels.

4. Encourage ambulation to stimulate bone recalcification.

Evaluation

Client maintains calcium values within normal range; experiences normal muscle functioning; follows prescribed diet.

Nursing Process: Hypofunction

Assessment (see Table 3-31)
Analysis (see p. 175)
Planning, Implementation, and Evaluation

> **Goal:** Client will be free from the complications of prolonged calcium imbalance.

Implementation

1. Acute stage
  a. Assess for symptoms of tetany frequently
  b. Keep calcium gluconate at bedside
2. Chronic stage
  a. Provide high-calcium, low-phosphorus diet
  b. Provide information about prescribed medications (i.e., name, dosage, side effects)
3. Teach client symptoms of calcium imbalance.

Evaluation

Client follows prescribed medication and diet regimen; is free from the symptoms of hypocalcemia.

☐ Hyperfunction of the Adrenal Glands
General Information

1. Definition: oversecretion of hormones from either the adrenal cortex or adrenal medulla
  a. Cushing's syndrome: excessive secretion of glucocorticoids and possibly androgens from the adrenal cortex
  b. Pheochromocytoma: catecholamine-producing tumor of the adrenal medulla (see Table 3-32)
  c. Hyperaldosteronism: excessive secretion of aldosterone from the cortex because of a tumor, adenoma, or a secondary response to chronic sodium loss (see Table 3-32)
2. Incidence
  a. True Cushing's syndrome is relatively rare, but occurs most frequently in women aged 20-60
  b. Can result from adrenal tumors or excessive pituitary secretion of ACTH from any cause
  c. A common result of the chronic use of exogenous steroids
3. Diagnosis: increased plasma cortisol, blood glucose, urinary 17-hydroxysteroids and 17-ketosteroids; decreased potassium
4. Complications
  a. Cardiac problems (e.g., CHF or hypertension)
  b. Skeletal fractures
  c. Opportunistic infections

Table 3-32   Other adrenal disorders

Disorder	Description	Symptoms	Medical management
Pheochromocytoma	A rare disorder that may occur in middle age in either sex and appears to have some familial patterns. They are highly vascular tumors that produce, store, and secrete catecholamines. Diagnosed through elevated metanephrine and catecholamine levels and urinary vanillylmandelic acid (VMA).	Paniclike hypermetabolic state. Sustained or paroxysmal hypertensive attacks associated with headache, palpitations, sweating, and anxiety. MI and CVA are significant risks.	Surgical adrenalectomy is treatment of choice after control of catecholamine release and blood pressure is established.
Hyperaldosteronism	The primary disorder affects mainly women in middle age and usually involves a benign adenoma, adrenal hyperplasia, or tumor. Secondary disease results from the activation of the renin angiotensin system by a nonadrenal stimulus like sodium loss, renal arteriolar narrowing, nephrosclerosis, and cirrhosis.	Usually asymptomatic but may have hypertension, headache, fatigue, and hypokalemia.	Options include surgical adrenalectomy and medications to control blood pressure and restore potassium levels.

5. Medical treatment
   a. Surgical adrenalectomy if tumor is present
   b. Hypophysectomy for tumor of pituitary
   c. Drug therapy with cortisol inhibitors
   d. Alteration in exogenous steroid dose if possible

Nursing Process

Assessment
1. Cushing's syndrome
   a. Abnormal fat distribution
      1. weight gain, thick trunk, thin legs
      2. moon face, buffalo hump (cervical dorsal fat pad)
   b. Skin changes
      1. thin fragile skin, red cheeks
      2. purple striae (stretch marks)
      3. bruises or acne
      4. body hirsutism
   c. Cardiovascular
      1. sodium and water retention, hypokalemia
      2. hypertension
      3. fluid overload, CHF
   d. Musculoskeletal
      1. muscle weakness, decreased muscle mass, fatigue
      2. osteoporosis, bone pain, fractures
   e. Increased susceptibility to infection
   f. Decreased resistance to stress
   g. Increased secretion of pepsin and HC1
   h. Hyperglycemia
   i. Mental changes and mood swings
   j. Changes in secondary sex characteristics, menstrual irregularities, amenorrhea

Analysis (see p. 175)

Planning, Implementation, and Evaluation

Goal 1: Client with Cushing's syndrome will have fewer symptoms.

Implementation
1. Provide diet low in calories and sodium, but high in protein, potassium, and calcium.
   a. Offer diet in small, frequent feedings.
   b. Monitor for signs of hyperglycemia, GI bleeding.
2. Protect client from unnecessary exposure to infection.
   a. Monitor vital signs regularly.
   b. Use strict hygiene and asepsis.
   c. Institute reverse isolation if needed.
3. Provide atmosphere conducive to rest; space activities and help with care as needed.
4. Observe for signs of CHF.
5. Monitor daily weights, I&O, blood and urine glucose measurements.
6. Offer needed support in dealing with changes in body image.

Evaluation
Client maintains or loses weight; experiences increased strength and stamina; is free from infection, accidental injury, or peptic ulceration; refers to self in a positive way.

Goal 2: Client treated with adrenalectomy will be free from complications.

Implementation
1. Measure urine output accurately and frequently.
2. Monitor vital signs frequently.
3. Watch for signs of adrenal crisis; have IV fluids, pressor drugs, corticosteroids readily available.
4. Minimize physiological and psychological stress.
5. Prevent thrombotic and respiratory problems.
6. Monitor wound healing carefully.
7. Teach regarding postdischarge self-care (e.g., diet, medications, activity level, and follow-up care).

Evaluation
Client maintains stable vital signs, adequate urine output and respiratory gas exchange postoperatively; states self-care needs to expect after discharge.

☐ Hyposecretion of the Adrenal Glands
General Information
1. Definition: Addison's disease: insufficient secretion of glucocorticoids, mineralocorticoids, and possibly androgens from the adrenal cortex
2. Incidence
   a. Rare disease occurring in 1 in 100,000; affects both sexes and usually occurs in middle age
   b. True Addison's disease is usually caused by autoimmune adrenalitis, but will occur after bilateral surgical removal of the adrenal glands or withdrawal of exogenous steroids after long-term suppression
3. Diagnosis
   a. Low serum cortisol levels
   b. Low serum sodium and glucose
   c. Elevated serum potassium
   d. ACTH stimulation tests
4. Complications: adrenal crisis—acute adrenal insufficiency with sudden, marked deprivation of adrenocortical hormones producing vascular collapse and hypoglycemia
5. Medical intervention: steroid replacement maintained throughout life
   a. Glucocorticoids
      1. hydrocortisone usually given for maintenance
      2. dose will need to be increased at any time of increased stress, including illness or surgery
   b. Mineralocorticoids: fludrocortisone (Florinef) 0.05-0.2 mg daily (if more needed, long-acting preparation may be given)

c. Periodic testosterone injections to support protein anabolism

Nursing Process

Assessment

(NOTE: The clinical picture from the history and symptoms is often vague.)

1. Lethargy, apathy, depression
2. Gastrointestinal symptoms: anorexia, nausea, weight loss, abdominal pain
3. Increased pigmentation of skin and mucous membranes
4. Muscle weakness and fatigue
5. Hypotension, fluid deficit
6. Hypoglycemia
7. Adrenal crisis
   a. Severe headache or abdominal pain
   b. Hypotension or shock
   c. Confusion, restlessness, or coma
   d. Fever
   e. Nausea and diarrhea

Analysis (see p. 175)

Planning, Implementation, and Evaluation

Goal 1: Client will recover from an adrenal crisis.

Implementation

1. Give large dose of glucocorticoids and vasopressors by IV infusion.
2. Encourage complete bed rest; prevent physical activity and emotional stress.
3. Monitor vital signs (especially BP for hypotension) fluid and electrolyte balance, and glucose levels until condition stabilizes.

Evaluation

Client maintains vital signs within normal limits; exercises and returns to normal activity levels gradually.

Goal 2: Client will maintain normal hormonal balance.

Implementation

1. Provide information about prescribed medications (i.e., name, dosage, or side effects) and the importance of ongoing medical supervision.
2. Teach to balance activity and rest, maintain a regular activity pattern.
3. Promote good nutrition; monitor weight, fluid status, and I&O.
4. Help client to deal effectively with stress.
5. Teach client the signs and symptoms of underdose or overdose of medications, and conditions that will require dosage adjustments (see Table 3-33).

Evaluation

Client is asymptomatic; takes and adjusts medications as indicated; maintains ongoing medical care.

☐ Hypofunction of the Pancreas: Diabetes Mellitus

General Information

1. Definition: a chronic, systemic disease producing disorders in carbohydrate, protein, and fat metabolism; results from disturbances in the production, action,

---

Table 3-33 Corticosteroid drugs

Common drugs	Common side effects	Client teaching
Dexamethasone (Decadron)	Weight gain, moon face, truncal obesity	Take medication with a meal or snack.
Hydrocortisone (Cortef, Solu-Cortef)	Muscle wasting and weakness	Never skip a dose or suddenly stop taking the drug.
Prednisone (Deltasone)	Osteoporosis	Maintain an adequate supply and keep the medication on hand during travel.
Methylprednisolone acetate (Medrol)	Sodium and fluid retention, edema	Maintain scrupulous hygiene and avoid persons with infections.
	Hypertension	
	Delayed wound healing	Eat a high-protein, low-sodium, and low-calorie diet.
	Increased risk of infection	Exercise regularly.
	Mood alterations, depression	Obtain and wear a Medic-Alert bracelet.
	Nausea	Tell all health care providers about medication regimen.
	Gastric hyperacidity	Report the presence of any of the following immediately:
	Hyperglycemia	edema.
	Menstrual cycle changes	black or bloody stools.
		sudden weight gain.
		increased thirst or urination.

or use of insulin; eventually produces destructive changes in a wide variety of organs and tissues. The insulin deficiency may be relative or absolute.

2. Incidence
   a. Most common endocrine disorder; more than 10 million diabetics in the United States
   b. Diabetes and its complications are among the leading causes of death and disability in the United States

3. Etiology
   a. Basic etiology remains unknown
   b. Considered to be a group of syndromes whose development is influenced by genetic factors, viruses, autoimmunity, and environmental factors such as stress and obesity

4. Types
   a. Insulin-dependent (IDD; type I): results from destruction of the beta cells of the pancreas resulting in little or no insulin production; requires daily insulin administration
   b. Non–insulin-dependent (NIDD; type II): probably results from a disturbance in insulin reception in the cells or loss of beta cell responsiveness to glucose; most common in middle-aged, overweight adults; 80% of all cases

5. Pathophysiology: type 1 (IDD)
   a. Normally blood-glucose levels are maintained in the homeostatic range of 60-100 mg/dl by a series of feedback mechanisms
   b. In the absence of insulin, glucose accumulates in blood and urine leading to
      1. hyperglycemia
      2. glycosuria
   c. Glucose is hypertonic and depletes the body of large amounts of water (from extracellular fluid) as it is excreted by the kidneys causing
      1. polyuria
      2. polydipsia
      3. loss of sodium and potassium
   d. Glucose is then not available for cellular nutrition, and this causes polyphagia
   e. Fat and protein stores are broken down and used for energy; fatty acid and triglyceride accumulation cause ketone build up with
      1. ketoacidosis
      2. ketonuria
      3. weakness
   f. Other metabolic effects
      1. microcirculatory and macrocirculatory changes producing atherosclerosis and arteriosclerosis (e.g., coronary artery disease, peripheral vascular disease, retinal and kidney damage)
      2. alteration in immune and inflammatory response
         a. glucose concentration in the skin creates an excellent medium for infection
         b. glucose inhibits the phagocytic action of leukocytes, leading to decreased resistance
      3. alterations in perception and coordination caused by developing neuropathies (a common complication the cause of which is not well understood)

6. Pathophysiology: type II (NIDD)
   a. Serum-insulin level may be low, normal, or even elevated
   b. Pathology thought to be a combination of
      1. slowed response in insulin release
      2. reduced number of insulin receptors
      3. receptor abnormality to insulin binding
      4. peripheral resistance to insulin

7. Medical treatment
   a. Drug therapy (see Table 3-34)
      1. insulin: short-, intermediate-, and long-acting forms
      2. oral hypoglycemic agents
   b. Diet: individually planned regimens based on the client's age, sex, weight, and usual life-style (see Table 3-35)
      1. diet is manipulated to distribute the nutrient intake appropriately over a 24-hour period
      2. diet is planned using the American Diabetic Association's (ADA) exchange method of meal planning
      3. diet is used to correct obesity when necessary
   c. Exercise

Nursing Process

Assessment

1. Type 1: initial symptoms
   a. Polyphagia, polyuria, polydipsia, weight loss
   b. Hyperglycemia, glycosuria, ketonuria
   c. Weakness, fatigue
2. Type 2: initial symptoms
   a. Initial symptoms may be less acute or unrecognized
   b. May have classic type 1 signs
   c. Weakness, chronic fatigue, weight gain
   d. Hyperglycemia, glycosuria
3. Fasting glucose greater than 140 mg/dl or random glucose greater than 200 mg/dl on at least two occasions
4. Abnormal glucose tolerance test

Analysis (see p. 175)

Planning, Implementation, and Evaluation

Goal 1: Client will demonstrate knowledge of the principles of diet control.

Implementation

1. Assess client's knowledge of a diabetic diet.
2. Reinforce teaching of the dietician as needed.
3. Encourage client to use the individualized meal plan.

Table 3-34   Hypoglycemic agents

Description	Drugs that act to either stimulate the islet cells in the pancreas to secrete more insulin (oral) or act as insulin replacement when pancreatic function ceases (parenteral)
Uses	Treatment of diabetes mellitus
Side effects	Hypoglycemic reactions, GI distress, neurological symptoms, alcohol intolerance (oral preparations), allergic reactions
Nursing implications	Know onset and duration of action for each agent and teach to client; monitor for and teach client to monitor for hypoglycemic reaction; stress compliance with total diabetic regimen; check for beef or pork allergy (insulin preparations); teach client self-administration of insulin including proper storage, care of equipment, site rotation, urine testing for sugar and acetone, and serum glucose checks (finger stick). Purified insulins are used infrequently as intermittent therapy or for clients with insulin allergy, lipodystrophy, gestational diabetes, or massive insulin resistance. They cannot be used interchangeably with standard-purity insulin.

Type of examples	Peak (hours)	Duration (hours)
ORAL AGENTS		
Acetohexamide (Dymelor)		12-24
Chlorpropamide (Diabinese)	3-6	24
Tolbutamide (Orinase)	5-8	6-12
Tolazamide (Tolinase)	10	16
Glipizide (Glucotrol)	1-3	up to 24
Glyburide (DiaBeta, Micronase)	2-8	24
INSULIN (USUALLY ARE STANDARD PURITY)		
Rapid acting (onset ½-1 hr)		
Crystalline zinc (Iletin)	2-4	5-8
Regular	2-4	4-6
Insulin zinc suspension prompt (Semilente)	6-10	12-16
Regular human (Humulin-R, Novolin-R)	1-3	3-5
Intermediate acting (onset 4 hr)		
Globin zinc (Iletin)	6-10	18-24
Isophane insulin suspension (NPH)	8-12	28-32
Insulin zinc suspension (Lente)	8-12	28-30
NPH human insulin isophane (Humulin-N, Novolin-N)	8-12	26-30
Long acting (onset 4-6 hr)		
Protamine zinc (PZI)	16-24	24-36
Insulin zinc suspension extended (Ultralente)	16-24	more than 36
Lente human insulin	16-24	24-30

4. Reinforce the importance of not skipping meals.
5. Measure foods accurately; do not estimate them.
6. Discuss with client the diet modifications needed to compensate for changes in life-style or illness.
7. Assist client with NIDD to lose weight as indicated.

Evaluation

Client makes appropriate selections from sample menus; maintains normal body weight; maintains fasting blood-glucose levels within normal ranges.

> **Goal 2:** Client will correctly administer insulin or other hypoglycemic agent as indicated.

Implementation
1. Assess client's knowledge of hypoglycemic agents.
2. Teach client preparation of injection, storage of insulin, and the principles of site rotation.

a. Insulin in current use may be stored at room temperature, all others in refrigerator or cool area.
b. Insulin must be at room temperature before administration.
c. Roll insulin to mix, double-check label concentration.
d. If client mixes insulin, do so in same sequence each day; e.g., always draw up regular or shorter-acting insulin first followed by longer-acting preparations (i.e., clear to cloudy).
e. Rotate sites so that no one site is used more frequently than once a month; know that switching from separate injections to a mixture of insulins in one injection may alter local response.
f. Inject at 45° or 90° angle.
g. Press (do not rub) the site after injection.
h. Avoid smoking for 30 minutes after injection (cigarette smoking decreases absorption).

Table 3-35   Diabetic meal planning

NUTRIENT BALANCE (PERCENT OF TOTAL CALORIES)

Carbohydrate	55%-60%
Fat	less than 30%
Protein	12%-20%

EXAMPLES OF FOODS IN EXCHANGE LISTS

Free foods	List 1 Milk exchanges (quantity 1 cup)	List 2 Vegetable exchanges (quantity ½ cup)	List 3 Fruit exchanges (quantity approx. ½ cup)	List 4 Bread exchanges (quantity 1 slice, ½ cup)	List 5 Meat exchanges (quantity 1 oz)	List 6 Fat exchanges (quantity 1 tsp or 1 tbs)
Coffee, tea	Whole milk	Asparagus	Apple	Bread	Meat and	Butter or
Clear broth	(omit 2 fat	Beets	Applesauce	Cereals	poultry	margarine
Gelatin	exchanges)	Broccoli	Banana	Spaghetti,	Cold cuts	Bacon (crisp)
(unsweetened)	Skim milk	Cabbage	Strawberries	noodles	Frankfurters	Cream
Pepper and other	Buttermilk	Cauliflower	Cantaloupe	Crackers	(high-fat	Mayonnaise
spices	made with	Cucumbers	Cherries	Beans and	meats re-	Nuts
	skim milk	Chard	Grapefruit	peas (dried	quire	Olives
		Collards	Orange juice	and cooked)	omitting	
		Mushrooms	Pear	Corn	½-1 fat	
		Onions	Pineapple	Potatoes	exchange)	
		Tomatoes	Prunes, dried		Eggs	
		Turnips	Watermelon		Fish	
		Raw vegetables			Shrimp	
		(quantity as			Cheese:	
		desired)			cheddar,	
		Chicory			cottage	
		Chinese cab-			Peanut	
		bage			butter	
		Endive				
		Escarole				
		Lettuce				
		Parsley				
		Radishes				
		Watercress				

GENERAL RULES (FOR ALL CLIENTS TO KNOW AND FOLLOW CAREFULLY)

1. Eat all meals about the same time daily. Do not skip meals.
2. Eat only those foods, in the amount given, on the diet list.
3. Do not eat between meals unless it is part of the dietary plan, unless replacing food not eaten at a previous meal, or unless an insulin reaction is "coming on."

REPLACEMENT MEALS FOR ILLNESS

1. Drink liquids hourly to replace losses.
2. Carbohydrates are necessary to prevent ketosis; use simple sugars for easy digestion, 50-70 g every 8 hr.

3. Provide opportunities for multiple return demonstrations.
4. Teach at least one family member to administer insulin.
5. Teach client factors that influence the body's need for insulin.
   a. Increased need: trauma, infection, fever, severe psychological or physiological stress, smoking marijuana.
   b. Decreased need: active exercise.

Evaluation

Client properly administers own insulin; shows no signs of lipodystrophy.

Goal 3: Client will monitor diabetic status regularly and correctly through the use of finger sticks or urine testing.

Implementation

1. Assess client's knowledge of glucose monitoring.

2. Teach client the principles of urine testing (used primarily for ketone monitoring since correlation with serum glucose is poor).
   a. Consistent use of one product.
   b. Test before meals and at bedtime using a fresh urine sample.
   c. Record results in percentages.
3. Teach client about common medications that interfere with urine test results (e.g., vitamin C, cephalosporin antibiotics).
4. Teach client proper technique for finger sticks.
   a. Follow product guide carefully for timing results.
   b. Use sides of fingers or earlobes.
5. Keep accurate date and time records for both urine and finger-stick testing.
6. Teach client to notify physician if urine tests greater than 1% or finger-stick results are greater than the physician-specified limit.

Evaluation

Client demonstrates accurate urine testing and/or finger-stick glucose measurements; correctly interprets the results; maintains consistent, accurate records of the results; knows when to contact physician.

Goal 4: Client will establish and maintain a pattern of regular exercise.

Implementation

1. Assess client's knowledge of the relationship between exercise and diabetes.
2. Individualize exercise plan for each client; instruct client with NIDD to have a cardiovascular evaluation before beginning an exercise program.
3. Tell client to perform exercise after meals to ensure an adequate level of blood glucose.
   a. Teach client with IDD to carry a rapid-acting source of glucose.
   b. Teach client that excessive or unplanned exercise may trigger hypoglycemia.
   c. Teach client to take insulin before active exercise.

Evaluation

Client engages in planned regular exercise without experiencing difficulties with hypoglycemia.

Goal 5: Client will practice good personal hygiene and positive health promotion to avoid diabetic complications.

Implementation

1. Assess client's knowledge of health promotion and complications.

2. Teach client diabetic foot care.
   a. Daily gentle cleansing and inspection.
   b. Properly fitting shoes.
   c. Use lanolin cream to prevent dryness and cracking of heels.
   d. Avoid going barefoot.
   e. Wear socks with shoes.
   f. Visit a podiatrist regularly for care of nails, calluses, and corns.
3. Teach client interventions to prevent peripheral vascular disease (refer to "Circulatory Problems," p. 141).
4. Teach client the adjustments that must be made in the event of minor illness (e.g., colds, flu).
   a. Continue taking insulin or oral hypoglycemic agent regularly (injection increases the body's need for insulin).
   b. Maintain fluid intake, replace diet with appropriate liquids if unable to eat solid food (see Table 3-35).
   c. Increase the frequency of blood/ketone testing.
   d. Contact physician if necessary.
5. Help client identify stressful situations in life-style that might interfere with good diabetic control.
6. Encourage good daily hygiene and regular checkups by dentist.
7. Advise regular eye exams.
8. Teach aggressive care for minor skin cuts and abrasions; avoid clothing and activities that cause chaffing and irritation.

Evaluation

Client maintains teeth and gums in good repair; maintains soft, intact skin; states adjustments that are to be made to maintain control during periods of minor illness.

Goal 6: Client will recognize the signs of hypoglycemia and ketoacidosis and take appropriate actions.

Implementation

1. Assess client's knowledge about hypoglycemia and hyperglycemia.
2. Teach signs of hypoglycemia and the situations that may trigger it (see Table 3-36 for symptoms).
   a. Too much insulin or too little food.
   b. Strenuous, unplanned exercise.
3. Teach client to reverse hypoglycemia if possible with 5-15 g of a rapid-acting carbohydrate.
4. Teach client signs of ketoacidosis and situations that may trigger it (see Table 3-36 for symptoms).

Table 3-36   Differentiating hypoglycemia from ketoacidosis (hyperglycemia)

	Hypoglycemia (insulin reaction)	Ketoacidosis (diabetic coma)
Causes	Delayed or missed meals, excess insulin, excess exercise	Inadequate insulin, too much food, infection, injury, physical or emotional stress
Symptoms	Anxiety, weakness, sweating, hunger, tremor, nausea (severe: headache, confusion, unconsciousness)	Thirst, increased urination, weakness, nausea, abdominal pain (classic: acetone breath odor, Kussmaul's respirations, decreased consciousness).

Treatment	5-15 g of carbohydrate as:
	  10 oz soft drink
	  6-8 Life Savers
	  1-1½ Tbs honey
	  1-2 Tbs jam
	Administer glucagon if unable to swallow. Give some complex carbohydrate from meal plan within 1 hr after initial treatment.
		Correct volume depletion with IV fluids.
		Administer regular insulin by infusion.
		Replace electrolytes as volume restored.
		Monitor vital signs, I&O, blood glucose, and level of consciousness.

  a. Failure to take insulin.
  b. Too much food.
  c. Episode of illness, infection, or stress.
5. Teach client that development of ketoacidosis requires immediate transport to a health care facility.
  a. Correct dehydration by administering IV fluids.
  b. Correct blood-glucose level with administration of insulin (usually low-dose insulin infusion).
  c. Record I&O accurately (Foley catheter is usually necessary).

  d. Assess for decreasing LOC and declining cardiopulmonary status at frequent intervals.
  e. Monitor ketones and blood glucose at frequent intervals.
  f. Replace electrolytes as ordered.
6. Tell client to wear a diabetic alert bracelet or tag at all times.

Evaluation

Client lists the symptoms of hypoglycemia and ketoacidosis and states appropriate actions to take for each; wears a diabetic alert tag.

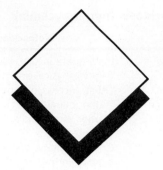

Elimination

The nursing care presented in this unit concerns selected health problems related to disturbances in the kidneys and the large bowel.

The Kidneys

GENERAL CONCEPTS
Overview/Physiology

1. Kidneys
   a. Location: paired organs that lie in the retroperitoneum at the costovertebral angle (CVA)
      1. upper border: T12
      2. lower border: L3
   b. Size: 120-170 g (4-6 oz) each
   c. Regions (see Fig. 3-15)
      1. cortex
         a. outer layer
         b. contains glomeruli, proximal and distal tubules
      2. medulla
         a. middle layer
         b. composed of 6-10 renal pyramids, formed by collecting ducts and tubules
         c. deepest part of loop of Henle
      3. pelvis
         a. innermost layer
         b. hollow collection area composed of calyces
         c. papillae move urine into ureter by peristaltic action
   d. Nephron (see Fig. 3-16)
      1. functional unit of kidney
      2. one million nephrons in each kidney
      3. composition
         a. glomerulus
         b. tubule
            ◆ Bowman's capsule
            ◆ proximal convoluted tubule
            ◆ loop of Henle
               • descending limb
               • ascending limb
            ◆ distal convoluted tubule
            ◆ collecting duct
      4. action: all elements to be excreted or conserved are acted on in the nephron by the processes of filtration, concentration, reabsorption, or secretion
2. Ureters
   a. Join with renal pelvis; distal end implanted in bladder
   b. Composed of smooth muscles that have peristaltic action
   c. Narrow at ureteropelvic junction, bifurcation of iliac vessels and join with bladder
3. Bladder
   a. Stores urine until eliminated
   b. Muscular organ (detrusor muscle)
4. Urethra
   a. Passageway for urine during excretion
   b. Surrounded by prostate gland in men
5. Functions of the kidney
   a. Fluid and electrolyte balance (see Tables 3-37 and 3-38)
      1. control of sodium balance
         a. intake in normal diet is usually greater than needed
         b. filtered by glomeruli
         c. reabsorption in tubules is controlled by active and passive processes and by the renin-angiotensin-aldosterone system
      2. control of chloride balance follows sodium
         a. intake in normal diet is usually greater than needed
         b. filtered by the glomeruli
         c. actively transported out of the ascending loop of Henle
      3. control of H_2O balance
         a. intake controlled by social habits and thirst
         b. reabsorption controlled by antidiuretic hormone (ADH) concentration in the collecting duct
      4. control of potassium balance

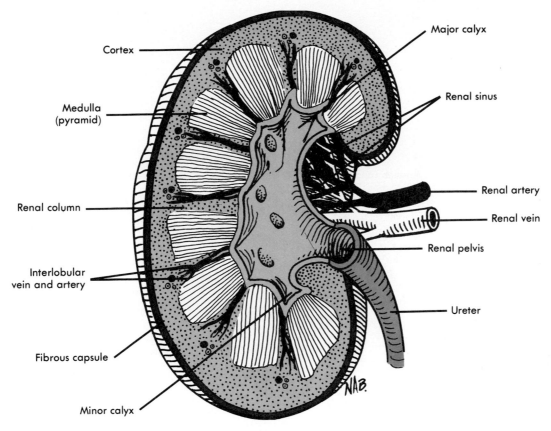

Fig. 3-15 Frontal section of kidney. (From: Long, B.C., & Phipps, W.J. [1989]. *Medical-surgical nursing: A nursing process approach* [2nd ed.]. St. Louis: Mosby–Year Book.)

Table 3-37 Fluid imbalance

Etiology	Assessment	Nursing implications
OVERHYDRATION		
Renal failure Excessive fluid intake Excess IVs Water intoxication (GU irrigation with hypotonic fluids) Hypernatremia	Level of consciousness, vital signs, weight (increases), peripheral edema, venous pressure (increases), pulmonary edema, symptoms of CHF or increased intracranial pressure	*Prevention* Monitor IV fluids closely. Monitor urine output, I&O, weight. *Treatment* Reduce edema (e.g., positioning). Give diuretics as ordered. Limit intake. Maintain low sodium intake.
DEHYDRATION		
Nausea and vomiting Increased urinary output Diuretics Insufficient intake (because of age, immobility, etc.) Inadequate replacement following excess fluid loss (diaphoresis, diarrhea)	Level of consciousness, vital signs, weight (may be decreased), skin turgor (poor), thirst, urine output	*Prevention* Monitor I&O. Replace lost fluids. Client teaching about excess perspiration. *Treatment* Replace fluids carefully. Monitor I&O and weight.

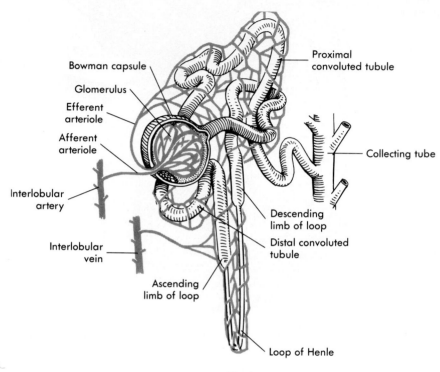

Bowman capsule

Glomerulus

Efferent arteriole

Afferent arteriole

Interlobular artery

Interlobular vein

Ascending limb of loop

Proximal convoluted tubule

Collecting tube

Descending limb of loop

Distal convoluted tubule

Loop of Henle

Nephron.

Part of Nephron	Function	Substance
Glomeruli	Filtration	H₂O and solute, electrolytes (Na, K, PO₄, Ca, Cl, Mg), urea, creatinine, uric acid, glucose, amino acids
Proximal tubules	Reabsorption, secretion	H₂O, electrolytes (Na, K, Mg, Ca, Cl, HCO₃), glucose, amino acids
Loop of Henle	Reabsorption	H₂O, electrolytes (Na, K)
Distal tubule	Acid-base balance, secretion	Hydrogen ions (H), Na
Collecting tubule	Concentration	H₂O

Fig. 3-16   Nephron. (From Long, B.C., & Phipps, W.J. [1989]. *Medical-surgical nursing: A nursing process approach* [2nd ed.]. St. Louis: Mosby–Year Book.)

Table 3-38 Electrolyte imbalances

Problem	Etiology	Assessment	Nursing implications
SODIUM			
Hypernatremia Na$^+$ >145 mEq/L	*Hyperosmolar* Sodium increased in relation to water, water loss without sodium loss, dehydration	Increased hemoglobin, signs of dehydration, thirst, decreased BP, concentrated urine with high specific gravity	Offer sodium-restricted diet and fluids. Maintain strict I&O. Prevent shock. Maintain adequate urine output. Monitor serum Na.
	Sodium excess Both sodium and water increased, renal failure, cirrhosis, steroid therapy, aldosterone excess	Edema, weight gain, hypertension, symptoms of fluid overload	Offer low-sodium diet, water restriction. Maintain strict I&O. Monitor for signs of CHF or increased intracranial pressure. Measure daily weight. Administer diuretics (Na-wasting) as ordered.
Hyponatremia Na$^+$ <136 mEq/L	*Hypoosmolar or "dilutional"* Water increased in relation to sodium, water intoxication, exercise, IVs without NaCl, sodium-restricted diet *Sodium deficit* Both sodium and water decreased, diuretics, GI losses, burns	Fluid volume excess, increased urine output with low specific gravity, no thirst, nausea/vomiting, weakness/cerebral dysfunction Decreased BP, poor skin turgor, dehydration/shock, oliguria	Restrict water. Monitor I&O, serum Na. Watch for circulatory overload. Replace Na carefully. Give high-Na diet. Monitor for shock. Provide good skin care. Give isotonic fluids. Monitor I&O, serum Na.
POTASSIUM			
Hyperkalemia K$^+$ >5.0 mEq/L	Severe burns, crush injuries, Addison's disease, renal failure, acidosis, excessive K intake (oral or IV)	ECG changes (high T wave), skeletal muscle weakness, bradycardia, cardiac arrest, oliguria, intestinal colic and diarrhea	Monitor cardiac function, serum K, neurological signs. Limit K intake. Give D$_{50}$ plus insulin as ordered. Give exchange-resins (sodium polystyrene sulfonate [Kayexalate] PO or enemas) as ordered. Give bicarbonate to correct acidosis. Dialysis (renal/peritoneal).
Hypokalemia K$^+$ <3.5 mEq/L	Diuretic therapy (thiazides), poor intake, GI loss, ulcerative colitis, Cushing's syndrome, alkalosis	Digitalis toxicity, muscle weakness and decreased reflexes, flaccid paralysis, paralytic ileus, CNS depression, lethargy, hypotension, anorexia, ECG changes (flattened T wave)	Administer K slowly IV. Monitor ECG. Teach adequate K replacement when taking diuretics. Administer PO K drugs/diet.

Continued.

Table 3-38 Electrolyte imbalances—cont'd

Problem	Etiology	Assessment	Nursing implications
CALCIUM			
Hypercalcemia Ca^{++} >10.5 mg	Immobility, hyperparathyroidism, bone metastasis, excess vitamin D intake, parathyroid tumor, osteoporosis, decreased renal excretion	Skeletal muscle weakness; bone pain; renal calculi; pathological fractures; CNS depression, altered level of consciousness (LOC); GI (constipation, nausea, vomiting, anorexia); decreased serum phosphorus	Limit intake. Client teaching. Prevent fractures. Give phosphorus. Maintain adequate I&O. Monitor neurological signs.
Hypocalcemia Ca^{++} <9 mg	Hypoparathyroidism, low vitamin D in diet, parathyroidectomy, pregnancy and lactation, postthyroidectomy, rickets, renal disease	Tetany, tingling, paresthesias of fingers and around mouth, muscle twitching, cramps; positive Chvostek's and Trousseau's signs; laryngospasm; increased phosphorus	Give Ca as needed. Monitor for early muscle spasms, neurological signs. Monitor those at risk. Give phosphate-binding antacids. Monitor serum Ca.
MAGNESIUM			
Hypermagnesemia Mg^{++} >3.0 mEq/L	Renal insufficiency, diabetic ketoacidosis, excess Mg intake (antacids), dehydration	CNS and neuromuscular depression, hypotension, sedation, or arrest	Monitor replacement carefully. Support respiration. Teach client correct antacid intake. Monitor neurological signs.
Hypomagnesemia Mg^{++} <1.6 mEq/L	Alcoholism, malnutrition, loss (GI, diuresis), low intake, hypercalcemia, diabetes, toxemia, renal disease	Tremors and neuromuscular irritability, disorientation, positive Chvostek's and Trousseau's signs, convulsions	Give Mg cautiously as ordered. Monitor closely for Mg excess. Teach adequate intake. Monitor neurological signs.

a. intake adequate in normal diet
b. filtered by glomeruli
c. almost all filtered potassium is reabsorbed in proximal tubules
d. secreted into distal tubules and into distal ducts where there is selective secretion or reabsorption
e. dependent upon hormonal influence
    ◆ increase of aldosterone causes increased potassium secretion
    ◆ decrease of aldosterone causes decreased potassium secretion
f. potassium also lost through GI tract
b. Control of acid-base balance (see Table 3-39)
    1. excretion of organic acids
        a. HPO_4 buffer system; $H + HPO_4 \rightarrow H_2PO_4$
        b. NH_3 buffer system

◆ $NH_3 + H \rightarrow NH_4$
◆ $NH_4 + NaCl \rightarrow NH_4Cl + Na$
    c. liberation of free hydrogen ions
    2. conservation of bicarbonate
c. Excretion of waste products (primarily products of protein metabolism: urea and creatinine)
d. Production and secretion of erythropoietin in response to hypoxia (stimulates bone marrow to produce hemoglobin)
e. Manufacture and activation of vitamin D (plays a role in calcium metabolism: active form of vitamin D must be available for parathormone to work)
f. Regulation of arterial blood pressure: renin and aldosterone
    1. kidneys secrete an enzyme called renin, which acts on plasma protein to cause the release of angiotensin (a vasoconstricting substance)

Table 3-39 **Acid-base imbalance**

Problem	Etiology	Assessment	Compensating mechanisms	Nursing implications
RESPIRATORY ACIDOSIS				
pH <7.35 Pco_2 >45 HCO_3 normal	Hypoventilation acute causes respiratory infections CNS depressant overdose paralysis of re s-piratory muscles atelectasis brain damage postoperative abdominal distension chronic causes obesity ascites pregnancy	Hypoventilation; tachycardia, irregular pulse; decreased chest excursion; headache, dizziness; cyanosis; drowsiness leading to coma	Kidneys retain and manufacture more bicarbonate leading to pH 7.4 Pco_2 >45 HCO_3 >28	Turn, cough, and deep-breathe qh. Suction as needed. Monitor vital signs. Give respiratory stimulants as ordered. Give bronchodilators. Give O_2 cautiously to prevent CO_2 narcosis.
RESPIRATORY ALKALOSIS				
pH >7.45 Pco_2 <35 HCO_3 normal	Hyperventilation emotions, hysteria O_2 lack fever salicylate poisoning CNS stimulation by drugs/disease	Hyperventilation light-headedness, tingling of hands and face (tetany) Convulsions, diaphoresis, low serum K^+	Kidneys excrete large amounts of bicarbonate leading to pH 7.4 Pco_2 <35 HCO_3 <22	Calm client. Slow the rate of ventilation. Use rebreather to increase Pco_2. Administer O_2 as needed.
METABOLIC ACIDOSIS				
pH <7.35 Pco_2 normal HCO_3 <22	Bicarbonate loss diarrhea GI fistula Acid gain diabetic ketoacidosis lactic acidosis renal failure salicylate intoxication K^+ excess	Headache, dizziness; Kussmaul's respiration; fruity breath odor; disoriented; coma; nausea/vomiting; high serum K^+	Lungs hyperventilate to blow off CO_2 and reduce plasma carbonic acid content leading to pH 7.4 Pco_2 <35 HCO_3 <22	Administer sodium bicarbonate as ordered. Give insulin as ordered. Monitor I&O, vital signs. Support client.
METABOLIC ALKALOSIS				
pH >7.35 Pco_2 normal HCO_3 >26	Acid loss vomiting or GI suction steroid therapy thiazide diuretics Bicarbonate retention excess use of bicarbonate (baking soda) as antacid excess infusion of Ringer's lactate citrated blood	Headache, numbness and tingling leading to tetany and convulsions, hypoventilation, confusion and agitation, low serum K^+	Lungs hypoventilate to retain CO_2 and increase plasma carbonic acid content leading to pH 7.4 Pco_2 >45 HCO_3 >26	Give IV ammonium chloride as ordered. Maintain K^+ level with diet or drugs. Teach client high K^+ diet if taking thiazide diuretics. Give acetazolamide (Diamox) as ordered. Maintain calm, quiet environment.

2. angiotensin increases total peripheral resistance leading to increased aldosterone secretion by adrenal cortex
3. increased aldosterone stimulates increased sodium reabsorption
4. increased sodium reabsorption leads to increased water retention and plasma volume, which increases arterial BP

Application of the Nursing Process to the Client with Kidney Problems

Assessment

1. Health history
   a. Urinary retention, stasis (e.g., associated with pregnancy, neurogenic bladder, immobility, diabetes)
   b. Bladder infections: caused by contamination from large intestine (especially young girls)
   c. Intrusive procedures (e.g., catheterization, cystoscopy, coitus)
   d. Bone demineralization
   e. Metabolic disease
   f. Changes in color of urine (e.g., hematuria)
   g. Changes in volume of urine
      1. polyuria: greater than 2500 ml/day
      2. oliguria: less than 400 ml/day
      3. anuria: less than 100 ml/day
   h. Changes in voiding pattern
      1. nocturia
      2. frequency
      3. hesitancy
      4. urgency
      5. change in urinary stream
      6. incontinence
         a. amount
         b. frequency of occurrence
         c. dribbling
   i. Medications
      1. diuretics
      2. antibiotics
      3. nephrotoxic agents: aspirin (ASA), acetaminophen, mercaptomerin sodium, phenylbutazone, sulfonamides, gentamicin
      4. cholinergics, anticholinergics
2. Physical examination
   a. Inspection of genitals
   b. Palpation of kidneys
   c. Palpation of prostate
   d. Pain
      1. back
      2. flank
      3. CVA tenderness
3. Diagnostic tests (see Table 3-40)
   a. Urine (visual inspection)
      1. color: pale to deep amber; changes with medication, food, or disease
      2. volume: 30 ml or more each hour
      3. appearance: clear
      4. odor: normally aromatic; strong ammonia after stored for a period of time

Table 3-40 Laboratory tests used to evaluate renal function

Test	Normal range	Usual range in renal disease	What it measures
Hemoglobin	12-18 g/dl	Lowered	Formation of red blood cells
Blood urea nitrogen (BUN)	5-20 mg/dl	Elevated	Renal excretory function
Electrolytes			
Sodium	136-145 mEq/L	Elevated (not necessarily) or lowered	Fluid and electrolyte balance
Potassium	3.5-5 mEq/L	Elevated or lowered	Electrolyte balance
Chloride	90-110 mEq/L	Elevated (not necessarily) or lowered; has partnership with sodium	Fluid and electrolyte balance
Serum creatinine	0.7-1.5 mg/dl	Elevated	Renal function
Serum osmolality	275-300 mOsm/kg	Elevated or lowered	Dissolved particles in the blood
Glucose	70-115 mg/dl	Slight hyperglycemia	
Blood pH	7.35-7.45	Usually lowered	Acidity vs. alkalinity of blood
Calcium	9.0-10.5 mg/dl	Usually lowered	Renal excretory function
Phosphorus	2.5-4.5 mg/dl	Elevated	Renal excretory function
Albumin	3.2-4.5 g/dl	Usually lowered	Albumin (helps maintain blood's osmotic pressure)

b. Urinalysis: microscopic exam for color, appearance, pH, protein, glucose, ketones, RBCs, WBCs, and casts
 1. specific gravity: 1.015-1.025 (random samples)
    a. reflects concentrating ability of kidneys
    b. increases (greater than 1.035) with glucosuria, proteinuria, and dehydration
    c. decreases (less than 1.002) with distal renal tubular disease, endocrine disorders associated with insufficiency of ADH, and overhydration
    d. fixed (1.010) with glomerulonephritis
 2. pH: 4.8-8.0
    a. reflects the acid-base balance
    b. greater than 8.0: alkaline; occurs with metabolic alkalosis, overuse of alkalizing medications, in presence of urinary tract infection (UTI)
    c. less than 4.8: acidic; occurs with metabolic acidosis, uncontrolled diabetes, some medications (e.g., ammonium chloride, high doses of vitamin C)
 3. glucose
    a. normally not present
    b. may occur after heavy meal, emotional stress, or with infusion of glucose
    c. occurs abnormally with diabetes mellitus, pancreatic disorders, impaired reabsorption in the proximal tubules
 4. ketones
    a. normally not present
    b. occur with uncontrolled diabetes, fasting, severe infections accompanied by nausea and vomiting
 5. protein
    a. normally not present
    b. occurs with serious kidney or proximal tubular disorders, nephrotic syndrome, toxemia
    c. may occur after heavy protein meal, strenuous exercise, or prolonged standing
 6. red blood cells
    a. normally 0-3/high-power field
    b. increase with kidney malfunction or trauma to urinary tract or tumor or infection in urinary tract
 7. white blood cells
    a. normally 0-4/high-power field
    b. increase with infection within urinary tract system
 8. hyaline casts
    a. normally not present
    b. indicate acute glomerulonephritis or pyelonephritis, chronic renal disease, or renal calculi

 9. granular casts
    a. normally not present
    b. indicates acute renal rejection (transplant), pyelonephritis, or chronic lead poisoning
c. Urine culture and sensitivity
 1. voided specimen (clean catch): bacterial count over 100,000 organisms/ml (if infection is cause)
 2. sterile, catheterized specimen: over 10,000 organisms/ml
d. Tests of filtration function
 1. creatinine clearance (the most important test of kidney function)
    a. amount of creatinine filtered by glomeruli (since creatinine is not reabsorbed and is only minimally secreted, this test is a measure of glomerular filtration rate)
    b. determined by 24-hour urine specimen
    c. normal values
       ◆ 115 ± 20 ml/min
       ◆ serum creatinine: 0.7-1.5 mg/dl
    d. as glomerular filtration rate falls, serum creatinine rises and 24-hour urine creatinine decreases
    e. advantage of serum creatinine: independent of protein metabolism
 2. blood urea nitrogen (BUN)
    a. normal: 5-20 mg/dl
    b. urea: end product of protein metabolism
    c. increases with decrease in glomerular filtration
    d. less reliable measure then serum creatinine because
       ◆ after being filtered, urea is reabsorbed back into renal tubular cells
       ◆ urea production varies according to the state of the liver function, and protein intake and breakdown
e. Radiological tests
 1. KUB: kidney, ureters, bladder
    a. simple x-ray without contrast medium
    b. results indicate size, position, and any radiopaque calcifications
 2. tomography
    a. x-ray at different angles: no contrast medium
    b. useful for clear picture when colon and other organs block kidney
    c. can distinguish solid tumors from cysts
 3. IVP: intravenous pyelogram (excretory urogram)
    a. injection of contrast medium that is excreted by kidneys
    b. allows visualization of kidneys, ureters, and bladder
    c. used to diagnose masses, cysts, obstruc-

tions, renal trauma, bladder dysfunction
   d. contraindicated in severe renal disease or dehydration and individuals allergic to shellfish or iodine
   e. nursing care pretest
      ◆ check for iodine allergies
      ◆ ensure informed written consent is on the chart
      ◆ tell client that a dye is injected and x-rays are taken at 2-, 5-, 10- 15-, 20-, 30-, and 60-minute intervals
      ◆ administer strong cathartic, enemas night before
      ◆ NPO after midnight
      ◆ have client void immediately before test
   f. nursing care posttest: check for signs and symptoms of allergic reaction to dye and signs of acute renal failure
4. nephrotomogram
   a. techniques of tomography with IVP
   b. provides a clearer visualization
5. retrograde pyelogram
   a. catheter is passed through urethra, urinary bladder, and into right or left ureter, where contrast medium is injected
   b. allows more detailed visualization of the urinary collecting system independent of the status of renal function
   c. disadvantages: increased chances of trauma (catheter manipulation) and infection
   d. nursing care pretest
      ◆ check for iodine allergies
      ◆ ensure informed written consent is on the chart
      ◆ teach client concerning procedure
      ◆ administer cathartics, enemas evening before
      ◆ keep NPO after midnight
   e. nursing care posttest
      ◆ observe amount of urine
      ◆ watch for hematuria
      ◆ watch for signs of urinary sepsis
      ◆ check for signs and symptoms of allergic reaction to dye
6. renal angiography, arteriography
   a. catheter is introduced through the femoral artery to the renal artery
   b. contrast medium is injected and 2-3 x-rays are taken at 2-second intervals
   c. allows visualization of renal arteries, capillaries, and venous system
   d. used to diagnose renal artery stenosis, renal masses, trauma, thrombosis, and obstructive uropathy
   e. risks: bleeding, thrombosis, damage to vessels, allergic reaction
   f. nursing care pretest
      ◆ check for iodine allergies
      ◆ ensure informed written consent is on the chart
      ◆ administer cathartics, enemas evening before
      ◆ ensure that chart contains hematological evaluation
      ◆ have client void immediately before test
   g. nursing care posttest
      ◆ maintain bed rest 12-24 hours; flat, no sitting
      ◆ check insertion site for hematoma formation
      ◆ check pressure dressing on insertion site
      ◆ monitor postoperative vital signs
      ◆ check peripheral pulses distal to insertion site
      ◆ measure urine output
7. cystography
   a. a flexible metal tube is inserted into the bladder and a dye is injected; x-rays are taken at 30-minute intervals
   b. assesses bladder function and explores the possible presence of stones in the bladder
   c. nursing care: same as retrograde pyelogram
8. cystoscopy
   a. a cystoscope is inserted into bladder through the urethra
   b. direct inspection of bladder to biopsy and resect tumors, to remove stones, cauterize bleeding areas, dilate ureters, and implant radium seeds
   c. nursing care pretest
      ◆ ensure written informed consent is on the chart
      ◆ administer prep as ordered
      ◆ teach client about procedure (e.g., position [lithotomy], darkened room)
      ◆ keep NPO if general anesthesia will be used
      ◆ administer preoperative medications as ordered
   d. nursing care posttest
      ◆ monitor urine output
      ◆ monitor urine color, blood-tinged is common
      ◆ provide comfort measures (back pain, bladder spasms, feeling of fullness are common) such as sitz baths and/or analgesics (e.g., belladonna and opium [B&O] suppository as ordered)
      ◆ check temperature and urine for signs of infection
      ◆ encourage increased fluid intake (unless contraindicated)

9. renal biopsy
   a. a specially designed needle is inserted percutaneously to obtain sample of kidney tissue
   b. determines histology of glomeruli and tubules
   c. contraindications: a single, functioning kidney; infection; tumors; hydronephrosis; coagulation disorders; or uncooperative client
   d. risks: uncontrolled bleeding, hematuria, loss of kidney function
   e. nursing care pretest
      ◆ ensure written informed consent is on the chart
      ◆ check results of coagulation studies and hematocrit
      ◆ teach client to hold breath during procedure
   f. nursing care posttest
      ◆ maintain bed rest for 24 hours with tight dressing or sandbag over insertion site
      ◆ force fluids
      ◆ monitor vital signs frequently
      ◆ monitor hematocrit frequently
      ◆ monitor urine
      ◆ teach to avoid strenuous activity for approximately 2 weeks

Analysis

1. Safe, effective care environment
   a. High risk for infection
   b. Knowledge deficit
2. Physiological integrity
   a. Pain
   b. High risk for fluid volume deficit
   c. Functional incontinence
3. Psychosocial integrity
   a. Ineffective individual coping
   b. Altered patterns of sexuality
   c. Anxiety
4. Health promotion/maintenance
   a. Impaired adjustment
   b. Altered health maintenance
   c. Knowledge deficit

General Nursing Planning, Implementation, and Evaluation

Goal 1: Client will be free from infection.

Implementation

1. Collect necessary urine specimen for culture and sensitivity.
2. Teach women proper perineal hygiene.
3. Use and teach client good hand-washing techniques.
4. Use strict sterile technique during catheterization procedures.
5. Provide daily Foley catheter care using proper techniques.
6. Administer antibiotics as ordered, for 10-14 days (see Table 3-41).
7. Increase fluid intake to 3000-5000 ml/day, if not contraindicated by renal or cardiovascular status.
8. Acidify urine through acid-ash diet (e.g., meats, eggs, cheese, fish, fowl, whole grains, cranberries, plums, prunes) or by administration of methenamine hippurate (Hiprex) or vitamin C if compatible with antibiotic therapy.
9. Teach good oral hygiene techniques.
10. Teach client with chronic kidney infections signs and symptoms of upper respiratory infections (URIs) and importance of seeking early treatment; screen client from staff or significant others with URIs; teach client to avoid exposure to persons with infections (streptococcal infections can lead to glomerulonephritis).
11. Monitor level of potential nephrotoxic agents (i.e., gentamicin, tetracycline, tobramycin).
12. Teach client potentially nephrotoxic agents.

Evaluation

Client is free from dysuria, frequency, fever, and other signs of infection; states procedure for proper perineal hygiene; takes medications as prescribed; has I&O of at least 3000-5000 ml/day; lists signs and symptoms of URI and need for early treatment; states potentially nephrotoxic agents to avoid in the future.

Goal 2: Client will be free from discomfort.

Implementation

1. Administer sitz baths to decrease urethral burning.
2. Administer phenazopyridine hydrochloride (Pyridium) or urinary antispasmodics if ordered (see Table 3-41)
3. Apply hot water bottle or heating pad to suprapubic region.

Evaluation

Client is free from pain, discomfort; reports no burning with urination.

Goal 3: Client's normal urinary function will be maintained.

Implementation

1. Measure urine output accurately.
2. Collect urine specimens for routine urinalysis.
3. Encourage adequate fluid intake.
4. Observe for early signs of renal failure.

Evaluation

Client's urine output remains equal to or greater than 30 ml/hr; client remains free from symptoms of renal failure.

Table 3-41   Drugs used to treat urinary tract infection

Generic name (trade name)	Action/use	Side effects	Nursing implications
URINARY ANALGESIC			
Phenazopyridine hydrochloride (Pyridium)	Exerts an anesthetic effect on the mucosa of the urinary tract as it is excreted in the urine. Used for relief of urinary tract pain.	Red-orange or rust discoloration of urine.	Inform that urine will be orange-colored. Take drug with food. Use Clinitest for urine testing.
URINARY ANTISEPTICS			
Cinoxacin (Cinobac) Methenamine hippurate (Hiprex) Nitrofurantoin (Furadantin, Macrodantin)	Act as disinfectants within the urinary tract. Concentrated by the kidneys and reach therapeutic levels only within the urinary tract. Used to treat UTIs.	Nausea, vomiting, GI upset, diarrhea, hypersensitivity reaction, and dizziness. Brown or rust discoloration of urine.	Keep urine acidic; give vitamin C (6-12 g/day) or cranberry, plum, prune, or apple juice. Give after meals to minimize GI upset. Warn that urine may be brown- or rust-colored. Monitor I&O; maintain fluid intake of 1500-2000 ml/day.
SULFONAMIDES			
Trimethoprim/sulfamethoxazole (Bactrim, Septra) Sulfasalazine (Azulfidine) Sulfisoxazole (Gantrisin)	Bacteriostatic against gram-positive and gram-negative organisms. Excreted unchanged and dissolves well in urine. Used to treat UTIs, acute otitis media, inflammatory bowel disease, chronic bronchitis, parasitic infections, and for preoperative bowel sterilization.	GI disorders, hypersensitivity reactions, headache, peripheral hearing loss, crystalluria, and hypoglycemia.	Force fluids to 3000-4000 ml/day. Keep urine alkaline. Give with at least 8 oz of water 1 hr before or 2 hr after meals for maximum absorption. Monitor I&O. Monitor clients with potential renal or hepatic impairment closely. Advise clients to complete drug course. Warn about potential increased effect of oral hypoglycemics and false-positive Clinitest results when appropriate.
OTHER ANTIINFECTIVES			
Ciprofloxacin (Cipro)	Broad-spectrum antibiotic used for mild to moderate UTIs.	GI disturbances, headache, and rash.	Give 2 hr before or after administration of antacids containing magnesium. Give 2 hr after meals. Drink plenty of fluids.

Goal 4: Client and significant others will receive emotional support.

Implementation
1. See Table 2-4 on p. 22.
2. Provide encouragement when client becomes frustrated with treatment and progression of illness.
3. Explain cause of disease and treatments to client and significant others as necessary.
4. Allow client and significant others to express fears, feelings, and questions.
5. Encourage discussion of diagnosis and ways to cope with problems (e.g., group session for families).
6. Prepare the client for possibility of hemodialysis or peritoneal dialysis.
7. Refer to social service or pastoral care as needed.

Evaluation
Client and significant others state necessity of treatments; show increasing acceptance of diagnosis and treatment; work through feelings and fears; discuss altered body image; and have plans to alter life-style.

SELECTED HEALTH PROBLEMS RESULTING IN ALTERATION IN URINARY ELIMINATION

☐ Cystitis/Pyelonephritis
General Information
1. Definitions
   a. *Cystitis:* inflammation of the bladder wall
   b. *Pyelonephritis:* inflammation of the kidney caused by a bacterial infection
      1. acute (short course): organisms gain access to the kidney by ascending from the lower urinary tract or via bloodstream; no permanent renal impairment
      2. chronic (slowly progressive): multiple, recurrent, acute attacks that scar the renal parenchyma, damaging tubules, vessels, glomeruli
2. Incidence: both more common in women
3. Risks/predisposing factors
   a. Cystitis
      1. prostatic hypertrophy with urinary retention (men)
      2. contamination from large intestine (women)
      3. intrusive procedures: catheterization, cystoscopy
      4. coitus (women)
      5. atonic bladder (spinal cord injury)
      6. chronic disease (e.g., diabetes)
      7. pregnancy (because of pressure of uterus on bladder and urethra)
      8. chronic stasis (e.g., atonic bladder, immobility, and infrequent voiding)
   b. Pyelonephritis

1. anomalies of the kidney
2. pregnancy
3. calculi
4. diabetes mellitus
5. neurogenic bladder
6. instrumentation (i.e., procedures)
7. bacterial infection elsewhere in the body

Nursing Process
Assessment
1. Cystitis (often asymptomatic)
   a. Burning
   b. Frequency
   c. Urgency
   d. Suprapubic pain
   e. Slight hematuria
2. Pyelonephritis
   a. Symptoms of cystitis may or may not be present
   b. Severe flank pain, CVA tenderness
   c. Hematuria, pyuria
   d. Fever
   e. Chills
3. Diagnostic tests
   a. Urinalysis, urine C&S: midstream urine specimen for evaluation of bacterial content
   b. CBC: leukocytosis
Analysis (see p. 197)
Planning, Implementation, and Evaluation
(refer to General Nursing Goals 1, 2, and 3, p. 197)

☐ Urinary Calculi
General Information
1. Types
   a. Calcium oxalate: hard, small; alkaline urine
   b. Calcium phosphate: large, soft; alkaline urine
   c. Cystine: metabolic, familial; acid urine
   d. Uric acid: may be accompanied by gout; acid urine
   e. Struvite: large, soft; associated with urinary tract infections, alkaline urine
2. Incidence: can occur at any age
3. Locations
   a. Bladder
   b. Ureter (especially at narrow points)
   c. Pelvis of the kidney
4. Risk factors
   a. Supersaturation of urine with poorly soluble crystalloids (calcium, uric acid, cystine)
   b. Infection: alkaline urine leads to precipitation of calcium and struvite
   c. Increased concentration of urine
   d. Stasis
   e. Bone demineralization leading to increased calcium phosphate in serum and urine
   f. Metabolic diseases (e.g., gout [increased uric acid])

g. Certain medications (e.g., corticosteroids, vitamin D [hypervitaminosis D])

5. Medical treatment
   a. Medical interventions
      1. ambulation to increase the likelihood of passing the stone
      2. fluids to decrease the concentration of substances involved in stone formation, to promote passage of the stone, and to prevent infection
   b. Surgical intervention (see Fig. 3-17)
      1. *ureterolithotomy:* incision into ureter through an abdominal or flank excision to extract stones from the ureter
         a. ureteral catheter is inserted to act as splint; ureter not sutured to avoid stricture; catheter is never irrigated to maintain patency
         b. Penrose drain inserted around ureter to collect any extra drainage
      2. *pyelolithotomy:* removal of a stone from renal pelvis through a flank incision; Penrose drain inserted outside renal pelvis
      3. lithotripsy

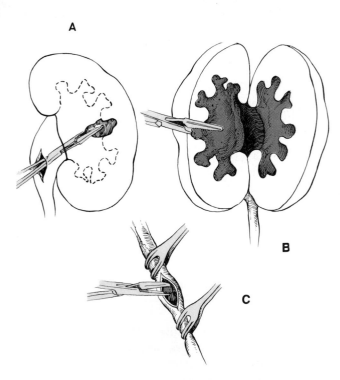

Fig. 3-17 Location and methods of removing renal calculi from upper urinary tract. **A,** Pyelolithotomy, removal of stone through renal pelvis. **B,** Nephrolithotomy, removal of staghorn calculus from renal parenchyma (kidney split). **C,** Ureterolithotomy, removal of stone from ureter. (From Long, B.C., & Phipps, W.J. [1989]. *Medical-surgical nursing: A nursing process approach* [2nd ed.]. St. Louis: Mosby–Year Book.)

a. percutaneous lithotripsy: percutaneous nephrostomy tract made through a small incision over the kidney; an endoscope is passed through this tract, and a basket is used to remove the calculi; if unable to remove the stone, ultrasonic lithotripsy is used to disintegrate the calculi
      b. transcutaneous shock wave lithotripsy: client is submerged in a large tub of water; ultrasonic shock waves are fired at the area of the calculi; results in disintegration of the calculi
   4. *nephrolithotomy:* parenchyma of kidney is cut and stone extracted through a flank incision
      a. nephrostomy tube placed to divert urine and drain pelvis to allow kidney to heal; never irrigated unless specifically ordered
      b. Penrose drain inserted
   5. *nephrectomy:* removal of kidney through a flank incision
      a. may be needed if stone and infection have caused extensive damage to kidney parenchyma
      b. Penrose drain inserted into renal bed

Nursing Process

Assessment
1. Pain
   a. Renal colic: sudden, sharp, severe; located in deep lumbar region; radiating to side
   b. Ureteral colic: same type pain radiating to genitalia and thigh
2. Renointestinal reflex: nausea and vomiting, diarrhea, constipation
3. Hematuria, frequency, altered pH of urine
4. Increased WBC
5. Fever, chills
6. Signs of paralytic ileus with right-sided renal colic
7. If stone is formed in renal pelvis, may be asymptomatic for years until signs of infection occur
8. IVP results
9. Urine for mineral precipitate
10. Blood levels of uric acid, calcium, and phosphorus if metabolic problems suspected

Analysis (see p. 197)

Planning, Implementation, and Evaluation

Goal 1: Client will be free from pain.

Implementation
1. Administer analgesics as ordered (often morphine is necessary because of severity of pain).
2. Administer anticholinergics, propantheline (Pro-Banthine) as ordered, to relax smooth muscles.
3. Encourage client to ambulate.
4. Strain all urine for stones.

Evaluation

Client is free from discomfort; ambulates; strains all urine for stones.

Goal 2: Client will be free from infection leading to urinary calculi (refer to General Nursing Goal 1, p. 197).

Goal 3: Client will decrease risk of stone formation.

Implementation

1. Teach client importance of maintaining adequate fluid intake (3000 ml/day).
2. Teach client about medications and reason for prescription (e.g., to maintain recommended urinary pH).
3. Teach client about any medication ordered to decrease levels of minerals (e.g., aluminum hydroxide + PO_3 → $AlPO_3$, eliminated through the GI tract).
4. Teach client how to measure urine pH.
5. Assess diet for excess intake of substances that contribute to stone formation.
6. Teach client about dietary restrictions.
7. Explain advantages of regular exercise and voiding at least every 2 hours (e.g., to prevent stasis calculi).

Evaluation

Client states importance of maintaining large urine output; lists actions and need for medication to maintain recommended pH; demonstrates ability to monitor urinary pH; demonstrates adherence to dietary restrictions.

Goal 4: Client will be free from postoperative complications.

Implementation

1. Refer to "Perioperative Period," p. 119.
2. Note urine: amount, color, and specific gravity.
3. Maintain adequate respiratory function following a flank incision.
4. Encourage early ambulation.
5. Monitor for
   a. Hypostatic pneumonia (client may be reluctant to deep-breathe and cough because of discomfort).
   b. Hemorrhage.
   c. Paralytic ileus (from reflex paralysis).
   d. Severe pain.
   e. Urinary tract infection.
   f. Redness or bruising at site of lithotripsy shock waves.
   g. Renal colic pain 3 or more days following lithotripsy and report to physician.
   h. Weight gain after lithotripsy (may indicate urinary retention).

6. Give urinary antiseptics and antiinfectives as ordered (see Table 3-41).

Evaluation

Client rests comfortably; is free from signs of UTI (e.g., no WBCs, culture less than 100,000 organisms/ml), complications of surgery.

Goal 5: Client will understand home care.

Implementation

1. Refer to General Nursing Goal 3, p. 197.
2. Teach client how and why to avoid upper respiratory tract infection.
3. Tell client to avoid heavy lifting for 4-8 weeks after operation.

Evaluation

Client lists home health measures.

☐ Cancer of the Bladder
General Information

1. Characteristics
   a. More than 66% of cases occur in men
   b. Most tumors start as benign papillomas or as leukoplakia
   c. Multiple tumors frequent
   d. Tumors often recur
2. Risk factors: probably a disease of multiple etiologies, not yet specifically identified; industrial carcinogens, smoking, aniline dyes, benzene, asbestos, and alcohol have been implicated
3. Medical treatment
   a. Surgical intervention
      1. transurethral bladder resection if tumors are of the trigone or posterior bladder wall (85%)
      2. complete cystectomy when cure highly probable
      3. urinary diversion
         a. *ileal conduit:* a portion of the ileum becomes a conduit; the ureters are transplanted into one end and the other end becomes an external stoma
         b. *cutaneous ureterostomy:* dissection of one or both ureters, bringing them to the skin, forming one or two stomas (for inoperable tumors)
   b. Radiation therapy
      1. preoperative irradiation improves survival in clients with high-grade tumors
      2. external or internal radiation therapy for non-operable tumors or clients who refuse surgery

Nursing Process
Assessment

1. Painless hematuria
2. Abnormal cystogram
3. Abnormal blood and urine studies

4. Cystoscopy, biopsy results
Analysis (see p. 197)
Planning, Implementation, and Evaluation

Goal 1: Client will be prepared for surgery.

Implementation
1. Refer to "Perioperative Period," p. 118.
2. Give or arrange for sexual counseling regarding impotence (in men).
3. Give bowel prep as ordered.
4. Arrange for introduction to diversionary appliance.
5. Ensure stoma site (RLQ) is marked.

Evaluation
Client discusses planned surgery and its implications; inspects diversionary appliance.

Goal 2: Client will remain free from postoperative complications.

Implementation
1. Refer to "Perioperative Period," p. 119.
2. Check ureteral splints for patency, output, and color of urine qh.
3. Monitor stoma for normal color (pink to red; dark purplish color indicates vascular compromise).
4. Record I&O for at least 3 days; encourage up to 3000 ml fluid intake/day.
5. Offer psychological support as needed.

Evaluation
Client maintains intake of 3000 ml/day; shows no signs of shock or hemorrhage (e.g., tachycardia, hypotension, apprehension, and cold clammy skin, decreased BP, and increased pulse).

Goal 3: Client will learn care of urinary diversion appliance and will begin to adjust to alteration in body image.

Implementation
1. Have enterostomal therapist orient client to appliance and its care.
2. Reinforce all teaching regarding skin care, cleanliness, and odor control.
3. Allow client an opportunity to express feelings and concerns regarding changed body image.
4. Encourage client to assume full care of appliance as soon as possible.

Evaluation
Client begins to adapt to body image change (e.g., discusses change, cares for appliance); achieves self-care management of appliance with successful odor control.

☐ Acute Renal Failure
General Information

1. Definition: a sudden and potentially reversible loss of kidney function

2. Categories and causes of renal failure
   a. *Prerenal* (outside kidney): poor perfusion, decrease in circulating volume
   b. *Renal:* structural damage to kidney resulting from acute tubular necrosis
   c. *Postrenal:* obstruction within urinary tract
3. Risk/predisposing factors
   a. Prerenal
      1. reduction in blood volume (shock)
      2. trauma
      3. septic shock
      4. dehydration
      5. cardiac failure
   b. Renal
      1. hypersensitivity (allergic disorders)
      2. obstruction of renal vessels (embolism, thrombosis)
      3. nephrotoxic agents (bacterial toxins and drugs)
      4. mismatched blood transfusion
      5. glomerulonephritis
   c. Postrenal
      1. kidney stones or tumors
      2. benign prostatic hypertrophy or obstruction

Nursing Process
Assessment
1. Oliguric phase (urine volume less than 400 ml/day)
   a. Decreased serum sodium and increased potassium; decreased calcium and bicarbonate
   b. Increased BUN, creatinine maintaining a 10:1 ratio (normally 20:1 ratio)
   c. Increased specific gravity
   d. Hypervolemia, hypertension
   e. Usually lasts 8 days-3 weeks
2. Diuretic phase (urine volume greater than 3000 ml/day)
   a. Serum sodium and potassium may return to normal, stay elevated, or decrease
   b. Increased BUN and serum creatinine
   c. Decreased specific gravity of urine
   d. Hypovolemia
   e. Weight loss
   f. Usually lasts several days to 1 week
3. Recovery phase: gradual return of normal function over period of 3-12 months
Analysis (see p. 197)
Planning, Implementation, and Evaluation

Goal 1 (if prerenal failure): Client will experience increased renal blood flow through an increased circulating blood volume.

Implementation
1. Monitor vital signs as ordered, especially BP and pulse.
2. Maintain strict I&O; monitor urinary output hourly.
3. Administer IV fluids as ordered.

Table 3-42 Diuretic drugs

Name	Action	Side effects	Nursing implications
OSMOTIC DIURETICS			
Mannitol (Osmitrol)	Draws water from the cells and extracellular spaces into the intravascular. Used to treat or prevent oliguric phase of acute renal failure. Reduces intraocular and cerebrospinal fluid.	Transient circulatory overload and edema, headache, confusion, blurred vision, thirst, nausea, vomiting, fluid/electrolyte imbalance, water intoxication, cellular dehydration	Monitor I&O. Check for electrolyte imbalance, water intoxication, cellular dehydration. Be aware of renal and cardiovascular function. Give frequent mouth care to relieve thirst.

THIAZIDE DIURETICS (see Table 3-16, p. 138)
POTENT DIURETICS (see Table 3-16, p. 138)
POTASSIUM-SPARING DIURETICS (see Table 3-16, p. 138)

4. Treat shock if present.
5. Administer prescribed medications to increase renal flow (e.g., dopamine 2-5 µg/kg/min).
6. Administer prescribed diuretics to increase production of urine (e.g., mannitol, furosemide) if client still has output (see Table 3-42)

Evaluation

Client has adequate circulation (normal BP, palpable pulse with regular rate and rhythm, skin warm, oriented in 3 spheres); urine output greater than 30 ml/hr.

Goal 2: Client will maintain fluid, electrolyte, and nitrogen balance.

Implementation (oliguric phase)
1. Weigh client daily.
2. Measure I&O carefully.
3. Administer only enough fluid to replace losses.
4. Include insensible losses in measurement of output.
   a. 500 ml/day if less than 5000 feet above sea level.
   b. 1000 ml/day if more than 5000 feet above sea level.
5. Observe for edema and electrolyte imbalance.
6. Monitor serum lab test results.
7. Administer 50% dextrose with 5-10 units regular insulin as ordered, to drive potassium into cells.
8. Administer ion-exchange resin Kayexalate enema as ordered, to lower high potassium levels.
9. Reduce potassium, sodium, and phosphorus in diet.
10. Administer IV sodium bicarbonate for acidosis.
11. Administer phosphate binders such as aluminum hydroxide (Amphojel) or aluminum carbonate (Basaljel) for hyperphosphatemia.
12. Reduce protein in diet and teach client rationale; provide high biological-value protein for diet (see Table 3-43).

Table 3-43 Low-protein diet sample menu

	Serving	Protein (g)
BREAKFAST		
Orange juice	½ glass	1
Farina	½ cup	1
Margarine	1 tbsp	trace
Sugar	1 tbsp	—
Low-protein bread	1 slice	1
Jelly	1 tbsp	—
Milk	½ cup	3.5
Coffee		—
LUNCH		
Fruit salad:		
Peaches (canned)	1	trace
Pears (canned)	1	trace
Apple (fresh)	1	trace
Low-protein bread, toasted	1 slice	1
Margarine	1 tbsp	trace
Jelly	1 tbsp	—
Sherbet	½ cup	1
Ginger ale with added sugar	1 glass	—
Tea		—
DINNER		
Omelette	2 eggs	13
Asparagus	½ cup	trace
Carrots	⅔ cup	1
Baked potato	1	3
Margarine	1 tbsp	trace
Ginger ale with added sugar	1 glass	—
Coffee	—	—
Cantaloupe	¼	½
	TOTAL	26 g

Usual protein intake: 40-60 g.

Implementation (diuretic phase)

1. Prevent dehydration; balance I&O.
2. Increase dietary sodium and potassium to normal levels.
3. Maintain positive nitrogen balance and sufficient calories to prevent body protein from being metabolized.
4. Prevent infection.

Evaluation

Client maintains approximately equal intake and output and stable weight; remains free from signs of electrolyte imbalance, edema, and dehydration; lists foods on a low-potassium, low-protein diet.

Goal 3: Client will be free from infection and further damage to kidneys (refer to General Nursing Goal 1, p. 197).

☐ Chronic Renal Failure
General Information

1. Definition: a progressive, irreversible deterioration of renal function that ends in fatal uremia unless kidney transplant or dialysis is performed
2. Risk/predisposing factors
   a. Urinary tract obstruction and infection
   b. Infectious diseases that cause hypertension and increased catabolism with retention of metabolites (glomerulonephritis)
   c. Metabolic disease (diabetes)
   d. Nephrotoxic agents (bacterial toxins, drugs)
   e. Acute renal failure
3. Pathophysiology
   a. Kidneys lose their ability to reabsorb electrolytes
   b. Urine output is decreased
   c. Anemia (thought to be caused by inadequate production of erythropoietin and depression of bone marrow as uremia increases)
   d. End products of protein metabolism accumulate in blood (BUN, creatinine)
   e. Reduced resistance to infection
   f. Complications: acidosis, pericarditis, and renal osteodystrophy (abnormal calcium metabolism)

Nursing Process

Assessment

1. Urine output: oliguria, anuria
2. Metabolic indicators
   a. Elevated BUN, creatinine
   b. Hyperphosphatemia
   c. Hyperkalemia
   d. Hypocalcemia
   e. Metabolic acidosis
   f. Elevated, normal, or decreased serum sodium depending on water retention
3. Cardiovascular indicators
   a. Hypertension
   b. Congestive heart failure
   c. Pericarditis
4. Hematological indicators
   a. Anemia (decreased renal production of erythropoietin)
   b. Alteration of platelet function leading to bleeding tendencies
   c. Susceptibility to infection (changes in leukocyte function)
5. Respiratory indicators
   a. Pulmonary edema
   b. Uremic pneumonitis
   c. Uremic pleurisy
6. Gastrointestinal indicators
   a. Mucosal irritation in GI tract
   b. Ammonia on breath (uremic fetor)
   c. Anorexia, nausea, vomiting, hiccoughs
7. Central nervous system indicators
   a. Early: mild deficit in mental functioning
   b. Late: altered sensorium, slurred speech, generalized seizures, encephalopathy with toxic psychosis, coma
8. Peripheral nervous system indicators
   a. Peripheral neuropathy involving all extremities
   b. Burning, painful paresthesias
9. Musculoskeletal indicators
   a. Renal osteodystrophy
   b. Bone pain in feet and legs upon walking and standing, pathological fractures
10. Dermatological indicators
    a. Pruritus
    b. Dry skin: caused by atrophy of sweat glands
    c. Easy bruising, petechiae, and purpura
    d. Pallor related to anemia
    e. Sallow, yellow-tan color to skin
    f. Brittle, dry hair
    g. Dry and ridged nails
    h. Uremic frost: crystallization of urea on skin (late sign)
11. Endocrine indicators
    a. Hypothyroidism
    b. Decreased T_4 level
12. Reproductive indicators
    a. Infertility
    b. Loss of libido
    c. Amenorrhea in women
    d. Decreased testosterone and sperm count in men

Analysis (see p. 197)

Planning, Implementation, and Evaluation

Goal 1: Client will maintain fluid and electrolyte balance (refer to "Acute Renal Failure" Goals 1 and 2, pp. 202 and 203).

Goal 2: Client will remain free from infection (refer to General Nursing Goal 1, p. 197).

Goal 3: Client will maintain adequate caloric intake to prevent muscle wasting and prevent own body stores from being metabolized.

Implementation
1. Initiate daily calorie count.
2. Give medication to control nausea and vomiting before meals.
3. Adjust level of protein in diet to client's serum levels of BUN and creatinine.
4. Encourage protein of high biological value (essential amino acids).
5. Serve food attractively and at appropriate temperature.

Evaluation
Client's BUN and creatinine levels remain within normal limits or stable; calorie count is 35-40 calories/kg body weight.

Goal 4: Client will be protected from self-injury during period of altered sensorium.

Implementation
1. Restrain if necessary.
2. Institute seizure precautions.
3. Perform neurological checks frequently.
4. Monitor BUN and creatinine closely.
5. Teach significant others about cause of altered sensorium.

Evaluation
Client is free from injury during periods of confusion; significant others state awareness of relationship between disease process and altered sensorium.

Goal 5: Client will be relieved of itching and maintain skin integrity.

Implementation
1. Avoid soap.
2. Use soft cloth.
3. Add oil to tepid bath water (baking soda in water may help).

Evaluation
Client's itching is relieved; skin remains intact.

Goal 6: Client and significant others will be supported emotionally (refer to General Nursing Goal 4, p. 199, and Table 2-4, p. 22).

Goal 7: Client will adapt to altered sexual functioning.

Implementation
1. Teach client and significant other about alterations in sexual functioning.
2. Provide or arrange sexual counseling if necessary.
3. Encourage client and significant other to discuss the problem.

Evaluation
Client and significant other discuss change and alteration in sexual expression.

☐ Dialysis

Dialysis is the passage of particles (ions) from an area of high concentration to an area of low concentration (diffusion) across a semipermeable membrane; simultaneously, water moves (osmosis) toward the solution in which the solute concentration is greater. When dialysis is used as a substitute for kidney function, the semipermeable membrane used is either the peritoneum (peritoneal dialysis) or an artificial membrane (hemodialysis). The principle of exchange is the same with both methods. The pores in the membrane are large enough to allow the passage of urea, electrolytes, and creatinine, but are too small to allow the passage of blood cells and other protein molecules (see Fig. 3-18).

General Information: peritoneal dialysis

1. Definition: placement of catheter through abdominal wall into peritoneal space
2. Procedure: body or room temperature dialysate is allowed to flow into the peritoneal cavity by gravity; the solution remains in the abdomen for exchange to occur and then is drained from the peritoneal cavity by gravity; it carries with it waste products and excess electrolytes and can last from 12-24 hours
3. Number of cycles: varies according to the client's problems, tolerance, response, and type of solution
4. Types (see Table 3-44)
   a. Intermittent manual
   b. Intermittent automatic
   c. Continuous ambulatory (CAPD)
      1. dialysate remains in peritoneum 24 hr/day with several dialysate exchanges each day
      2. advantages
         a. lower BP (9 out of 10 clients can discontinue BP medications)
         b. increased Hct and Hgb
         c. less expensive
         d. greater freedom for client
         e. weight gain from glucose absorbed from dialysate (later can become a disadvantage)
      3. disadvantages and risks
         a. peritonitis

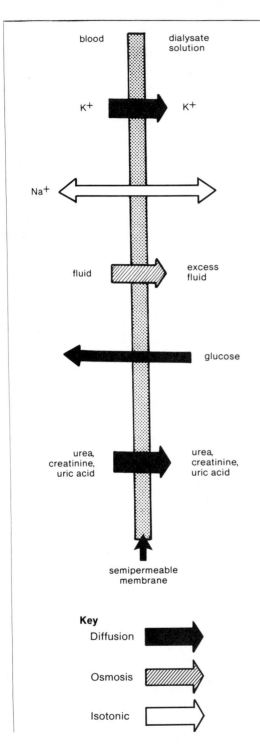

Fig. 3-18 Schematic representation of dialysis.

b. infection at catheter exit site
c. dialysate leakage
d. hypotension
e. hypoalbuminemia (caused by increased loss of protein from repeated peritonitis and large pores in peritoneum)
5. Peritoneal access (e.g., Tenckhoff peritoneal catheter extends access to the peritoneal cavity for weeks to months)

Nursing Process

Assessment
1. Temperature, pulse, respirations, and blood pressure
2. Blood chemistries (electrolytes, BUN, creatinine, glucose)
3. Daily I&O
4. Daily weight (after fluid is drained from cavity)
5. Catheter site for signs of infection or leakage (redness, tenderness, pain, or exudate)

Analysis (see p. 197)

Planning, Implementation, and Evaluation

Goal 1: Client will be protected from peritonitis.

Implementation
1. Use scrupulous aseptic technique throughout dialysis.
2. Check dialysate for cloudiness (sign of infection).
3. Notify physician immediately if peritonitis is suspected (cloudy peritoneal fluid, fever, chills).
4. Obtain peritoneal fluid sample for fluid analysis, culture and sensitivity.
5. Initiate antibiotic therapy as ordered (cephalosporins or aminoglycosides either systemically or instilled into dialysate).
6. Take temperature q4h.
7. Change catheter site dressing at least daily; cleanse with iodine solution and apply topical antibiotic ointment.

Evaluation
Client's peritoneal fluid remains clear; temperature remains within normal limits.

Goal 2: Client will experience successful intermittent dialysis and maintain optimal concentrations of serum electrolytes.

Implementation
1. Weigh client daily before dialysis.
2. Have client empty bladder and bowel prior to paracentesis.
3. Place client in comfortable supine position.
4. Warm dialysate to body temperature using warming pads before instilling.
5. Permit 2 L of dialysate to flow unrestricted into peritoneal cavity (inflow).
6. Leave fluid in peritoneal cavity for 20-30 minutes so that solution can equilibrate (dwell time).

Table 3-44   Comparison of peritoneal dialysis and continuous ambulatory peritoneal dialysis (CAPD)

	Peritoneal dialysis	CAPD
Type of catheter	Tenckhoff	Tenckhoff
Number of exchanges per day	Average of 24	3 during day 1 at night
Dwell time	20-30 min per exchange	Day: 4-5 hr Night: 8 hr
Amout of dialysate	1500-2000 ml per exchange	Average 2000 ml per exchange
Type of dialysate	1.5%, 2.5%, 4.25% (4.25% is most concentrated and will remove most fluid)	Day: 1.5%, 2.5% Night: 4.25%
Activity of client	Usually bed rest—may turn from side to side	Ambulatory as desired
Diet of client	Increase protein to 1 g/kg/day 40 kilocalories/kg/day Restrict fluids to 400-500 ml/day Restrict sodium to 1-2 g/day Restrict potassium to 1500-2000 mg/day Limit phosphorus Take daily water-soluble vitamin supplement	Increase protein to 1.2-1.5 g/kg/day Limit phosphorus Include liberal potassium Include liberal fluids Avoid fats and sweets to control cholesterol level and HDL levels

From Williams, S.R. (1990). *Essentials of nutrition and diet therapy* (5th ed.). St. Louis: Mosby—Year Book.

7. Drain equilibrated fluid from peritoneal cavity.
8. Record amount of fluid loss or gain; outflow should be approximately 100-200 ml more than inflow; have client turn on sides to localize fluid and promote drainage; if retention continues, notify physician.
9. Repeat cycle as ordered.
10. Perform blood chemistries as ordered.
11. Maintain client comfort during dialysis.

Evaluation

Client's weight decreases after each dialysis session; has larger output than inflow.

Goal 3: Client will be free from hypertension.

Implementation

1. Monitor BP standing and sitting.
2. Monitor BP during dialysis (should decrease as fluid volume is reduced).
3. Use a more hypertonic dialysate if hypertension persists.
4. Restrict fluid and sodium intake.
5. Give antihypertensive medications as ordered.
6. Notify physician if symptoms of hypotension occur during procedure; treat by administering normal saline directly into the arterial or venous line and slowing the dialyzing procedures.

Evaluation

Client's BP remains within predetermined guidelines.

Goal 4: Client will be successful with CAPD at home if client's condition requires chronic dialysis.

Implementation

1. Educate client and significant others in the principles, process, and techniques of CAPD.
   a. Instill 2 L of room-temperature dialysate.
   b. Leave in peritoneal cavity 4-8 hours.
   c. Go about daily activities.
   d. Drain fluid and discard.
   e. Replace with 2 L of fresh dialysate.
   f. Repeat procedure 4 times/day.
   g. Leave dialysate in peritoneal cavity overnight.
2. Educate about sterile technique and its importance in preventing peritonitis.
3. Have client keep a written record of daily weight and BP.
4. Provide diet instruction to replace lost protein; liberalize protein, potassium, salt, and water intake.
5. Teach the importance of regular medical and nursing follow-up for lab work, catheter change, evaluation of dialysis technique, monitoring of weight and BP, and any other problems.

Evaluation

Client uses CAPD at home free from any problems; explains proper diet and the importance of follow-up.

Goal 5: Client will be assisted in coping psychologically with ongoing dialysis treatments (refer to "Hemodialysis" Goal 3, p. 210).

General Information: Hemodialysis

1. Definition: passage of heparinized blood from client through a tube consisting of a semipermeable membrane immersed in a dialysate bath composed of all

Access to client's circulation	Advantages/Disadvantages	Nursing implications
Arteriovenous shunt 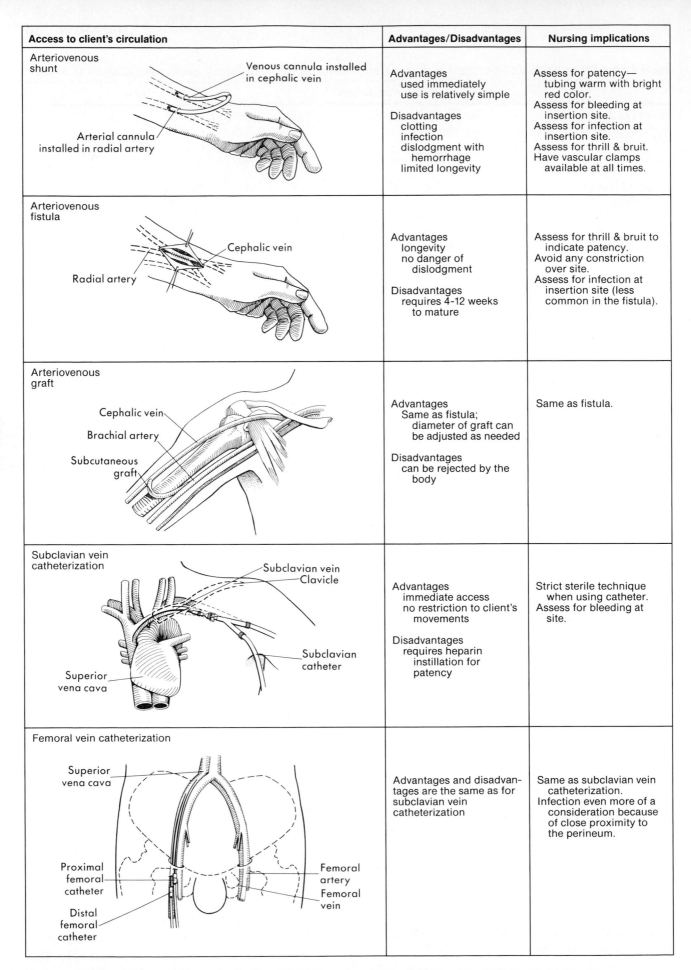 Venous cannula installed in cephalic vein Arterial cannula installed in radial artery	Advantages used immediately use is relatively simple Disadvantages clotting infection dislodgment with hemorrhage limited longevity	Assess for patency— tubing warm with bright red color. Assess for bleeding at insertion site. Assess for infection at insertion site. Assess for thrill & bruit. Have vascular clamps available at all times.
Arteriovenous fistula Cephalic vein Radial artery	Advantages longevity no danger of dislodgment Disadvantages requires 4-12 weeks to mature	Assess for thrill & bruit to indicate patency. Avoid any constriction over site. Assess for infection at insertion site (less common in the fistula).
Arteriovenous graft Cephalic vein Brachial artery Subcutaneous graft	Advantages Same as fistula; diameter of graft can be adjusted as needed Disadvantages can be rejected by the body	Same as fistula.
Subclavian vein catheterization Subclavian vein Clavicle Subclavian catheter Superior vena cava	Advantages immediate access no restriction to client's movements Disadvantages requires heparin instillation for patency	Strict sterile technique when using catheter. Assess for bleeding at site.
Femoral vein catheterization Superior vena cava Proximal femoral catheter Distal femoral catheter Femoral artery Femoral vein	Advantages and disadvantages are the same as for subclavian vein catheterization	Same as subclavian vein catheterization. Infection even more of a consideration because of close proximity to the perineum.

Fig. 3-19 Access to client's circulation. (From Long, B.C., & Phipps, W.J. [1989]. *Medical-surgical nursing: A nursing process approach* [2nd ed.]. St. Louis: Mosby—Year Book.)

important electrolytes in their ideal concentration. Diffusion and ultrafiltration occur between the client's blood and the dialysate. Protamine sulfate may be used to counteract the heparin effects.

2. Procedure: fresh dialysate is used continuously until the client's electrolyte and fluid balances are within safe levels.
3. Schedule varies with clinical condition and type of dialyzer
   a. Up to 3 times/week
   b. 4-6 hr/day is possible for coil and hollow-fiber dialyzers; 10-12 hr/day is necessary for plate-type dialyzers
4. Access to client's circulation (see Fig. 3-19)
   a. Arteriovenous (AV) shunt
      1. external device
         a. composed of two nonthrombogenic Silastic rubber tubes or cannulas with Teflon tips, one sutured in artery, the other in vein
         b. between dialysis, the two tubes are joined by Teflon connector
         c. most commonly used vessels are the radial artery and cephalic vein of forearm
      2. advantages
         a. can be used immediately after insertion
         b. use is relatively simple
      3. disadvantages
         a. clotting
         b. infection
         c. accidental dislodgement with hemorrhage
         d. limited longevity
   b. Arteriovenous (AV) fistula: access of choice for hemodialysis
      1. internal access
         a. created by side-to-side or end-to-end anastomosis between adjacent vein and artery (often radial artery and cephalic vein)
         b. creates enlarged superficial vein with easy access for venipuncture
      2. advantages
         a. longevity
         b. no danger of disconnection
      3. disadvantages
         a. must be constructed 4-12 weeks in advance
         b. needs time to mature
         c. complications
            ◆ thrombosis
            ◆ venous hypertension distal to anastomosis
            ◆ ischemia of extremity
            ◆ infection (less frequent than AV shunts)
   c. Graft
      1. internal access (e.g., piece of bovine carotid artery or Gore-Tex material)
      2. usually done when client's vessels are unsuitable to be used as a fistula

3. advantages
   a. not dependent on adequate client circulation for placement
   b. diameter is predetermined
4. disadvantages
   a. does not have healing properties (e.g., more chance of bleeding, infection, aneurysm formation)
   b. cannot be used for several weeks
   c. not used for clients awaiting transplants since bovine grafts can be rejected

Nursing Process

Assessment
1. Arterial flow of AV shunt, AV fistula, or graft
   a. Palpate for thrill
   b. Listen for bruit
   c. Check skin temperature and pulses distal to access site
   d. Color of blood should be bright, cranberry red (shunt only)
2. Check client's temperature and BP
3. Check dialysate composition and temperature
4. Client's psychological reaction to dialysis
   a. Reaction to physical condition
   b. Predialysis personality
   c. Family support system
   d. Financial status
   e. Signs of depression, fear, anxiety, denial, and regression
   f. Noncompliance with diet or fluid restrictions
   g. Verbalization of self-deprecation
   h. Relinquishment of decision making to family or staff
   i. Suicidal ideation
   j. Reaction to sexual dysfunction

Analysis (see p. 197)

Planning, Implementation, and Evaluation

> **Goal 1:** Client will have access site protected from trauma.

Implementation
1. Keep extremity elevated several hours after insertion.
2. Instruct client to keep affected arm or leg as straight as possible at all times.
3. Have clamps or tourniquet available at all times to control any severe bleeding from accidental dislodgement of shunt.
4. Notify physician immediately of severe bleeding or clotting of cannula.
5. Instruct client to avoid lifting heavy objects with affected arm.
6. Do not use affected arm for BP or venipuncture.
7. Instruct client to avoid constrictive clothing over shunt site.

8. Instruct client to avoid exposing access site to extreme cold.

Evaluation

Client's blood flow to access site remains cranberry red with palpable thrill, audible bruit, and warm temperature.

> **Goal 2:** Client will remain free from infection at access site.

Implementation

1. Check site frequently for signs of infection (pain, redness, tenderness, or increase of temperature).
2. Perform suture line care (10-14 days until sutures are removed).
  a. Remove old dressing.
  b. Clean suture line with povidone-iodine solution.
  c. Apply new sterile dressing.
3. Instruct client not to irritate scabs that form over needle insertion sites.
4. Apply skin softening cream to scabs.
5. Wash the affected limb with antibacterial soap (e.g., Dial, Safeguard) and water daily.

Evaluation

Client remains free from pain, redness, and tenderness at site of shunt.

> **Goal 3:** Client will cope with ongoing dialysis treatments.

Implementation

1. See Table 2-4 on p. 22.
2. Encourage client to express concerns, feelings, and to ask questions about procedures and life-style adaptations.
3. Educate client concerning treatments and rationale behind restrictions.
4. Give consistent information to client and significant others.
5. Encourage client to maintain as active and productive a life as possible, and to plan daily activities around treatments.
6. Encourage client to be as independent and responsible for care as possible.
7. Encourage significant others to express their feelings.
8. Counsel significant others to avoid unrealistic expectations and overprotectiveness.
9. Help client move from depression, despair, and defeat to acceptance of illness by exhibiting hope and planning for realistic goals.
10. Refer for vocational rehabilitation, sheltered workshops, or special services as needed (e.g., financial).
11. Provide marital or sexual counseling.
12. Conduct regular team conferences to discuss care of clients.

Evaluation

Client leads as active and productive a life as possible within the constraints of the illness; shows acceptance of disease by managing care and setting realistic goals.

☐ Kidney Transplantation
General Information

1. Definition: the surgical implantation of a donated, allogenic kidney to restore kidney function in a client with end-stage renal failure
2. Donor
  a. Live
  b. Cadaver
3. Rejection of the grafted kidney is a significant problem
  a. Attempts to minimize: tissue typing before transplantation (must indicate high degree of histocompatibility)
  b. Types of rejection
    1. *hyperacute:* occurs on the operating room table
    2. *acute:* first episode can occur 5-7 days after transplant; subsequent episodes can occur within the first year
    3. *chronic:* rejection continues despite repeated attempts at immunosuppression
    4. rejection rates
      a. 20%-25% of cadaver grafts
      b. 5%-10% of live donor grafts
      c. greatly increased by the presence of diabetes
4. Immunosuppressive drugs are given to all transplant recipients; see Table 3-45.

Nursing Process
Assessment

1. Metabolic state
2. Tissue histocompatibility
3. Immunological defense status
4. Psychological and emotional status
5. Potential sources of postoperative infection (carious teeth, infected donor kidneys) since client will be immunosuppressed
6. Age; desires of the client regarding this risk-filled procedure

Analysis (see p. 197)
Planning, Implementation, and Evaluation

> **Goal 1:** Client will be adequately prepared pre-operatively to maximize the chances of a successful outcome.

Implementation

1. Refer to "Perioperative Period," p. 118.
2. Maintain accurate I&O; adhere to fluid restriction.
3. Know that the client may need to undergo preoperative hemodialysis to achieve an optimal metabolic state.

Table 3-45 Immunosuppressive drugs

Generic name (trade name)	Action	Side effects	Nursing implications
Azathioprine (Imuran)	Inhibits RNA and DNA synthesis. Inhibits lymphoid tissue (where cells divide rapidly during the rejection process) thereby diminishing the rejection process.	Skin rash, alopecia, nausea, vomiting, leukopenia, thrombocytopenia	Begin drug 1-5 days before surgery and continue afterward. Monitor hematological status. Institute reverse isolation if needed. Monitor for fever, chills, unusual bleeding, bruising, and sore throat.
Cyclosporin (Sandimmune)	Strongly inhibits the antibody production that leads to graft rejection. Use should be accompanied by adjunct steroid administration.	Nephrotoxicity, hypertension, tremor, gum hyperplasia, hepatotoxicity, hirsutism	Monitor kidney and liver function. Dilute oral solution with milk or orange juice and give at room temperature. Observe for anaphylaxis for at least 30 minutes after start of IV infusion of drug.
Lymphocyte immune globulin (Atgam)	Inhibits cell-mediated immune response.	Hypotension, chest pain, nausea, vomiting, anaphylaxis	Monitor for signs and symptoms of infection. Refrigerate drug. Do not use drug if more than 12 hours old. Skin test before first dose. Do not give if allergic to equine products.
Muromonab-CD3 (Orthoclone OKT3)	Restores function of allograft and reverses rejection.	Chest pain, nausea, vomiting, fever, chills, tremors, dyspnea	Use only one time (an antibody preparation). Obtain chest x-ray before treatment (risk of pulmonary edema). Give antipyretics before a dose to decrease incidence of fever or chills.
Corticosteroids (see Table 3-33)			

4. Protect client from possible sources of infection (reverse isolation).

Evaluation

Client is able to describe the postoperative routine.

Goal 2: Client will be psychologically prepared for the surgery.

Implementation

1. Refer to "Perioperative Period," p. 118.
2. Allow client the opportunity to discuss feelings and concerns regarding the surgery and its chances of success.
3. Answer client's questions as honestly and completely as possible.
4. Allow client an opportunity to discuss any ambivalent feelings about the donor (may be a very close relative).
5. Know that significant others also need support and information.

Evaluation

Client experiences only a moderate level of anxiety preoperatively; expresses realistic hope regarding outcome of transplant.

Goal 3: Client will be free from postoperative complications.

Implementation

1. Refer to "Perioperative Period," p. 119.
2. Assess fluid and electrolyte balance carefully.
   a. Measure urine output (may range from massive diuresis [live donor] to aneuresis [cadaver donor]).
   b. May require hemodialysis.
3. Protect client from infection.
   a. Give Foley catheter care.
   b. May be in reverse isolation.
   c. Monitor temperature.
4. Observe for signs of acute rejection of transplant.
   a. Oliguria, anuria

b. Fever (temperature greater than 37.7° C)

c. Increased blood pressure

d. Swollen, tender kidney

e. Flu symptoms

5. Maintain integrity of venous access.

Evaluation

Client has vital signs within normal limits; output equivalent to fluid intake; remains free from infection.

Goal 4: Client will take medications correctly.

Implementation

1. Teach client that immunosuppressive drugs are the main defense against transplant rejection.

2. Teach side effects and complications of these drugs and that withdrawal (if it is ever appropriate) must be done gradually.

3. Tell client that he is more susceptible to infection while taking these drugs and to notify physician at the first sign of a cold or infection.

4. Teach client how to avoid or at least decrease exposure to sources of infection.

Evaluation

Client lists side effects of all drugs; know when to call physician regarding drug-related problems; states an awareness of administration schedule and importance of maintaining it.

☐ Benign Prostatic Hypertrophy (BPH)
General Information

1. Incidence: more than 50% of all men over 50

2. Predisposing factors: unknown

3. Medical treatment: surgical intervention

   a. Transurethral resection of prostate (TURP) is most common

   b. Suprapubic and retropubic approaches also used

Nursing Process

Assessment

1. Urinary dysfunction

2. Symmetrical, smooth enlargement of prostate

3. Signs and symptoms of hydronephrosis followed by renal failure (late)

Analysis (see p. 197).

Planning, Implementation, and Evaluation

Goal 1: Client will have adequate urinary flow preoperatively.

Implementation

1. Insert Foley catheter.

   a. On initial insertion: prevent bladder collapse by clamping draining tube after 1000 ml urine is drained.

   b. Unclamp tube after 1 hour and repeat protocol.

2. Measure I&O.

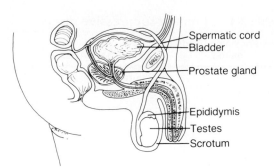

Fig. 3-20   Normal male anatomy.

3. Know that a suprapubic catheter may be necessary.

Evaluation

Client's intake and output remains balanced.

Goal 2: Client will be able to describe surgical approach and postoperative care (see Table 3-46 and Fig. 3-21).

Implementation

1. Teach client that vasectomy is usually done to reduce chance of epididymitis.

2. Know that most prostatectomies produce retrograde ejaculation and sterility.

Evaluation

Client describes a TURP; knows what to expect postoperatively (e.g., pain and discomfort, ambulation).

Goal 3: Client will have normal urinary drainage, clear to lightly pink-tinged in color; will be free from hemorrhage.

Implementation

1. Know that a 3-way Foley catheter with 30 ml balloon will be inserted postoperatively.

2. Ensure Foley catheter is patent.

3. Apply traction on the Foley catheter for 24 hours (puts pressure on prostatic bed).

4. Maintain constant bladder irrigation (CBI).

5. Increase speed of irrigation if increased blood seen; notify physician if this is not effective.

6. Measure I&O each shift.

7. Monitor urinary output after Foley catheter is removed (2-3 days).

8. Care for dressing around suprapubic catheter if suprapubic prostatectomy done.

Evaluation

Client's urine remains clear and amber-colored.

Goal 4: Client will have minimal discomfort from bladder spasms.

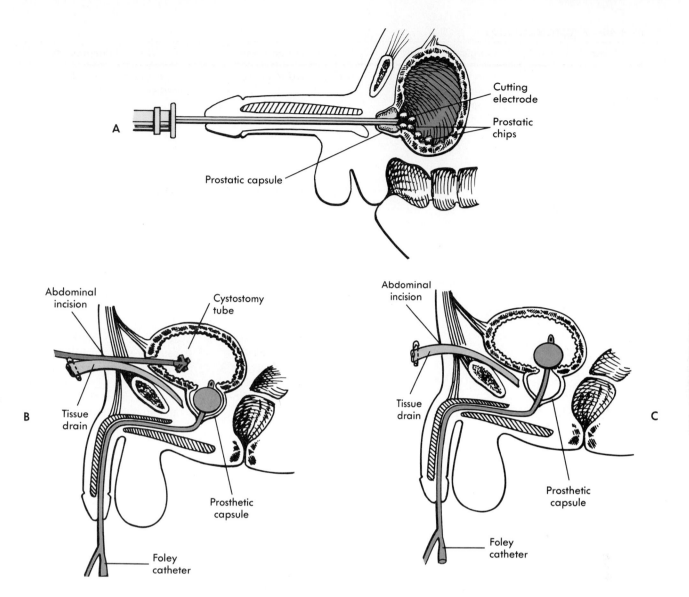

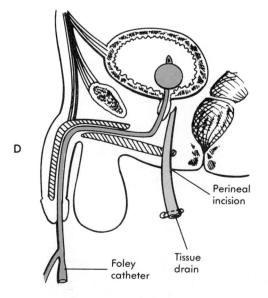

Fig. 3-21 Types of prostatectomies. **A,** Transurethral prostatectomy. **B,** Suprapubic prostatectomy. **C,** Retropubic prostatectomy. **D,** Radical perineal prostatectomy. (From Long, B.C., & Phipps, W.J. [1989]. *Medical-surgical nursing: A nursing process approach* [2nd ed.]. St. Louis: Mosby—Year Book.)

Table 3-46 Prostatectomies

Type	Surgical approach	Common problems	Nursing implications
Transurethral resection (TUR)	Client in lithotomy position Gland removed through resecting cystoscope Most common approach	Not all gland removed	Explain that benign prostatic hypertrophy can recur.
		Constant bladder irrigation to decrease bleeding	Ensure catheter patency. Run irrigant at rate to keep urine light pink. Use only isotonic solution to prevent water intoxication.
		May damage internal sphincter leading to incontinence or bladder-neck strictures	Teach perineal exercises.
		May or may not cause sterility	Reassure client potency *not* affected.
Suprapubic	Abdominal approach Bladder is opened Allows abdominal exploration	Suprapubic catheter or drain with urinary drainage	Do frequent dressing changes. Prevent infection or irritation.
		Hemorrhage common: large-balloon Foley catheter with traction is used to stop bleeding	Watch closely for bleeding. Check catheter patency. Irrigate with saline prn to prevent clots.
		Bladder spasms common	Reposition client. Give propantheline bromide (Pro-Banthine).
		Causes sterility	Reassure client potency *not* affected.
Retropubic	Low abdominal incision; no bladder incision Allows complete, direct removal of gland with less bleeding	Can be done for cancer or BPH	Reassure client potency *not* affected.
		Causes sterility	
		Less chance of bleeding; sometimes constant bladder irrigation is ordered for 24 hours	Watch for bleeding.
		Few spasms	Medicate prn.
Perineal, radical (for cancer)	Incision in perineum between scrotum and rectum Client in lithotomy position	Causes impotence, sterility, and some incontinence	Allow expression of feelings. Teach perineal exercises.
		Large perineal wound with risk of infection and bleeding	Clean well. Check and change dressing prn.
		Straining or rectal trauma may increase bleeding	Avoid rectal temperature or tubes. Give stool softeners.
		May be done for castration for carcinoma	Talk to client. Explain changes.

Implementation

1. Know that a large balloon on the Foley catheter can stimulate spasms (more likely to be used with TURP).
2. Administer narcotics plus anticholinergic drugs as ordered.
3. Administer belladonna and opium suppositories as ordered.
4. Institute strategies to prevent thrombophlebitis.
5. Know that incisional infection is more frequent with suprapubic prostatectomy.
6. Observe for signs of epididymitis (swelling, pain of scrotum, testes) if vasectomy was not done.
7. For epididymitis place ice pack under testes and scrotum.

Evaluation

Client is free from postoperative infections, signs of epididymitis.

Goal 5: Client will understand activities allowed after discharge.

Implementation

1. Tell client to refrain from postoperative sexual activity for approximately 6 weeks.
2. Have client avoid heavy lifting, straining, driving car for approximately 6 weeks.
3. Monitor urine: should be continually clear.
4. Teach client to increase fluid intake (i.e., 1 glass of liquid qh).
5. Teach client to avoid alcohol for 6 weeks.
6. Teach client that dribbling may occur after removal of catheter and that pubococcygeal exercises can help increase sphincter tone.

Evaluation

Client describes activity restrictions; states intent to monitor urine at home.

☐ Cancer of the Prostate
General Information

1. Incidence
   a. Increasing
   b. Second most common cancer in men
   c. Most frequent in 50-plus age group
2. Predisposing factors
   a. Family tendency
   b. Environmental risks and oncogenic virus suspected
3. Other information
   a. Usually starts in posterior lobe
   b. Most commonly adenocarcinoma
   c. Usually palpable on rectal exam
4. Medical treatment: surgical intervention
   a. Radical perineal prostatectomy
   b. Radical retropubic prostatectomy
   c. TURP for palliation followed by hormonal manipulation (DES or bilateral orchiectomy)

Nursing Process

Assessment (findings depend on size of tumor)
1. Prostatic specific antigen (PSA) for early detection
2. Rectal exam: if small tumor, hard nodule on prostate
3. Positive biopsy of prostate
4. BPH resulting from large tumor
5. Signs of metastasis (usually spine): low back and leg pain
6. Increased acid phosphatase with spread beyond capsule
7. Increased alkaline phosphatase with bone metastasis

Analysis (see p. 197).

Planning, Implementation, and Evaluation

Goal 1: Client will understand the planned surgery and what to expect postoperatively.

Implementation

1. Refer to "Perioperative Period," p. 118.
2. Counsel client regarding impotence and/or available penile prosthetic devices.
3. Include significant others in preoperative discussion.

Evaluation

Client describes planned surgery in own words.

Goal 2: Client's incision will be kept clean and remain intact.

Implementation

1. Do not take rectal temperatures or insert rectal tubes.
2. Use T-binder if indicated.
3. Give sitz baths after drains removed.
4. Maintain patency of Foley catheter.

Evaluation

Client's incision heals well.

Goal 3: Client will remain free from postoperative complications.

Implementation

1. Refer to "Perioperative Period," p. 119.
2. Monitor for lymphedema if pelvic lymph nodes removed.

Evaluation

Client is afebrile, maintains clear lung sounds; is free from leg edema.

Goal 4: Client will regain perineal muscle tone and urinary continence.

Implementation

1. Teach pubococcygeal exercises.
2. Institute exercises 48 hours postoperatively; have client do them qh.
3. Reassure client that some urinary control can be obtained.

Evaluation

Client demonstrates perineal exercises; expresses a positive attitude about regaining continence.

Goal 5: Client will be able to explain alternate ways of sexual expression.

Implementation

1. Encourage client to discuss concerns/fears.
2. Encourage client to discuss sexuality with significant other; have them explore different ways to satisfy each other sexually.

Evaluation

Client shows a willingness to discuss sexual concerns.

Goal 6: Client and significant other will understand the therapy for advanced disease.

Implementation

1. Explain hormonal manipulation and side effects of female hormones.
2. Prepare client for bilateral orchiectomy if indicated. Answer questions concerning prosthetic devices and the inguinal incision.
3. Prepare client for TURP if cancer is causing obstruction but is not surgically treatable.

Evaluation

Client describes future care needs.

THE LARGE BOWEL

GENERAL CONCEPTS

Overview/Physiology

1. The large intestine extends from the ileocecal valve to the anus (cecum, ascending colon, transverse colon, descending colon, sigmoid colon, rectum, and anal canal).
2. The major functions of the colon are the absorption of water and electrolytes in the proximal half of the large intestine and storage of feces in the distal half until defecation occurs.
3. Bacterial action in the large bowel not only provides gases to increase the bulk of and propel the feces but also facilitates synthesis of vitamin K, thiamin, riboflavin, vitamin B_{12}, folic acid, biotin, and nicotinic acid.

Application of the Nursing Process to the Client with Large Bowel Problems

Assessment

1. Health history
   a. Bowel habits: frequency and character of stool patterns
   b. Changes in bowel habits: decrease or increase in frequency, change in consistency (more liquid leads to diarrhea; less liquid leads to constipation)
   c. Presence of blood or change in color of stool
   d. Use of laxatives or other methods that affect elimination
   e. Effect of dietary habits on elimination
   f. Presence of abdominal or rectal pain
   g. Altered weight
2. Physical examination
   a. Inspection
      1. abdomen
         a. scars, striae, wounds, fistulas, ostomy
         b. engorged veins
         c. skin characteristics
         d. visible peristalsis and pulsations
         e. visible masses and altered contour
      2. anus
         a. presence of dilated veins
         b. constipation
         c. breaks in skin, fissures
   b. Auscultation
      1. bowel sounds
      2. bruit
      3. hum and friction rub
   c. Percussion
      1. liver size
      2. presence of fluid
   d. Palpation
      1. masses
      2. rigidity of abdominal muscles
      3. pain/tenderness
      4. fluid waves
3. Diagnostic tests
   a. Stool examinations
      1. odor, consistency, color
      2. presence or absence of mucus
      3. occult blood (by guaiac exam)
      4. ova and parasites
   b. Barium enema
      1. definition: barium is instilled in the rectum through a rectal catheter
         a. permits x-ray visualization of large intestine
         b. used to detect polyps, tumors, diverticula, positional abnormalities (e.g., malrotation)
      2. nursing care pretest
         a. explain procedure
         b. administer cathartics as ordered the day before procedure
         c. administer a suppository if ordered on the day of the procedure
         d. may restrict diet to clear liquids for 24 hours before exam
         e. keep NPO after midnight
      3. nursing care posttest
         a. administer laxatives following procedure as ordered to prevent impaction
         b. instruct client that stool will remain light-colored for 24-72 hours
   c. Proctoscopy, sigmoidoscopy, colonoscopy
      1. definition: visualization of inside of entire colon (colonoscopy), sigmoid colon (sigmoidoscopy) or rectum (proctoscopy) through a lighted scope
         a. proctoscopy and sigmoidoscopy: rigid scope
         b. colonoscopy: flexible scope
      2. nursing care pretest
         a. explain procedure
         b. give clear liquids 24-48 hours before exam

c. prepare bowel with laxatives, enemas, or suppositories as ordered
3. nursing care posttest
   a. observe for hemorrhage, abdominal distension, pain
   b. check for return of normal bowel function following procedure
d. Biopsy
   1. definition: removal of polyps or biopsy specimens through a specialized piece of equipment inserted during endoscopy
   2. nursing care
      a. same as for proctoscopy
      b. monitor carefully for hemorrhage

Analysis

1. Safe, effective care environment
   a. High risk for infection
   b. Knowledge deficit
2. Physiological integrity
   a. Constipation, diarrhea, bowel incontinence
   b. Altered nutrition: less than body requirements
3. Psychosocial integrity
   a. Anxiety
   b. Body image disturbance
   c. Altered pattern of sexuality
4. Health promotion/maintenance
   a. Altered health maintenance
   b. Knowledge deficit
   c. Impaired adjustment

General Nursing Planning, Implementation, and Evaluation

Goal 1: Client's bowel elimination will follow a normal pattern.

Implementation

1. Instruct client how to promote proper bowel function; adjust teaching if client has an ileostomy or colostomy.
2. Teach client to respond to defecation reflex since holding feces can contribute to constipation.
3. Instruct client on the use of foods high in bulk and roughage: skin and fibers of fruits and vegetables.
4. Increase fluid intake if allowed.
5. Encourage regular exercise to aid in elimination.
6. Teach about the relationship of stress to altered bowel function.
7. Prevent diarrhea thorough proper sanitation and hygiene.
8. Restrict fruit juices and raw fruits and vegetables that contribute to diarrhea.
9. Observe client with diarrhea for signs of fluid and electrolyte imbalance.
10. Administer antidiarrheals (see Table 3-47).
11. Encourage intake of electrolyte-containing drinks (e.g., Gatorade).

Evaluation

Client establishes a normal pattern of bowel elimination; lists and consumes foods that promote bowel evacuation; establishes a pattern of regular exercise; passes stool of normal consistency.

Goal 2: Client's dietary intake will follow prescribed restrictions yet provide all needed nutrients.

Implementation

1. Increase or decrease dietary nutrients as ordered.
2. Teach client rationale for restrictions.
3. Explore with client means of fostering compliance.
4. Provide needed support and encouragement.

Evaluation

Client selects appropriate diet from sample menus; verbalizes rationale for restrictions; expresses a positive attitude toward diet alteration.

Goal 3: Client will be knowledgeable about disease process, medications, and the prevention of complications.

Implementation

1. Explain disease process and its relationship to medications.
2. Discuss rationale for ordered treatment regimen.
3. Provide data concerning the administration and side effects of all medications.
4. Help client identify potential stressors in life-style that might trigger complications of the disease; discuss appropriate client actions.

Evaluation

Client takes medications as ordered, returns for follow-up care; remains free from preventable complications.

SELECTED HEALTH PROBLEMS RESULTING IN ALTERATION IN LARGE BOWEL ELIMINATION

☐ Alteration in Normal Bowel Evacuation

General Information

1. Definitions
   a. *Constipation:* difficult or infrequent defecation with passage of unduly hard and dry fecal material
   b. *Diarrhea:* frequent passage of abnormally watery bowel movements
   c. Normal bowel evacuation: 2-3 movements/day to 2/week; varies in healthy individuals
2. Precipitating factors
   a. Constipation: worry, anxiety, fear, improper diet, intestinal obstruction, tumors, excessive use of laxatives, use of certain drugs, atony or spasticity of intestinal musculature
   b. Diarrhea: diet, inflammation or irritation of intestinal mucosa, GI infections, use of certain drugs, psychogenic factors

Table 3-47 Antidiarrheal and laxative drugs

Drug	Action	Use	Side effects	Nursing implications
ANTIDIARRHEALS				
Local acting				
Kaolin and pectin (Kaopectate) Bismuth subsalicylate (Pepto-Bismol)	Reduce liquidity of feces. Act within the bowel to soothe the intestinal tract and increase the absorption of water, electrolytes, and nutrients.	Treat acute and chronic diarrhea	Constipation Intestinal obstruction in chronic use Drug absorbs nutrients	Advice client to stop the medication and notify physician if drug is not effective in 48 hours. Advise to maintain fluid intake during diarrhea. Instruct to shake well before taking a liquid drug. Check for presence of glaucoma; if present do not give medications containing atropine. Hold drug and call physician if abdomen becomes distended, if bowel sounds diminish or are absent, or if impaction is suspected.
Systemic acting				
Diphenoxylate hydrochloride with atropine sulfate (Lomotil) Loperamide (Imodium) Camphorated tincture of opium (Paregoric)	Act systemically to inhibit the peristaltic reflex and reduce GI motility.	Same as above	CNS: drowsiness, headache, sedation, dizziness CV: tachycardia GU: urinary retention GI: dry mouth, nausea or vomiting, constipation	
LAXATIVES				
Bulk formers				
Psyllium (Metamucil) Methylcellulose (Citrucel) Bran	Produce soft stool by retaining fluid. Working time: 1-3 days	Prophylaxis and treatment of functional constipation	GI: abdominal cramps, diarrhea, nausea or vomiting; intestinal obstruction if taken dry or chewed	Discontinue drug if abdominal pain occurs. Advise to take 1 hour apart from other oral medications to prevent absorption of drugs by laxative.

Table 3-47 Antidiarrheal and laxative drugs—cont'd

Drug	Action	Use	Side effects	Nursing implications
LAXATIVES— cont'd				
Emollients Docusate sodium (Colace) Docusate calcium (Surfak) Docusate potassium (Dialose)	Docusate salts act as detergents in the intestine, reduce surface tension of interfacing liquids, thus promoting incorporation of fat and additional liquid, softening the stool.	For clients who must avoid straining at stool	Increased absorption if used with mineral oil. Throat irritation if liquid used. Mild abdominal cramping	Advise loss of effectiveness with long-term use. Dilute liquid, but not the syrup preparations, to improve taste. Discontinue if severe abdominal cramping occurs.
Irritants Cascara (Cas-Evac) Senna (Senokot) Castor oil (Alphamul) Bisacodyl (Dulcolax)	Stimulates intestine, promotes peristalsis. Working time: 1-3 hours	Preoperative cleansing, diagnostic studies; treat constipation unresponsive to other agents	Abdominal cramps, diarrhea. In excessive use: electrolyte imbalance. Constipation after catharsis. Laxative dependence.	Advise cascara may color urine reddish-pink or brown depending on urine pH. Monitor for electrolyte imbalance or laxative dependence.
Lubricant Mineral oil	Acts in the colon, lubricates the intestine, and retards colonic fluid absorption. Working time: 6-8 hours	Cleansing enema, preparation for bowel studies, constipation	Impaired absorption of fat-soluble vitamins, digitalis glycosides, sulfonamides, anticoagulants, oral contraceptives. Potential toxic absorption levels of mineral oil if taken with stool softeners. Nausea, vomiting.	Prevent aspiration by not allowing the client to lie flat during or after drug administration. Monitor clients for impaired absorption of medications or vitamins. Obtain detailed history if client takes mineral oil as a regular laxative.
Saline/osmotics Milk of magnesia Magnesium sulfate Magnesium citrate (Epsom salt) Lactulose (Cephulac)	Produce watery stools that distend the bowel. This promotes peristalsis and bowel evacuation. Working time: 1-6 hours	Preprocedure cleansing, constipation	Abdominal cramps. Flatulence. Diarrhea with dehydration and loss of electrolytes.	Monitor for fluid and electrolyte balance and dehydration.
For all laxatives	1. Teach clients the importance of exercise, proper fluid intake, and high-fiber diet to promote regular bowel elimination patterns. 2. Do not use any laxative if obstruction is suspected. 3. Avoid routine use of laxatives.			

Nursing Process

Assessment

1. Stool consistency, appearance
2. Acute or chronic pain, rebound tenderness
3. Weight loss, malnutrition
4. Dehydration
5. Nausea, vomiting; projectile vomiting
6. Electrolyte imbalance, especially sodium, potassium, chloride
7. Aggravation by certain foods and milk products
8. Drug history
9. Malabsorption of foods
10. Mass in abdomen
11. Low-grade fever
12. Anemia
13. Anorexia
14. Presence of bowel sounds: increased or decreased
15. Abdominal distension
16. Decreased flatus

Analysis (see p. 217)

Planning, Implementation, and Evaluation
(refer to General Nursing Goal 1, p. 217)

☐ Chronic Inflammatory Bowel Disease (Regional Enteritis, Ulcerative Colitis)
General Information

1. Definition
   a. *Regional enteritis* (Crohn's disease) is a small-bowel, segmental, transmural inflammatory process that may involve any part of the alimentary tract; the ileum is the principal site
   b. *Ulcerative colitis* is a large-bowel, continuous inflammatory process of the mucosa, primarily of the colon and rectum
2. Incidence: young people between 20 and 40 years of age
3. Etiology: unknown: possibly result of infection, stress, and/or autoimmunity; familial tendency
4. Pathophysiology
   a. Regional enteritis symptoms include marked thickening of the submucosa with lymphedema, hyperplasia, granulomas, ulcerations, and fissures; the longitudinal ulcers and transverse fissures produce a cobblestone effect; in the later stages, full-thickness penetration of the intestinal wall results in the formation of fistulas and abscesses
   b. Ulcerative colitis symptoms include congestion, edema, multiple superficial ulcerations, and crypt abscesses in the rectum and distal colon and spread upward; characterized by profuse watery diarrhea containing blood, mucus, and pus
5. Diagnostic test
   a. Stool for blood, fat, and culture
   b. Proctosigmoidoscopy with biopsy

Table 3-48 Comparison of chronic inflammatory bowel diseases

	Regional enteritis (Crohn's disease)	Ulcerative colitis
General appearance	Usually normal	May feel and look ill
Age	Bimodal: 20-30 yr and 40-50 yr	Mostly young adults
Area affected	Mainly terminal ileum, cecum, and ascending colon (right side)	Colon only, primarily the descending colon (left side)
Extent of involvement	Segmental areas of involvement	Continuous, diffuse areas of involvement
Inflammation	Mostly submucosal	Mostly mucosal
Mucosal appearance	Cobblestone effect; granulomas	Ulcerations
Cancer potential	Normal incidence	Increased incidence
Character of stools	No blood; may have some fat; 3-4 semisoft/day	Blood present; no fat; frequent liquid stools
Reasons for surgery	Fistulas; intestinal obstruction	Poor response to medical therapy; hemorrhage; perforation
Complications	Fistulas; perianal disease; strictures; vitamin and iron deficiencies; fistulas to other organs	Pseudopolyps; hemorrhage; toxic megacolon; cachexia; perforation less often, causes peritonitis

From *Mosby's medical, nursing, and allied health dictionary* (1990). St. Louis: Mosby–Year Book.

   c. Barium enema (cathartics are contraindicated as a prep)

Nursing Process

Assessment

1. Rectal bleeding
2. Diarrhea: frequent liquid stools with tenesmus; may contain blood, mucus, or pus
3. Abdominal cramps before bowel movement; colicky cramping with urgency to defecate
4. Pain, usually located in the left lower quadrant, with ulcerative colitis
5. Anorexia, nausea, vomiting

Table 3-49   Foods to be *avoided* on low-residue diets

Types of food	Foods to be avoided
Beverages	Milk in excess of 2 cups
Breads and cereals	Whole grain or bran
Desserts	Any containing fruits and nuts
Fruits	Any with seeds or skins, raw fruits except bananas
Meats, fish, poultry, cheese, and eggs	Tough meats, pork, fried or highly seasoned meats, fish, cheese
Vegetables	Raw vegetables

6. Dehydration
7. Electrolyte imbalance (e.g., decreased potassium and sodium, metabolic acidosis)
8. Weight loss
9. Weakness, debilitation, malnutrition
10. Anemia
11. Fever
12. Emotional concerns, immature and dependent personality
13. Dietary habits
Analysis (see p. 217)
Planning, Implementation, and Evaluation

Goal 1: Client will be well nourished and hydrated.

Implementation
1. Weigh client daily.
2. Keep NPO in acute stage; give parenteral fluids with vitamins and minerals as ordered.
3. Administer total parenteral nutrition (TPN) as ordered.
4. Initiate high-protein, high-calorie, bland, low-residue diet as tolerated (see Table 3-49).
5. Avoid gas-producing or irritating foods and milk products.
6. Offer small feedings as necessary.
7. Replace deficiency of fat-soluble vitamins (A, D, E, and K).
8. Record caloric intake.
9. Avoid too hot or too cold foods.
10. Urge up to 3000 ml fluid intake/day (if not contraindicated); keep I&O (include measurement of liquid stools).
11. Involve client and significant others with dietitian for proper diet instructions.
Evaluation
    Client maintains weight; states meal plan utilizing high-protein, low-residue, high-calorie, bland diet; maintains at least 2500 ml fluid intake daily.

Goal 2: Client will experience reduced physical and psychological stress.

Implementation
1. Enforce bed rest to decrease intestinal motility in acute stage.
2. Maintain quiet, comfortable, nonstressful environment.
3. Keep room odor-free.
4. Empty bedpan promptly and have within easy reach of client during acute episodes.
5. Keep perianal area clean and dry, applying lubricant or ointments as necessary.
6. Administer pain medications as ordered.
7. Give sitz baths at least 3 times/day or as needed.
Evaluation
    Client states relief of pain; rests comfortably.

Goal 3: Client will be free from infection.

Implementation
1. Prevent and treat secondary infection through use of sulfonamides (e.g., sulfasalazine [Azulfidine]) as ordered (see Table 3-41).
2. Help and teach client to turn, cough, and deep-breathe q2-4h (during acute stage).
3. Check temperature q4h, avoid taking rectal temperature if anus is excoriated.
4. Administer oral hygiene as necessary.
5. Provide good skin care.
Evaluation
    Client remains free from signs of infection (e.g., increased temperature, infiltrate in lungs, or secondary infection in mucous membranes of mouth, skin, or colon).

Goal 4: Client will have fewer bowel movements than when admitted.

Implementation
1. Administer antidiarrheal medications as ordered (see Table 3-47).
    a. Opium alkaloids (Paregoric)
    b. Diphenoxylate (Lomotil)
    c. Anticholinergic drugs (tincture of belladonna, Donnatal)
    d. Kaolin and pectin (Kaopectate)
2. Reduce inflammation by administration of
    a. Azathioprine (Imuran) (immunosuppressive agent)
    b. 6-mercaptopurine (see Table 5-22)
    c. Corticosteroids
    d. See Table 3-45
3. Check bowel sounds q2-4h; report increase or decrease to physician.
4. Note frequency, color, and amount of stools.

5. Report increase in abdominal distension to physician.
6. Reduce emotional stress (direct influence on course of illness).
Evaluation
Client has a decrease in frequency and amount of stools; has no increase in abdominal distension.

Goal 5: Client will maintain a balance of adequate rest and exercise.

Implementation
1. Encourage rest after meals.
2. Do not confine to bed unless very weak.
3. Provide calm, reassuring environment.
4. Give sedation as necessary to provide adequate night's sleep.
5. Initiate ambulation at short, frequent intervals.
6. Allow for frequent rest periods.
Evaluation
Client verbalizes feeling rested; sleeps through the night; increases periods of ambulation as strength returns.

Goal 6: Client will accept alteration of life-style imposed by chronic illness.

Implementation
1. Provide teaching regarding
　a. How to live with chronic disease.
　b. Factors in environment that aggravate colitis (emotional stress, dietary indiscretion, ingestion of irritants, overfatigue, infections, or pregnancy).
　c. How to maintain nutrition.
　d. Importance of medical management of the disease.
　e. Need for biannual sigmoidoscopy and barium enema (increased incidence of carcinoma of large intestines).
2. Provide emotional counseling and support as needed.
3. Encourage verbalization of anxieties.
4. Provide diversional activities.
Evaluation
Client verbalizes acceptance of disease; lists life-style modifications to be initiated.

☐ Total Colectomy with Ileostomy
General Information
1. Definition: surgical removal of the entire colon, rectum, and anus with the construction of permanent ileostomy to provide for passage of feces
2. Indications: when medical management fails and constant relapses with intractability occur; occurrence of complications (e.g., perforation, hemorrhage, obstruction, toxic megacolon, abscess, and fistula); more effective as treatment for ulcerative colitis

Nursing Process
Assessment
1. Physical status
2. Emotional status
3. Acceptance of ostomy
4. Understanding of ostomy function
5. Ability to verbalize feelings
Analysis (see p. 217)
Planning, Implementation, and Evaluation

Goal 1: Client will be physically and psychologically prepared for surgery.

Implementation
1. Refer to "Perioperative Period," p. 118.
2. Give TPN as ordered, to improve preoperative nutritional status.
3. Prepare bowel for surgery: low-residue diet, clear liquids, oral antibiotics, cathartics, enema.
4. Obtain help of an enterostomal therapist, if available, to plan site of stoma placement and to introduce client to appliance.
5. Encourage client to express fears and concerns regarding change in body image.
6. Introduce client to concept of ostomy support groups; obtain volunteer if desired.
Evaluation
Client views appliances; expresses positive reaction to outcomes of surgery.

Goal 2: Client will remain free from infection and complications postoperatively.

Implementation
1. Refer to "Perioperative Period," p. 119.
2. Observe stoma size, color.
Evaluation
Client remains free from any signs of postoperative infection or complications (e.g., has normal temperature, clear lungs).

Goal 3: Client will maintain normal fluid and electrolyte balance.

Implementation
1. Monitor I&O, weigh daily, NG tube drainage.
2. Monitor state of hydration (skin turgor and condition of mucous membranes), urine output.
3. Monitor serum electrolyte levels.
4. Monitor ileal output; postoperative drainage begins immediately.
5. Administer IV fluids as ordered, until client can take oral nourishment.
Evaluation
Client's I&O, electrolytes remain within normal limits.

Goal 4: Client will understand dietary restrictions.

Implementation

1. Teach client that food ingested will pass through the ileostomy within 4-6 hours.
2. Teach client that each individual has different food tolerances.
3. Provide diet information: most ostomy clients are discharged on a low-residue, high-protein, high-carbohydrate diet rich in high-potassium foods and low in gas-producing, highly seasoned, or fried foods.
4. Know that vitamin supplements A, D, E, K, and B_{12} may be necessary.
5. Prepare client for possible weight gain resulting from increased food tolerance postoperatively.
6. Refer to dietitian as necessary.

Evaluation

Client states dietary changes; verbalizes intent to work out a diet plan within the limits of the individual variations.

Goal 5: Client will achieve self-care management.

Implementation

1. Instruct client (step by step) and receive return demonstration on stoma care including
   a. Equipment: type, how to use, and where to purchase.
   b. Skin care: ileostomy drainage is erosive and continuous.
   c. Application of appliance.
   d. Odor control.
   e. Use services of enterostomal therapist if available.
2. Refer to visiting nurses (VNA) for home follow-up or continue following up by enterostomal therapist.

Evaluation

Client successfully manages self-care of ileostomy.

Goal 6: Client will successfully cope with altered body image.

Implementation

1. Encourage verbalization of concerns.
2. Assure client that major change in life-style is not necessary.
3. Encourage involvement in ostomy club.
4. Provide emotional support to the significant other in adjusting to ostomy.
5. Obtain sexual counseling for client, if needed.

Evaluation

Client discusses altered body image; shows evidence of coping with change and resumption of normal activity.

☐ Mechanical Obstruction of the Colon
General Information

1. Pathophysiology
   a. Obstruction can be partial or complete
   b. Emergency situation if blood supply is compromised
   c. If blood supply is not compromised, fluid and electrolyte deficiency becomes the major problem
   d. Absorption decreases and fluids and electrolytes accumulate in GI tract
   e. Fluid will either stay in GI tract or be lost through vomiting
   f. Subsequent decrease in extracellular fluid volume (dehydration)
   g. Metabolic acidosis results
2. Risk/causative factors
   a. Small intestine: adhesions, hernia, volvulus
   b. Large intestine: neoplasm, stricture, diverticulitis
3. Medical treatment
   a. Medical intervention
      1. decompression with intestinal tubes
         a. Cantor tube: permanent mercury-weighted tip
         b. Miller-Abbott tube: has port for injection of mercury
         c. length to be passed is determined by physician
      2. fluid and electrolyte replacement
   b. Surgical intervention
      1. colon resection with end-to-end anastomosis or temporary/permanent colostomy
      2. abdominoperineal resection with permanent colostomy

Nursing Process

Assessment

1. Abdomen distended; altered bowel habits; most common with large intestine obstruction
2. Projectile vomiting and severe pain, most common with small intestine obstruction
3. Decreased or increased bowel sounds
4. Decreased fluids

Analysis (see p. 217)

Planning, Implementation, and Evaluation

Goals 1 through 4: (refer to "Total Colectomy with Ileostomy," p. 222.)

Implementation

1. Attach NG tube to intermittent suction.
2. Care for intestinal tube if ordered.
   a. After the tube is passed, tell client to lie 2 hours in each of the following positions in order: right side, back, left side; this will facilitate passage of the tube into the intestine (usually passes at a rate of 2-3 inches/hr.

b. Do not allow tube to pass rapidly since twisting and knotting may result.

c. Monitor for correct tube placement by testing for pH of aspiration contents (>7 = tube is in small intestine; <7 = tube is in stomach).

d. DO NOT tape tube until it has passed into the small intestine.

e. If massive stomach content loss occurs, monitor for metabolic alkalosis (see Table 3-39); if massive intestinal loss, monitor for acidosis.

f. Remove slowly when ordered to prevent twisting the intestine.

3. Know that the client additionally will undergo preoperative bowel preparation that will include
   a. Clear liquids several days preoperatively; then NPO
   b. Bowel sterilization routine as ordered with neomycin and sulfonamides
   c. Several enemas and cathartics

4. Monitor I&O, urine specific gravity, and gastric output.

5. Give narcotics sparingly (may mask symptoms); avoid morphine (decreases intestinal motility).

Evaluation

Client's bowel is clean and prepared for surgery.

Goal 5: Client will cope successfully with altered body image.

Implementation

1. See "Total Colectomy with Ileostomy" Goal 6, p. 223.

2. Instruct client about irrigation and dietary management for regulation of colostomy (see Fig. 3-22).
   a. Most physicians advocate colostomy regulation with diet.

b. If irrigation is required
   1. allow 1 hour for the process
   2. remove old pouch and clean skin around stoma
   3. use 1000 ml of warm water; hang bag no higher than shoulder level.
   4. insert irrigating cone into stoma (use of cone is safer than inserting tube)
   5. let water run in slowly
   6. remove cone and allow solution to drain
   7. apply clean pouch

3. If the colostomy is to be closed at a future date, encourage client to work for that day while at the same time reinforcing the importance of good daily care and adjustment to a temporarily changed body image.

Evaluation

Client discusses altered body image; expresses a willingness to adjust and to maintain colostomy until closure can be accomplished.

☐ Cancer of the Colon
General Information

1. Definition: malignant neoplasm of the large bowel; 70% of cases occur in the rectosigmoid area

2. Incidence
   a. Second most common malignancy in adults
   b. Equal in both sexes
   c. Occurs after fourth decade; peaks in the seventh decade
   d. Most are adenocarcinoma

3. Risk factors
   a. Family history
   b. History of ulcerative colitis, polyps
   c. Possibly related to increased fat in diet, food additives, low-fiber diet, or chronic constipation

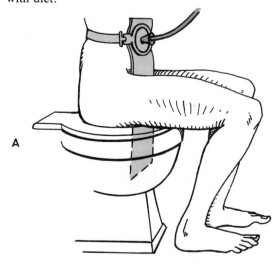

A

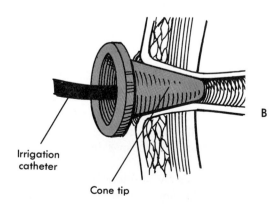

B

Irrigation catheter

Cone tip

Fig. 3-22 Colostomy irrigation. **A,** Colostomy irrigation with person sitting on toilet: irrigating sleeve drains into toilet. **B,** Cone irrigating tip inserted in stoma. (From Long, B.C., & Phipps, W.J. [1989]. *Medical-surgical nursing: A nursing process approach.* [2nd ed.]. St. Louis: Mosby–Year Book.)

4. Metastasis
   a. Lymph nodes
   b. Liver by way of the bloodstream
5. Diagnostic tests
   a. Rectal exam (almost 50% of these tumors are palpable on digital exam)
   b. Sigmoidoscopy, colonoscopy
   c. Barium enema
   d. Stool exam for occult blood
   e. Alkaline phosphatase and SGOT: metastasis to liver
   f. Carcinoembryonic antigen (CEA) level: elevated in advanced adenocarcinoma
6. Medical treatment
   a. Surgical intervention: colon resection
      1. colectomy with anastomosis of the remaining colon or colostomy
      2. abdominal-perineal resection (removal of anus and rectum) with a permanent colostomy
   b. Medical intervention
      1. radiation therapy
      2. chemotherapy

Nursing Process

Assessment
1. Change in bowel habits; blood in stool (more likely with left colon and rectal involvement)
2. Vague, dull pain (more likely with ascending-colon involvement)
3. Anorexia, weight loss, weakness, and anemia
4. Signs of obstruction
5. Hemorrhage
6. Perforation with peritonitis, abscess and fistula formation

Analysis (see p. 217)
Planning, Implementation, and Evaluation
(Refer to "Total Colectomy with Ileostomy," p. 222, and "Mechanical Obstruction of the Colon," p. 223. Refer to *Cellular Aberration* for information and goals pertinent to chemotherapy and radiation therapy.)

☐ Diverticulosis/Diverticulitis
General Information
1. Definitions
   a. Diverticulum: outpouching of the musculature of the intestine
   b. Diverticulosis: the condition of being afflicted with diverticulum
   c. Diverticulitis: inflammation of the diverticulum
   d. Fiber and roughage: plants or foodstuff not digested by the body
   e. Residue: that part of foodstuff left after digestion, eventually collected in the large intestine
2. Most common is the sigmoid colon
3. Risk factors
   a. Diet low in fiber and high in refined and processed foods
   b. Age (frequently over 40 years of age)
   c. Chronic constipation
4. Medical treatment
   a. Medical intervention
      1. acute episodes: NPO, antibiotics, IV fluids; if eating a low-fiber, low-roughage, low-residue diet
      2. ongoing care: high-fiber, high-roughage diet, high or low in residue (MD choice), bulk laxatives, antispasmodics
   b. Surgical intervention: bowel resection with or without a temporary colostomy

Nursing Process
Assessment
1. Diverticulosis is usually asymptomatic
2. Diverticulitis
   a. Crampy pain in left lower quadrant
   b. Constipation, possibly alternating with diarrhea
   c. Fever and leukocytosis
Analysis (see p. 217)
Planning, Implementation, and Evaluation

Goal 1: Client's acute episode will subside without complications.

Implementaiton
1. Give antibiotics, IV fluids, electrolytes as ordered.
2. Keep client NPO until pain subsides, then advance to liquid diet.
3. Keep on bed rest to decrease intestinal motility.
4. Observe for complications of perforation or peritonitis.
Evaluation
Client remains free from pain and complications; has normal bowel function; tolerates diet.

Goal 2: Client will recover from any necessary surgery (e.g., bowel resection, colostomy) without complications. Refer to "Total Colectomy," p. 222.

Goal 3: Client will take measures to control diverticulosis.

Implementation
1. Teach client
   a. To eat a high-fiber, high-roughage diet (see Table 3-50).
   b. To take bulk laxatives (e.g., psyllium hydrophilic [Metamucil]) as ordered.
   c. About use of ordered antispasmodics (e.g., propantheline [Pro-Banthine], oxyphencyclimine [Daricon]).

Table 3-50   High-fiber, high-roughage diet

Food groups	Recommended foods
Fruits	Fresh fruits with skin
Vegetables	Raw vegetables
Breads	Whole wheat and whole grain Bran-type cereals
Grains and flour	Wheat germ, cornmeal, rice, buckwheat
Protein substitutes	Legumes

  d. Ways to decrease stress in life and life-style.
  e. To increase daily fluid intake.
  f. To avoid activities that increase intra-abdominal pressure.
  g. To avoid all nuts or fruits and vegetables with seeds to prevent the seeds from lodging in the intestinal pouches and causing infection.

Evaluation

Client remains free from symptoms of diverticulitis; tolerates high-fiber, high-roughage diet; decreases stress.

☐ Hemorrhoids or Anal Fissure
General Information

1. Definitions
  a. *Hemorrhoids:* dilated veins under the mucous membranes in the anal area; may be either internal or external
  b. *Anal fissure:* linear ulceration on the margin of the anus
2. Predisposing factors
  a. Straining at stool
  b. Pregnancy
  c. Portal hypertension
  d. Congestive heart failure
3. Complications
  a. Bleeding
  b. Thrombosis
  c. Strangulation
  d. Infection
4. Medical treatment
  a. Medical intervention
    1. high-roughage diet and 6-8 glasses of fluid/day
    2. stool softeners
    3. ointments or suppositories to shrink hemorrhoids
    4. warm sitz bath
    5. injection of a sclerosing substance into the tissues at the base of the vein
    6. rubber-band ligation
  b. Surgical intervention
    1. hemorrhoidectomy: excision of dilated veins
    2. fissurectomy: excision of fissure

Nursing Process
Assessment
1. Pain and pruritus around anus
2. Character and amount of rectal drainage
3. Usual bowel habits
4. Abdominal distension
5. Urinary retention
6. Anemia caused by chronic bleeding
Analysis (see p. 217)
Planning, Implementation, and Evaluation

Goal 1: Client will remain free from postoperative complications.

Implementation
1. Refer to "Perioperative Period," p. 119.
2. Avoid sitting for prolonged periods; while sitting, use flotation pad.
3. Prevent infection.
  a. Initiate procedures as ordered for thorough preoperative bowel cleansing.
  b. DO NOT take rectal temperature.
  c. Administer perineal care with antiseptic solution after each stool.
  d. Administer sitz baths as necessary to clean incision.

Evaluation

Client remains free from complications (e.g., infection).

Goal 2: Client will experience relief of pain.

Implementation
1. Give analgesics as ordered.
2. Avoid supine position; if supine position is unavoidable, use flotation pad under buttocks.
3. Apply ice packs or warm, moist compresses if ordered.
4. DO NOT use rubber rings.
5. Administer topical anesthetic as ordered.

Evaluation

Client states pain is controlled; is comfortable in all positions.

Goal 3: Client's bowel function will return to normal.

Implementation
1. Give low-residue, soft diet as tolerated for first week postoperatively; then advance diet to include roughage and fresh fruits.
2. Force fluids to 2500-3000 ml/day unless contraindicated.
3. Administer stool softener/lubricant or laxative as ordered (see Table 3-47).

4. Provide support during initial BM, noting presence of blood in stool; be alert for vertigo; and administer analgesic as necessary.

5. Teach client how to avoid constipation after discharge.

6. Watch for and teach client symptoms of anal stricture (and report to physician).

    a. Increased pain with BM

    b. Difficulty passing stool

Evaluation

Client passes soft, brown, formed stool on third post-operative day with minimal discomfort; lists ways to prevent constipation; states signs of anal stricture.

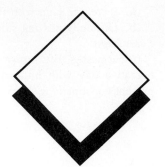

Sensation and Perception

The nursing care presented in this unit concerns selected health problems related to disturbances in the nervous system, eye, ear, nose, and throat.

GENERAL CONCEPTS
Overview/Physiology

1. Nervous system: like an electrical conduction system; coordinates and controls all activities of the body
   a. Receives stimuli or information from internal and external environments over varied sensory pathways
   b. Communicates information between distant parts of body (periphery and central nervous system)
   c. Computes or processes information received at various reflex (spinal cord) and conscious (higher brain) levels to determine responses appropriate to existing situations
   d. Transmits information rapidly over varied motor pathways to effector organs for body-action control or modification
2. Central nervous system
   a. Brain
      1. cerebrum or cerebral cortex
         a. hemispheres: right and left; speech is function of dominant hemisphere (i.e., left for all right-handed and most left-handed people)
         b. frontal lobe: functions
            ◆ personality
            ◆ higher intellectual functions (e.g., learning, problem solving)
            ◆ ethical, social, and moral behavior
            ◆ posterior edge of frontal lobe: center for initiation of motor function
         c. parietal lobe: responsible for interpretation of sensory input
         d. temporal lobe: center for hearing, taste, and smell
         e. occipital lobe: visual center
         f. structure

            ◆ skull
            ◆ meninges: connective tissue covering brain and spinal cord
            ◆ layers of brain
               • dura mater: extradural, epidural, tentorial, and subdural layers
               • arachnoid
               • pia mater
            ◆ blood-brain barrier
            ◆ brain tissue
      2. brainstem: contains midbrain, pons, and medulla oblongata
         a. relays impulses from spinal cord to cerebrum
         b. controls basic body functions (cardiac, respiratory, and vasomotor centers [medulla])
      3. cerebellum
         a. orientation of body in space (equilibrium)
         b. coordination and inhibition of movement
         c. control of antigravity muscles
         d. coordination of muscle tone
   b. Spinal cord
      1. 31 segments (do not correspond in name to the vertebral segments)
         a. 8 cervical: supply neck and upper extremities, diaphragm, and intercostals
         b. 12 thoracic: supply thoracic and abdominal areas
         c. 5 lumbar: supply lower extremities
         d. 5 sacral: supply lower extremities; urinary tract and bowel control
         e. 1 coccygeal
      2. anterior portion of cord carries motor information (descending tracts)
      3. posterior section of cord carries sensory information (ascending tracts)
      4. lateral columns contain preganglionic fibers for autonomic nervous system
3. Peripheral nervous system
   a. Cranial nerves (12): classified in order of their

arising from the brain (number) and by describing their nature, function, and distribution (name) (see Table 3-51)
  b. Spinal nerves (31 pairs)
4. Autonomic nervous system: concerned with the control of involuntary bodily functions; divided into parasympathetic (craniosacral) and sympathetic (thoracolumbar) divisions (see Table 3-52)
  a. Divisions
    1. parasympathetic or craniosacral division controls normal body functioning
    2. sympathetic or thoracolumbar division prepares body for fight or flight
  b. Most effector organs receive innervation from both sympathetic and parasympathetic fibers
  c. Vascular supply of skeletal muscle receives only sympathetic innervation
5. Vision
  a. Major function of eyes is to produce vision: light-waves→cornea→lens→retina→optic nerve (II)→occipital lobe of brain

  b. Cranial nerves of the eye
    1. optic (II): vision
    2. oculomotor (III), trochlear (IV), abducent (VI): external muscles of the eye
    3. oculomotor (III) also controls pupil size
  c. Exterior of eye
    1. tears secreted by lacrimal glands to lubricate lids and keep corneas moist; excess tears drain through lacrimal ducts into nasal cavity
    2. six extrinsic eye muscles produce movements of eyeball
    3. outer layer of eye
      a. cornea: nonvascular transparent fibrous covering of eye
      b. sclera: white, dense connective tissue covering all of eye except cornea
      c. canal of Schlemm: venous sinus at the junction of the sclera and cornea
  d. Interior of eye (see Fig. 3-23)
    1. iris: circular muscle that constricts or dilates pupil
    2. lens: focuses image accurately on retina
    3. aqueous humor and vitreous humor: liquids acting along with lens as refracting media
    4. aqueous humor production: secreted continuously by ciliary process of ciliary body behind iris into posterior chamber→through pupil→anterior chamber→drained off into canal of Schlemm→bloodstream
    5. choroid: black, inner surface of eye that prevents scattering of light rays
    6. retina: light-sensitive layer of eye; sensations of vision result from retina's focused response to image
    7. optic disk: entrance of optic nerve into eyeball
    8. optic pathway: transmits visual data to occipital lobe of the cerebrum (see Fig. 3-26)
6. Hearing
  a. The major functions of the ears are balance and hearing; hearing pathway: sound waves→pinna→external ear canal→tympanic membrane

Table 3-51 Cranial nerves

Number	Name	Type
I	Olfactory	Sensory
II	Optic	Sensory
III	Oculomotor	Motor, parasympathetic
IV	Trochlear	Motor
V	Trigeminal	Sensory, motor
VI	Abducent	Motor
VII	Facial	Sensory, motor parasympathetic
VIII	Acoustic or auditory	Sensory
IX	Glossopharyngeal	Sensory, motor, parasympathetic
X	Vagus	Sensory, motor, parasympathetic
XI	Accessory	Motor
XII	Hypoglossal	Motor

Table 3-52 Parasympathetic and sympathetic effects of the autonomic nervous system

Site	Parasympathetic effects	Sympathetic effects
Eye	Pupils constricted	Pupils dilated
	Far-vision accommodation	Near-vision accommodation
Lungs	Bronchoconstriction	Bronchodilation
Heart	Cardiac rate slowed	Cardiac rate increased
	Contraction force decreased	Contraction force increased
	Coronary vessels constrict	Coronary vessels dilate
Liver	Hepatic glycogenesis	Hepatic glycogenolysis and lipolysis
Stomach and intestine	Secretion and peristalsis stimulated	Secretion and peristalsis inhibited
Urinary bladder	Bladder contracted	Bladder relaxed
	Sphincter open	Sphincter closed
Adrenal medulla		Epinephrine and norepinephrine secretion
Penis	Erection	Ejaculation

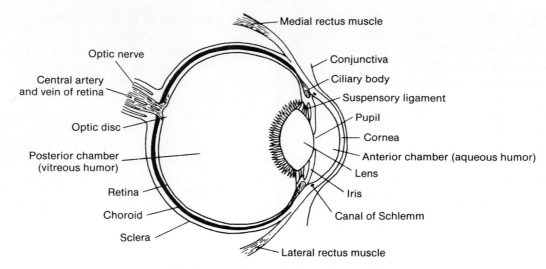

Fig. 3-23   The eye (horizontal section).

→ossicles in middle ear→cochlea→auditory nerve (VIII)→auditory cortex in temporal lobe
  b. External ear
    1. pinna: external flap of cartilage covered with skin that gathers and concentrates sound waves
    2. external ear canal (auditory meatus): cavity in skull lined with skin; ceruminous glands produce cerumen (wax) to assist in protecting the canal from small foreign particles; conveys sound waves from pinna to tympanic membrane
    3. tympanic membrane: flexible membrane that closes distal end of external auditory canal; membrane vibrates in response to sound, transmitting vibrations to middle ear
  c. Middle ear
    1. ossicles: malleus, incus, and stapes
    2. set into motion by sound waves from tympanic membrane
    3. amplifies sound waves and transmits them to inner ear
    4. connected with nasopharynx by eustachian tube
  d. Inner ear
    1. cochlea: organ of sound perception
    2. innervated by the auditory nerve VIII
      a. cochlear branch: transmits auditory impulses from the cochlea to auditory cortex of brain
      b. vestibular branch: controls balance
  e. Auditory portion of cerebral cortex interprets auditory information (temporal lobe) (see Fig. 3-26)
7. Nose
  a. Air passageway
  b. Contains sensory receptors for smell
  c. Lined with mucosa, hair
    1. secretes mucus
    2. filters, warms, and humidifies inspired air
  d. Paranasal sinuses drain into nasal cavity

Application of the Nursing Process to the Client with Problems of Sensation and Perception

Assessment
1. Health history
  a. Family history
  b. History of problem: date of onset, precipitating factors, extent, duration or frequency, interventions that have been effective, location, any changes in description
  c. Headaches
  d. Seizures
  e. Medications: prescription and nonprescription
  f. Recent change in behavior or personality
2. Physical examination
  a. Neurological examination
    1. cognitive function
      a. general behavior, emotional status
      b. level of consciousness (LOC): major index of client's neurological status
      c. attention span
      d. ability to follow commands
      e. memory: short- and long-term
      f. arithmetic ability
      g. abstract thinking
      h. language/speech
        ◆ *motor aphasia* (expressive): inability to speak or write words

◆ *sensory aphasia* (receptive): inability to comprehend written words (visual) or spoken words (auditory)

◆ *dysarthria:* difficult speech caused by paralysis of muscles

2. cerebellar function
   a. balance
   b. coordination
3. motor function
   a. muscle size, tone, and strength
   b. involuntary movements (e.g., tremors)
   c. coordination and accuracy of movement
   d. motor integration
   e. bowel and bladder function
4. sensory function
   a. superficial sensation: touch and pressure
   b. superficial pain
   c. sensitivity to temperature and vibration
   d. deep pressure, pain
   e. motion and position sense
   f. vision
      ◆ amount of sight with or without glasses or contact lenses
      ◆ distortion
         • halos around lights
         • difficulty adjusting to dark room
         • diplopia
         • floaters
   g. hearing
      ◆ amount of hearing
         • use of hearing aid
         • tinnitus or other noises
      ◆ conductive deafness (common causes: otosclerosis, otitis media)
         • impairment of outer- and middle-ear conduction of sound waves
         • causes problems of perception of volume, not discrimination of sounds
         • can benefit from hearing aid
         • benefits from increased decibels (dB) and high frequencies (cps)
      ◆ sensorineural deafness (common causes: old age, noise, drug toxicity)
         • impairment of inner-ear nerve conduction
         • causes problems of loss of sensitivity to and discrimination of high-frequency sounds
         • hearing aid not beneficial
         • benefits from decreased decibels and low frequencies
      ◆ combined (conductive and sensorineural)
      ◆ general speech pattern
      ◆ indications of hearing loss

Table 3-53 Levels of consciousness

Level	Description
1	Consciousness (oriented to person, place, and time)
2	Lethargy, somnolence, drowsiness, or obtundation
3	Stupor (can be aroused by verbal stimuli but responds poorly or inappropriately)
4	Light coma, semicoma (no response to verbal stimuli but responds to painful stimuli)
5	Deep coma (no reaction to painful stimuli)

   • says "huh" frequently
   • asks you to repeat what you said
   • does not respond to questions or conversation
   • responds inappropriately to questions or comments

5. reflexes: superficial and deep tendon
6. cranial nerves (see Table 3-51)

b. Neurological check
   1. LOC: *most reliable indicator of neurological status* (see Table 3-53)
   2. vital signs
   3. pupils: size and reaction to light
   4. motor function
      a. move all extremities
      b. muscle strength (grip)
   5. sensory function: response to touch or painful stimuli
   6. seizures
   7. blood or cerebrospinal fluid (CSF) leakage from nose or ear(s)
   8. posturing (pathological motor responses)
      a. decorticate posture (corticospinal tract): rigid flexion of arms, wrists, and fingers with adduction of upper extremities, and extension with internal rotation of legs (see Fig. 3-24)
      b. decerebrate posture (midbrain and pons): rigid extension of neck, back, arms, and legs, with hyperpronation of arms and plantar flexion of feet (see Fig. 3-25); prognosis grave

3. Diagnostic tests
   a. Lumbar puncture (LP)
      1. description
         a. collection of CSF, measurement of pressure and characteristics of spinal fluid
         b. Queckenstedt's test can be done during LP: with manometer still in place, compress jugular veins for 10 seconds
            ◆ normal response: increase in spinal fluid

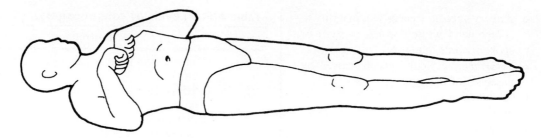

Fig. 3-24 Decorticate posturing.

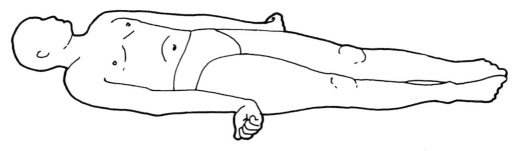

Fig. 3-25 Decerebrate posturing.

pressure of approximately 100 mm H$_2$O within 10 seconds and return to normal within 30 seconds after compression is removed

◆ abnormal response: drop in spinal fluid pressure or no rise in pressure; indicates complete obstruction of flow of spinal fluid

2. nursing care
   a. explain procedure carefully to client before procedure
   b. position client on side with legs flexed onto abdomen and head bent down
   c. keep client flat in bed up to 24 hours after test to avoid a headache caused by fluid-tension change
   d. review CSF characteristics
   e. force fluids to replace loss and restore fluid balance
   f. observe for headache

b. Radiological exams
   1. x-rays of skull and spine
   2. computerized axial tomogram (CAT scan)
      a. description: 360° photographed view of brain in 1° angles; provides data on integrity of intracranial structures and precise location of abnormalities; used with or without contrast medium

   b. nursing care
      ◆ explain procedure to client beforehand
      ◆ client needs to lie still on table for 30-60 minutes
   3. magnetic resonance imaging (MRI)
   4. myelogram (see *Mobility*, p. 256)
   5. brain scan
      a. description: following administration of oral or IV radiopharmaceutical, the head is scanned and uptake of the material is recorded
      b. nursing care
         ◆ explain procedure to client
         ◆ reassure about radioactivity
   6. cerebral arteriogram
      a. description: injection of a radiopaque dye through a catheter inserted into femoral, carotid, or vertebral artery; aortic arch; or brachial vessels to study cerebral circulation
      b. nursing care
         ◆ explain procedure and posttest routine to client before test
         ◆ ensure that pretest baseline neurological status is documented
         ◆ check for allergies to iodine and report if present
         ◆ remove hairpins and dentures as ordered
         ◆ bed rest 8-24 hours after test, with head of bed elevated 30°

- ◆ check incision for hemorrhage frequently
- ◆ maintain pressure dressing to incision site if femoral or brachial artery used; apply ice bag to reduce swelling
- ◆ watch for symptoms of sensitivity to dye (urticaria, pallor, respiratory difficulty) and report immediately
- ◆ watch for neurological changes that indicate emboli in cerebrovascular system (limb weakness or paralysis; facial paralysis; speech difficulty; disorientation; change in level of of consciousness) and report immediately
- ◆ observe and record vital signs and neurological signs according to protocol (usually q15min until stable, then qh for several hours, then q4h)

c. Electroencephalogram (EEG)
1. description: study of electrical activity of brain
2. nursing care
   a. give information to client to allay fear of being electrocuted
   b. clean client's hair before the test
   c. continue anticonvulsants
   d. have client remain on anticonvulsant
   e. have client eat meal before test (fasting affects electrical pattern) but avoid stimulants (e.g., coffee, tea, cola, cocoa)
   f. tell client to remain calm and quiet during the test
   g. remove EEG paste from hair after test

d. Eye tests
1. Snellen test (eye chart) (see *Nursing Care of the Child*, p. 436)
2. ophthalmoscopic exam
3. intraocular pressure (normal: 12-20 mm Hg)

e. Ear/hearing tests
1. otoscopic exam
2. whisper test for gross hearing: cover the ear not being tested and whisper words into the other ear or hold a ticking watch near the ear
3. audiogram
   a. client wears earphones in soundproof room and signals when tone is heard, when tone disappears, and in which ear the tone is heard
   b. hearing is measured in *intensity* (dB = decibels) and *frequency* (cps = cycles per second)
4. Weber and Rinne tests (see *Nursing Care of the Child*, p. 436)

f. Nose/sense of smell tests: provide various scents for client to identify with eyes closed (e.g., alcohol, chocolate, tobacco)

g. Mouth and throat/sense of taste tests: provide various things for client to taste with eyes closed (e.g., chocolate, peppermint)

Analysis

1. Safe, effective care environment
   a. High risk for injury
   b. High risk for knowledge deficit
   c. High risk for sensory-perceptual alteration (specify)

2. Physiological integrity
   a. High risk for activity tolerance
   b. High risk for aspiration
   c. Pain
   d. Impaired physical mobility
   e. Ineffective breathing pattern
   f. Impaired verbal communication
   g. Hyperthermia

3. Psychosocial integrity
   a. Fear
   b. Altered thought processes
   c. Social isolation

4. Health promotion/maintenance
   a. Ineffective family coping: disabled
   b. Altered health maintenance
   c. Knowledge deficit
   d. Self-care deficit

General Nursing Planning, Implementation, and Evaluation

Goal 1: Client will be free from increased intracranial pressure.

Implementation

1. Monitor for early signs of increased intracranial pressure
   a. Changes in level of consciousness (see Table 3-53).
   b. Vital signs changes
      1. BP: widening of pulse pressure; systolic increases, diastolic remains the same
      2. rise in temperature with failing thermoregulator
      3. bradycardia
      4. slow, deep, irregular respirations
   c. Pupils: unequal, progressing to fixed and dilated.
   d. Other clinical signs and symptoms (classic triad)
      1. headache (generalized)
      2. projectile vomiting
      3. papilledema

2. Assess at least q15min.

3. Administer osmotic diuretics (e.g., mannitol) as ordered (see Table 3-42) and then monitor urine output qh.

4. Keep client slightly dehydrated to reduce or prevent cerebral edema.

5. Administer corticosteroid therapy, if ordered.
6. Prevent transient increases in intracranial pressure.
   a. Elevate head of bed 15°-30°.
   b. Avoid neck flexion.
   c. Maintain calm environment.
   d. Avoid Valsalva maneuver (straining).
   e. Administer stool softeners, and teach client not to strain with bowel evacuation.
   f. Avoid bending over, coughing, sneezing, or vomiting.
   g. Avoid isometric contraction of muscles (e.g., pushing up in bed on elbows, pressing feet against a footboard).

Evaluation

Client's intracranial pressure remains within normal limits (5-10 mm Hg).

Goal 2: Client will remain free from complications of unconsciousness.

Implementation

1. See General Nursing Goal 4, *Mobility*, p. 256.
2. Prevent contractures and immobile joints (e.g., use range-of-motion exercises).
3. Keep skin clean, dry, and intact.
4. Keep mucous membranes clean, moist, and intact.
5. Maintain adequate bowel and bladder function.
6. Ensure normal respiratory function (e.g., turn client frequently).
7. Provide safe environment (e.g., bed side rails).
8. Administer feedings through NG tube as ordered.
   a. Put client in high-Fowler's position if allowed.
   b. Check to be sure tube is in stomach and not lungs (aspirate stomach contents; inject 5 ml of air while listening with a stethoscope over the gastric area for a swishing sound).
   c. Give feeding at slow rate.
   d. Observe for regurgitation during and after feeding.
   e. Observe for gastric retention.
   f. Give feedings at room temperature.
   g. Know that client will probably be given no more than 2 L/day of a liquid feeding with a concentration of 0.5-1 kilocalorie/ml.
9. Administer total parenteral nutrition (TPN) as ordered (see Table 3-27).
10. Check tissue hydration.
11. Monitor fluid and electrolyte balance.
12. Prevent corneal damage (e.g., use eye patches as needed).
13. Maintain communication with client.

Evaluation

Client is free from contractures, immobile joints, pressure sores, fecal impactions, respiratory distress, injuries, malnutrition, and fluid and electrolyte imbalances.

Goal 3: Client with aphasia will maximize ability to use and understand written and spoken words.

Implementation

1. Determine client's level of understanding.
2. Determine client's use of speech or communication skills.
3. Use gestures if client understands that best.
4. Use aids to increase and improve communication: word cards, pictures, slate boards, and audiotapes.
5. Talk slowly using natural tone (do not abbreviate, reducing sentences to a shorter, incomplete form; it does not help comprehension).
6. Use simple words and phrases.
7. Allow client time to respond; be patient.
8. Listen and watch carefully when the client attempts to communicate.
9. Keep distractions to a minimum.
10. Maintain a calm, accepting manner.
11. Sit level with client and maintain eye contact.
12. Arrange for referral to speech therapist as needed.

Evaluation

Client attempts to communicate using written and spoken words.

Goal 4: Disabled client will function as independently as possible.

Implementation

1. Determine client's strengths and deficits.
2. Establish realistic, long-range goals with client and significant other.
3. Devise measures with client to achieve goals.
   a. Institute measures for gaining bowel and bladder control if necessary.
   b. Arrange for physical therapy.
   c. Arrange for occupational and recreational therapy.
   d. Give client and significant others emotional support (e.g., adapting to altered body image, see *Loss and Death and Dying*, p. 27).
   e. Refer to appropriate community agency.

Evaluation

Client performs ADL, to extent possible, without assistance.

Goal 5: Client will adapt to visual deficits.

Implementation

1. Call client by name when approaching.
2. Identify yourself when approaching client.
3. Communicate in usual manner.
4. Ambulate with client.
5. Teach client
   a. How to summon staff.

b. Where possessions are.

c. Physical layout of room.

d. Placement of food on tray.

e. Arrangement of food on plate.

f. Use of cane to aid in walking.

6. Provide meaningful sensory input.

a. Interaction with staff and significant others.

b. Radio, records, and TV.

c. Physical exercise.

7. Provide safe environment (e.g., remove unnecessary equipment).

8. Refer to appropriate community agencies.

9. Encourage and reinforce client's independence.

Evaluation

Client functions in hospital environment without difficulty.

Goal 6: Client will adapt to hearing loss.

Implementation

1. Face client when speaking.

2. Keep light on your own face so client can watch your mouth.

3. Speak with normal speech pattern.

4. Allow more time than usual for communication.

5. Help client get a hearing aid if appropriate.

Evaluation

Client responds to directions appropriately.

SELECTED HEALTH PROBLEMS RESULTING IN AN INTERFERENCE WITH SENSATION AND PERCEPTION

☐ Acute Head Injury

General Information

1. Clients with acute head trauma need close scrutiny immediately following trauma; shock is rarely seen

2. Types

a. *Concussion:* no structural alteration, but immediate and transitory impairment of neurological function resulting from mechanical force and release of enzymes

b. *Contusion:* structural alteration (bruised cortex) characterized by extravasation of blood

c. *Laceration:* a tear in brain or blood vessel

d. *Hemorrhage*

1. extradural or epidural: arterial blood collects between skull and dura rapidly; usually results from a tear in an artery

a. may lose consciousness and regain it temporarily

b. within a few hours, rapid deterioration: lethargy, coma, hemiplegia

2. subdural: venous bleeding (hematoma) below dura accompanied by manifestations of increased ICP

a. acute: develops within few days after injury; surgical intervention needed

b. subacute: develops between few days to 3 weeks; surgical intervention follows

c. chronic: develops weeks to months after injury

Nursing Process

Assessment (refer to neurological exam, p. 230)

Analysis (see p. 233)

Planning, Implementation, and Evaluation

Goal 1: Client will have an open airway at all times.

Implementation

1. Establish and maintain airway.

2. Position client for optimum ventilation.

3. Maintain adequate O_2 level through use of respiratory aids as necessary.

Evaluation

Client's airway remains unobstructed; color is normal; arterial blood gases are within normal limits.

Goal 2: Client will be protected from increasing intracranial pressure.

Implementation

1. Refer to General Nursing Goal 1, p. 233.

Evaluation

Client is free from papilledema; maintains normal vital signs and stable LOC.

Goal 3: Client will maintain optimal fluid and electrolyte status.

Implementation

1. Monitor and record I&O.

2. Administer IV fluids as ordered (fluids are usually restricted because of fear of increased intracranial pressure).

3. Give osmotic diuretics (e.g., mannitol) as ordered (see Table 3-42).

4. Monitor serum electrolyte levels.

Evaluation

Client's output remains greater than intake.

Goal 4: Client will have any CSF or blood draining from nose or ears detected.

Implementation

1. Observe and record at least qh any leak of blood or clear fluid from nose or ears.

2. Do not pack nose or ear; have fluid drain onto sterile towel or dressing.

3. Report to physician immediately if any drainage is found.

Evaluation

Client remains free from CSF or blood leakage from nose and ears.

Goal 5: Client will be free from infection or injuries.

Implementation

1. Protect from chilling.
2. Take seizure precautions: use bed with padded side rails, a nonmetal airway, and a suction apparatus at bedside. (See "Seizure Disorders," p. 470.)
3. Employ aseptic technique during all invasive procedures.
4. Do not permit visitors with colds.

Evaluation

Client remains afebrile; has skin and mucous membranes free from cuts, ecchymosis, and abrasions.

☐ Intracranial Surgery
General Information

1. Definitions: surgery performed inside the cranial cavity
   a. *Craniotomy:* any operation on the cranium
      1. tentorium: fold of dura mater between cerebellum and occipital lobes
      2. supratentorial: above the cerebellum (e.g., cerebrum, anterior two thirds of brain)
      3. infratentorial: posterior cranial fossa (e.g., cerebellum, brainstem, posterior third of brain)
   b. *Cranioplasty:* repair of cranial defect by inserting a bone graft or a plate made of a synthetic substance; protects the brain from trauma
2. Reasons for surgery
   a. To debride or repair any trauma to the skull and underlying structures
   b. To control intracranial hemorrhage (e.g., aneurysms)
   c. To remove space-occupying lesions (e.g., scar tissue, abscess, tumor)
   d. Intracranial neoplasms
      1. all potentially fatal unless treated, because of lack of space within skull
      2. more than 50% are malignant
      3. types
         a. gliomas (within brain substance)
         b. meningiomas (external to brain substance)

Nursing Process

Assessment

1. Establish baseline data preoperatively (refer to neurological exam, p. 230)
2. Client and significant others' knowledge of procedure and expected outcome

Analysis (see p. 233)
Planning, Implementation, and Evaluation

Goal 1: Client and significant others will be able to explain preoperative and postoperative care, and OR-RR-ICU environment and care.

Implementation

1. Refer to "Perioperative Period," p. 117.
2. Prepare client for the likelihood of postoperative periocular edema and photophobia.

Evaluation

Client and significant others describe planned procedure and postoperative routine.

Goal 2: Client will be physically prepared for surgery.

Implementation

1. Refer to "Perioperative Period," p. 117.
2. Know that narcotics are contraindicated preoperatively.
3. Prepare scalp.
   a. Wash hair.
   b. Cut hair (save according to agency policy); shave scalp.
   c. Wash head and cover with clean towel.
4. Carry out any special order (e.g., insert indwelling Foley catheter, give enemas slowly to avoid straining and increased intracranial pressure).

Evaluation

Client's scalp is prepared for surgery without nicks or cuts.

Goal 3: Client will remain free from respiratory, circulatory, renal, neurological, or psychological complications or any infections postoperatively.

Implementation

1. Refer to "Perioperative Period," p. 117.
2. Perform frequent neurological checks; compare with preoperative baseline (refer to neurological exam, p. 230).
3. Observe for seizures.
4. Monitor breathing; client must not cough.
5. Support head when turning client.
6. Position properly and frequently.
   a. Supratentorial craniotomy: do not position on operative site if large tumor was excised; elevate head 45°.
   b. Infratentorial craniotomy: keep head of bed flat and client's head aligned with vertebral column at all times; position on either side for first 24 hours, not on back; avoid flexion of neck (danger is brainstem compression).
7. Do not use suction through nose.

8. Do not use central nervous system depressants (e.g., opiates, sedatives).
9. Check ears, nose, and dressing for drainage (blood or CSF leakage).
10. Change dressings only when ordered; reinforce as needed.
11. Use strict aseptic technique for all dressings and other procedures.
12. Assess periocular edema; relieve with ice packs.
13. Administer steroids (e.g., dexamethasone sodium [Decadron]) as ordered to prevent or relieve cerebral edema (see Table 3-33).
14. Do not take oral temperatures.
15. Give passive ROM exercises q8h.

Evaluation

Client remains free from complications in the postoperative period.

Goal 4: Client and significant others will accept lengthy rehabilitation period.

Implementation

1. See General Nursing Goal 4, p. 234.
2. Inform client of residual effects that may be temporary (e.g., diplopia) or permanent (e.g., aphasia, paralysis).

3. Inform client of cosmetic aids available when indicated (e.g., hairpiece, wig).
4. Prevent client from striking or bumping head.

Evaluation

Client and significant others express willingness to participate in rehabilitation program; verbalize understanding of the need for patience and persistence.

☐ Cerebrovascular Accident (CVA)
General Information

1. Definition: severe, sudden decrease in cerebral circulation caused by either a thrombus or hemorrhage resulting in a cerebral infarct (i.e., tissue death); also called a stroke
2. Incidence
   a. Third leading cause of death in the United States
   b. Ages 60-69: most frequent cause is thrombosis
   c. Ages 30-60: most frequent cause is a ruptured aneurysm with hemorrhage
3. Symptoms depend upon
   a. Location of the infarct (Fig. 3-26)
   b. Amount of collateral circulation to affected area of the brain
   c. Type of pathophysiology involved
4. Risk factors
   a. Hypertension

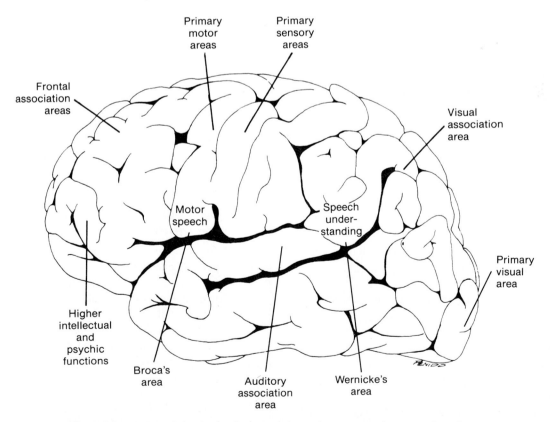

Fig. 3-26 Areas of the brain that control certain motor and sensory functions.

b. Arteriosclerosis/atherosclerosis
c. Intracranial aneurysms
d. Diabetes mellitus
e. Peripheral vascular disease
5. Etiology
   a. Rupture of the wall of a cerebral artery or an aneurysm
   b. Trauma to a cerebral artery
   c. Severe spasm of the cerebral artery
   d. Embolus or thrombus blocking cerebral arterial system

Nursing Process

Assessment
1. Refer to neurological exam, p. 230, and areas of the brain that control certain motor and sensory functions (see Fig. 3-26)
2. Hemiplegia (paralysis) or hemiparesis (muscular weakness) of half of body
3. Aphasia (most common with left cerebral infarct and right-handedness)
4. Ataxia (staggering gait)
5. Nuchal rigidity (with hemorrhage)
6. Perceptual deficit
7. Emotional lability
8. Emotional needs of clients and significant others
9. Results of diagnostic studies
   a. CAT scan
   b. MRI
   c. Cerebral arteriogram
   d. Lumbar puncture

Analysis (see p. 233)
Planning, Implementation, and Evaluation

> **Goal 1:** Client will be free from any additional cerebral damage.

Implementation
1. Monitor neurological status frequently until stable.
2. Do not stimulate cough.
3. Give passive ROM.
4. If thrombus is cause of CVA: administer vasodilators and anticoagulants as ordered.
5. If hemorrhage is cause of CVA
   a. Elevate head of bed 30°-45° (to improve venous drainage).
   b. Turn *gently* to *unaffected* side.
   c. Decrease environmental stimuli (e.g., keep room in semidarkness).
   d. Maintain complete bed rest until bleeding has been controlled and client's condition is stable.

Evaluation
Client remains stable, free from additional cerebral damage.

> **Goal 2:** Client will ingest adequate fluids and food.

Implementation
1. Help client feed self as needed.
2. Provide adequate fluids to maintain skin turgor and sufficient output.
3. Give small, frequent feedings as indicated (more easily tolerated than three large meals).
4. Administer tube feedings if client is unable to take food and fluids orally (see General Nursing Goal 2, p. 234).
5. Monitor electrolyte levels.

Evaluation
Client's weight remains stable; skin turgor is firm; urinary output is greater than 30 ml/hr; urine is clear, straw-colored, free from pus and blood.

> **Goal 3:** If unconscious, client will remain free from complications (refer to General Nursing Goal 2, p. 234).

> **Goal 4:** Client will become as independent as possible.

Implementation
1. Refer to General Nursing Goals 3 and 4, p. 234.
2. Explain prognosis: lengthy rehabilitation, potential lifetime implications.
3. Expect labile emotions (depression is common).
4. Prevent deformities.
5. Make referral to speech therapist as indicated.
6. Arrange for gait training; if fatigued from exercises, monitor for potential injury.

Evaluation
Client begins rehabilitation; participates in rehabilitation activities.

☐ **Meningitis** (refer to *Nursing Care of the Child,* p. 472)
☐ **Spinal Cord Injuries (SCI)**
General Information

1. Definition: fracture or displacement of one or more vertebrae, causing damage to spinal cord and nerve roots with resulting neurological deficit and altered sensory perception or paralysis or both. There will be total or partial absence of motor and/or sensory function below the level of the injury.
2. Incidence: estimated 10,000-20,000 people affected annually; usually younger age group
3. Predisposing factors
   a. Trauma: car or motorcycle accidents, falls, or diving accidents

b. Tumors

c. Congenital defects; spina bifida

d. Infectious and degenerative diseases

e. Ruptured intervertebral disks

4. Types of injuries

a. Fracture of vertebral body (excessive vertical compression)

b. Compression of vertebral body (excessive flexion of vertebral column)

c. Spinal malalignment or vertebral body displacement (rotational injury)

d. Partial or complete dislocation of one vertebra onto another

e. Disruption of intervertebral disk and compressed interspinous ligament (hyperextension injury)

5. Most common sites: cervical and lumbar vertebrae

6. Immediately after an accident, care must be taken to prevent further neurological damage while patent airway and circulation are maintained

Nursing Process

Assessment

1. Respiratory function

2. Cardiovascular function

3. Loss of sensation and motor function in body parts below injury level (see Table 3-54)

4. Loss of perspiration below injury level with resultant inability to cool body (autonomic responses become unpredictable)

5. Bowel and bladder control (assess for paralytic ileus and urine retention)

6. Pain

7. Edema

8. Nutritional status

9. Fever

10. Psychological needs

11. Remaining sensory and motor function

12. Diagnostic tests

a. Neurological exam

b. X-ray of spine

Analysis (see p. 233)

Planning, Implementation, and Evaluation

Goal 1: Client will be free from further injury to spinal cord.

Implementation

1. Immobilize the head and entire spine.

2. Keep client's body and head in alignment.

3. "Log-roll" client if moving is necessary.

4. Use specialized equipment for turning: Stryker frame, Foster frame, or CircOlectric bed.

5. Apply cervical traction for cervical lesion.

6. Know that a laminectomy may be done to prevent further compression of spinal cord.

7. Administer steroids (dexamethasone sodium [Decadron]) or osmotic diuretic (e.g., mannitol) IV as ordered, to reduce cerebral and spinal cord edema (see Tables 3-33 and 3-42).

Evaluation

Client shows no signs of progression of paralysis.

Goal 2: Client will maintain adequate respiratory function.

Implementation

1. Observe respirations frequently (client may have spontaneous respirations after an accident but lose them later).

2. Maintain respiratory function through use of a respirator if necessary.

3. If respirations are spontaneous, have client deep-breathe and cough qh.

4. Care for and suction secretions from tracheostomy tube if in place.

Evaluation

Client's respiratory rate remains within normal limits.

Goal 3: Client will be free from undetected spinal shock.

Implementation

1. Expect spinal shock to develop 30-60 minutes after injury and to last 2-3 days to 3 months.

Table 3-54 Spinal cord

Area of spinal cord	Gross movements controlled
Upper cervical	Neck and head movement; elevation of the shoulders.
Middle cervical	Movement of the upper arms and forearms; diaphragmatic breathing.
Lower cervical	Movements of fingers and hands.
Thoracic	Intercostal muscles involved in respiration; muscles involved in abdominal contractions.
Upper lumbar	Leg flexion at hip; adduction of thigh.
Lower lumbar	Remaining thigh movements; movements in lower legs.
Sacral	Foot and toe movements; sphincter and perineal muscle contraction.

2. Observe for signs and symptoms caused by suppression of reflexes at all spinal segments below the level of injury.
   a. Hypotension
   b. Dyspnea
   c. Flaccid paralysis
   d. Urinary retention
   e. Absence of sweating
3. Administer colloid fluids and analgesics prn as ordered.

Evaluation
Client's spinal shock is detected promptly.

Goal 4: Client with cervical or high-thoracic injury will remain free from autonomic dysreflexia.

Implementation
1. Observe for signs and symptoms caused by marked sympathetic stimulation.
   a. Rapidly increasing BP
   b. Bradycardia
   c. Severe headache
   d. Flushing
   e. Profuse sweating
   f. Goose pimples
2. Take preventive measures.
   a. Prevent bowel and bladder distension (chief causes of this phenomenon).
   b. Observe urinary drainage from catheter frequently.
   c. Prevent pressure sores, pain in lower extremities, or pressure on penis or testes when client is in prone position.
3. Initiate treatment immediately (medical emergency).
   a. Check the bladder for distension.
   b. Look for stimuli other than bladder distension (e.g., cold air, drafts, sharp objects pressing on skin below level of injury).
   c. Remove the cause (e.g., empty bladder by catheterization or irrigation of Foley catheter).
   d. Elevate head of bed to lower blood pressure.
   e. Administer ganglionic-blocking agents (e.g., hexamethonium chloride) as ordered.

Evaluation
Client remains free from signs of autonomic dysreflexia; maintains bowel and bladder function.

Goal 5: Client will ingest adequate fluids and nutrition.

Implementation
1. Give liquid diet until possibility of paralytic ileus has passed, then diet as tolerated.
2. Administer vitamin supplements as ordered.
3. Encourage fluid intake.
4. Monitor I&O.

Evaluation
Client's weight remains within desired range; skin turgor is firm.

Goal 6: Client will be free from urinary tract infection.

Implementation
1. Insert Foley catheter, or use intermittent catheterization as ordered, using sterile technique.
2. Give aseptic care to Foley catheter.
3. Observe client for signs of bladder infection (e.g., fever; abnormal UA, urine C&S).
4. Encourage fluid intake to 3 L/day.
5. Observe odor, appearance, and amount of urine.
6. Monitor I&O carefully.

Evaluation
Client drains normal urine; has no fever.

Goal 7: Client will be free from stress ulcer.

Implementation
1. Monitor for complaints of ulcerlike pain.
2. Observe for melena, hematemesis.
3. Administer antacids frequently as ordered to prevent gastric irritation (see Table 3-25).

Evaluation
Client offers no complaints of abdominal pain; has stools negative for occult blood.

Goal 8: Client will be free from pain in paralyzed limbs.

Implementation
1. Handle the affected limbs gently to avoid muscle spasms.
2. Identify and eliminate stimuli that cause spasms.
3. Medicate as ordered to control spasms and pain.

Evaluation
Client experiences relief of pain.

Goal 9: Client will become as independent as possible. Refer to General Nursing Goal 4, p. 234.

☐ Parkinson's Syndrome (Parkinsonism)
General Information

1. Definition: a progressive debilitating syndrome in which there is degeneration of nerve cells in the basal ganglia that impairs
   a. Important centers of coordination, especially control of associated automatic movements
   b. Control of muscle tone to produce finely coordinated movements
   c. Control of initiation and inhibition of gross, intentional movements

2. Incidence: one of the major causes of neurological disability; estimated to affect more than a half-million people in the United States; more common in men

3. Onset: usually 50-60 years of age

4. Etiology
  a. Unknown
  b. It is hypothesized that these clients have a deficiency of dopamine, which is required for normal functioning of the basal ganglia; drug therapy aims at returning dopamine levels to normal to control symptoms of the syndrome

5. Precipitating factors
  a. Drug induced: phenothiazines and rauwolfia alkaloids
  b. Atherosclerosis
  c. Trauma (e.g., midbrain compression)
  d. Encephalitis
  e. Toxic poisoning: carbon monoxide

Nursing Process

Assessment
1. Muscle rigidity

Table 3-55   Comparison of chronic degenerative neurological diseases

	Parkinsonism	Multiple sclerosis	Amyotrophic lateral sclerosis	Myasthenia gravis
Onset age	50-60 years	20-40 years	40-70 years	20-50 years
Sex	Male >female	Female >male	Male >female	Female >male
Etiology	Unknown	Unknown; virus/autoimmune origin suspected	Unknown; virus/autoimmune origin suspected	Unknown; autoimmune origin suspected; occurs in cool climates
Area affected	Substantia nigra cells in basal ganglia	Disseminated demyelinated plaques in white matter of brain and spinal cord	Motor neurons in brain and spinal cord	Myoneural junction of voluntary muscle
Pathophysiology	Impaired coordinated muscle movement and autonomic dysfunction because of deficiency of dopamine	Impaired nerve impulse conduction because of destruction of myelin	Impaired nerve impulse conduction because of degeneration of motor neurons	Impaired transmission of nerve impulse to skeletal muscle possibly because of acetylcholine deficiency
Signs and symptoms	Rigidity Slow movements Nonintentional tremor Autonomic dysfunction	Depends on site of plaque: Visual problems Spastic weakness/paralysis Poor coordination Paresthesias Speech defects Intentional tremor Bowel/bladder dysfunction Emotional disorders Exacerbations and remissions	Twitching Muscle weakness, progressing to atrophy and paralysis of upper and lower extremities Usually fatal 2-15 years after onset	Profound muscle weakness and fatigue Can progress to respiratory failure (myasthenic crisis)
Treatment	Supportive Medication	Symptomatic	Symptomatic	Supportive Medication Surgery sometimes: thymectomy
Medication	Levodopa Carbidopa/levodopa (Sinemet)	Muscle relaxants Antiinflammatory (steroid) during exacerbation	Antibiotics for respiratory and urinary tract infections	Anticholinesterase: Diagnosis—Edrophonium chloride (Tensilon) Maintenance—Pyridostigmine bromide (Mestinon) Antiinflammatory (steroids) during acute phase

Table 3-56 Drugs used to treat parkinsonism

Name	Action	Side effects	Nursing implications
Levodopa (Larodopa)	Converts to dopamine in basal ganglia	Gastrointestinal irritation (e.g., nausea, anorexia, vomiting); gastrointestinal hemorrhage; psychiatric symptoms; orthostatic hypotension	Begin with low dosage; gradually increase to therapeutic level. Give medications with meals. Use cautiously in clients with cardiovascular, respiratory, endocrine, or hepatic peptic ulcer disease. Avoid vitamin B_6 (reverses effects of levodopa).
Carbidopa and levodopa (Sinemet)	Combined drugs provide same action as above at lower levels	Same as levodopa	Same as levodopa.
Amantadine (Symmetrel)	Unknown	Restlessness; mental and emotional changes	Well tolerated (less effective than levodopa).
Trihexyphenidyl (Artane)	Anticholinergic: blocks muscarinic receptors at cholinergic synapses with CNS; relieves tremor, rigidity. Minimal effect on akinesia	Dry mouth; blurred vision; constipation; urinary retention; mental dullness, confusion. Sudden withdrawal precipitates sudden, incapacitating increase in symptoms	Begin using small doses; increase dosages gradually. Avoid sudden withdrawal of medications; withdrawal of drug reverses side effects. Monitor client with psychosis, wide-angle glaucoma, diabetes. Administer after meals to avoid GI irritation.
Procyclidine (Kemadrin)	Same as trihexyphenidyl	Same as trihexyphenidyl	Same as trihexyphenidyl.
Benztropine mesylate (Cogentin)	Same as trihexyphenidyl	Same as trihexyphenidyl	Same as trihexyphenidyl.
Selegirine hydrochloride (L-deprenyl or Eldepryl)	Irreversibly, selectively inhibits monoamine oxidase type B	May exacerbate parkinsonism manifestations. Toxicity: nausea, dizziness, fainting	Used to delay the onset of severe disability in clients in early stages of parkinsonism; can be given with Sinemet. Avoid concurrent use of meperidine; interacts with deprenyl; rapidly absorbed and metabolized.

   a. Major disability
   b. Bradykinesia and akinesia
2. Tremors at rest (nonintentional)
   a. Especially of hands (pill rolling), arms, and head
   b. Rhythmic: regular and rapid
3. Facial mask
4. Speech difficulty
5. Loss of automatic movements (e.g., blinking of eyes)
6. Propulsive gait, shuffling in nature

7. Emotional changes (mood disturbances), depression, and confusion
8. Autonomic nervous system dysfunction
   a. Decreased salivation
   b. Perspiration
   c. Lacrimation
   d. Constipation
   e. Incontinence
   f. Decreased sexual activity

Analysis (see p. 233)
Planning, Implementation, and Evaluation

> **Goal 1:** Client will have optimal function of muscles and joints.

Implementation
1. Administer prescribed medications (see Table 3-56).
2. Observe for side effects of medications.
3. Help client remain as active as possible (see General Nursing Goal 4, p. 234).
   a. Frequent ambulation
   b. Attention to grooming

Evaluation
Client maintains movement in muscles and joints; continues to ambulate and participate in ADL.

> **Goal 2:** Client will be free from injury.

Implementation
1. Use ambulatory aids such as hand rails in all rooms and near bathtub or shower.
2. Instruct client to walk slowly and carefully.
3. Balance activity and rest to avoid fatigue.

Evaluation
Client is free from cuts, abrasions, and falls.

> **Goal 3:** Client will maintain gastrointestinal integrity.

Implementation
1. Provide adequate fluid intake.
2. Give high-fiber diet.
3. Restrict protein as indicated.
4. Observe for constipation.
5. Administer stool softeners or laxatives as ordered prn (see Table 3-47).
6. Give oral hygiene to relieve dryness of the mouth.
7. Keep urinal and bedpan available in case client is unable to reach bathroom in time.

Evaluation
Client is free from constipation and impactions; has adequate bowel function.

> **Goal 4:** Client will maintain positive body image and self-concept.

Implementation
1. Provide devices to assist in ADL.
2. Teach about or provide clothes that are simple and easy to put on.
3. Allow sufficient time for meals.
4. In general, do *not* hurry client.
5. Supervise and assist in skin care and personal hygiene.

6. Allow expression of depression and hopelessness (see "Depression," p. 48).
7. Reward attempts at activity that the client makes.
8. Arrange for speech therapy for dysarthria.
9. Refer to community agency (e.g., American Parkinson's Disease Association).

Evaluation
Client's grooming projects positive self-concept; accepts responsibility for ADL to the extent possible.

> **Goal 5:** Client and significant others will express fears and other feelings about present and future.

Implementation
1. Assess level of anxiety.
2. Give emotional support and relieve anxiety (see *Anxious Behavior,* p. 31).
3. Explain disease and drug therapy.
4. Clarify misconceptions and lack of information.
5. Explain prognosis.

Evaluation
Client and significant others express feelings (e.g., fear, sadness, anger); state realistic expectations for the future.

☐ Multiple Sclerosis
General Information
1. Definition: chronic progressive disease of the central nervous system characterized by unpredictable exacerbations and remissions; typically, demyelinization of the white matter of the spinal cord and brain occurs in multiple areas
2. Incidence
   a. Disease of young adults
   b. More common in women
3. Risk factors
   a. Living in the temperate zone 40°-60° north or south of the equator
   b. Higher incidence among higher socioeconomic classes
4. Etiology
   a. Unknown
   b. May be a virus that is latent for months or years before some other factor initiates disease
   c. Possibly an autoimmune disorder
   d. Mineral deficiency or toxic substances

Nursing Process
Assessment
1. At onset: vague symptoms
   a. Diplopia
   b. Awkwardness in handling articles and frequent dropping of articles
   c. Stumbling or falling with no apparent cause
2. Symptoms vary depending on location of myelin or nerve fiber destruction

  a. Classic symptoms
    1. nystagmus (rapid, involuntary movements of eyes)
    2. intention tremors, absent at rest
    3. scanning speech (slow enunciation with tendency to hesitate at beginning of a word or syllable, speech with pauses between syllables)
  b. Sensory disorders
    1. paresthesias (numbness, tingling, "dead" feeling, "pins and needles")
    2. diminished vibration sense
    3. impaired proprioception
  c. Visual disorders
    1. optic neuritis
    2. diplopia
    3. scotomas (blind spots)
  d. Motor disorders: spastic weakness or paralysis of limbs
  e. Cerebellar dysfunction: cerebellar ataxia
  f. Bowel and bladder dysfunction
    1. hesitancy, urgency, frequency
    2. retention, incontinence
    3. constipation
  g. Emotional disorders: euphoria, mood swings
3. Long-term effects of progressive disease
  a. Spasticity
  b. Paraplegia
  c. Speech defects
  d. Eating difficulties
  e. Extreme fatigue
  f. Vision difficulties
  g. Complete paralysis
Analysis (see p. 233)
Planning, Implementation, and Evaluation

Goal 1: Client will have optimal function of muscles and joints.

Implementation
1. Arrange for physical therapy (muscle stretching and strengthening).
2. Assist with gait retraining if ataxic.
3. Encourage client to remain active and to do as many ADL as possible.
Evaluation
  Client's joints and muscles function well; participate in ADL.

Goal 2: Client will maintain health-promoting habits in daily living.

Implementation
1. Determine and encourage optimal activity level.
2. Promote adequate rest periods to prevent exhaustion.
3. Use safety devices such as hand rails and walkers to prevent falls.

4. Maintain good nutrition and fluid intake.
5. Supply self-help devices for eating, ambulation, and reading.
6. Provide pain medication and muscle relaxants (e.g., baclofen [Lioresal]) as ordered.
7. Attend to incontinence and pressure areas to maintain integrity of skin and mucous membranes.
8. Make referral to community agencies (e.g., VNA, local branch of National Multiple Sclerosis Society) to help client and significant others in long-term management.
9. Educate client and significant others about these aspects of care.
Evaluation
  Client maintains good personal hygiene; eats a nutritious, well-balanced diet.

Goal 3: Client will maintain positive body image and self-concept.

Implementation
1. Provide devices to assist in ADL.
2. Promote as much independence in client as possible; teach significant others to do the same.
3. Encourage hobbies and other pleasurable distractions.
4. DO NOT hurry client.
5. Supervise and assist in skin care and personal hygiene.
6. Reward client's attempts at activity.
7. Encourage and reinforce perseverance and hope.
8. Help client identify realistic goals.
Evaluation
  Client's grooming projects positive self-image; performs ADL within own limits.

Goal 4: Client and significant others will express fears about present and future.

Implementation
1. Set aside time to talk to client and significant others together and separately.
2. Encourage expression of feelings.
3. Clarify misconceptions and lack of information about present status and prognosis.
4. Allow expression of depression and hopelessness.
5. Emphasize what the client can still do.
Evaluation
  Client and significant others express fear about the diesase; state what to realistically expect in the future.

Goal 5: Client and significant others will learn to cope with illness-related problems and prevent complications.

Implementation
1. Evaluate knowledge and skills that client and signif-

icant others have and go over areas where they have not retained information.

2. Teach knowledge and skills related to Goals 1 and 2.

Evaluation

Client and significant others describe care needed because of disabilities; explain how to avoid complications related to disabilities.

☐ **Epilepsy** (see "Seizure Disorders" in *Nursing Care of the Child*, p. 470)

☐ **Amyotrophic Lateral Sclerosis (ALS)**

General Information

1. Definition: progressive, degenerative disorder of motor neurons in the brain, spinal cord, and motor cortex; remissions are uncommon; death occurs 2-15 years after onset.
2. Incidence
   a. Disease of middle age
   b. More common in men
   c. 3000 new cases in United States annually
3. Major complication: aspiration pneumonia
4. Etiology: unknown
5. Diagnosis
   a. Electromyography (EMG)
   b. Muscle biopsy to confirm diagnosis
   c. Elevated serum creatinine phosphokinase (CPK)

Nursing Process

Assessment

1. At onset
   a. Awkward fine–hand movements
   b. Weakness, wasting of hand muscles
   c. Twitching, cramping
2. Atrophy of hand, forearms; hyperactive reflexes
3. Progresses to upper arms, neck, shoulders
4. Late stage: weakness involves lower extremities
5. Remains alert and oriented
6. Bulbar palsy may be accompanied by erratic affective behavior (e.g., uncontrollable crying outbursts)
7. Impaired swallowing, palate, tongue, and pharynx

Analysis (see p. 233)

Planning, Implementation, and Evaluation

Refer to "Multiple Sclerosis" Goals 1-5, p. 244.

☐ **Myasthenia Gravis**

General Information

1. Definition: a chronic, progressive neuromuscular disorder characterized by rapid exhaustion of voluntary muscles; caused by a defect at the myoneural junction
2. Pathophysiology: transmission of impulse from nerve to muscle is impaired because of inadequate acetylcholine at the myoneural junction; contractions of voluntary muscles become progressively weaker and cease when the muscle is stimulated
3. Etiology
   a. Unknown
   b. Possibly an autoimmune disorder
   c. Client may have a genetic predisposition

Nursing Process

Assessment

1. Onset of symptoms insidious and gradual
2. Progressive voluntary-muscle weakness
3. Incapacitating fatigue
4. Ocular symptoms: ptosis, inability to open eyes, diplopia
5. Expressionless appearance with facial muscle involvement; characteristic "snarl" when client attempts to smile
6. Respiratory distress
7. Diagnostic test: positive Tensilon test (anticholinesterase): edrophonium chloride (Tensilon) injected IV produces increase in strength (see Table 3-57)

Analysis (see p. 233)

Planning, Implementation, and Evaluation

> **Goal 1:** Client will have control of voluntary muscles.

Implementation

1. Administer anticholinesterase medications to control symptoms (e.g., neostigmine methylsulfate [Prostigmin], pyridostigmine bromide [Mestinon]); see Table 3-57.
2. Administer medications on individually adjusted schedule.

Evaluation

Client has control of voluntary muscles.

> **Goal 2:** Client will remain free from respiratory impairment.

Implementation

1. Observe respiratory status.
2. Use postural drainage; turn frequently.
3. Give prophylactic antibiotics to prevent respiratory infections.
4. Instruct client to avoid exposure to people with upper respiratory infections (URIs).
5. Teach client diaphragmatic breathing exercises, to maintain strength with maximum ventilation and minimum energy expenditure.
6. Balance physical activities with rest.
7. Put client in a rocking bed.
8. Know that client may require mechanical ventilation.

Evaluation

Client's lungs are clear; no respiratory distress.

> **Goal 3:** Client will remain well nourished.

Implementation

1. Give anticholinesterase medications (e.g., pyridostig-

Table 3-57   Drugs used to treat myasthenia gravis

Name	Action	Side effects	Nursing implications
Neostigmine bromide Neostigmine methylsulfate (Prostigmin)	Anticholinesterase: blocks breakdown of acetylcholine at myoneural junction	Nausea, vomiting, diarrhea, abdominal cramps, muscle twitching, weakness, hypotension *Toxic effect:* cholinergic crisis—increased myasthenia symptoms, vomiting, perspiration, salivation, bradycardia, muscle tightness, fasciculations May cause skin rash	Give smallest dose that provides greatest strength; may give anticholinergics (e.g., atropine sulfate) to prevent side and toxic effects Monitor vital signs; note CNS, irritability Increased potassium levels potentiate drug's effects
Pyridostigmine bromide (Mestinon)	As above	As above	Give 20-30 minutes before meals
Ambenonium chloride (Mytelase)	As above	As above	Less commonly used than above drugs; drug of choice if client is sensitive to bromides
Edrophonium chloride (Tensilon)	As above Short duration of action	As above	Useful in emergency treatment and as diagnostic agent Differentiates disease from cholinergic crisis—watch for immediate relief of symptoms vs. increased weakness because of medication overdose

mine bromide [Mestinon]) 20-30 minutes *before* meals for full advantage (see Table 3-57).
2. Provide small, frequent, semisolid, or fluid meals that are nutritious and high in potassium (adequate serum levels of potassium potentiate anticholinesterase effect).
3. Provide IV or NG feedings if needed.
4. Observe for aspiration; have suction equipment available.
5. Allow client to eat meals without rushing.
6. Observe for anorexia, nausea, diarrhea, abdominal cramping (common side effects of anticholinesterase drugs).

Evaluation
Client's weight remains stable.

Goal 4: Client will receive psychological and rehabilitative support.

Implementation
1. Evaluate client and significant others' attitudes toward and knowledge of disease.
2. Provide careful explanations of disorder.
3. Offer opportunities for expressions of feelings.
4. Promote a balance of rest and activities.
5. Encourage healthy life-style.

6. Refer to Myasthenia Gravis Foundation for information and support.

Evaluation
Client expresses positive outlook for future; has a plan for balancing activities with adequate rest periods.

Goal 5: Client remains free from an undetected "cholinergic crisis."

Implementation
1. Know that a "cholinergic crisis" (medical emergency) occurs when client cannot tolerate the dosage of anticholinesterase medications (see Table 3-57).
2. Carefully monitor vital signs, including pupil checks, of client receiving increasing doses of anticholinesterase agents.
3. Observe for signs and symptoms of excessive parasympathetic stimulation (see toxic effect: cholinergic crisis, Table 3-57).
4. Discontinue medications and give IV anticholinergic drug as ordered (e.g., atropine sulfate); see Table 3-58.

Evaluation
Client is free from symptoms of cholinergic crisis (no diarrhea, pallor).

Table 3-58   Eye medications

Name	Action	Side effects	Nursing implications
CYCLOPLEGICS			
Atropine sulfate	Parasympatholytic (anticholinergic) Dilation of pupil and paralysis of accommodation	Dryness of mouth, tachycardia, light sensitivity, inability to focus on near objects	Used to correct refractive errors, inflammations of the eye. Monitor for side effects, increased intraocular pressure (e.g., nausea, vomiting, pain). Inform of inability to accommodate for close-by objects, long duration of action, and photophobia. Contraindicated in glaucoma. Store in safe place out of reach of children.
Homatropine hydrobromide	As above Slow onset; prolonged action	As above	As above, plus use cautiously with older adults.
MIOTICS			
Pilocarpine hydrochloride	Cholinergic causes: contraction of sphincter muscle of the iris, resulting in pupil constriction (miosis); spasms of ciliary muscle and deepening of the anterior chamber; and vasodilation of vessels where intraocular fluids leave the eye	Headache	Drug of choice in treatment of glaucoma. Monitor for side effects, individual duration of action and tolerance and/or resistance. Inform of difficult adjustment to changes in illumination. Instruct regarding frequent instillation.
Carbachol (Carbacel, Isopto Carbachol, Miostat)	As above Produces intense and prolonged miosis	Headache, conjunctival hyperemia	Used for glaucoma if pilocarpine is ineffective. As above.
Physostigmine salicylate (Eserine)	Anticholinesterase Pupil constriction Spasm of accommodation Short duration of action	Conjunctivitis, allergic reactions	As above, plus give every 4-6 hr for wide-angle glaucoma.
Isoflurophate (Floropryl)	Anticholinesterase Pupil constriction Spasm of accommodation	Vomiting and diarrhea, tenesmus	Used for wide-angle glaucoma; plus above.
Neostigimine bromide (Prostigmin)	As above Short duration of action	Conjunctivitis	As above.
BETA-BLOCKING AGENT			
Timolol maleate (Timoptic)	Beta-adrenergic receptor blocking agent Reduces intraocular pressure by decreasing aqueous formation Acts in ½ hour	Headache, bronchospasm, cardiac failure, hypotension, muscle weakness, dizziness	Generally well tolerated. Contraindicated in clients with COPD; used cautiously in those with hyperthyroidism. Monitor for side effects.

Continued.

Table 3-58   Eye medications—cont'd

Name	Action	Side effects	Nursing implications
CARBONIC ANHYDRASE INHIBITORS			
Acetazolamide (Diamox) Ethoxzolamide (Cardase) Methazolamide (Neptazane) Dichlorphenamide (Daranide)	Inhibit carbonic anhydrase, an enzyme necessary for formation of aqueous humor Result in reduced intraocular pressure	Lethargy, anorexia, numbness, tingling of face and extremities, acidosis, ureteral stones	Used for treatment of glaucoma. Monitor for side effects. Prohibit use in first trimester of pregnancy.
OSMOTIC AGENTS (see Table 3-42) **Antiinfectives**			
Bacitracin ophthalmic ointment* (Baciguent)	Bactericidal antibiotic; effective against gram-positive bacteria	No systemic effects	Preserve solutions with refrigeration; potency remains for 3 weeks. Ointment stable for 1 year at room temperature.
Neomycin sulfate (Myciguent)	Broad-spectrum bactericidal antibiotic	Minimal allergenic effects	Use cautiously with other systemically used antibiotics due to cross-sensitivity reactions. Effective for conjunctival and corneal infections.
Polymyxin B sulfate* (Aerosporin)	Bactericidal antibiotic; effective against gram-negative bacteria	Minimal	Often used in combination with above two to produce broader effects.
Tetracyclines (Achromycin) (Aureomycin) (Terramycin)	Bacteriostatic antibiotic for superficial infections	Rare	Monitor for effects.
Sulfacetamide sodium (Bleph-10)	Bacteriostatic sulfonamide for surface infections	Local irritation	Monitor for ocular purulent drainage or exudate (interferes with sulfonamide's action).
ANTIINFLAMMATORIES			
Cortisone acetate Fludrocortisone acetate	Decrease defense mechanisms and reduce resistance to pathogenic organisms Inhibit inflammatory response	Prolonged use increases susceptibility to glaucoma, cataracts, and fungus infection	Indicated for all allergenic reactions, nonpyogenic inflammation, and severe injury. Use for limited period. Monitor for increased intraocular pressure and secondary fungus function.

*See Table 3-20.

☐ Cataracts
General Information
1. Definition: total or partial opacity of the normally transparent crystalline lens; the opacity of the lens interferes with light passage through the lens to the retina
2. Incidence
   a. Common after age 55
   b. Third leading cause of blindness
3. Etiology: unknown
4. Risk factors
   a. Aging
   b. Diabetes mellitus
   c. Intraocular surgery
   d. Previous injury to the eye
5. Medical treatment: surgical removal of lens, one eye at a time
   a. Intracapsular extraction by cryosurgery or extracapsular extraction by ultrasound fragmentation (phacoemulsification)

b. Partial iridectomy commonly done with lens extraction to prevent acute secondary glaucoma

c. Lens implantation commonly done

Nursing Process

Assessment

1. Distorted, blurred vision
2. Gradual and painless loss of vision
3. Absence of red reflex (the red reflection seen when the retina is viewed through an ophthalmoscope)
4. Knowledge of treatment modalities
5. Knowledge of procedure and expected outcome

Analysis (see p. 233)

Planning, Implementation, and Evaluation

Goal 1: Client and significant others will be able to explain preoperative and postoperative care and the OR-RR environment.

Implementation

1. Refer to "Perioperative Period," p. 117.
2. Prepare client for preoperative instillation of eye medications (mydriatics and cycloplegics) as ordered (see Table 3-58).
3. Teach about postoperative procedures.
   a. Bed position varies with type of surgery (usually head of bed up 30°).
   b. No turning or turn only to *unaffected* side postoperatively.
   c. Prevent falls (e.g., bed rails up, assist with ambulation).
   d. Keeps hands away from eyes to prevent infection (eye patch often used on first two postoperative days).
   e. Perform ROM exercise routine.

Evaluation

Client describes plan of treatment and postoperative care; explains what will happen in OR-RR.

Goal 2: Client will be able, preoperatively, to explain how to prevent increasing intraocular pressure.

Implementation

1. Teach client before surgery
   a. No straining.
   b. No coughing or sneezing.
   c. No bending or heavy lifting.
   d. To prevent vomiting.
   e. No squeezing eyelids shut.
2. Evaluate client knowledge after teaching.
3. Continue to explain areas client does not remember or understand.

Evaluation

Client explains how to prevent increased intraocular pressure.

Goal 3: Client will remain free from postoperative complications.

Implementation

1. Refer to "Perioperative Period," p. 117.
2. Provide adequate fluids.
3. Deep-breath qh; no coughing.
4. Elevate head of bed 30°-45°.
5. Turn only to *unaffected* side if turning is permitted.
6. Check dressing frequently for bleeding (q15min for 2h, then qh for 8h).
7. Prevent increased intraocular pressure.
8. Give antiemetics (Table 3-64) and laxatives or stool softeners (Table 3-47) prn.
9. Observe and report severe eye pain immediately.

Evaluation

Client's vital signs are stable; has no complaints of pain.

Goal 4: Client will know the characteristics of the type of lenses or glasses to be used after surgery for optimal vision.

Implementation

1. Teach according to client's situation.
   a. Cataract glasses (wear old glasses until curvature changes are complete: 12-14 weeks postoperatively)
      1. magnify objects by one third
      2. clear vision only through center of lens
   b. Contact lenses (less vision distortion than glasses; more costly)
   c. Intraocular lens
      1. synthetic lens implanted in eye
      2. designed for distance vision
      3. for near vision, needs corrective glasses
2. Discuss a plan for obtaining new glasses or contact lenses.

Evaluation

Client correctly describes type of corrective eyewear prescribed.

Goal 5: Client will be discharged with a written rehabilitation plan and a physician's appointment for follow-up.

Implementation

1. Refer to "Perioperative Period," p. 117.
2. Develop a written plan that explains
   a. Strenuous activity restrictions for 6-8 weeks
   b. Progressively increased activity
   c. Return to sexual activity
   d. Driving
   e. Dressing changes as required
   f. Eye medications as ordered

g. Dark glasses when exposed to bright sunlight
3. Instruct significant others in dressing change and medication administration.
4. Secure physician or clinic appointment for client.
Evaluation
Client correctly states activity limitations upon discharge; significant others administer eye medications correctly.

☐ Retinal Detachment
General Information

1. Definition: actual splitting of the retina between the rod and cone layers of the retina and the pigment epithelial layer. Partial separation becomes complete (if untreated) with subsequent total loss of vision.
2. Pathophysiology: vitreous humor seeps through opening and separates retina from pigment epithelium and choroid. Blindness results.
3. Types
   a. Primary: from a break in the continuity of retina
   b. Secondary: from intraocular disorders (e.g., postcataract extraction, perforating injuries, severe myopia)
4. Medical treatment: early surgical repair imperative to avoid irreparable damage and irreversible blindness
   a. Cryosurgery: freezing stimulates inflammatory response leading to adhesions
   b. Photocoagulation: laser beam stimulates inflammatory response
   c. Electrodiathermy: creates inflammatory response
   d. Scleral buckling

Nursing Process
Assessment
1. Gradual or sudden onset
2. Sudden flashes of light
3. Blurred vision that becomes progressively worse
4. Loss of portion of visual field
5. Ophthalmological examination: retina hangs like a grey cloud; one or more tears
Analysis (see p. 233)
Planning, Implementation, and Evaluation

> **Goal 1:** Client will be able to explain preoperative and postoperative care, and the OR-RR environment.

Implementation
1. Prepare client for surgery (see "Perioperative Period," p. 117)
   a. Apply bilateral eye patches preopertively
   b. Protect client from injury
   c. Minimize stress on eye (e.g., avoid sneezing, coughing, sudden jarring)

   d. Instill preoperative medications as ordered (cycloplegics, mydriatics) (see Table 3-58)
2. Teach client postoperative positions and care.
Evaluation
Client explains surgical plan, preoperative and postoperative care, and the OR-RR environment.

> **Goal 2:** Client will be able, preoperatively, to explain how to prevent increasing intraocular pressure (see "Cataracts" Goal 2, p. 249).

> **Goal 3:** Client will recover free from postoperative complications.

Implementation
1. Refer to "Perioperative Period," p. 117.
2. Have client avoid prone position.
3. Speak before approaching client.
4. Check eye patches frequently.
5. Give antiemetics (see Table 3-64), analgestics (see Table 3-7) prn.
Evaluation
Client is stable and free from postoperative complications.

> **Goal 4:** Client will be discharged with a written plan for rehabilitation.

Implementation
1. Refer to "Perioperative Period," p. 117.
2. Inform client of activities upon discharge.
   a. May watch television.
   b. Avoid reading for 2-3 weeks.
   c. Continue to avoid straining, injury to head.
   d. May shave, comb hair, bathe, and ambulate.
3. If pinhole glasses are prescribed, provide client with instructions for use.
Evaluation
Client correctly describes activities and limitations upon discharge.

☐ Glaucoma
General Information

1. Definition: abnormal increase in intraocular pressure caused by any obstruction of the outflow channels of aqueous humor; uncontrolled glaucoma causes irreversible blindness as a result of atrophy of the optic nerve
2. Types
   a. *Chronic* (wide angle): most common
      1. resistance to flow because of thickening of collecting channels, trabecular network, and canal of Schlemm

2. insidious onset characterized by a decrease in peripheral vision
  b. *Acute* (narrow angle)
    1. occurs when iris is abnormally structured in an anterior position
    2. exerts pressure on collecting channels and decreases size of anterior chamber
    3. sudden onset characterized by severe eye pain and rapid loss of vision
3. Risk factors
  a. Heredity
  b. Trauma
  c. Tumor or inflammation of the eye
  d. Vascular disorders
  e. Diabetes
  f. Prior eye surgery
4. Other information
  a. One of leading causes of blindness
  b. Early detection is crucial (vision destroyed by optic nerve atrophy cannot be restored)
  c. Regular eye exams that include tonometry (measure of intraocular pressure) are recommended for persons over age 35

Nursing Process

Assessment
1. Difficulty adjusting to dark rooms (early symptom)
2. Difficulty focusing on close work
3. Halos around lights
4. Loss of peripheral vision; loss of central vision with progression
5. Increased intraocular pressure (normal = 12-20 mm Hg)
6. Client's support system
7. Client's and significant others' coping mechanisms

Analysis (see p. 233)

Planning, Implementation, and Evaluation

> **Goal 1:** Client's intraocular pressure will remain within normal limits.

Implementation
1. Teach client
  a. How to instill eyedrops correctly (e.g., timolol maleate).
  b. How miotic eyedrops decrease intraocular pressure (e.g., pilocarpine); see Table 3-49.
  c. That emotional or stressful events can increase intraocular pressure.
  d. To avoid lifting, shoveling, wearing constrictive clothing around the neck.

Evaluation
Client's intraocular pressure remains between 12-20 mm Hg with medication.

> **Goal 2:** Client will be free from further visual impairment.

Implementation
1. Teach client that ocular damage that has already occurred is not reversible, but further visual impairment can be prevented by compliance with prescribed regimen.
2. Emphasize importance of routine eye exams and follow-up care.

Evaluation
Client develops no further visual impairment.

☐ Nasal Problems Requiring Surgery
General Information
1. Definition: bone and soft tissue deformities requiring corrective surgery (usually under local anesthesia)
2. Precipitating factors
  a. Fracture
  b. Tumor
  c. Foreign body
  d. Deviated septum
  e. Polyps
  f. Cosmetic problems
3. Types of surgery
  a. Submucous resection (rhinoplasty)
  b. Reduction of a nasal fracture
  c. Removal of polyps, tumors, foreign bodies

Nursing Process

Assessment
1. Nasal obstruction
2. Pain (fractures)
3. Nasal congestion
4. Bleeding
5. Allergies
6. Self-concept/body image

Analysis (see p. 233)

Planning, Implementation, and Evaluation

> **Goal 1:** Client and significant others will understand preoperative and postoperative care, and the OR-RR environment.

Implementation
1. Refer to "Perioperative Period," p. 117.
2. Teach about postoperative procedures
  a. Mouth breathing (nasal packing)
  b. No nose blowing
  c. Fowler's position
  d. Ice packs
3. Prepare for postoperative appearance (black eyes, dressing).

Evaluation

Client and significant others describe the surgery and postoperative course.

Goal 2: Client will remain free from any postoperative complications.

Implementation

1. Refer to "Perioperative Period," p. 117.
2. Observe for frequent swallowing (hemorrhage).
3. Check dressing frequently for bleeding.
4. Change gauze pad under nose when saturated and note amount of bleeding.
5. Apply ice continously to the area for first 24 hours.
6. Give frequent oral hygiene.
7. Maintain Fowler's position to prevent aspiration.

Evaluation

Client has vital signs within normal limits; minimal periorbital edema and discoloration.

☐ Epistaxis
General Information

1. Definition: nosebleed
2. Risk factors
   a. Trauma
   b. Hypertension
   c. Acute sinusitis
   d. Deviated nasal septum
   e. Nasal surgery

Nursing Process

Assessment

1. Bleeding from nose
2. Frequent swallowing
3. Bright red vomitus

Analysis (see p. 233)

Planning, Implementation, and Evaluation

Goal 1: Client will experience control of epistaxis.

Implementation

1. Use first-aid interventions: direct pressure, Fowler's position, and ice pack.
2. Know that cautery may be used.
3. Monitor anterior and posterior nasal packing (removed in 48-96 hours to prevent infection).
4. Give vasoconstrictors as ordered (e.g., topical phenylephrine hydrochloride [Neo-Synephrine]).
5. Observe frequently for bleeding.

Evaluation

Client has no further bleeding from nose.

Goal 2: Client will remain free from future attacks.

Implementation

1. Teach client and significant others first-aid measures to use in event of future attack.
2. Demonstrate proper nasal care.
3. Help client identify precipitating factors.
4. Monitor BP for hypertension.

Evaluation

Client states methods to prevent future attacks.

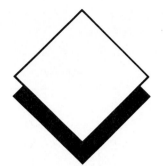

Mobility

The nursing care presented in this unit concerns selected health problems related to disturbances in the musculoskeletal system. The nurse plays an important role in maintaining musculoskeletal function by assessment, range-of-motion techniques, exercise, and early progressive ambulation.

GENERAL CONCEPTS
Overview/Physiology

1. Musculoskeletal system
   a. Muscles: contract and relax under the control of the nervous system to produce movement of the body as a whole or of its parts
      1. *fascia:* surrounds and divides muscles, main blood vessels, and nerves
      2. *tendons:* fibrous attachment between muscles and bones
      3. *ligaments:* fibrous connective tissue connecting bones and cartilage and serving as support for or attachment of muscles and fascia
   b. Bones: for support and protection
      1. *joints:* junction between two bones
         a. synovium: lining of joints that secretes fluid to lubricate
         b. bursa: a closed cavity containing a gliding joint
      2. *cartilage:* dense connective tissue covering the ends of bones and at other sites where flexibility is needed
2. Terminology (see Fig. 3-23)
   a. *Adduction:* movement toward the main axis of the body
   b. *Abduction:* movement away from the main axis of the body
   c. *Flexion:* act of bending
   d. *Extension:* stretching out into a straightened position
   e. *Strain:* trauma to the muscle caused by violent contraction or excessive forcible stretch

   f. *Sprain:* trauma to a joint with some degree of injury to the ligaments
3. Range-of-motion (ROM) exercises (see Fig. 3-27)
   a. Uses
      1. prevent atrophy
      2. prevent weakness
      3. prevent contracture
      4. prevent degeneration of muscles and joints
   b. Types
      1. active
      2. passive
   c. Procedure
      1. stress importance of performing full ROM exercises
      2. perform ROM exercises at least twice daily, especially for clients on bed rest
      3. breathing should be as normal as possible (e.g., client should not hold breath)
      4. perform movements slowly and gently, especially with active ROM
      5. provide rest between each exercise
      6. perform each exercise same number of times on both sides of body; initially do each exercise three times, then work up to five times
      7. teach significant others to do ROM exercises for client
         a. demonstrate exercises
         b. allow return demonstration
         c. provide written instructions
4. Massage (centripetal: toward the heart)
   a. Uses
      1. increases circulation
      2. reduces edema
      3. relieves spasm
   b. May be used with heat
5. Isometric exercises
   a. Definition: alternately tightening and relaxing muscles without moving the joints
   b. Uses

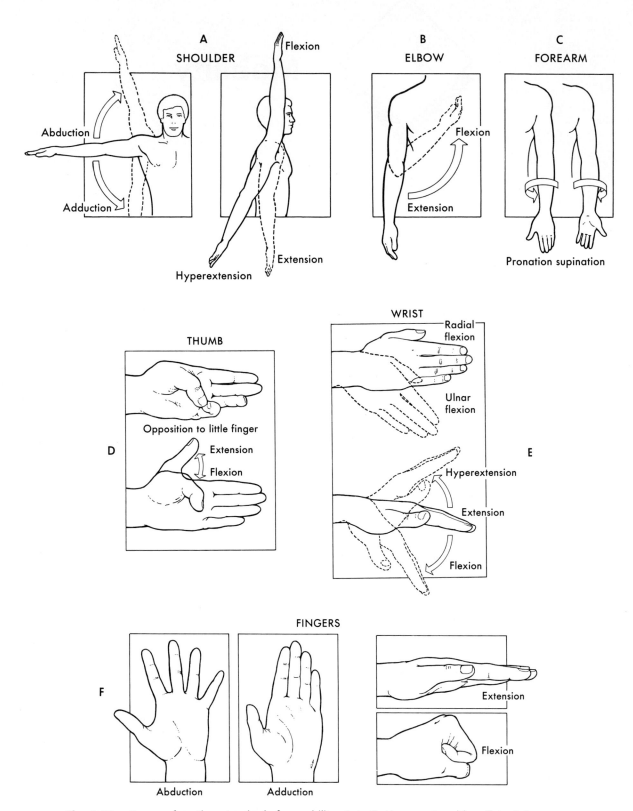

Fig. 3-27 Range-of-motion standards for mobility. **A** to **F,** Upper extremities. **G** to **J,** Lower extremities. (From Beare P., & Myers, J. [1990]. *The principles and practice of adult health nursing.* St. Louis: Mosby—Year Book.)

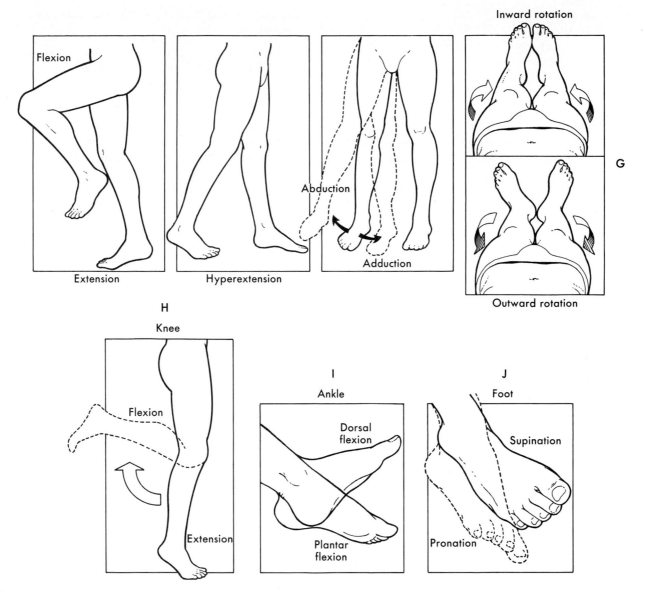

Fig. 3-27, cont'd   For legend see opposite page.

1. maintain muscle tone
2. increase muscle strength

Application of the Nursing Process to the Client with Mobility Problems

Assessment

1. Health history
   a. Current health status
   b. History of present complaint (e.g., weakness, stiffness, pain, or swelling)
   c. Usual activities (e.g., work, social and recreational pursuits)
   d. Diet and sleep patterns
2. Physical examination
   a. General inspection

1. symmetry of the two sides of the body
2. presence of spinal deformities, skin lesions, masses
3. posture
   b. Gait and balance: watch for specific gait patterns associated with specific disorders
   c. Joints: active and passive ROM
   d. Muscle strength and bulk
   e. Vascular system of extremities
      1. pulses
      2. varicosities
      3. edema
   f. Deep-tendon reflex testing (do not test in painful or arthritic joints)
      1. upper extremities

a. biceps
b. triceps
c. radial
2. lower extremities
a. patellar
b. Achilles
3. Diagnostic tests
   a. Radiological studies
   1. x-rays: detection of bone and soft-tissue injury
   2. bone scan: detection of bone tumors
   3. myelogram
      a. inspection of the spinal column
      b. radiopaque medium injected into subarachnoid space of the spine
      c. nursing care pretest:
         ◆ check for iodine allergy
         ◆ teach client regarding spinal tap and x-ray procedure
      d. nursing care posttest:
         ◆ keep flat in bed for 6-8 hours if client complains of a headache or if an oil-based medium was used
         ◆ keep head of bed elevated at least 20° if a water-based medium was used
         ◆ force fluids
   4. CAT scan
   5. MRI
   b. Hematological studies
   1. increased sedimentation rate and serum globulin (nonspecific for inflammatory process)
   2. C-reactive protein (CRP): arthritis
   3. elevated serum uric acid: gouty arthritis
   4. CBC (increased WBC with gouty arthritis)
   5. antinuclear antibodies (ANA): positive with systemic lupus erythematosus (SLE)
   c. Electromyogram (EMG): a graphic record of the contraction of a muscle as a result of electrical stimulation

Analysis
1. Safe, effective care environment
   a. High risk for trauma
   b. Impaired physical mobility
   c. Knowledge deficit
2. Physiological integrity
   a. Pain
   b. Impaired physical mobility
   c. High risk for disuse syndrome
3. Psychosocial integrity
   a. Anxiety
   b. Ineffective individual coping
   c. Body image disturbance
4. Health promotion/maintenance
   a. Altered health maintenance
   b. Impaired adjustment
   c. Diversional activity deficit

General Nursing Planning, Implementation, and Evaluation

Goal 1: Client will achieve and maintain maximum physical mobility.

Implementation
1. Teach client the proper use of assistive devices.
2. Help client learn proper use of prosthetic devices.
3. Provide needed support and encouragement.

Evaluation
Client expresses and demonstrates proper use of assistive devices; maintains maximum physical mobility.

Goal 2: Client will adapt to changes in body image.

Implementation
1. Encourage client to verbalize concerns.
2. Provide client with correct information about extent of body image alteration.

Evaluation
Client expresses self-acceptance; engages in usual social activities.

Goal 3: Client will be knowledgeable about disease process, medications, and the prevention of complications.

Implementation
1. Outline symptoms of disease.
2. Outline progression of disease if applicable.
3. Explain the rationale for ordered treatment regimen.
4. Provide information regarding the administration and side effects of all medications.
5. Discuss interventions that prevent the development of complications, including musculoskeletal damage and deficits.

Evaluation
Client takes medications as prescribed, returns for follow-up appointments; remains free from preventable complications.

Goal 4: Client will be free from complications of immobility.

Implementation
1. See *Sensation and Perception*, General Nursing Goal 2, p. 234.
2. Prevent constipation.
   a. Increase fluid intake, unless contraindicated.
   b. Increase dietary roughage.
3. Assist with active ROM exercises as appropriate. (see Fig. 3-27)
4. Prevent urinary calculi with increased fluids.

5. Prevent pressure sores.
   a. Turn q2h.
   b. Gently massage skin.
   c. Keep skin clean and dry.
6. Prevent thrombophlebitis.
   a. Apply antiembolic hose.
   b. Encourage isometric exercises.
   c. Avoid pillows behind the knees.
7. Prevent atelectasis by having client cough and deep-breathe.

Evaluation
   Client remains free from complications of immobility.

SELECTED HEALTH PROBLEMS RESULTING IN AN INTERFERENCE WITH MOBILITY

☐ Fractures

General Information
1. Types (can be assigned both classifications)
   a. Classified according to severity
      1. *compound:* open
      2. *closed:* simple
      3. *complete*
      4. *comminuted:* fragmented
      5. *compression:* depressed
      6. *stress:* fatigue or sudden violent force
      7. *pathological:* disease related, spontaneous
   b. Classified according to direction of fracture line
      1. *linear, longitudinal (vertical):* fracture runs parallel to long axis of the bone
      2. *transverse, horizontal:* fracture line runs straight across the bone
      3. *spiral:* twisted along shaft of the bone
      4. *oblique:* 45° angle
2. Risk factors
   a. Old age
   b. Active sports
   c. Accidents
   d. Osteoporosis from disease or steroid therapy
3. Medical treatment
   a. Closed reduction (external fixation)
      1. manual manipulation of bone fragments into anatomic alignment
      2. immobilized in cast/traction
   b. Open reduction (internal fixation)
      1. surgical procedure with direct visualization
      2. realignment of fracture fragments and immobilization with metallic device (e.g., plate, intramedullary rod)
      3. advantages: allows early weight bearing
      4. complications include postoperative infections and delayed union
   c. Ambulation with assistive devices
      1. crutches (see Table 3-59)
         a. non–weight bearing: 3-point gait
         b. weight bearing

Table 3-59   Common crutch-walking gaits

WEIGHT BEARING

Two-point gait—crutch on one side moves forward simultaneously with opposite leg; same motion is repeated on other side.

Four-point gait—two-point gait is broken down and performed more slowly. Crutch is placed and then followed by the opposite leg. Both motions are then repeated with the opposite side.

Swing-through gait—both crutches are moved forward together, then both legs are swung past the crutches by lifting both lower limbs.

NON–WEIGHT BEARING

Three-point gait—both crutches are moved forward together. Then the body swings forward to that position by lifting placed leg. Second limb is held off the ground at all times.

From Phipps, W., Long, B., & Woods, N. (1987). *Clinical handbook of medical-surgical nursing.* St. Louis: Mosby–Year Book.

   ◆ 2-point gait
   ◆ 4-point gait
   ◆ swing-through gait
      2. cane carried in hand opposite affected leg for support
      3. walker
      4. sling for arm
   d. Traction (refer to *Nursing Care of the Child,* p. 513)
4. Emergency care of suspected fractures
   a. Control of evident hemorrhage (most important problem); sterile bandage to open wound
   b. Immobilize affected part (splint) before moving client
   c. Do not attempt to reduce fracture
   d. Apply ice pack to reduce swelling, hematoma, pain
   e. Transport to medical facility as soon as possible

Nursing Process

Assessment
1. Age, developmental consideration
2. Usual activity, recreational needs
3. Circumstances of fracture occurrence (most result from accidents)
4. Concurrent health problems (will affect healing)
Analysis (see p. 256)
Planning, Implementation, and Evaluation

Goal 1: If closed reduction is used, client's cast will dry properly.

Implementation
1. Support cast on pillows along length of cast until dry (usually 24 hours).

2. Know that drying creates heat, which causes cast to harden; heat should be uniform in nature, not felt as isolated hot spots.
3. Use fan to stir air, but do not direct fan on the cast.
4. *Never* use heat lamp or hair dryer on plaster cast.
5. Do not completely cover the cast; when dry it is porous and will allow skin underneath to "breathe."
6. Avoid bearing weight on cast for 48 hours.
7. Do not handle cast when wet, if possible; handle with palms, not fingertips.
8. Do not place on hard surface while drying.
9. Know that x-ray will be taken after cast application to ensure proper alignment.

Evaluation

Client's cast dries completely with fracture in proper alignment.

Goal 2: Client will maintain good circulation after cast is applied.

Implementation

1. Observe for the five Ps of neurovascular assessment for muscle ischemia.
   a. Pain: progressive pain on movement of the affected extremity
   b. Pallor: in the affected extremity
   c. Paralysis: inability to move the affected part
   d. Paresthesia: numbness and tingling
   e. Pulselessness
2. Observe circulatory status in exposed fingers or toes frequently during each shift.
   a. Color: normal
   b. Temperature: warm and dry
   c. Swelling: minimal or none
   d. Circulation: good blanching; nail beds fill rapidly; adequate pulses
3. Observe for neurological impairment.
   a. Presence of persistent, localized pain
   b. Ability to move digits
   c. Degree of sensation
4. Avoid pressure areas on extremity.
   a. Position client away from side on which he has a cast.
   b. Support cast on pillow in a nondependent position.
   c. "Petal" cast edges to eliminate rough, abrasive edges (see Fig. 5-5, p. 516).

Evaluation

Client's toes (fingers) are warm, color good, blanch well.

Goal 3: Client's activity level will be safe and maintained to the extent allowed.

Implementation

1. Know the instruction client has been given for crutch walking and reinforce teaching.

2. Reinforce the principles of non–weight bearing or use of affected extremity.
3. Instruct client in principles of safe movement (e.g., no hopping around).
4. Instruct client in isometric, ROM exercises as appropriate.

Evaluation

Client uses crutches correctly and safely.

Goal 4: Client will experience relief of pain.

Implementation

1. Administer pain medications as ordered.
2. Know that pain should decrease after fracture is set (increasing pain may indicate that the cast is too tight or infection is beginning).
3. Instruct client to notify nurse of any new pain or pain unrelieved by analgesics.
4. Have client on crutches ambulate only with assistance after administration of pain medication.

Evaluation

Client is free from discomfort.

Goal 5: Client's rehabilitation course will remain free from complications.

Implementation

1. Teach client signs and symptoms of complications (e.g., poor circulation, infection, nerve damage).
   a. Check for "hot spots," which indicate an area of inflammation beneath them.
   b. Note odor under cast (necrotic tissue will produce malodor).
2. Teach client principles of cast care (see Table 3-60).
   a. Keep clean and dry.
   b. Do not put objects (e.g., for scratching) down the cast.
3. Alert client to possible side effects of decreased mobility (e.g., weight gain, constipation).
   a. Increase fluids.
   b. Readjust diet to include more protein and roughage, fewer carbohydrates.

Evaluation

Client demonstrates methods of cast care; maintains weight; remains free from infection and constipation.

Goal 6: If open reduction with a cast or skeletal traction is used, client will be free from postoperative complications.

Implementation

1. Observe for postoperative bleeding.
   a. Draw circle around evidence of bleeding on cast; mark with date and time.
   b. Check frequently.

Table 3-60   Client education guide to cast care

PLASTER OF PARIS CAST

Do not wash the cast, because washing can weaken the cast and allow mildew to form. A slightly damp rag with cleanser may be used if moisture is wiped away afterward.

Protect the cast with a plastic wrap during bathing or if in rain or snow.

Remove loose plaster crumbs from under cast edges and brush them away from the area.

SYNTHETIC CAST

Cover any rough edges by petaling, or smooth them by lightly filing with a nail file or emery board.

Use only a small amount of mild soap in the area of the cast if getting the cast wet is allowed; rinse the cast well after bathing.

Try to keep all particles, such as dirt or sand, out of the cast; rinse out any particles that may get into the cast.

After swimming in a chlorinated pool or lake, flush the cast thoroughly with water.

Thoroughly dry padding and stockinette each time the cast gets wet, so that skin maceration will not result:

1. Remove excess water by blotting cast with a towel.
2. Use a hand-held hair dryer (on cool or warm setting) in sweeping motion over cast surface to reduce drying time.
3. Continue drying cast for about 1 hour; the cast will be dry when it no longer feels cold and clammy.

From Beare, P., & Myers, J. (1990). *Principles and practice of adult health nursing.* St. Louis: Mosby—Year Book.

2. Apply ice pack if ordered to reduce swelling and pain (protect cast from moisture).
3. Administer analgesics as ordered.
4. Maintain traction in proper alignment, with correct amount of weight.
5. Prevent complications of immobilization.
   a. Give frequent skin care over bony prominences to prevent decubitus ulcers; use sheepskin or egg-crate mattress.
   b. Perform isometric and ROM exercises on unaffected extremities to prevent contractures, thrombophlebitis, footdrop.
   c. Know that if the fracture occurred in the middle third of the femur, client may exercise ankle; if fracture is in the lower third, no ankle exercise.
   d. Increase fluids, roughage to prevent constipation, urinary calculi.
6. Observe carefully for postoperative would infection.
   a. Provide pin care q8h if in skeletal traction.
   b. If client has a cast, observe for increased pain, swelling, or a malodor coming from cast.
7. Provide bedridden client with age-appropriate diversions or activities, if possible.
   a. Arrange for schoolwork for child or adolescent.

b. Arrange private time for adult clients and their visitors.
8. Be aware that prolonged bed rest may lead to sleep disturbances, sensory deprivation.

Evaluation

Client is free from complications during the recovery phase (maintains proper alignment, skin integrity); performs ROM exercises on unaffected extremities.

☐ Fractured Hip (Proximal End of Femur)

General Information

1. Definition: "broken hips" include fractures that are within the head of the femur, associated with osteoporosis and minor trauma; extracapsular fractures that occur below the capsule and are caused by severe trauma or a fall; and those of the greater or lesser trochanter
2. Incidence
   a. Increases after age 60
   b. More common in women than men
3. Precipitating factors
   a. Falls associated with osteoporotic and degenerative changes of the bone
   b. Age-related physiological changes in balance and perception
4. Medical treatment
   a. Medical intervention: closed reduction achieved with traction (rare in older clients)
   b. Surgical intervention: open reduction and internal fixation, or a prosthetic head-of-the-femur

Nursing Process

Assessment

1. Affected leg
   a. Shortened
   b. Externally rotated
   c. Abducted
   d. Severe pain and tenderness
2. Age of client and circumstances of injury
3. Current health and mental status, including degree of orientation
4. Availability of family support mechanisms

Analysis (see p. 256)

Planning, Implementation, and Evaluation

Goal 1: Preoperatively, client will experience relief of symptoms and be protected from further injury.

Implementation

1. Administer analgesics as ordered.
2. Use skin traction (Buck's) to relieve muscle spasms and reduce edema.
3. Turn only 45° to affected side; may turn only slightly to unaffected side, with or without traction.
4. Use fracture pan for elimination.
5. Prevent external rotation of affected hip.

6. Assess and monitor coexisting medical problems.
Evaluation

Client remains free from preoperative pain with affected leg in good alignment.

Goal 2: Postoperatively, client will maintain the proper position for functional healing of the hip.

Implementation
1. Prepare client's bed (e.g., firm mattress, bed board, overhead trapeze, adjustable footboard, bed rails, and other decubitus ulcer–prevention aids).
2. Know that rapid onset of sharp hip pain may indicate dislocation.
3. For femoral head prosthesis: prevent internal rotation and maintain abduction of affected leg at all times (e.g., use an abductor splint or pillows between legs).
4. For internal fixation with nails or pins: prevent external rotation by placing a trochanter roll along affected side.
5. Turn every 2 hours alternating unaffected side and back.
6. Apply an antiembolic stocking from toes to groin on unaffected leg.
7. Monitor Hemovac drainage; ensure that tubes remain patent.
8. Prevent acute flexion of hip by keeping bed low (e.g., not higher than 35°-40°); elevate only for meals.
Evaluation

Client is afebrile postoperatively; has minimal pain; maintains affected leg in abduction.

Goal 3: Client will remain free from complications of immobility.

Implementation
1. See General Nursing Goal 4, p. 256.
Evaluation

Client's postoperative course is free from complications (e.g., no fever, skin in good condition).

Goal 4: Client's activity level will increase progressively (depending on type of surgery and degree of bone healing).

Implementation
1. Internal fixation with nails or pins
   a. Have client stand first.
   b. Get client up in chair 1-2 days postoperatively.
   c. Allow only partial weight bearing for 3 months.
   d. Allow full weight bearing in 6 months.
2. Femoral-head prosthesis:
   a. Use measures to prevent dislocation at all times.
   b. Have client stand at side of bed, starting 2-4 days postoperatively.

c. Allow partial weight bearing 4-10 days postoperatively.
   d. Allow full weight bearing 2-6 months postoperatively.
   e. Do not use wheelchair for 2 weeks to aid rising to a standing position and to prevent hyperflexion.
   f. Prevent flexion greater than 90°.
3. Consult physician regarding muscle-setting exercises for gluteal and quadriceps muscles, movements of the affected leg, ambulation, and weight bearing on the unaffected leg.
4. Work with physical therapist to coordinate exercise and mobilization regimen.
5. Perform full ROM exercises at least twice daily on unaffected limbs.
6. Lead with *unaffected* leg when using transfer techniques.
Evaluation

Client ambulates with or without assistance and with or without partial weight bearing, depending on surgical intervention.

Goal 5: Client will remain free from psychosocial complications of hospitalization and immobility.

Implementation
1. Refer to "Depression," p. 48, and "Confused Behavior," p. 42.
Evaluation

Client maintains contact with reality; is minimally confused, disoriented, and dependent.

Goal 6: Client will regain use of joint to the maximum degree possible.

Implementation
1. Refer to General Nursing Goal 4, p. 256.
2. Teach client and family about precautions after discharge.
   a. Avoid sleeping on operative side.
   b. Use cane, walker, or crutches for support and partial weight bearing; wear sturdy shoes when walking.
   c. Do not cross or twist legs.
   d. Do not lift heavy objects.
   e. Observe carefully for signs of wound infection.
3. Reinforce need for continued exercise and maintenance of normal activities as possible.
Evaluation

Client uses rehabilitative measures to enhance recovery; pursues activities within range of ability, age, and level of interest.

Goal 7: Client will develop a workable plan for long-term convalescence.

Implementation

1. Help client and significant others decide about home care or where client will go upon discharge (e.g., home, extended-care facility).
2. Teach client and significant others about
   a. Length of convalescence and progress of weight-bearing ambulation.
   b. General health measures to be followed (e.g., medications, exercise, diet).
   c. Correct safety precautions for use of cane, walker, or wheelchair.
   d. Persons and agencies who can be contacted for services.
3. Help client and significant others develop a plan to eliminate unsafe environmental conditions that may have contributed to fracture.

Evaluation

Client makes adequate arrangements for long-term convalescence.

☐ Amputation
General Information

1. Definition: removal of an appendage or limb
2. Indications
   a. Certain tumors
   b. Severe traumatic injuries (usually affects upper extremities)
   c. Problems related to peripheral vascular disease (e.g., gangrene); usually affects lower extremities

Nursing Process

Assessment

1. Physical and psychological strengths of client
2. Support systems (e.g., family and friends)
3. Health status, high-risk factors (i.e., smoking habits, cardiovascular disease, diabetes, cancer)
4. Condition of affected appendage or limb
   a. Color of skin
      1. necrotic tissue may be blue or gray-blue
      2. turns dark brown or black
   b. Presence of infection
      1. red streaks along lymphatic channels
      2. systemic symptoms

Analysis (see p. 256)
Planning, Implementation, and Evaluation

> **Goal 1:** Client will be physically and emotionally prepared for surgical outcome.

Implementation

1. Refer to "Perioperative Period," p. 117.
2. Explain that surgery is performed above level of healthy tissue.
3. Explain that grieving is normal.
4. Allow client and significant others opportunities to express anger and fears.

5. Initiate exercises to develop strength in muscles that will be used in rehabilitation.
6. Prepare client for postoperative stump care and prosthesis if appropriate.
7. Give prophylactic antibiotics as ordered.

Evaluation

Client expresses grief over anticipated loss.

> **Goal 2:** Client's stump will remain free from contractures and will be reduced in size.

Implementation

1. Elevate stump for 24 hours (to hasten venous return and prevent edema).
2. Avoid elevation of stump after first 48 hours postoperatively to prevent hip contracture (most common postoperative complication).
3. Keep stump in an extended position; have client with a leg amputation lie prone for short periods 2-3 times daily to prevent flexion contractures.
4. Use "shrinker sock" or elastic bandage if prosthetic fitting is delayed; apply in a *figure-eight* fashion to reduce size of stump in preparation for prosthesis; teach client how to apply properly (elastic bandages applied to above-the-knee amputations are also wrapped around the waist).
5. Know that an immediate prosthetic fit reduces the incidence of postoperative complications, particularly incisional pain and phantom limb sensation.

Evaluation

Client applies shrinker sock properly; stump is clean, free from contractures; experiences minimal pain.

> **Goal 3:** Client will recover from surgery free from complications.

Implementation

1. Refer to "Perioperative Period," p. 117.
2. Know that pain may be sharp and acute in the incisional area.
3. Assess for phantom limb sensation vs. phantom limb pain (limb sensation subsides with time).

> **Goal 4:** Client will adapt to altered body image.

Implementation

1. Refer to General Nursing Goal 2, p. 256.

> **Goal 5:** Client will use prescribed prosthetic device.

Implementation

1. See General Nursing Goal 1, p. 256.
2. Know that a good prosthetic fit takes time and adjustments.
3. Reinforce teaching done by the prosthetist.

4. Teach client to observe stump for signs of infection, irritation.
5. Teach client proper skin care: wash and dry daily, avoid use of skin creams.
6. Continue to offer encouragement and support to client and significant others throughout the rehabilitation process.
7. Reinforce client's efforts at maintaining balance and posture, and increasing auxiliary muscle strength.
8. If prosthesis is not an option, instruct client in safe use of wheelchair, transfer techniques.

Evaluation

Client adapts to prosthesis with few problems; transfers from bed to wheelchair safely.

☐ Arthritis
General Information

1. Rheumatoid arthritis
   a. Definition: a chronic, systemic, diffuse, collagen disease characterized by inflammatory changes in joints and related structures, resulting in crippling deformities
   b. Incidence
      1. occurs three times more frequently in women
      2. peak incidence between 30 and 40 years of age
      3. primarily affects proximal joints and synovial membranes before involving larger weight-bearing joints
   c. Predisposing factors
      1. possibly an autoimmune disorder
      2. stress, obesity, aggravation are implicated
   d. Pathophysiological sequence: synovitis → pannus formation → fibrous ankylosis → bony ankylosis (frozen joint)
   e. Osteoporosis is common
2. Osteoarthritis
   a. Definition: a chronic disease involving the weight-bearing joints; nonsystemic
   b. Incidence
      1. occurs five times more frequently in women
      2. peak incidence between 50 and 70 years of age
   c. Predisposing factors
      1. aging
      2. trauma
      3. excessive use of joint (e.g., worker who sews)
      4. obesity
   d. Pathophysiological sequence: degeneration of articular cartilage → new bone formation: Heberden's nodes (bony nodules or spurs on the dorsolateral aspects of distal joints of fingers)
3. Gouty arthritis
   a. Definition: inflammation of a joint caused by gout (uric acid crystals deposited in joint)
   b. Incidence
      1. 19 times more frequent in men
      2. peak incidence between ages 20 and 40
      3. often affects a terminal joint (e.g., great toe)
   c. Predisposing factors
      1. hyperuricemia
      2. several metabolic disorders
   d. Pathophysiology
      1. metabolic disorders of purine metabolism
      2. urate deposits in and around joints
4. Surgical interventions: for rheumatoid arthritis, osteoarthritis
   a. *Tendon transplant:* from a normal muscle to another location to assume function of a damaged muscle
   b. *Osteotomy:* cutting bone to correct bone or joint deformity
   c. *Synovectomy:* removal of synovial membrane; helps prevent recurrent inflammation
   d. *Arthroplasty*
      1. hemiarthroplasty: one part of a joint is replaced (e.g., head of femur)
      2. total hip replacement: head of the femur and the acetabulum are replaced
      3. total knee replacement: both articular surfaces of the knee are replaced
      4. interphalangeal joint replacement

Nursing Process: Rheumatoid Arthritis and Osteoarthritis

Assessment
1. Rheumatoid arthritis
   a. Stiffness, especially in morning
   b. Proximal joint pain that decreases with use; fingers usually involved
   c. Swollen joint
   d. Limitation of muscle strength and atrophy; functional impairment caused by pain and muscle irritation
   e. Acute and chronic episodes with remissions and exacerbations
   f. Systemic symptoms (e.g., anemia, fatigue, elevated body temperature)
   g. Elevated sedimentation rate, serum rheumatoid factors
2. Osteoarthritis
   a. Stiffness, especially in morning
   b. Joint pain that increases with use
   c. Limitation of joint motion; no systemic symptoms
   d. Aggravation of symptoms with temperature, humidity change, and weight bearing

Analysis (see p. 256)
Planning, Implementation, and Evaluation

Goal 1: Client will function as comfortably and as normally as possible.

Implementation

1. Teach client to balance rest and activity.
   a. Encourage to optimum level of functioning.
   b. Exercise joint to point of pain—never beyond.
   c. Perform PT and OT activities as prescribed.
   d. During acute phase maintain complete bed rest and wear splints on affected joints as prescribed.
2. Apply heat to provide analgesia and relax muscles.
3. Teach client about medications and their side effects; see Tables 3-33 and 3-61.
4. Help client modify environment to accomplish activities easily.

Evaluation

Client maintains activity without undue stress; can state side effects of ordered medications.

Goal 2: Client will adjust to the chronicity of the condition.

Implementation

1. Allow client to express fear and concerns.
2. Encourage as much activity as possible.
3. Teach client that continuous immobilization may cause increased pain.

4. Teach client to avoid sudden jarring movements of joints.
5. Warn client about "quacks" who promise miracle cures.
6. Encourage continued follow-up to reevaluate progression of disease and efficacy of drug therapy.
7. Counsel client and family regarding the need for a well-balanced diet and, if obesity is a problem, weight reduction.

Evaluation

Client states a willingness to continue with therapeutic regimen as prescribed; expresses concerns about chronicity of the disease; maintains maximum activity level.

Goal 3: Client will be prepared for surgery.

Implementation

1. Refer to "Perioperative Period," p. 117.
2. Usually joint surgeries require multiple preps, then covering with a sterile towel.

Evaluation

Client describes what to expect in immediate postoperative period.

Table 3-61   Antiinflammatory drugs

Type	Side effects	Nursing implications
Acetylsalicylic acid (aspirin)	Tinnitus, GI distress, nausea, vomiting, prolonged bleeding time	Give with food, milk, or antacids. Avoid use with oral or parenteral anticoagulants.
Phenylbutazone (Butazolidin)	Nausea, vomiting, diarrhea, bone marrow depression, cardiac decompensation, salt and water retention, liver damage	Give with food, milk, or antacids. Monitor client for fever, sore throat, mouth ulcers, bleeding, and weight gain. Monitor CBC. Record client's weight and I&O daily.
Ibuprofen (Motrin)	Epigastric distress, nausea, vomiting, occult blood loss	Give with food, milk, or antacids. Monitor for GI distress, weight gain. Check renal and hepatic function in long-term therapy.
Indomethacin (Indocin)	Headaches, dizziness, blurred vision, nausea, vomiting, severe GI bleeding, hemolytic anemia, bone marrow depression	Give with food, milk, or antacids. Contraindicated for clients with aspirin allergy and GI disorders. In long-term drug therapy, monitor CBC and renal function, and encourage eye examinations.
Naproxen (Naprosyn)	Epigastric distress, nausea, occult blood loss	Monitor for GI distress.
Sulindac (Clinoril)	Epigastric distress, nausea, occult blood loss, aplastic anemia	Give with food, milk, or antacids. Monitor for bleeding. Watch for edema and periodically check blood pressure.
Piroxicam (Feldene)	Same as indomethacin (Indocin)	Same as indomethacin.
Gold salts (Myochrysine)	Renal and hepatic damage, corneal deposits, ulcerations in mouth, dermatitis	Monitor for skin eruptions, metallic taste in mouth, oral lesions.
Corticosteroids (see Table 3-33)		

Goal 4: If surgery is performed on the affected hip, client will remain free from postoperative complications.

Implementation
1. Refer to "Perioperative Period," p. 117.
2. See Goal 2, "Fractured Hip," p. 260.

Goal 5: Client will regain use of joint to the maximum degree possible.

Implementation
1. Refer to Goal 6, "Fractured Hip," p. 260.

Nursing Process: Gouty Arthritis

Assessment
1. Pain, swelling, and inflammation of affected joint (usually great toe)
2. Increased serum uric acid, sedimentation rate, WBC count

Analysis (see p. 256)

Planning, Implementation, and Evaluation

Goal 1 and 2: Refer to "Rheumatoid Arthritis," p. 262.

Goal 3: Client will adjust diet and life-style to prevent future attacks.

Implementation
1. Teach client about use of medications and their side effects.
2. Obtain dietary counseling for client; instruct in a low-purine diet (i.e., restrict meats, especially organ meats, and legumes).
3. Encourage daily high intake of fluids to prevent precipitation of uric acid crystals in the kidney.
4. Advise regarding weight control as needed.

Evaluation

Client lists foods to be avoided; has a plan for weight reduction, if indicated.

☐ Collagen Disease
General Information

1. Definition: a group of diseases characterized by widespread pathological changes in connective tissue; these are difficult to diagnose, have no cure, and cannot be prevented
2. Systemic lupus erythematosus (SLE): generalized connective tissue disorder
   a. Incidence
      1. affects women four times more frequently than men
      2. more likely to occur in young adults and adolescents
   b. Etiology and risk factors are unknown; an autoimmune disease
3. Medical treatment: aim is temporary remission or slowing of collagen destruction
   a. High doses of steroids for exacerbation
   b. Aspirin for pain
   c. Nonsteroidal antiinflammatory drugs
   d. Plasmapheresis (plasma exchange)

Nursing Process

Assessment
1. Arthritis-like symptoms

Table 3-62   Antigout medications

Types	Uses	Action	Side effects	Nursing implications
Colchicine	Gout	Inhibits renal tubular reabsorption of urate	Nausea, vomiting, abdominal pain, diarrhea, aplastic anemia, and agranulocytosis with prolonged use	Monitor for GI distress. Monitor fluid I&O. Keep daily output at 2000 ml; force fluids (6-8 glasses/day).
Allopurinol (Zyloprim)	Gout	Reduces the production of uric acid	GI distress, drowsiness, headache, dizziness, agranulocytosis, aplastic anemia, and skin rash	Monitor for rash (may be first sign of severe hypersensitivity reaction). Give with or immediately after meals. Monitor I&O. Keep daily output at 2000 ml; force fluids (6-8 glasses/day). Periodically check CBC, hepatic and renal function.
Phenylbutazone (Butazolidin)	Acute gout	Antiinflammatory, antipyretic analgesic	See Table 3-61.	See Table 3-61.

2. Sensitivity to sun
3. Presence of erythematous "butterfly" rash across bridge of nose
4. Alopecia
5. Involvement of other organ systems
   a. Renal (leading cause of death)
   b. Cardiovascular
   c. Peripheral vascular
   d. Nervous
   e. Respiratory
6. Polymyositis (inflammation of skeletal muscle)
7. Raynaud's phenomenon
8. Diagnostic test results
   a. Positive lupus erythematosus (LE) prep
   b. Anemia
   c. Proteinuria

Analysis (see p. 256)

Planning, Implementation, and Evaluation

Goal 1: Client will follow correct medication regimen.

Implementation
1. Outline plan for steroid therapy.
2. Minimize side effects through diet modification, time of administration, etc.
3. Teach client safety precautions for steroid therapy (see Table 3-33).

Evaluation
Client describes medications, expected side effects, and ways to minimize them.

Goal 2: Client will understand disease and its complications.

Implementation
1. See General Nursing Goal 3, p. 256.

☐ Lumbar Herniated Nucleus Pulposus (Ruptured Disk)

General Information
1. Definition: a protrusion of the gelatinous cushion between the vertebrae (intervertebral disk) through the surrounding cartilage causing pressure on nerve roots with resultant pain; most common sites are L3-4, L4-5, L5-S1
2. Incidence: more frequent in men
3. Predisposing/risk factors
   a. Sedentary occupations
   b. Long-term driving (e.g., truck driver)
   c. Infrequent physical exercise, certain sports (e.g., bowling, baseball)
4. Medical treatment
   a. Medical intervention
      1. bed rest on a firm mattress with bed board

2. pelvic traction
3. proper body alignment (e.g., no prone position)
4. medications
   a. muscle relaxants
   b. analgesics
   c. nonsteroidal antiinflammatory agents
   d. steroids
5. physical therapy
   a. diathermy
   b. back exercises
   c. braces
6. weight reduction as needed
   b. Surgical intervention
      1. indications
         a. prevention of further nerve damage and deficits
         b. severe back and leg pain that does not respond to conservative therapy
         c. a totally extruded disk that causes sensory and motor deficits in the lower extremities, bowel, and bladder (an emergency)
      2. procedures
         a. *laminectomy:* removal of the posterior arch of the vertebra to relieve pressure on the nerve root
         b. *spinal fusion* (for additional stability): bone graft from iliac crest used to fuse two or more vertebrae together
         c. *chemonucleolysis:* relieves pressure if pain persists (check for allergies to meat tenderizer or papaya)
      3. success rate ranges from 50%-90%

Nursing Process

Assessment
1. Low-back pain radiating down posterior thigh (sciatic nerve involvement)
2. Paresthesia of affected nerve roots
3. Muscle weakness, muscle spasm in lumbar region
4. Numbness, weakness, paralysis, or decreased reflexes along affected nerve pathway of leg, ankle, and foot
5. Character of pain
   a. Intermittent; more frequent and severe depending on degree of herniation
   b. May be related to a single traumatic event
   c. Gets progressively worse
   d. Worsened by anterior and lateral flexion of the spine; rotational movements, laughing, sneezing, coughing, straining; straight leg raising to 80° or 90° while supine
6. Client's occupation, exercise routine, physical status
7. Diagnostic tests
   a. CAT scan
   b. MRI scan

Analysis (see p. 256)
Planning, Implementation, and Evaluation

Goal 1: Client will be relieved of pain.

Implementation
1. Place on bed rest on a firm mattress with bed board; traction as ordered.
2. Administer analgesics, muscle relaxants as ordered, noting client's response.
3. Prevent twisting and straining.
4. Use noninvasive methods to relieve pain (e.g., frequent back rubs, diversion).

Evaluation
Client experiences decreased pain; requires infrequent analgesia; maintains bed rest.

Goal 2: Client will learn how to care for back to prevent future episodes.

Implementation
1. Observe and reinforce physical therapy regimens.
2. Give warm bath and muscle relaxants prn prior to exercise sessions.
3. Help client apply back supports in a side lying position and observe for any signs of skin irritation.
4. Teach client to use appropriate body mechanics.
   a. Use broad base of support.
   b. Use large body muscles.
   c. Maintain good posture.
   d. Bring object close to the body before moving.
   e. Pull rather than push an object.
   f. Do not lift items.
   g. Squat, do not bend over.
5. Walk rather than stand, but stand rather than sit.

Evaluation
Client demonstrates back exercises correctly and states a willingness to do them regularly; demonstrates use of appropriate body mechanics.

Goal 3: If surgery is required, client will be physically and psychologically prepared for surgery.

Implementation
1. Refer to "Perioperative Period," p. 117.
2. Explain importance and demonstrate postoperative positioning, log roll turning, and body alignment.
3. Explain that if spinal fusion is to be done, a turning frame may be used.
4. Tell client about incision needed for bone graft and Hemovac that may be in place.
5. Obtain preoperative neurological assessment for postoperative comparison.

Evaluation
Client verbalizes a positive attitude toward the surgical outcome; demonstrates understanding of planned procedure and immediate postoperative care.

Goal 4: Client will remain free from postoperative complications.

Implementation
1. Refer to "Perioperative Period," p. 117.
2. Keep client flat in bed for first 12 hours; then may raise head of bed to 30°.
3. Know that client will usually get out of bed on first or second postoperative day (unless spinal fusion done).
4. Use turning sheet and turn client by log rolling.
5. Tell client to report numbness or tingling in feet or legs.
6. Give medications as ordered for pain and frequent muscle spasms.
7. Provide laxative to avoid straining.
8. When client is allowed to be up, have client stand and not sit.
9. Apply antiembolic stockings and have client do leg exercises to prevent thrombophlebitis.
10. For better support when client is ambulating, have client wear shoes and not slippers.
11. Prepare client for 3-6 months with body cast or brace postoperatively if fusion was done.

Evaluation
Client has uneventful postoperative course; maintains dry and intact dressing; has adequate sensation in toes; ambulates frequently with minimal discomfort.

Goal 5: Client and significant others will be adequately prepared for discharge.

Implementation
1. Refer to General Nursing Goal 3, p. 256.
2. Provide client and significant others with written instructions regarding care of operation site, back care regimen, and back exercises.
3. Ensure that client knows proper application of back brace, if ordered.
4. Provide client with a list of instructions or a timetable to resume activities such as driving, sexual intercourse, sports, housework, or job responsibilities.
5. Ensure that client knows to report signs of illness, fever, increasing back pain, or muscle spasms to physician.

Evaluation
Client states schedule for exercising; applies back brace correctly; knows when to resume additional activities.

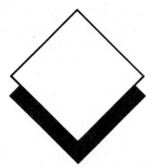

Cellular Aberration

The nursing care presented in this unit contains selected health problems related to neoplastic disease.

GENERAL CONCEPTS
Overview/Physiology

1. Terms pertaining to neoplasia
   a. *Cancer:* a group of diseases characterized by uncontrolled growth and spread of abnormal cells
   b. *Neoplasia:* uncontrolled cell growth that follows no physiological demand
   c. *Carcinoma:* a malignant tumor arising from epithelial tissue
   d. *Sarcoma:* a malignant tumor arising from nonepithelial tissue (connective, muscle, and osseous tissue)
   e. *Differentiation:* degree to which neoplastic tissue resembles the parent tissue
   f. *Metastasis:* spread of cancer from its original site to other parts of the body
   g. *Adjuvant therapy:* therapy designed to be adjunctive or supplemental to primary therapy
   h. *Palliation:* relief or alleviation of symptoms without cure
   i. *Dysplasia:* bizarre cell growth resulting in cells that differ in size, shape, or arrangement from other cells of the same type of tissue
2. Tumors are characterized by tissue of origin
   a. Adeno: glandular tissue
   b. Angio: blood vessels
   c. Basal cell: epithelium, mainly sun-exposed areas
   d. Embryonal: gonads
   e. Fibro: fibrous tissue
   f. Lympho: lymphoid tissue
   g. Melano: pigmented cells of epithelium
   h. Myo: muscle tissue
   i. Osteo: bone
   j. Squamous cell: epithelium
3. Incidence
   a. Second leading cause of death in the United States (after cardiovascular disease)
   b. One of every four Americans can expect to develop cancer
   c. Occurs in all age groups; incidence increases with age
   d. Most cancer occurs in adults age 65 or older
4. Etiology: no *single* cause
5. Risk factors (American Cancer Society)
   a. Tobacco: smoking or chewing
   b. Alcohol: excessive intake
   c. Hormones (e.g., estrogen, diethylstilbestrol [DES])
   d. Genetic predisposition
   e. Immune deficiency
   f. Age
   g. Occupational: exposure to carcinogens (e.g., asbestos, vinyl chloride, or benzene)
   h. X-rays: overexposure
   i. Sunlight: long exposure
   j. Diet: high fat or high total calories, lack of fiber
6. Characteristics of malignant cells
   a. Anaplastic (loss of differentiation)
   b. Disorderly division
   c. Uncontrolled growth pattern
   d. Loss of normal growth-limiting mechanisms (expands in all directions)
   e. Nonencapsulated
   f. Tend to metastasize
   g. May be necrotic from poor vascular supply
   h. Often recur after treatment
7. Metastasis
   a. Modes
      1. lymphatic
      2. vascular
      3. direct extension
      4. seeding
   b. Site(s)
      1. usually determined by the lymph and blood drainage patterns of the original cancer site (e.g., primary tumors entering systemic venous circulation are apt to lodge in the lung)

2. most common: lung, liver, bone, and brain
8. Classification
   a. Grading: tumor cells are classified from Grade 1 to Grade 4 (the higher the grade, the poorer the prognosis)
   b. TNM classification: a widely used classification system that stages the primary tumor, regional nodes, and evidence of metastasis
9. Prognosis depends on
   a. Tumor size
   b. Nodal involvement
   c. Metastasis

Application of the Nursing Process to the Client with Cancer

Assessment

1. Health history
   a. Seven warning signs (CAUTION)
      1. *C*hange in usual bowel and bladder function
      2. *A* sore that does not heal
      3. *U*nusual bleeding or discharge: hematuria, tarry stools, ecchymosis, bleeding mole
      4. *T*hickening or a lump in the breast or elsewhere
      5. *I*ndigestion or dysphagia
      6. *O*bvious change in a wart or mole
      7. *N*agging cough or hoarseness
   b. Family history
   c. Presenting symptoms
      1. appetite
      2. weight loss
      3. energy level
      4. pain (severe pain is *not* a common early problem)
2. Physical exam
   a. General appearance
   b. Percussion
      1. fluid waves (ascites)
      2. chest percussion
   c. Palpation
      1. masses (breast/testicular exam)
      2. lymph nodes
3. Diagnostic tests
   a. Lab tests
      1. CBC, platelet count
      2. blood chemistries
      3. CEA (carcinoembryonic antigen): a tumor marker
      4. AFP titer (alpha-fetoprotein): presence suggests testicular, ovarian, gastric, or pancreatic cancer
      5. specific tests depending on suspected site of cancer
   b. Cytological studies (microscopic exam of body secretions for cancer cells) (e.g., Pap smear, sputum cytology)
   c. Biopsy of mass

   d. Radiological studies
      1. x-rays (e.g., mammogram)
      2. computerized axial tomography (CAT) scans
      3. radioisotope scanning
      4. ultrasound
      5. thermography
   e. Endoscopic examinations (e.g., bronchoscopy, gastroscopy)
   f. Magnetic resonance imaging (MRI)
4. Medical treatment
   a. Surgery
      1. principles
         a. excision/radical excision: tumor plus margin of healthy tissue must be excised
         b. often results in some significant defect or loss of function
      2. uses
         a. diagnosis
         b. cure
         c. palliation
            ◆ remove obstruction
            ◆ debulk large unresectable tumors
            ◆ control pain (e.g., cordotomies, nerve blocks)
         d. ablation: removal of hormone-producing organs to effect a response in hormone-dependent tumor
         e. reconstruction
         f. prophylaxis: removal of lesions that are likely to develop into cancer (e.g., polyps)
   b. Radiation
      1. definition: the use of ionizing radiation to cause damage and destruction to cancerous growths
      2. effect: radiation causes damage at the cellular level
         a. indirectly: water molecules within the cell are ionized
         b. directly: causes strand breakage in the double helix of DNA
         c. not every cell is damaged beyond repair
      3. uses
         a. cure
         b. palliation
         c. combined with surgery
            ◆ preoperatively: to reduce size of the tumor
            ◆ postoperatively: to retard/control metastasis of tumors cells
         d. combined with chemotherapy
      4. administration
         a. external
            ◆ orthovoltage machines: delivers radiation dose to superficial lesions
            ◆ megavoltage (cobalt-60): delivers radiation to deeper body structures
            ◆ linear accelerators: delivers radiation

dosage to deep lesions without harming skin and with less scattering of radiation within body tissues

    b. internal (e.g., implants)

5. side effects

    a. radiation syndrome: systemic effects not related to site treated

- fatigue, malaise
- headache
- anorexia, nausea, vomiting

    b. specific side effects: related to site treated

- cranium: transitory or permanent hair loss (i.e., alopecia)
- mouth, rectum: mucositis, stomatitis
- mouth, head, and neck: taste alteration, reduced saliva production (xerostomia), dental caries
- throat, esophagus: dysphagia
- GI tract: nausea, vomiting, diarrhea
- abdomen: malnutrition, anorexia
- pelvis, long bones, sternum: bone marrow suppression
  - thrombocytopenia (decrease in platelets), which leads to bleeding
  - leukopenia (decrease in WBCs), which leads to infection
  - erythropenia (decrease in RBCs), which leads to anemia
- bladder, pelvis: cystitis
- testicles, ovaries: sterility
- rectum: proctitis
- lungs, chest wall: pneumonitis
- skin: dry desquamation
- vagina: shortening and narrowing, loss of lubrication

c. Chemotherapy

1. definition: the use of drugs to retard the growth of or destroy cancerous cells
2. classification/effect (see Table 5-23, p. 520).

    a. antineoplastics

- cell-cycle specific: attack cells at a specific point in the process of cell division
- cell-cycle nonspecific: act at one time during cell division

    b. hormones

- alter the hormone balance
- modify the growth of some hormone-dependent tumors

3. combination chemotherapy

    a. two or more drugs used simultaneously

    b. each drug has different effect

    c. increases the effectiveness of the destruction or retardation of cancerous cells

4. uses

    a. cure

    b. palliation

    c. combined with surgery

    d. combined with radiation

5. administration

    a. intravenous infusion

- most common route
- diffuses drug throughout the entire body

    b. arterial infusion

- drug is introduced through a catheter directly into the tumor via the main artery that supplies it
- advantage: high proportion of drug is absorbed by tumor before it reaches systemic circulation

    c. regional perfusion

- one extremity is isolated from the general circulation
- advantage: systemic circulation of drug is diminished, thus systemic toxic effects are reduced

    d. intraperitoneal chemotherapy

- allows for high drug concentration in the peritoneal cavity for treatment of ovarian cancer and some colorectal cancers
- advantage: keeps systemic toxicity at a lower level because of the peritoneal cavity's cellular barrier
- procedure is time consuming: requires infusion of chemotherapy diluted in 2 L of warmed normal saline, a 4-hour dwell time, and 2 hours for drainage

    e. oral, IM (less common)

6. drug-specific side effects (see Table 5-23)

    a. nausea and vomiting

    b. bone marrow depression

    c. alopecia

    d. fatigue, anorexia

    e. stomatitis

    f. menstrual irregularities, aspermatogenesis

    g. renal damage

d. Biological response modifiers

1. definition: treatments that have the ability to alter the immunological relationship between a tumor and the client with cancer to provide a therapeutic benefit
2. types

    a. interferons

- have antiviral and antitumor properties
- help restore and strengthen immune mechanisms
- effective on hairy-cell leukemia

    b. monoclonal antibodies: the growth and production of specific antibodies to fight specific malignant cells

c. lymphokines and cytokines (interleukin-2)
- ◆ stimulate the production and activation of T lymphocytes
- ◆ help improve the cell-killing activity of the killer cells and cytotoxic T cells

e. Bone marrow transplant (BMT)
  1. used to treat
     a. acute lymphoblastic leukemia
     b. acute myelogenous leukemia
     c. aplastic anemia
     d. chronic myelogenous leukemia
  2. types
     a. allogeneic BMT: bone marrow comes from a healthy donor (usually an immediate family member)
     b. autologous BMT: client is given own bone marrow
f. Supportive (e.g., nutrition, comfort measures)

Analysis
1. Safe, effective care environment
   a. High risk for infection
   b. High risk for injury
   c. Sensory-perceptual alterations: visual, auditory, kinesthetic, gustatory, tactile, olfactory
2. Physiological integrity
   a. Pain
   b. Fatigue
   c. Altered nutrition: less than body requirements
   d. Altered oral mucous membranes

3. Psychosocial integrity
   a. Anxiety
   b. Body image disturbance
   c. Ineffective individual coping
   d. Anticipatory grieving
4. Health promotion/maintenance
   a. Knowledge deficit
   b. Ineffective family coping: compromised
   c. Diversional activity deficit

General Nursing Planning, Implementation, and Evaluation

> **Goal 1:** Client will know guidelines for early detection of cancer.

Implementation
1. Use detection or screening services.
2. Explain importance of American Cancer Society guidelines for early detection in asymptomatic individuals (see Table 3-63).
3. Refer client to American Cancer Society for information.

Evaluation
Client lists guidelines for early detection of cancer.

> **Goal 2:** Client undergoing cancer surgery will be physically and psychologically prepared.

Table 3-63   American Cancer Society Guidelines for Early Detection of Cancer

	Age		
Exam	20-40	40-50	51-plus
CANCER-RELATED CHECKUP	Every 3 years	Every year	Every year
BREAST EXAM:			
Self-exam	Monthly	Monthly	Monthly
Physician exam	Every 3 years	Every year	Every year
Mammogram	Single baseline between 35-39	Every 1-2 years *(or as directed by physician)*	Every year
UTERUS			
Pelvic exam	Every 3 years	Every year	Every year
PAP smear	Every 3 years *after 3 initial negative tests that are 1 year apart* (from onset of sexual activity)	Every 3 years *(or as directed by physician)*	Every 3 years *(or as directed by physician)*
COLON AND RECTUM			
Digital rectal	—	Yearly	Yearly
Guaiac test	—	—	Yearly
Proctosigmoidoscopy	—	—	Every 3-5 years *after 2 initial negative exams that are 1 year apart*

Implementation
1. Refer to "Perioperative Period," p. 117.
2. Help client deal with body image changes.
3. Arrange referral to appropriate agency (e.g., Lost Chord, Reach-to-Recovery).

Evaluation

Client describes surgery in own terms; expresses fears and concerns.

> **Goal 3:** Client and staff will be knowledgeable about planned radiation treatment and how to minimize side effects.

Implementation
1. Discuss reasons for radiation therapy and type to be used (e.g., external or internal).
2. External radiation
   a. Tell client that although he or she will be alone during the treatment, someone will be watching closely.
   b. Explain that skin markings must not be washed off for duration of therapy.
   c. Teach proper skin care.
      1. avoid soaps and bathing the area unless approved by physician
      2. avoid exposing area to sun, temperature extremes, and heat lamps
      3. expose area to air
      4. wear nonconstrictive clothing
      5. do not apply cosmetics, lotions, or powder to area unless directed to do so
      6. do not rub area
      7. do not apply tape over area
   d. Maintain or improve client's nutritional status
      1. administer antiemetics as needed before vomiting occurs; see Table 3-64
      2. obtain nutritional counseling
      3. observe for signs of mucositis
      4. teach good oral hygiene; perform every 2 hours with a soft toothbrush and toothpaste for sensitive gums
      5. teach use of prescribed medications (e.g., viscous lidocaine [Xylocaine], oral antibiotics [nystatin (Mycostatin)] suspension)
      6. record daily weights
      7. avoid the use of commercial mouthwashes that contain alcohol
      8. advise small, low-residue meals if diarrhea develops
      9. encourage fluid intake
      10. advise sweet foods if taste is altered
   e. Protect client from bleeding and infection.
   f. Help client balance activity with rest.
3. Internal radiation
   a. *Intracavitary irradiation* for cancer of the endometrium, vagina, or cervix (a radioactive substance is put into a sealed metal capsule and placed into a body cavity to deliver radiation)
      1. place client in a private room
      2. restrict visitors: no pregnant women or children under the age of 18; others are allowed one 15-minute visit each day.
      3. wear radiation badges when giving direct care
      4. explain radiation precautions of *time, distance,* and *shielding*
      5. mark room with signs regarding radiation therapy
      6. monitor for displacement of radiation source every 4-6 hours; use long forceps to handle a dislodged implant and place in a lead-lined container
      7. place client on strict bed rest while implant is in place
      8. keep head of bed in low position to prevent dislodging cervical implant
      9. maintain Foley catheter
      10. give low-residue diet
      11. monitor for uterine cramping if the implant extends into the uretus
      12. change perineal pads frequently (may have foul-smelling discharge)
      13. instruct client in the use of a vaginal dilator twice a week (adhesions and shortening of the vagina may occur)
      14. tell client that sexual intercourse may be resumed 3 weeks after the implant is removed; advise use of a water-soluble lubricant because of loss of natural vaginal lubrication
   b. *Interstitial radiotherapy:* implant of radioactive needles, wires, or seeds into the tissues; holding tubes for the radioactive source are inserted while the client is under local or general anesthesia
      1. follow routine precautions for individuals receiving irradiation (implant remains in place for 2-3 days)
      2. limit to quiet activity
      3. know that lead aprons do not provide adequate protection against the high radiation emitted by implant sources
      4. place lead shields strategically around the bed
      5. assess for possible esophagitis and pneumonitis with breast implants
      6. avoid use of deodorants with breast implants

Evaluation

Client states reason for and undergoes radiation therapy with minimal side effects.

> **Goal 4:** Client will understand the goals of chemotherapy, names of drugs, anticipated side effects, and treatment of side effects.

Implementation
1. Discuss treatment plans with client.
2. Tell client names of drugs prescribed and probable side effects.

Table 3-64   Antiemetic Drugs

Generic name (trade name)	Action	Side effects	Nursing implications
PHENOTHIAZINES			
Prochlorperazine (Compazine)	Acts on chemoreceptor trigger zone to inhibit nausea and vomiting	Drowsiness, dizziness, extrapyramidal symptoms, orthostatic hypotension, blurred vision, dry mouth	Dilute oral solution with juice etc. Give deep IM only. Obtain baseline BP before administration. Monitor BP carefully.
Perphenazine (Trilafon)	Same as above	Same as above	Same as above.
Thiethylperazine (Torecan)	Same as above	Same as above	Same as above.
NONPHENOTHIAZINES			
Dimenhydrinate (Dramamine)	Inhibits nausea and vomiting by means of unknown mechanism	Drowsiness	Warn client of decreased alertness. Dilute (very irritating to veins).
Benzquinamide (Emete-con)	Acts on chemoreceptor trigger zone to inhibit nausea and vomiting	Drowsiness	Do not give IV in clients with cardiovascular disease or with preanesthetic drugs. Do not reconstitute with 0.9% saline. Use large muscle for IM injection.
Trimethobenzamide (Tigan)	Same as above	Drowsiness	Do not give to children with viral illness (may contribute to Reye's syndrome). Warn client of drowsiness. Give deep IM.
Diphenidol (Vontrol)	Inhibits vestibular cerebellar pathways and possibly chemoreceptor trigger zone to inhibit nausea and vomiting	Drowsiness, dry mouth, confusion	Monitor BP carefully. Use only on hospitalized client. Observe for visual and auditory hallucinations.
Metoclopramide (Reglan)	Stimulates motility of upper GI tract; blocks dopamine receptors at chemoreceptor trigger zone to inhibit nausea and vomiting	Restlessness, anxiety, drowsiness, extrapyramidal symptoms, headache, and dry mouth	Give IV slowly over 15 min. Warn client of decreased alertness. Avoid alcohol and other depressants. Give oral dose ½-1 hr before meals for better absorption.

3. Maintain integrity of veins.
   a. Use arm veins.
   b. Discontinue infusion at first sign of infiltration, check patency by aspirating every 2-3 ml during IV push drugs.
   c. Know drugs that are vesicants (e.g., nitrogen mustard, doxorubicin).
4. Avoid prolonged, severe nausea and vomiting.
   a. Use antiemetics preventatively.
   b. Advise light food intake before treatments.
   c. Avoid dairy products and red meats.
   d. Encourage dry, bulky foods, sweet foods, clear fluids, and noncarbonated cola.

5. Prevent infection.
   a. Monitor client's bone marrow function.
   b. Monitor CBC.
   c. Hold chemotherapy if WBC falls below 3000 mm³.
   d. Hold chemotherapy if granulocyte count falls below 2000 mm³.
   e. Monitor for increased temperature.
   f. Institute reverse isolation if needed.
   g. Employ strict hand washing.
   h. Screen visitors for colds or other infectious diseases.
6. Prevent bleeding.

a. Monitor platelet count daily.

b. Institute bleeding precautions for a platelet count below 100,000.

c. Assess frequently for hematuria, bruising, and bleeding into joints.

d. Avoid IM injections whenever possible.

e. Use soft toothbrush or foam cleaner for oral hygiene.

f. Use electric razor for shaving.

g. Test all excreta for occult blood.

h. Administer platelet transfusion as ordered.

7. Prepare client for possible hair loss.

a. Explain that all body hair is susceptible to effects of chemotherapy but that the fastest growing hair is most affected.

b. Advise client to purchase a wig, hats, or scarves before losing hair.

c. Tell client that hair will grow back after chemotherapy is discontinued, but color and texture may be different.

8. Maintain good oral hygiene.

a. Teach client good oral hygiene.

b. Teach client signs and symptoms of stomatitis.

c. Teach client what to do if stomatitis develops.

Evaluation

Client states the goals of chemotherapy and lists the drugs and measures to minimize side effects.

SELECTED HEALTH PROBLEMS

☐ **Cancer of the Lung** see p. 153

☐ **Cancer of the Bladder** see p. 201

☐ **Cancer of the Prostate** see p. 215

☐ **Cancer of the Colon** see p. 224

☐ **Cancer of the Larynx** see p. 154

☐ **Hodgkin's Disease**

General Information

1. Definition: malignancy of the lymphoid system characterized by a generalized painless lymphadenopathy; unknown etiology

2. Incidence

a. Peak incidence between 15-30 years of age and after age 50

b. More common in males

c. Non-Hodgkin's lymphomas (lymphosarcoma, reticulum cell sarcoma) are more common in children under age 15

d. 5-year survival rate is 90%; late recurrences (after 5-10 years) are not uncommon

3. Medical treatment

a. Diagnostic tests

1. lymphangiography

2. inferior venacavogram

a. erythrocyte sedimentation rate (ESR): elevated

b. serum copper: elevated

3. biopsies

a. bone marrow

b. liver

c. spleen

b. Clinical staging: surgical laparotomy to determine stage of the disease and best course of treatment; staging determines prognosis

1. lymph node biopsy for characteristic cell (Reed-Sternberg cell)

2. surgical clips are used to outline area for irradiation

3. splenectomy

c. Chemotherapy: combination drug MOPP (mechlorethamine [Mustargen], vincristine [Oncovin], prednisone, procarbazine) for 6-18 months

d. Radiation therapy

Nursing Process

Assessment

1. Enlarged lymph nodes (most common sites: cervical, inguinal, mediastinal, axillary, retroperitoneal regions)

2. Anemia

3. Fever, infection (increased susceptibility to infection)

4. Anorexia, weight loss

5. Malaise

6. Night sweats

7. Pruritus

Analysis (see p. 270)

Planning, Implementation, and Evaluation

Goal 1: Client will be prepared for lymphangiography; will be free from complications.

Implementation

Pretest

1. Explain the procedure in terms of what the client and client's family can expect.

a. Food and drink are usually not restricted.

b. Procedure lasts approximately 4 hours, may last longer.

c. Feet are anesthetized and immobilized for lymphatic vessel catheterization.

d. Client must lie still during procedure, sedation usually given.

e. The dye may cause the following normal reactions

1. unusual taste sensations

2. fever

3. headache

4. insomnia

5. retrosternal burning sensation

6. bluish-green discoloration of urine or stools for several days

7. Evans blue dye will stain the skin for up to 48 hours, occasionally a few weeks or longer

2. Check for allergies to iodine or seafood.

3. Ensure consent is on chart.
4. Have client void before test.

Posttest

5. Monitor for signs of complications.
   a. Bleeding or infection from cutdown site
   b. Oil embolism (from oil-based dye)
      1. fever, chills
      2. dyspnea
      3. cough
      4. chest pain, soreness
      5. hypotension
6. Maintain bed rest for 24 hours or as ordered.
7. Monitor vital signs frequently until stable, then every 4 hours for 48 hours.
8. Assess incision site for infection; dressing is usually not changed for 48 hours.
9. Do not get original dressing wet.
10. Check for leg edema; elevate lower extremities as necessary.
11. Report numbness or discomfort distal to the incision to the physician.
12. Repeat x-ray in 24 hours.

Evaluation

Client is prepared for procedure and develops no complications.

Goal 2: Client and family are prepared for staging and splenectomy.

Implementation

1. Refer to "Perioperative Period," p. 117.
2. Inform client of effects of splenectomy: increased susceptibility to infection.

Evaluation

Client and family states effects of splenectomy and implications for life-style (minimizing exposure to infection).

☐ Cancer of the Cervix
General Information

1. Incidence
   a. Second most common cancer location in women
   b. Usually occurs in women between 30-50 years of age
   c. 100% cure if detected early (stage 0)
   d. Squamous cell most common cell type
2. Classification: clinical stages
   a. Stage 0: carcinoma in situ
   b. Stage I: confined to cervix
   c. Stage II: spread from cervix to vagina
   d. Stage III: involves lower one-third of vagina and has invaded paracervical tissue to pelvic wall on one or both sides and is associated with palpable lymph nodes in pelvic wall
   e. Stage IV: involves bladder and rectum and extends outside true pelvis
3. Predisposing factors
   a. Early, frequent coital exposure to multiple partners
   b. Pregnancy at young age
   c. History of sexually transmitted disease/herpes
   d. Venereal warts caused by human papilloma virus
4. Medical treatment
   a. Stage 0: conization of the cervix
   b. Stage I: hysterectomy or possible conization
   c. Stage II or III: intracavitary and external beam irradiation; possible radical hysterectomy
   d. Stage IV: radiation therapy followed by pelvic exenteration when there is persistent disease

Nursing Process
Assessment

1. Menstrual history
2. Pain in back, flank, and legs
3. Vaginal discharge
4. Pain after coitus, bleeding
5. Diagnostic tests: positive cytological results (Pap smear), cervical biopsy, colposcopy

Analysis (see p. 270)
Planning, Implementation, and Evaluation

Goal: Refer to "Uterine Fibroids," p. 317.

☐ Cancer of the Endometrium of the Uterus
General Information

1. Incidence
   a. Most common in postmenopausal women between the ages of 50 and 60
   b. Ratio of cervical to endometrial cancer is 3:1
   c. About 50% of clients with postmenopausal bleeding have endometrial carcinoma
   d. Diagnosis is made only after development of overt symptoms
2. Predisposing factors
   a. History of infertility
   b. Dysfunctional uterine bleeding
   c. Long-term estrogen therapy
   d. Obesity
3. Medical treatment
   a. Total abdominal hysterectomy (removal of uterine body and cervix), bilateral salpingo-oophorectomy, and saline wash of the peritoneal cavity
   b. More advanced endometrial cancer may require a radical hysterectomy (removal of uterus, supporting tissue, uppermost section of vagina, and pelvic lymph nodes), with pelvic lymph node dissection and irradiation
   c. Chemotherapy may be used in advanced cancer

Nursing Process
Assessment

1. Menstrual history

2. Irregular uterine bleeding
3. Diagnostic tests: aspiration curettage; dilation and curettage; endometrial, cervical, and endocervical biopsies

Analysis (see p. 270)

Planning, Implementation, and Evaluation

> **Goals:** Refer to "Vaginal Wall Changes," p. 317.

☐ Cancer of the Breast

General Information

1. Incidence
   a. Most common cancer in women
   b. Can be bilateral
   c. Highest incidence in ages 40-49 and 65 and older
   d. Incidence increasing, especially in women under age 40
2. Predisposing factors
   a. Family history of breast cancer on maternal side (sister, mother)
   b. Chronic irritation; fibrocystic disease
   c. Menarche before age 11; menopause after age 50
   d. No children or first child after age 30
   e. Previous breast cancer
   f. Uterine cancer
3. Breast cancer in men
   a. Incidence: 900 men each year in the United States
   b. Risk factors: history of gynecomastia, increased age
   c. Treatment: mastectomy
4. Surgical and medical treatment
   a. Surgical intervention
      1. modified radical mastectomy: breast, axillary contents
         a. most commonly performed surgery
         b. suitable for palpable, nonfixed tumors
      2. wedge (quadrant) resection of breast
         a. a wide local excision
         b. suitable for small (less than 1 cm) or nonpalpable tumors
         c. usually followed by radiation and chemotherapy, hormonal manipulation
         d. often done in combination with axillary lymph node dissection or sampling
         e. remains somewhat controversial
      3. Halsted radical mastectomy; breast, axillary contents, pectoralis muscle
         a. for advanced, fixed tumors
         b. infrequently used
      4. lumpectomy: removal of only the tumor and some surrounding tissue
         a. indicated when tumors are well defined, less than 5 cm in size, no involvement of nipple, and no metastasis
         b. usually involves dissection of the axillary

lymph node closest to the affected breast
      c. radiation therapy follows lymphectomy to eliminate any remaining cancer cells; usually begins 2 weeks after surgery; a second dose of radiation is given 2 weeks after initial dosage
      d. iridium implants (^{192}Ir) may be used to seed the cancer site
   b. Adjuvant therapy
      1. chemotherapy: specifics of therapy vary from institution to institution
      2. hormonal manipulation done if tumor is known to be estrogen-receptor–positive
         a. premenopausal women: antiestrogen therapy (tamoxifen)
         b. postmenopausal women: estrogen therapy
5. Sequence of surgery
   a. One-step: biopsy, frozen section, and mastectomy if positive; one anesthetic
   b. Two-step: biopsy under local or general anesthetic; client is awakened and when pathology results are available (2-3 days), treatment options are discussed; mastectomy or definitive surgery under a second anesthetic

Nursing Process

Assessment

1. Dimpling of skin
2. Retraction of nipple
3. Hard lump; not freely movable
4. Change in skin color
5. Change in skin texture (peau d'orange)
6. Alterations of contour of breast
7. Discharge from nipple
8. Pain (late sign)
9. Ulcerations (late sign)
10. Diagnostic tests: positive mammography, biopsy, and frozen section
11. Hormonal receptor assay: determines if tumor is estrogen or progesterone dependent
12. Symptoms of bone, lung, and brain involvement (common areas of metastasis)

Analysis (see p. 270)

Planning, Implementation, and Evaluation

> **Goal 1:** Client will be able to explain proposed surgery, effects of surgery, and preoperative and postoperative care.

Implementation

1. Refer to "Perioperative Period," p. 117.
2. Explore client's expectations of what surgical site will look like.
3. Discuss possibility of reconstructive surgery.

Evaluation

Client describes treatment options and expresses satisfaction with treatment decision.

Goal 2: Client will remain free from postoperative complications.

Implementation

1. Refer to "Perioperative Period," p. 117, for common complications.
2. Check under dressing, Hemovac, and under client's back for bleeding.
3. Expect sanguinous drainage during first 4 hours, turning to serous drainage thereafter.

Evaluation

Client is free from postoperative complications, evidence of bleeding.

Goal 3: Client will regain use of arm and joint movement on side of surgery.

Implementation

1. Position arm to decrease incidence of lymphedema; if the arm is not incorporated into the dressing, then elevate hand higher than the arm and keep arm elevated above the level of the right atrium.
2. Teach exercises when allowed to prevent contracture of the shoulder and to promote lymphatic flow.
3. Position arm on operative side on a pillow.
4. Encourage hand activity (e.g., squeeze small ball).
5. Have client use arm and hand for daily activities (e.g., brush hair).
6. Consult with physician regarding additional exercises.
7. Instruct client in postoperative exercises (e.g., wall climbing).

Evaluation

Client demonstrates appropriate postoperative exercises; knows schedule for exercising.

Goal 4: Client will be able to explain incision care, prosthetic devices available.

Implementation

1. Encourage client to look at incision.
2. On discharge, have client wear own bra with cotton padding or Reach-to-Recovery prosthesis.
3. Discuss with client plans for obtaining a permanent prosthesis.
4. Teach client to wash incision with soft cloth using soap and water.

Evaluation

Client has viewed incision; explains wound care.

Goal 5: Client will describe lymphedema and list ways to prevent it.

Implementation

1. Teach client reasons for lymphedema.
2. Have client sleep with arm elevated on pillows.
3. Elevate arm throughout day.
4. Avoid any constriction around arm.
5. Apply elastic bandage, arm stocking as needed.
6. Decrease sodium and fluid intake.
7. Obtain an order for a Jobst pressure machine if above methods are ineffective.

Evaluation

Client describes measures to prevent lymphedema, keeps arm elevated at rest.

Goal 6: Client will describe precautions necessary to prevent infections in arm on side of surgery.

Implementation

1. Avoid BP measurements, injections, blood drawing in affected arm.
2. Wear gloves when gardening etc.
3. Attend to any small cut or scrape immediately.
4. Avoid biting or chewing nails.
5. Prevent sunburn and any kind of regular burn.
6. Do not shave axilla on affected side.
7. Avoid carrying heavy objects with affected arm.

Evaluation

Client lists measures to avoid arm infection.

Goal 7: Client will demonstrate positive self-concept.

Implementation

1. Encourage return to normal activities.
2. Help plan for prosthesis fitting and discuss types of clothes she can wear.
3. Discuss reconstruction possibilities.
4. Encourage client to discuss operation and diagnosis with significant others.
5. Spend time with significant others to allow discussion of concerns and fears, so they can provide support for client's needs.
6. Arrange Reach-to-Recovery visit.

Evaluation

Client has Reach-to-Recovery visit; discusses self in positive terms; has plans to obtain prosthesis.

Goal 8: Client will experience normal grieving.

Implementation

1. Allow client to cry, withdraw, etc.
2. Explain that these feelings are usual and expected, that other women in a similar situation feel the same way.
3. Help client focus on future, but discuss loss.
4. Let client know that sometimes grief is delayed 2 or 3 months, and that it is a normal experience nonetheless.

Evaluation

Client expresses grief over loss of breast, diagnosis.

> **Goal 9:** Client and significant other can describe additional treatment when appropriate.

Implementation

1. Refer to General Nursing Goals 3 and 4, p. 271.

Evaluation

Client lists anticipated side effects of planned adjuvant therapy.

☐ Acquired Immunodeficiency Syndrome (AIDS)
General Information

1. Definition: A syndrome characterized by a defect in cell-mediated immunity; may have a long incubation period (from 6 months to 7-15 years). As the cell-mediated immunity becomes more impaired, the client becomes more likely to develop any of the opportunistic infections characteristically seen with the syndrome. To date there is no known cure and the syndrome is predominantly fatal.

2. Incidence: approximately 74% of adult AIDS clients are homosexual or bisexual males, 16% are men or women who have abused IV drugs; the remaining 10% is composed of persons with hemophilia who have received clotting factor products, newborns of high-risk or infected mothers, and sex partners of infected persons.

3. Causative agent: human immunodeficiency virus (HIV), a retrovirus that destroys T4 lymphocytes

4. Mode of transmission
   a. Sexual contact
   b. Exposure to HIV-infected blood or blood products
   c. Perinatally from mother to child
   d. HIV found in blood, semen, vaginal secretions, saliva, tears, breast milk, cerebrospinal fluid, amniotic fluid, and urine; but studies to date have implicated only blood, semen, vaginal secretions, and possibly breast milk in transmission.

5. Diagnostic tests
   a. Diagnosis of AIDS requires presence of cellular immunodeficiency, opportunistic infection, or cancer and positive test result for antibody to HIV
   b. HIV antibody tests
      1. enzyme-linked immunosorbent assay (ELISA)
      2. Western blot assay: confirms positive ELISA test
      3. positive results indicate that the client has been exposed to HIV and has produced antibodies; it does not mean that client has the disease of AIDS
      4. negative results do not necessarily indicate that a client is free of HIV (if the test was done immediately before exposure to HIV, then detectable levels of antibodies may not be present)
   c. Antigen tests
      1. HIVAGEN test: detects antigens to HIV as early as 2 weeks after infection
      2. presence of the HIV antigen along with the HIV antibody indicates the virus is replicating
   d. HIV culture: detects live HIV
   e. CBC and differential
   f. Immune profile (T cell assay)
      1. measures the number of T cells
      2. there is usually an increase in number and percentage of T suppressor cells (T8 lymphocytes) and a decrease in T helper cells (T4 lymphocytes)

6. Opportunistic infections seen in HIV
   a. Protozoal diseases
      1. *Pneumocystis carinii* pneumonia (PCP)
      2. *Toxoplasma gondii*
      3. *Cryptosporidium muris*
   b. Mycobacterial diseases
      1. *Mycobacterium tuberculosis*
      2. *Mycobacterium avium intracellulare*
   c. Fungal diseases
      1. *Candida albicans*
      2. *Cryptococcus neoformans*
      3. *Histoplasma capsulatum*
      4. *Aspergillus*
   d. Viral diseases
      1. herpesviruses
      2. herpes simplex virus
      3. varicella zoster virus (VZV)
      4. cytomegalovirus (CMV)

7. Cancers in HIV infection
   a. Kaposi's sarcoma
   b. Lymphomas
   c. Non–Hodgkin's lymphoma
   d. Primary central nervous system lymphoma

8. Medical treatment
   a. Zidovudine (Retrovir), once known as azidothymidine (AZT), is the only drug that has received FDA approval for treating AIDS
      1. slows the rate of virus reproduction so that additional cells will not become infected
      2. does not eliminate the virus from the body; the person infected still has the virus and can transmit it
      3. dosage: 200 mg po q4h
      4. side effects: low WBC, nausea, headache, muscle pain, low RBC, and low hematocrit
      5. cost of drug therapy averages $600 a month
   b. Drug therapy to treat HIV infections
      1. antimicrobial therapy
      2. chemotherapy
   c. Supportive care

d. Other drugs (including a vaccine for HIV) are being researched
9. Universal blood and plasma precautions
   a. Based on the risk of exposure to body fluids rather than on a diagnosed disease state
   b. Eliminates the need to follow blood and body-fluid precautions (isolation) previously recommended by the Centers for Disease Control (CDC) for clients with known or suspected infections
   c. CDC recommends that *all* clients be treated as though they were HIV-positive

Nursing Process

Assessment
1. Fever
2. Weight loss
3. Fatigue
4. Lymphadenopathy
5. Diarrhea
6. Night sweats
7. Signs and symptoms of opportunistic infections or cancer

Analysis (see p. 270)

Planning, Implementation, and Evaluation

Goal 1: Significant others and staff will be protected from client's infection.

1. Ensure implementation of universal precautions.
2. Use additional precautions as necessary for associated infections such as tuberculosis, cytomegalovirus, and infectious diarrhea.
3. Use protective barriers to prevent skin and mucous membrane exposure to blood and body fluids (e.g., gloves, masks, protective eyewear, gowns, and face shields).
4. Wash hands after removing gloves and between client contact.
5. Exercise care when handling sharp instruments.
   a. Do not recap needles.
   b. Do not clip or bend needles.
   c. Dispose of sharps in a puncture-resistant container
6. Use disposable mouthpieces and airways instead of mouth-to-mouth resuscitation.
7. Do not rewash gloves to use with another client.
8. Use gloves when inserting or discontinuing an IV or NG tube or when drawing blood.

Evaluation
Significant others and staff remain free from the client's infection.

Goal 2: Client will be free from respiratory infection and subsequent respiratory distress.

Implementation
1. Provide oxygen as needed
2. Place in comfortable position for best respiratory effort.
3. Pace activities so as not to cause or increase fatigue.
4. Assess for signs and symptoms of respiratory infection, distress, and failure.
5. Administer pharmacological therapy as ordered for PCP.
   a. pentamidine isethionate (Pentam 300)
   b. sulfamethoxazole (Septra, Bactrim)
6. Teach client and family signs and symptoms of respiratory complications.

Evaluation
Client breathes easily, remains afebrile; paces daily activities; reports early signs of respiratory problems.

Goal 3: Client will have adequate nutrition and hydration.

Implementation
1. Monitor I&O, nutritional status, and electrolyte balance closely.
2. Provide appropriate calorie intake if oral nutrition is tolerated.
3. Provide antidiarrheal drugs prn.
4. Administer TPN as ordered.
5. Provide meticulous mouth care.
6. Provide pain relief from mouth lesions if present, before attempts at oral feedings.

Evaluation
Client eats prescribed diet, has adequate calorie intake; maintains good urine output and moist mucous membranes; maintains desired weight.

Goal 4: Client will understand goals of therapy, anticipated side effects of drugs, and methods to prevent HIV transmission to others.

Implementation
1. Assess client's knowledge of syndrome.
2. Encourage client to discuss feelings, concerns about plan of therapy, changes in work, home, and lifestyle environment.
3. Use a nonjudgmental approach during care.
4. Tell client names of drugs prescribed and possible side effects.
5. Teach signs and symptoms of infection and what steps to take if these symptoms occur.
6. Teach how to avoid transmission of the illness.
7. Warn not to share toilet articles or donate blood or organs.
8. Advise client to inform physicians, dentists, and sexual partners of diagnosis and required precautions.

Evaluation
Client discusses goals of therapy, lists side effects of

prescribed drugs; employs methods to prevent spread of virus.

Goal 5: Client will accept psychosocial support throughout illness.

Implementation

1. Allow client to express fear and grief regarding the fact that illness is incurable.
2. Assess client's adjustment to altered body image and self-concept.
3. Spend time listening to concerns and feelings.
4. Refer client to appropriate community agency for financial support as necessary.
5. Encourage acceptance of support from significant others during illness.
6. Teach significant others what they can do to help and support client, and to protect themselves from the virus.

Evaluation

Client expresses feelings, acknowledges support throughout diagnosis and treatment.

BIBLIOGRAPHY
The healthy adult

Berliner, H. (1986). Aging skin. *American Journal of Nursing, 86,* 1138-1141.

Berliner, H. (1986). Aging skin: Part 2. *American Journal of Nursing, 86,* 1259-1261.

Burnside, I. (1988). *Nursing and the aged* (3rd ed.). St. Louis: Mosby–Year Book.

Carnevali, F., & Patrick, M. (Eds.). (1986). *Nursing management for the elderly* (2nd ed.). Philadelphia: Lippincott.

Dychtwald, D. (Ed.). (1986). *Wellness and health promotion for the elderly.* Rockville, MD: Aspen.

Ebersole, P., & Hess, P. (1990). *Toward healthy aging: human needs and nursing response* (3rd ed.). St. Louis: Mosby–Year Book.

Edelman, C.L., & Mandle, C.L. (1990). *Health promotion throughout the lifespan* (2nd ed.). St. Louis: Mosby–Year Book.

Eliopoulos, C. (1987). *Gerontological nursing.* Philadelphia: Lippincott.

Malasanos, L., Barkauskas, V., & Stoltenberg-Allen, K. (1990). *Health assessment* (4th ed.). St. Louis: Mosby–Year Book.

Matteson, M.A., & McConnell, E.S. (1988). *Gerontological nursing: concepts and practice.* Philadelphia: W.B. Saunders.

Phipps, W., Long, B., & Woods, N. (Eds.). (1991). *Medical surgical nursing: Concepts and clinical practice* (4th ed.). St. Louis: Mosby–Year Book.

Seidel, H.M., Ball, J.W., Dains, J.E., & Benedict, W. (1991). *Mosby's Guide to Physical Examination* (2nd ed.). St. Louis: Mosby–Year Book.

Williams, S.R. (1989). *Essentials of nutrition and diet therapy.* (5th ed.). St. Louis: Mosby–Year Book.

The adult client undergoing surgery

*American Pain Society. (1988). CE: Relieving pain: An analgesic guide. *American Journal of Nursing, 88,* 816-826.

Blackwood, S. (1986). Back to basics: The preoperative exam. *American Journal of Nursing, 86,* 39-44.

Bray, C.A. (1986). Postoperative pain: Altering the patient's experience through education. *Association of Operating Room Nurses Journal (AORNJ), 43,* 672-683.

Copp, L.A. (1990). The spectrum of suffering. *American Journal of Nursing, 90*(9), 35-39.

Coyle, N. (1987). Analgesics and pain: Current concepts. *The Nursing Clinics of North America, 22*(3), 727-741.

Fitzgerald, J.J., & Shamy, P. (1987). Let your patient control his analgesic. *Nursing 1987, 17*(7), 48-51.

Kleinman, R., Lipman, A., Hare, B., & MacDonald, S. (1987). PCA versus regular IM injections for severe post-op pain. *American Journal of Nursing, 87,* 1491-1492.

Kneedler, J.A., & Dodge, G.W. (1987). *Perioperative patient care* (2nd ed.). St. Louis: Mosby–Year Book.

Long, B., & Phipps, W. (Eds.). (1989). *Medical-surgical nursing: A Nursing process approach,* (2nd ed.). St. Louis: Mosby–Year Book.

McCaffery, M. & Beebe, A. (1989). *Pain: Clinical manual for nursing practice.* St. Louis: Mosby–Year Book.

McEntyre, R.L. (1989). *Practical guide to care of the surgical patient* (3rd ed.). St. Louis: Mosby–Year Book.

McConnell, E. (1987). *Clinical considerations in perioperative nursing.* Philadelphia: Lippincott.

Meeker, M., & Rothrock, J.C. (1991). *Alexander's care of the patient in surgery,* (9th ed.). St. Louis: Mosby–Year Book.

Montanari, J. (1986). Action STAT: Wound dehiscence. *Nursing 86, 16*(2), 33-36.

Rowland, M.A. (1990). Myths and facts about postoperative discomfort. *American Journal of Nursing, 90*(5), 60-64.

Oxygenation

Anderson, S. (1990). ABGs: Six easy steps to interpreting blood gases. *American Journal of Nursing, 90*(8), 42-45.

Andreoli, K. et al. (Eds.). (1987). *Comprehensive cardiac care: A text for nurses, physicians, and other health personnel* (2nd ed.). St. Louis: Mosby–Year Book.

Beavers, B. (1986). Health education and the patient with peripheral vascular disease. *Nursing Clinics of North America, 21*(2), 265-271.

Becker, D., et al. (1989). Cholesterol: Interpreting the new guidelines. *American Journal of Nursing, 89*(12), 1622-1624.

Bolgiano, C., et al. (1990). Administering oxygen therapy: what you need to know. *Nursing 90, 20*(6), 47-51.

Carroll, P. (1986). The ins and outs of chest drainage systems. *Nursing 86, 16*(12), 26-33.

Caruthers, D. (1990). Infectious pneumonia in the elderly. *American Journal of Nursing, 90*(2), 56-60.

Cornell, E. (1988). Tuberculosis in hospital employees. *American Journal of Nursing, 88,* 484-485.

Dennison, R. (1986). Cardiopulmonary assessment. *Nursing 86, 16*(4), 34-42.

Dennison, R. (1987). Upper airway obstruction. *Nursing 87, 17*(10), 34-41.

Donner, C., & Cooper K. (1988). The critical difference: pulmonary edema. *American Journal of Nursing, 88,* 59.

Doyle, J. (1986). Treatment modalities in peripheral vascular disease. *Nursing Clinics of North America, 21*(2), 241-253.

Erickson, R. (1989). Mastering the ins and outs of chest drainage, Part 1. *Nursing 89, 19*(5), 37-44.

Erickson, R. (1989). Mastering the ins and outs of chest drainage, Part 2. *Nursing 89, 19*(6), 46-50.

Goodman, A.G., et al. (Eds.). (1990). *Goodman & Gilman's the pharmacological basis of therapeutics.* New York: Macmillan.

Herman, J. (1986). Nursing assessment and nursing diagnosis in patients with peripheral vascular disease. *Nursing Clinics of North America, 21*(2), 219-231.

*Reprint.
†Highly recommended.

Hill, M., & Cunningham, S. (1989). The latest wards for high BP. *American Journal of Nursing, 89*(4), 504-510.

Holloway, N. (1988). *Nursing the critically ill adult* (3rd ed.). Menlo Park, CA: Addison-Wesley Publishing Company.

How to work with chest tubes (programmed instruction). (1980). *American Journal of Nursing, 80*, 685-712.

Jones, S., & A. Bagg (1988). LEAD-drugs for cardiac arrest. *Nursing 88, 18*(1), 34-42.

Kersten, L. (1989). *Comprehensive respiratory nursing: a decision-making approach*. Philadelphia: W.B. Saunders Company.

Krosky, N. & Vanscoy, G. (1989). Running an anticoagulant clinic. *American Journal of Nursing, 89*(10), 1304-1306.

Lancaster, E. (1988). Tuberculosis on the rise. *American Journal of Nursing, 88*, 485.

Lung cancer. (1987). *American Journal of Nursing, 87*, 1427-1446.

Malasanos, L., et al. (1989). *Health assessment* (4th ed.). St. Louis: Mosby–Year Book.

McCann, M. (1989). Sexual healing after heart attack. *American Journal of Nursing, 89*(9), 1132-1140.

McCormac, M. (1990). Managing hemorrhagic shock. *American Journal of Nursing, 90*(8), 22-29.

Moore, L., & Pulliam, C. (1986). An on the spot guide to antihypertensive drugs. *Nursing 86, 16*(1), 54-57.

New CPR guidelines: Bicarbonate now a last resort. (1986). *American Journal of Nursing, 86*, 889.

Pagana, K., & Pagana, T. (1988). *Pocket nurse guide to laboratory and diagnostic tests*. St. Louis: Mosby–Year Book.

Rodriguez, S., & Reed, R. (1987). Thrombolytic therapy for MI. *American Journal of Nursing, 87*(5), 631-640.

Sawyer, D., & Bruya, M. (1990). Care of the patient having radical neck surgery or permanent laryngostomy: a nursing diagnostic approach. *Focus on Critical Care, 17*(2), 167-173.

Smith, C. (1988). Assessing chest pain quickly and accurately. *Nursing 88, 18*(5), 52-60.

Standards and guidelines for cardiopulmonary resuscitation (CPR) and emergency cardiac care (ECC). (1986). *Journal of the American Medical Association, 255*(21), 2905-2984, and *256*(13), 1727.

Stoy, D. (1989). Controlling cholesterol with diet. *American Journal of Nursing, 89*(12), 162-1627.

Turner, J. (1986). Nursing intervention in patients with peripheral vascular disease. *Nursing Clinics of North America, 21*(2), 233-240.

Viall, C. (1990). Your complete guide to central venous catheters. *Nursing 90, 20*(2), 34-42.

Wagner, M. (1986). Pathophysiology related to peripheral vascular disease. *Nursing Clinics of North America, 21*(2), 195-205.

Nutrition and metabolism

Adinaro, D. (1987). Liver failure and pancreatitis: Fluid and electrolyte concerns. *Nursing Clinics of North America, 22*(4), 843.

Anderson F.D. (1986). Portal systemic encephalopathy in the chronic alcoholic. *Critical Care Quarterly, 8*(4), 76.

Anderson, F.D. (1986). The cirrhotic process in the alcoholic. *Critical Care Quarterly, 8*(4), 74.

Atkins, J., & Oakley, C. (1986). A nurse's guide to TPN. *RN, 49*(6), 20-24.

Brockstein, A.J. (1986). Peptic ulcer disease: New concepts, new and current therapies. *Consultant*, April, pp. 157-176.

Bryant, R. (1986). Diverticular disease. *Journal of Enterostomal Therapy, 13*(3), 114-117.

Buckingham, A. (1986). Arterial blood gases made simple. *Nursing Life, 5*(6), 48-51.

Caine, R., & Bufalino, P. (1987). *Nursing care planning guides for adults*. Baltimore: Williams & Wilkins.

Cerrato, P.L. (1990). Diarrhea: The usual suspect may not be to blame. *RN*, August, 73-75.

Chandler, W., et al. (1987). Surgical treatment of Cushing's disease. *Journal of Neurosurgery, 66*(2), 204.

Cohen, D.J., & Starling, J.R. (1986). Surgery for reflux esophagitis: experience with the antireflux prosthesis. *AORN Journal, 43*, 858.

Dobberstein, K. (1987). The liver: To know it is to love it. *Nursing, 87*(1), 74.

*Gavin, J. (1988). Diabetes and exercise. *American Journal of Nursing, 88*, 178-181.

Green-Hernandez, C. (1987). Surgery and diabetes. *American Journal of Nursing, 87*, 788-793.

Haire-Joshu, D., Flavin, K., & Clutter, W. (1986). Controlling the insulin balance: Contrasting Type I and Type II diabetes. *American Journal of Nursing, 86*, 1239.

Hartshorn, J., & Hartshorn, E. (1988). Vasopressin in the treatment of diabetes insipidus. *Journal of Neuroscience Nursing, 56*(2), 58.

Hauser, S.C. (1987). Answers to questions on gall bladder disease. *Hospital Medicine, 23*(6), 44.

Jermier, B.J., & Treloar, D.M. (1986). Bringing your patient through gallbladder surgery. *RN, 49*(11), 18.

MacKowiak, L., & McCarthy, R. (1989). Managing diabetes on sick days. *American Journal of Nursing, 89*(7), 950-953.

McAdams, R., & Birmingham, D. (1986). When diabetes races out of control. *RN, 49*(5), 46-53.

Robertson, C. (1986). When an insulin dependent diabetic must be NPO. *Nursing 86, 16*(6), 30-31.

Rowland, G.A., Marks, D.A., & Torres, W.E. (1989). The new gallstone destroyers and dissolvers. *American Journal of Nursing, 89*(11), 1473-1476.

Sabesin, S. (1987). Countering the dangers of acute pancreatitis. *Emergency Medicine, 19*(17), 71.

Staren, E., et al. (1986). Surgical intervention for pheochromocytoma. *AORN Journal, 44*(5), 764.

Steil, C.F., & Deakins, D.A. (1990). Today's insulins: What you and your patient need to know. *Nursing 90*, August, 34-40.

Stone, M.B. (1987). Questions that diabetes patients ask. *Diabetes Educator, 13*(3), 298.

Trourson, L. (1986). Nursing diagnosis and the syndrome of inappropriate antidiuretic hormone. *Journal of Post Anesthesia Nursing, 1*(4), 244.

Wilkinson, M. (1990). Your role in needle biopsy of the liver. *RN*, August, 62-66.

Elimination

Baer, C.L. (1990). Acute kidney failure: Recognizing and reversing its deadly course. *Nursing 90, 20*(6) 34-40.

Becker, K. (1988). Performing in-depth abdominal assessment. *Nursing 88, 18*(6), 59-63.

Booth, L.S., et al. (1989). Living without kidneys. *American Journal of Nursing, 89*(2), 270.

Bristoll, S.L., et al. (1989). The mythical danger of rapid urinary drainage. *American Journal of Nursing, 89*(3), 344-345.

Brogna, L., & Lakaszawski, M. (1986). The continent urostomy. *American Journal of Nursing, 85*, 160-163.

Frank, A., & Murray, S. (1988). A no guess guide for urinary color assessment. *RN, 51*(6), 46-51.

Ghiotto, S. (1988). A full range of care for nephrostomy patients. *RN, 51*(4), 72-77.

Gloeckner, M. (1984). Perceptions of sexual attractiveness following ostomy surgery. *Research in Nursing and Health, 7*, 87-92.

Mallette, C. (1990). What those "difficult" renal patients need from you. *RN, 53*(4), 25-27.

Malti, J., et al. CAPD: a dialysis breakthrough with its own burdens. *RN, 51*(1), 46-53.

McConnell, E.A. (1989). Discovering a post TURP complication. *Nursing 89, 19*(9), 96-98.

McConnell, E.A. (1987). Meeting the challenge of intestinal obstruction. *Nursing 87, 17*(7), 34-42

Monroe, D. (1990). Patient teaching for x-ray and other diagnostics. *RN, 53*(4), 52-56.

Newman, D.K., et al. (1989). Incontinence: The problem patients won't talk about. *RN, 52*(3), 42-45.

Office of Medical Applications of Research. (1988). Prevention and treatment of kidney stones. *JAMA, 260*, 977-981.

Pagana, K. (1987). Preventing complications in jejunostomy tube feedings. *Dimensions of Critical Care Nursing, 6*(1), 28-38.

Pagana, K., & Pagana, T. (1989). *Diagnostic testing and nursing implications: A case study approach* (3rd ed.). St. Louis: Mosby–Year Book.

Preshlock, K. (1989). Detecting the hidden UTI. *RN, 52*(1), 65-66, 68-69.

Pritchard, V. (1988). Geriatric infections: The urinary tract. *RN, 51*(5), 36-38.

Questions and answers about ulcerative colitis and Crohn's disease. (1988). *Patient Care, 22*(15), 169-170.

Reilly, N., & Torosian, L. (1988). The new wave in lithotripsy: Implications for nursing, *RN, 51*(3), 44-50.

Ruge, C. (1987). Catheter-related UTIs: What's the best way to prevent them? *Nursing 87, 17*(12), 50-51.

Snyder, T.E. (1989). An exercise program for dialysis patients. *American Journal of Nursing, 89*(3), 362-364.

Stark, J. (1988). A quick guide to urinary tract assessment. *Nursing 88, 18*(7), 56-58.

Strangio, L. (1988). Believe it or not: Peritoneal dialysis made easy. *Nursing 88, 18*(1), 43-46.

Sensation and perception

Carver, J. (1987). Cataract care made plain. *American Journal of Nursing, 87*, 626-630.

Clark, J.B., Queener, S.F., & Karb, V.B. (1990). Pharmacological basis of nursing practice (3rd ed.). St. Louis: Mosby–Year Book.

Coburn, K.L., Hodson, C., & Hundley, J. (1988). High-tech maps of the brain. *American Journal of Nursing, 88*, 1500-1501.

†Coma (Continuing Education). (1986). *American Journal of Nursing, 86*, 541-556.

†Finocchiaro, D.N. & Herzfeld, S.T. (1990). Understanding autonomic dysreflexia. *American Journal of Nursing, 90*, 56-59.

†Fode, N.C. (1988). Subarachnoid hemorrhage from ruptured intracranial aneurysm. *American Journal of Nursing, 88*(5), 673-680.

Olson, E.V., et al. (1990). The hazards of immobility. *American Journal of Nursing, 90*(3), 43-48.

Passarella, P., & Gee, Z. (1987). Starting right after stroke. *American Journal of Nursing, 87*, 802-807.

Rhynsburger, J. (1989). How to fight MG fatigue. *American Journal of Nursing, 89*, 337-340.

Rubin, M. (1988). The physiology of bedrest. *American Journal of Nursing, 88*, 50-55.

Shovein, J.T., Land, L.P., & Leedom, D.L. (1989). Near-drowning, *American Journal of Nursing, 89*, 680-686.

Topp, B. (1987). Toward a better understanding of Parkinson's disease. *Geriatric Nursing, 8*(4), 180-182.

Van Oteghen, S.L. (1987). An exercise program for those with Parkinson's disease. *Geriatric Nursing, 8*(4), 183-184.

†Yen, P.K. (1990). Does a low-protein diet help with Parkinson's? *Geriatric Nursing, 11*(1), 48.

Mobility

Gamron R. (1988). Taking the pressure out of compartment syndrome. *American Journal of Nursing, 88*, 1076-1080.

Henning, L., & Burrows, S. (1986). Keeping up on arthritis meds. *RN, 49*(2), 32-38.

Miller, R. & Evans, W. (1987). Immediate post-op prosthesis. *American Journal of Nursing, 87*, 310-311.

Phipps W., et al. (1987). *Clinical handbook of medical-surgical nursing.* St. Louis: Mosby–Year Book.

Rubin, M. The physiology of bed rest. *American Journal of Nursing, 88*, 50-56.

Stinger, K. & Metzgar E. (1989). A systematic approach to patient assessment. *Nursing 89, 19*, 32O-32Q.

Cellular aberration

Abernathy, E. (1987). Biological response modifiers. *American Journal of Nursing, 87*, 458-459.

Abernathy, E. (1987). How the immune system works. *American Journal of Nursing, 87*, 456-459.

Armstrong, D.A. (1987). The diagnostic workup. *American Journal of Nursing, 87*, 1433.

Baird, S.B. (1988). *Decision making in oncology nursing.* Toronto: B.C. Decker.

Barrick, B. (1988). Caring for A.I.D.S. patients: A challenge you can meet. *Nursing 88, 18*(11), 50-59.

Cancer update. (1990). *Nursing 90, 20*(4), 61-64.

D'Agostino, N.S. (1989). Managing nutrition problems in advanced cancer. *American Journal of Nursing, 89*, 50-56.

Doane, L.S., Fischer, L.M., & McDonald, T.W. (1990). How to give peritoneal chemotherapy. *American Journal of Nursing, 90*(4), 58-64.

Engelking, C. (1987). Teaching, counseling, and caring. *American Journal of Nursing, 87*, 1439-1441.

Engelking, C. (1987). The language of staging. *American Journal of Nursing, 87*, 1434-1437.

Engelking, C. (1987). Chemotherapy. *American Journal of Nursing, 87*, 1438-1441.

Frank-Stromberg, M., Krafka, B., Gale, D., & Porter, N. (1986), Carcinogens: Are some risks acceptable? *American Journal of Nursing, 86*, 814-817.

Gee, G., & Moran, T.A. (Eds.). (1988). *AIDS: Concepts in nursing practice.* Baltimore: Williams and Wilkins.

Gerberding, J.L. (1988). Occupational health issues for providers of care to patients with HIV infection. *Infectious Disease Clinics of North America, 2*(2), 321-328.

Haylock, P.J. (1987). Radiation therapy. *American Journal of Nursing, 87*, 1441-1446.

Hollander, H. (1988). Work-up of the HIV-infected patient. *Infectious Disease Clinics of North America, 2*, 353-358.

Hood, L.E. (1987). Interferon. *American Journal of Nursing, 87*, 459-464.

Hughes, C.B. (1986). Giving cancer drugs IV: Some guidelines. *American Journal of Nursing, 86*, 34-38.

Jaffe, H.W., & Lifson, A.R. (1988). Acquisition and transmission of HIV. *Infectious Disease Clinics of North America, 2*, 299-306.

Jassak, P.F., & Spiewak, P.L. (1987). Interleukin-2. *American Journal of Nursing, 87*, 464-467.

Jenkins, B. (1986). Sexual healing after pelvic irradiation. *American Journal of Nursing, 86*, 920-922.

Klug, R.M. (1986). AIDS beyond the hospital. *American Journal of Nursing, 86*, 1016-1021.

LaCharite, C.L., & Meisenhelder, J.B. (1989). Zidovudine: Flawed champion against AIDS. *RN, 52*(1), 35-38.

Laufman, J.K. (1989). AIDS, ethics, and the truth. *American Journal of Nursing, 89*, 924, 929, 930.

Levy, J.A. (1988). The human immunodeficiency virus and its pathogenesis. *Infectious Disease Clinics of North America, 2,* 285-297.

Lewis, A. (1988). *Nursing care of the person with AIDS/ARC.* Rockville, MD: Aspen.

McNaull, F.W. (1987). What are the odds? *American Journal of Nursing, 87,* 1428-1429.

McNaull, F.W. (1987). Tobaccoism in America. *American Journal of Nursing, 87,* 1430-1433.

Rieger, P.T. (1987). Monoclonal antibodies. *American Journal of Nursing, 87,* 469-473.

Rust, D.L., & Dloppenborg, E.M. (1990). Don't underestimate the lumpectomy patient's needs. *RN, 53*(3), 58-64.

Scherer, P. (1990). How AIDS attacks the brain. *American Journal of Nursing, 90*(1), 44-53.

Stam, H.J., & Challis, G.B. (1988). Rating the toxicities of cancer drugs. *American Journal of Nursing, 88,* 1362-1363.

Sticklin, L.A. (1987). Interleukin-2 and killer T cells. *American Journal of Nursing, 87,* 468-469.

Taber, J. (1989). Nutrition in HIV infection. *American Journal of Nursing, 89,* 1446-1451.

Volberding, P.A. (1988). Caring for the patient with AIDS. *Infectious Disease Clinics of North America, 2,* 543-550.

Wikle, T., Coyle, K., & Shapiro, D. (1990). Bone marrow transplant: Today and tomorrow. *American Journal of Nursing, 90*(5), 48-56.

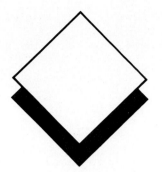

Reprints

Nursing Care of the Adult

ARRHYTHMIA MIMICS

By Lauren Saul
Reprinted from American Journal of Nursing March, 1991

Sometimes it seems that the more you know, the more you know you don't know. That piece of wisdom certainly applies to interpreting cardiac rhythm strips. A cursory glance at what appears to be a familiar rhythm can yield a quick interpretation that just misses the mark. Often misinterpreted are multifocal atrial tachycardia, atrial fibrillation, and atrial tachycardia.

Multifocal atrial tachycardia (MAT), also called *chaotic atrial tachycardia* or *chaotic atrial mechanism,* is commonly misinterpreted as atrial fibrillation, or occasionally, as atrial tachycardia[1]. Often triggered by premature atrial contractions (PACs), MAT shows up on a cardiac rhythm strip as an ectopic atrial rate between 100 and 250 beats per minute, with a slightly irregular atrial rhythm (observed by measuring P-P intervals). The P waves have two or more distinct configurations—peaked or tent-shaped waves as well as notched waves are most likely to show up clearly in Leads II and MCL$_1$ (monitored chest lead V$_1$). The baseline between P-P in-

Lauren Saul, RN, MSN, CCRN, is a cardiovascular clinical nurse specialist at Shadyside Hospital, Pittsburgh, PA. The author thanks Juan Estrada, MD, and Connie Richless, RN, MSN, CCRN, for reviewing the manuscript.

tervals is isoelectric (flat) and, although the P-R intervals vary slightly, they are usually of normal duration. These atrial variations occur because multiple foci in the atria are discharging impulses. The ventricular rate and rhythm depend on the atrioventricular (AV) conduction of the arrhythmia[1].

MAT is often seen in critically ill patients who have chronic obstructive pulmonary disease (COPD) or some form of chronic hypoxia. Moreover, many patients with MAT also have chronic cor pulmonale (right-sided heart failure from COPD). Other causes of MAT include digitalis toxicity, coronary artery disease with refractory congestive heart failure, and postanesthesia hypoxemia. Occasionally, MAT results from pulmonary embolism, septicemia, hypertension, valvular heart disease, or electrolyte imbalance, especially hypokalemia.

MAT is treated with oxygen therapy and pulmonary treatments, both of which are more helpful than antiarrhythmic drugs such as propranolol (Inderal) and quinidine. However, when MAT coincides with congestive heart failure (CHF), digitalis is effective. Of course, the drug must be stopped if the patient is found to have digitalis toxicity. When MAT causes hemodynamic compromise, cardioversion (synchronized coun-

tershock), beginning with 50 to 100 joules, is the treatment of choice.

Atrial fibrillation is characterized by rapid, chaotic atrial activity and an irregularly irregular ventricular response. No distinct P waves appear on the rhythm strip, thus you cannot measure the P-R intervals. Instead, you see f waves—coarse, medium, or fine atrial oscillations.

With AF, the atrial rate is difficult to measure, but usually falls between 400 and 650 beats per minute. As the rapid atrial activity bombards the AV junction, it interferes with the AV junction's conduction of atrial impulses to the ventricles. This phenomenon, called **concealed AV conduction,** is responsible for the irregularly irregular ventricular rhythm.

Unless the patient is taking digitalis, beta blockers, or calcium antagonists, the ventricular rate is rapid (120 to 200 beats per minute). Elderly patients who develop AF but do not take cardiovascular drugs tend to have slow ventricular rates, usually due either to advanced AV block or to underlying sick sinus rhythm[1, 2].

The many theories about the cause of AF include multiple reentry circuits and ectopic-impulse formation. Reentry occurs because an impulse depolarizes an area and returns to activate the same area in a repetitive sequence. A single PAC may initiate AF, or AF may follow atrial flutter or atrial tachycardia. AF is often associated with coronary artery disease, rheumatic heart disease, mitral stenosis, hypertension, thyrotoxicosis, and Wolff-Parkinson-White (WPW) Syndrome (1, 2).

Unless the ventricles are slow to respond, digitalis is the drug of choice for AF, whether or not the patient has CHF. Also effective are propranolol (Inderal), quinidine, procainamide (Pronestyl), and verapamil (Calan, Isoptin). When the arrhythmia first occurs, if drug therapy does not work, then elective cardioversion is recommended, because AF responds best to cardioversion in the first few weeks and months of the arrhythmia.

Several key features help distinguish **multifocal atrial tachycardia** and **atrial fibrillation**. While atrial fibrillation is a rapid atrial rhythm that creates a chaotic, undulating baseline, MAT's rhythm demonstrates a flat baseline between atrial activity. AF's atrial rate cannot be counted, whereas MAT's atrial rate of 120 to 200 beats per minute can be. If a rhythm looks like AF but has unusual P waves and the patient has some form of COPD, inspect the strip more closely for MAT.

Atrial tachycardia (AT), although in the same family of arrhythmias as MAT, has different ECG criteria. AT's atrial rate ranges from 160 to 250 beats per minute. The P waves differ from a sinus-rhythm P wave, but are all of the same configuration because this arrhythmia originates in one atrial focus. Like MAT, the baseline between AT's P waves is flat and the P-R intervals are within the normal range. At faster rates, AT's P waves often merge with T waves, making it difficult to identify the atrial activity.

The rate of ventricular response and regularity of ventricular rhythm are affected by conduction through the AV node. Usually, conduction takes the form of one P for every QRS; however, a preexisting AV block or digitalis toxicity may alter conduction (i.e., two or three P waves for every QRS). Varying conduction helps with interpretation, because it makes the P waves more apparent.

The mechanism of AT is either reentry or enhanced automaticity of an atrial ectopic focus. Reentrant atrial tachycardia that is suddenly initiated by a premature atrial contraction and terminates abruptly is called **paroxysmal atrial tachycardia (PAT).** When an atrial ectopic focus begins to depolarize rapidly, the resulting atrial tachycardia is called **automatic** or **ectopic atrial tachycardia.**

Examples of MAT

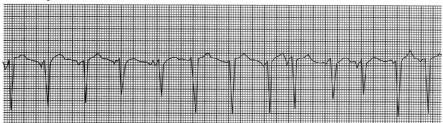

Rhythm strip reveals multifocal atrial tachycardia (MAT) with 1:1 conduction. Note the atrial rate is between 100-250 (about 110 in this example). The different-shaped P waves are prominent with slightly varying P-R intervals.

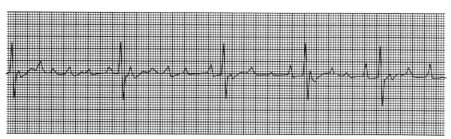

This MAT has varying conduction (more than one P wave for every QRS) that reveals the isoelectric (flat) baseline. Note the different P-wave morphology; some are notched while others are peaked.

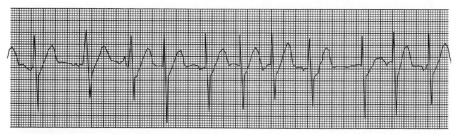

This MAT looks very much like atrial fibrillation, but note the varying-shaped P waves in front of the QRSs.

Differentiating Atrial Arrhythmias

Multifocal atrial tachycardia has a variety of P-wave shapes and slightly irregular rhythm, a flat baseline, varying P-R intervals, and a slightly irregular ventricular response.

Atrial fibrillation has no distinct P waves; a chaotic, undulating baseline; and an irregularly irregular ventricular response.

Atrial tachycardia has P waves that are uniform in shape and regular in rhythm, a flat baseline, and a frequently regular ventricular response.

Rapid Atrial Fibrillation

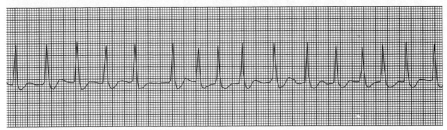

This rhythm strip shows rapid atrial fibrillation. Note the irregularly irregular ventricular response (R-R). The fine atrial oscillations (f waves) almost give an appearance of an isoelectric baseline.

Atrial Fibrillation with Slow Ventricular Response

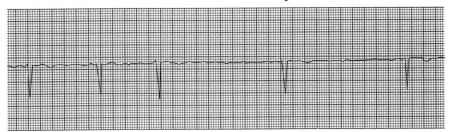

This atrial fibrillation has a slow ventricular response revealing the f waves. This patient may be taking digitalis, beta blockers or calcium antagonists, or the patient may have advanced AV block.

Atrial Tachycardia

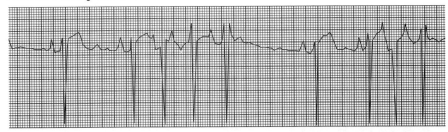

This rhythm strip reveals two episodes of a three-beat run of PAT. Note the different-shaped P wave (ectopic P) from the sinus P wave. The ectopic P waves are superimposed on the previous T waves.

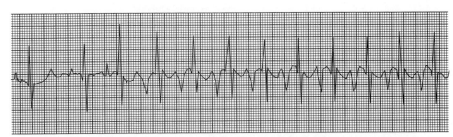

This rhythm strip begins with two sinus beats, followed by a PAC and a run of supraventricular tachycardia (SVT). SVT is a term used for a rapid rhythm that occurs above the ventricles in which P waves cannot be easily discerned. (Some examples of SVT are rapid atrial fibrillation, atrial flutter with 1:1 conduction, junctional tachycardia and atrial tachycardia.) This SVT is most likely atrial tachycardia. Note the difficulty in assessing the P waves, because they are superimposed on the previous T waves. This atrial tachycardia begins abruptly (with a PAC) and terminates spontaneously. Therefore, it can be called paroxysmal atrial tachycardia (PAT). The PAT ends abruptly and is followed by an atrial beat (note ectopic tent-shaped P wave) followed by two sinus beats.

Often seen in healthy adults, AT is a result of overstimulation of the sympathetic nervous system from fatigue, smoking cigarettes, or drinking alcohol. AT is also seen in patients who have coronary artery disease, valvular heart disease, or CHF(3).

Healthy people who have paroxysmal atrial tachycardia can usually slow or stop the arrhythmia with vagal maneuvers. These maneuvers can be done at home and include yawning, breath holding, or bearing down against a closed glottis (the Vasalva maneuver). Another effective intervention is immersing the face in cold water, thus triggering a strong vagal response(4). Carotid massage is an option only when the patient has no bruits, and only when the patient is on a cardiac monitor, because baroreceptor response by the carotid artery could cause asystole or profound blocking at the AV junction.

Drug therapy with verapamil (Calan, Isoptin) has been most effective for slowing or terminating AT; digoxin (Lanoxin), quinidine, propranolol (Inderal), procainamide (Pronestyl), and disopyramide (Norpace) can also be used. Newer drugs being used for AT and other supraventricular tachycardias are propafenone (Rythmol), esmolol (Brevibloc), and adenosine (Adenocard).

Cardioversion with 50 to 100 joules is recommended for patients with AT who develop hemodynamic compromise(3).

So, to differentiate **multifocal atrial tachycardia** from **atrial tachycardia**, remember that MAT's P waves are of two different configurations, while AT's P waves are uniform. Also, MAT's rhythm is irregular due to the different atrial foci, whereas AT has one focus with a regular rate of discharge.

REFERENCES

1. Chung, E. *Principles of Cardiac Arrhythmias,* 4th ed. Baltimore, Williams & Wilkins, 1988.
2. Marriott, H. J. *Practical Electrocardiography,* 8th ed. Baltimore, Williams & Wilkins, 1988.
3. Ordonez, R. V. Monitoring the patient with supraventricular dysrhythmias. *Nurs.Clin.North Am.* 22(1):49-59, Mar. 1987.
4. Phillips, R. E., and Feeney, M. K. *Cardiac Rhythms: A Systematic Approach to Interpretation.* 2d ed. Philadelphia, W.B. Saunders Co., 1980.

HOW HIV ATTACKS THE PERIPHERAL NERVOUS SYSTEM

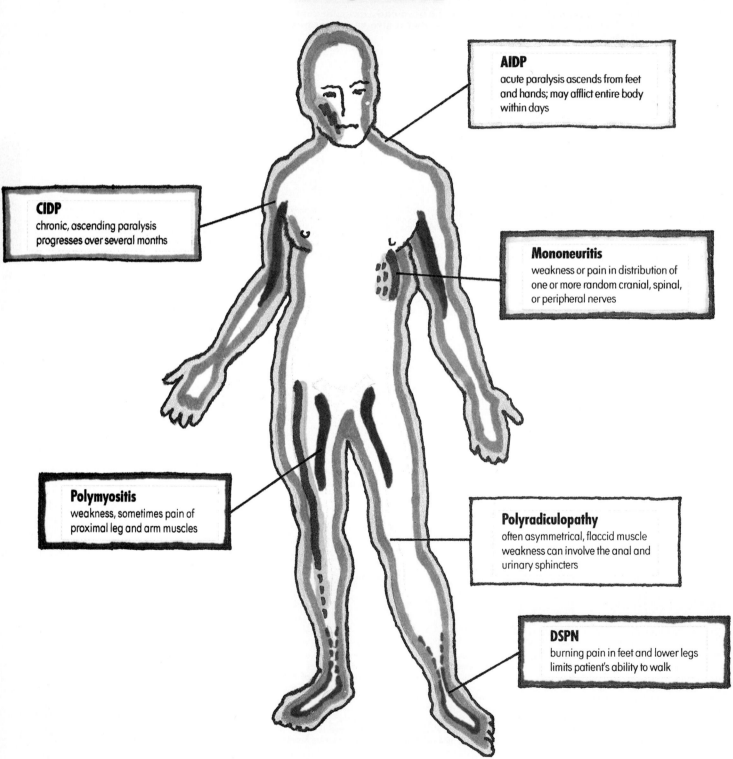

AIDP
acute paralysis ascends from feet and hands; may afflict entire body within days

CIDP
chronic, ascending paralysis progresses over several months

Mononeuritis
weakness or pain in distribution of one or more random cranial, spinal, or peripheral nerves

Polymyositis
weakness, sometimes pain of proximal leg and arm muscles

Polyradiculopathy
often asymmetrical, flaccid muscle weakness can involve the anal and urinary sphincters

DSPN
burning pain in feet and lower legs limits patient's ability to walk

By Priscilla Scherer
Reprinted from American Journal of Nursing May, 1990

As HIV-infected patients live longer, new and different HIV-related illnesses are beginning to surface. What happens to these patients' peripheral nervous systems over time?

One of the cruel ironies of human immunodeficiency virus (HIV) is that as successfully treated patients live longer HIV-related opportunistic illnesses continue to emerge. And some conditions, once obscured by fiercely debilitating and often fatal bouts with *Pneumocystis carinii* pneumonia, are now taking center stage. Such is the case with HIV-associated peripheral nervous system (PNS) disease.

The neuromuscular manifestations of HIV are perhaps the least understood of all HIV-related phenomena. By some reports, as many as 80 percent of people with HIV disease suffer some neurological symptoms, ranging from minor, nonprogressing numbness of the fingertips to, less commonly, quadriplegia[1-4]. Some asymptomatic HIV-positive people have white blood cells in their cerebrospinal fluid (a condition called CSF pleocytosis); they may remain asymptomatic or they may develop PNS symptoms at any time during the course of infection.

Studies have shown that 25 to 60 percent of HIV-infected people who have no neurological symptoms have demonstrated electrophysiologic evidence of neuromuscular dysfunction[2,5]. PNS disease can also crop up as a result of the malnutrition, wasting, and immobility associated with advanced HIV disease, namely, AIDS[2]. And making matters even worse is the fact that some of the very drugs used to fight HIV-related illness can also cause sensory and motor neuropathies[6].

Priscilla Scherer, RN, BA, is a contributing editor of AJN *and an education consultant at the Momentum Project, Inc., and the Gay Men's Health Crisis, New York, NY. She thanks JoAnne Bennett, RN, MA, for her expert advice.*

BRENDA BOOTH

The neuropathies

Acute inflammatory demyelinating sensorimotor polyradiculopathy (AIDP), also called Guillain-Barré syndrome, can and does occur anywhere along the continuum of HIV disease. The syndrome has been seen at seroconversion, sometimes even before HIV antibodies can be detected in the blood, but more often it flares later, during the long period of otherwise asymptomatic HIV infection[2-4].

HIV-related AIDP develops much like the seronegative forms—10 to 15 days after a bout with a viral illness (in this case, HIV) and the associated fever, swollen glands, rash, and diarrhea. Symptoms of AIDP include an ascending paralysis, primarily motor, that starts in the hands and feet but gradually overtakes arms, legs, abdomen, chest, and head[2-4]. These symptoms usually develop and peak within days of onset. Sometimes AIDP will only involve the lower body, but more often, the syndrome progresses to quadriplegia and patients need ventilatory support. Gradually, the paralysis subsides—first from the head and trunk and eventually from the hands and feet.

Most patients recover from AIDP, but by some reports, at a slower rate than do HIV-negative patients[3]. Plasmapheresis can help speed recovery, although some patients recover spontaneously. For a few, however, the course is sudden and intense and ends in death[2].

Because early treatment can blunt the severity of the symptoms of AIDP, keep close watch on any HIV-positive person who begins to feel sensorimotor symptoms in his (her) hands or feet. Since AIDP develops rapidly, alert the patient and those

By some reports, as many as 80 percent of HIV-infected people suffer some neurological symptoms, ranging from minor tingling of the fingertips all the way to quadriplegia.

around him to signs of disease progression. Refer him for diagnosis and treatment. And refer anyone not known to be HIV-positive who presents with early symptoms of AIDP for HIV screening.

Because most patients with AIDP fear they'll stop breathing and die when no one is paying attention, they may seem demanding. All they really want, however, is the reassurance that someone is watching out for them. Ideally, such patients would be admitted to intensive care for around-the-clock monitoring. Short of one-on-one nursing care, you might try respiratory monitoring and care schedules that promote frequent contact with staff. Far less than ideal is a private room, where the patient may feel too isolated.

As the weakness and numbness ascend the arms, **watch for signs of respiratory involvement,** such as easy fatigability, air hunger, and abdominal breathing. The HIV patient who needs mechanical ventilation will require more attention than usual to prevent pulmonary infection.

To forestall atrophy from lack of use of already weakened muscles and to head off later functional disability, arrange for the patient to have physical therapy as soon as symptoms appear. If only his feet are involved, urge him to flex and extend them hourly while awake to prevent foot drop and to enhance vascular return. If the patient is too weak for active exercise, incorporate passive range of motion exercises and position changes into his daily care routine.

Preventing skin breakdown is important for anyone confined to bed, but for the immunocompromised person, intact skin is vital for holding potentially lethal infections at bay. Keep the patient well nourished and

hydrated and his skin clean and dry. Massage his skin often to stimulate circulation and reposition him at least every two hours. Since energy needs rise with HIV infection and since the patient with AIDP may not be able to swallow, he may need enteral and parenteral supplements.

Chronic inflammatory demyelinating polyneuropathy (CIDP) can also occur before or after other symptoms of HIV disease appear. Chronic IDP resembles acute IDP except that after onset the chronic type proceeds slowly over several months instead of over several days(2,3). Typically, patients develop muscle weakness or paralysis with some sensory deficits and their deep tendon reflexes disappear.

CIDP improves spontaneously in some patients, but most become progressively weaker over time. Plasmapheresis reverses the syndrome, but it may have to be repeated since CIDP can relapse. Prednisone relieves the symptoms, but it can also compound immune dysfunction, making it risky therapy for patients who are HIV-positive(2,4).

How do acute and chronic IDP develop? Theories include direct infection of the spinal nerves and nerve roots with either HIV or cytomegalovirus (CMV) or both; an immune-system attack on the myelin surrounding the nerves (a theory also proposed for HIV-seronegative Guillain Barré syndrome); and an autoimmune response against specific cells of the myelin sheath. This autoimmune response might be triggered by HIV-induced B-cell dysfunctions(2,3,7).

Distal sensory polyneuropathy (DSPN), also called distal axonopathy, is the most common neuropathy seen in people with AIDS, although it can emerge earlier in the course of

HIV disease. The exact cause of DSPN is not known; theories include toxic, metabolic, and nutritional factors, as well as direct infection of the nerves by HIV and other viruses such as CMV(2-4).

Symptoms begin in the foot, where burning pain and hypersensitivity make it difficult for the person to walk. Soon the entire foot becomes weak, sensitivity to touch becomes exaggerated, and Achilles tendon reflexes disappear(2,3). DSPN progresses relentlessly, responding neither to steroids nor to plasmapheresis. Treatment focuses on symptom relief—with tricyclic antidepressants, anticonvulsants, salicylates, cannabis (marijuana), and narcotic analgesics(2,3). Zidovudine (AZT, Retrovir) has improved symptoms and nerve conduction in a limited number of patients(2,4,8).

For nurses, managing these symptoms can be frustrating since the person's pain may be unremitting despite drug therapies. To head off the pain with analgesics before it becomes intractable, monitor changes in pain intensity and teach the patient to do the same. Give analgesics around-the-clock instead of PRN to sustain steady pain relief. Encourage the patient to try relaxation techniques, imagery, and meditation to help alleviate the pain(9).

If the patient can walk, suggest he wear loose-fitting shoes made of a soft material that "gives"—canvas, for example—and thick Orlon-and-cotton athletic socks to cushion the feet. A cradle over the foot of the bed keeps sheets and blankets from rubbing against the feet and aggravating the pain.

Progressive polyradiculopathy is commonly seen in people with AIDS, although it can occur earlier in the

DRUGS, FOOD, AND THE PNS

Drugs and nutritional derangements can cause peripheral nervous system (PNS) symptoms that mimic organic syndromes. While the experimental nucleoside analogue dideoxyinosine (ddI) may be the most notorious culprit, a number of other drugs used to treat HIV itself or related opportunistic infections may also produce PNS symptoms. Below is a partial list. Because our experience with most treatments is limited and still evolving, any drug should be suspect when neurologic symptoms emerge in HIV disease.

DRUG	SYMPTOM
amphotericin B (Fungizone)	paresthesia, muscle cramps, extreme fatigue
diaminodiphenylsulfone (Dapsone)	predominantly motor neuropathy
dideoxyinosine (ddI)	painful paresthesia
DHPG (Ganciclovir)	myalgia
etoposide (VePesid)	ataxia, paresthesia
phenytoin (Dilantin)	ataxia, nystagmus
pyrimethamine (Daraprim)	ataxia
sulfadoxine/pyrimethamine (Fansidar)	peripheral pain, ataxia, muscle weakness
sulfamethoxazole/trimethoprim (Bactrim)	myalgia, arthralgia
vinblastine (Velban)	ataxia, paresthesia, myalgia, muscle weakness
zidovudine (Retrovir, AZT)	myalgia, generalized weakness

NUTRITIONAL DEFICIENCY	SYMPTOM
calories	muscle wasting, weakness
protein	muscle wasting, weakness
vitamin B1 (Thiamine)	distal muscle weakness, painful peripheral neuropathy
vitamin B6 (Pyridoxine)	painful peripheral neuropathy, muscle twitching
vitamin B12	numbness, paresthesia, ataxia, weakness
biotin	muscle pain
pantothenic acid	impaired coordination
phosphorus	muscle weakness, pain, paresthesia
potassium (K+ excess: muscle weakness)	muscle weakness
sodium	muscle weakness, cramps
tryptophan	ataxia

Sources: AIDS-HIV Infection: A Reference Guide for Nursing Professionals, ed. by J. H. Flaskerud. Philadelphia, W. B. Saunders Co., 1988.

Harrison's Principles of Internal Medicine 10th ed., New York, McGraw Hill Book Co., 1988.

Physician's Desk Reference, Oradell, NJ, Medical Economics Co., 1989.

course of HIV disease. The syndrome affects the legs as well as the anal and urinary sphincters. It causes an often asymmetrical flaccid muscle weakness, obliterates deep tendon reflexes, and blunts sensation in the legs. This neuropathy does not respond to treatment and inevitably leads to death(2,4).

Infection of the nerve roots in the spinal cord, probably with CMV, is a likely cause of polyradiculopathy(4). One case report, however, describes a patient with the syndrome who improved slightly with AZT therapy, suggesting that the syndrome is directly related to HIV(10).

Mononeuritis multiplex is an inflammation of random individual spinal, cranial, or peripheral nerves. The inflammation leads to sensory or motor deficits—isolated facial nerve paralysis (Bell's palsy), for example, or lower leg pain and weakness from inflammation of the sciatic nerve. These symptoms are typically seen during the early stages of symptomatic HIV infection(2-4).

Some cases resolve spontaneously and some patients respond to plasmapheresis, but for others, nerve involvement progresses and takes over many peripheral nerves, leading to chronic deficits and even death(2,3). It's important to distinguish mononeuritis multiplex from other syndromes that cause similar symptoms but that might respond to therapy (varicella-zoster and HIV or CMV meningitis, for example).

The myopathies
Polymyositis is the most common muscle disease seen in HIV-infected people(2). It can appear before other symptoms of HIV infection or not until the later stages of AIDS. Patients experience a subacute onset of

weakness and sometimes pain in the proximal muscles of the thighs and upper arms.

What causes polymyositis is not certain, but it seems that muscle fibers infiltrated with phagocytes (possibly engulfing an infectious agent such as HIV) become inflamed and eventually degenerate and die.

Although immunosuppressants have proved successful in treating non-HIV-related polymyositis, only about half the HIV-positive patients with the syndrome have responded. Because immunosuppressants may aggravate the disease process, they must be used with extreme caution in HIV-positive patients(2,3).

A variety of other neuromuscular disorders have been reported in people who have HIV disease, among them syndromes associated with malnutrition, rapid weight loss, prolonged bed rest; **amyotrophic lateral sclerosis** (ALS) with acute onset at seroconversion; and subclinical neuromuscular disease(2,5). **Vacuolar myelopathy** with ataxia and leg weakness is often associated with the AIDS dementia complex(11). (See "How AIDS Attacks the Brain," AJN, January 1990.) As our experience with HIV broadens, the list is sure to lengthen.

Immobility's other toll
Since HIV most often strikes during the prime of life, the debilitation and loss of control are especially devastating. We spend a great deal of energy helping these patients ward off the physical hazards of immobility; meanwhile, the emotional hazards are demanding equal attention.

Toward that end, try to bolster the patient's abilities by letting him do as much as he can. Temper your expectations with an understanding of

what he can actually achieve physically. Emphasize accomplishments without setting unrealistic goals. Reinforce the patient's opportunities to make decisions and to express preferences(9).

False optimism can only do a disservice to the person with HIV-related PNS disease. It can undermine his trust in you and erode his self-esteem as he recognizes his progressive decline. On the other hand, helping him to confront his disability may trigger self-discovery and guide him toward previously untapped strengths.

REFERENCES

1. Jansen, R. S., and others. Human immunodeficiency virus (HIV) infection and the nervous system: report from the American Academy of Neurology AIDS Task Force. *Neurology* 39:119–122, Jan. 1989.
2. Dalakas, M. C., and Pezeshkpour, G. H. Neuromuscular diseases associated with human immunodeficiency virus infection. *Ann.Neurol.* 23(Suppl):S38–S48, Nov. 1988.
3. Cornblath, D. R. Treatment of the neuromuscular complications of human immunodeficiency virus infection. *Ann.Neurol.* 23(Suppl):S88–S91, Nov. 1988.
4. Parry, G. J. Peripheral neuropathies associated with human immunodeficiency virus infection. *Ann.Neurol.* 23(Suppl):S49–S53, Nov. 1988.
5. Chavenet, P., and others. Infraclinical neuropathies related to immunodeficiency virus infection associated with higher T-helper cell count. *J.Acquired Immune Def.Synd.* 2:564–569, Nov. 1989.
6. Flaskerud, J. H., ed. *AIDS/HIV Infection: A Reference Guide for Nursing Professionals.* Philadelphia, W. B. Saunders Co., 1988, pp. 58–73.
7. *Ibid.*, pp. 37–57.
8. Yarchoan, R., and others. Long-term administration of 3′-azido-2′, 3′-dideoxythymidine to patients with AIDS-related neurological disease. *Ann.Neurol.* 23(Suppl):S82–S87, Nov. 1988.
9. Bennett, J. Helping people with AIDS live well at home. *Nurs.Clin.North.Am.* 23:731–748, Dec. 1988.
10. Dalakas, M. C., and others. Treatment of human immunodeficiency virus-related polyneuropathy with 3′-azido-2′, 3′-dideoxythymidine. *Ann.Neurol.* 23(Suppl):S92–S94, Nov. 1988.
11. Navia, B. A., and others. The AIDS dementia complex. Part 1, clinical features. *Ann.Neurol.* 19:517–524, June 1986.

CARDIOVASCULAR

LASERS

A LOOK INTO THE FUTURE

By Laura T. Hall

Reprinted from American Journal of Nursing July, 1990

Since their development in the early 1960s, lasers have received some sensational press. Movie makers depict the ultimate weapon as a bright ray that cuts through anything. Remember James Bond in the movie *Goldfinger*—strapped to a metal table that was slowly being bisected by a laser? Lasers, of course, have a therapeutic side as well. Their preciseness and diversity make them ideal for surgery, particularly cardiovascular procedures, such as laser angioplasty.

Although long-term results of laser angioplasty are not yet in, so far it seems that using a laser to open occlusions and relieve stenosis of coronary arteries does work. One study cited a 5% to 7% reocclusion rate at one year—possibly so low because the smooth arterial surface the laser leaves discourages thrombus formation[1,2].

Successful laser angioplasty selectively ablates plaque without embolization, perforation, burns, or shock-wave effects that cause vessels to spasm[3]. When followed by balloon angioplasty the procedure is called *laser-assisted balloon angioplasty* (LABA).

Lasers can be used on total occlusions that cannot be opened by balloon angioplasty alone. Patients who otherwise would have no choice but bypass are now being treated percutaneously. And, laser therapy without subsequent balloon dilation makes it possible to relieve long, calcified and/or eccentric lesions and stenoses and occlusions in the left main coronary artery or at bifurcations—all of which are risky subjects for balloon treatment[4].

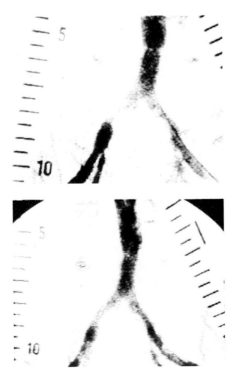

Dramatic evidence of stenosis in iliac artery (top) opened by laser angioplasty (bottom).

The smooth, thrombus-resistant finish may be a main advantage of another new procedure: using lasers just after standard balloon angioplasty to weld intimal flaps (created as plaque is disrupted) to the artery wall. With this technique, arteries of all 13 patients in one study were still open one month later[5].

Plaque can also be removed from arteries with laser endarterectomy. Intraoperatively, a hand-held CO_2 laser is used to remove plaque distal to bypass sites. Since the energy delivery system is introduced via a small incision in the artery, the need for excessive dissection is eliminated. Laser endarterectomy cleans out the plaque more completely than standard endarterectomy techniques do, but early thrombosis has been seen in 24% of cases[6].

Preparing the patient

Percutaneous laser angioplasty is usually done in the angiography suite or cath lab, but it can also be done in the O.R. using general anesthesia. Preoperatively, the patient needs to know how the laser works and what to expect. Understanding terminology and seeing the laser equipment beforehand may relieve the shock of being wheeled into a cath lab housing a noisy laser machine—and hearing staff drop words like "fire."

The hazards of deflected laser beams include eye and skin damage

Laura T. Hall, RN, MSN, is coordinator of the cardiovascular laser center at the University of California at Los Angeles Medical Center.

and burns. During the procedure, protect the patient's eyes either by goggles that do not absorb the specific wavelength the laser emits or by saline-soaked eye pads. Wet drapes and nonflammable prep solutions are also used to prevent burns. (For more information about protection, see "Hospital Hazards," part I, Feb., and part II, Apr.)

During laser emission, it is not unusual for patients to feel a slight burning in the target area; some patients feel chest pain as their coronary arteries are treated(7). Transient reperfusion arrhythmias sometimes occur just after a coronary artery is opened. They usually respond to lidocaine or other antiarrhythmics.

Heparin is often given during laser surgery to keep clots from forming on the catheter. If direct anticoagulation therapy is needed to keep the artery open or to dissolve newly formed thrombi, the femoral sheath used to maintain arterial access is sutured in place and an anticoagulant drug infused(8).

After laser surgery

Check the access site for frank bleeding or hematoma after the laser surgery is completed. If the site bleeds, apply direct pressure above the puncture site until the bleeding stops (it may take 15 to 30 minutes if the patient is on anticoagulant therapy). Encourage the patient to drink liquids and give IV fluids as prescribed.

Keep an accurate intake and output record. The contrast medium used for fluoroscopy acts as an osmotic diuretic and can be toxic to the kidneys, so monitor the renal function tests. To check for hidden blood loss, monitor the patient's hemoglobin and hematocrit.

Have the patient lie flat in bed (less than a 30° elevation) with the leg (the arm is rarely used as the access site) held straight for six to eight hours after the procedure or until the

femoral sheath is removed. If the patient needs continued anticoagulant therapy, check that the sheath's position is intact and monitor partial thromboplastin levels(8). Monitor patients for cardiac arrhythmias.

Most patients undergoing cardiovascular laser procedures that use the percutaneous approach can resume near-normal activities safely the day after discharge. The hospital stay is usually only 24 to 36 hours—a distinct advantage over the six-week-

recovery period coronary bypass patients need.

On the horizon

Cardiovascular use of lasers is still in its infancy, and many new applications are under evaluation. Laser techniques for microvascular anastomosis, for direct myocardial revascularization, and for aberrant conduction pathway repair of dissecting aneurysms are just some of the areas being investigated(7,9).

The Evolving Cardiovascular Laser

The direct-beam laser. The earliest clinical trials of cardiovascular (CV) laser therapy used direct laser energy, guided by fluoroscopy. The direct beam burned or perforated whatever it fired on—plaque, blood, or a healthy arterial wall. But because the channel the direct beam drives through the occlusion is very narrow, reocclusion rates were high.

One of the first studies of CV laser therapy described using an Nd:YAG laser with a bare-tipped optical fiber to recanalize two totally occluded arteries and one severely stenosed artery(12). Researchers concluded that the technique had limited use because they could only create a narrow tunnel (leaving plaque behind) and that, whenever a laser was used, arterial walls were burned.

Another early study reported successful use of direct laser energy to open peripheral arteries in eight of 16 patients(13). The researchers reported shock-wave–induced arterial spasm when higher energy settings were used. The spasms did not respond to drug therapy, but the arteries reopened spontaneously shortly afterward and were successfully dilated via balloon.

The hot-tipped or thermal probe laser. The next step in removing arteriosclerotic plaques was using a rounded, metal-tipped catheter to create a larger channel through the obstruction. The procedure uses the energy of either an Nd:YAG or an argon laser to heat the tip of the catheter to more than 400° C (752° F). Under fluoroscopy, the lesion is crossed as the tip melts through the occlusion, creating a channel wide enough to admit a balloon catheter, which widens the channel even further. A study of 129 patients undergoing hot-tipped laser angioplasty reported an initial success rate and a one-year success rate of 77%(14). However, a more recent study involving 47 patients reported an initial success rate of only 55%(15).

The hot-tipped laser can adhere to a vessel wall or to plaque, causing arterial burns, although the risk of this complication can be reduced by keeping the tip in motion. Incidence of perforation is lower than with a direct beam and any debris produced is small enough to be filtered out by the kidneys(16).

The eximer laser emits a short-duration, high-energy pulse of ultra-

Anastomosing small vessels by laser is faster than the typical eight-suture anastomosis—and reduces the risk of foreign bodies entering the wound. Less scar tissue forms after laser anastomosis; the incidence of pseudo-aneurysms is low; and animal studies have shown that laser anastomoses are strong, discourage thrombus formation, and heal well(9,10).

In Japan and in the Soviet Union, myocardial revascularization has also been attempted on animals. Using an

violet light that has a shorter wavelength than that of an argon laser. It creates a crater with a smooth edge and seems to ablate tissue without burning adjacent tissue(17). One group of researchers reported that the eximer laser seems safe and effective for recanalizing arteries(18). Another group reported an initial success rate of 77%, with a 28% reocclusion rate at three months(19). That study also reported that the eximer is especially useful for removing hard or calcified plaque.

The 'smart' laser was developed in an attempt to avoid damaging healthy tissue by better directing laser energy. This laser uses a computerized system that identifies tissue based on its fluorescence, that is, the specific wavelength at which a given tissue readmits light(20). The system consists of a computer, a low-powered diagnostic laser, a high-power treatment laser, and a fiber-optic energy delivery system (Laserwire ™).

In brief, the laser wire is advanced to the occlusion and the diagnostic laser fires. If the computer identifies the tissue as plaque or thrombus, the treatment laser fires *into* a portion of the tissue the diagnostic laser has penetrated, thus eliminating the risk

of burning healthy tissue that may be thinly covered by plaque or thrombus. FDA-approved in 1988 for clinical trials, this laser has shown an initial success rate of 100% (in 19 patients), and when followed by balloon dilation, a success rate of 94%(21).

Clearing coronary arteries. The first published study of using lasers in coronary arteries described treating proximal coronary artery stenosis with an argon laser during bypass surgery(22). All five of the treated patients had patent arteries immediately after surgery, but only one had a patent native coronary artery 25 days later.

A case study described using a hot-tipped laser to reduce a 90% occlusion of a left anterior descending artery to a 50% occlusion(15). Bal-

loon angioplasty subsequently reduced the stenosis to 10%, and the patient was asymptomatic four weeks later. Reported complications of the thermal-probe approach include transient chest pain during laser emission, arterial wall dissection, slight postprocedure CPK elevations, and evidence of myocardial infarction (possibly due to spasm or thrombus formation at the site of an arterial wall injury)(23).

In another study, stenosis was reduced in two patients who underwent percutaneous eximer laser therapy(24). One restenosed four weeks after the procedure, but the second was still symptom-free eight months later. Another study of 30 patients treated with an eximer laser reported a 90% immediate success rate with only one early reocclusion(25).

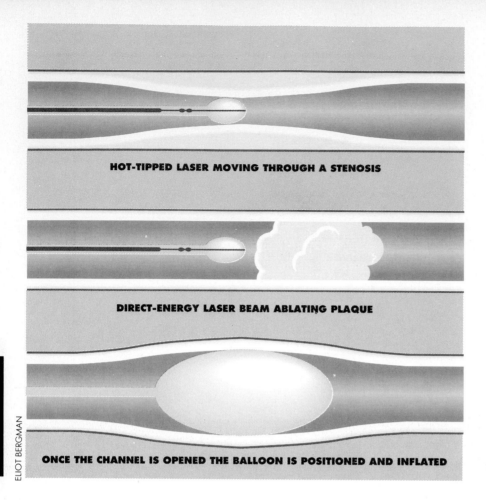

HOT-TIPPED LASER MOVING THROUGH A STENOSIS

DIRECT-ENERGY LASER BEAM ABLATING PLAQUE

ONCE THE CHANNEL IS OPENED THE BALLOON IS POSITIONED AND INFLATED

ELIOT BERGMAN

argon laser to drill miniature holes into ischemic left ventricular myocardium, the researchers reestablished perfusion to the compromised muscle(10). Five months postop, the laser channels were still patent, channel walls had endothelialized, and the adjacent muscle was healthy.

Resecting aberrant conduction pathways percutaneously in a full beating heart poses a technical challenge; in fact, the surgery carries a 10% mortality rate. Animal studies suggest that using a laser percutaneously to interrupt and/or ablate the circuit may lower that mortality rate and may even obviate surgery(7,11).

Also on the horizon are valvular calcium resection with lasers, control of arrhythmias by irradiating ectopic foci, and laser myomectomy for hypertrophic obstructive cardiomyopathy(7,11).

Of course, laser technology has yet to be perfected and many questions need to be answered. For example, is perforation less likely with a plastic tip than with a metal one? And which is best for recanalizing arteries—the hot-tipped laser, direct energy, or a combination of both?

We need lengthy follow-up studies to see how long the arteries opened with lasers stay open—and how cost-effective it is to use lasers. Why do arteries reocclude in some patients and not others? What we can do to stop occlusions before they occur?

Many of the laser therapies discussed in this article are still experimental. Some may prove ineffective; others undoubtedly will be standard treatment in the near future.

REFERENCES

1. Sanborn, T. A. Laser angioplasty. *Circulation* 78:769–774, Sept. 1988.
2. _____, and others. Percutaneous laser thermal angioplasty: initial results and 1-year follow-up in 129 femoropopliteal lesions. *Radiology* 168:121–125, July 1988.
3. White, G. H. Angioscopy and lasers in cardiovascular surgery: current applications and future prospects. *Aust.N.Z.J.Surg.* 58:271–274, Apr. 1988.
4. Eldar, M. Laser angioplasty: a review. *Isr.J.Med.Sci.* 25:222–228, Apr. 1989.
5. Jenkins, R., and Spears, R. Laser welding as an adjunct to endovascular intervention. IN *Endovascular Surgery*, ed. by W. S. Moore and S. S. Ahn. Philadelphia, W. B. Saunders Co., 1989, pp. 278–288.
6. Livesay, J. J. Laser technique for coronary endarterectomy. *Adv.Cardiol.* 36:54–61, 1988.
7. Sakallaris, B. Laser therapy for cardiovascular disease. *Heart Lung* 16:465–471, 1987.
8. Webber, M., and Jenkins, N. Laser treatment in peripheral vascular disease. *Prog.Cardiovasc.Dis.* 30:81–88, 1988.
9. Hunter, J. G., and Dixon, J. A. Lasers in cardiovascular surgery—current status. *West.J.Med.* 142:506–510, Apr. 1985.
10. Robertson, T. L. Overview of laser applications in the treatment of cardiovascular disease. IN *Lasers in Cardiovascular Disease*, ed. by R. A. White and W. S. Grundfest. Chicago, Year Book Medical Publishers, 1989, pp. 64–74.
11. Bohigian, G., and others. Laser applications today and tomorrow. *Patient Care* 87:62–79, 1987.
12. Geschwind, H. J., and others. Conditions for effective Nd-YAG laser angioplasty. *Br.Heart J.* 52:484–489, Nov. 1984.
13. Ginsburg, R., and others. Percutaneous transluminal laser angioplasty for treatment of peripheral vascular disease. *Radiology* 156:619–624, Sept. 1985.
14. Sanborn, T. A., and others. Percutaneous coronary laser thermal angioplasty. *J.Am.Coll.Cardiol.* 8:1437–1440, Dec. 1986.
15. Brown, E. Laser advancements spur debate on role in angioplasty. *Amer.Med.News*, Apr. 20, 1990, pp. 17–18.
16. Cox, J. L., and Jacobs, C. P. Laser-assisted angioplasty. *AORN J.* 46:835–846, Nov. 1987.
17. Higginson, L. A., and others. Arterial response to eximer and argon laser irradiation in the atherosclerotic swine. *Lasers Med.Sci.* 4:85–92, 1988.
18. Selzer, P. M., and others. Optimizing strategies for laser angioplasty. *Invest.Radiol.* 20:860–866, Nov. 1985.
19. Grundfest, and others. Eximer laser angioplasty: from basic science to clinical trials. IN *Endovascular Surgery*, ed. by W. S. Moore and S. S. Ahn. Philadelphia, W. B. Saunders Co., 1989, pp. 432–441.
20. Mok, W. Construction of the MCM smart laser. IN *Endovascular Surgery*, ed. by W. S. Moore and S. S. Ahn. Philadelphia, W. B. Saunders Co., 1989, pp. 453–465.
21. Geschwind, H. J., and others. Percutaneous pulsed laser-assisted balloon angioplasty guided by spectroscopy. *Am.Heart J.* 117:1147–1152, May 1989.
22. Choy, D. S., and others. Human coronary laser recanalization. *Clin.Cardio.* 7:377–381, July 1984.
23. Cumberland, D. C., and others. Percutaneous laser-assisted coronary angioplasty. (Letter) *Lancet* 2:214, July 26, 1986.
24. Litvack, F., and others. Percutaneous eximer laser angioplasty of aortocoronary saphenous vein grafts. *J.Am.Coll.Cardiol.* 14:803–808, Sept. 1989.
25. Karsch, K. R., and others. Percutaneous coronary eximer laser angioplasty: initial clinical results. *Lancet* 2:647–650, Sept. 16, 1989.

UNDERSTANDING AUTONOMIC DYSREFLEXIA

By Darlene N. Finocchiaro/Shari T. Herzfeld

Reprinted from American Journal of Nursing September, 1990

Mitch was severely sunburned at the beach yesterday. Since then, he's been in medical ICU receiving IV antihypertensives.

Every time David has a full bladder, he gets a headache and his BP rises 20 mm Hg.

Lucy is in labor. As the baby's head crowns, Lucy's blood pressure shoots up precipitously.

What do these three people have in common? They are all spinal-cord injured, and they are all experiencing autonomic dysreflexia—a life-threatening complication of high thoracic and cervical spinal-cord injuries. Besides causing paralysis, the spinal-cord lesion interrupts the feedback loop of the autonomic nervous system. Without that feedback, any irritation below the level of the injury stimulates an exaggerated, unopposed, autonomic response.

Classic manifestations of dysreflexia include elevated blood pressure, pounding headache, bradycardia, sweating, and piloerection (gooseflesh). If the dysreflexic cycle continues unchecked, it may result in a stroke, cardiac arrest, blindness, or even death.

The ANS and spinal injury

The autonomic nervous system (ANS) has two branches—the sympathetic and the parasympathetic.

The parasympathetic branch is responsible for energy-conserving, maintenance functions such as digestion and elimination, whereas the sympathetic branch evokes a high-energy response in the face of danger—the "fight-or-flight" response.

The two branches of the ANS have complementary roles; as either is activated, the other is suppressed in a negative-feedback system. For example, in a stressful situation, the sympathetic effects of rapid pulse and respiration and elevated BP dominate, while parasympathetic functions such as digestion shut down. That is why a person under stress often becomes nauseated or loses his (her) appetite. Once the stress is relieved, the parasympathetic response returns the body to a calmer state.

The sympathetic and parasympathetic branches follow different routes from the central nervous system (CNS) to the periphery. The parasympathetic branch exits the CNS via the vagus nerve and the sacral segments at the end of the spinal cord; the sympathetic branch exits from the thoracic and lumbar regions of the spinal cord.

A spinal-cord injury above the thoracic sympathetic outflow—above the area of T5 and T6—separates the two branches of the ANS by disconnecting the feedback loop. Thus, dysreflexia is almost always seen in patients who have lesions above T6, although it has also been seen in patients with lesions as low as the T8 level(1). Because the syndrome is life-threatening, it is safer to err on the side of caution and consider any episode of paroxysmal hypertension in a patient with a lesion at T8 or above

Your 'stable' patient with a spinal-cord injury above T8 suddenly complains of a pounding headache. Here's why you should act fast.

to be autonomic dysreflexia.

In isolation, that is, without an intact feedback loop, the two branches of the ANS function independently. An irritant such as a full bladder or bowel can stimulate the sympathetic system with no opposition from the parasympathetic system. Without any opposition, systolic BP can reach 300 mm Hg, possibly causing cerebral or ocular hemorrhage or death. The sympathetic discharge can also cause pallor and piloerection below

When a spinal cord injury is at T8 or higher, an irritant below the level of injury can stimulate the autonomic nervous system to an exaggerated, dangerously unopposed response. Here, a full bladder triggers a sympathetic response (red line). The sympathetic response causes vasoconstriction, so the BP rises. The patient may also notice gooseflesh or pallor below the level of injury. The sympathetic response also constricts the bladder neck. However, the sympathetic response cannot cross the injured area of the cord to communicate with the parasympathetic system, so the BP continues to rise dangerously. Meanwhile, the baroreceptors in the carotids detect the rising BP and try to compensate by stimulating a parasympathetic response (blue line). The vagus nerve responds to the parasympathetic signals and slows the heart rate. Above the level of injury, the patient feels other parasympathetic effects: vasodilation, headache, flushing, sweating, and nasal congestion.

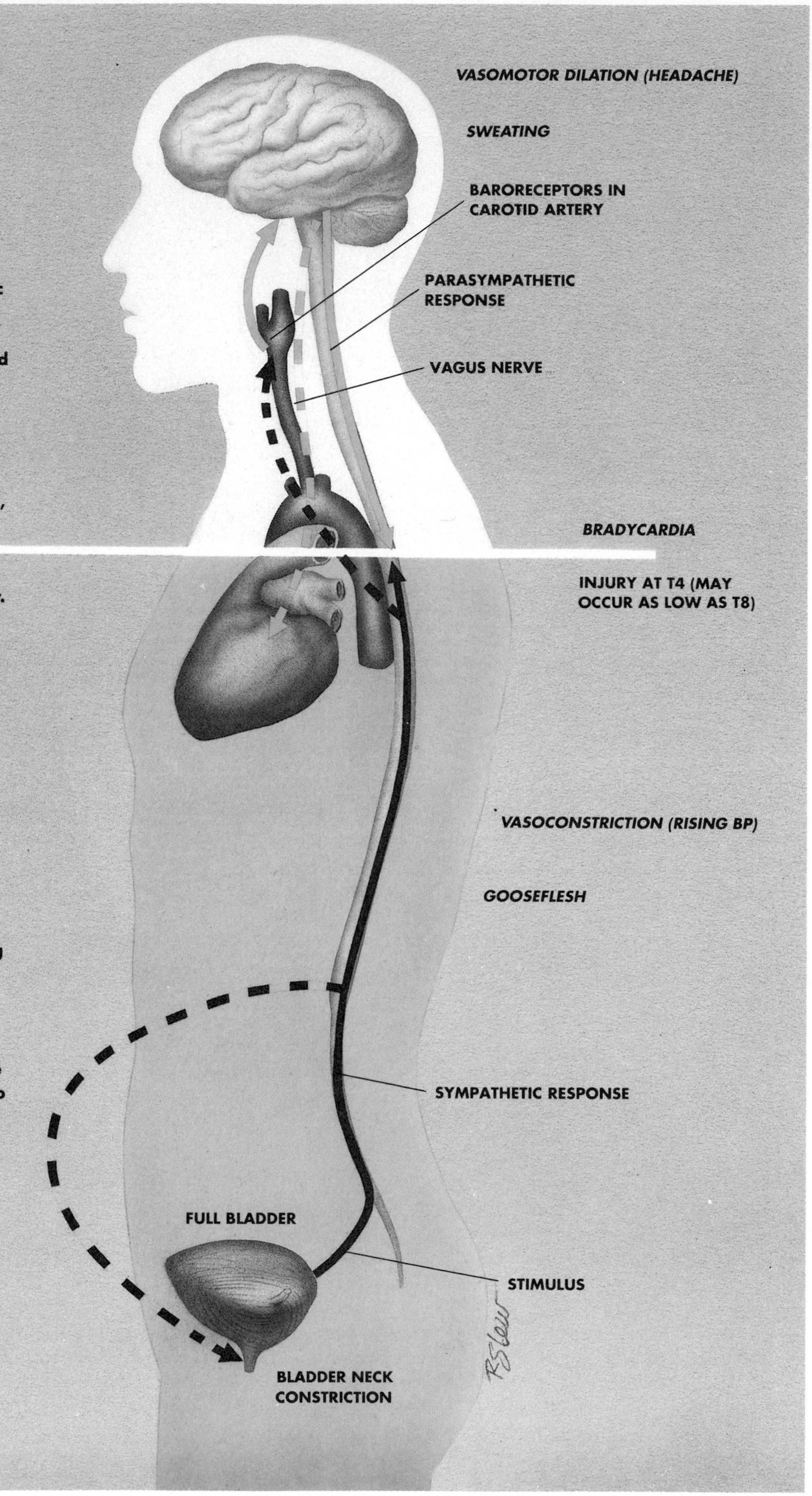

VASOMOTOR DILATION (HEADACHE)

SWEATING

BARORECEPTORS IN CAROTID ARTERY

PARASYMPATHETIC RESPONSE

VAGUS NERVE

BRADYCARDIA

INJURY AT T4 (MAY OCCUR AS LOW AS T8)

VASOCONSTRICTION (RISING BP)

GOOSEFLESH

SYMPATHETIC RESPONSE

STIMULUS

FULL BLADDER

BLADDER NECK CONSTRICTION

the level of injury as well as urinary retention, which, interestingly enough, is also the most common stimulus of dysreflexia.

When a sympathetic response is triggered, the body attempts to compensate in several ways. As the carotid bodies in the neck detect a rise in blood pressure, they stimulate a parasympathetic response of vasodilation above the level of injury. This accounts for the pounding headache, the profuse sweating and flushing above the level of injury, and the nasal congestion. The vagus nerve, a cranial nerve unaffected by spinal-cord injury, responds by triggering bradycardia, which, unchecked, can lead to cardiac arrest. But the parasympathetic response cannot cross the spinal lesion and is not strong enough to lower the BP. Meanwhile, the sympathetic system continues to raise the BP as long as the noxious stimulus continues. Fortunately, removing the noxious stimulus relieves the symptoms immediately.

Dysreflexia may not necessarily trigger the classic symptoms, but anyone who has had dysreflexia knows how his body responds. Therefore, listen to the patient. Some dysreflexia-prone patients wear a medical ID band or carry an alert card.

When to worry, what to do

When a spinal-cord-injured patient complains of pounding headache or diaphoresis, suspect autonomic dysreflexia. First, check his BP. If it is 20 mm Hg higher than usual and the patient's spinal lesion is above T8, dysreflexia is probably the reason. Stay with the patient and call for help. If the symptoms are severe, make sure the physician is notified. If the patient is not in a hospital, consider transporting him to the nearest emergency department.

Meanwhile, elevate the patient's head 90° if it can be done safely and quickly. This action will cause orthostatic hypotension and the BP will begin to drop.

Next, try to find out what triggered the episode. Pain, pressure,

sunburn, sexual intercourse, and surgical manipulation are possible causes, but the most common is bladder stimulation, which accounts for 76% of cases, followed by a full bowel, which accounts for 19%(2). Look for the source systematically, beginning with the most likely one, the bladder.

Whether the patient uses an external or an indwelling catheter, check that the drainage system is kink-free and working. Empty the collection bag to alleviate any back pressure in the system.

urine specimen for culture and sensitivity tests.

If the BP does not drop when the bladder is drained (and retained urine is not the problem), check the bowel—the next likely source of the dysreflexic episode.

Only an X ray can ascertain whether the bowel is full, but this is an impractical step in a hypertensive emergency. Instead, gently insert one-half to one ounce of anesthetic jelly such as dibucaine (Nupercainal) or Xylocaine ointment into the patient's rectum. Wait for the anesthetic to take

With 250,000 spinal-cord-injury survivors living in the United States today, dysreflexia is no longer confined to neuro or rehab units.

If no urine is draining and the catheter is indwelling, it may be plugged. Replacing the catheter is the best option; irrigating it at this point might further irritate the already distended bladder. But if you cannot change the catheter right away, irrigate it gently with no more than 30 mL of saline solution.

If the catheter is external or if the patient does not have a catheter in place, stimulate the bladder to empty reflexively by lightly tapping the area just over the symphysis pubis, by stroking the inside of the thigh, or by gently pulling the pubic hair. Perform these techniques gently because too much stimulation can further raise the BP. If the bladder does not empty, catheterize it with a Robinson catheter. Drain the bladder slowly and recheck the BP. When help arrives, have one person check the BP every two minutes, while the other continues the pressure-lowering techniques.

Sometimes as little as 200 mL of urine can cause dysreflexia in a sensitive patient who has a small bladder capacity. However, when a relatively small volume of urine causes a dysreflexic episode, the problem may be due to a urinary tract infection. In such situations, be sure to send a

effect, and then manually check for impaction and remove any retained feces.

If neither bladder nor bowel stimuli are the cause of dysreflexia, look for another source of pressure or irritation. If you cannot relieve the patient's symptoms, notify the physician. Have an IV line ready to deliver antihypertensive drugs and continue monitoring the BP every two minutes.

If drugs are needed

If the BP does not drop after the irritant is removed, or if the irritant is not easily removed (a pressure sore, for example), the patient needs antihypertensive drug therapy with hydralazine hydrochloride (Apresoline), diazoxide (Hyperstat), nifedipine (Procardia), atropine sulfate, or trimethaphan camsylate (Arfonad). Nitroglycerine paste is also sometimes used.

Hydralazine is often preferred because of its rapid onset, but it requires IV access. Nifedipine is popular because of its easy sublingual administration. A ganglionic-blocking agent such as mecamylamine (Inversine) is not recommended; besides interfering with nerve impulses that trigger vasoconstriction, it also blocks baroreceptors that would otherwise help raise the heart rate to its normal range. It is important to consider which drugs are safe to use to treat dysreflexic episodes, since the rise in BP is often accompanied by a drop in pulse rate.

The antihypertensives phenoxybenzamine (Dibenzyline) and prazosin hydrochloride (Minipress) are good choices for preventing dysreflexic episodes because, over time, they relax the bladder neck, thus promoting emptying.

Relief and results: three happy endings

Mitch, a C6 quadriplegic, cannot feel the pain of his sunburn; yet his sympathetic nervous system still registers the pain and responds accordingly. Generally, anything that is painful to a neurologically intact person can cause dysreflexia in a susceptible spinal-cord-injured person.

As soon as Mitch feels the pounding headache and is sweating above the level of injury, it's time to take action. First, take his vital signs. Mitch's usual BP is 96/50; now it is 180/110. His usual pulse rate is 78; now it is 56. To encourage orthostatic hypotension, raise his head and put his legs in a dependent position.

Next, find the cause of the episode of dysreflexia. The obvious trigger is the sunburn, but you catheterize him to keep urinary retention from further aggravating the episode. Continue checking his BP every two minutes to evaluate the effectiveness of your actions.

A severe sunburn doesn't just go away; so Mitch will need antihypertensive drug therapy, cooling baths, topical pain-relieving agents, and close monitoring until the sunburn heals. These same strategies—immediate attention to symptoms, quick action to identify and remove the precipitating cause of the episode, close monitoring of blood pressure and, if the cause cannot be eliminated, drug therapy—hold true for autonomic dysreflexia due to infection, a pressure ulcer, or an overdistended bladder or bowel.

David, a C7 quadriplegic, develops relatively mild dysreflexic symptoms every time he has a full bladder. Correcting the problem begins with a careful evaluation of his bladder function and a bladder program aimed at improving emptying without triggering dysreflexia.

Antihypertensive drugs such as phenoxybenzamine (Dibenzyline) are another option for patients prone to chronic, mild episodes of dysreflexia. When diaphoresis is severe, low doses of oxybutynin (Ditropan) may help. Oxybutynin must be given with caution since it can also cause urinary retention, which would only aggravate the dysreflexia.

Because of the risk of complications, long-term catheterization is not recommended for patients such as David. If catheterization is necessary, anticholinergics such as propantheline bromide (Pro-Banthine) or oxybutynin (Ditropan) can be given to quell the dysreflexic irritation the catheter might otherwise cause.

A better alternative may be an intermittent catheterization (IC) program. With IC, the bladder is emptied without the irritation reflexive emptying generates. IC has an obvious drawback, though: because these patients do not have hand control, they need reliable help. Another alternative is surgical widening of the bladder sphincter, after which less force and pressure are required for the patient to void.

If a full bowel had been the source of David's dysreflexia, he would have undergone a program that begins with an irritant laxative, followed ten to 12 hours later by fluids, a high-fiber diet, and stool softeners. By eliminating the risk of constipation, bowel emptying becomes less irritating to the autonomic nervous system. A well-managed program of bladder and bowel emptying is the best prevention for autonomic dysreflexia.

Lucy, a pregnant T4 paraplegic at term, started feeling pain between her shoulders and sensed that "something wasn't right inside her." Suddenly, her membranes ruptured—possibly Lucy's only indication that she was in labor. A pregnant quadriplegic or high paraplegic (like Lucy) may feel abdominal spasms, pain referred to the shoulder, or dysreflexia, but rarely the uterine contractions.

As Lucy reaches the second stage of labor and her baby is about to be delivered, the forceful stimulation in the pelvic region triggers dysreflexia. It's vitally important to distinguish dysreflexia from pregnancy-induced hypertension. The wrong treatment can be as dangerous as either disorder to mother and child.

As with Mitch and David, you monitor Lucy's BP carefully and establish IV access. You give an antihypertensive drug as prescribed. Hydralazine (Apresoline) is a good choice because its side effects are minimal and it works immediately.

Even though her spinal injury keeps her from feeling the pain of labor, Lucy may need epidural anesthesia to block the sympathetic stimulation and prevent dysreflexia from occurring at delivery. Only when dysreflexia is uncontrollable is a cesarean section warranted; spinal-cord injury itself is not an indication for cesarean section(3). As soon as her dysreflexia is under control, Lucy is ready to deliver her baby vaginally.

By the way, Mitch's sunburn has faded and he's now working on a gradual golden tan. David had an external sphincterotomy and is now voiding reflexively without any headaches or rises in BP. And Lucy has a beautiful daughter.

Darlene N. Finocchiaro, RN, MS, certified in rehabilitation (CRRN), is a staff nurse at Rancho Los Amigos Medical Center, Downey, CA, and staff development officer for the U. S. Air Force Reserve, March AFB. Shari T. Herzfeld, RN, MN, CRRN, is clinical nurse educator for the spinal injury service at Rancho Los Amigos and clinical assistant professor of nursing at the University of Southern California, Los Angeles.

REFERENCES

1. Comarr, A. E. Personal communication. Oct. 26, 1989.
2. Kewalramani, L. S. Autonomic dysreflexia in traumatic myelopathy. *Am.J.Phys.Med.* 59:1–21, Feb. 1980.
3. Verduyn, W. H. Spinal cord injured women, pregnancy and delivery. *Paraplegia* 24:231–240, Aug. 1986.

Is It Really Alzheimer's?

How your careful assessment can reduce the risk of a self-fulfilling misdiagnosis

By Virginia B. Newbern
Reprinted from American Journal of Nursing February, 1991

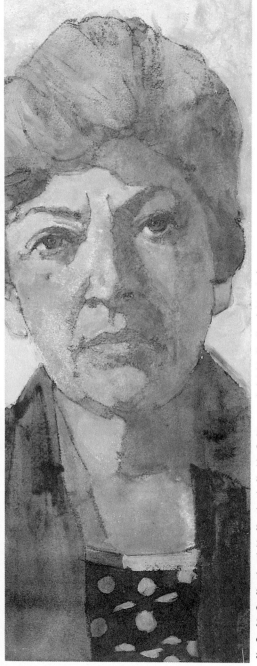

Mr. A, a 72-year-old widower who lives alone, had been active in various social organizations and often traveled with tour groups. His daughter became concerned when he gave up his club memberships and stopped traveling. He gained weight and complained of feeling "bone-weary" most of the time. She noticed, too, that his memory seemed to be failing and that he appeared confused at times.

Ms. B, 80 years old, lives in a congregate living facility in a large city. A widow for 10 years, she'd moved to the city five years earlier to be near her only son and his family. She'd been a member of the facility's planning committee and active at her church. Recently, though, her son had been promoted and had to move to a distant city. Then, two members of her bridge club were transferred to nursing homes and a third died. Soon after, she gave up her position on the committee and stopped going to church. She lost weight, her personal appearance deteriorated, and she seemed confused and apathetic. The staff noticed that she'd become withdrawn.

Virginia B. Newbern, RNC, PhD, is an associate professor and director of the gerontological nursing specialty project at the University of North Carolina, Greensboro.

Ms. C, a 68-year-old retired college professor, had been active all her life. After a year or two of retirement, she'd gained weight, so she put herself on a 1,200-calorie diet and stayed on it for a year. She also embarked on a systematic exercise program, playing at least nine holes of golf twice a week, swimming 30 laps a day in a nearby pool, and taking a dance/exercise class in winter. Her husband noticed, however, that, despite her healthy pursuits, she was tiring easily. She also was becoming more and more forgetful and she seemed confused and paranoid at times.

"There is nothing more emotionally devastating than knowing you're losing your mind," in the words of one Alzheimer's disease specialist[1]. Indeed, it seems safe to say that *fearing* you're losing your mind can be almost as devastating.

Older people who begin having problems with memory loss or confusion tend to think that such difficulties are simply a natural part of aging and that nothing can be done to help them. They may try to hide their problems by withdrawing, by becoming angry, or, more constructively, by devising coping mechanisms such as lists or other memory triggers.

COMMON DRUG INTERACTIONS
THAT CAN PRODUCE CONFUSION

DRUG TYPE	INTERACTING WITH...	CAUSES...
Alcohol	CNS depressants	Additive CNS effect
	Oral hypoglycemics	Potentiated effects of both
Antacids	Cimetidine	Interference with cimetidine metabolism
	Morphine, propranolol	Reduced clearance
Anticholinergics	Other drugs with anticholinergic properties	Potentiated CNS problems
Antidepressants (tricyclics)	Alcohol	Additive effects
	Beta blockers	Reduced antidepressant effect
	Barbiturates	Increased barbiturate effect
Barbiturates	CNS depressants	Additive effects
	Antidepressants (tricyclics)	Interference with antidepressant effect
Beta-adrenergic blockers	Antidiabetic agents	Prolonged hypoglycemic episodes
	Furosemide	Increased propranolol effect
Cimetidine	Propranolol	Increased propranolol effect
Corticosteroids	Antidiabetic agents	Reduced antidiabetic drug effect
	Potassium-depleting diuretics	Further potassium depletion
Diuretics (potassium–depleting)	Digitalis	Digitalis toxicity due to hypokalemia
Phenylbutazone	Antidiabetic agents	Potentiated hypoglycemia
Quinidine	Digoxin	Enhanced risk of digoxin toxicity
Salicylates	Antidiabetic agents	Increased hypoglycemic effects

Source: Burnside, I.M., Nursing Care and the Aged. New York, McGraw-Hill, 1988, pp. 615-618. Adapted with permission.

Each of these three elders was first diagnosed as having organic brain syndrome of the Alzheimer's type. But actually, each was a victim of an acute episode either of delirium or pseudodelirium. Mr. A had developed hypothyroidism, Ms. B was severely depressed, and Ms. C had a vitamin B_{12} deficiency. All three problems are reversible when discovered in time, but each might also progress to dementia or even to death if not reversed(2).

An early warning sign

Often, the first sign of a dementia-like problem is agitated behavior. Possible causes of such behavior include physical disorders, paranoia, schizophrenia, depression, dementia, environmental factors, and, simply, any upsetting situation. Agitation usually accompanies both delirium and pseudodelirium.

Acute delirium, for many years called *acute organic brain syndrome,* is an acute confusion of sudden onset, characterized by impaired thinking, disturbed perceptions, incoherent speech, and an altered sleep-wake cycle(3). The acronym TITMEND refers to the underlying causes of delirium, some of which are reversible: **t**umor, **i**nfection, **t**hyroid, **m**etabolic problems, **e**ndocrine problems, **n**eoplasms, and **d**ementia.

Pseudodelirium is most often a manifestation of depression in people who have experienced profound or accumulated losses; pseudodelirium may also occur in people who have histories of affective disorders or alcohol abuse(4).

Insidious dementia is a description of a clinical syndrome of acquired, persistent intellectual impairment with decrements in at least three of the following: language, memory, visuospatial skills, personality/affect, or cognition(5). Such a definition suggests that dementia is actually a "constellation of signs of intellectual compromise that must be investigated to rule out reversible as well as irreversible causes"(6).

Estimates indicate that 6.1% of people over the age of 65 have symptoms of dementia; yet, in one in five of those people, the symptoms may be reversed if the underlying cause is treated(7). Possible causes of *reversible* dementias overlap the causes of delirium, but these conditions may also cause gradual changes in mental status. They include neurosyphilis, vitamin deficiencies, hydrocephalus, tumors, infections, metabolic disorders, endocrine disorders, pernicious anemia, and hyponatremia. *Untreatable* dementias include Alzheimer's disease, Down's syndrome, Huntington's chorea, alcoholic encephalitis, neoplasms, arteriosclerosis, and senile and presenile dementia.

Looking for clues

Ask the patient (or family member, close friend, or caregiver) questions that elicit specific information about the onset, duration, and course of the patient's symptoms. Ask about changes in sleep cycle, sensorium, perception and speech. For example, inquire: How is your sight? Does glare bother you? Any changes in your sense of smell? (Some research reveals that loss of smell is an early indicator of Alzheimer's.) Are you involved with community or family activities or with friends? Do you think their attitudes toward you have changed? Do you manage your own finances?

Explore changes in the patient's lifestyle, home environment, diet, drugs taken (including nonprescription drugs), personal habits, appearance, job, and leisure activities.

Question the patient sensitively about losses in the past year—family, friends, neighbors, pets, home, personal possessions, assets, job, driver's license, and the like. Don't overlook long-standing relationships, such as a maid, the family physician, or the "Mom and Pop" grocery store that had occupied a nearby corner for 30 years.

Identify physical changes, such as visual and hearing losses, strength and stamina decrements, coordination and proprioception deficits, and impaired mobility associated with arthritis or other musculoskeletal disorders.

Next, examine the patient, keeping in mind the possibility that what appear to be age-related changes might, in fact, be changes that suggest disease. Blurred vision, for example, could be the result of the normal, age-related thickening of the lens, or cataracts or glaucoma, but it might also be a sign that digitalis is causing an episode of confusion.

To evaluate the patient's mental sta-

THE MINI-MENTAL STATUS EXAMINATION*

The Mini-Mental Status Examination is useful for differentiating dementia from depression. The test formally measures memory and orientation, as well as cognitive abilities. Out of a possible score of 32, depressed but nondemented patients usually score between 24 and 30. Patients who have Alzheimer's or senile dementia generally score below 20. The test is administered as follows:

• Ask the patient for the date. To score five points, the patient must tell you correctly the year, season, day, date, and month. Ask specifically for any element omitted.

• Ask the patient to name the place where he is right now. To score five points, she must tell you the name of the state, city, street, hospital, and floor. If you are not in a hospital, substitute other orientation questions, such as asking for the name of the nursing home or the county.

• Ask the patient if you may test his memory. Name three unrelated objects, clearly and slowly, allowing about one second for each. After you have said all three words, ask the patient to repeat them. The first attempt determines the score (0-3), but repeat the test for up to six trials if the patient is not successful.

• Ask the patient to begin with 100 and count backward by sevens. Stop after five subtractions (93, 86, 79, 72, 65) and score the total number of correct answers for a maximum of five points. If the patient cannot perform this task, ask him instead to spell the word *world* backward. The score is the number of letters in correct order (d-l-r-o-w = 5, d-l-o-r-w = 3).

• Ask the patient to recall the three words you asked him to remember previously, for a score of 0 to 3.

• Show the patient a wristwatch and ask him what it is. Repeat with a pencil. Score 0 to 2.

• Ask the patient to repeat the phrase, "No ifs, ands, or buts." Allow only one trial and score 0 or 1.

• Hand the patient a sheet of paper and give a three-stage command: "Take the paper in your right hand, fold it in half, and put it on the floor." Score one point for each step carried out correctly.

• On a blank sheet of paper, print the sentence, "Close your eyes" in letters large enough for the patient to see clearly. Ask him to read it and to do what it says. Score one point only if he actually closes his eyes.

• Give the patient a blank sheet of paper and ask him to write a sentence for you. It must contain a subject and a verb and make sense to score one point. Correct grammar and punctuation are not necessary.

• On a sheet of paper, draw two pentagons, each side about one inch, with two angles intersected and ask him to copy the drawing exactly as it is. All ten angles must be present and two angles must intersect to score one point. (Ignore other issues, such as tremor or rotation of the paper.)

---

*Folstein, M., and others. The meaning of cognitive impairment in the elderly. *J.Am.Geriatr.Soc.* 33:228-235, Apr. 1985.)

PHYSIOLOGICAL
PRIMARY CEREBRAL DISEASE

NONSTRUCTURAL FACTORS	• Vascular insufficiency—transient ischemic attacks, cerebral vascular accidents, thrombosis • Central nervous system infection—acute and chronic meningitis, neurosyphilis, brain abscess
STRUCTURAL FACTORS	• Trauma—subdural hematoma, concussion, contusion, intracranial hemorrhage • Tumors—primary and metastatic • Normal-pressure hydrocephalus

EXTRACRANIAL DISEASE

CARDIOVASCULAR ABNORMALITIES	• Decreased cardiac output states—myocardial infarction, arrhythmias, congestive heart failure, cardiogenic shock • Alterations in peripheral vascular resistance—increased and decreased states • Vascular occlusion—disseminated intravascular coagulopathy, emboli
PULMONARY ABNORMALITIES	• Inadequate gas exchange states—pulmonary disease, alveolar hypoventilation • Infection—pneumonias
SYSTEMIC INFECTIVE PROCESSES (ACUTE AND CHRONIC)	• Viral • Bacterial—endocarditis, pyelonephritis, cystitis
METABOLIC DISTURBANCES	• Electrolyte abnormalities—hypercalcemia, hypo- and hypernatremia, hypo- and hyperkalemia, hypo- and hyperchloremia, hyperphosphatemia • Acidosis/alkalosis • Hypo- and hyperglycemia • Acute and chronic renal failure • Volume depletion—hemorrhage, inadequate fluid intake, diuretics • Hepatic failure • Porphyria
DRUG INTOXICATIONS (THERAPEUTIC AND SUBSTANCE ABUSE)	• Misuse of prescribed medications • Side effects of therapeutic medications • Drug interactions • Improper use of over-the-counter medications • Ingestion of heavy metals and industrial poisons
NUTRITIONAL DEFICIENCIES	• B vitamins • Vitamin C • Hypoproteinemia
PHYSIOLOGIC STRESS	• Pain, surgery
ALTERATIONS IN TEMPERATURE REGULATION	• (Hypo- and hyperthermia)
UNKNOWN PHYSIOLOGIC ABNORMALITY	• (Sometimes defined as pseudodelirium)

PSYCHOLOGICAL

• Severe emotional stress—postoperative states, relocation, hospitalization
• Depression
• Anxiety
• Pain—acute and chronic
• Fatigue
• Grief
• Sensory/perceptual deficits—noise, alteration in functioning of senses
• Mania
• Paranoia
• Situational disturbances

ENVIRONMENTAL

• Unfamiliar environment creating a lack of meaning in the environment
• Sensory deprivation/environmental monotony creating a lack of meaning in the environment
• Sensory overload
• Immobilization—therapeutic, physical, pharmacologic
• Sleep deprivation
• Lack of temporal/spatial reference points

Source: Foreman, M. D. Acute confusional states in hospitalized elderly: A research dilemma. Nurs.Res. 35(1): 35, Jan.-Feb. 1986.

tus, any of a number of mental examinations may be used. A popular one is the Mini-Mental Status (MMS) Examination (see sidebar), because it takes only five to ten minutes to administer anywhere, yet it is comprehensive, reliable, and valid.

Once all the data have been collected, look for patterns. Ms. B, for example, exhibited a classic pattern of depression.

Look for drug interactions and potentiations. A hypertensive patient being treated with beta blockers, for example, may become confused when she begins taking timolol maleate (Timoptic) eye drops (another beta blocker) for glaucoma.

The effects of drugs on elderly people are as varied as the people for whom they are prescribed. Many factors come into play, such as advancing age, sex, other chronic conditions, other drugs.

In fact, whenever you work with elders, keep the *rule of five* in mind—taking more than five medicines at one time dramatically raises the chances of adverse drug interactions.

Report the results of your nursing assessment to the patient's physician, who will then eliminate the various reversible possibilities of dementia before making a final diagnosis.

Only after reversible causes of organic brain syndrome are eliminated and careful evaluation is done for untreatable conditions should a patient be labeled as suffering from Alzheimer's disease. To do less may condemn a patient to madness or death, causing anguish and sorrow that need not be.

REFERENCES

1. Reisburg, B. Alzheimer's Disease: Clinical Diagnosis and Assessment. Paper presented at a symposium held at Lenoir-Rhyne College, Hickory, NC, Oct. 1987.
2. Gomez, G. E., and Gomez, E. A. Delirium. *Geriatr.Nurs.* 8:330-332, Nov.-Dec. 1987.
3. Godschalk, M. F. Delirium: a confusing diagnosis. *Age in Action* 2:1, 14, Jun. 1989.
4. Gomez, G. E., and Gomez, E. A. Dementia? or delirium? Here's help in sorting it out. *Geriatr.Nurs.* 10:141-142, May-Jun., 1987.
5. Cummings, J. Reversible dementia: illustrative cases, definition, and review.*JAMA* 243:2434-2439.
6. Shapira, J., and others. Distinguishing dementias. *Am.J.Nurs.* 86:698-702, Jun. 1986.
7. Folstein, M., and others. The meaning of cognitive impairment in the elderly. *J.Am.Geriatr.Soc.* 33:228-235, Apr. 1985.
8. Foreman, M. D. Complexities of acute confusion. *Geriatr.Nurs.*11:136-139, May-Jun. 1990.

DIABETES AND EXERCISE

By James R. Gavin III

Reprinted from American Journal of Nursing February, 1988

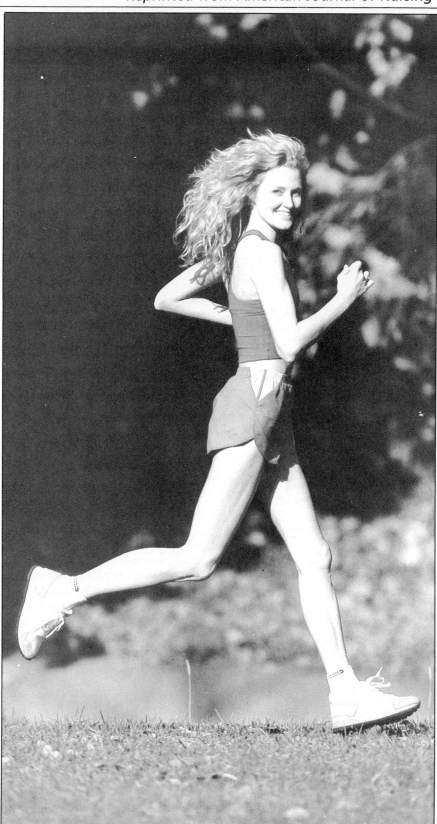

Regularly performed aerobic exercise—exercise that involves the use of large numbers of muscles and that elevates the pulse to 70 to 80 percent of its maximum attainable rate—can be as complex to prescribe as it is crucial in both insulin-dependent (IDDM) and non-insulin-dependent (NIDDM) diabetes mellitus.

One must draw a fundamental distinction between the effects of random physical activity—for example, running to catch the bus or walking up one flight of stairs because the elevator just left—versus regular exercise or exercise training. The former produces acute, short-lived responses by muscles and other organ systems, but confers little in the way of lasting benefits.

Endurance training, on the other hand, lowers triglycerides and blood glucose, heightens sensitivity to insulin, and lowers blood pressure. Many of these changes are exactly the types of modifications that would be expected to reduce the risk of atherosclerosis, a desirable goal in diabetes mellitus.

WHETS THE APPETITE

When a person begins to exercise, muscle glycogen is the primary fuel. After 5 to 10 minutes, glucose uptake from blood is 7 to 20 times the resting rate, depending on how strenuous the exercise is. By 40 minutes or so of continuous exercise, blood glucose provides 75 to 90 percent of the total carbohydrate consumed by muscle, since muscle glycogen is depleted.

Patients with diabetes can benefit from this uptake of glucose from the blood during exercise—but

James R. Gavin III, MD, PhD, is presently professor of medicine and chief, diabetes section, Division of Endocrinology, Metabolism and Hypertension of Oklahoma University Health Sciences Center, Oklahoma City, OK.

Without enough insulin, exercise can make a diabetic ketotic and hyperglycemic.

only if they have adequate insulin available. Without adequate circulating insulin levels, insulin-dependent diabetics actually become *more* ketotic and *more* hyperglycemic with vigorous exercise.

How is it that blood sugar can actually rise, instead of fall, in the insulin-deficient person? During the early phases of exercise, the liver steps up its rate of glycogen breakdown to keep pace with muscle uptake of glucose. With prolonged exercise, gluconeogenesis from circulating substrates including alanine, lactate, pyruvate, and glycerol provides more of the glucose produced.

Insulin promotes uptake of glucose by muscles and prevents excessive glycogen breakdown and gluconeogenesis in the liver. If a person is insulin deficient, exercise can paradoxically create an overload of glucose in the blood. Without sufficient insulin, the muscles are not able to use as much glucose and the liver has no check on its glucose production.

EXERCISE AND IDDM

The absolute requirement for exogenous insulin means that IDDM patients must carefully coordinate the dose and the timing of insulin injections with the exercise program. Exercise works almost like insulin. Taken to the extreme, diabetics participating in marathons or triathlons need only two to five units of insulin *per day* during competition to maintain normal blood sugar levels. The key is to ensure adequate insulin levels so the exercise can be beneficial.

Unfortunately, one cannot look to blanket guidelines for determining how to adjust the insulin.

Since vigorous exercise of the injection site can speed the rate of insulin absorption, the patient is taught to avoid injections into the arms or legs before vigorous physical activity. Absorption also can be faster when blood flow to and from the injection site increases, such as when exercising in warm outdoor temperatures or in vinyl clothing. The problem with rapid absorption of insulin is the high probability of transient hypoglycemia.

IDDM diabetics must check their blood glucose within 30 minutes before exercise and an hour after exercise.

Before exercise, if the blood sugar exceeds 225 mg/dl and the person has not taken a short-acting insulin in the last two hours or an intermediate-acting drug in the last five to six hours, he should take Regular insulin to reduce blood sugar below 200 mg/dl before exercising. However, if Regular insulin has been taken within the last 1½ hours, or intermediate-acting insulin within the past five hours, the person should just delay exercise until the blood sugar responds to the insulin.

Of course, some patients become so adept at recognizing their own response patterns that they can exercise safely even when their blood sugars fall outside these guidelines.

At the other extreme is the blood sugar below, for example, 100 mg/dl. In this case, extra carbohydrate should be consumed or carried to prevent exercise-induced hypoglycemia. Since hypoglycemia may occur or persist several hours after exercise, the diabetic needs to ingest enough carbohydrates to replenish expended stores within the first few hours after exercise.

Patients with proliferative retinopathy should avoid exercises that jar the body (jumping rope, jogging, aerobic dancing) or that require a head-down position or the Valsalva maneuver (bench-pressing, floor exercises for abdominal muscle strengthening). These exercises may result in reti-nal detachment or increased intraretinal vascular pressure with subsequent hemorrhage.

Patients with significant nephropathy may spill more protein into their urine with vigorous, high-impact physical activities. Diabetics with peripheral neuropathy should exercise with caution because their impaired sensations can mask lower-extremity injuries. Patients with autonomic neuropathies should avoid vigorous exercise that elevates heart rate or increases sweat response—functions that may be impaired in such patients. In these patients, the benefits of vigorous aerobic exercise are likely to be outweighed by the risks involved.

EXERCISE FOR NIDDM

Because insulin resistance is a problem, any therapeutic exercise for NIDDM patients must overcome this resistance. For many with NIDDM, regular physical exercise eliminates the need for an intense campaign of food restriction for weight loss—not to mention the way exercise improves blood lipid levels, hypertension, and overall well-being.

All diabetics need a physical examination before starting an exercise program. For NIDDM patients, who are older, more obese, sedentary, and in a high-risk group for cardiac disease, this is especially important. They need to be checked for ischemia, angina pectoris, and arrhythmias.

Patients—especially those who have heart-disease symptoms, elevated blood lipids, or strong family histories of heart disease—should be assessed for exercise tolerance as they do graded exercise tests.

Patients who have not been exercising must build up their exercise intensity gradually, monitoring their heart rates to measure progress. The patient is taught to stop for 15 seconds at the peak of exercise, counting the pulse for 10 seconds, and multiply by six. Comparing the pulse at peak with the target pulse rate (usually 65 to 80 percent of maximum) set with the clinician determines whether or not the intensity of the patient's exercise is appropriate.

Studies have shown that the target pulse must be maintained for 15 to 30 minutes three to four times per week for exercise to be beneficial. Also, the effects of exercise on sensitivity to insulin are lost if exercise is stopped for 72 hours. Those effects are quickly regained when exercise is resumed. Our studies of sedentary NIDDM patients showed that they needed 10 to 12 weeks of slowly progressing exercise before they could exercise at recommended intensity and duration. Attempts to shorten the time resulted in sore joints and muscles, fatigue, and failure to continue the program.

NIDDM patients on insulin or oral hypoglycemic drugs are taught to monitor their pre- and postexercise blood sugars and adjust drug timing and dose accordingly. NIDDM patients on small doses of insulin or oral drugs can often stop the drugs entirely once regular exercise is established.

PRESCRIBING EXERCISE

A 26-year-old IDDM woman with no known complications decides to exercise. She takes 15 units NPH and 8 units Regular insulin every morning, plus 10 units NPH and 5 units Regular insulin every evening.

She prefers running, so a jogging program is prescribed. She is told to begin with a walk/run routine for 15 minutes and gradually increase duration and intensity over four to six weeks.

She is instructed to check her blood sugar just before exercise. If it is 220 mg/dl or higher, she takes three to four units Regular insulin in an abdominal injection site. If her pre-exercise glucose is 100 mg/

dl or less, she is to take some concentrated carbohydrate, such as a fast-dissolving mint, along during the run. If blood glucose is 80 mg/dl or less, she ingests 20 to 30 g of carbohydrate before the run.

After jogging, she is advised to check her BS within an hour. Deciding whether she needs extra calories or extra insulin is done on the basis of her blood glucose pre- and postexercise. Since she will exercise prior to the evening meal, her insulin requirements at this time will be expected to decrease as the intensity and duration of her

> **Be precise in the exercise prescription: type, mode, intensity, duration, and frequency.**

exercise sessions increase.

The symptoms of hypoglycemia are carefully reviewed with her and she is advised that if such symptoms occur during or after exercise, she must stop immediately and ingest some carbohydrate (or the most immediately available fuel). She is reminded that such symptoms may occur for several hours postexercise. She learns to keep a diary of her exercise activity, her blood glucose readings, and any symptoms of hypoglycemia.

Contrast this to NIDDM. For example, a 49-year-old man with NIDDM elects to increase his exercise and reduce his calories to lower his blood sugar and body weight. He is in good general health except for diabetes, obesity, and his sedentary life-style.

After a discussion of the various options for aerobic exercise, he chooses an exercise bicycle. The

staff teach him to take his pulse and give him a booklet that describes warm-up routines. For the first week he is advised to do stretch/flex exercises for 10 to 15 minutes and to begin low-intensity cycling for 10-minute periods at a workload of 60 to 65 percent of his maximum heart rate (MHR). His MHR is calculated by subtracting his age from 220: $220 - 49 = 171$. Multiplying his MHR by 0.65, his pulse rate at peak exercise ought to be about 110.

He is provided a three-times-a-week schedule in which his exercise periods are increased by three to five minutes per session with a workload of 70 to 75 percent of maximum heart rate by the end of week three. By the end of week six, he is advised to have reached a duration of 30 to 45 minutes of cycling activity with a peak pulse rate of 80 to 85 percent of MHR.

He maintains a diary containing results of SMBG, weights, and any reports of incidents that may be of interest or concern to the patient. Data from the diary is reviewed with the clinician by telephone biweekly and during visits.

When you teach a patient to exercise, give him a regimen no less detailed than one for a drug. Specify the type, mode, intensity, frequency, and duration, and discuss the benefits and risks. With reasonable goals, the patient can soon learn that exercise is one of the very few forms of therapy that is certain to work and that can also be fun.

BIBLIOGRAPHY

Felig, P., and Wahren, J. Fuel homeostasis in exercise. *N.Engl.J.Med.* 293:1078–1084, Nov. 20, 1975.

Vranic, M., and Berger, M. Exercise and diabetes mellitus. *Diabetes* 28:147–163, Feb. 1979.

Zinman, B., and others. Comparison of the acute and long-term effects of exercise on glucose control in Type I diabetes. *Diabetes Care* 7:515–519, Nov.–Dec. 1984.

Zinman, B., and others. The role of insulin in the metabolic response to exercise in diabetic man. *Diabetes* 28(Suppl. 1):76–81, Jan. 1979.

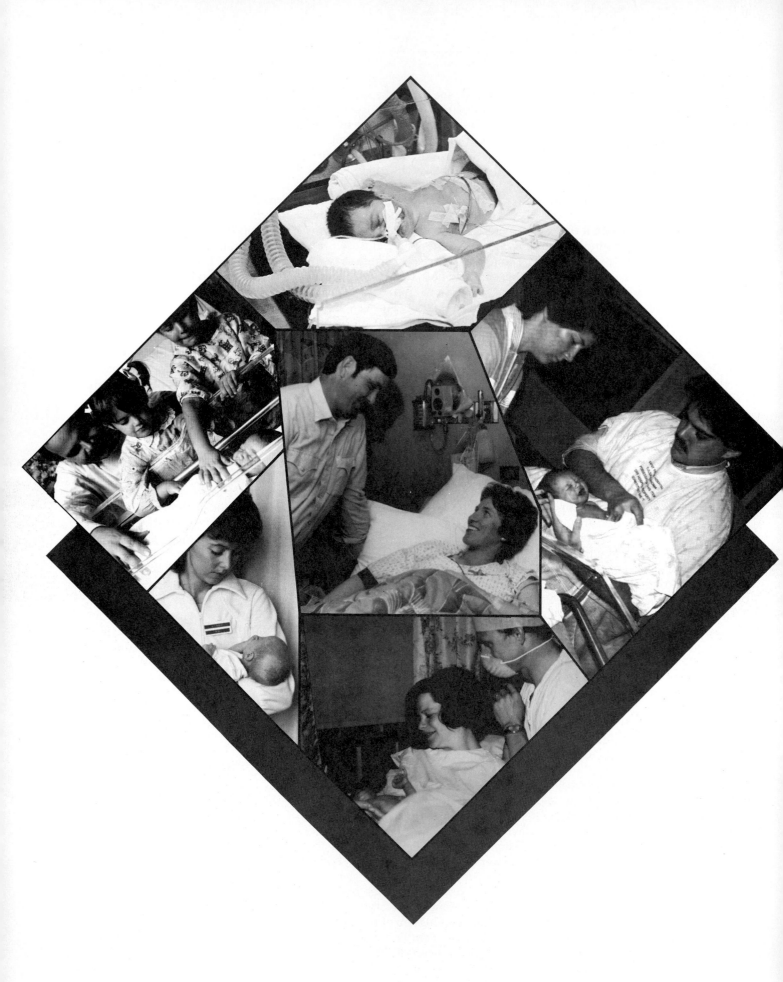

Nursing Care of the Childbearing Family

Coordinator

Marybeth Young, PhD, MSN, RNC

Contributors

Quilla D. Bell-Turner, PhD, RN
Gita Dhillon, CNM, MA, MS, MEd, RNC
Kathleen Haubrich, MSN, RNC
Roberta A. Kordish, MSN, RN
Marianne Scharbo-DeHaan, CNM, MN, RN

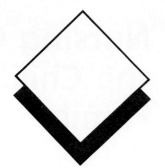

Women's Health Care

GENERAL CONCEPTS

NOTE: The concept development in the sections on the adult, child, and the client with psychosocial problems also applies to the mother and her newborn. However, this section has been organized according to the normal childbearing cycle, from conception to postpartum.

Overview/Physiology

1. Structure of the female pelvis (see Fig. 4-1)
   a. Pelvic structure (four united bones): two hip bones (right and left innominate), the sacrum, and the coccyx
   b. Pelvic divisions: two parts divided by the inlet or brim
      1. false pelvis: upper portion above brim; supports uterus during late pregnancy
      2. true pelvis: located below brim; composed of three parts: the pelvic inlet, the midcavity, and the pelvic outlet; forms birth canal through which fetus passes during parturition
   c. Pelvic variations: pelvic structures differ in shape and size
      1. android: normal male type; heart-shaped inlet, narrow pubic arch; influence on labor and delivery is not favorable
      2. gynecoid: true female type; slightly ovoid or rounded inlet; influence on labor and delivery *most favorable*
      3. platypelloid: flattened anteroposteriorly, oval-shaped inlet; influence on labor and delivery not favorable
      4. anthropoid: apelike type; oval-shaped inlet; influence on labor and delivery favorable
   d. Pelvic measurements
      1. diagonal conjugate (DC): distance between sacral promontory and lower margin (inferior border) of symphysis pubis; adequate size for childbirth is 12.5 cm more, depending on fetal size, position *estimated on pelvic exam*
      2. true conjugate or conjugate vera (CV): distance between upper margin, superior border of sym-

physis pubis to sacral promontory; adequate size for childbirth 11 cm or more (1.5-2 cm less than diagonal conjugate); *measured accurately by x-ray*
      3. obstetrical conjugate: the shortest distance between the inner surface of the symphysis and the sacral promontory; *measured by x-ray*
      4. tuber-ischial diameter: transverse diameter of the outlet, the distance between the ischial tuberosities; adequate size for childbirth 9-11 cm or more; *estimated on pelvic exam*
      5. assessment of size
         a. estimate of pelvic dimensions: diagonal conjugate and tuber-ischial diameter on pelvic exam
         b. x-ray or internal pelvimetry: use is limited to suspected pelvic bony contractions and suspected cephalopelvic disproportion (most accurate measurement of pelvic size)

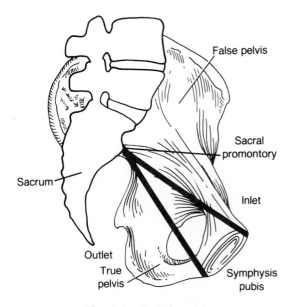

Fig. 4-1 Female pelvis.

c. ultrasonography: employs use of high-frequency sound waves for determination of gestational age

2. Female external organs
   a. Mons veneris or pubis: rounded, soft, fatty pad over symphysis pubis, covered by coarse hair in adult
   b. Labia majora: two folds of skin containing fat and covered with hair; located on either side of the vaginal opening
   c. Labia minora: two thin folds of delicate tissue without hair; located within labia majora
   d. Glans clitoris: a small body of erectile tissue partially hidden between the anterior ends of the labia minora; highly sensitive to touch, temperature, and pressure
   e. Hymen: thin mucous membrane; located at the opening of the vagina, can be stretched or torn during intercourse, physical activity, tampon insertion, or vaginal examination
   f. Urinary meatus: external opening of the urethra
   g. Openings of vulvovaginal or Bartholin's glands: two small glands situated between the vestibula on either side of the vaginal orifice; secrete alkaline mucus during coitus
   h. Openings of Skene's ducts: two paraurethral glands open onto posterior urethral wall
   i. Perineum: area between vagina and rectum consisting of fibromuscular tissue

3. Female internal organs (see Fig. 4-2)
   a. Ovaries: two oval-shaped organs located on either side of the uterus in the upper pelvic cavity; responsible for producing the ovum and the female hormones estrogen and progesterone
   b. Fallopian or uterine tubes: two thin, muscular canals extending from the cornua of the uterus to the ovaries; responsible for transport of the ovum from the ovaries to the uterus; fertilization occurs in middle third (ampulla) of either fallopian tube
   c. Uterus: a hollow muscular organ that is the site of implantation, retainment, and nourishment of the products of conception. It is also the organ of menstruation in the nonpregnant female. The larger, upper portion of the uterus is known as the *body* and the smaller, lower segment is called the *cervix*. The convex, upper part between the insertion of fallopian tubes is the *fundus*. In the nonpregnant female, the uterus is located in the pelvic cavity between the bladder and rectum and weighs approximately 60 g. The uterus is composed of smooth muscle (myometrium) and an inner mucoid lining (the endometrium) that responds to estrogen and progesterone during the menstrual cycle.
   d. Vagina: a thin-walled, dilatable canal located between the bladder and rectum that serves as the passageway for menstrual discharge, copulation, and the fetus
   e. Accessory structures (breasts): two mammary glands composed of glandular tissue and fat, which are capable of producing and secreting milk for nourishment of the infant

4. Menstrual cycle

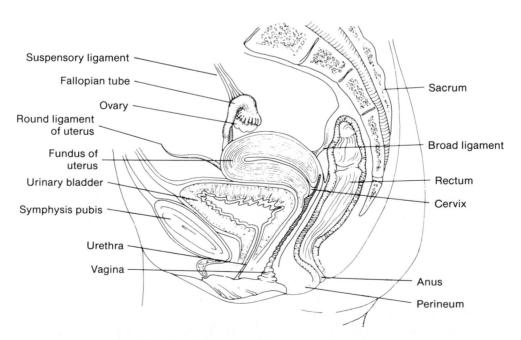

Fig. 4-2   Female internal reproductive organs (side view).

a. Reproductive hormones (all are affected by thyroid function)
   1. follicle-stimulating hormone (FSH): secreted by anterior pituitary gland during the first half of the menstrual cycle; stimulates development of graafian follicles and thins the endometrium
   2. interstitial cell–stimulating hormone (ICSH) or luteinizing hormone (LH): secreted by the pituitary gland; stimulates ovulation and development of the corpus luteum; causes the endometrium to thicken
   3. estrogen: secreted primarily by the ovaries, by the adrenal cortex (in small amounts), and by the placenta in pregnancy; assists in maturation of ovarian follicles, stimulates thickening of the endometrium, causes suppression of FSH secretion, and is responsible for development of secondary sex characteristics; in pregnancy, it maintains the endometrium, causes fatigue, and stimulates contraction of smooth muscle
   4. progesterone: secreted by corpus luteum and by the placenta during pregnancy; supplements estrogen effect on endometrium by facilitating secretory changes; relaxes smooth muscle; decreases uterine motility; has thermogenic effect (i.e., increases temperature); causes cervical secretion of thick viscous mucus; allows pregnancy to be maintained
   5. prostaglandins: fatty acids categorized as hormones, produced by many organs of the body, including the endometrium; affect the menstrual cycle and may influence the onset and maintenance of labor
b. Ovulation: growth and release of a nonfertilized ovum from the ovary after puberty; generally occurs 13-15 days before next menses in regular cycle; presence of stretchable cervical mucus (spinnbarkeit) observed at ovulation; purpose to enhance sperm motility and permit fertilization
c. Menstruation: cyclic vaginal discharge of blood and superficial fragments of endometrium and other secretions in response to falling levels of estrogen and progesterone after puberty
   1. amenorrhea: absence or abnormal cessation of the menses
      a. primary (menses have never occurred)
      b. secondary (menses occurred at puberty but have since stopped)
   2. hypomenorrhea: abnormally short menstruation
   3. hypermenorrhea: abnormally long menstruation
   4. oligomenorrhea: infrequent menstruation
   5. polymenorrhea: too frequent menstruation
   6. dysmenorrhea: painful menstruation

5. Fertilization: impregnation of an ovum by a spermatozoon, occurring in the ampulla of the fallopian tube; egg life span is 24-36 hours after ovulation; sperm life span is 48-72 hours or more after ejaculation; usual sperm count is 250-400 million
6. Implantation: the imbedding of the fertilized ovum into the uterine mucosa (usually in the upper segment); occurs approximately 7-10 days after ovulation (also known as nidation)
7. Menopause: cessation of menses at end of fertility cycle
   a. Occurrence: normal developmental process that occurs naturally between the ages of 35 and 60 (average age is 53)
   b. Alterations: early menopause may be stimulated by
      1. multiple, frequent pregnancies or abortions
      2. hypothyroidism with obesity
      3. surgical removal of ovaries
      4. hard physical work or very active exercise
      5. overexposure to radiation
   c. Medical treatment: for symptom relief
      1. estrogen replacement therapy: often controversial
      2. vitamins: increased doses of B complex and vitamin E for symptoms such as hot flashes
      3. hormonal vaginal creams and water-soluble lubricants for painful intercourse (dyspareunia)
      4. emotional support during this developmental change/crisis

Application of the Nursing Process to Reproductive Health Maintenance/Health Promotion of Adult Women

Assessment
1. Health history: onset of menarche, duration of menstrual periods, menstrual problems, premenstrual tension, osteoporosis (decrease in skeletal bone mass), use of family planning, past and current pregnancies, infertility problems (see Table 4-1), symptoms such as hot flashes, dizzy spells, palpitations; identification of risk factors
2. External reproductive organs (by physician or nurse); breast palpation for masses; bimanual internal examination; and observation of cervical-vaginal discharge
3. Knowledge of progesterone-to-estrogen ratio, hormonal effects (mild or severe episodes of irritability, depression, anxiety, fatigue, exhaustion, or food cravings)

Analysis
1. Safe, effective care environment
   a. Knowledge deficit
   b. High risk for infection
2. Physiological integrity

Table 4-1   Assessment of fertility/infertility

Test	Purpose	Nursing implications
MALE Semen analysis	To determine sperm count, motility	Take careful history of both partners chronic health problems medications
FEMALE (simplest to more complex) Basal body temperature Cervical-mucus examination (self-performed, basis for natural family planning)	To determine time of ovulation To determine elasticity for sperm motility	drug use exposure to chemicals, radiation Provide detailed explanation of all tests to couple.
Pelvic examination (bimanual)	To identify obvious reproductive problems	Know that process of assessment of fertility and subsequent interventions may be lengthy and, for the couple, frustrating.
Blood hormone levels and thyroid function tests	To measure levels of estrogen and progesterone, and influence of the thyroid	
Sims-Huhner test (postcoital cervical mucus test)	To determine pH of cervical mucus, effects of hormones	
Tubal patency tests hysterosalpingogram (x-ray) laparoscopic exam (direct visualization)	To determine condition, patency of fallopian tubes	
Endometrial biopsy	To determine condition of endometrium	
Culdoscopy (examination through cul-de-sac with dye injection)	To determine function of fallopian tubes	

a. Altered nutrition: less than body requirements
b. Sleep pattern disturbance
c. Stress incontinence
3. Psychosocial integrity
   a. Fear
   b. Anxiety
   c. Self-esteem disturbance
   d. Altered sexuality patterns
4. Health promotion/maintenance
   a. Health-seeking behaviors
   b. Impaired adjustment

General Nursing Planning, Implementation, and Evaluation

Goal 1: Client will understand her reproductive system; will report gynecological problems to the physician.

Implementation
1. Discuss anatomy and physiology of female reproductive system.
2. Review menstrual cycle, ovulation, and fertilization.
3. Teach client reportable problems.

Evaluation
Client gives a basic explanation of reproductive anatomy and physiology; explains relationship of menstrual cycle, ovulation, and fertilization; reports problems to health care provider.

Goal 2: Client will be knowledgeable about various methods of family planning.

Implementation
1. Assess client's learning needs.
2. Provide information as needed (see Table 4-2).

Evaluation
Client describes family planning options; asks questions about them; uses chosen method consistently according to directions; lists potential problems with specific method; reports problems associated with use.

Goal 3: Client will understand the importance of periodic examinations in reproductive health maintenance.

Implementation
1. Explain the need for periodic Papanicolaou (Pap) smears (cells taken from squamocolumnar junction) to detect cancer of the uterus and abnormalities of cervical, vaginal cells (frequency varies according to sexual activity, age, and risk).
2. Explain importance of regular breast self-examination after cessation of menstrual period (days 5-7 of menstrual cycle) or after menopause on regular monthly basis.
3. Demonstrate breast self-examination (palpation and inspection of breasts and nipples while standing and

Table 4-2   Family planning

Method and mode of action	Characteristics	Nursing implications
TEMPORARY METHODS		
Oral contraceptives (birth control pills): May be single hormone or combination of estrogen and progesterone prevent ovulation by inhibiting FSH change cervical mucus	*Effectiveness:* 99% if used as directed *Advantages:* convenient, effective *Disadvantages:* increased risk over age 35; smokers; women with risk/history of vascular disease, hypertension, respiratory problems, breast cancer in family	Teach proper and regular use. action to take if one or more pills are missed side effects; reportable signs (e.g., headaches, chest or calf pain, heavy bleeding). Recommend regular Pap smears Caution against use of antibiotics unless physician is aware that client uses oral contraceptives. Increase folic acid, vitamins B and C. Advise client to notify physician and discontinue oral contraceptives if pregnancy is suspected.
Intrauterine device (IUD) causes local inflammatory response inhibiting implantation several IUD products have been withdrawn by manufacturers	*Effectiveness:* 90%-99% *Advantages:* convenient, long term, effective *Disadvantages:* increased risk for pelvic infection, ectopic pregnancy; subsequent infertility	Teach compliance with regular health care visits reportable signs (e.g., abdominal pain, foul discharge) to check for presence of string before coitus. Must be removed by health care provider.
Diaphragm barrier to seminal fluid, sperm when used with spermicidal cream	*Effectiveness:* 83%-95% if correctly fit and properly used *Advantages:* side effects are rare *Disadvantages:* requires motivation and planning; may interfere with spontaneity; must remain in place several hours after coitus	Teach proper use with spermicide (not KY jelly). Suggest that client be refitted after pregnancy, weight changes. Report problems with fit, removal, vaginal discharge.
Vaginal contraceptive sponge	*Effectiveness:* 84%-97% *Advantages:* convenient; no additional creams needed; may leave in place up to 24 hours; barrier to seminal fluid, sperm; economical *Disadvantages:* increased risk of allergies, toxic shock; removal may be difficult	Teach proper use and insertion. Avoid use for over 30 hours. Avoid use during menses. Urge immediate reporting of problems/symptoms.
Cervical cap barrier to seminal fluid and sperm FDA approved for research used with spermicidal cream	*Advantages:* side effects are rare; unlikely to dislodge during coitus *Disadvantages:* increased risk of cervical erosion, inflammation; may be difficult to remove	Teach proper use. Report signs of vaginal infection or other problems. Seek regular health care.
Condom barrier to passage of sperm when slipped over erecct penis	*Effectiveness:* 64%-98% when used with spermicides *Advantages:* Involves male in family planning; protects against some sexually transmitted diseases; easily available *Disadvantages:* Requires motivation and planning; may tear during use; rare allergic reactions	Teach proper use. Discuss role in prevention of transmission of sexually transmitted diseases, AIDS.

Table 4-2   Family planning—cont'd

Method and mode of action	Characteristics	Nursing implications
Spermicides immobilizes or destroys sperm	*Effectiveness:* 70%-98% depending on use; more effective with other methods (e.g., condom, diaphragm) *Advantages:* Easily available; few side effects *Disadvantages:* Inconvenient; may cause allergic reaction; there is concern (unproven) about potential risk of birth defects in some users	Teach proper use after reading specific product directions. Avoid douching after coitus. Report problems (e.g., itching, burning).

Natural family planning
  abstinence from coitus during the fertile (ovulation) phase of the menstrual cycle (the couple trying to conceive may also plan optimal time for coitus to achieve pregnancy)
  assessment of ovulation if based on
    daily basal body temperature (BBT) (Fig. 4-3) to monitor changes before and at ovulation (slight drop, then rise after ovulation)
    cervical mucus characteristics: clear, slippery, elastic at ovulation (Billings method)
    calendar recording based on usual menstrual pattern
    symptothermal method: a combination of calendar tracking of monthly fertility cycle, BBT, and cervical mucus self-exam
  research has led to development of several OTC products for self-assessment of ovulation
	Effectiveness: 75%-98% depending on accuracy of observations, motivation of both partners
	Advantages: Inexpensive; involves both partners; no chemical or mechanical barrier to sperm movement; no health risk
	Disadvantages: Requires motivation of both partners; may be less effective in presence of infection or during menopause
		Teach and reinforce information to both partners.

PERMANENT METHODS

Method and mode of action	Characteristics	Nursing implications
Tubal ligation/vasectomy ligation/severance of fallopian tube or vas deferens for permanent sterilization	*Effectiveness:* Greater than 99.5% (reversing the procedure is difficult, outcome is not guaranteed) *Advantages:* Prevents pregnancy permanently *Disadvantages:* Requires informed consent; rare complications	Teach couple alternative methods if permanent sterility is not desired. Caution that pregnancy is still possible for a short period of time following vasectomy.

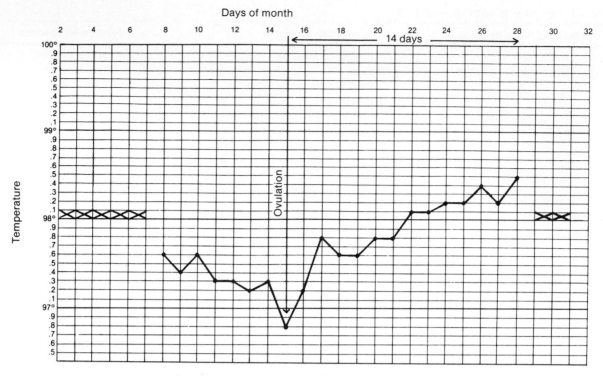

Fig. 4-3 Basal body temperature (30-day cycle).

reclining); ask client for return demonstration; emphasize reporting any changes or suspicious findings immediately.
4. Tell client to see physician for regular breast examination.
5. Explain value of mammography.
6. Discuss meaning, purposes, and interpretation of various tests (see Table 4-3).
7. Provide supplemental reading materials to increase client's knowledge.

Evaluation
Client performs breast self-examination regularly at end of each menstrual cycle; schedules appointments for periodic checkups and Pap smears.

> **Goal 4:** Client will be knowledgeable about premenstrual tension syndrome; will discuss any concerns with health care provider.

Implementation
1. Assess client's learning needs.
2. Provide information as needed.
3. Review hormones and their effects.

Evaluation
Client gives basic description of hormones and their effects; asks questions; uses a method to relieve symptoms.

Table 4-3   Interpretation of Pap test results

Class I	No abnormal cells
Class II	Atypical cells (rule out inflammation)
Class III	Suspicious abnormal cells
Class IV	Malignant cells may be in situ
Class V	Invasive cancer

> **Goal 5:** Client will be physically and psychologically prepared for menopause; will make informed choices and comply with treatment.

Implementation
1. Allow client to voice feelings about menopause.
2. Teach client how to maintain and promote health and prevent osteoporosis (see Table 4-4).
3. Discuss normal developmental changes that occur with menopause.
4. Dispel "myths" concerning menopause.
5. Discuss sexuality needs and family planning until ovulation ceases.
6. Provide emotional support, anticipatory guidance.

Evaluation
Client lists the signs and symptoms of menopause; participates in decisions about treatment as an informed consumer.

Table 4-4 Health teaching to reduce risk of osteoporosis

ALL ADULT WOMEN SHOULD

Eat a balanced diet to ensure adequate vitamin and mineral intake.

Increase daily food sources of calcium (dairy products, seafood, yogurt, greens) to prevent or compensate for bone loss.

Decrease excess phosphorus intake (animal proteins, dairy products, diet soda) to prevent calcium excretion. (Aluminum antacids may be suggested as phosphorus binders.)

Maintain adequate vitamin D intake (sunlight, fortified milk products) to balance calcium and phosphorus.

Exercise regularly to strengthen bones.

MENOPAUSAL AND POSTMENOPAUSAL WOMEN SHOULD

Take calcium carbonate or calcium gluconate supplements as prescribed by a physician.

Avoid calcium preparations purchased in health food stores that contain lead, bone meal, and dolomite.

Follow physician recommendations on estrogen replacement therapy to prevent further bone loss.

SELECTED HEALTH PROBLEMS

☐ Uterine Fibroids

General Information

1. Definition: benign uterine tumors of connective tissue and muscle
2. Incidence
   a. 20%-25% of women over age 30 have myomas
   b. Higher incidence in black women
3. Predisposing factors
   a. Infertility
   b. Hormone usage
   c. Age (myomas often disappear with menopause)
4. Medical treatment: depends on symptoms such as bleeding, pressure, and client's age and reproductive status
   a. Medical intervention
      1. close supervision
      2. no hormone administration
      3. reassess after menopause
   b. Surgical intervention
      1. simple myomectomy (subsequent pregnancies may require delivery by cesarean section)
      2. hysterectomy
         a. vaginal approach
         b. abdominal approach

Nursing Process

Assessment

1. Menorrhagia
2. Dysmenorrhea
3. Low-back and pelvic pain
4. Constipation
5. Uterine enlargement
6. History of infertility or miscarriage
7. Presence of predisposing factors

Analysis (see p. 312)

Planning, Implementation, and Evaluation

> **Goal:** Client will be free from problems during conservative management until pregnancy and birth are achieved.

Implementation

1. Discourage hormone usage.
2. Support client's decision for immediate pregnancy.
3. Monitor for increased severity of symptoms.

Evaluation

Client experiences no increase in symptoms; is able to conceive and sustain a pregnancy with minimal difficulty.

☐ Vaginal Wall Changes Associated with Childbearing or Aging

General Information

1. Definitions
   a. *Cystocele:* relaxation of the anterior vaginal wall with prolapse of the bladder
   b. *Rectocele:* relaxation of the posterior vaginal wall with prolapse of the rectum
   c. *Uterine prolapse:* downward displacement
2. Predisposing factors
   a. Multiparity
   b. Pelvic tearing during childbirth
   c. Inappropriate bearing down during labor
   d. Congenital weakness
   e. Vaginal-muscle weakness associated with aging
   f. Less common in ethnic women of color
3. Medical treatment
   a. Preventive
      1. correctly performed episiotomy
      2. postpartum perineal exercises
      3. spaced pregnancies
   b. Surgical intervention
      1. vaginal hysterectomy
      2. anterior and/or posterior vaginal repair (colporrhaphy)
   c. Postoperative care
      1. no hormones needed
      2. evaluate success of repair

Nursing Process

Assessment

1. Cystocele
   a. Incontinence or dribbling with cough, sneeze, or any activity that increases intraabdominal pressure
   b. Retention
   c. Cystitis

2. Rectocele
   a. Constipation
   b. Hemorrhoids
   c. Sensation of pressure
3. Uterine prolapse
   a. Dysmenorrhea
   b. Cervical ulceration
   c. Pelvic pain
   d. Dragging sensation in pelvis and back

Analysis (see p. 312)

Planning, Implementation, and Evaluation

> **Goal:** Client will remain free from undetected complications following anterior and posterior colporrhaphy or vaginal hysterectomy; will regain normal urinary and bowel control.

Implementation
1. Refer to general preoperative and postoperative care, p. 117.
2. Administer cleansing douche and enema preoperatively as ordered.
3. Instruct client to refrain from coughing, sneezing, or straining postoperatively.
4. Promote perineal healing as in postpartal care (see p. 368).
5. Note amount and character of vaginal drainage.
6. Avoid rectal tubes and taking rectal temperatures.
7. Apply vaginal creams as ordered.
8. Check Homan's sign.
9. Monitor urinary output.
10. Provide Foley catheter care.
11. Teach perineal (Kegel) exercises qh and gradual bladder training (i.e., when urinating, stop the stream and then let it resume; performed with every voiding and hourly).
12. Observe for abdominal distension.
13. Ambulate as soon as possible.
14. Instruct on gradual increase of residue in diet.
15. Administer stool softeners and mineral oil before first bowel movement.
16. Provide emotional support.

Evaluation

Client heals postoperatively free from complications; demonstrates normal control and elimination patterns.

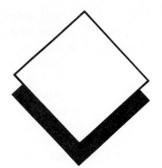

Antepartal Care

GENERAL CONCEPTS
Normal Childbearing

1. Definition: care provided to a woman and her family during pregnancy
2. Normal adaptations: changes that occur in body systems of childbearing women because of the influence of hormones and growth of the embryo/fetus
   a. Integumentary system
      1. changes in skin pigmentation stimulated by elevated levels of melanocyte-stimulating hormone
         a. chloasma (mask of pregnancy): brown blotches that appear on face and neck, often visible in second trimester; usually fade after delivery
         b. linea nigra: a dark line that extends from umbilicus to mons veneris; will lighten after delivery
      2. striae gravidarum: pink or slightly reddish streaks on abdomen, thighs, or breasts, resulting from stretching of underlying connective tissue because of adrenal cortex hypertropy; grow lighter after delivery but never disappear completely
      3. vascular spider angiomas and palmar erythema
   b. Reproductive system
      1. changes in the uterus
         a. size: increases in length (6-32 cm), width (4-24 cm), and depth (2.5-22 cm)
         b. weight increase: 60-1000 g
         c. shape: from globular to oval; wall thickens and then becomes thin at term
         d. location: rises out of pelvis at twelfth week; near xiphoid process at term
         e. structure
            ◆ body of uterus
               • three distinct uterine segments in pregnancy
               • vascularity increases
               • muscle fiber changes, mainly enlargement of preexisting fibers; longitudinal fibers will shorten with contraction of labor to cause effacement; middle-layer fibers constrict blood vessels in labor; add to force of labor; inner fibers exert pressure on blood vessels in lower uterus; prevent hemorrhage
               • new fibroelastic tissue develops and strengthens uterine wall
            ◆ softening of the lower uterine segment *(Hegar's sign)*
            ◆ cervix: softens *(Goodell's sign)* and increases in vascularity
            ◆ formation of mucus plug (prevents bacterial contamination)
         f. contractility: *Braxton Hicks contractions* occur intermittently throughout pregnancy
      2. changes in the vagina
         a. increased vascularization, which results in purplish discoloration *(Chadwick's sign)* beginning in sixth week of pregnancy
         b. thickening of mucosa
         c. loosening of connective tissue
         d. increased vaginal discharge (thick, whitish) without signs of itching or burning
      3. changes in the breasts
         a. enlargement and prominence of superficial veins
         b. increase in size and firmness
         c. Montgomery's glands in areola enlarge
         d. nipples become more prominent, areolas darken and increase in diameter
         e. colostrum may be secreted in fourth or fifth month (16-20 weeks) and subsequently in small amounts until delivery
         f. alveoli and duct system enlarge
      4. changes in joints and ligaments
         a. relaxation of pelvic joints and ligaments

b. hypertrophy and elongation of
   - broad, round ligaments (stabilize uterus)
   - uterosacral ligaments (support cervix)
5. changes in abdomen: occur to accommodate progressive growth in uterine size
   a. at end of twelfth week the uterus is at level of symphysis pubis
   b. by 22-24 weeks uterus is at level of umbilicus
   c. by 38 weeks the uterus is at level of xiphoid process until lightening occurs
   d. decrease in fundal height after lightening in primiparous women

c. Endocrine system (placenta)
1. function of placenta
   a. secretes hormones from early weeks of pregnancy: estrogen, progesterone, human chorionic gonadotropin (HCG), and human placental lactogen (HPL), also called human chorionic somatomammotropin
   b. acts as a barrier to some substances and organisms (e.g., heparin in large doses does not cross; bacteria are less likely to cross placenta than a virus is); barrier not effective for nicotine, alcohol, depressants, stimulants, antibiotics, etc.
   c. nutrition: transports nutrients and water-soluble vitamins to fetus and eliminates wastes
   d. exchanges: fluid and gas transport
      - diffusion, e.g., O_2 and CO_2, water, electrolytes (low molecular weight)
      - facilitated transport (e.g., glucose)
      - active transport: amino acids, calcium, iron (high molecular weight)
      - pinocytosis (e.g., gamma globulin, albumin, fat particles)
      - leakage because of slight placental defects allows fetal and maternal blood cells to mix slightly
2. dimensions
   a. 15×3 cm
   b. discoid
   c. 400-600 g at term
   d. covers quarter of uterine wall
   e. fetal-placental weight ratio at term at 6:1
3. structure and development
   a. fully developed by twelfth week from the decidua basalis and chorion of the embryo; functions most effectively through 40-41 weeks; may be dysfunctional after maturity
   b. normally develops in the posterior surface of the upper uterine segment
   c. two surfaces
      - fetal (amniotic) surface: chorionic villi

and their circulation; membranes: amnion (inner) and chorion (outer) fused
   - maternal surface: decidua basalis (hypertrophied endometrium of pregnancy) and its circulation; cotyledons present
d. umbilical cord: 55 cm at term; most commonly is inserted centrally into fetal surface of placenta; contains one vein to oxygenate fetus and two arteries to carry deoxygenated blood from fetus to placenta to mother
4. hormones
   a. estrogen and progesterone: after first 2 months of gestation, placenta is major source of production; responsible for growth of uterus and development of breasts
   b. human chorionic gonadotropin (HCG): secreted by third week after fertilization, detected in urine 10 days after missed period (basis for simple pregnancy tests); HCG prolongs life of corpus luteum; radioimmunoassay (RIA) for HCG will be positive the second day after implantation
   c. human chorionic somatomammotropin (human placental lactogen): secreted by third week after ovulation; prepares breasts for lactation, influences somatic cell growth of fetus; antagonist to insulin, considered principal maternal diabetogenic factor

d. Musculoskeletal system
1. relaxation and increased mobility of pelvic joints result in a waddling gait and instability
2. increase in normal lumbosacral curve because of enlarging uterus; poor posture may increase problem
3. stress on ligaments and muscles of middle and lower spine
4. backache and leg cramps may occur

e. Cardiovascular system
1. heart and vessels
   a. heart rate increases 10-15 beats/min in second trimester; persists to term
   b. blood pressure should remain constant during pregnancy with a decrease in the second trimester
   c. increase in vasculature: dilation of pelvic veins, varicose veins, varicosities of the vulva, hemorrhoids
2. cardiac output increases 20%-30% during first and second trimesters to meet increased tissue demands
3. blood volume altered in pregnancy; total increase approximately 20%-30%, peaking in third trimester; increases immediately after delivery because of fluid shift
   a. plasma volume increases out of proportion to the red-cell increase resulting in hemo-

dilution; this causes normal physiological anemia

    b. hemoglobin range 10-16 g/dl; may decrease; problematic if it falls below 10 g/dl

    c. hematocrit range 35%-42%; may decrease approximately 10% in second and third trimesters; anemia if it falls below 35%

    d. average WBC count 5000-11,000/mm^3 (higher than normal)

  4. palpitations: common in early and late pregnancy because of sympathetic nervous system disturbance and increased intra-abdominal pressure

f. Renal system

  1. elimination/fluid transport greatly increased because of circulatory changes and need to excrete fetal waste products

  2. glomerular filtration rate increases 50%

  3. renal functioning is compromised in standing or sitting position; lateral recumbent position enhances kidney function

  4. reduced renal threshold for glucose glycosuria may occur; reflection of kidneys' inability to absorb glucose; appears to have little relationship to serum glucose

  5. increased amount of urine; decreased specific gravity

  6. dilatation of ureters, especially on the right, may lead to urinary stasis

  7. decreased bladder tone, caused by progesterone effect

  8. increased pressure on bladder by enlarging uterus (first and third trimesters), therefore decreased capacity and increased frequency

g. Respiratory system

  1. diaphragm rises as much as 1 inch; dyspnea may occur until lightening (60% of pregnant women)

  2. thoracic cage is pushed upward and widened

  3. increased vital capacity, tidal volume, respiratory minute volume to supply maternal and fetal needs

  4. increased vascularization because of elevated estrogen can cause nasal stuffiness; nosebleed, voice changes, eustachian tube blockage

h. Digestive system

  1. gastrointestinal motility and digestion slowed because of progesterone effects

  2. delayed emptying time of stomach; reflux of food

  3. upward displacement and compression of stomach

  4. displacement of intestines as fetus develops

  5. decreased secretion of HCl

  6. slower emptying of gallbladder may lead to gallstone formation

  7. common problems

    a. nausea and vomiting (morning sickness, 50%-75% of pregnant women)

    b. pica; food or substance cravings (e.g., laundry starch, clay)

    c. acid indigestion or heartburn

    d. constipation

    e. hemorrhoids

    f. bleeding, swollen gums because of estrogen

i. Psychosocial adaptations in pregnancy

  1. factors influencing a woman's response to pregnancy (varies with developmental stage)

    a. memories of her own childhood

    b. cultural background

    c. existing support systems

    d. socioeconomic conditions

    e. perceptions of maternal role

    f. impact of mass media

    g. coping mechanisms

  2. maternal adaptations to pregnancy

    a. first trimester: initial ambivalence about pregnancy; pregnant woman places main focus upon self (i.e., physical changes associated with pregnancy and emotional reactions to pregnancy)

    b. second trimester: relatively tranquil period; acceptance of reality of pregnancy; increased awareness and interest in fetus; introversion and feeling of well-being

    c. third trimester: anticipation of labor and delivery and assuming mothering role, viewing infant as reality vs. fantasy; fears, fantasies, and dreams about labor are common; "nesting" behaviors (e.g., preparing layette)

  3. psychological tasks of pregnancy (Rubin, 1961)

    a. acceptance of pregnancy as a reality and incorporation of fetus into body image

    b. preparation for physical separation from fetus (birth)

    c. attainment of maternal role

  4. developmental tasks of pregnancy

    a. accept the biological fact of pregnancy (i.e., "I am pregnant")

    b. accept the growing fetus as distinct from self and as a person to care for (i.e., "I am going to have a baby")

    c. prepare realistically for the birth and parenting of the child (i.e., "I am going to be a mother")

  5. paternal reactions to pregnancy

    a. vary with developmental stage, sociocultural factors (as with woman), and involvement

    b. first trimester: ambivalence and anxiety

Table 4-5 Signs and symptoms of pregnancy

Symptoms	Signs
PRESUMPTIVE	
Amenorrhea	Chadwick's sign
Breast sensitivity	Breast enlargement
Nausea, vomiting	Skin pigmentation, striae
Urinary frequency	
Fatigue	
Quickening	
PROBABLE	
Enlarged abdomen	Ballottement
Hegar's sign	Braxton Hicks contractions
Goodell's sign	Positive pregnancy tests
POSITIVE	
	By examiner
	fetal movements
	fetal outline—sonography
	x-ray
	fetal heart tones

about role change; concern or identification with mother's discomforts

 c. second trimester: increased confidence and interest in mother's care; difficulty relating to fetus; "jealousy"

 d. third trimester: changing self-concept; active involvement common; fears about delivery, mutilation or death of partner or fetus

 6. sibling reactions to pregnancy

  a. normal rivalry dependent on developmental stage

  b. may need increased affection and attention

  c. regression in behavior (may appear in bedwetting and thumbsucking)

3. Signs and symptoms of pregnancy (see Table 4-5)

 a. Presumptive symptoms (subjective)

  1. amenorrhea (approximately 2 weeks after conception)

  2. breast sensitivity and fullness (as early as fourth week)

  3. nausea and vomiting (primarily 5-12 weeks)

  4. increased urinary frequency (6-12 weeks)

  5. fatigue (first trimester)

  6. quickening: maternal perception of fetal movement 18-20 weeks in primipara, 16 weeks in multipara

 b. Presumptive signs (objective)

  1. dark-blue discoloration of the vaginal mucosa (Chadwick's sign; 8-12 weeks)

  2. skin pigmentation and striae

 c. Probable signs (objective)

  1. enlargement of abdomen

  2. changes in the uterus: size, shape, and consistency (Hegar's sign) (5-7 weeks)

  3. softening of the cervical tip (Goodell's sign) (sixth week)

  4. ballottement: movement of the fetus in the pregnant uterus by the examiner (16-32 weeks)

  5. Braxton Hicks contractions (early as 8 weeks throughout pregnancy)

  6. positive pregnancy test: biological and immunological tests based on secretion of HCG in maternal urine or in serum (7-14 days)

 d. Positive signs (objective)

  1. fetal outline and movements felt by examiner (about 20 weeks)

  2. presence of fetal heart sounds detected by fetoscope at 16 weeks (Doppler, 10 weeks)

  3. confirmation of pregnancy by ultrasonography

  4. x-ray outline of fetal skeleton (rarely used)

4. Fetal development

 a. During first lunar month (1 lunar month = 4 weeks)

  1. following fertilization, the ovum (zygote) begins a process of rapid cell division (mitosis or cleavage) leading to formation of *blastomeres*, which eventually become a ball-like structure called the morula

  2. the *morula* changes into a *blastocyst* after entering the uterus

  3. implantation occurs within 1-2 days, when the exposed cells of the trophoblast (cellular walls of the blastocyst) implant in the anterior or posterior fundal portion of the uterus

  4. the cells of the embryo will differentiate into three main groups: an outer covering (ectoderm), a middle layer (mesoderm), and an internal layer (entoderm)

   a. ectoderm: later differentiates into epithelium of skin, hair, nails, nasal and oral passages, sebaceous and sweat glands, mucous membranes of mouth and nose, salivary glands, the nervous system

   b. mesoderm: later differentiates into muscles; bones; circulatory, renal, and reproductive organs; connective tissue

   c. entoderm: differentiates into epithelium of gastrointestinal and respiratory tracts, the bladder, thyroid

 b. Subsequent lunar months

  1. end of first lunar month (4 weeks): heart functions; beginning formation of eyes, nose, digestive tract; arm and leg buds

  2. end of second lunar month (8 weeks): recognizable human face, rapid brain development, appearance of external genitalia

3. end of third lunar month (12 weeks): placenta fully formed and functioning; sex determination apparent; bones begin to ossify; less danger of teratogenic effects after this time; length: 3½ inches (9 cm), weight: ½ oz (2 g)

4. end of fourth lunar month (16 weeks): external genitalia obvious; meconium present in intestinal tract; eye, ear, and nose formed; fetal heartbeat heard with fetoscope; length: 6½ inches, weight: 4 oz

5. end of fifth lunar month (20 weeks): lanugo present; fetus sucks and swallows amniotic fluid; quickening (mother can feel movement); length: 10 inches, weight: 8 oz

6. end of sixth lunar month (24 weeks): vernix present; skin reddish and wrinkled; considered viable, but usually doesn't survive if born now; length: 12 inches, weight: 1 lb 5 oz

7. end of seventh lunar month (28 weeks): iron stored; surfactant production begins; nails appear; better chance of survival if delivered than in earlier gestation; length: 15 inches, weight: 2 lb 8 oz (1000 g)

8. end of eighth lunar month (32 weeks): iron, calcium stored; more reflexes present; good chance of survival if delivered preterm

9. end of ninth lunar month (36 weeks): well-padded with subcutaneous fat; survival same as term

10. end of tenth lunar month (39-40 weeks or full term): lanugo shed, nails firm, testes fully descended; length: 18-22 inches (45-55 cm), weight: average 7 lb 8 oz (3400 g)

c. Fetal circulation

1. fetus receives oxygen through placenta (see Fig. 4-21)

2. oxygenated blood enters fetal circulation through umbilical vein of cord to the ductus venosus and liver; ductus venosus attaches to inferior vena cava and allows blood to bypass liver

3. from inferior vena cava, blood flows into right atrium and goes directly to the left atrium through the foramen ovale

4. blood enters right atrium through superior vena cava, flows to right ventricle, to pulmonary artery (small amount enters lungs for nourishment); the ductus arteriosus shunts blood from pulmonary artery into the aorta, allows bypass of fetal lungs

5. two umbilical arteries return deoxygenated blood from fetus to placenta

d. Amniotic fluid

1. multiple origins; composition changes in pregnancy; from maternal serum to fetal urine towards term

2. appearance: clear, pale, straw colored, with faint characteristic odor; neutral to slightly alkaline (pH 7.0-7.25) while vaginal secretions are normally acidic

3. volume: about 30 ml at 10 weeks, 350 ml at 20 weeks, approximately 1000 ml at term; specific gravity 1.007 to 1.025

   a. *oligohydramnios* is less than 300-500 ml of fluid

   b. *polyhydramnios* is greater than 1500-2000 ml of fluid

4. contains albumin, urea, uric acid, creatinine, lecithin, sphingomyelin, bilirubin, epithelial cells, fat, fructose, leukocytes, enzymes, lanugo

5. functions

   a. protects fetus from injury

   b. separates fetus from fetal membrane

   c. allows fetus freedom of movement

   d. provides source of oral fluids

   e. serves as excretion-collection system

   f. exchanges at rate of 500 ml/hr (at term)

   g. regulates fetal body temperature

Overview of Management

1. Interdisciplinary health team: nurses, nurse practitioners, midwives, physicians, social workers, dietitians, and other health care providers

2. Schedule of visits

   a. Routine if no complications

   1. every 4 weeks, up to 32 weeks

   2. every 2 weeks from 32-36 weeks (more frequently if problems exist)

   3. every week from 36-40 weeks

   b. Initial visit

   1. obtain family and obstetrical history

      a. personal and social profiles of childbearing family, including cultural patterns, education, support systems, coping methods, economic level (low income level may mean little or no antenatal care, inadequate nutrition, or high risk for preeclampsia)

      b. maternal factors affecting course of pregnancy: smoking, use of alcohol or drugs, activities of daily living, sleep patterns, bowel habits, nutrition (inadequate diet increases risk of anemia, preeclampsia), weight, age, and living at high altitude (increased hemoglobin)

      c. preexisting medical disorders: diabetes mellitus, cardiac disease, anemia, hypertension, thyroid disorders

      d. family planning measures; health history during pregnancies; history of infertility

e. attitudes toward present pregnancy

f. history of preceding pregnancies and perinatal outcomes (TPAL)
- ◆ T: number of term births (i.e., born at 37 weeks gestation or beyond)
- ◆ P: number of premature births
- ◆ A: number of abortions (spontaneous or induced)
- ◆ L: number of living children
- ◆ *gravida:* all pregnancies regardless of duration or outcome, including present pregnancy
- ◆ *parity:* past pregnancies resulting in viable fetus (20-24 weeks), whether born dead or alive (twins considered as one)
- ◆ cesarean births
- ◆ Rh or ABO sensitization
- ◆ serious emotional or psychological distress
- ◆ stillborns

g. past personal and family medical history

2. calculate expected date of delivery (or confinement [EDC]) using Nägele's rule: count back three calendar months from the first day of the last regular menstrual period (LMP) and add seven days (see Table 4-6)

c. Initial and subsequent visits

1. assess vital signs and blood pressure for normal range or baseline

2. check urine for albumin and glucose: ideally not more than 1+ glucose with protein negative

3. monitor weight gain: a total gain of 25-30 lb is recommended, depending on prepregnant nutritional state
   a. 2-4 lb in the first trimester
   b. 11-14 lb in the second trimester
   c. 8-11 lb in the third trimester (i.e., 0.5 lb weekly)

4. assess fetal growth and development over duration of pregnancy
   a. fetal heart rate (FHR)
   b. abdominal palpation
   c. fundal height

5. allow time for client to express concerns, problems or discomfort, and learning needs

6. document accurately

Table 4-6 Nägele's rule

If first day of last menstrual period was
January 17
subtract 3 months
+
add 7 days
Estimated date of delivery is October 24

Application of the Nursing Process to Normal Childbearing, Antepartal Care

Assessment

1. Refer to "Initial and Subsequent Visits"

Analysis

1. Safe, effective care environment
   a. High risk for injury
   b. Knowledge deficit
2. Physiological integrity
   a. Fatigue
   b. Altered nutrition; less than body requirements
3. Psychosocial integrity
   a. Self-esteem disturbance
   b. Altered role performance
4. Health promotion/maintenance
   a. Health-seeking behaviors
   b. Altered family processes

Planning, Implementation, and Evaluation

> **Goal 1:** Client will maintain optimal health through preventive health measures and regular antepartal and prenatal care; fetus will be well oxygenated and nourished throughout gestation.

Implementation

1. Measure vital signs, including temperature, blood pressure, pulse, and respiration.
2. Assess client: general physical assessment including height and weight (initial visit).
3. Help with physical examination and bimanual pelvic examination.
   a. Prepare and arrange necessary equipment (gloves, lubricant [for digital exam], vaginal speculum, materials for Pap smear [no lubricant used], light, and pelvimeter).
   b. Prepare client for procedure by providing explanation, instructing her to empty bladder, and placing her in lithotomy position, position hands across chest.
   c. Provide emotional support and maintain comfort of client before and during examination (using relaxation, breathing, and focusing techniques).
4. Measure fundal height using McDonald's rule (in second and third trimester): symphysis pubis to fundus (see Table 4-7).
5. Estimate fetal weight (EFW): rump-to-crown length in utero in centimeters × 100 = EFW (g)
6. Check for fetal heartbeat, detectable as early as 16 weeks with fetoscope and by 10-12 weeks with Doppler device.

Table 4-7 McDonald's rule

Height of fundus (cm)
× 2/7 = duration of pregnancy in *lunar months*
× 8/7 = duration of pregnancy in *weeks*

7. Assist in obtaining samples for laboratory studies.
   a. Clean-catch urine for urinalysis, albumin, glucose, and asymptomatic bacteriuria.
   b. Blood for hemoglobin, hematocrit, type, Rh, rubella titer (greater than 1:8 shows immunity).
   c. Sickle cell disease or trait in black women.
   d. Standard tests for sexually transmitted diseases (serology for syphilis; smears for gonorrhea, herpes).
   e. Schedule glucose tolerance test during 24-28 weeks
8. Encourage regular antepartal care.
   a. Explain need for continuity.
   b. Describe *"danger signals"* (e.g., vaginal bleeding, dizziness or visual spots, swelling of face or fingers, epigastric pain, physical trauma) or reportable signs that require immediate medical care.
9. Promote health through anticipatory guidance: rest and exercise, personal hygiene, sexual activity, dental care, clothing, travel, immunizations, smoking, alcohol use, substance abuse.
   a. Tell couple to expect an increased need for sleep during entire pregnancy, with fatigue common in first trimester; needs vary among individuals; plan rest times during day.
   b. Teach relaxation methods in preparing for sleep.
   c. Advise to continue usual exercise regimen; avoid introduction of strenuous sports; avoid exercise leading to fatigue, exhaustion, overheating, dehydration.
   d. Explain exercise limitations related to the changing center of gravity (e.g., high-impact aerobics, jogging).
   e. Avoid sauna/whirlpool activities.
   f. Suggest that client may continue to work except if exposed to toxic chemicals, radiation, biological or safety hazards (if job requires sitting for long period, encourage frequent position changes).
   g. Teach hygiene and skin care; daily baths if desired (caution on safely getting into and out of bathtub); avoid soap on nipples; towel-dry breasts; for vaginal discharge: daily bathing, wear cotton underwear (douching not recommended).
   h. Suggest that changes in sexual desire/response may occur, related to discomforts or anxieties of pregnancy; encourage couple to share their concerns and feelings; alternative coital positions may be helpful, as may be other methods of satisfying sexual needs; coitus may be continued throughout pregnancy unless premature labor, rupture of membranes, or bleeding occur.
   i. Encourage dental checkup early in pregnancy and delay extensive dental work and x-ray examinations when possible; hypertrophy and tenderness of gums is a common problem.
   j. Recommend comfortable, nonrestricting maternity clothing, well-fitting bra, and low-heeled, supportive shoes.
   k. Advise client to stop or reduce cigarette consumption; *maternal smoking is associated with low birth weight.*
   l. Advise client to *avoid alcohol consumption* during pregnancy because alcohol, even in minimal to moderate amounts, is harmful to fetus; linked to fetal alcohol syndrome.
   m. Warn client to avoid medication, particularly in the first trimester (over-the-counter and prescription drugs may cross placental barrier); physicians must weigh advantages vs. risks of medications for individual clients.
   n. Suggest that while traveling long distances by auto, walk frequently; use seat belts for safety.
   o. Teach couple that attenuated, live vaccines (e.g., mumps, rubella) are contraindicated for immunizations during pregnancy.

Evaluation

Client receives initial and regular antepartal care to prevent or detect any early complications; avoids substances that may potentially harm the fetus; fetus maintains a growth and development pattern appropriate for gestational age as evidenced by maternal weight gain, fundal height, activity level, and other antenatal screening techniques; is protected from environmental hazards and stresses (e.g., alcohol, nicotine).

> **Goal 2:** Client will be aware of common discomforts of pregnancy and know how to relieve them.

Implementation

1. Teach health maintenance and relief of common discomforts.
   a. *Morning sickness:* eat dry crackers or toast before slowly arising; eat small, frequent meals; avoid greasy, highly seasoned food; take adequate fluids between meals.
   b. *Breast tenderness:* wear a well-fitted, supportive bra with wide, adjustable straps.
   c. *Heartburn and indigestion:* avoid overeating, ingesting fatty or fried food; take small, frequent meals; avoid taking sodium bicarbonate; remain upright 3-4 hours after eating.
   d. *Backache:* maintain proper body alignment (pelvic tilt) and use good body mechanics; use maternity girdle in selected situations; wear comfortable shoes; use proper mattress; rest frequently; do pelvic-rock exercise and tailor sitting.
   e. *Leg cramps:* stretch involved muscles (i.e., extension of leg with dorsiflexion of the foot); may be related to alterations in calcium, phosphorus.
   f. *Varicose veins:* elevate legs frequently when sitting or lying down in bed; avoid sitting or standing

for prolonged periods or crossing legs at the knees; avoid tight or constricting hosiery or garters (physician may suggest wearing supportive hose).

g. *Hemorrhoids:* apply warm compresses; upon recommendation of physician, reinsert hemorrhoids (place client in a side-lying or knee-chest position; use gentle pressure and a lubricant), avoid constipation; take sitz baths.

h. *Constipation:* increase fluid intake (ideal is 6-8 glasses/day), roughage; develop good daily bowel movement habits; exercise.

i. *Urinary frequency:* empty bladder regularly; report any burning, dysuria, cloudiness, or blood in urine.

j. *Ankle edema:* change position, lie on left side; rest with legs and hips elevated (report any edema in face and in hands).

k. *Uterine contractions* (Braxton Hicks): normal during late pregnancy; report if they progressively increase and are accompanied by signs of labor.

l. *Faintness:* avoid staying in one position over a long period; arise from bed from a lateral position (to prevent supine hypotension).

m. *Shortness of breath:* use proper posture when erect; sleep with head elevated by several pillows (left lateral position preferred).

Evaluation

Client identifies own basic discomforts of pregnancy and appropriately relieves them.

Goal 3: Client will have adequate knowledge of nutrition to meet her own developmental needs, the physical requirements of pregnancy and lactation, and fetal growth and development.

Implementation

1. Obtain complete nutritional profile (suggest client use 24-hour recall).
   a. Prepregnant and current nutritional status (e.g., overweight, underweight, anemic)
   b. Physical symptoms possibly indicative of poor nutrition (e.g., dry scaly skin, lack of skin turgor, fatigue)
   c. Socioeconomic status: available finances for a balanced diet; customs and cultural/religious restrictions
   d. Dietary habits: regularity of meals, junk-food intake, pica, peer pressure
   e. Knowledge of nutritional needs, basic four food groups, recommended allowances during pregnancy.
2. Assess for nutritional risk factors at the onset of pregnancy.
   a. Adolescence
   b. Frequent pregnancies
   c. Poor reproductive history

d. Economic deprivation
e. Bizarre food patterns
f. Vegetarian diet
g. Smoking, drug addiction, or alcoholism
h. Chronic systemic disease
i. Prepregnant weight problems, including anorexia and bulimia

3. Assess for nutritional risk factors during pregnancy.
   a. Anemia of pregnancy
   b. Pregnancy-induced hypertension
   c. Inadequate or excessive weight gain
   d. Demands of lactation
4. Teach based on consideration of mother's age, routine activity, developmental needs, cultural dietary patterns, and risk factors.
5. Encourage good nutritional practices; see Tables 4-4 and 4-8 to 4-10.
   a. Discuss well-balanced diet, including basic four groups as adapted during pregnancy.
   b. Recommend that pregnant adolescents take in additional calories, protein, and calcium for own developmental needs.
   c. Suggest a minimum fluid intake of 6-8 glasses of fluids or water each day.
   d. Discuss possible vitamin and mineral supplements (e.g., iron or folic acid).
   e. Caution against overdose of vitamins A and D (may cause fetal deformities).
   f. Monitor weight gain each antepartal visit; a total weight gain of 25-30 lb is usually recommended.
   g. Recognize when restrictions in salt may be indicated (e.g., high-sodium foods such as carrots, spinach, celery, carbonated beverages, canned soup, bacon, ham, monosodium glutamate, pickles, and olives).
   h. Refer to nutritionist for additional teaching/counseling as needed.

Evaluation

Client identifies the basic four food groups and their components; knows the nutrients and calories needed each day; follows a balanced diet; gradually and steadily gains 25-30 lb during the pregnancy; fetus maintains a growth and development pattern appropriate for gestational age.

Goal 4: Client and family will verbalize a familiarity with the relaxation techniques and exercises that are part of childbirth education; will experience reduced anxiety about childbirth and parenting.

Implementation

1. Explain the purpose and scope of childbirth education (decrease fear and anxiety through knowledge, effective use of relaxation techniques to reduce pain perception during labor and delivery).
2. Discuss various methods (see Table 4-11).

Table 4-8 Recommended dietary allowances for females age 11-50

Nutrients	Age (yr): Weight (lb):	Nonpregnant girls and women 11-14 (101)	15-18 (120)	19-22 (120)	23-50 (120)	Pregnant women	Lactating women
Energy (kcal) (mean)		2200	2100	2100	2000	+300	+500
Protein (g)		46	46	44	44	+ 30	+ 20
Vitamin A (μg)		800	800	800	800	+200	+400
Vitamin D (μg)		10	10	7.5	5	+ 5	+ 5
Vitamin E (mg)		8	8	8	8	+ 2	+ 3
Vitamin C (mg)		50	60	60	60	+ 20	+ 40
Thiamin (mg)		1.1	1.1	1.1	1.0	+ .04	+ 0.5
Riboflavin (mg)		1.3	1.3	1.3	1.2	+ 0.3	+ 0.5
Niacin (mg)		15	14	14	13	+ 2	+ 5
Vitamin B_6 (mg)		1.8	2.0	2.0	2.0	+ 0.6	+ 0.5
Folacin (μg)		400	400	400	400	+400	+100
Vitamin B_{12} (mcg)		3	3	3	3	+ 1	+ 1
Calcium (mg)		1200	1200	800	800	+400	+400
Phosphorus (mg)		1200	1200	800	800	+400	+400
Magnesium (mg)		300	300	300	300	+150	+150
Iron (mg)		18	18	18	18	Suppl*	*
Zinc (mg)		15	15	15	15	+ 5	+ 10
Iodine (mg)		150	150	150	150	+ 25	+ 50

From the Committee on Dietary Allowances, Food and Nutrition Board, Division of Biological Sciences; Assembly of Life Sciences, National Research Council. (1980.) *Recommended dietary allowances* (9th rev. ed.). Washington, D.C.: National Academy of Sciences.
*Recommendation: Iron supplement of 30-60 mg during pregnancy and for 2-3 months postpartum. Iron needs during lactation do not differ substantially from those of nonpregnant women. The supplement is to replenish stores depleted by pregnancy.

Table 4-9 Selected nutrients essential for health in pregnancy and lactation

Nutrient	Food source
Iron	Liver, meat, eggs, whole enriched grains, leafy vegetables, nuts, legumes, dried fruits, oysters, and clams
Calcium	Milk, cheese, ice cream, whole grains, leafy vegetables, egg yolks, and dried beans
Vitamin C	Citrus fruits, tomatoes, cantaloupe, strawberries, potatoes, broccoli, and leafy greens
Protein	Milk, pudding, custard, yogurt, cheese, meat, poultry, fish, eggs, legumes, and nuts

3. Offer direct instructions (Leboyer) or referral to appropriate resources (e.g., La Leche League or International Childbirth Education Association).

Evaluation

Couple expresses a positive attitude toward pregnancy and is adequately prepared for birth experience; openly expresses concerns and provides emotional support to each other; begins the role transition to parenthood.

High-Risk Childbearing

1. Definition: any existing or developing condition or factor that prevents or impedes the normal progress of pregnancy to the delivery of a viable, healthy, term infant.
2. Assessment of risk factors
   a. Age: under 17 or over 35 (greater risk over 40)
      1. pregnant adolescents have a higher incidence of prematurity, pregnancy-induced hypertension, cephalopelvic disproportion, poor nutrition, and inadequate antepartal care

Table 4-10 Pregnant woman's daily food intake

Food group	Recommended daily amount
Dairy products	Three to four 8-oz cups
Meat group	Two 6-8–oz servings; 1 egg
Grain products, whole grain or enriched	4-5 servings
Fruits/fruit juices	1-2 servings; include 4 oz of orange or grapefruit juice
Vegetables/vegetable juices	4-6 servings (1 or 2 servings raw; 1 serving of dark green or deep yellow)
Fluids	4-6 glasses (8 oz) water plus other fluids to equal 8-10 cups/day

From Bobak, I., et al. (1989). *Maternity and gynecologic care* (4th ed.). St. Louis: Mosby–Year Book.

Table 4-11   Childbirth preparation

Method	Chief focus	Breathing/relaxation techniques
G.D. Read	Earliest modern physician to identify fear-tension-pain cycle Avoidance of medication; removed childbirth from illness orientation	
Gamper	Based on Read; use of uterus as focal point	Abdominal/natural breathing
Bradley	Based on Read/Gamper Focus on individual relaxation methods Mother-centered; coached by partner Emphasis of client decision making	Diaphragmatic breathing
Lamaze (psychoprophylactic)	Conscious application of conditioned responses to stimuli Use of focal point outside mother's body	Chest breathing in early labor Increasing rate as labor progresses Cleansing breaths

2. women over 35 are at increased risk for chromosomal disorders in infants (e.g., Down syndrome), pregnancy-induced hypertension, and cesarean delivery
  b. Parity
    1. multiparity: two or more pregnancies (may not be significant)
    2. grand multiparity: six or more pregnancies
    3. interval between pregnancies
  c. Past health history
    1. diabetes
    2. heart disease
    3. renal conditions
    4. essential hypertension
    5. anemia
    6. thyroid disorder
    7. physical abuse
  d. Past obstetrical history
    1. lack of antepartal care; poor compliance with visit schedule (may be a factor in late detection of health problems); contributes to high infant mortality rate in this country
    2. abortions: spontaneous
    3. ectopic pregnancy
    4. preterm labor and delivery
    5. intrauterine growth retardation
    6. congenital malformations: result of genetic disorders
    7. cesarean births
    8. previous fetal loss
    9. pregnancy-induced hypertension
    10. diabetes
    11. vaginal bleeding in pregnancy
    12. isoimmunization
    13. multiple gestation
    14. large infants
  e. Current obstetrical history
    1. pregnancy-induced hypertension (21% of maternal deaths)

    2. infections (18% of maternal deaths)
      a. sexually transmitted diseases
      b. TORCH syndrome (*T*oxoplasmosis, *O*ther, *R*ubella, *C*ytomegalovirus infection, *H*erpes)
      c. other viral diseases (e.g., hepatitis or AIDS)
      d. bacterial infections (e.g., tuberculosis)
    3. hemorrhage (14% of maternal deaths)
    4. exposure to toxic environmental agents
    5. use of drugs
    6. multiple gestation
    7. abnormal presentation
    8. premature rupture of membranes
    9. chronic health problems (e.g., diabetes, cardiac disease, anemia)
    10. coexisting medical problems
    11. abnormal antenatal test results (e.g., on amniotic-fluid analysis, ultrasound)
  f. Socioeconomic-cultural status
    1. low socioeconomic status: often associated with
      a. inadequate nutrition
      b. lack of general knowledge about health care needs
    2. incidence of small-for-gestational-age babies is common in some Asian and black women and adolescents
  g. Malnutrition or deprivation: less than 4 kg weight gain by 30 weeks of gestation; may be related to eating disorders
  h. Drug or alcohol addiction: associated with congenital anomalies, intrauterine growth retardation, and numerous other problems
  i. Smoking: associated with low-birth-weight infants
3. Diagnostic tests, biophysical and biochemical, to evaluate fetal-placental function or fetal maturity; critical in high-risk pregnancy
  a. Fetal movement or fetal kick count

1. definition: daily recording of fetal movements to assess active and passive fetal states in normal pregnancies, as well as in those with complications
2. procedure: a noninvasive test that may be done directly by pregnant woman
3. interpretation (optimal number of fetal movements varies with source)
   a. normally three or more movements felt in an hour; fetal states normally vary (cyclic periods of rest and activity)
   b. marked decrease in fetal activity (unrelated to sleep) of two or less movements/hr should be reported and a nonstress test (NST) may be scheduled
4. reassure client that there are fetal rest and sleep states with minimal or no fetal movement

b. Nonstress testing (NST)
1. definition: observation of fetal heart rate (FHR) related to fetal movement (accelerations suggest fetal well-being with good prognosis)
2. indications: for fetal evaluation, especially in postterm pregnancies, uteroplacental insufficiency, poor fetal history
3. procedure
   a. performed in an ambulatory setting or in the hospital obstetrical unit by nurse trained in test administration
   b. requires external electronic monitoring (indirect) using ultrasound transducer to measure FHR and tokodynamometer to trace fetal activity or spontaneous uterine activity
   c. pregnant woman placed in semi-Fowler's or left lateral position
   d. maternal BP recorded initially
   e. requires 30-50 minutes to administer test (10- to 12-minute tracing obtained)
   f. client must activate "mark button" with each fetal movement
4. interpretation
   a. reactive (normal): two FHR accelerations (greater than 15 beats per minute) above baseline—lasting 15 seconds or more— occur with fetal movement in a 10- or 20-minute period
   b. nonreactive (abnormal): failure to meet the reactive criteria indicates the need for additional evaluation, perhaps using contraction stress test (CST) or oxytocin challenge test (OCT)
   c. unsatisfactory result: uninterpretable FHR or fetal activity recording; additional testing performed in 24 hours or OCT done

c. Contraction stress test (CST) or oxytocin challenge test (OCT)
1. definition: the response of the fetus (FHR pattern) to induced uterine contractions is observed as an indicator of uteroplacental and fetal physiological integrity
2. indications: pregnancies at risk for placental insufficiency or fetal compromise
3. procedure
   a. performed on an outpatient basis in or near the labor and delivery unit
   b. requires external electronic monitoring (indirect) using ultrasound transducer to measure FHR and tokodynamometer to trace uterine activity
   c. pregnant woman placed in semi-Fowler's or left lateral position
   d. maternal blood pressure recorded initially and at intervals during test
   e. requires 60 minutes to 3 hours to complete test
   f. increasing doses of oxytocin are administered as a dilute intravenous infusion according to hospital protocol or physician's orders until uterine contractions occur
4. interpretation
   a. negative (normal): the absence of late decelerations of FHR with each of three contractions during a 10-minute interval; known as "negative window"
   b. positive (abnormal): the presence of late decelerations of FHR with three contractions during a 10-minute interval; known as "positive window"
   c. equivocal or suspicious: the absence of a positive or negative window (i.e., criterion of three contractions in a 10-minute interval is not achieved)
   d. unsatisfactory tests occur when interpretable tracings are not obtained or adequate uterine contractions are not achieved
   e. high-risk pregnancies are usually allowed to continue if a negative OCT is obtained; test is repeated weekly for these clients

d. Nipple stimulation-contraction stress test
1. baseline data obtained through monitoring as in CST procedure
2. breast stimulated by warm towel application or nipple rolling, causing release of oxytocin and producing uterine contractions
3. interpretation: as with CST, uterine contraction with absence of late decelerations is the desired result

e. Ultrasonography
1. definition: a noninvasive procedure involving the passage of high-frequency sound waves through the uterus in order to obtain an outline of the fetus, placenta, uterine cavity, or any other area under examination

2. purposes
   a. confirm pregnancy (first trimester)
   b. determine fetal viability
   c. estimate fetal age through measuring the biparietal diameter of the fetal head; most accurate at 12-24 weeks
   d. monitor fetal growth
   e. determine fetal position
   f. locate placenta
   g. detect fetal abnormalities
   h. identify multiple gestation
   i. confirm fetal death
   j. fetal biophysical profile
3. procedure
   a. advise pregnant woman to consume 1 quart of water 2 hours before procedure and avoid emptying bladder; scanning is done when the bladder is full (exception: before amniocentesis)
   b. transmission gel spread over maternal abdomen
   c. sonographer scans vertically and horizontally in sections across abdomen
4. possible risk
   a. none known with brief, infrequent exposure to high-intensity sound
   b. couple and physician should discuss indications, benefits, and potential risks

f. Chorionic villi sampling
   1. definition: removal of a small sample of chorionic villi for examination
   2. purposes
      a. detect chromosomal defects
      b. detect biochemical abnormalities
   3. procedure
      a. done at 8-10 weeks' gestation
      b. catheter passed through cervix into the uterus (guided by sonography)
      c. sample aspirated under negative pressure
   4. advantages
      a. early detection of abnormalities allowing for first-trimester termination of the pregnancy if desired
      b. results available within 2-10 days
   5. disadvantages
      a. risk of abortion
      b. infection

g. Amniocentesis
   1. definition: an invasive procedure for amniotic fluid analysis to assess fetal health and maturity; done from 14 weeks of gestation
   2. procedure
      a. ultrasonography is first performed to locate the placenta
      b. pregnant woman must empty bladder before

procedure if greater than 20 weeks' gestation
   c. baseline vital signs and FHR are assessed; monitor every 15 minutes
   d. pregnant woman is placed in supine position and given an abdominal prep
   e. a needle is passed through the abdominal and uterine walls into the amniotic sac, and a small amount of amniotic fluid is withdrawn
3. possible risks: overall, less than 1%
   a. maternal: hemorrhage, infection, Rh isoimmunization, abruptio placentae, labor
   b. fetal: death, infection, hemorrhage, abortion, premature labor, injury from needle
4. observe client closely for 30-40 minutes following procedure; instruct client to report any side effects (e.g., unusual fetal activity, vaginal bleeding, leakage of amniotic fluid, uterine contractions, fever, or chills)

h. Laboratory studies
   1. urinary or serum estriol determination: to assess placental functioning
      a. steroid precursor produced by the adrenals of the fetus is synthesized into estriols in the placenta and is excreted by the maternal kidneys; mother's levels normally rise during pregnancy
      b. serial estriol determinations are obtained with repeat blood samples or 24-hour urine collections after 20 weeks of gestation (preferably after 32 weeks); instruct regarding 24-hour urine collection (i.e., discard first specimen, then save all urine; refrigerate)
      c. a sudden drop in estriol level is associated with fetal hypoxia; continuous low levels associated with compromise of fetus
   2. Serum placental lactogen
      a. hormone produced by placenta; levels rise through 36 weeks of gestation, then stabilize
      b. low values indicate possible fetal distress, values low in threatened abortion, toxemia, intrauterine growth retardation, and postmaturity
   3. analysis of amniotic fluid (see Table 4-12)
      a. chromosomal studies to assess genetic disorders (e.g., Down syndrome, cell culture for karyotype)
      b. determination of sex chromatin in fetal cells to assess sex-linked disorders
      c. biochemical analysis of fetal-cell enzymes to assess inborn errors of metabolism
      d. determination of lecithin-to-sphingomyelin

Table 4-12   Laboratory studies of fetal well-being

Study	Purpose/Indication	Interpretation
Urinary/serum estriol	Assess placental functioning	Sudden drop = fetal hypoxia Continuous low levels = fetal compromise
Amniotic fluid analysis	Chromosomal studies	Detection of genetic disorders
	Determination of sex chromatin	Detection of sex-linked disorders
	Biochemical analysis of fetal-cell enzymes	Detection of inborn errors of metabolism
	Fetal lung maturity (lecithin/sphingomyelin ratios)	L/S ratio of 2:1 or greater = fetal lung maturity
	Alpha-fetoprotein (AFP) levels	High levels = neural-tube defects, anencephaly
	Creatinine levels	More than 2.0 mg = fetal age greater than 36 wk
	Identification and evaluation of Rh incompatibility	Increased bilirubin = evaluate for intrauterine transfusion and/or delivery
	Lipid cells (Nile blue stain)	20% of cells stained orange = fetal weight at least 2500 g
	Meconium presence	Fetal hypoxia (except with breech)

ratios (L/S ratios) to assess fetal lung maturity (most reliable)

- ◆ lecithin and sphingomyelin are important components of surfactant, a phosphoprotein that lowers surface tension in the fetal lungs and facilitates extrauterine expiration
- ◆ an L/S ratio of 2:1 or greater is generally associated with fetal lung maturity except for selected high-risk neonates (e.g., infants of diabetic mothers)

e. evaluation of phospholipids (PG) (Nile blue stain); useful if membranes have ruptured prematurely

f. determination of creatinine level: 2.0 mg or greater suggests fetal age greater than 36 weeks

g. identification and evaluation of isoimmune disease; usually done after 24 weeks to assess bilirubin levels and optical density

h. determination of alpha-fetoprotein (AFP) levels to assess neural-tube defects such as anencephaly and spina bifida; high levels also associated with congenital nephrosis, esophageal atresia, fetal demise

i. identification of meconium (often indicative of fetal hypoxia)

Application of the Nursing Process to the High-Risk Pregnant Client

Assessment
1. Risk factors (see p. 327)
2. Results of diagnostic tests

Analysis
1. Safe, effective care environment
   a. High risk for trauma
   b. High risk for infection
2. Physiological integrity
   a. Ineffective airway clearance/high risk for aspiration
   b. Actual/high risk for fluid volume deficit
3. Psychosocial integrity
   a. Anxiety
   b. Anticipatory grieving
4. Health promotion/maintenance
   a. Altered family processes
   b. Actual/high risk for altered parenting
   c. Knowledge deficit

Planning, Implementation, and Evaluation

Goal: The pregnant woman and partner will verbalize an understanding of symptoms (danger signals) of high-risk conditions to be reported immediately.

Implementation
1. Teach woman and partner to immediately report any of the following danger signals.
   a. Infection
   b. Vaginal bleeding
   c. Generalized edema
   d. Trauma
   e. Leaking amniotic fluid
   f. Elevated temperature
   g. Headache
   h. Visual changes (e.g., spotting before eyes)
   i. Abdominal, epigastric pain
   j. Projectile vomiting
   k. Decreased fetal activity
2. Reinforce the importance of keeping appointments as scheduled and of complying with therapeutic regimen.
3. Provide emotional support.

4. Assess client and fetal heart rate at each subsequent visit for potential or actual problems.

5. Document accurately.

Evaluation

The pregnant woman or partner reports danger signals immediately upon detection.

SELECTED HEALTH PROBLEMS IN THE ANTEPARTAL PERIOD

☐ Abortion
General Information

1. Definition: one of the bleeding disorders of pregnancy, it is termination of pregnancy before viability (fetus less than 20 weeks' gestation or less than 500 g) as a result of elective procedures or reproductive failure. Approximately 75% of all spontaneous abortions occur during the second and third month of gestation.

2. Types
   a. *Therapeutic* (or induced): pregnancy that has been purposely terminated
   b. *Spontaneous:* natural termination of pregnancy without therapeutic intervention
   c. *Threatened:* possible loss of the products of conception; slight bleeding, mild uterine cramping, cervical os closed, no passage of tissue
   d. *Inevitable:* threatened loss of the products of conception that cannot be prevented or stopped; moderate bleeding, cramping; open cervical os; no passage of tissue
   e. *Incomplete:* the expulsion of part of the products of conception and the retention of other parts in utero; heavy bleeding, severe cramping, open cervical os, passage of tissue
   f. *Complete:* the expulsion of all the products of conception, slight bleeding, mild cramping, closed cervical os, passage of tissue
   g. *Missed:* retention of the products of conception in utero after the fetus dies, slight bleeding, no cramping, closed cervical os, no passage of tissue
   h. *Habitual:* spontaneous abortion in three or more successive pregnancies

3. Predisposing factors (spontaneous abortion): often unknown (20%-25%), may be associated with
   a. Embryonic/fetal problems (50%-60%): disorganization of germ plasma, ovular defects, chromosomal aberration, faulty placental development
   b. Maternal problems (15%-20%): systemic infections, severe nutritional deprivation, abnormal pathological conditions of the reproductive tract, endocrine dysfunction, trauma, medical diseases

Nursing Process
Assessment

1. Identify symptoms (spontaneous vaginal bleeding, uterine cramping, contractions)

2. Evaluate blood loss: save pads; assess saturation, frequency of change

3. Recognize signs and symptoms of shock (see p. 128)

Analysis (see p. 331)
Planning, Implementation, and Evaluation

> **Goal:** Client will be free from complications.

Implementation

1. Note and record blood and tissue loss.

2. Institute nursing measures to treat shock if necessary (see "Shock," p. 128).

3. Monitor I&O.

4. Replace fluids as ordered.

5. Prepare for dilatation and curettage (D&C) as necessary (incomplete abortion).

6. Provide emotional support of grieving process (refer to *Loss and Death and Dying,* p. 26).

Evaluation

Client is free from excessive blood loss, fluid imbalance, and infection.

☐ Incompetent Cervical Os/Premature Dilatation of the Cervix
General Information

1. Definition: mechanical defect in the cervix, often a cause of habitual second trimester abortions or preterm labor (premature cervical dilatation)

2. Predisposing factors: anatomical deviation of the cervix, cervical trauma from D&C, conization, cauterization, or cervical lacerations with previous pregnancies

3. Medical treatment: physician determines preferred surgical intervention, suturing of cervix during 14-18 weeks of gestation, or before next pregnancy
   a. Permanent suture (Shirodkar procedure); subsequent delivery by cesarean section
   b. Temporary purse string (McDonald procedure); suture removed at term, with vaginal delivery

Nursing Process
Assessment

1. History of miscarriages or abortions

2. Relaxed cervical os on pelvic examination

Analysis (see p. 331)
Planning, Implementation, and Evaluation

> **Goal:** Client with an incompetent cervical os will report problems, seek treatment, and comply with restricted activity; will maintain gestation to term.

Implementation (postoperative)

1. Suggest limited activity for 2 or more weeks following this procedure.
2. Tell client to report signs of labor.
3. Monitor fetal growth to term and continue prenatal assessment and care as needed.
4. Observe for signs of labor, infection, and premature rupture of the membranes.

Evaluation

Client complies with activity restrictions after treatment; carries fetus to term.

☐ Ectopic Pregnancy
General Information

1. Definition: an *extrauterine* pregnancy, implantation occurring most often in ampulla of the fallopian tubes (see Fig. 4-4)
2. Incidence: 1 in 80 to 1 in 200 live births, seventh highest cause of maternal mortality (from rupture of tube leading to hemorrhage, infection, and shock)
3. Predisposing factors: any condition that causes constriction of the fallopian tube (e.g., pelvic inflammatory disease, puerperal and postabortion sepsis, developmental defects, prolonged use of an IUD)
4. Medical treatment: diagnosis, ultrasound, surgical intervention (laparoscopy, laparotomy with salpingectomy, salpingostomy)

Nursing Process
Assessment

1. Signs and symptoms
   a. Lower unilateral abdominal tenderness, cramps related to stretching of the tube
   b. Knifelike pain in lower quadrant (only when tube has ruptured)
   c. Profound shock, if ruptured
   d. Vaginal spotting (may be inconsistent with degrees of shock observed)
2. History: last menstrual period
3. Prior history of infection, IUD use

Analysis (see p. 331)

Planning, Implementation, and Evaluation

> **Goal:** Client will report early signs of ectopic pregnancy; will be free from complications following surgery; will return to a homeostatic state.

Implementation

1. Monitor vital signs; carry out an ongoing assessment for shock.
2. Maintain intravenous infusion for administration of plasma/blood, antibiotics, or other required medication.
3. Prepare client for surgery, physically and emotionally.
4. Postoperatively, continue to monitor vital signs, I&O; have client cough and deep-breathe q2h.
5. Support grieving process.

Evaluation

Client seeks treatment before rupture of tube, is free from other complications; regains postoperative homeostasis.

☐ Hydatidiform Mole
General Information

1. Definition: a developmental anomaly of the chorion causing degeneration of the villi and formation of grapelike vesicles; fertilized ovum is initially present but usually no embryo develops (see Fig. 4-5)
2. Incidence: 1 in 1500 pregnancies
3. Predisposing factors: unknown; however, it is associated with induction of ovulation by clomiphene therapy and adolescence or maternal age greater than 40 years
4. Medical treatment
   a. Surgical intervention (D&C or, in women over 45 or with profuse bleeding, hysterectomy)
   b. Medical intervention: monitor HCG levels; chemotherapy, if indicated
   c. Close supervision for 1 year

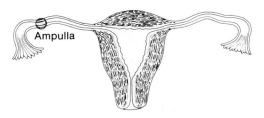

Fig. 4-4   Common site of ectopic pregnancy.

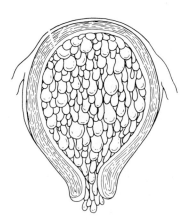

Fig. 4-5   Hydatidiform mole.

Nursing Process

Assessment

1. Signs and symptoms
   a. Initially appears as a normal pregnancy
   b. Uterus larger than expected for reported gestational age
   c. Lower uterine segment soft and full upon palpation
   d. Excessive nausea and vomiting (hyperemesis gravidarum)
   e. Brownish discharge or vaginal spotting; passing of vesicles; onset around 12 weeks of gestation
   f. Hypertension and other symptoms of preeclampsia (e.g., proteinuria)
2. Pregnancy test: HCG often very high

Analysis (see p. 331)

Planning, Implementation, and Evaluation

> **Goal:** Client will report abnormal signs, seek treatment; will comply with physician's plan for supervision for 1 year to detect signs of choriocarcinoma; will delay subsequent pregnancy.

Implementation

1. Administer plasma or blood replacement as ordered.
2. Maintain fluid and electrolyte balance through replacement.
3. Emphasize need for follow-up supervision for 1 year with HCG measurement, examination to detect choriocarcinoma, chemotherapy if indicated.
4. Emphasize that pregnancy should be avoided for at least 1 year.
5. Provide emotional support.

Evaluation

Client has hydatidiform mole removed; complies with regular schedule of visits following therapy; avoids pregnancy until cleared by physician.

☐ Placenta Previa
General Information

1. Definition: abnormal implantation of placenta in lower uterine segment
2. Incidence: 1 in 170 pregnancies; most common cause of bleeding in late pregnancy
3. Predisposing factors: decreased vascularity of upper uterine segment, multiparity, scarring from prior surgery
4. Degrees of placenta previa (see Fig. 4-6)
   a. *Partial:* placenta partially covers the internal cervical os
   b. *Complete:* placenta totally covers the cervical os (cesarean birth necessary)
   c. *Low-lying or marginal:* placenta encroaches on margin of internal cervical os
5. Placental abnormalities in formation or implantation: associated with maternal bleeding during the third trimester or intrapartum period; hemorrhage is the leading cause of maternal mortality
6. Medical intervention: diagnosis; blood and fluid replacement and cesarean birth if placental placement prevents vaginal birth of fetus

Nursing Process

Assessment

1. Signs and symptoms
   a. Painless, bright red, vaginal bleeding in the third trimester (often begins in seventh month); early episodes may have small amount of bleeding; several episodes of profuse bleeding may occur
   b. Soft uterus
   c. Manifestations of hemorrhage, shock
2. Diagnosis is confirmed by ultrasound

Analysis (see p. 331)

Planning, Implementation, and Evaluation

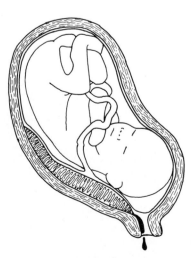

Marginal implantation

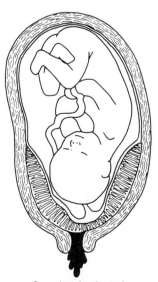

Complete implantation

Fig. 4-6 Placenta previa.

Goal: Client will report signs of bleeding from abnormal placental implantation; will maintain fluid balance, experience minimal blood loss; will understand need for cesarean birth for total placenta previa; will deliver healthy newborn.

Implementation

1. Maintain bed rest, avoid vaginal examinations, and observe carefully (conservative management).
2. Monitor blood loss closely.
3. Assess maternal vital signs and FHR frequently.
4. Institute appropriate nursing measures if shock develops (i.e., administer fluids, transfusions).
5. Give physical and emotional preparation for possible cesarean birth; physician may perform "double setup."
6. Observe for associated problems (e.g., prematurity of newborn, disseminated intravascular coagulation [DIC]).

Evaluation

Couple is adequately prepared for possible cesarean birth; client is free from frank hemorrhage and shock; delivers a healthy newborn at or near term.

☐ Abruptio Placentae

General Information

1. Definition: premature partial or complete separation of normally implanted placenta; also known as accidental hemorrhage or ablatio placentae
2. Incidence: 1 in 80 to 1 in 200 pregnancies
3. Predisposing factors: pregnancy-induced hypertension, fibrin defects; associated with older multigravidas
4. Types (see Fig. 4-7)
   a. *Marginal* (overt): evident external bleeding; placenta separates at margin
   b. *Central* (concealed): bleeding not evident or inconsistent with extent of shock observed; placenta separates at the center
5. Medical intervention: diagnosis; blood and fluids replacement; cesarean birth as necessary to save fetal or maternal lives

Nursing Process

Assessment

1. Bleeding: third trimester; amount of bleeding is not an accurate indicator of degree of separation
   a. Mild to moderate bleeding: uterine irritability
   b. Severe bleeding
      1. severe abdominal pain
      2. rigid, distended uterus
      3. enlarged uterus
      4. shock
      5. associated problems (e.g., renal failure, hypofibrinogenemia, DIC)
2. Diagnosis: ultrasound

Analysis (see p. 331)

Planning, Implementation, and Evaluation

Goal: Client will maintain homeostasis despite signs of placental separation; will maintain fluid balance, have blood loss replaced; couple will understand the need for emergency surgery or vaginal delivery as indicated; will deliver a viable, well-oxygenated newborn.

Implementation

1. Maintain bed rest.
2. Monitor FHR and maternal vital signs.
3. Assess blood loss and uterine pain.
4. Administer blood replacement as ordered by physician.

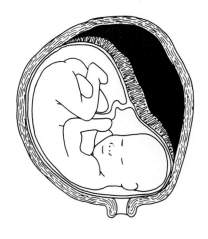

Concealed bleeding

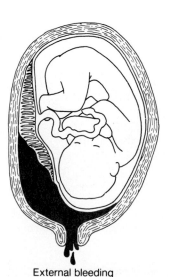

External bleeding

Fig. 4-7 Abruptio placentae.

5. Measure I&O.
6. Institute nursing measures for shock (e.g., flat in bed, monitor vital signs frequently, keep warm, increase IV fluids); see also "Shock," p. 128.
7. Provide emotional support; explain what is happening and all procedures; encourage expression of feelings.
8. Prepare physically and emotionally for emergency cesarean birth or prompt delivery.
9. Observe for associated problems after delivery (e.g., DIC, poorly contracted uterus, fetal neonatal hypoxia).

Evaluation

Couple is prepared for emergency birth; client delivers a viable newborn; has blood loss controlled; maintains fluid balance.

☐ Pregnancy-Induced Hypertension (Hypertensive Disorders)
General Information

1. Definition: a group of disorders characterized by presence of hypertension, with onset during last 10 weeks of pregnancy or in preceding pregnancy
2. Incidence: 6%-7% of all gravidas; one of three major causes of maternal mortality and a significant cause of fetal and neonatal deaths
3. Common types
   a. Pregnancy-induced hypertension (toxemia)
      1. preeclampsia
      2. eclampsia
   b. chronic essential hypertension
      1. antecedent to pregnancy
      2. with superimposed preeclampsia (coincidental with pregnancy)

4. Predisposing factors: age (less than 17 or more than 35 years), primiparity, low socioeconomic class, inadequate protein intake, diabetes, previous history of hypertension; absence of early or regular antepartal care is a factor in late detection and treatment
5. Etiology: unknown
   a. Vasospasm and ischemia believed to be underlying mechanism
   b. Impaired placental function may result from vasospasm
   c. Development of uteroplacental changes leading to decreased oxygen and nutrition to fetus
   d. May lead to degenerative changes in renal, endocrine, and hematological systems and the brain
6. HELLP syndrome (hemolysis, elevated liver enzymes, low platelet count)
   a. 2%-12% of women with untreated or uncontrolled preeclampsia will develop this syndrome
   b. Maternal mortality: 0%-24%
   c. Perinatal mortality: 8%-60%
7. Medical interventions: bed rest, increased protein in diet, possible salt reduction, medications to prevent convulsions and reduce blood pressure
8. The only cure for preeclampsia is delivery of all of the products of conception

Nursing Process
Assessment
1. Third trimester onset of hypertension, edema, rapid weight gain, and proteinuria
2. Classification (see Table 4-13)
Analysis (see p. 331)
Planning, Implementation, and Evaluation

Table 4-13 Classification of pregnancy-induced hypertension

MILD PREECLAMPSIA

Elevated BP	A systolic increase of 30 mm Hg and diastolic increase of 15 mm Hg or more above baseline × 2 at least 6 hours apart or a BP above 140/90
Weight gain	More than 1 lb/wk in the third trimester
Edema	Hands and in front of tibia (1+ or 2+)
Proteinuria	≥ 1 g/24 hr (1+ or 2+ on qualitative testing)
Hyperreflexia	3+

SEVERE PREECLAMPSIA

All changes associated with mild preeclampsia, plus

Elevated BP	Systolic ≥ 160 mm Hg or diastolic ≥ 110 mm Hg × 2 at least 6 hours apart with client restricted to bed rest
Weight gain	More than 5 lb/wk
Edema	Generalized edema, puffiness of face (3+ or 4+)
Proteinuria	≥ 5 g/24 hr (3+ or 4+ on qualitative testing)
Hyperreflexia	4+, clonus
Oliguria	≤ 400-500 ml
Other	Severe headaches, dizziness, blurred vision, retinal arteriolar spasm, spots before eyes, nausea and vomiting, epigastric pain, irritability, pulmonary edema, elevated liver enzymes, hemolysis

ECLAMPSIA

All changes associated with preeclampsia, plus tonic and clonic convulsions, coma, and hypertensive shock or crisis

Goal 1: Client will comply with schedule for care; will verbalize an understanding of a balanced diet and other care; will not develop marked BP changes; will report potential or actual problems immediately; will maintain a stable BP after delivery; will deliver a well-oxygenated newborn.

Implementation
1. Detect preeclampsia through early and regular antepartal care.
2. Prevent severe preeclampsia/eclampsia by promoting regular antepartal care and good nutrition (with adequate protein).
3. Monitor BP, weight, edema, urine, and reflexes (each antepartal visit).
4. Instruct to take daily weight at home.
5. Provide bed rest lying on left side if signs of pregnancy-induced or preexisting hypertension occur (at home for milder forms of preeclampsia; hospitalization for severe preeclampsia).
6. Provide specific dietary information; may include reduced sodium.
7. Monitor I&O, BP, weight, urine for protein, FHR for hospitalized client.
8. Monitor administration of magnesium sulfate (anticonvulsant and sedative) if ordered, see Table 4-14; assess for signs of toxicity.
    a. Symptoms of CNS depression (anxiety followed by drowsiness or lethargy)
    b. Respirations less than 12/min
    c. Reduced BP
    d. Deep-tendon reflexes absent or less than 1+
    e. Signs of paralysis
    f. Stop administration if there are signs of toxicity or if urinary output less than 30 ml/hr; antidote is calcium gluconate (10%) solution
9. Administer sedatives, antihypertensives, and anticonvulsants (e.g., phenobarbital, diazepam [Valium], hydralazine [Apresoline]) as ordered by physician to control symptoms and to prevent eclampsia and CVAs.
10. Monitor progress of labor.
11. Provide emotional support to couple.

Evaluation
Client complies with prenatal teaching; maintains pregnancy as long as possible without compromising self or fetus; is safely delivered of a healthy newborn; has blood pressure controlled before and after delivery.

Goal 2: Client will be free from physical injury in the event of seizure; will regain homeostasis; will maintain fetal oxygenation.

Implementation (if convulsion occurs)
1. Maintain patent airway.
2. Use suction to prevent aspiration.
3. Protect mother from injury.
4. Note nature, onset, and progression of seizure.
5. Monitor for signs of abruptio placentae.
6. Administer O_2.
7. Monitor FHR.
8. Administer medications as ordered.

Evaluation
Client recovers from convulsion(s) without physical injury; remains stable; FHR is within normal limits.

☐ Diabetes
General Information
1. Definition: an inherited metabolic disorder characterized by a deficiency in insulin production from the

Table 4-14 Magnesium sulfate

Action	Side effects	Nursing implications
Anticonvulsant that decreases amount of acetylcholine (IV or IM) liberated with nerve impulse, relaxes smooth muscle, depresses CNS, lowers BP Especially valuable in lowering seizure threshold in women with pregnancy-induced hypertension; may be used in preterm labor to decrease uterine activity (no FDA approval for this use at this time)	*Maternal:* severe CNS depression, hyporeflexia, flushing, confusion *Fetal:* tachycardia, hypoglycemia, hypocalcemia, hypomagnesemia	Monitor for seizures. Observe for signs of CNS depression. Monitor fetal heart rate. Monitor magnesium levels regularly. Have calcium gluconate available to counteract toxicity of magnesium sulfate. Discontinue infusion if respirations are below 12/min, reflexes are severely hypotonic, output is below 20-30 ml/hr, or in event of mental confusion or lethargy or fetal distress.

beta cells of the islets of Langerhans in the pancreas (see also p. 182)
2. Incidence: 1 in 100 pregnancies; the condition may be a concurrent disease in pregnancy or have its first onset during gestation
3. Predisposing factors
   a. Family history of diabetes
   b. Glucosuria
   c. Obesity
   d. History of repeated spontaneous abortions or fetal loss (stillbirth)
   e. History of delivery of infants over 10 lb
4. Classes (White's classification, currently used in high-risk OB management): according to age at onset and pathological changes
   a. Class A: diabetes that can often be controlled by diet; includes gestational diabetes (90% of all pregnant diabetics)
      1. onset or first recognition during pregnancy
      2. often indicated by family history
      3. insulin may be needed; severity of symptoms varies
   b. Class B: onset after age 20; duration 0-9 years; no vascular involvement
   c. Class C: onset at age 10-19; duration 10-19 years; no vascular involvement
   d. Class D: onset before age 10; duration 20 or more years; calcification present in legs; retinitis
   e. Class E: presence of calcified pelvic vessels
   f. Class F: presence of nephritis
5. Effects of diabetes: maternal risk and fetal loss increase as classes change from A to E
   a. Effects of maternal diabetes on the fetus/infant
      1. overall perinatal mortality increases when mother has diabetes
      2. as classes change from A to E, increased incidence of ketoacidosis for mother resulting in high risk for fetus
      3. greater risk (3-4 times) of congenital abnormalities that may result in neonatal death
      4. hypoxia and fetal death more common
      5. infants large for gestational age (classes A, B, C)
      6. neonatal hypoglycemia common as a result of fetal response to hyperglycemia of mother
   b. Effects of diabetes on the mother
      1. uteroplacental insufficiency often complicates pregnancy
      2. higher incidence of dystocia
      3. susceptibility to infections
6. Effects of pregnancy on diabetes
   a. Insulin resistance progressively increases in most pregnant diabetics
   b. Blood glucose less easily controlled
   c. Insulin shock common
7. Medical treatment

a. Diagnostic tests (with *criteria* for *high risk* as seen in gestational diabetes or insulin-dependent diabetes)
   1. screening of all pregnant women at 24-28 weeks' gestation for gestational diabetes
      a. 50 g oral glucose: >140 mg/dl at 1 hour
   2. 100 g glucose tolerance test (GTT): highly sensitive, used if screening is abnormal
      a. fasting blood glucose: >105 mg/dl
      b. 1 hour: >190 mg/dl
      c. 2 hours: >165 mg/dl
      d. 3 hours: >145 mg/dl
   3. 2-hour postprandial blood glucose
      a. >120 mg/dl
      b. used to randomly evaluate diet and compliance
   4. mean blood glucose test (HbA$_{1c}$ [glycosylated hemoglobin]): at risk over 8.8%; indicates recent hyperglycemia
   5. chem strip blood-glucose testing may be advised
   6. urine glucose monitoring inaccurate during pregnancy
   7. repeat GTT on gestational diabetics at 6 weeks postpartum to evaluate status
   b. Nutritional counseling with calories and sucrose ingestion altered
   c. Insulin therapy as indicated based on blood glucose; use of oral hypoglycemics is contraindicated
   d. Hospitalization to stabilize condition if necessary
   e. Monitoring of fetal/placental oxygenation with nonstress testing, CST, ultrasound, biophysical profile, L/S ratio, estriol levels
   f. Cesarean birth or induction at 36-37 weeks if evidence of fetal compromise; attempt made to maintain pregnancy until fetal lungs are mature

Nursing Process

Assessment
1. Signs and symptoms of hypoglycemia and hyperglycemia (refer to Table 3-36, p. 187)
2. Indications of hydramnios, preeclampsia, infection
3. History of large-for-gestational-age (LGA) newborns
4. Insulin requirements

Analysis (see p. 331)

Planning, Implementation, and Evaluation

> **Goal:** Client will follow prescribed diet/insulin; will detect problems and report them immediately; will carry gestation to near-term; will adequately oxygenate fetus.

Implementation
1. Stress importance of ongoing, regular, and more frequent antepartal care.
2. Assist in performing diagnostic tests.

3. Demonstrate accurate glucose-testing technique; have client return demonstration.
4. Educate client regarding nutritional needs: strict adherence to prescribed dietary regimen.
5. Teach to give own insulin (regular insulin preferred); observe for accuracy and correct as necessary.
6. Regulate insulin dose as prescribed by blood glucose levels, not by urine tests, because of lowered renal threshold; expect altered requirements in intrapartal and postpartal periods.
7. Recognize and share changes in diabetic state with client.
   a. As pregnancy develops, insulin need increases.
   b. Insulin need will decrease postpartum.
8. Promote good personal hygiene to prevent infection.
9. Monitor for early signs of infection.
10. Assure mother that she will be able to breastfeed her infant, if she wishes.
11. Initiate ophthalmological referral.

Evaluation

Client complies with diet and insulin regimen during pregnancy; prevents complications of diabetes during pregnancy and the puerperium; carries pregnancy as close to term as possible; delivers a newborn with minimal problems.

☐ Cardiac Disorders
General Information

1. Definition: includes a number of heart diseases/defects, which include both congenital and acquired conditions. Pregnant women with heart disease are seen more frequently today because of better care, screening, and surgical correction of defects. Refer also to "Congestive Heart Failure," p. 136
2. Effects of pregnancy on heart disease: alters heart rate, blood pressure, and volume of cardiac output
3. Incidence: 0.5%-2% of all pregnant women
4. Predisposing factors: syphilis, arteriosclerosis, renal and pulmonary disease, rheumatic fever, congenital defects of the heart, surgical repair of defects
5. Types: New York Heart Association's functional classification system for clients with heart disease (based on client history of past and present disability and uninfluenced by presence or absence of physical signs); used in current obstetrical management
   a. Class 1: no limitation of activity; no symptoms of cardiac insufficiency
   b. Class 2: slight limitation of activity; asymptomatic at rest; ordinary activities cause fatigue, palpitations, dyspnea, or angina
   c. Class 3: marked limitation of activities; comfortable at rest; less than ordinary activities cause discomfort
   d. Class 4: unable to perform any physical activity without discomfort; may have symptoms even at rest

6. Prognosis depends on
   a. Functional capacity of heart
   b. Complications that further increase cardiac load
   c. Quality of health care provided
   d. Maternal and fetal risk (increases from Classes 1 to 4; women in Classes 3 and 4 will have serious problems in pregnancy)
      1. maternal heart failure
      2. spontaneous abortion or premature labor, caused by maternal hypoxia
      3. maternal dysrhythmias
      4. intrauterine growth retardation
7. Medical treatment
   a. Confirm diagnosis
      1. difficult to differentiate heart disease because of normal cardiac changes that occur with pregnancy
         a. functional systolic murmurs common
         b. edema and some dyspnea frequently present in last trimester
         c. changes in position of heart suggest cardiac enlargement
      2. criteria for establishment of diagnosis of heart disease
         a. continuous diastolic or presystolic heart murmur
         b. a loud, harsh systolic murmur, especially if associated with a thrill
         c. unequivocal cardiac enlargement
         d. severe dysrhythmia
   b. Hospitalization: may be necessary 1-4 weeks before delivery
   c. Prophylactic antibiotic treatment to prevent subacute bacterial endocarditis
   d. Vaginal delivery (method of choice, using regional anesthesia and forceps)

Nursing Process
Assessment
1. Fetal heart rate; maternal vital signs
2. Compliance with prescribed therapeutic regimen
3. Cardiac and respiratory status both at rest and with activity

Analysis (see p. 331)
Planning, Implementation, and Evaluation

> **Goal:** Client will comply with treatment and will notify physician of problems; will be free from complications; will regain homeostasis after delivery; will maintain optimal fetal oxygenation.

Implementation
1. Encourage early and more frequent antepartal care; monitor vital signs, FHR, and weight.
2. Promote compliance with therapeutic regimen.
3. Teach proper nutrition with adequate iron intake to prevent anemia.

4. Stress need for additional rest.
   a. Classes 1 and 2: some limits on strenuous activity
   b. Classes 3 and 4: bed rest with expert medical supervision
   c. Semi-Fowler's position in bed if helpful for breathing; left lateral preferred
5. Prevent exposure to persons with upper respiratory tract infections; provide early treatment of URIs.
6. Observe the subtle changes in condition indicative of congestive heart failure (e.g., rales with cough, decreased ability to carry out household tasks, increased dyspnea on exertion, hemoptysis, tachycardia, progressive edema).
7. Administer medications as ordered by physician (e.g., diuretics, digitalis); explain actions, side effects to woman and significant other.
8. Maintain continuous maternal and fetal monitoring during the intrapartum period; advise client to avoid pushing; position in semi-Fowler's.
9. Postpartum, assess for signs of hemorrhage, puerperal infection, thromboembolism, and congestive heart failure; avoid giving ergonovine and other oxytocics.

Evaluation

Client complies with regimen of rest, exercise, and care; is free from complications of cardiac disease during pregnancy/puerperium; delivers a healthy newborn.

☐ Anemia
General Information

1. Definition: decrease in the oxygen-carrying capacity of the blood
2. Cause: often because of low iron stores and reduced dietary intake
3. Incidence: 20% of all pregnant women; 90% of anemias are caused by iron deficiency; it is the most frequently encountered complication of pregnancy
4. Predisposing factors: heredity and malnutrition
5. Prognosis: maternal and fetal mortality and morbidity rates are increased; specifically
   a. Anemia aggravates existing problems such as cardiac disease during pregnancy
   b. Anemic women have increased incidence of abortion, premature labor, infection, pregnancy-induced hypertension, and postpartum hemorrhage
   c. Maternal anemia is associated with intrauterine growth retardation
   d. Severe anemia may cause heart failure
6. Types of disorders
   a. Iron deficiency: most common
   b. Folic acid deficiency (megaloblastic anemia): less than 3% of all gravidas; caused by poor diet and malabsorption
   c. Hemoglobinopathies (e.g., sickle cell anemia [higher mortality in pregnancy; crises common; refer to *Nursing Care of the Child*, p. 488]), thalassemia

Nursing Process
Assessment

1. Signs and symptoms are usually absent in mild to moderate iron-deficiency anemia
2. Diagnosis based upon
   a. Hgb < 11 g/dl or HCT < 37%
   b. Hgb < 10.5 g/dl or HCT < 35% in second trimester
   c. Hgb < 10 g/dl or HCT < 33% in third trimester
3. Nutritional intake

Analysis (see p. 331)
Planning, Implementation, and Evaluation

> **Goal:** Client will maintain an optimal Hgb and HCT; will be free from severe anemia; will comply with diet, treatments, and medication; will maintain adequate fetal oxygenation.

Implementation

1. Monitor Hgb or HCT levels at initial antepartal visit and in later pregnancy.
2. Provide dietary counseling regarding importance of iron-rich diet (minimum of 18 mg/day).
3. Instruct to take oral iron compounds (ferrous sulfate or gluconate) as daily supplement as ordered; teach regarding side effects.
   a. Change in color of stools (become black)
   b. Take with a source of vitamin C to facilitate absorption
   c. Take with food only if gastric distress occurs (better absorbed between meals)
4. Provide folic acid supplement of 5 mg/24 hr orally for folate deficiency, as ordered.
5. Observe for symptoms of hemolytic crisis (e.g., chills, fever, pain in back and abdomen, prostration, shock) with hemoglobinopathies.
6. Refer for genetic counseling (women with inherited disorders).

Evaluation

Client eats a balanced, adequate, iron-rich diet during pregnancy; takes prescribed iron medications; maintains health; delivers newborn of appropriate size for gestational age.

☐ Hyperemesis Gravidarum (Pernicious Vomiting of Pregnancy)
General Information

1. Definition: excessive vomiting during pregnancy, leading to dehydration, starvation, and electrolyte imbalance
2. Cause: not always clear; may be psychological, or result from multiple pregnancy, hormonal abnormalities, or hydatidiform mole
3. Prognosis: severe cases may lead to dehydration and fluid-electrolyte complications

Nursing Process

Assessment (signs and symptoms are related to severity)
1. Mild: slight dehydration and weight loss
2. Severe: metabolic acidosis, hypoproteinemia, hypovitaminosis, jaundice, hemorrhage

Analysis (see p. 331)

Planning, Implementation, and Evaluation

> **Goal:** Client will retain food and fluids; will maintain hydration.

Implementation (hospitalization may be necessary)
1. Administer parenteral fluids.
2. Promote a quiet environment.
3. Provide frequent, small meals when oral feedings are tolerated.
4. Refer to psychological consultant if necessary.

Evaluation

Client is free from vomiting; maintains fluid and electrolyte balance; eats adequate diet; begins to gain weight.

☐ Infections
General Information

1. Definition: a variety of infectious agents can affect maternal and fetal health, leading to increased morbidity and mortality. Maternal disease that is mild or even asymptomatic can cause severe anomalies or death in the embryo/fetus/neonate.
2. Types of infectious diseases
   a. The TORCH syndrome (*T*oxoplasmosis, *O*ther, *R*ubella, *C*ytomegalovirus infection, *H*erpes)
      1. *toxoplasmosis* (protozoa)
         a. transmitted through ingestion of raw or undercooked meat; through improper hand washing after handling cat litter that has been contaminated with infected cat's feces
         b. maternal symptoms may be absent or nonspecific
         c. possible to detect by serological screening
         d. organism readily crosses placenta
         e. fetal effects include hydrocephaly, chorioretinitis, mental retardation, neurological damage
      2. *other*
         a. *beta-hemolytic streptococcal* infection: streptococci estimated to be present in genital tract of approximately 15% of women of childbearing age; associated with urinary tract infection; premature rupture of the membranes, premature labor, chorioamnionitis; may cross placenta and cause septic abortion, puerperal sepsis, stillbirth, neonatal sepsis, meningitis, sensory impairment, retardation

   b. *syphilis:* prenatal serological screening test is important for prevention of congenital syphilis; associated with late abortion, stillbirth, prematurity, severe anemia, and congenital syphilis
   c. *gonorrhea:* may cause postpartum infection, pelvic inflammatory disease, sterility; danger to newborn is ophthalmia neonatorum, sepsis, pneumonia; refer to "Sexually Transmitted Diseases," p. 449
   d. *acquired immunodeficiency syndrome* (AIDS): viral infection with severe depression of immune system; perinatal transmission from infected mother to fetus; high mortality rate; precautions as for hepatitis B (see also "Newborn Care," p. 394)
   e. *nongonococcal urethritis* (NGU)
      ◆ mild; may be asymptomatic
      ◆ increasingly common STD
      ◆ organism: chlamydia
      ◆ partner should be treated; erythromycin often used for pregnant client
      ◆ may cause stillbirth, pneumonia, conjunctivitis in newborn
3. *rubella:* extremely teratogenic in first trimester
   a. transmitted transplacentally
   b. congenital rubella syndrome in the neonate includes cataracts, hemolytic anemia, heart defects, mental retardation, deafness (first-trimester exposure)
   c. exposure after the first trimester can lead to intrauterine growth retardation, sepsis
   d. infected infant can shed live viruses for many months after birth
   e. women with low titers should receive vaccine in early postpartum period and avoid pregnancy for at least 2 months
4. *cytomegalovirus* (CMV); also called cytomegalic inclusion disease (CMID): member of herpesvirus group
   a. adult usually asymptomatic or has mononucleosis-like symptoms; very common
   b. transmission in adults is respiratory, possibly venereal
   c. transmission to fetus is transplacental; occasionally may be transmitted during passage through birth canal
   d. no effective treatment
   e. effects on neonate include mental retardation, intrauterine growth retardation, congenital heart defects, deafness, microcephaly
5. *herpes simplex virus* (HSV II)
   a. sexually transmitted, painful vesicles present on cervix, vaginal wall, vulva, and

thighs; last 10 days to 2 weeks; remissions, exacerbations
   b. usual mode of transmission to neonate is passage through birth canal; may occur transplacentally in rare cases
   c. infection results in high infant mortality, preterm births
   d. cesarean birth, if pregnant woman has active herpesvirus, type 2
 b. Tuberculosis
   1. rarely transmitted to fetus
   2. may be asymptomatic
   3. disease must be arrested by usual methods of care for client with TB
   4. infant usually kept from close contact with mother, if the disease is active, to protect from infection
 c. Urinary tract infections
   1. affect approximately 10% of gravidas, generally as a result of *E. coli;* may be asymptomatic
   2. predisposing factors: urinary stasis, related to anatomical changes during pregnancy; poor hygiene
   3. increased incidence of pyelonephritis if bacteria present
   4. associated with increased incidence of premature labor
   5. treated with appropriate antibiotic after culture
 d. Condylomas (genital warts)
   1. viral transmission
   2. may be transmitted to fetus at birth
   3. should be treated with laster beam, antibiotics, cautery, cryosurgery
   4. biopsy indicated for large warts (potential malignancy)
 e. Candidal infections
   1. caused by fungus *Candida albicans*
   2. present in about 20% of pregnant women
   3. fetus may contract thrush if infection not cured before delivery
 f. *Trichomonas vaginalis*
   1. protozoan
   2. treated with metronidazole (Flagyl), which may possibly be teratogenic and should not be used during first half of pregnancy
 g. Hepatitis
   1. may cause abortion, preterm birth, fetal or newborn hepatitis
   2. precautions depending on type A or B; refer to "Hepatitis," p. 169

Nursing Process
Assessment
1. Routine smears, cultures, serological studies for sexually transmitted disease; selected laboratory tests as indicated

2. Signs and symptoms of infectious diseases
Analysis (see p. 331)
Planning, Implementation, and Evaluation

> **Goal:** Client will be free from infection in pregnancy; will seek medical care and will comply with treatment if exposed to infection; when indicated, partner will comply with treatment; fetal effects will be minimized.

Implementation
1. Review precautions in order to minimize exposure to infection.
2. Teach client to report any symptoms (e.g., vesicles, discharge, rash, elevated temperature).
3. Administer drugs as ordered for sexually transmitted diseases (e.g., penicillin for syphilis).
4. Promote compliance of partner.
5. Instruct to take drugs as ordered (e.g., isoniazid [INH], streptomycin, PAS); explain expected actions, side effects; avoid self-medication.
Evaluation
Client is free from infectious disease; maternal or fetal risks are minimized; client and partner comply with therapeutic regimen.

☐ Multiple Gestation
General Information
1. Definition: gestation of two or more fetuses. Twins may be produced from a single ovum (monozygotic or identical twins) or from separate ova (dizygotic or fraternal). Fraternal twinning is an inherited autosomal recessive trait and is more common (70%) than identical twins (30%). Triplets result from one, two, or three separate ova.
2. Incidence: 2%-3% of all viable births
3. Predisposing factors
   a. Black women have higher incidence of multiple pregnancies than white women
   b. Family history of dizygotic twins
4. Prognosis
   a. Increased risk of premature labor, pregnancy-induced hypertension (25%), hemorrhage, placenta previa
   b. Increased risk of delivery of low-birth-weight infants, often premature (50%)
   c. Increased risk of maternal anemia (40%-50%)
   d. Increased risk of uterine inertia (10%), hydramnios (5%-10%), intrauterine asphyxia (5%)
   e. Increased risk of secondary cessation or weakening of effective uterine contractions
   f. Monozygotic twins have higher mortality and morbidity rates than dizygotic twins because of increased congenital anomalies, twin-to-twin transfusion syndrome, and intrauterine growth retardation

Nursing Process

Assessment

1. Early identification of multiple pregnancy based upon
   a. History
   b. Weight gain
   c. Abdominal palpation
   d. Fundal height greater than expected for dates
   e. Asynchronous fetal heartbeats
   f. Ultrasonography
2. Maternal and fetal status: prenatal visits every 2 weeks
3. Nutritional status

Analysis (see p. 331)

Planning, Implementation, and Evaluation

> **Goal:** Client with a multiple pregnancy will report early signs of health problems; will comply with health regimen and keep regular antepartal appointments; will deliver as close to term as possible.

Implementation

1. Advise frequent rest periods; left lateral position provides oxygenation for fetal/placental unit.
2. Teach balanced diet, with adequate protein; iron and vitamin supplements as ordered.
3. Monitor FHR carefully for indication of fetal distress.
4. Prepare for vaginal delivery unless complications arise (e.g., fetal distress, cephalopelvic disproportion).
5. Administer oxytocic agent as ordered immediately following birth to prevent postpartum hemorrhage (very important because of overdistension of the uterus).

Evaluation

Client is free from complications (e.g., anemia); carries multiple pregnancy to term (or close to term), with delivery of healthy newborns.

☐ Adolescent Pregnancy
General Information

1. Definition: pregnancy in a female under 17 years of age (see also "The Healthy Child," p. 435)
2. Incidence: worldwide, one-third of all births are to girls under 17 years of age; one million teenage pregnancies each year (10% of all teenagers) (World Health Organization 1987)
3. Predisposing factors: teenage pregnancies are associated with
   a. Earlier onset of menarche
   b. Changing sexual behavior
   c. Poor family relationships
   d. Poverty

4. Prognosis
   a. For pregnant girls under 15 years, a high risk of stillbirths, low-birth-weight infants, neonatal mortality, and cephalopelvic disproportion
   b. Increased maternal risk of pregnancy-induced hypertension, prolonged labor, iron-deficiency anemia, and urinary tract infections

Nursing Process

Assessment

1. Nutrition status
2. Knowledge of physiology of pregnancy
3. Emotional status
4. Support systems

Analysis (see p. 331)

Planning, Implementation, and Evaluation

> **Goal:** The pregnant teen will maintain good health; will eat a balanced diet with adequate protein; will prepare for birth and care of newborn; will achieve developmental tasks of adolescence and pregnancy; fetus will develop appropriately for gestation.

Implementation

1. Help pregnant teen achieve developmental tasks of adolescence (in addition to those of pregnancy).
   a. Develop sense of identity.
   b. Accept changing body image.
   c. Develop close, mature relations with peers (male and female).
   d. Socialize into appropriate gender role.
   e. Establish an independent and satisfying lifestyle.
2. Provide dietary counseling regarding
   a. Importance of well-balanced meals.
   b. Selection of nutritionally valuable yet acceptable food.
   c. Increased protein, calcium, and iron intake.
3. Prepare for childbirth; arrange for coaching assistance.
4. Refer to social service for
   a. Career and educational counseling.
   b. Options regarding child care/adoption.
   c. Support services in community (i.e., parenting classes, supplemental food programs).
5. Instruct in child care.
6. Teach family planning.

Evaluation

Client is free from preventable complications; has a positive birth experience; delivers a healthy newborn; cares safely for newborn or arranges for alternate placement; achieves appropriate developmental tasks.

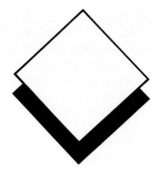

Intrapartal Care

GENERAL CONCEPTS
Normal Childbearing

1. Definitions
   a. Labor: a series of processes by which the products of conception are expelled from the maternal body
   b. Delivery: the actual event of birth
2. Essential factors in labor: the four *P*'s
   a. *Powers:* uterine contractions, voluntary bearing down, abdominal muscle contractions, and contractions of levator ani muscle
   b. *Passageway:* bones, tissues, ligaments
      1. type of pelvis: gynecoid, android, anthropoid, and platypelloid; refer to "The Structure of the Female Pelvis," p. 310
      2. adequacy of planes of true pelvis
         a. true pelvis forms the birth canal through which fetus must pass
         b. three distinct levels
            ◆ plane of inlet
            ◆ midplane (plane of least dimensions)
            ◆ plane of outlet
      3. condition of soft tissues (lower uterine segment, cervix, and vaginal canal)
   c. *Passenger:* the fetus
      1. attitude (habitus or posture): the relation of the fetal parts to its own trunk; normal attitude of the fetus in utero is complete flexion
      2. engagement: the entrance of the greatest diameter of the presenting part through the plane of inlet and the beginning of the descent through the pelvic canal (biparietal diameter of head is fixed in pelvis)
      3. lie: the relation of the long axis of the fetus to the long axis of the mother; it is either transverse, longitudinal, or oblique
         a. transverse lie: long axis of fetus is at right angle to mother's long axis; it is a pathological lie if present at term
         b. longitudinal lie: long axis of the fetus is parallel to mother's long axis; it has two alternatives

   ◆ cephalic presentation (head first)
   ◆ breech presentation (buttocks first)
   4. presentation and presenting part: that part of the fetal body that enters the true pelvis and presents itself at the internal cervical os for delivery; the presentation is dependent upon the attitude of the fetal extremities to its body and the fetal lie
      a. in cephalic presentations (95% of term deliveries), the fetal head is the presenting part: the head may be
         ◆ completely flexed upon the fetal chest (vertex presentation)
         ◆ moderately flexed (sinciput presentation)
         ◆ partially extended (brow presentation)
         ◆ hyperextended with chin presenting (face presentation)
      b. in breech presentations (3% of term births)
         ◆ the fetus' knees and hips both may be flexed, positioning the thighs on the abdomen and calves on the posterior thighs (complete breech)
         ◆ the hips may be flexed and the knees extended (frank breech)
         ◆ extension of the knees and hips (footling breech)
         ◆ shoulder presentation is commonly known as a transverse lie
   5. position: the relationship of a specific established point (i.e., occiput, sacrum, shoulder, chin, brow, mentum, or face) of the fetus to one of the quadrants of the mother's pelvis (see Fig. 4-8)
      a. breech presentation: sacrum (S)
      b. cephalic presentation: occiput (O)
      c. shoulder presentation: scapula (Sc)
      d. six different positions are thus possible for each of the above by relating the established point to the right or left side of the mother's pelvis and to the anterior or posterior aspect

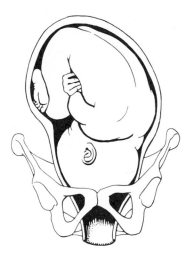
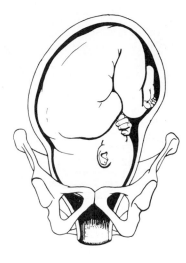
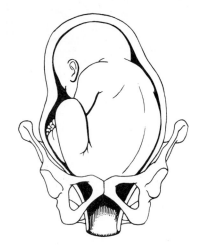

Left occipital anterior   Right occipital anterior   Left sacral anterior

Fig. 4-8   Selected categories of presentation. (From *Clinical education aids.* Columbus, Ohio: Ross Laboratories.)

6. station: the relationship of the presenting part of the fetus to the ischial spines of the mother (i.e., the degree of engagement); measured in centimeters above or below the pelvic midplane from the presenting part to the ischial spines (see Fig. 4-9)

d. *Person:* pregnant woman's general behavior and influences upon her (psyche)
   1. maternal response to uterine contractions
   2. cultural influences and perceptions about labor and delivery
   3. antepartal and/or childbirth education
   4. ability to communicate feelings to significant other(s) and staff
   5. support system

3. Signs of labor
   a. Premonitory signs of labor: changes indicating that labor will be approaching shortly
      1. increased Braxton Hicks contractions: intermittent contractions of the uterus occurring throughout pregnancy; generally painless but may cause discomfort in late pregnancy
      2. lightening or engagement: the descent of the fetus into the pelvic cavity; generally occurs 2-3 weeks before the onset of labor in primigravidas; causes increased bladder pressure and reduced diaphragm pressure
      3. show: blood-tinged mucus discharged from cervix shortly before or during labor
      4. sudden burst of energy
      5. weight loss resulting from fluid loss and electrolyte shifts
      6. increased backache and sacroiliac pressure due to fetal pressure

7. spontaneous rupture of membranes may occur; woman will be advised to enter hospital immediately
   b. True vs. false labor
      1. true labor
         a. contractions increase progressively in strength, duration, and frequency
         b. regular pattern, not relieved by walking (walking may increase the strength of the contractions)
         c. felt in back or radiating toward front
         d. *effacement and dilatation of the cervix*
         e. fetal membranes
            ◆ intact: generally in early labor, indicated by negative nitrazine paper test (yellow to yellow-olive paper) or negative ferning
            ◆ ruptured: generally in active labor, indicated by positive nitrazine paper test (blue-green to blue paper or positive ferning); false readings may be obtained if contaminated by blood; meconium staining may indicate fetal distress, except in breech presentation
      2. false labor
         a. an exaggeration of the periodic uterine contractions normally occurring during pregnancy
         b. does not produce progressive dilatation, effacement, or descent
         c. contractions are irregular and do not increase in frequency, duration, or intensity
         d. walking has no effect on contractions
         e. discomfort felt in lower abdomen and groin

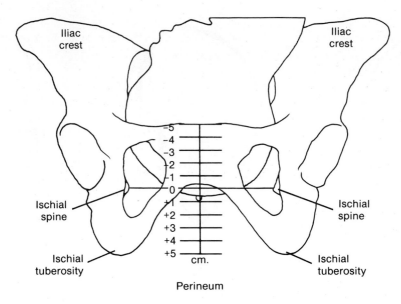

Fig. 4-9 Station. (From *Clinical education aids.* Columbus, Ohio: Ross Laboratories.)

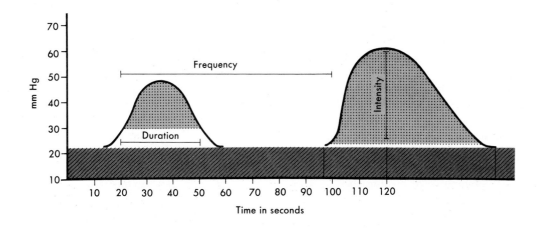

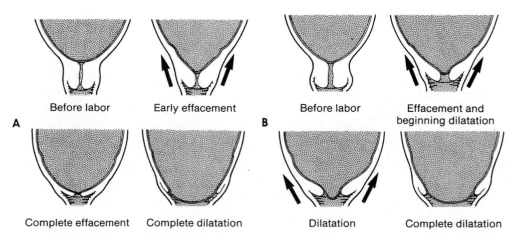

Fig. 4-10 Cervical dilatation and effacement. **A,** Primigravida; **B,** multigravida. (From *Clinical education aids.* Columbus, Ohio: Ross Laboratories.)

f. absence of bloody show
4. Labor onset theories
   a. Oxytocin stimulation: alone or in combination with other factors
   b. Progesterone withdrawal: allowing uterine contractions to progress
   c. Estrogen stimulation: causing hypertrophy of myometrium and increased production of contractile proteins
   d. Prostaglandin secretion: effect on uterine muscle (increased uterine irritability)
   e. Fetal endocrine secretion of cortical steroids
   f. Distension of uterus: with subsequent pressure on nerve endings stimulating contractions and increased irritability of uterine musculature
5. Physiological alterations occurring during labor (see Fig. 4-10)
   a. Dilatation to 10 cm: the process by which the cervix opens
   b. Effacement: thinning, shortening, and obliteration of cervix
   c. Physiological retraction ring: the separation of the upper (active, thicker) and lower (passive, thinner) uterine segments in labor
6. Fetal positional response to labor (mechanisms of labor)
   a. Engagement: descent of fetus into true pelvis
   b. Descent: the passage of the presenting part through the pelvis
   c. Flexion: further flexion of the fetal head when it meets resistance from the pelvic floor
   d. Internal rotation: the process by which the long axis of the fetal skull changes from the transverse diameter to an anteroposterior diameter at the outlet
   e. Extension of the head as it leaves the outlet
   f. External rotation of the head (restitution): in order to rotate the shoulders and leave the outlet
   g. Expulsion of the total baby
7. Fetal heart rate (FHR) during labor
   a. Baseline fetal heart rate: fetal heart rate when there are no contractions or in between contractions; normally between 120-160/min; see Fig. 4-11 and Table 4-15
   b. Baseline variability: normal irregularities of FHR caused by autonomic nervous system stimuli; may be altered in normal fetal sleep, prematurity, medications (NOTE: true beat-to-beat variability can be determined only by direct fetal or internal monitoring); see Fig. 4-11

Table 4-15   Baseline fetal heart rate (normal range: 102-160 beats/min)

	Tachycardia	Bradycardia
Mild	161-180 beats/min	100-119 beats/min
Marked	Greater than 180 beats/min	Less than 100 beats/min
Causes	Maternal fever	Maternal hypotension
	Early fetal hypoxia	Late fetal hypoxia
	Drugs	Drugs
	Amnionitis	

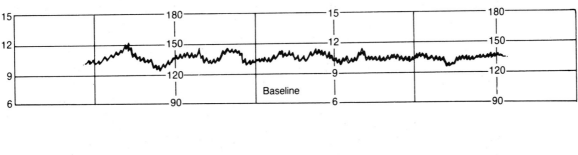
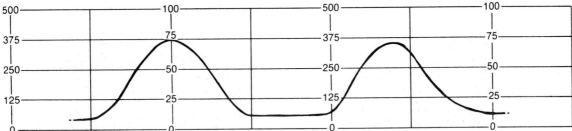

Fig. 4-11   Tracing of normal fetal heart rate.

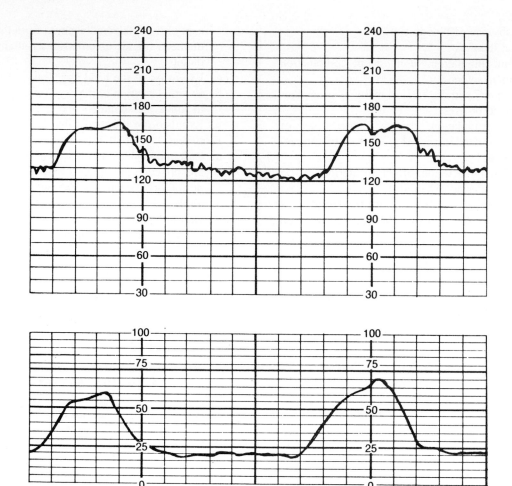

Fig. 4-12 Acceleration of fetal heart rate in response to uterine activity.

Table 4-16   Decelerations in fetal heart rate (see Fig. 4-13)

TYPE 1 (EARLY DECELERATIONS)

Cause: fetal head compression
FHR decreases with onset of contraction and mirrors the pattern of contractions
FHR returns to baseline as the contraction ends
Range of drop in FHR within normal parameters
Has a uniform shape
Innocuous
Nursing implications: continue observation

TYPE 2 (LATE DECELERATIONS)

Cause: uteroplacental insufficiency causing fetal hypoxia
FHR decreases *after* the onset of contraction
FHR deceleration persists beyond completion of contraction
Range of drop in FHR within normal

Has a uniform shape
Ominous
Nursing implications: turn client to left side, give O_2, and summon physician

TYPE 3 (VARIABLE DECELERATIONS)

Cause: umbilical cord compression
FHR decreases at any point *during* or *between* contractions
Decelerations may be jagged V or U shape
Range of drop in FHR is large and extends below normal
Not uniform in shape
Ominous
Nursing implications: turn client to left side, give O_2 and summon physician

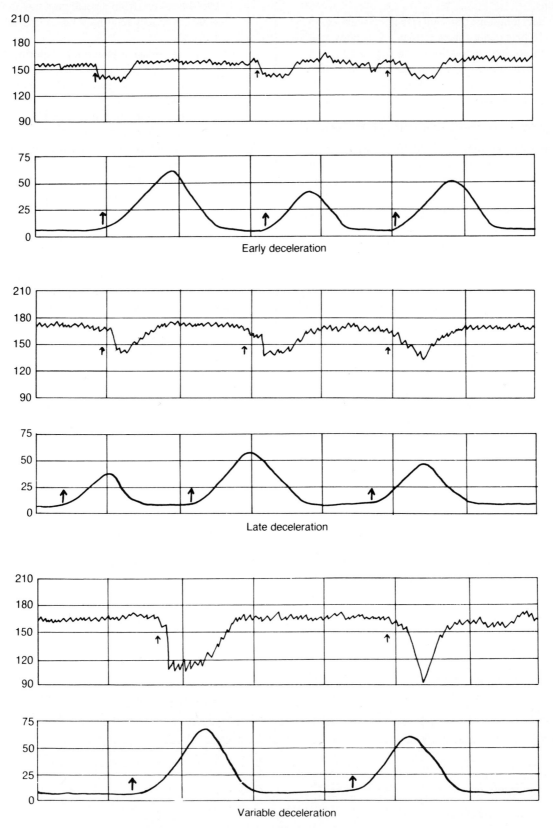

Fig. 4-13 Types of deceleration in fetal heart rate.

c. Periodic changes: FHR changes during contractions
1. accelerations: transient rise in FHR greater than 15 beats/min for more than 15 seconds related to uterine contractions; see Fig. 4-12
2. decelerations: transient decrease in FHR related to uterine contractions; see classifications in Table 4-16

Ongoing Management and Nursing Care

1. Fetal monitoring: monitor FHR by either
   a. Periodic auscultation: count for 1 full minute during and immediately after uterine contractions
   b. Electronic fetal monitor
      1. external or indirect electronic monitoring: applied when membranes intact
         a. *tokodynamometer:* disk attached over fundus and secured with belt; provides continuous record of external pressure created by contractions, allows measurement of frequency and duration of contractions
         b. *ultrasonic transducer:* applied at site of loudest fetal heartbeat, secured with belt (conducting gel is spread over transducer); provides continuous FHR recording, which is interpreted in relation to uterine activity; phonocardiography also may be used for indirect fetal electrocardiography
      2. internal or direct monitoring: applied when membranes have ruptured and cervix has dilated 2-3 cm
         a. *pressure transducer:* an intrauterine catheter filled with water is inserted beyond presenting part; allows measurement of frequency, duration, and intensity of contractions
         b. *internal spiral electrode:* applied to fetal scalp; provides continuous measurement of FHR, baseline variability, and periodic changes

   c. Fetal blood sampling: a small volume of fetal blood is taken (from a small puncture into the fetal scalp) to assess fetal hypoxia during labor
      1. procedure
         a. an invasive technique requiring rupture of the fetal membranes and cervical dilatation (3-4 cm); performed when fetus is in jeopardy
         b. pregnant woman generally placed in a lithotomy position
         c. an amnioscope (truncated plastic or metal cone) is employed for visualization of presenting part of fetus during the procedure
         d. electronic fetal monitoring is desirable during the procedure
         e. after procedure, observe for vaginal bleeding (of fetal origin) and fetal tachycardia
      2. laboratory analysis of fetal pH, Po_2, and Pco_2 is done from blood sample (normal pH: 7.25-7.35; pH of 7.20 is associated with hypoxia)
2. Uterine contractions: refer to Table 4-17 and Fig. 4-14; monitor
   a. Frequency: timed from beginning of one to beginning of next contraction
   b. Duration: timed from beginning to end of one contraction
   c. Intensity: degree of muscle contraction; may be mild, moderate, or strong (50-100 mm Hg)
   d. Tonus: pressure within the uterus in between contractions; only measurable with an intrauterine catheter (10-12 mm Hg)
3. Analgesics: drugs that relieve pain or alter its perception may alter level of consciousness and reflex activity; administer as ordered and monitor effects; common obstetrical analgesics include
   a. Sedatives
      1. produce sedation; may depress fetus
      2. examples: secobarbital sodium (Seconal) and pentobarbital sodium (Nembutal) may be given in early labor

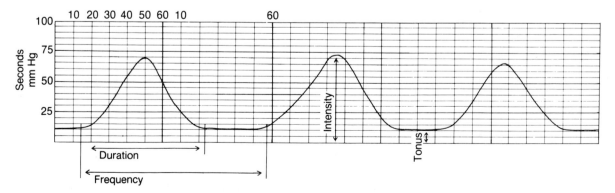

Fig. 4-14 Assessment of uterine contractions.

   b. Narcotics (e.g., meperidine [Demerol])
   1. may initially slow labor, have depressive effect on neonatal respirations
   2. administered when client is in active labor (4-5 cm); avoid use in transition
   c. Tranquilizers
   1. produce sedation and relaxation; often given with narcotics because of potentiating effects; when given alone, there may be little or no analgesia; may cause excitement and disorientation in presence of pain

   2. examples: promethazine hydrochloride (Phenergan), hydroxyzine pamoate (Vistaril), promazine hydrochloride (Sparine) and diazepam (Valium)
   3. effects
      a. peak action within 60 minutes
      b. may last 6-8 hours depending on stage of labor and activity of client
   d. Amnesics (rarely used today)
   1. produce sedation and alter memory
   2. example: scopolamine (belladonna alkaloid)

Table 4-17 Stages and phases of labor

First stage (onset of regular contractions to complete dilatation)

	LATENT: PHASE I	ACTIVE: PHASE II	TRANSITION: PHASE III
Time			
Primipara	8½ hours	4 hours	1 hour
Multipara	5½ hours	2 hours	10-15 minutes
Cervix			
Effacement	0-50%	Completed	
Dilatation	0-3 cm	4-7 cm	8-10 cm
Contractions			
Frequency	More than 10 minutes apart	3-5 minutes	2-3 minutes
Duration	30 seconds	45 seconds	60-90 seconds
Intensity	Mild: less than 50 mm Hg	Moderate: 50-75 mm Hg	Hard: 75-100 mm Hg
Manifestations	Abdominal cramps; backache; client generally excited, alert, talkative, and in control; may rupture membranes	Show; moderate increase in pain; client more apprehensive; fear of losing control; focusing on self; skin warm and flushed	Client may be irritable and panicky; may lose control; amnesic between contractions; perspiring, nausea and vomiting common; trembling of legs; pressure on bladder and rectum; backache; increased show; circumoral pallor

Second stage (complete dilatation of birth to newborn)

Time	
Primipara	30-50 minutes
Multipara	20 minutes
Contractions	
Frequency	2-3 minutes
Duration	60-90 minutes
Intensity	Very hard; 100 mm Hg
Manifestation	Decrease in pain from transitional level; increased bloody show; pressure on rectum; urge to bear down; bulging perineum; client excited, eager, and in control

Third stage (delivery of newborn to delivery of placenta)

Time	5-30 minutes
Contractions	Strong uterus changing to globular shape
Manifestation	Gush of blood; apparent lengthening of cord; client focuses on newborn; excited about birth; feeling of relief

Fourth stage (delivery of placenta to homeostasis)

Time	Usually defined as first hour postpartum
Uterus	Firm, at midline, 2 finger breaths above umbilicus
Manifestation	Lochia rubra; exploration of newborn; parent-infant bonding begins; newborn alert and responsive; first period of reactivity

3. may cause dysrhythmias and fetal tachycardia
4. **Anesthetics:** produce a local, regionalized, or generalized loss of sensation
   a. Local infiltration
      1. examples: lidocaine hydrochloride (Xylocaine), chloroprocaine (Nesacaine)
      2. used for pain relief during second stage of labor: episiotomy and perineal repair
      3. temporarily interrupts nerve impulses and pain in the perineum
      4. any agent may cause an allergic response
   b. Regional blocks
      1. paracervical block
         a. agent: a dilute, local anesthetic solution
         b. used during first stage, active phase of labor to produce rapid relief of contraction pain; no perineal effect
         c. blocks nerves to lower uterine segment, cervix, and upper vagina for about 1 hour
         d. may cause fetal intoxication: bradycardia or CNS depression and apnea at delivery
      2. pudendal block
         a. agent: a dilute, local anesthetic solution
         b. used during second stage of labor to relieve vaginal and perineal pain
         c. blocks nerves at the cervix for about 30 minutes
         d. safe for newborn; does not affect contractions, but diminishes bearing-down reflex
      3. peridural block
         a. agent: a suitable local anesthetic or morphine
         b. used during first stage, active phase, and during second stage of labor to relieve uterine and perineal pain; used to prevent pain during and after cesarean birth
         c. may be single injection or repeated doses (continuous) through an indwelling catheter
         d. types
            ◆ epidural
               • site: between lumbar vertebrae into epidural space; does *not* pierce dura mater of spinal cord
               • possible untoward effects: maternal hypotension, depression of contractions, fetal distress, diminished bearing-down reflex
            ◆ caudal
               • site: through the sacral hiatus and the sacral canal into the lowest part of the peridural space
               • possible untoward effects: same as for epidural
      4. intradural block
         a. agent: local anesthetic mixed with dextrose solution

b. used during second stage of labor or for abdominal surgery to produce instant loss of sensation and muscle relaxation; loss of bearing-down reflex
c. injected between lumbar vertebrae, *through* dura mater of spinal cord, *between contractions,* and mixes with cerebrospinal fluid; duration of 1-3 hours
d. possible untoward effects: maternal hypotension, respiratory inadequacy from high level, spinal headache from leakage of cerebrospinal fluid at puncture site; mother remains flat for 8-12 hours after dose to prevent leakage (limited value)
e. types
   ◆ spinal block: into third, fourth, or fifth lumbar interspace
   ◆ saddle block or low spinal block: dermal anesthetic level at or below umbilicus; anesthetizes low back, pudendum, symphysis pubis, and pelvic viscera
   c. General—inhalation
      1. examples: thiopental sodium (Pentothal), halothane (Fluothane) inhalation, combination (thiopental, nitrous oxide and oxygen, succinylcholine)
      2. rarely used for uncomplicated vaginal births; can be used to relax the uterus for intrauterine manipulation or version or for cesarean birth
      3. produces sleep and general loss of sensitivity to touch, pain, and stimulation
      4. possible untoward effects: aspiration, respiratory depression, newborn depression

Application of the Nursing Process to Normal Childbearing, Intrapartal Care

Assessment
1. Premonitory signs of labor
2. Labor status: true labor; stage and phase of labor (refer to Table 4-17)
3. Uterine contractions
4. Due date
5. Membranes intact or ruptured
6. Fetal response to labor
7. Psychological factors: preparation for childbirth; support systems; culture and religious beliefs
8. Newborn adaptation at birth
9. Maternal homeostasis after delivery

Analysis
1. Safe, effective care environment
   a. High risk for injury
   b. High risk for infection
   c. Knowledge deficit
2. Physiological integrity
   a. Pain
   b. Fatigue

c. Impaired skin integrity
3. Psychosocial integrity
   a. Anxiety
   b. Ineffective individual coping
   c. Powerlessness
4. Health promotion/maintenance
   a. Impaired adjustment
   b. Self-care deficit: bathing/hygiene

Planning, Implementation, and Evaluation

> **Goal 1:** The client will experience minimal anxiety on admission to the labor and delivery unit; will be knowledgeable about the birth process and procedures performed.

Implementation

1. Orient client to physical setting and review basic procedures to be performed.
2. Determine onset, duration, and frequency of contractions.
3. Determine client's knowledge of the labor and delivery process, childbirth preparation.
4. Obtain baseline vital signs and BP.
5. Perform Leopold's maneuver (see Fig. 4-15): have client empty bladder and flex knees for abdominal relaxation; warm hands, then:
   a. Proceed with fundus palpation: note breech or cephalic presentation.
   b. Proceed with lateral palpation: note back and small parts of fetus.

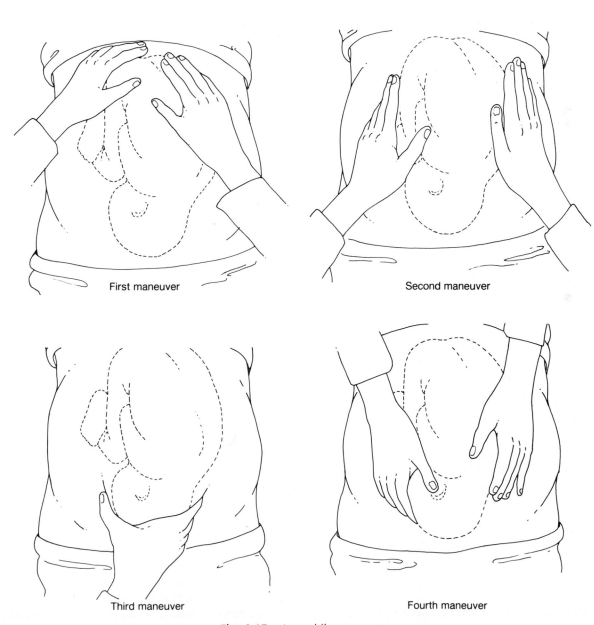

First maneuver

Second maneuver

Third maneuver

Fourth maneuver

Fig. 4-15 Leopold's maneuvers.

c. Just above symphysis pubis, note position and mobility of fetal head.

d. Midline about 2 inches above Poupart's ligaments, note position and descent of head, location of back.

6. Observe FHR and pattern changes in relation to contractions (NOTE: the use of electronic fetal monitoring for every woman is determined by hospital policy or physician. Obtain consent to use an internal electrode).

7. Prepare and position client appropriately for initial vaginal exam and reinforce the rationale for exam; explain the results of exam.

8. Note color, consistency, amount, and gross appearance of amniotic fluid.

9. Obtain laboratory specimens: urine for protein (normally negative), glucose (normally negative), and ketones (normally negative); blood for Hgb (normal range 12-16 g/dl), Hct (normal range 38%-45%), WBC (normal range 4500-11,000 ml), Veneral Disease Research Laboratory (VDRL) test.

10. Determine time of last food ingestion.

11. Document all assessments.

12. Review process of labor.

13. Provide emotional support to client and coach.

14. Perform vulvar and/or perineal preparation as ordered.

15. Administer cleansing enema if ordered by physician; check FHR after procedure.

Evaluation

Client is admitted to labor and delivery unit; verbalizes an understanding of status; displays minimal anxiety.

> **Goal 2:** Client will be comfortable and safe during the first stage of labor; will be supported by coach; will maintain optimal fetal oxygenation.

Implementation

1. Take maternal vital signs qh, if stable and within normal limits.

2. Monitor temperature q2h if membranes ruptured more than 24 hours previously or if temperature is greater than 37.5° C (may indicate infection or dehydration).

3. Observe blood pressure between contractions q1-2h.

4. Watch for supine-hypotensive syndrome caused by pressure of enlarged uterus on vena cava (decreased BP, pulse, pallor, clammy skin); condition may be prevented or corrected by placing client in left lateral position.

5. Monitor fetal status.

   a. Auscultate FHR using a stethoscope q30min (early labor) to q5min (transition) (see Fig. 4-16); count rate for 1 full minute (normal is 120-160/min) or observe FHR tracing from electronic monitor for baseline changes, variability, and periodic changes related to contractions.

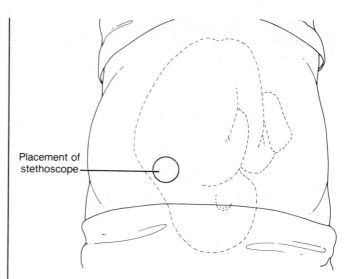

Fig. 4-16 Site of auscultation of FHR with fetus in ROA position.

Placement of stethoscope

   b. Check FHR immediately after rupture of membranes.

   c. Check for prolapse of cord; client may feel cord slither down vagina, nurse may see cord outside vagina or palpate cord on vaginal examination; if cord is prolapsed, place in Trendelenburg's or knee-chest position (to minimize pressure of presenting part on cord), give O_2, and notify physician immediately; grave danger of fetal hypoxia because of cord compression; prepare for immediate delivery.

6. Monitor uterine contractions through abdominal palpations q30min (in early labor) to q5min (in transition); note regularity, frequency, intensity, and duration, or observe uterine tracings from electronic monitor for tonus, frequency, duration, and intensity of contractions.

7. Document all assessments.

8. Assist with or perform periodic vaginal examination to assess dilatation and effacement of cervix, fetal descent, presentation, and lie.

9. Monitor fluid and electrolyte balance.

   a. Record I&O.

   b. Encourage voiding q2h; catheterize for bladder distension.

   c. Observe for signs of dehydration.

   d. Note diaphoresis.

   e. Monitor parenteral therapy; specific use determined by medical regimen and duration of labor.

10. Provide sufficient nourishment according to medical policy and client need.

    a. NPO routine in many hospitals, especially if client is receiving medication; observe for signs of hypoglycemia.

b. Ice chips or liquid diet may be given in some settings (NOTE: GI absorption and motility are decreased during labor).

c. Observe for nausea and vomiting during transition (common).

11. Maintain a safe environment.

    a. Client may ambulate in early labor if desired, unless there are contraindications (e.g., membranes ruptured, medications, or IV infusion).

    b. Keep side rails up as necessary to prevent injury during active labor.

    c. Advise client and coach not to smoke.

12. Administer basic comfort measures: pillows to support body; frequent position change; bathe face and body as necessary; back rubs; effleurage for abdominal discomfort; change linen and pads frequently.

13. Assist client with breathing techniques or provide direct coaching as necessary.

    a. Use appropriate techniques taught in antepartal or childbirth classes or instruct as necessary (e.g., abdominal breathing, shallow chest breathing, panting).

    b. Advise client to rest between contractions but wake client and begin breathing techniques at onset of next contraction.

    c. Observe for symptoms of hyperventilation (light-headedness, dizziness, and tingling and numbness of lips); if it occurs, slow breathing; have client breathe into paper bag or cupped hands.

    d. Support coach by giving periodic relief for a break and nourishment.

    e. Praise efforts and keep client and significant other informed about progress in labor.

14. Assess ability to manage pain, desire for medications.

15. Administer analgesics (or assist with anesthetic administration) as ordered by physician, in accordance with client's preference or decision.

    a. Provide relaxing environment by maintaining calm manner and reducing external stimuli.

    b. Administer and record administration of medications ordered.

    c. Note client and fetal response to medication; report any undesired side effects.

    d. Monitor client's vital signs and FHR q5-15min, depending on drug given.

    e. Place client in appropriate position for administration of anesthetic.

    f. Place client in lateral position, increase IV fluids if hypotension develops.

    g. Administer 6-8 L of O_2 per minute for maternal hypotension or late decelerations in FHR.

Evaluation

During the first stage of labor, the client maintains homeostasis, is as comfortable as possible; is supported effectively by coach or nurse; fetal heart rate is normal in response to contractions.

Goal 3: Client will be maintained during the second stage of labor; will assist with birth by effective pushing, supported by coach; a healthy newborn will be delivered with minimal trauma.

Implementation

1. Maintain a safe environment.

    a. If transfer to delivery room is required, plan move between uterine contractions (multiparas may be transported 8-9 cm dilatation, primiparas at full dilatation with perineal bulging).

    b. Wear appropriate apparel and assist significant other in proper hand washing and obtaining appropriate scrub attire for delivery room; birthing room regulations may be flexible.

    c. Place client in optimal position on delivery table for birth of newborn.

        1. for lithotomy position: pad stirrups; maintain equal height of legs; ensure no pressure on popliteal space

        2. alternate positions may include semi-Fowler's on birthing table, side lying, and squatting

2. Prep vulvar and perineal area wearing sterile gloves.

3. Palpate fundus for uterine contractions, or assess electronically.

4. Monitor FHR by either auscultation with a fetoscope or electronically.

5. Monitor BP at intervals.

6. Encourage strong pushing with contractions.

    a. Instruct client to begin by taking two short breaths, then hold and bear down; legs should be spread with knees slightly flexed.

    b. Show the client which muscles are to be used by showing or touching those muscles in the pelvic floor.

    c. Use blow-blow breathing pattern to prevent pushing between contractions.

7. Assist physician or midwife as necessary.

8. Promote emotional well-being of client and coach.

    a. Inform them about progress and all procedures.

    b. Position mirror so delivery may be viewed.

    c. Encourage rest and relaxation between contractions.

    d. Praise frequently for efforts.

Evaluation

Client is positioned appropriately and safely for delivery; pushes and bears down effectively; is supported by coach; delivers fetus with minimal trauma.

Goal 4: Client will remain stable during the third stage; will expel placenta intact; will be free from excessive bleeding; newborn will remain stable and have early contact with mother.

Implementation

1. Note time of delivery of infant.

2. Provide immediate newborn care; refer to p. 385.

3. Place newborn close to client, on uncovered abdomen if possible.
4. Allow client to touch and explore infant after cord is cut.
5. Assess for signs that placenta has separated.
   a. Uterus rises up in abdomen.
   b. Uterus changes to globular shape.
   c. Sudden trickle of blood appears.
   d. Umbilical cord lengthens.
6. Observe time and mechanism of placental delivery; chart on delivery record.
   a. Duncan mechanism: maternal surface of the placenta presents upon delivery; appears dark and rough; increased risk of retained placental fragments.
   b. Schultze mechanism: fetal surface of the placenta presents upon delivery; appears shiny, smooth.
7. Inspect placenta for intactness and three blood vessels.
8. Palpate uterus to check for muscle tone at frequent intervals (firm and contracted).
9. Administer and document oxytocic agents as ordered (see Tables 4-18 and 4-20).
   a. Drug and dose determined by individual need and physician's order; may be given IM or added to existing IV
   b. Used to prevent or control postpartum hemorrhage by stimulating uterine contractility
   c. Very important with overdistension or poor muscle tone
10. Measure BP at 5- to 15-minute intervals (decreases in BP are often associated with blood loss and administration of oxytocic drugs).
11. Give antilactation agents if appropriate (see Table 4-25)
12. Send cord blood to lab if client is Rh negative or O positive (for direct Coombs' test).
13. Allow client (and significant other if present) opportunity to see and directly touch newborn (promotes bonding) after initial stabilization.
14. Initiate breastfeeding (hospital policies may vary).

Evaluation

Client remains stable during the third stage of labor; delivers placenta intact; maintains firmly contracted uterus; has minimal bleeding; parent-infant bonding begins.

> **Goal 5:** Client will remain stable during recovery period; will be free from complications; will maintain homeostasis; will bond with newborn.

Implementation

1. Take vital signs q15min until stable (take temperature upon admission and subsequently as indicated).
2. Check height of fundus.
   a. Palpate q15min during first hour.
   b. Note position in relation to umbilicus (at or just above umbilicus, 1-2 finger-breadths).
   c. Note consistency: should be firmly contracted; if boggy, massage until firm (avoid overmassaging).
3. Palpate bladder for distension; measure initial voiding; catheterize if necessary (full bladder displaces the uterus).
4. Observe lochia q15min during first hour; note amount (small, moderate, or heavy), color (rubra), consistency; presence of large clots may indicate retained placental fragments; flow is considered excessive if bleeding saturates pad within 15 minutes (flow may increase as oxytocics wear off); keep pad count.
5. Check perineum: note general appearance, any swelling, redness, bruising, drainage, or condition of episiotomy; assess for pain.
6. Assess for afterpains.
7. Promote general comfort.
8. Provide contact with newborn, if not possible in delivery room.
9. Assist with breastfeeding if client desires.
10. Perform and teach perineal care (see p. 368); reinforce that pad should be applied from front to back.
11. Maintain adequate fluid intake; state specific amounts of fluids to be taken in 8-hour period.
12. If transfer to recovery room required, ensure that both client and baby are stabilized.
    a. Monitor client's vital signs q15min until stable.
    b. Palpate position, firmness, and consistency of fundus.

Table 4-18 Uterine smooth muscle stimulants

Drug name	Action	Side effects	Nursing implications
Ergonovine maleate (Ergotrate)	Reduces risk of or treats postpartum hemorrhage by stimulating uterine contraction	Nausea, vomiting, dizziness, hypotension, hypertension	Monitor BP before and during administration. Palpate fundus and note lochia.
Methylergonovine maleate (Methergine)	Stimulates uterine contraction, increases uterine muscle tone, prevents/controls postpartum hemorrhage	Nausea, vomiting, dizziness, slight changes in BP (less likely than with ergonovine maleate), headaches	Monitor contractions, lochia.

c. Observe lochia for quantity, color, and consistency.

13. Transfer to postpartum care when condition stable (usually within 1-2 hours); may remain in birthing room.

Evaluation

Client is physiologically and psychologically stable; couple gazes at, holds, touches, and cuddles newborn.

Application of the Nursing Process to the High-Risk Intrapartal Client

Assessment

1. Risk factors in pregnancy
2. Problems identified in the intrapartal period
3. Alterations of labor progress

Analysis

1. Safe, effective care environment
   a. High risk for infection
   b. High risk for injury
2. Physiological integrity
   a. Pain
   b. Impaired gas exchange
3. Psychosocial integrity
   a. Anxiety
   b. Ineffective individual coping
4. Health promotion/maintenance
   a. Knowledge deficit

Planning, Implementation, and Evaluation

> **Goal:** Client and fetus will experience no undetected complications; will receive immediate treatment for problems; will have a safe birth experience. Newborn and mother will maintain physiological and psychosocial integrity.

Implementation

1. Observe for potential and actual problems in labor and delivery.
2. Act immediately to maintain fetal and maternal well-being.
3. Report problems to physician.
4. Administer therapy and medications as ordered.
5. Document assessments and care.
6. Support couple in difficult birth situation.

Evaluation

Client and fetus at risk have problems detected and treated immediately; return to a homeostatic state following a safe delivery.

SELECTED HEALTH PROBLEMS IN THE INTRAPARTAL PERIOD

☐ Dystocia

General Information

1. Definition: difficult, painful labor and/or delivery characterized by abnormally slow progress
2. Incidence: approximately 5% of intrapartum women

Table 4-19 Uterine dysfunction in labor

	Hypertonic	Hypotonic
Contractions	Intense, high tonus	Weak, ineffective
Symptoms	Painful	Painless
Fetal distress	Fetal hypoxia	Tendency for sepsis
Treatment	Sedation	Stimulation of labor

(largely primigravidas) experience some type of dystocia

3. Types: fall into four categories, which may exist alone or in combination
   a. The *powers* (or forces): the main ones are
     1. hypertonic uterine dysfunction (primary inertia); see Table 4-19
       a. the uterine muscle is in a state of greater than normal muscle tension; contractions are of poor quality, and the force of the contraction is distorted
       b. increased tonus
       c. no cervical changes
       d. treatment: sedation
     2. hypotonic uterine dysfunction
       a. the tone or tension of the muscle is defective or inadequate, resulting in failure of cervical dilatation and effacement
        ◆ primary inertia: inefficient contractions from onset of labor
        ◆ secondary inertia: well-established contractions become weak, inefficient, or stop
     3. inadequate voluntary expulsive forces
       a. may be a result of exhaustion, position, etc.
       b. treatment: coach woman in bearing down; cesarean delivery if necessary
   b. The *passageway:* abnormalities in the size or character of the birth canal that form an obstacle to the descent of the fetus
     1. cephalopelvic disproportion (CPD): disproportion between the size of the fetal head and that of the birth canal
       a. most frequently caused by a contracted pelvis: slight irregularities in the structure of the pelvis may delay the progress of labor; marked deformities often make delivery through the natural passages impossible
        ◆ contraction of the inlet
        ◆ contraction of the midpelvis
        ◆ contraction of the outlet
        ◆ a combination
     2. soft-tissue dystocia: obstruction of birth passage by an anatomical abnormality (e.g., myoma or tumor)
   c. The *passenger:* variations in position, presentation, or development of the fetus; includes a va-

riety of conditions that are associated with pro-longed labor, failure to progress, lack of engage-ment

1. abnormal position: persistent occiput posterior position (25% of pregnancies)
2. faulty presentation
   a. shoulder or face presentation
   b. breech presentation
3. excessive size of fetus
   a. a fetus over 4000 g (8 lb 13½ oz) may be too large to pass through the birth canal of some pregnant women; the fetal head also becomes less malleable when fetal weight increases
   b. hydrocephalus (internus): excessive accumulation of cerebrospinal fluid in the ventricles of the brain with consequent enlargement of the cranium; incidence: 1 in 2000 births
   c. enlargement of the body of the fetus (e.g., abdominal distension, tumors)
   d. The *person*
   1. position of mother: upright, walking, etc.
   2. psychological response: emotional readiness, educational preparation, support, environment

Nursing Process

Assessment

1. Vaginal exam, pelvimetry, or ultrasound to establish diagnosis
2. False labor vs. true labor
3. Fetal status
4. Cause of dystocia
5. Complications of uterine dysfunction
   a. Maternal exhaustion
   b. Intrapartum infection
   c. Traumatic operative delivery
   d. Uterine rupture
   e. Fetal death and injury
6. Presentation of fetus by palpation (Leopold's maneuver)
7. Meconium staining of amniotic fluid (normal when associated with breech presentation)
8. Anxiety

Analysis (see p. 357)

Planning, Implementation, and Evaluation

> **Goal 1:** Client will have dystocia detected; the client with dystocia will remain stable during the intrapartal period; will not experience undetected complications; fetal distress will be identified.

Implementation

1. Assess uterine contractions/pattern.
2. Plot individual labor pattern, compare to Friedman curve (average labor curve of cervical dilatation and hours in labor; see Fig. 4-17)

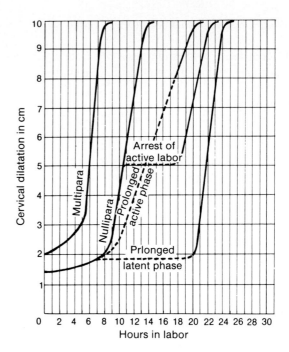

Fig. 4-17   Friedman curve.

3. Assist with ultrasonographic or radiographic studies for laboring woman who has previously suspected CPD.
4. Immediately assess FHR when fetal membranes rupture (spontaneously or artificially); observe for cord prolapse (see p. 354).
5. Monitor IV therapy and electrolyte replacement.
6. Administer broad-spectrum antibiotics as ordered for treatment of intrauterine infection.
7. Promote rest and pain relief.
8. Support family.

Evaluation

Abnormalities in the powers, passageway, or passenger are identified during the antepartal or early intrapartal period; client with dystocia is promptly treated; client and fetus remain stable during difficult labor; healthy newborn is delivered.

> **Goal 2:** Client will be stable during oxytocin augmentation or prostaglandin (PGE) administration.

Implementation

1. Administer oxytocin (Pitocin) according to physician's order or hospital's protocol and client's condition (see Table 4-20); the physician must consider the following criteria before administration
   a. There must be true hypotonic dysfunction; oxytocin ABSOLUTELY CONTRAINDICATED for *hypertonic* uterine dysfunction.
   b. The client must be in true labor (progressed to at

Table 4-20 Oxytocin (Pitocin)

Action	Side effects	Nursing implications
Stimulates uterine smooth muscle to contract; increases intracellular calcium. Used in dilute concentrations IV (10 units in 500 or 1000 ml normal saline or D$_5$W); infusion rate gradually increased to induce or augment labor contractions and stimulate cervical effacement and dilatation before delivery. After delivery acts to stimulate uterine contraction and prevent hemorrhage as a result of atony.	**IN LABOR** Maternal: overstimulation of uterus resulting in rapid labor, delivery; tetany and uterine rupture; abruptio placentae, water intoxication Fetal: hypoxia, distress, trauma with precipitous delivery **FOLLOWING DELIVERY** Water intoxication, uterine atony (if overused)	Monitor and record vital signs and contractions (frequency, duration, and strength). Discontinue infusion if contractions exceed 70-90 seconds, for signs of tetany or abruptio placentae. Record I&O. Monitor FHR; discontinue infusion if distress; turn client to left side. Report problems immediately to responsible physician. Monitor BP, uterine contraction, lochia, output.

least 3 cm dilatation and cervix thinning).

  c. No mechanical obstructions to safe delivery exist (e.g., cephalopelvic disproportion).

  d. The condition of the fetus must be good: regular fetal heart rate, no meconium staining.

  e. The client usually must be less than a para 5 (greater parity increases the risk of uterine rupture).

  f. The uterus must not be overdistended because of a large infant (weighing 4000 g or more) or multiple gestation.

  g. No previous history of cesarean births or uterine surgery.

2. Monitor administration of oxytocin.
  a. Use infusion pump.
  b. Increase infusion rate as ordered.
  c. Monitor vital signs, infusion rate frequently.
  d. Continue electronic fetal monitoring; observe and document fetal heart rate pattern with contractions (duration, intensity, tonus, and frequency).
  e. Place client in a left lateral position to maximize uterine blood flow by reducing pressure on vena cava and aorta.
  f. Never leave client unattended (physician must be available).
  g. Assess for problems (e.g., rigid abdomen, intense pain).
  h. If uterine tetany occurs, or contractions exceed 70-90 seconds in duration, or there is fetal distress or bradycardia, discontinue oxytocin.
  i. Give O$_2$ for signs of fetal distress.
  j. Monitor for abruptio placentae.

3. Monitor client receiving PGE
  a. Perform maternal and fetal assessments as with oxytocin.
  b. Maintain bed rest for 1 hour after PGE administration.
  c. Observe for diarrhea (common side effect).

Evaluation

Client is free from complications related to oxytocin or PGE administration; has effective uterine contractions; maintains optimal fetal status.

> **Goal 3:** Client will experience minimal anxiety; will be supported and comforted during labor.

Implementation

1. Inform client about her status and measures taken to help her.
2. Provide basic comfort measures as in normal labor.
3. Assess level of fatigue and ability to cope with pain.
4. Provide emotional support to client and significant other.
5. Assist with administration of anesthetic to relax uterus (hyperactive uterine contractions).
6. Discuss rationale and expected outcomes with client and partner if cesarean birth indicated.

Evaluation

Client experiences minimal anxiety; knows the status of labor and the fetus; rests comfortably between contractions, treatments; is supported by coach and nurse.

> **Goal 4:** Client with fetus in abnormal position or presentation will be free from complications and will be safely delivered of a newborn in stable condition.

Implementation

1. Assist with vaginal or rectal exam to determine presenting fetal part.
2. Explain and prepare client for ultrasonic or radiographic studies to confirm previously unsuspected malpositions (anomalies often undetected before intrapartum period).
3. Assess effectiveness of labor and fetal well-being by continuous electronic monitoring.

4. Encourage left lateral position.
5. Provide emotional support and coaching as indicated (labors are often prolonged).
6. Support significant other.
7. Apply sacral pressure and frequent back rubs to keep pressure of fetal occiput off client's sacrum (occiput posterior presentation).
8. Observe for cord prolapse (occurs in 1 in every 400 births) when membranes rupture (see p. 354).
9. Assist with vaginal delivery or cesarean birth as indicated by fetal presentation, labor progression, and maternal well-being.

Evaluation

Client safely is delivered of a healthy newborn; has problems such as abnormal fetal position identified early.

□ Premature Labor
General Information

1. Definition: onset of labor before completion of 37 weeks of gestation
2. Predisposing factors that may cause premature labor; pregnancy complications that may necessitate delivery of preterm infant
   a. Maternal
      1. diabetes
      2. cardiovascular and/or renal disease
      3. pregnancy-induced or chronic hypertension
      4. infection: chorioamnionitis
      5. uncontrolled hemorrhage associated with placenta previa or abruptio placentae
      6. prematurely ruptured membranes
      7. incompetent cervix
      8. smoking
      9. severe isoimmunization
      10. DES exposure
      11. abdominal surgery during pregnancy
      12. iatrogenic causes
   b. Fetal
      1. multiple pregnancy
      2. hydramnios
      3. infection
      4. intrauterine growth retardation (IUGR)
3. Prognosis: fetal/neonatal mortality is less than 5% in pregnancies when gestation has lasted 35 or more weeks and fetus is larger than 2000 g

Nursing Process

Assessment
1. Identify women at risk
2. Assess for true labor (contractions of increased frequency and duration, effacement and dilatation of cervix)
3. Estimate gestation
Analysis (see p. 357)
Planning, Implementation, and Evaluation

> **Goal:** Client in preterm labor will experience a cessation of labor; will carry fetus as close to term as possible.

Implementation
1. Maintain bed rest, lateral recumbent position in a quiet environment.
2. Administer selected tocolytic agents to suppress labor as prescribed by physician (e.g., isoxsuprine [Vasodilan], ritodrine, terbutaline, magnesium sulfate).
   a. Assess the effects of drugs upon the pattern of labor (uterine contractions) and fetal well-being with electronic monitoring system.
   b. Avoid these drugs for control of premature labor if contraindicated (e.g., client has a cardiac condition, gestation less than 20 weeks).
   c. If administering ritodrine: assess for specific cardiovascular side effects (see Table 4-21).
   d. If administering magnesium sulfate: assess BP, reflexes, respirations, and urinary output before and during administration (see Table 4-14).
3. Document response to therapy; alter dose as ordered.
4. Maintain adequate hydration through oral or parenteral intake.
5. Monitor I&O.
6. Monitor client's vital signs.
7. Provide emotional support to client and significant other.
8. Administer glucocorticoid therapy (betamethasone) if indicated to prevent respiratory distress syndrome in newborn.
   a. Drug is effective if delivery can be delayed 48 or more hours.
   b. Avoid use if delivery is imminent or if maternal hypertensive or cardiovascular disorders exist.
   c. Observe for signs of pulmonary edema (reported in rare cases when ritodrine and corticosteroids are used together).
9. Administer minimal analgesics for pain during labor and delivery.
10. Prepare for preterm delivery if maternal complications are present (e.g., diabetes, hemorrhage, eclampsia) or dilatation progresses.
Evaluation
Client carries the pregnancy as close to term as possible and is safely delivered of the newborn.

□ Emergency Birth (unassisted by physician, nurse, or midwife)
General Information

1. May occur in a hospital or community setting
2. Predisposing factors: precipitate labor, environmental problems, absence of physician and midwife
3. Prognosis: increased maternal and fetal risk associated with possible

Table 4-21   Ritodrine hydrochloride

Drug name	Action	Side effects	Nursing implications
Ritodrine hydrochloride IV (Yutopar—oral) (only drug with current FDA approval for preterm labor)	Relaxes arterioles in uterine muscle; vasodilator As a beta-sympathetic agent, stops uterine contractions in preterm labor of at least 20 weeks (membranes should be intact) IV solution (150 mg to 500 ml fluid) is given at increasing rates until desired effect is achieved	Maternal: tachycardia, tremors, palpitations, PVCs; pulmonary edema, widening pulse pressure, headache, hyperglycemia, hypokalemia, anxiety, diarrhea (contraindicated if history of CV, thyroid disease; asthma) Fetal: tachycardia, hypoxia, acidosis	Maintain infusion rate; increase as ordered. Monitor apical pulse; report and document pulse above 120; check BP frequently. Record I&O; observe for side effects. Monitor glucose and potassium levels. Teach client to expect responses such as nervousness. Explain that the value of therapy is to allow time for fetal lung development (glucocorticoids may be ordered to stimulate surfactant). Monitor for signs of pulmonary edema. Have antidote (propranolol) available. Monitor and document FHR.

a. Intrauterine hypoxia (precipitate labor or delivery)
b. Laceration of the perineum
c. Infection

Nursing Process

Assessment

1. Fetal status
2. Stage and phase of labor

Analysis (see p. 357)

Planning, Implementation, and Evaluation

> **Goal:** Client is safely delivered of newborn, free from complications, despite an emergency situation.

Implementation

1. Remain with client; have another adult (if present) call for assistance; remain calm.
2. Provide as clean an environment as possible.
3. Instruct client to pant when head crowns.
4. Rupture amniotic sac (if intact) when fetal head crowns.
5. Apply gentle pressure on fetal head to prevent head from "popping out," damaging fetal head, and causing maternal lacerations.
6. Deliver fetal head between contractions.
7. Check for cord around neck; if wrapped around neck, slip cord over newborn's head.
8. Clear airway and facilitate mucus drainage; do not hold upside down by feet or ankles.
9. Dry newborn rapidly (maintain at level of uterus).

10. Cover newborn with blanket or towel to prevent heat loss.
11. Clamp cord in two places and cut between the two clamps; use sterile or clean scissors or knife; leave intact if medical assistance will be available shortly or if clamps/scissors are not available.
    a. Do not pull on cord.
    b. Instruct client to gently push out placenta.
13. Place newborn on client's abdomen or to breast to stimulate uterine contractions.
14. Assess client following birth.

Evaluation

Client is safely delivered of a healthy newborn; is free from complications.

NOTE: The next four selected health problems are classified as "Operative Obstetrics."

☐ Episiotomy
General Information

1. Definition: an incision made into the perineum to facilitate delivery
2. Indications: any condition that places the woman at risk for perineal tearing, such as
   a. Rapid labor
   b. Large baby
   c. Malposition of the fetus
3. Prognosis: generally heals within 2-4 weeks following delivery; may cause mild to moderate discomfort in the postpartum period
4. Types (see Fig. 4-18)
   a. Median (midline)

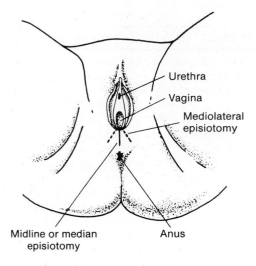

Fig. 4-18 Types of episiotomies.

1. advantages: easily repaired; generally less painful; minimal blood loss
2. disadvantages: increased risk of third- or fourth-degree extension
   b. Mediolateral (right or left)
1. advantage: minimal risk of extension into rectum
2. disadvantages: greater blood loss; repair more difficult; area more painful during healing; possible damage to pubococcygeal muscle

Nursing Process (see *Postpartal Care*, Nursing Goal 1, p. 368)

☐ Forceps
General Information

1. Definition: obstetrical instruments that are used to extract the fetal head during delivery. Each consists of a blade, shank, handle, and lock.
2. Predisposing factors
   a. Maternal
1. to shorten second stage of labor in dystocia
2. expulsive efforts that are ineffective or deficient because of anesthesia or maternal exhaustion
3. if pushing is contraindicated because of a chronic disease or cardiac problem
   b. Fetal
1. premature labor (to protect fetal head)
2. fetal distress
3. arrested descent
4. abnormal presentation
3. Prognosis
   a. Perineal lacerations may occur with a difficult forceps delivery or may follow a precipitate delivery
1. first-degree laceration involves fourchette, perineal skin, and vaginal mucosa

2. second-degree laceration involves skin, mucous membrane, muscles of perineal body
3. third-degree laceration involves skin, mucous membranes, muscles of perineal body, and rectal sphincter
4. fourth-degree laceration involves all features of third-degree lacerations plus tearing into the lumen of the rectum
   b. Pressure by forceps on fetus' facial nerve may cause temporary paralysis of one side of the face
   c. Perinatal morbidity and mortality increased, particularly with midforceps delivery
   d. Increased risk of postpartum hemorrhage with midforceps delivery
   e. Maternal complications following forceps or other traumatic delivery may include cystocele, rectocele, or uterine prolapse later in life
4. Types of forceps deliveries
   a. Outlet or low forceps: fetal head on perineal floor
   b. Midforceps: fetal head at the level of ischial spines

Nursing Process
Assessment

1. Cervix fully dilated before use of forceps
2. Head engaged
3. Fetus in vertex presentation (or face with mentum anterior)
4. Membranes ruptured
5. No cephalopelvic disproportion
6. Bowel and bladder empty

Analysis (see p. 357)
Planning, Implementation, and Evaluation

> **Goal:** Client and fetus will experience minimal trauma despite forceps delivery.

Implementation

1. Explain procedure to client and significant other.
2. Provide physician with selected forceps.
3. Monitor fetal heart rate continuously during procedure.
4. Assess newborn for forceps bruises.

Evaluation

Client is free from complications of forceps delivery; is delivered of a healthy newborn with minimal trauma.

☐ Vacuum Extraction (used infrequently in current practice)
General Information

1. Definition: the use of an obstetrical instrument consisting of a suction cup attached to a suction pump for extraction of the fetal head; it employs negative pressure and traction
2. Predisposing factors
   a. Prolonged labor
   b. Fetal distress

c. Fetal malposition

d. Chronic maternal disease or complications that contraindicate pushing

3. Prognosis

    a. Increased risk of tissue necrosis of the fetal head, cephalhematoma, and cerebral trauma

    b. Increased risk of trauma to vagina and cervix

    c. Increased risk of postpartum hemorrhage

Nursing Process

Assessment

1. Fetal status
2. Fetal position

Analysis (see p. 357)

Planning, Implementation, and Evaluation

> **Goal:** Client will verbalize understanding of the procedure; experiences no undetected complications.

Implementation

1. Clarify procedure following physician's explanation.
2. Assemble and set up necessary equipment.
3. Monitor fetal heart rate continuously.
4. Assist the physician with the suction apparatus.
5. Assess newborn for caput and cerebral swelling.

Evaluation

Newborn is delivered safely; mother is free from undetected problems.

☐ Cesarean Birth
General Information

1. Definition: delivery of a newborn through abdominal wall and uterine incisions. The procedure may be prearranged and performed before the onset of labor (elective) or unplanned and initiated after the onset of labor (emergency).

2. Indications

    a. Cephalopelvic disproportion

    b. Weakened or defective uterine scar, caused by previous cesarean birth or other uterine surgery (VBAC, or vaginal birth after cesarean, may be an option for selected women); refer to p. 364

    c. Severe preeclampsia, eclampsia, or poorly controlled diabetes

    d. Placenta previa or premature separation

    e. Dystocia

    f. Pelvic tumors

    g. Maternal vaginal infection (e.g., active herpes lesions)

    h. Fetal distress

    i. Prolapsed cord

    j. Fetal abnormalities (e.g., hydrocephalus)

    k. Abnormal presentations (e.g., breech)

    l. Multiple birth

3. Prognosis

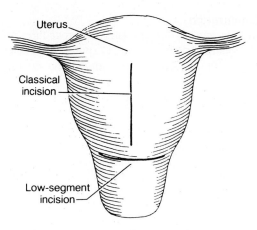

Fig. 4-19 Types of cesarean incisions.

    a. Related to the reasons the cesarean delivery was performed, the type of procedure used, length of time membranes were ruptured, and the nature of complications occurring

    b. Perinatal mortality increases with fetal immaturity and complications compromising uteroplacental blood exchange

4. Types (see Fig. 4-19)

    a. Classical: vertical incision is made through the visceral peritoneum and into the full body of the uterus above the bladder; performed infrequently

        1. advantages: simple and rapid to perform, useful when there is an anterior placenta previa

        2. disadvantages

            a. potential for rupture of the scar with subsequent pregnancy

            b. increased risk of small bowel adhesion to the suture line

    b. Lower segment: incision made into the lower segment of the uterus

    c. Extraperitoneal: incision is made into the lower uterine segment without entering the peritoneal cavity

Nursing Process

Assessment

1. Indications
2. Maternal and fetal well-being
3. Pain and anxiety

Analysis (see p. 357)

Planning, Implementation, and Evaluation

> **Goal 1:** Preoperatively, client and fetus will be free from problems; client will be physically and emotionally prepared for the cesarean birth.

Implementation

1. Provide care as for any surgical procedure; refer to "Perioperative Period," p. 117 (preoperative care will vary with an elective vs. an emergency cesarean birth).
2. Perform or request laboratory studies: type and cross-match, CBC, Hgb, and Hct, Rh.
3. Insert Foley catheter.
4. Monitor fetal heart rate.
5. Administer atropine or antacid as ordered.
6. Prepare emergency equipment for resuscitation of mother and newborn.

Evaluation

Client and fetus are in no distress; couple is prepared for cesarean birth.

> **Goal 2:** Client will tolerate surgery; will achieve postoperative homeostasis; will initiate maternal-infant bonding; newborn will be free from preventable complications.

Implementation

1. Refer to "Perioperative Period," p. 117; Goal 5, p. 356; and "Postpartal Care," p. 366.
2. Assist physician with surgical procedure as necessary.
3. Monitor maternal-fetal status.
4. Assess for signs and symptoms of hemorrhage.
5. Administer oxytocic agents as ordered by physician.
6. Provide assistance as necessary during mother-infant interactions.
7. Monitor recovery from anesthesia.
8. Anticipate client's possible feelings of failure and grief response.
9. Provide emotional support to help mother and significant other integrate the experience.

Evaluation

Client is free from complications; remains stable and comfortable during the postoperative period; initiates bonding; newborn is in good condition.

☐ Vaginal Birth After Cesarean Delivery (VBAC)
General Information

1. Incidence: VBAC is increasing: 60%-65% of women who attempt vaginal deliveries after cesarean births are successful
2. Contraindications
   a. Upper segment uterine incision
   b. Any contraindication for vaginal delivery (e.g., CPD, complete previa)

Nursing Process
Assessment
1. Maternal status
2. Fetal responses to contractions
Analysis (see p. 357)
Planning, Implementation, and Evaluation

> **Goal:** Client will be free of complications with labor and vaginal delivery after previous cesarean birth; is delivered of a newborn in good condition.

Implementation

1. Monitor uterine contractions very frequently.
2. Monitor fetal status continuously.
3. Assess for threatened rupture or rupture of uterus (see "Rupture of the Uterus" below).

Evaluation

Client experiences normal labor free from complications; client and newborn are in satisfactory condition.

☐ Rupture of the Uterus
General Information

1. Definition: the uterus ruptures from the stress of labor; rupture may be complete or partial
2. Occurrence: rare, 1 in every 2000 births
3. Predisposing factors
   a. Previous surgery of myometrium or cesarean birth
   b. Oxytocin (Pitocin) induction (second most common cause)
   c. Nonprogressive labor
   d. Very intense contractions
   e. Faulty position or fetal abnormalities
   f. Injudicious use of forceps
   g. Trauma
4. Prognosis
   a. Maternal mortality 5%-10%
   b. Fetal mortality is high: 50%-75%

Nursing Process
Assessment
1. Sharp abdominal pain (during contractions); onset sudden
2. Tachypnea, tachycardia, anxiety, cool and clammy skin, confusion (shock), rapid change in condition
3. Sudden absence of uterine contractions (with complete rupture)
4. Uterus palpated as a hard mass adjacent to fetus
5. Hemorrhage into the abdominal cavity or vagina
6. Abdominal tenderness

Analysis (see p. 357)
Planning, Implementation, and Evaluation

> **Goal:** Client will be free from hemorrhage or uterine rupture; will maintain fluid and electrolyte balance; will verbalize an understanding of the need for emergency surgery; will maintain oxygenation of fetus.

Implementation

1. Assess carefully during labor; report any signs of an impending rupture.
2. Monitor fetal status.
3. Implement appropriate measure for failure to progress.
4. Provide immediate treatment for shock.
5. Prepare client and significant other for possible emergency cesarean birth or hysterectomy.
6. Provide emotional support to couple.

Evaluation

Client is delivered of a newborn in stable condition before rupture of uterus; has hemorrhage controlled; is in good condition following emergency surgery.

☐ Amniotic Fluid Embolism
General Information

1. Definition: the entrance of amniotic fluid into the maternal circulation through the placental site and venous sinuses
2. Occurrence: extremely rare complication that occurs in the intrapartum or early postpartum period
3. Predisposing factors: rapid, intense contractions from oxytocin infusion; multiparity with large fetus
4. Prognosis
   a. Fetal death will result if delivery is not implemented immediately
   b. Maternal death may occur within 1-2 hours if emergency interventions are ineffective
   c. Presence of meconium and/or mucus in amniotic fluid is indicative of increased lethality, graver outlook

Nursing Process (Refer to "Pulmonary Embolus," p. 150.)

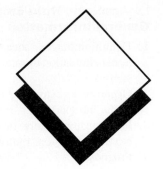

Postpartal Care

GENERAL CONCEPTS
Normal Childbearing

1. Definition: the postpartum period (puerperium) starts immediately after delivery and is completed when the reproductive tract has returned to the nearly prepregnant state and family readjustment has occurred (usually defined as 6 weeks)
2. Restoration to pregravid status
   a. Uterine involution
      1. process of involution takes 4-6 weeks to complete
         a. weight of uterus decreases from 2 pounds to 2 ounces
         b. hormones decrease
         c. autolysis occurs (enzyme action)
         d. contractions increase muscle tone
         e. vasoconstriction occurs at placental site
         f. endometrium regenerates
         g. fundus steadily descends into true pelvis; fundal height decreases about 1 finger-breadth (1 cm) per day; by 10 days postpartum, cannot be palpated abdominally
      2. factors delaying involution
         a. multiparity
         b. conditions causing overdistension of uterus
         c. infection
         d. retained placenta or membranes
         e. hormonal deficiencies
      3. cervical involution
         a. after 1 week, muscle begins to regenerate
         b. small lacerations may heal or need cauterization
         c. external cervical os remains wider than in a nonparous woman
         d. internal cervical os closed after 1 week
      4. lochia (see Table 4-22)
         a. constituents: blood, mucus, particles of decidua, cellular debris, leukocytes, RBCs
         b. changes from rubra (delivery day to day 3: bright red) to serosa (days 4-10: brownish pink) to alba (days 10-14: white, as a result of increased leukocytes); normally has fleshy odor; decreases daily in amount; increases with ambulation; lochia disappearance coincides with healed internal reproductive tract
         c. signs of abnormal lochia
            ◆ foul smell
            ◆ excessive amount (any stage)
            ◆ scant (during rubra stage)
            ◆ return to rubra after serosa and/or alba
      5. afterbirth pains resulting from contraction of uterus occur primarily in multiparas as well as in mothers who
         a. have a history of blood clots
         b. were treated with oxytocic drugs
         c. breastfeed their infant
         d. had an overdistended uterus during pregnancy (large baby, multiple gestation, polyhydramnios)
   b. Perineal healing
      1. vaginal distension decreases although muscle tone is never restored completely to its pregravid state
      2. vaginal rugae begin to reappear around third week
      3. lacerations or episiotomy suture line gradually heals
      4. hemorrhoids common; generally subside
   c. Bladder and bowel function: physiological adaptations include
      1. increased urinary output resulting from normal diuresis
      2. increased bladder capacity; trauma to the bladder during delivery may diminish urge to void

Table 4-22 Lochia changes

Time postpartum	Characteristics
Delivery-day 3	Lochia rubra (red)
4-10 days	Lochia serosa (brownish to pink)
10-14 days	Lochia alba (white)

3. urine may show increased acetone, nitrogen, albumin, and lactose
4. edema of the urethra and vulva
5. GI tract motility sluggish because of
   a. relaxed abdominal and intestinal muscles
   b. decreased intraabdominal pressure because of distension of the abdominal wall
   d. **Restoration of abdominal wall**
1. abdomen may be soft and flabby; usually returns to normal state by 6-8 weeks
2. striae fade to silvery-white; linea nigra fades
   e. **Breast changes:** condition of breasts during pregnancy maintained for first 2 days postpartum; physiological adaptations include
1. establishment of lactation
   a. colostrum secreted during first 2-3 days postpartum
   b. prolactin released from anterior pituitary gland
   c. oxytocin (released from posterior pituitary) causes let-down reflex
2. engorgement
   a. onset usually day 3
   b. lasts 24-48 hours
   c. caused by venous and lymphatic stasis of the breasts
3. mechanism of lactation: sucking activates nerve impulses from nipple to spinal cord to pituitary gland
   a. anterior pituitary gland produces prolactin only if breasts are emptied; seems to inhibit FSH and LH
   b. posterior pituitary gland secretes oxytocin, causing let-down reflex when milk is ejected from ducts
4. effect on mother
   a. increased metabolic-system stress
   b. loss of large amounts of stored protein and fats
   c. increased need for calcium, phosphorus, and all nutrients and fluids; see Table 4-8 (note the increased need of the lactating woman)
   d. hastens involution of uterus, may decrease incidence of breast cancer
   e. enhances physical closeness with infant (usually pleasurable)
5. infant's sucking stimulates milk production of 200-300 ml (6-10 oz) by day 4; by end of 6 weeks; about 600 ml/day
   f. **General physiological status**
1. restoration of energy reserves
   a. immediate need for sleep
   b. subsequent need for sleep and rest increased
2. blood
   a. decreased in volume
   b. moderate anemia if excessive blood loss at delivery
   c. leukocytosis immediately after delivery
   d. elevated fibrinogen levels during first week postpartum; may contribute to thrombophlebitis
3. weight loss
   a. usually 11-15 pounds immediately because of baby, placenta, amniotic fluid, and diuresis
   b. 5 pounds in following week
4. vital signs
   a. temperature first day may be 38° C (100.4° F)
   b. pulse: initially decreases postpartum, range 50-70
   c. blood pressure: normal limits
   3. **Maternal psychological adaptation** (see Table 4-23)
   a. Adaptive responses to parental role (Rubin, 1961)
1. taking-in phase: first 2-3 days postpartum
   a. passive and dependent behavior

Table 4-23 Maternal psychological adaptation (Rubin)

Phase	Characteristics	Nursing implications
Taking in (1-2 days postpartum)	Mother passive, dependent, concerned with own needs; verbalizes delivery experience	Assist mother in meeting physical needs. Begin teaching to prepare for possible early discharge.
Taking hold (3-10 days postpartum)	Mother strives for independence; strong anxiety element; maximal stage of learning readiness; mood swings may occur	Provide positive reinforcement of parenting abilities.
Letting go (10 days to 6 weeks postpartum)	Mother achieves interdependence; realistic regarding role transition; accepts baby as separate person; new norms established for self	Assist mother in providing for her increased energy requirements; provide positive reinforcement as she identifies her roles with her support system. Allow her to verbalize her new role.

b. mother focuses upon own needs rather than baby's (e.g., sleeping and eating)

c. verbalizations center on reactions to delivery (help integrate experience)

d. beginning to recognize child as an individual

2. taking-hold phase: third to tenth day postpartum

a. mother strives for independence; wants to care for self and child

b. strong element of anxiety
   ◆ unsure of mothering role (primipara)
   ◆ unsure of own ability to physically care for child

c. stage of maximum readiness for learning

d. interested in learning baby care

e. may show mood swings

3. letting-go phase: 10 days to 6 weeks

a. achieves independent, realistic role transition

b. learns to accept baby as separate person and establishes new norms for self

b. Postpartum blues (see Table 4-23 and "Postpartum Depression," p. 375).

Application of the Nursing Process to Normal Childbearing, Postpartal Care

Assessment

1. Degree of homeostasis achieved
2. Vital signs
3. Fundus: height, consistency, and position
4. Lochia: amount, color, consistency, and odor
5. Perineum: REEDA, comfort, hemorrhoids
6. Bladder: distension and displacement
7. Bowel: constipation
8. Breasts/nipples: secretions, engorgement; nipple variations/condition; color, support
9. Psychological status
10. Homans' sign: thrombophlebitis
11. Costovertebral angle (CVA) tenderness: kidney infection

Analysis

1. Safe, effective care environment
   a. High risk for infection
   b. Knowledge deficit
2. Physiological integrity
   a. Effective breastfeeding
   b. Altered comfort
3. Psychosocial integrity
   a. Altered sexuality patterns
   b. Anxiety
4. Health promotion maintenance
   a. Altered family processes
   b. Altered parenting

Planning, Implementation, and Evaluation

> **Goal 1:** Client will achieve homeostasis; will be comfortable; will be knowledgeable about self-care.

Implementation

1. Review antepartum and intrapartum records for history.
   a. Antepartal care, labor and delivery, and chronic conditions
   b. Lab values: Hgb, HCT, VDRL, blood type, Rh factor, rubella titer

2. Monitor vital signs on admission to postpartum unit, then every 4-8 hours.
   a. BP may drop initially after birth, then returns to normal.
   b. Bradycardia (50-70 beats per minute) common first 10 days postpartum
   c. Temperature may be elevated within first 24 hours because of dehydration.
   d. Temperature of 38° C (100.4° F) or above on any 2 consecutive days is considered febrile (excluding first 24 hours); possible causes: endometritis, urinary tract infection.

3. Monitor ongoing postpartal progress by daily assessment.

4. Promote perineal healing and relief of perineal and hemorrhoidal discomfort.
   a. Inspect episiotomy daily for normal healing; observe for *r*edness, *e*dema, *e*cchymosis, *d*ischarge, *a*pproximation (REEDA), and hematoma.
   b. Apply ice pack during first 12-24 hours to reduce edema (as ordered).
   c. Encourage use of sitz baths, cool astringent compresses, and topical anesthetic creams as ordered to promote comfort and healing.
   d. Teach proper technique for frequent perineal care (e.g., dry perineal area from front to back, blot rather than wipe; apply perineal pad carefully; cleanse area front to back in shower daily).
   e. Reinforce teaching of perineal care and comfort measures.

5. Treat afterbirth pains.
   a. Encourage frequent voiding.
   b. Advise mother to lie on her abdomen.
   c. Give analgesics as ordered.

6. Administer Rho(D)immune globulin (RhoGAM) if ordered; indicated for unsensitized (negative Coombs' test) Rh-negative women bearing an Rh-positive child; given within 72 hours of delivery (antepartal RhoGAM is used for selected clients) (see Table 4-24).

7. Observe abdomen for muscle tone, diastasis recti abdominis; measure degree of any diastasis; teach corrective exercise to client.

Table 4-24 Rh$_o$ (D) human immune globulin

Drug name	Action	Side effects	Nursing implications
RhoGAM	Provides transient passive immunity by preparing RBCs containing Rh-positive antigens for lysis by phagocytes	Transfusion reaction	Explain protection is for next pregnancy. Teach to carry identification card and to inform physician of RhoGAM history.
Anti Rh$_o$ (D) gamma globulin	Prevents antibody formation in unsensitized Rh-negative women with negative newborn cord blood Coombs' test (these antibodies cause hemolysis of fetal RBCs) Effective if administered to woman during pregnancy or within 72 hours of abortion or miscarriage or delivery of each Rh-positive infant	Contraindicated if antibodies are present	Instruct that woman will need additional dose during subsequent pregnancies and following each miscarriage/abortion or delivery of Rh-positive infant if antibodies remain negative (Coombs' test).

8. Promote bowel and bladder function.
   a. Encourage usual voiding patterns.
   b. Recognize signs of bladder distension and catheterize if necessary.
   c. Ambulate to bathroom.
   d. Measure initial voidings.
   e. Check for signs of urinary infection (e.g., frequency, burning).
   f. Encourage adequate fluid intake and a balanced diet, high in fiber to avoid constipation.
   g. Use stool softeners, cathartics, and enemas as ordered by physician.
9. Teach self-assessment and self-care.
10. Document accurately.

Evaluation

Client has stable vital signs, adequate intake and output; experiences no more than minimal pain and discomfort; performs self-care.

> **Goal 2:** Client will verbalize and demonstrate knowledge of breast changes, breast care, lactation, or suppression of lactation.

Implementation

1. Teach daily cleansing of breast; breastfeeding mother should wash nipples with clear water only (nipples are cleansed by natural antiseptic lysozyme).
2. Encourage air-drying of nipples for 15-30 minutes after breastfeeding.
3. Apply bland cream or ointment (e.g., lanolin, A&D ointment) to sore nipples after feeding.
4. Explain mechanisms of lactation.
5. Help mother place infant to breast; demonstrate proper positioning.

6. Teach lactating mother to relieve breast engorgement (e.g., frequent emptying of breasts by nursing, manual expression, breast pump).
7. Apply warm packs before feeding for discomfort; ice packs may be used in between feedings for engorgement (varies with physician's suggestions).
8. Promote comfort with use of supportive nursing bra.
9. Give analgesics as ordered.
10. Observe breasts for
    a. Colostrum secretion
    b. Engorgement
    c. Nipple inversion or cracking
    d. Inflammation and/or pain
11. Instruct mother to safely remove infant from breast: squeeze infant's cheeks, place finger in infant's mouth.
12. Promote comfort of nonlactating client with use of supportive bra, ice packs, limited fluids; do not express milk or pump breasts; give medication if prescribed (see Table 4-25).

Evaluation

Lactating client demonstrates correct care of breasts, wears a supportive bra; feeds newborn comfortably, knows how to express milk (manually and via pump); nonnursing client lists measures to suppress lactation.

> **Goal 3:** Client will verbalize knowledge of nutrition to meet own needs and supply calories/nutrients for lactation.

Implementation

1. Review basic four food groups.
2. Encourage nutritious snacks and increased fluids.
3. Teach lactating client to increase amount of protein, calcium, iron, phosphorus, and vitamins (see Table 4-8).

Table 4-25 **Lactation suppressant agents**

Drug name	Action	Side effects	Nursing implications
Bromocriptine mesylate (Parlodel)	Ergot derivative; reduces prolactin level and inhibits lactation	Hypotension, nausea, dizziness, vomiting, vasospasm, GI bleeding	Stabilize BP before administering. Teach to continue use for 14 days. Observe for drowsiness and dizziness.
Chlorotrianisene (TACE) (seldom used)	Synthetic estrogen, prevents postpartum breast engorgement	Thromboembolism	Obtain informed consent. Teach risks vs. benefits.

4. Advise increased intake of iron-rich foods for mothers with low hemoglobin or history of hemorrhage.
5. Teach client to avoid medications that are transmitted by way of breast milk.

Evaluation

Client verbalizes understanding of dietary recommendations; selects foods from the basic four food groups to meet postpartal and lactation needs.

Goal 4: Client will be knowledgeable about rest and exercise in the immediate postpartal period.

Implementation

1. Encourage early ambulation to prevent thrombophlebitis and constipation. NOTE: if client had regional or spinal anesthesia, maintain recumbent position as ordered (e.g., 8-12 hours).
2. Restrict dangling of feet for long periods while sitting on side of bed (constricts popliteal arteries and veins).
3. Encourage frequent rest periods during day with minimal interruptions.
4. Teach postpartum exercises to strengthen muscles of back, pelvic floor, and abdomen; Kegel or pelvic-floor exercises increase vaginal tone.
5. Advise client to consult physician before resuming strenuous activities.

Evaluation

Client takes several rest periods during the day; performs postpartum exercises correctly.

Goal 5: Parents will continue to bond and attach to the newborn.

Implementation

1. Encourage physical closeness between newborn and parents; teach them to use eye-to-eye contact and an en face position.
2. Encourage physical examination: exploration with fingertips/palms, touching, and stroking.
3. Compare newborn's likeness to and differences from other family members.
4. Encourage addressing newborn by name.

5. Explain how normal newborn appears.
6. Allow parents to verbalize their positive feelings, concerns, and questions about newborn.
7. Stay with parents during initial feeding and care activities as needed.
8. Identify newborn behavioral cues and responses.
9. Teach newborn care.
10. Provide positive reinforcement of parenting abilities.

Evaluation

Parents exhibit bonding/attachment behaviors (e.g., gaze at, cuddle, fondle, talk to newborn); make positive statements about newborn.

Goal 6: Client will verbalize an understanding of common maternal role conflicts.

Implementation

1. Explain that conflicts are common.
   a. Independence vs. dependence
   b. Idealized vs. realistic role
   c. Love vs. resentment of newborn
   d. Self-fulfillment vs. motherhood
   e. Love for significant other vs. love for newborn
2. Promote maternal psychological adaptation.
   a. Listen to mother and help her to interpret events of labor and delivery.
   b. Clarify any misconceptions about the birth experience.
   c. Encourage rooming-in with newborn.
   d. Obtain information for evaluating the future parent-child relationship (i.e., plans to integrate newborn into family).
   e. Act as a role model in assisting the mother with maternal tasks.

Evaluation

Client discusses conflicts about maternal role; asks questions; shares feelings and concerns about caring for baby and incorporating newborn into family.

Goal 7: Parents will verbalize understanding about home care of mother and newborn.

Implementation
1. Provide discharge planning and teaching information about
   a. Normal physiological changes
   b. Expected weight loss
   c. Lochia: may last up to 3-6 weeks
   d. Changes in abdominal wall
   e. Perineal healing: episiotomy sutures absorb in about 3 weeks
   f. Diaphoresis common in first 2-3 weeks ("night sweats")
   g. Maintaining lactation
   h. Return of menses and ovulation (if mother not nursing, menses return within 6-12 weeks; in nursing mother, menses return within 4-18 months)
2. Teach maternal self-care, needs (e.g., rest, sleep, balanced diet, and increased fluids if nursing); proceed slowly with activities.
3. Instruct to report any of the following
   a. Increased temperature
   b. Increased lochia or reverse in trend in lochia characteristics
   c. Signs of bladder infection (e.g, frequency, burning)
   d. Pain in calf
4. Discuss and demonstrate newborn care (see p. 385).
5. Provide opportunity for client to care for newborn in hospital.
6. Review feeding technique.
7. Discuss concerns and questions about newborn care, behavior, and basic needs.
8. Review approaches to manage sibling rivalry: extra attention and special times needed for other children.
9. Discuss family planning.
   a. Review methods (see Table 4-2).
   b. Discuss methods previously used.
   c. Emphasize that breastfeeding is not a form of contraception.
10. Discuss sexual adjustment; encourage open communication between partners.
    a. Sexual intercourse may be resumed after cessation of lochia and when comfort permits (except if hematoma or infection); physician may suggest delay until postpartal examination in 2-3 weeks.
    b. Breastfeeding mothers may experience decreased vaginal lubrication or breasts leaking/spurting milk during orgasm.
    c. Fatigue and hormonal changes may influence desires.
    d. Altered body image may affect satisfaction.
    e. Birth-control measures should be used as soon as coitus is resumed.
    f. Consult physician before resuming use of birth control pills, diaphragm.
11. Review need for follow-up medical care to
    a. Assess involution
    b. Determine family planning needs
    c. Provide early treatment of problems

Evaluation

Parents describe and demonstrate skills for maternal self-care, newborn care; describe plans to set aside separate and special times for newborn's siblings; have an appointment for follow-up care.

Application of the Nursing Process to the High-Risk Postpartal Client

Assessment
1. Risk factors in pregnancy, labor, and delivery
2. Potential/actual problems following delivery

Analysis
1. Safe, effective care environment
   a. High risk for injury
   b. High risk for infection
   c. Knowledge deficit
2. Physiological integrity
   a. Altered tissue perfusion
   b. High risk for fluid volume deficit
   c. Pain
3. Psychosocial integrity
   a. Anxiety
   b. Powerlessness
   c. Altered role performance
4. Health promotion/maintenance
   a. High risk for altered parenting
   b. Altered health maintenance
   c. Impaired adjustment

Planning, Implementation, and Evaluation

> **Goal:** Client will be free from undetected problems; will maintain physiological and psychosocial integrity.

Implementation
1. Teach client normal postpartal adaptation.
2. Observe for actual/potential problems in immediate postpartal period (e.g., signs of developing hemorrhage/hematoma, infection).
3. Instruct on reportable signs at discharge.
4. Discuss possible problems of delayed involution.
5. Administer treatment or medication as ordered.
6. Reinforce importance of complying with postpartal check-up.

Evaluation

Client reports abnormal findings to physician; complies with treatment; maintains homeostasis.

SELECTED HEALTH PROBLEMS IN THE POSTPARTAL PERIOD

☐ Postpartum Hemorrhage

General Information

1. Definition: postpartum *bleeding of more than 500 ml after delivery*

2. Incidence: third highest cause of maternal mortality
3. Predisposing factors
   a. *Uterine atony:* most common cause, often associated with
      1. conditions that overdistend the uterus
         a. delivery of a large infant
         b. multiple gestation
         c. hydramnios
      2. multiparity
      3. use of deep general anesthesia
      4. premature separation of the placenta
      5. obstetrical trauma
      6. abnormal labor pattern (e.g., prolonged labor)
      7. oxytocin stimulation or augmentation during labor
      8. overmassage of an already contracted uterus
   b. *Lacerations:* more common after operative obstetrics
      1. perineum
      2. vagina
      3. cervix
   c. *Retained placenta fragments:* predicted by Duncan mechanism or manual removal by physician; associated with
      1. entrapment by uterine constriction ring
      2. premature uterine contraction by massage or ergot administration
      3. abnormal adherence of all or part of placenta to uterine wall (e.g., placenta accreta)
4. Prognosis: 14% of all maternal deaths are from hemorrhagic complications
5. Types
   a. *Early* postpartum hemorrhage occurs within the first 24 hours after birth; incidence is 1 in 200 births
   b. *Late* postpartum hemorrhage occurs between the second day and sixth week postpartum; incidence is 1 in 1000 births; more common in women with history of abortions or uterine bleeding during pregnancy

Nursing Process

Assessment
1. Inspection of placenta to determine intactness
2. Evaluation of vaginal bleeding after delivery
   a. May be slow and continuous (most common) or rapid and profuse
   b. Blood may escape from the vagina or accumulate in the uterus or maternal tissues
   c. Bleeding from a laceration appears often as bright-red vaginal bleeding in presence of a well-contracted uterus
3. Palpate fundus for firmness, height, and position
4. Recognize signs of shock; see "Shock," p. 128
5. Assess bladder distension

Analysis (see p. 371)
Planning, Implementation, and Evaluation

> **Goal:** Client will be free from undetected hemorrhage and shock; will have blood volume restored; will regain homeostasis; will comply with discharge teaching.

Implementation
1. Remain with the client.
2. Massage boggy fundus gently but firmly, cupping uterus between two hands; avoid overmassage.
3. Administer oxytocic agents in fourth stage of labor as prescribed by physician (see Tables 4-18 and 4-20).
4. Monitor closely during acute phase of hemorrhage (e.g., vital signs, intake, output, level of consciousness, fundal firmness, bleeding, and CVP).
5. Encourage frequent voiding.
6. Replace fluid and blood as ordered.
7. Administer O_2 through face mask at 4-7 L.
8. Maintain asepsis, since hemorrhage predisposes to infection.
9. Give prophylactic antibiotics as ordered.
10. Support significant other.
11. Assist with preoperative preparation (for surgical removal of retained placental fragments), suturing as indicated.
12. Before discharge, teach client signs of possible late hemorrhage (critical because of increasingly early discharge).
13. Counsel client to increase iron in diet; iron supplements; administer iron dextran (Imferon) if ordered.
14. Arrange for follow-up care.

Evaluation
Client is free from hemorrhage or complications of excessive blood loss; regains homeostasis; lists signs and symptoms of late hemorrhage; selects foods high in iron with daily diet.

☐ Hematoma
General Information
1. Definition: a collection of blood, often on the external genitalia, as a result of injury to a blood vessel during spontaneous or forceps delivery; occurs once in every 500-1000 deliveries; most common site of a genital tract hematoma is the lateral wall in the area of the ischial spines
2. Predisposing factors: prolonged pressure of fetal head on vaginal mucosa; forceps delivery

Nursing Process
Assessment
1. Complaints of *severe perineal pain or intense rectal pressure*

2. Visible large mass at the introitus or labia majora
3. Bruising, ecchymosis
4. Pain upon palpation
5. Inability to void owing to pressure of hematoma on the urethra
6. Signs and symptoms of shock in presence of well-contracted uterus and no visible vaginal bleeding

Analysis (see p. 371)

Planning, Implementation, and Evaluation

Goal: Client will experience minimal discomfort while the hematoma is treated/absorbed.

Implementation
1. Monitor changes/enlargement of hematoma.
2. Notify physician of condition.
3. Promote general comfort.
   a. Apply cold to site.
   b. Administer analgesics as ordered.
4. Prepare woman for surgery, if indicated, to evacuate the hematoma.
5. Assess for further vaginal bleeding.

Evaluation

Client's hematoma does not enlarge; client experiences only minimal discomfort; is free from additional complications.

☐ Pulmonary Embolus
General Information

1. Definition: the passage of a thrombus, often originating in one of the uterine or other pelvic veins, into a lung, where it obstructs the circulation of blood; usually occurs at end of first week postpartum
2. Predisposing factors
   a. Infection
   b. Hemorrhage
   c. Thrombosis
3. Prognosis: maternal mortality high with large and undetected clots (refer to "Pulmonary Embolus," p. 150)

☐ Puerperal Infection
General Information

1. Definition: any inflammatory process in the genital tract within 28 days following abortion or delivery of a newborn
2. Incidence: second highest risk of maternal mortality (18%)
3. Criterion: an elevation in temperature to 38° C (100.4° F) for two consecutive days, with the onset after the first 24 hours postpartum
4. Origin
   a. *Endogenous:* infection from within or other preexisting infection/sexually transmitted disease
   b. *Exogenous:* infection introduced by others and/or poor technique

5. Predisposing factors
   a. Debilitating antepartal conditions
      1. anemia
      2. malnutrition
   b. Debilitating conditions related to labor and delivery
      1. prolonged labor after membranes rupture
      2. soft-tissue trauma and/or hemorrhage
      3. operative obstetrical procedures (e.g., cesarean delivery, forceps delivery)
      4. invasive procedures (e.g., multiple vaginal examinations)
      5. prolonged labor resulting in weakness and exhaustion of client
   c. Retention of placental fragments
6. Prognosis
   a. One of three leading causes of maternal mortality
   b. Outcome improved with early detection and appropriate medical and nursing management
7. Types of infection
   a. Localized lesions of perineum, vulva, and vagina
   b. Endometritis: localized infection of lining of uterus, usually beginning at placental site
   c. Local infection may extend through venous circulation, resulting in
      1. infectious thrombophlebitis
      2. septicemia
   d. Local infection may extend through lymphatic vessels to cause
      1. peritonitis
      2. parametritis
      3. salpingitis
8. Bacterial causative agents
   a. *Streptococcus hemolyticus:* very virulent, early onset and rapid progression; less common today
   b. *E. coli*
   c. Mixed aerobic-anaerobic infection: low virulence, two or more species of bacteria present

Nursing Process
Assessment
1. Temperature greater than 38° C (100.4° F)
2. Lochia is abnormal
   a. Remains rubra longer or becomes brown
   b. May have foul odor
   c. Scant or profuse in amount
3. Tachycardia (may be 100-120 beats per minute)
4. Delayed involution
   a. Fundal height does not descend as rapidly
   b. Uterus may feel larger and softer
   c. Client may have pain and/or tenderness over the uterus
5. Pain, tenderness, or inflammation of perineum
6. Malaise
7. Fatigue
8. Chills

9. Abnormal lab results: leukocytosis, increased sedimentation rate
10. Calf tenderness, positive Homans' sign

Analysis (see p. 371)

Planning, Implementation, and Evaluation

> **Goal:** Client will be free from local or systemic infection; will have infection treated early; will comply with prescribed treatment; will have homeostasis restored.

Implementation

1. Determine source of infection and take measures to prevent further problems.
2. Use universal precautions when handling body fluids.
3. Obtain specimens for culture and sensitivity as ordered.
4. Take vital signs frequently.
5. Isolate client if indicated (may be separated from newborn).
6. Encourage semi-Fowler's position to facilitate lochia drainage.
7. Change perineal pads frequently.
8. Reinforce perineal hygiene techniques; encourage hand washing.
9. Provide comfort measures (e.g., sitz baths to promote perineal healing).
10. Administer analgesics as ordered.
11. Maintain adequate hydration with oral or intravenous fluids (2000-4000 ml/day).
12. Administer antibiotic therapy as prescribed by physician.
13. Administer oxytocic medications as prescribed by phsycian.
14. Encourage high–caloric fluid intake; high-protein diet.
15. Inform client about condition of newborn if separated.
16. Maintain bed rest with leg elevated for suspected thrombophlebitis; give anticoagulants if prescribed.

Evaluation

Client complies with and responds to treatment for infection (e.g., falling temperature, negative cultures, relief of symptoms, increasing energy).

☐ Mastitis
General Information

1. Definition: an inflammation of the breast as a result of an infection, usually caused by *Staphylococcus aureus* or *Streptococcus hemolyticus;* mainly seen in breastfeeding mothers
2. Predisposing factors: nipple fissure, erosion of the aerola; overdistension, milk stasis
3. Prognosis: condition is generally preventable; prompt and appropriate treatment with antibiotic therapy significantly decreases maternal morbidity

Nursing Process
Assessment

1. Blocked milk duct: hard, warm, reddened, and tender site; often in the outer, upper quadrant of the breast
2. Mastitis
   a. Fever
   b. Breast may have red area, be warm to touch, and be tender; lump may be visible
   c. Pain, chills
   d. Engorgement
   e. Axillary adenopathy
   f. Tachycardia often present (usual time of occurrence is 2-4 weeks after delivery)
   g. Headache

Analysis (see p. 371)

Planning, Implementation, and Evaluation

> **Goal:** Client will be free from undetected mastitis; will comply with treatment to prevent further complications; will maintain lactation, if desired.

Implementation

1. Administer antibiotics as ordered by physician.
2. Promote comfort.
   a. Suggest supportive bra.
   b. Apply local heat or cold.
   c. Administer analgesics as prescribed by physician.
3. Maintain lactation in breastfeeding mothers.
   a. Regular nursing of infant (controversial, will vary with physician)
   b. Manual expression of breast milk
   c. Use of a breast pump
4. Encourage good hand washing and breast hygiene.
5. Offer emotional support.
6. Prepare client for incision and drainage of abscess if necessary.

Evaluation

Client is free from symptoms of mastitis; maintains milk supply; resumes lactation as able.

☐ Postpartum Cystitis
General Information

1. Definition: an infection of the bladder occurring in about 5% of postpartum women; usually caused by coliform bacteria
2. Predisposing factors: trauma to the bladder during vaginal delivery or cesarean birth; catheterization during and/or after labor

Table 4-26 Postpartum depression

Type	Characteristics	Incidence
Blues	Mild, brief; orginates 2-10 days after birth	80%
Atypical	Moderate, longer lasting; physical as well as psychological symptoms	10%
Psychosis	Severe; may be long-term risks of suicide, infanticide	0.5%-3.0%

Nursing Process (refer to "Cystitis," p. 199)
☐ Psychological Maladaptations
General Information

Postpartum depression occurs in some new mothers; physical as well as psychological symptoms may be evident; usually benign and self-limiting, but can last for years in most severe form

1. Definitions on continuum (see Table 4-26)
   a. *Postpartum blues:* mild and brief; originates 2-10 days after birth; affects up to 80% of new mothers
   b. *Atypical depression:* moderate and longer lasting; more disabling; affects 10% or more of new mothers
   c. *Psychosis:* severe and long-term risks of suicide and infanticide; affects 0.5%-3.0% of new mothers
2. Manifestations (see also *Elated-Depressive Behavior*, p. 44)
   a. Feelings of sadness, guilt, or irritation
   b. Tearfulness, crying
   c. Decreased energy, decision-making ability
   d. Insomnia
   e. Decreased appetite, anorexia
3. Theories of etiology
   a. Hormonal changes
   b. Fatigue, discomfort
   c. Immaturity
   d. Sensory deprivation or overload
   e. Nonsupportive environment

Nursing Process
Assessment
1. Behavioral and psychological responses (e.g., depression, anger, blues that persist)
2. Maladaptations in attachment
3. Delusions, hallucinations
Analysis (see p. 371)
Planning, Implementation, and Evaluation

> **Goal:** Client and family will recognize common postpartum psychological changes; client will be free from psychological maladaptation or psychosis postpartum; will seek medical care and will comply with treatment; will function adequately as a parent.

Implementation
1. Recognize early signs of problems.
2. Refer client to obstetrician to evaluate physiological status.
3. Support positive parenting behaviors.
4. Refer client to resource: psychiatrist, nurse psychotherapist, pediatrician, support group, public health nurse.
Evaluation
Client and family list expected emotional changes; report deviations in normal responses; client receives prompt treatment and support for maladaptive responses or psychosis; shows signs of attachment to newborn and increased feelings of self-worth.

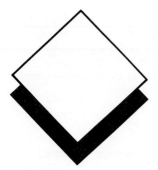

Newborn Care

THE NORMAL NEWBORN

1. Definition: full-term newborn
2. Gestational age: 38-41 weeks; between 10th and 90th percentiles on growth curves
3. A newborn may have a higher-than-normal risk of morbidity and mortality related to a maternal condition during the antepartal or intrapartal period (e.g., bleeding; poor nutritional status; maternal drug, smoking, and alcohol history; hypertension; infection; complications of labor and birth; and use of anesthetic/analgesic)
4. Risk of morbidity and mortality may also be increased; related to problems at birth or to the transition from intrauterine to extrauterine life

General Characteristics

1. Transition period
   a. Phase one: first period of reactivity
      1. birth through first 30 minutes
      2. awake, alert, active
      3. strong sucking reflex
      4. rapid and irregular respirations and heart rate
      5. falling body temperature
   b. Sleep period
   c. Phase two: second period of reactivity
      1. onset 4-8 hours after birth; variable duration in first 24 hours
      2. awakens; alert; mild cyanosis may occur
      3. frequent gagging with mucus regurgitation
      4. frequently passes first meconium stool
2. Stabilization with wakeful periods about every 3-4 hours
3. Behavior
   a. Sleeping and waking (Brazelton, 1973)
      1. individuality from birth: each normal newborn has unique, *usually predictable* behavioral responses in the first days of life
      2. state patterns
         a. pattern is a predictor of newborn's receptivity and cognitive response to stimuli
         b. sleep-wake states (alternate periods of physiological state and behavior)

- ◆ deep or light sleep states
- ◆ awake states
- ◆ drowsiness
- ◆ quiet alert (best for learning)
- ◆ active alert (high activity level)
- ◆ crying
      3. unique ability to "comfort" self by finger or thumbsucking (self-quieting) and to shut out stimuli (habituation)
   b. Sensory responses to environmental stimuli
      1. sight (response to visual stimulation)
         a. pupillary and blink reflexes present
         b. vision present; optimal range for visual acuity is 7-8 inches
         c. some degree of color and pattern discrimination: prefers complex stimuli
         d. can fixate and tract for short distance to midline
         e. focuses on human face
         f. prefers bright colors over black and white
      2. hearing (response to auditory stimulation)
         a. *in utero:* responds to music and to sound of mother's voice
         b. *in newborn:* within hours of birth, responds to sound by generalized activity depending on reactive state
            - ◆ loud sounds elicit Moro's reflex
            - ◆ prefers appealing sounds
      3. *taste:* response to feeding
         a. differentiates between sweet and bitter
         b. vigor of sucking may vary with arousal
      4. *smell:* response to olfactory stimulation
         a. present as soon as nose is cleared of mucus and amniotic fluid
         b. sensitive, discriminates (e.g., odor of mother's breast milk)
      5. *touch:* response to tactile stimulation
         a. well developed
         b. reacts to painful and soothing stimuli
4. Posture
   a. May assume prenatal position
   b. Assumes partially flexed position

c. Resists having extremities extended
5. Size (compared for length, weight, and weeks of gestation on growth curves)
   a. Length
      1. normal ranges 45-55 cm (18-22 inches)
      2. average: 50 cm (20 inches)
      3. rapid growth in first 6 months
   b. Weight
      1. normal range 2500-4000 g (5 lb 8 oz to 8 lb 13 oz)
      2. average weight 3400 g (7 lb 8 oz)
      3. 5%-10% of birth weight may be lost in first few days of life because of
         a. minimal intake of nutrients
         b. fluid shift
         c. loss of excess fluid (70% of newborn's body weight is fluid)
         d. passage of meconium
      4. regains birth weight within first 2 weeks
   c. Head circumference
      1. normal range 33-35 cm (13-14 inches)
      2. approximately 1-2 cm more than chest circumference
      3. essential assessment for suspected hydrocephalus
   d. Chest circumference
      1. normal range 30-32 cm (12-13 inches)
      2. shape and measurements change as newborn grows
   e. Symmetry
      1. face symmetrical
      2. ears symmetrical; placed opposite outer canthus of eyes
      3. bilateral, asynchronous movements of extremities
6. Vital signs
   a. Blood pressure: normal range 60-80/40-50 mm Hg
   b. Pulse: normal range 120-150/min (apical) if newborn is quiet
   c. Respirations
      1. normal range 30-50/min
      2. irregular and shallow
      3. diaphragmatic and abdominal breathing normal
   d. Temperature
      1. normal axillary range 36.5° C-37° C (97.6° F-98.6° F)
      2. temperature should stabilize within several hours of birth

Specific Body Parts: Usual Findings and Common Variations

1. Skin
   a. Texture: smooth, elastic
   b. Color
      1. pinkish or ruddy color over face and most of body
      2. color varies with ethnic background
   c. Erythema toxicum (newborn rash)
      1. pink papular rash anywhere on the body, appearing within 24-48 hours of birth
      2. harmless and disappears within a few days
      3. must be differentiated from rashes found in infections
   d. Localized cyanosis of extremities (acrocyanosis): peripheral circulation not well established
   e. Mottling (irregular discoloration of skin): resulting from vasoconstriction, lack of fat, and hypoxia
   f. Birthmarks (e.g., port-wine stain, strawberry) may or may not disappear with age, depending on type and location
   g. Vernix caseosa
      1. white, odorless, cheeselike substance on skin, usually found in folds of axillae, groin
      2. produced in utero; diminishes close to term
      3. is gradually absorbed or washed off after birth
   h. Lanugo
      1. fine, downy hair on shoulders, back, upper arms, forehead, and cheeks
      2. gradually disappears close to term
   i. Desquamation
      1. dry peeling of skin, particularly on palms and soles
      2. requires no treatment
      3. more pronounced in postmature newborn
   j. Milia
      1. pinpoint white papules on cheeks, across bridge of nose, or on chin; caused by blocked sebaceous glands
      2. require no treatment
      3. disappear in a few weeks
   k. Nevi (stork bite): red spots found on back of neck and eyelids; usually disappear spontaneously between first and second years of life
   l. Mongolian spots: areas of grayish-blue pigmentation most often found on buttocks and sacrum; increased frequency in specific racial groups; may disappear by school age
   m. Physiological jaundice (icterus neonatorum)
      1. yellowish discoloration of newborn skin/sclera often appearing 48-72 hours after birth (refer to "Neonatal Jaundice," p. 388)
      2. is common and appears in 50%-70% of newborns
      3. disappears in 7-10 days
2. Head
   a. Appears round and symmetrical; full movement to right and left, up and down; may be covered by silky hair in varying amounts

b. Molding: the shaping of the fetal head to accommodate passage through the birth canal as a result of overriding of the cranial bones; the head will return to its normal shape in about 2-3 days

c. Cephalhematoma: a collection of blood between the periosteum and the bone of the skull
1. caused by rupture of blood vessels from pressure during the birth process
2. swelling usually severe but does not cross suture lines
3. spontaneously resolves in 3-6 weeks

d. Caput succedaneum
1. localized, edematous area of the scalp, usually caused by birth process
2. extends across suture lines
3. is absorbed and disappears in 3-4 days

e. Fontanels (soft spots) (Fig. 4-20)
1. anterior
a. diamond shaped, palpable
b. 3-4 cm long, 2-3 cm wide
c. found between frontal and parietal bones
d. closes within 18 months
2. posterior
a. triangular, usually palpable
b. 1-2 cm
c. found between occipital and parietal bones
d. closes within 3 months

3. Eyes
a. Appearance
1. blue or grey-blue
2. bright and clear
3. pupils equal in size
4. eyes evenly placed on face
5. lacrimation in 50% of neonates not evident until 2-4 weeks old

b. Movement
1. to all directions
2. poor neuromuscular control

c. Common variations
1. subconjunctival hemorrhage: red spot on sclera, rupture of small capillaries during delivery; will be absorbed in about 2 weeks
2. chemical conjunctivitis: inflammation with discharge, resulting from reaction of silver nitrate or other chemical agents (must be differentiated from infectious process)

d. Vision (refer to "Sensory Responses," p. 376)

4. Mouth
a. Lips: appear equal on both sides of facial midline; symmetry of movement
b. Tongue
1. in midline; moves freely in all directions
2. size proportional to mouth
3. color pink (varies with ethnic group); white, cheesy coating may indicate thrush (related to maternal candidal vaginal infection)

c. Palate: intact
d. Epstein's pearls: small epithelial cysts on hard palate or gums; will disappear in 1-2 weeks
e. Saliva: small quantity present

5. Ears
a. Well-formed cartilage by term; recoil rapidly; may be flattened against skull because of pressure during birth

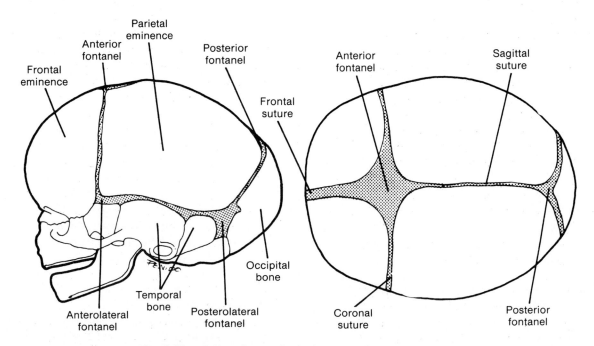

Fig. 4-20 Bones, fontanels, and sutures of newborn's skull.

b. Placement: same level and position on both sides of head (low-set ears are associated with trisomy 13 or 18 and renal agenesis)

c. Hearing: refer to "Sensory Responses," p. 376

6. Nose

a. Shape: varies; may appear flattened because of delivery process

b. Placement: evenly placed in relation to eyes and mouth

c. Nares: bilateral patency; newborns are nose-breathers

d. Sneezing common

7. Neck

a. Appears short; head moves freely

b. Skin folds present; no webbing

8. Chest

a. Shoulders: sloping; width greater than length

b. Chest movements: bilateral expansion equal with respiration; no retractions

c. Breath sounds: loud and equal bilaterally; clear on crying

d. Cough reflex: absent; appears by second or third day of life

e. Heart: rhythm regular, normal rate; usually heard to left of midclavicular space at third or fourth interspace; may have functional murmurs (refer to p. 377 for normal vital-sign values)

f. Breasts

1. flat; nipples symmetrical; breast-tissue diameter greater than 5 mm

2. breast engorgement common in both sexes; occurs by third day of life and may last up to 2 weeks; may have some nipple discharge resulting from maternal hormonal influence in utero and subsequent withdrawal after birth

9. Abdomen

a. Prominent: cylindrical; movements synchronous with respirations

b. Umbilical cord stump

1. two arteries and one vein apparent at birth, surrounded by Wharton's jelly

2. cord begins drying within 1-2 hours after birth, shed by 7-10 days after birth

3. protrusion of umbilicus often apparent in black newborns; assess for umbilical hernia

c. Diastasis recti (separation of rectus muscles): common in black or preterm neonates

d. Bowel sounds: audible

e. Femoral pulses: palpable and equal bilaterally

10. Genitalia

a. Female

1. labia majora cover labia minora; symmetrical, slightly edematous

2. clitoris enlarged

3. vaginal tag (hymen) may be evident

4. a mucoid, vaginal discharge is common

5. pseudomenstruation: blood-tinged discharge is normal

6. some vernix caseosa may be between labia

b. Male

1. urethral meatus evident at tip of penis

2. foreskin covers glans; prepuce not easily retractable

3. extensive rugae on scrotum

4. testes descended and palpable bilaterally in scrotal sac; if not, check inguinal, femoral, or abdominal areas for undescended testes

11. Buttocks and anus

a. Buttocks: symmetrical; anus patent

b. Gluteal folds: symmetrical

12. Extremities and trunk

a. Muscle tone: good

b. Position: extremities slightly flexed

c. Arms and legs: arms equal in length; legs equal in length; legs shorter than arms

d. Five digits on each hand and foot; freely movable, nails present

e. Normal palmar crease (simian line indicative of Down syndrome)

f. Spine: straight and flat (prone position)

g. Fat pads and creases covering soles of infant's feet

Systems Adaptations

1. Neuromuscular: normal neonatal reflexes

a. Sucking: newborn's tendency to suck any object that comes in contact with lips; essential for nutritional intake, oral satisfaction; begins to disappear at 12 months

b. Rooting: newborn's tendency to turn head in direction of stimulus and open lips to suck when object touches cheek or mouth; disappears at 7 months

c. Spontaneous reflexes

1. swallowing: usually follows sucking

2. gagging: lifelong reflex

3. yawning

4. stretching

5. sneezing

6. hiccoughing

d. Moro: newborn's tendency to symmetrically extend both arms and legs and then draw them up in normal flexed position in response to sudden movement or loud noise; most significant reflex indicative of CNS status; disappears by 6 months

e. Grasp

1. palmar grasp; newborn's tendency to grasp an examiner's finger when palm is stimulated; lessens at 3-4 months

2. plantar grasp: newborn's tendency to curl toes downward when sole of foot is stimulated; lessens at 8 months

f. Tonic neck: newborn's tendency to assume a fencer's position when head is turned to one side; the extremities on the same side extend, while flexion occurs on opposite side; response sometimes more dominant in leg than arm; disappears at 3-4 months

g. Stepping or walking: newborn's tendency when held upright to take steps in response to feet touching a hard surface; disappears at 4 weeks

h. Babinski's: newborn's tendency to hyperextend toes with dorsiflexion of big toe when one side of sole is stimulated from heel upward across ball of foot; disappears at 1 year

i. Motor function: head may be maintained erect for short periods of time; head lag less than 45°; movement of extremities may be jerky

2. Cardiorespiratory
   a. Circulatory adaptations occurring after birth and ligation of umbilical cord (Fig. 4-21)
      1. closure of ductus arteriosus, foramen ovale, and ductus venosus
         a. caused by changes in pressure in the first days of life
         b. allows oxygenation of all body systems
      2. closure of umbilical vessels after clamping of cord
   b. Pulses (reflect systemic circulation)
      1. femoral, brachial; easily palpable
      2. radial, temporal; more difficult to palpate
   c. Respirations
      1. initiation of respirations
         a. first breath; inflation of lungs in response to increased P_{CO_2} and lower pH
         b. reduction of pulmonary-vascular resistance
         c. increased pulmonary blood flow
         d. recoil of chest causing replacement of fluids
         e. surfactant reduces alveolar surface tension
      2. respiratory secretions may be abundant
      3. may be irregular with short periods of apnea
   d. Blood pressure
      1. highest immediately after birth; at lowest level at 3 hours
      2. crying and moving cause changes in BP (up to 20 mm Hg)

3. Hematological
   a. Blood values (venous samples): average ranges for a normal, full-term newborn

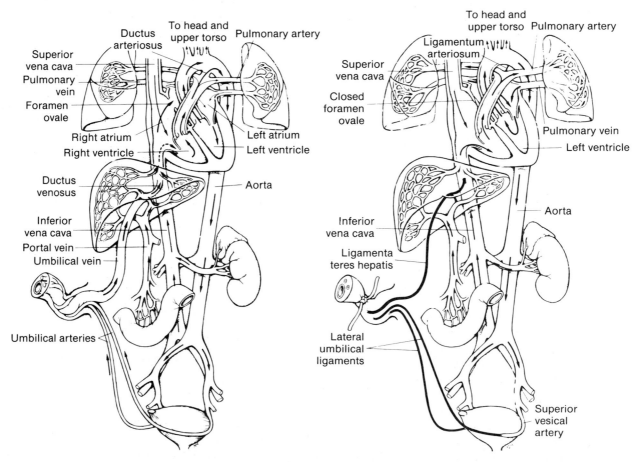

Fig. 4-21 Fetal circulation.

1. hemoglobin: 14-20 g/dL (reflects oxygenation of tissues); broken down to bilirubin
2. hematocrit: 42%-61%
3. RBC: 5-7.5 million/mm^3
4. WBC: approximately 20,000/mm^3 (10,000-30,000/mm^3)
5. platelets: 100,000-280,000
6. blood volume: 78-98 ml/kg depending on cord clamping

  b. Leukocytosis: normal; related to birth trauma
  c. Fetal RBCs: have short life (80-100 days); hemolyzed RBCs deposit bilirubin in body tissues
  d. Neonatal jaundice (physiological jaundice): common in 50% of newborns on second or third day of life because of deposits of bilirubin
  e. Coagulation
    1. inability to synthesize vitamin K because of absence of intestinal flora normal in older people
    2. supplementary injection of vitamin K (e.g., AquaMEPHYTON, given prophylactically to promote normal clotting)

4. Thermoregulation (temperature regulation)
  a. Adaptive factors
    1. newborn responds to cold with increased motor activity and restlessness
    2. increased metabolism compensates for cold stress, since newborn does not shiver
    3. brown fat (or brown adipose tissue) is the newborn's major source of thermogenesis (2%-6% of body weight) (located between scapulae, around kidneys, sternum, adrenals, and in the axillae); reserves are rapidly depleted with cold stress
  b. Heat loss: disproportionate to adult because of large skin surface to body mass; mechanisms of heat loss include
    1. *convection:* loss of heat from body surface to cooler surrounding air (e.g., newborn placed in cool incubator)
    2. *evaporation:* loss of heat from body occurring when fluid converts to vapor (e.g., wet newborn loses heat immediately after birth in delivery room)
    3. *conduction:* transfer of heat from warm object to a cooler surface (e.g., newborn placed on a cold object)
    4. *radiation:* indirect transfer of heat from a warmer object to a cooler one (e.g., newborn loses heat to cool wall of incubator)

5. Elimination (gastrointestinal and renal)
  a. Stools: change according to feeding
    1. meconium stool: viscous, dark-green or black; formed of mucus, vernix, lanugo, hormones, carbohydrates; first one usually passed within 24-48 hours (if no stool passed, assess for imperforate anus, intestinal obstruction)
    2. second to sixth day, transition stools: loose, green-brown, seedy
    3. breastfed newborns: golden-yellow, mushy stools, often after each feeding
    4. bottlefed newborns: soft, yellow-brown stools; more formed; 4-6/day
  b. Stomach capacity: 50-60 ml; empties in about 3 hours
  c. Urination: newborn usually urinates in first 24 hours; if newborn unable to void, assess for fluid intake and distension
    1. frequency: initially 6-10/day, then up to 20/day
    2. color: pale yellow (immature kidneys cannot concentrate); may appear cloudy if decreased fluid intake
    3. uric acid excretion is high; appears as red spots on diaper ("brick spots")

6. Immunological
  a. In utero: full-term fetus has had IgG (immunoglobulins) transferred; maternal antibodies may be present (depending on mother's immunity) for tetanus, diphtheria, pertussis, measles, mumps, rubella
  b. At birth: immunological system immature
    1. capable of some antibody response to immunizing agents
    2. phagocytosis ineffective
    3. cannot localize infection or respond with a well-defined, recognizable inflammatory response, as can older child
    4. breast milk: contains IgA; gives immunological protection from some infections
    5. elevated temperature may not reflect infection in newborn

7. Nutrition
  a. Sucks, swallows, and digests feedings; these reflexes may be weak in premature infants
  b. Digestion
    1. unable to digest complete carbohydrates because of insufficient quantities of amylase
    2. can absorb simple carbohydrates and protein
    3. fat absorption poor because of insufficient lipase
  c. Regurgitation is common
    1. cardiac sphincter is immature, nervous control of stomach incomplete
    2. newborns often spit up mucus in first 24 hours after birth
  d. Blood sugar normally 30-50 mg/dl (full term)
  e. Benefits from immunoglobulins, enzymes, and lactobacilli in breast milk
  f. Psychological factors
    1. both bottlefeeding and breastfeeding can be satisfying

Estimation of Gestational Age by Maturity Rating
Symbols: X–1st Exam   O–2nd Exam

Neuromuscular Maturity

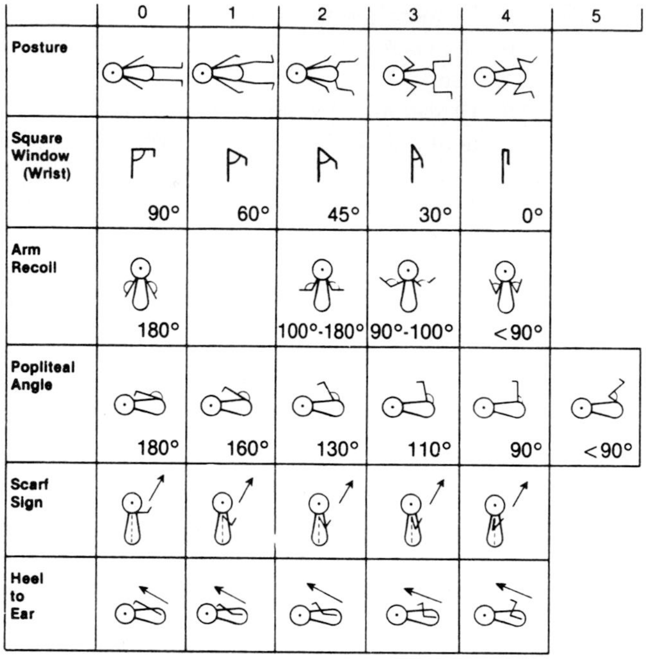

	0	1	2	3	4	5
Posture						
Square Window (Wrist)	90°	60°	45°	30°	0°	
Arm Recoil	180°		100°-180°	90°-100°	<90°	
Popliteal Angle	180°	160°	130°	110°	90°	<90°
Scarf Sign						
Heel to Ear						

Gestation by Dates _____ wks

Birth Date_____ Hour_____ am / pm
APGAR _____ 1 min _____ 5 min
Weight _____   Length _____
    Head _____   Chest _____

Maturity Rating

Score	Wks
5	26
10	28
15	30
20	32
25	34
30	36
35	38
40	40
45	42
50	44

Physical Maturity

	0	1	2	3	4	5
Skin	gelatinous red, transparent	smooth pink, visible veins	superficial peeling &/or rash, few veins	cracking pale area, rare veins	parchment, deep cracking, no vessels	leathery, cracked, wrinkled
Lanugo	none	abundant	thinning	bald areas	mostly bald	
Plantar Creases	no crease	faint red marks	anterior transverse crease only	creases ant. 2/3	creases cover entire sole	
Breast	barely percept.	flat areola, no bud	stippled areola, 1-2 mm bud	raised areola, 3-4 mm bud	full areola 5-10 mm bud	
Ear	pinna flat, stays folded	sl. curved pinna, soft with slow recoil	well-curv. pinna, soft but ready recoil	formed & firm with instant recoil	thick cartilage, ear stiff	
Genitals Male	scrotum empty, no rugae		testes descending, few rugae	testes down, good rugae	testes pendulous, deep rugae	
Genitals Female	prominent clitoris & labia minora		majora & minora equally prominent	majora large, minora small	clitoris & minora completely covered	

Scoring Section

	1st Exam = X	2nd Exam = O
Estimating Gest. Age by Maturity Rating	_____ Weeks	_____ Weeks
Time of Exam	Date _____ Hour_____ am/pm	Date _____ Hour_____ am/pm
Age at Exam	_____ Hours	_____ Hours
Signature of Examiner	_____ M.D.	_____ M.D.

Fig. 4-22   Newborn maturity rating and classification. (From Mead Johnson & Co., Evansville, Indiana. Scoring section adapted from Ballard, J.L., [1977]. *Pediatric Research* 11:374. Figures modified from Sweet, A.Y.: *Classification of the low-birth weight infant.* In Klaus, M.H., & Fanaroff, A.A. [1977]. *Care of the high-risk infant,* Philadelphia: W.B. Saunders Co.)

Table 4-27 Nutritional comparison of human and cow's milk

Nutrients	Amounts per liter		
	Human milk (breast)	Cow's milk* (whole)	Common formulas†
Protein (g)	10.12	32‡	15
Carbohydrate (g)	67.82§	45.4	72
Lipid	43.12	35.7	36
Calories	684.00	626.0	640

*Not given to newborns.
†Examples are Similac, Enfamil.
‡Because of the higher percentage of protein, cow's milk must be diluted to avoid kidney overload.
§Breast milk is higher in lactose, which limits pathogenic growth.

2. attachment facilitated by breastfeeding
3. stress can inhibit successful breastfeeding
g. Initial feedings: breast milk or sterile water given 4-6 hours after birth to assess sucking reflex and absence of structural anomalies
h. Subsequent feedings
   1. bottlefed newborns: q3-4h or on demand
   2. breastfed newborns: q2-3h or on demand
i. Fluid needs vary with age and size of newborn; average intake of 17½ oz/day for 7-lb baby
j. Calories: 80-120 cal/kg/day (birth to 5 months); most commercial formulas contain 20 calories/oz (see Table 4-27)

Gestational Age Variations Based on Neuromuscular Responses and External Physical Characteristics (see Fig. 4-22)

1. Premature newborn
   a. Definition: born before 38 weeks' gestation, regardless of birth weight
   b. Etiology: associated with chronic hypertensive disease, toxemia, placenta previa, abruptio placentae, incompetent cervix, infections, smoking, multiple gestation, inadequate maternal nutrition, maternal age under 20; premature rupture of membranes
   c. General appearance: will vary with gestational age
      1. head large in proportion to body
      2. transparent appearance to skin
      3. lack of subcutaneous fat
      4. excessive lanugo
      5. immature neurological system
      6. minimal flexion of extremities
      7. fontanels large; sutures prominent
   d. Associated problems (see Table 4-28)
      1. *high mortality rate*
      2. *respiratory distress syndrome* (RDS), related to immaturity of lungs and deficiency of surfactant (NOTE: L/S ratio determined by amniocentesis is helpful before delivery to determine lung maturity)
      3. *infection:* low WBC count, increased polymorphonuclear cells

4. *feeding problems*
   a. regurgitates food easily
   b. may aspirate because of weak or absent suck-swallow reflexes
   c. may require gavage feedings
   d. breast milk or 24-calorie/ml formula advised
5. *hypoglycemia* (glucose less than 20 mg/dl), caused by decreased glycogen and fat stores, decreased glyconeogenesis
6. *hypothermia* and cold stress, owing to poor temperature control, increased surface area for cooling, extension of extremities, lack of brown fat
7. *jaundice* because of impaired bilirubin conjugation in liver
8. *intracranial hemorrhage,* related to birth trauma or hypoxia after birth
9. *apnea,* related to fatigue or immaturity of respiratory mechanism
10. *oxygen therapy complications:* retrolental fibroplasia, bronchopulmonary dysplasia (alveolar-bronchial necrosis)

2. Postmature newborn
   a. Definition: born after 42 weeks of gestation (specific reference to potential intrauterine growth retardation)
   b. General appearance: related to advanced gestational age and placental insufficiency
      1. thin, long newborn
      2. dry, parchmentlike skin
      3. decreased or absent vernix
      4. little subcutaneous tissue; loose skin
      5. meconium staining of amniotic fluid (nails and skin stained yellow) related to hypoxia
      6. lanugo absent
      7. alert, wide-eyed (sign of hypoxia)
      8. nails lengthened
   c. Associated problems: higher morbidity and mortality (see Table 4-28)
      1. *hypoxia:* may be related to placental insufficiency

Table 4-28   High-risk conditions for newborns by gestational age and growth classifications

Growth class	Gestational age		
	SGA	Average	LGA
PRETERM			
Apnea of prematurity	X	X	X
Brain damage	X		
Congenital abnormalities	X	X	X
Hyperbilirubinemia	X	X	X
Hypoglycemia	X	X	X
Infection	X	X	X
Intracranial hemorrhage	X	X	X
Meconium aspiration	X		
Neonatal asphyxia	X		
Polycythemia	X		X
Pulmonary hemorrhage	X		
Respiratory distress syndrome	X	X	X
Temperature instability	X	X	X
TERM			
Brain damage	X		
Birth injuries			X
Congenital abnormalities	X		X
Hypoglycemia	X		X
Polycythemia	X		X
Infection	X		
Meconium aspiration	X		
Neonatal asphyxia	X		
Pulmonary hemorrhage	X		
Temperature instability	X		
POSTTERM			
Brain damage	X	X	X
Congenital abnormalities	X		X
Hypoglycemia	X		X
Infection	X		
Meconium aspiration	X	X	X
Neonatal asphyxia	X	X	X
Polycythemia	X	X	X
Pulmonary hemorrhage	X		
Temperature instability	X		

2. *hypoglycemia:* caused by decreased glycogen stores
3. *postmaturity syndrome* with intrauterine asphyxia and fetal distress
4. *polycythemia:* response to hypoxia
5. *seizure disorders:* related to hypoxia (chronic)
6. *cold stress* related to minimal subcutaneous fat
7. *meconium aspiration*

3. Small-for-gestational-age (SGA) newborn
 a. Definition: significantly underweight for gestational age (i.e., birth weight at or below the 10th percentile on intrauterine growth Denver curve); also known as intrauterine-growth-retardation or small-for-dates newborn
 b. Etiology: associated with maternal malnutrition,

pregnancy-induced hypertension, diabetes, drug addiction, alcoholism, smoking, maternal viral infections, prescribed or over-the-counter drugs, placental abnormalities or acute hypoxia, and other conditions affecting uteroplacental sufficiency
 c. General appearance
 1. little subcutaneous tissue
 2. loose, dry skin
 3. loss of muscle mass in trunk and extremities
 4. desquamation
 5. length often normal, yet weight decreased
 6. polycythemia: may be related to intrauterine hypoxia
 7. meconium staining of nails, skin

Table 4-29   Apgar scoring chart

	Score		
Sign	**0**	**1**	**2**
Heart rate	Absent	slow (below 100 beats/min)	Over 100 beats/min
Respiratory effort	Absent	Slow, irregular, weak cry	Good, strong cry
Muscle tone	Flaccid	Some flexion of extremities	Well flexed
Reflex irritability			
catheter in nostril	No response	Grimace	Cough or sneeze
slap to sole of foot	No response	Grimace	Cry and withdrawal of foot
Color	Blue, pale	Body pink, extremities blue	Completely pink

        8. appears alert because of hypoxia
   d. Associated problems (see Table 4-28)
      1. *intrauterine infection* if exposed to organisms while in utero
      2. *asphyxia at birth:* associated with intrauterine hypoxia
      3. *hypoglycemia:* caused by decreased glycogen stores and decreased glyconeogenesis (increased metabolic rate resulting from heat loss)
      4. *hypothermia:* related to decreased subcutaneous tissue and fat and poor thermal regulation
      5. *congenital anomalies* (10-20 times more frequent)
      6. *respiratory distress:* often follows perinatal asphyxia
      7. *hypocalcemia:* may be related to asphyxia and respiratory diseases
      8. *meconium aspiration:* subsequent possible minimal brain dysfunction
4. Large-for-gestational age (LGA) newborn
   a. Definition: significantly overweight for gestational age (birth weight at or above 90th percentile on intrauterine growth curve; usually over 9 lb 15 oz)
   b. Etiology: unclear; may be genetic predisposition associated with multiparity and maternal diabetes
   c. General appearance
      1. fat and puffy
      2. may be edematous
      3. poor muscle tone
   d. Associated problems (see Table 4-28)
      1. *birth trauma* because of CPD
      2. *hypoglycemia* related to lack of maternal glucose (after birth)
      3. *hypocalcemia*
      4. *polycythemia*
      5. *congenital birth defects*

Application of the Nursing Process to the Normal Newborn

Assessment
1. Immediate (in delivery room, birthing room, or other setting)

   a. Airway
      1. patency
      2. secretions: may contain mucus, blood, and amniotic fluid
   b. Apgar score: provides index of infant's initial condition at 1 minute and baseline for subsequent assessment at 5 minutes; the 5-minute score is the better indicator of adaptation (see Table 4-29)
      1. 0-2: severe asphyxia, extremely poor condition
      2. 3-6: mild to moderate asphyxia, fair condition
      3. 7-10: very mild or no distress, good condition
   c. Gross appearance: appears to be free from obvious birth defects
   d. Umbilical cord
      1. early clamping: less possibility of placental transfusion
      2. late clamping: expansion of newborn's blood volume, high systolic BP, higher Hgb
      3. blood vessels: two arteries, one vein
2. Ongoing
   a. Vital signs
   b. Passage of meconium and/or urine
   c. Umbilical cord
   d. Tracheoesophageal fistula or esophageal atresia, manifested by
      1. cyanosis during feeding
      2. immediate regurgitation
      3. inability to swallow feeding
   e. Parent-infant bonding

Analysis
1. Safe, effective care environment
   a. High risk for injury
   b. High risk for infection
2. Physiological integrity
   a. Decreased cardiac output
   b. Impaired gas exchange
   c. Ineffective airway clearance
   d. High risk for altered nutrition: less than body requirements
   e. Ineffective thermoregulation
3. Psychosocial integrity
   a. Anxiety (parental)
   b. Parental role conflict

4. Health promotion/maintenance
   a. Effective breastfeeding
   b. Knowledge deficit

Planning, Implementation, and Evaluation

> **Goal 1:** Newborn will adapt successfully to extrauterine life during the immediate period following birth; will have early contact with mother/father.

Implementation
1. Facilitate the immediate establishment of respiration.
   a. Clear air passages before onset of respirations (suction with DeLee or bulb syringe).
   b. Provide gentle tactile stimulation that aids breathing.
   c. Assist physician with resuscitation as necessary (ratio of heartbeat to respiratory ventilation rate is 5:1).
2. Prevent hypothermia: maintain newborn's body temperature and minimize heat loss; metabolic rate and O_2 consumption are minimized.
   a. Dry rapidly.
   b. Place on mother's skin, in warmed Isolette, under radiant heater, or in warm blanket.
   c. Leboyer or admission bath may be given when temperature becomes stable.
3. Provide prophylactic treatment of eyes with a 1% silver nitrate or other antibacterial agent such as erythromycin (0.5%) for protection against opthalmia neonatorum, which may be caused by gonococcal or chlamydial infection.
4. Promote bonding/attachment.
5. Place appropriate identification bands on newborn and mother; footprint may be taken.
6. Weigh and measure newborn.
7. Administer a single dose of vitamin K IM, as ordered, to prevent hypoprothrombinemia.
8. Send cord blood to lab as ordered.

Evaluation
Newborn maintains adequate oxygenation, breathes normally; maintains body temperature; is held by parent.

> **Goal 2:** Newborn will continue to maintain homeostasis free from respiratory, cardiovascular, nutritional, and elimination difficulties.

Implementation
1. Check identification on admission to nursery.
2. Monitor newborn's condition (frequency of assessment determined by condition).
   a. Assess apical pulse and respiration for 1 full minute.
   b. Note periods of apnea (should not exceed 20 seconds).
   c. Use suction if mucus is excessive.
   d. Position on side to promote drainage, especially after feedings.
   e. Observe skin, sclera, mucosa color (jaundice or cyanosis).
   f. Observe for respiratory changes or fatigue during feedings.
   g. Maintain adequate nutrition by assisting new mother with bottle feeding or breastfeeding.
3. Note time of first urination and passage of meconium; then monitor elimination.
4. Weigh daily or every other day and record on chart; newborn may take up to 10 days to regain birth weight after initial 5%-10% loss.
5. Obtain blood sample for phenylketonuria (PKU) (Guthrie test).
   a. A recessive hereditary disorder characterized by deficiency in the liver enzyme phenylalanine hydroxylase that is needed for conversion of phenylalanine into tyrosine
   b. Leads to mental retardation if undetected
   c. Newborn must have protein feedings 24-48 hours before test; with early discharge, parents must bring newborn back to lab for blood test in 2 days
   NOTE: in some states, screening for hypothyroidism and other metabolic tests may be required.

Evaluation
Newborn has vital signs within normal range; ingests nutritional fluids appropriate for size; voids and passes meconium.

> **Goal 3:** Newborn will remain infection free.

Implementation
1. Prevent infections from developing in newborn and spreading within nursery and mother-baby unit.
   a. Use proper hand-washing and scrub techniques to prevent staff-to-newborn and newborn-to-newborn infections.
   b. Exclude personnel with known infections from caring for newborns.
   c. Instruct parents about importance of handwashing and proper technique.
   d. Isolate newborns with any signs of infection or risk.
   e. Assess/clean newborn's cord daily with alcohol and a designated antibacterial agent.
2. Bathe newborn and maintain newborn's personal hygiene.
   a. Use plain water on face and mild soap on body for daily care.
   b. Proceed from clean to dirty areas (i.e., eyes to face to genitals).
3. Assess condition of circumcised penis: keep clean and observe for bleeding; a sterile petroleum jelly or antibiotic ointment may be applied uring first 24 hours; check for voiding

NOTE: currently, pediatricians discourage routine circumcision for health/medical reasons; cultural/religious practices should be considered in decision making.

Evaluation

Newborn has normal temperature; no signs of infection; is protected from exposure to infectious agents.

> **Goal 4:** Parents will verbalize an understanding of principles and techniques of newborn care; will demonstrate proper, safe care and feeding.

Implementation

1. Assess parents' knowledge and past experience with child care.
2. Offer modified or complete rooming-in.
3. Encourage new parent's involvement in newborn care (to foster bonding/attachment).
4. Demonstrate techniques of bathing and daily care.
   a. Emphasize safety and asepsis.
   b. Suggest timing of care (before feeding).
   c. Teach cord care.
   d. Emphasize frequent cleansing of diaper area to prevent rash.
5. Allow mother to give care in hospital.
6. Reinforce knowledge of caregiving.
7. Discuss the importance of touch and stimulation in developing trust.
8. Reinforce knowledge of feeding.
   a. Benefits of breastfeeding vs. bottle feeding (should be discussed in antepartal classes)
   b. Frequency of nursing (every 2-3 hours on demand)
   c. Length of nursing time (newborn obtains greatest quantity in 20-25 minutes)
   d. Importance of emptying breasts
   e. Position of newborn for nursing
   f. Common feeding problems (e.g., burping, regurgitation, constipation, hiccoughs)
   g. Position on side or abdomen after feeding

Evaluation

Parents demonstrate correct feeding, bathing, holding, and daily care of newborn.

> **Goal 5:** Parents will know what to expect at home regarding newborn's behavior, sleep patterns, stools, weight gain, feeding; will verbalize an understanding of reportable problems; will discuss adjustments of siblings.

Implementation

NOTE: criteria for discharge teaching vary with gestational age, weight, early discharge, general health status of newborn and mother, home environment, ages of siblings, and available resources.

1. Share common characteristics/variations of newborns.
2. Identify unique characteristics of newborn with parents and siblings.
3. Counsel on breastfeeding or formula preparation at home.
   a. Discuss common concerns (sore nipples, supplementary feedings, expression of milk).
   b. Review methods of formula preparation, care of bottles and nipples (aseptic and terminal methods, dishwashing).
   c. Discuss bottle-fed newborn's daily needs: intake approximately 3 oz, 6 times/day initially.
   d. Delay solids until 6 months.
   e. Avoid cow's milk until 12 months.
4. Discuss expected weight gain (birth weight doubles by 5-6 months, triples by 1 year).
5. Counsel on sibling adjustments to newborn.
6. Discuss newborn behavior and development in discharge teaching.
   a. Sleep needs: average 20 hr/day with wide variations; intermittent alertness
   b. Crying: newborn's method of communicating basic needs
   c. Discuss plans for health-care follow-up of newborn (with clinic, physician, or nurse practitioner)
   d. Refer to resource such as the community health nurse for assistance
   e. Teach *reportable signs* of problems (e.g., constipation, diarrhea, fever, vomiting, and behavioral changes)

Evaluation

Parents demonstrate knowledge of correct newborn care; describe adequate equipment for home care; express confidence in ability to care for newborn; list reportable signs; discuss plans for dealing with sibling adjustments.

Application of the Nursing Process to the Newborn at Risk

Assessment

1. Maternal risk factors
2. Actual/potential problems identified during fetal life
3. Immediate adaptation to extrauterine life
4. Actual/potential problems noted after birth

Analysis

1. Safe, effective care environment
   a. High risk for injury
   b. High risk for infection
2. Physiological integrity
   a. Impaired gas exchange
   b. Ineffective airway clearance
   c. High risk for altered nutrition; less than body requirements
   d. Ineffective thermoregulation
3. Psychological integrity
   a. Anxiety (parental)
   b. Altered role performance
4. Health promotion/maintenance

a. High risk for ineffective family coping

b. Knowledge deficit

Planning, Implementation, and Evaluation

Goal: Newborn will be free from undetected problems; will have problems treated immediately and will maintain physiological integrity. Family will comply with teaching for health maintenance and promotion.

Implementation

1. Perform ongoing assessment.
2. Notify physician of problems/changes in status.
3. Document altered condition.
4. Implement specific therapy as ordered.
5. Share information with family.
6. Maintain a safe environment.
7. Promote asepsis.
8. Teach parents specific care for problem.

Evaluation

Newborn has problems detected and treated immediately; has homeostasis maintained. Family complies with recommended follow-up care.

SELECTED HEALTH PROBLEMS IN THE NEWBORN

☐ Hypothermia

General Information

1. Definition: a drop in the newborn's body temperature below 36.5° C (97.7° F), produced by rapid heat loss to the environment. All newborns are at risk for heat loss because of their limited subcutaneous fat and large surface area in relation to body weight
2. Predisposing factors
   a. Newborns with reduced stores of subcutaneous fat (e.g., premature, postmature, SGA newborns)
   b. Newborns with reduced glycogen reserves (e.g., premature, nutritionally deprived, SGA newborns)

Nursing Process

Assessment

1. Newborn's body temperature
2. Signs of cold stress
   a. Increased activity level
   b. Crying
   c. Increased respiratory rate
   d. Cyanosis
   e. Mottling of skin

Analysis (see p. 387)

Planning, Implementation, and Evaluation

Goal: Newborn will expend a minimum amount of extra energy in the production of heat; will be free from periods of hypothermia.

Implementation

1. Prevent heat loss in delivery room (refer to Goal 1, p. 386.
2. Administer warmed air or O$_2$ to newborn prn.
3. Monitor newborn's temperature frequently; maintain axillary temperature at 36.5° C (97.8° F), abdominal skin temperature at 36.1° C-36.7° C (97° F-98° F).
4. Place crib or incubator away from draft and windows.
5. Keep portholes of incubator/Isolette closed.

Evaluation

Newborn maintains a skin temperature of 36.1° C-36.7° C.

☐ Neonatal Jaundice
General Information

1. Definition: excessive levels of bilirubin in the blood and tissues of the newborn (bilirubin is a product derived from the breakdown of erthryocytes and hemoglobin)
2. Expected levels of serum bilirubin (in mg/dl)
   a. *Full term*
      1. day 1: 2-6
      2. day 2: 6-7
      3. days 3-5: 4-12
   b. *Premature*
      1. day 1: 1-6
      2. day 2: 6-8
      3. days 3-5: 10-15
3. Predisposing factors
   a. Prematurity
   b. Isoimmunizations: maternal red blood cell–destroying antibodies are transferred to the fetus, resulting in fetal erythrocyte destruction; after initial maternal sensitization occurs, the effects upon subsequent pregnancies with blood incompatibilities increase in severity
      1. Rh-negative mother and Rh-positive father may produce an Rh-positive fetus; this leads to antigen-antibody response affecting subsequent fetus
      2. mother with type O blood and father (see Fig. 4-23) with type A, B, or AB produce a fetus with type A, B, or AB (generally results in less severe disease than Rh incompatibility)
   c. Polycythemia
   d. Exposure to drugs in utero
   e. Sepsis
4. Common forms
   a. Physiological jaundice
      1. onset
         a. full-term newborn: jaundice appears after 24 hours and disappears by end of seventh day
         b. preterm newborn: jaundice appears after 48 hours and disappears by ninth or tenth day
      2. lab values

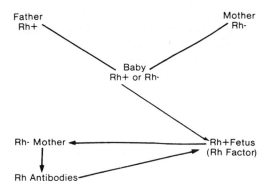

Fig. 4-23   Rh sensitization.

a. bilirubin is unconjugated (indirect); below 6 mg/dl, and newborn is without evidence of hemolytic disease or infection
b. RBCs and WBCs are normal

b. Pathological jaundice (hyperbilirubinemia)
1. onset: occurs within first 24 hours after birth
2. lab values: characterized by rising bilirubin level in excess of normal
   a. in full-term newborn: rises 6 mg/dl in 24 hours or value exceeds 12 mg/dl or persists beyond 7 days
   b. in premature newborn: exceeds 15 mg/dl; persists beyond 10 days
   c. direct bilirubin greater than 1.0 mg/dl
3. severe sequela is kernicterus (deposit of unconjugated bilirubin in basal ganglia of brain) when bilirubin levels rise over 20 mg/dl in full-term newborns and over 9-10 mg/dl in preterm newborns; signs and symptoms include
   a. lack of interest in feeding
   b. sluggish Moro's reflex wtih incomplete flexion of extremities
   c. opisthotonic posturing
   d. vomiting
   e. bulging fontanels
   f. twitching convulsions (late symptom)

c. Breast milk jaundice: yellowing of newborn's skin caused by high concentration of enzyme lipoprotein lipase, which breaks down lipids to form free fatty acids and glycerol; increasing the amount of free fatty acids is thought to inhibit conjugation of bilirubin; may affect 1%-2% of breastfed newborns
1. onset: after mature milk is secreted; 48-96 hours after delivery
2. lab values: bilirubin level begins to rise on about fourth day, peaks at 10-15 days of age, returning to normal between 3 and 12 weeks of age

5. Associated problems

a. Hydrops fetalis (erythroblastosis fetalis) related to Rh or ABO incompatibility: generalized edema, pleural and pericardial effusions, ascites
b. Hepatosplenomegaly
c. Progressive hemolytic anemia

Nursing Process
Assessment
1. Prenatal history
   a. Positive hemantigen test (maternal blood serum)
   b. Positive indirect Coombs' (maternal blood serum)
   c. No prior history of RhoGAM use
2. Early identification of newborns at risk; includes those with
   a. Predisposing factors (e.g., prematurity, birth trauma)
   b. Delayed passage of meconium
   c. Placental enlargement (may weigh one half to three fourths of newborn's weight)
   d. Visible jaundice of skin (bilirubin greater than 7 mg/dl): blanch bridge of nose or chest
   e. Abnormal bleeding (e.g., extensive bruising or cephalhematoma)
   f. Positive direct Coombs' test (neonatal cord blood)
   g. Yellow-stained vernix on cord
3. Signs and symptoms of polycythemia, especially in large-for-gestational-age newborns
   a. Decrease in peripheral pulses
   b. Redness of hands and feet
   c. Tachycardia
   d. Respiratory distress
4. Newborn pallor with jaundice, appearing within 24-36 hours after birth
5. Increased optical density of amniotic fluid

Analysis (see p. 387)
Planning, Implementation, and Evaluation

> **Goal:** Newborn at risk for jaundice will be identified; will be free from kernicterus.

Implementation
1. Interpret laboratory values and recognize deviations from normal (i.e, rise in serum bilirubin, Hgb decrease, rapid decrease in hematocrit, positive Coombs').
2. Offer early feedings (prevent reabsorption of bilirubin).
3. Give appropriate dose of vitamin K as ordered (decreases prothrombin time).
4. Give appropriate care to newborn undergoing phototherapy (method of treatment in which bilirubin is transported from skin to blood to bile and excreted).
   a. Remove clothing.
   b. Protect eyes with eye patches (to prevent retinal damage).
   c. Turn every 2 hours for maximum skin exposure.

d. Provide adequate fluids.

e. Feed q2-3h to prevent metabolic disorders (may be removed from light for feedings).

f. Assess for signs of dehydration (e.g., sunken fontanels).

g. Maintain lights 16 inches away.

h. Monitor temperature every 2 hours.

i. Monitor weight gain and loss.

j. Observe for side effects (e.g., bronze skin, peripheral vasodilatation, temperature and metabolic disturbances, diminished activity, loose stools).

5. Assist with exchange transfusion as indicated (newborn receives negative blood if problem related to Rh incompatibility since no A, B, or Rh antigens are present in negative blood. Antibodies remaining are gradually removed; no further hemolysis occurs).

a. Observe for signs of transfusion reaction.

b. Educate parents about procedure.

Evaluation

Newborn shows signs of decreasing jaundice (e.g., falling serum bilirubin level, decreasing yellowing of skin); is free from kernicterus.

☐ Respiratory Distress
General Information

1. Definition: difficulty in maintaining respiratory function adequate to meet oxygen needs; caused by a variety of problems

2. Predisposing factors

   a. Dysmaturity (SGA newborns)

   b. Prematurity

   c. Postmaturity

   d. Maternal diabetes

   e. Maternal bleeding

   f. Fetal asphyxia

   g. Birth asphyxia

   h. Pregnancy-induced hypertension

   i. Prolonged labor after rupture of the amniotic membranes

   j. Meconium-stained amniotic fluid

   k. Low Apgar score

   l. Cesarean birth

3. Common respiratory disorders

   a. Respiratory distress syndrome (RDS), also known as hyaline membrane disease (HMD)

      1. definition: deficiency of surfactant activity leading to atelectasis, which prevents adequate gas exchange

      2. characterized by collapse of the alveoli

      3. most frequently affects preterm newborns, especially those weighing between 1000 and 1500 g, it is also observed in newborns of diabetic mothers and newborns of mothers whose pregnancies were complicated by antepartum vaginal bleeding

   b. Meconium-aspiration syndrome

      1. aspiration of meconium-stained amniotic fluid into the lungs may occur with asphyxic or placental disturbances in utero

      2. associated with intrauterine growth retardation (SGA newborns) and postmaturity (postterm newborns)

4. Associated problems

   a. Hypoxia

   b. Atelectasis

   c. Bronchopulmonary dysplasia, retrolental fibroplasia (complications of O_2 administration)

Nursing Process
Assessment

1. Use *Silverman-Andersen scale:* index of respiratory distress (scores of 0 are indication of good respiratory function) (see Fig. 4-24)

   a. Grunting: sound of air pushing past partially closed glottis, heard during expiration

   b. Retractions: sternal and intercostal; resulting from use of accessory muscles to aid in breathing

   c. Flaring nares: resulting from newborn's effort to lessen resistance in narrow nasal passages

   d. Seesaw respirations: flattening of chest with inspiration and bulging of abdomen, caused by use of abdominal muscles during prolonged, forced respirations

2. Cyanosis

3. Alterations in respiratory rate, rhythm, and depth

   a. Tachypnea: respiratory rate greater than 60/min or greater than 15/min over baseline

   b. Bradypnea: respiratory rate less than 30/min

   c. Apneic spells: absence of respiration for 20 seconds or more

4. Falling body temperature

Analysis (see p. 387)
Planning, Implementation, and Evaluation

> **Goal:** Newborn will maintain adequate oxygen levels to meet physiological demands; will be free from undetected respiratory distress or further complications.

Implementation

1. Collect blood-gas samples and pH from umbilical line; interpret results of studies.

2. Administer prescribed oxygen (dependent on results of blood-gas study).

   a. Give warmed and humidified oxygen.

   b. Monitor concentration and pressure of oxygen.

3. Monitor oxygen concentration through oximeter, blood gas and pH studies, and transcutaneous oxygen tension.

4. Maintain newborn in supine position, with head slightly extended to improve respiratory function, or leave newborn flat.

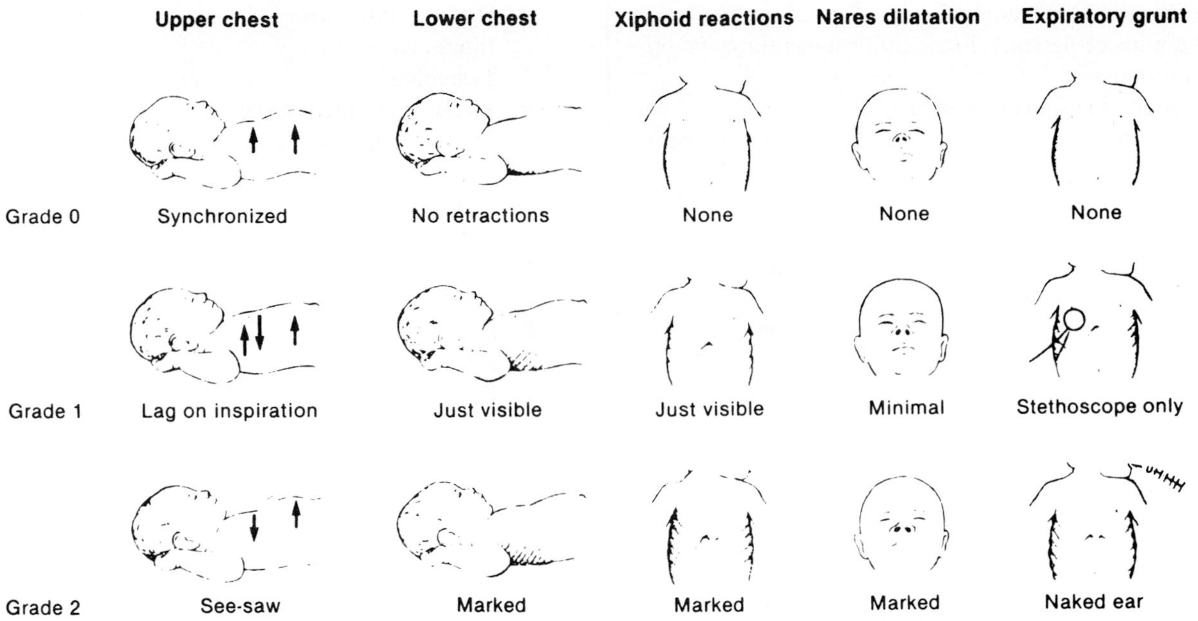

Upper chest	Lower chest	Xiphoid reactions	Nares dilatation	Expiratory grunt
Grade 0 Synchronized	No retractions	None	None	None
Grade 1 Lag on inspiration	Just visible	Just visible	Minimal	Stethoscope only
Grade 2 See-saw	Marked	Marked	Marked	Naked ear

Fig. 4-24   Silverman-Andersen scale. (From *Nursing inservice aid #2.* Columbus, Ohio: Ross Laboratories; Silverman, W., & Andersen, D. [1956]. *Peidatrics, 17:1.* American Academy of Pediatrics.)

5. Evaluate skin color.
   a. Pallor
   b. Plethora
   c. Cyanosis: circumoral, generalized, at rest or with activity
6. Maintain thermoneutral environment.
7. Minimize energy expenditure by keeping newborn warm.
8. Facilitate newborn's respiratory efforts.
   a. Continuous positive airway pressure (CPAP): controlled pressure exerted upon expiration to prevent collapse of alveoli
   b. Oxygen hood (to provide controlled oxygen and humidity)
9. Suction endotracheal tube q1-2h as needed; protect from extubation.
10. Protect skin on nasal septum from breakdown and undue pressure from endotracheal tube.
11. Provide for nutritional needs (IV, gavage, hyperalimentation) with minimal energy expenditure.
12. Prevent and detect complications.
13. Give supportive care to parents.

Evaluation

Newborn adequately meets oxygen needs of body; maintains respiratory rate between 30 and 60 without dyspnea; is free from complications from therapy.

☐ Neonatal Necrotizing Enterocolitis (NEC)
General Information

1. Definition: a disorder of vascular ischemia, affecting the gastrointestinal mucosa, often associated with perforation

2. Incidence: approximately 5% of all newborns in intensive care nurseries; morbidity and mortality can be reduced by early detection and treatment of asphyxia (within 30 minutes of birth)
3. Predisposing factors
   a. Neonatal asphyxia and hypoxia
   b. Pregnancy-induced hypertension
   c. Maternal vaginal bleeding
   d. Excessive amounts of feeding
   e. Immature immunological system
   f. Prematurity
4. Associated problem: sepsis

Nursing Process
Assessment
1. Abdominal distension
2. Pallor
3. Poor feeding
4. Gastric residuals (2 ml or more) before feedings
5. Occult blood in stool (positive guaiac test)
6. Increased apneic periods
Analysis (see p. 387)
Planning, Implementation, and Evaluation

> **Goal:** Newborn will be free from necrotizing enterocolitis, or complications from NEC.

Implementation
1. Check bowel sounds.
2. Monitor stools and gastric secretions for blood.
3. Monitor abdominal distension.

4. Record I&O, nature and type of gastric secretion.
5. Administer parenteral therapy or hyperalimentation as ordered.
6. Monitor for signs of dehydration.
7. Maintain nasogastric suction on low, intermittent suction.
8. Test urine for glucose to monitor tolerance for hyperalimentation solution.
9. Administer antibiotic therapy as indicated.
10. Provide appropriate preoperative and postoperative care when surgery is required (resection or colostomy).

Evaluation

Newborn receives prompt and appropriate treatment of any abnormalities (e.g., asphyxia, feeding problems); is free from sepsis and other complications of NEC.

☐ Hypoglycemia
General Information

1. Definition: decreased blood glucose level: less than 30 mg/dl (full-term) in first 72 hours of life or 45 mg/dl thereafter; less than 20 mg/dl in premature infants (NOTE: Dextrostix below 45 mg in term newborn, at 1 hour, warrants further testing)
2. Etiology: the beta cells in the fetal pancreas become overstimulated in utero because of high levels of circulating maternal glucose; after birth, insulin production remains higher than circulating glucose
3. Predisposing factors
   a. Malnourished newborns
      1. prematurity
      2. intrauterine growth retardation
      3. postmaturity
      4. twin pregnancy (smaller newborn affected)
   b. Newborns of diabetic mothers (usually LGA)
   c. Large-for-gestational age newborns (i.e., greater than 8.8 lb)
   d. Newborns of mothers with pregnancy-induced hypertension
   e. Severe Rh incompatibility
   f. Severely stressed newborns (e.g., newborns with cold stress, infections, respiratory distress)
4. Associated problems
   a. Jaundice
   b. Hypocalcemia (serum calcium less than 7-7.5 mg/dl); those at risk include premature infants, newborns of diabetic mothers, newborns with birth trauma and perinatal asphyxia

Nursing Process

Assessment
1. Note if any of predisposing factors are present
2. Signs and symptoms of hypoglycemia
   a. Apnea
   b. Lethargy
   c. Irregular respiration
   d. Feeding difficulties
   e. Jitteriness
   f. Twitching
   g. Weak, high-pitched cry
3. Signs and symptoms of hypocalcemia
   a. Neonatal tetany
   b. Twitching from central nervous system irritability
   c. Jerking tremors
   d. Seizures
   e. Cyanosis
   f. High-pitched cry
   g. Respiratory distress
   h. Poor feeding
4. Laboratory values for deviations from normal
5. Behavior and reflexes
   a. Daily weight
   b. Note frequency and amount of urination and stools

Analysis (see p. 387)

Planning, Implementation, and Evaluation

> **Goal:** Newborn will maintain normal blood glucose level for gestational age; will have hypoglycemic reactions detected before complications develop; will maintain adequate nutrition and fluid and electrolyte balance.

Implementation
1. Perform Dextrostix or laboratory blood glucose test on admission to nursery, and for newborns at risk for hypoglycemia, q30min 6 times, then qh 3 times, then q2h 6 times until stable; notify physician if Dextrostix result is less than 45 mg (full term) and less than 20 mg (preterm).
2. Provide adequate calories for all newborns.
3. Feed newborns at risk for hypoglycemia sterile water within first hour after birth, followed with glucose water, formula (oral or tube feeding as indicated), or breast milk.
4. Administer 10%-25% glucose, IV or orally, as ordered.
5. Minimize handling of newborn.
6. Observe carefully for signs of seizure related to low blood glucose.
7. Recommend regular pediatric care throughout childhood.

Evaluation
Newborn maintains normal blood-glucose level; has hypoglycemic reactions detected early; ingests calories appropriate for size; maintains fluid and electrolyte balance (e.g., moist mucous membranes, good skin turgor).

☐ Newborn Infection
General Information

1. Definition: an invasion of the fetus or newborn by bacterial or viral microorganisms during pregnancy or during or following birth

2. Predisposing factors
   a. Poor maternal nutrition
   b. TORCH (*t*oxoplasmosis, *o*ther, *r*ubella, *c*ytomegalovirus, *h*erpesvirus) syndrome
   c. Intrauterine growth retardation (SGA)
   d. Prematurity, especially gestational age less than 34 weeks
   e. Prolonged labor after rupture of membranes
3. Modes of transmission
   a. Chronic transplacental infection, acquired in utero through the placenta
      1. usually resulting from viruses; others include bacteria, protozoa
      2. onset early in gestation
      3. may lead to growth retardation
   b. Ascending intrauterine infection, acquired through the cervix after rupture of membranes
      1. onset late in gestation
      2. usually resulting form bacteria, often *E. coli;* herpesvirus
      3. may lead to premature labor and subsequent premature birth
   c. Newborn infection, acquired after birth from organisms in the environment by way of transmission from another person or newborn (sepsis is most common infection seen in newborn)
      1. often resulting from staphylococcus, streptococcus, or *E. coli*
      2. preterm newborns at greatest risk for infection because of lower immunological defenses
      3. more common in boys than in girls
4. Associated problems
   a. Generalized sepsis
   b. Septic sock (evidenced by fall in BP and tachypnea)
   c. Hyperbilirubinemia
   d. Meningitis (evidenced by bulging anterior fontanel)
   e. Increased mortality rate, especially in premature newborns

Nursing Process

Assessment
1. Antenatal and intrapartal history to identify newborns at risk
2. Septic workup if infection suspected (blood culture, lumbar puncture, gastric aspiration, umbilical-stump culture, stool culture, amniotic-membrane culture)
3. Signs and symptoms
   a. Lethargy
   b. Newborn does not "look right"
   c. Poor feeding and sucking
   d. Increased respiratory rate
   e. Jaundice
   f. WBC increase
   g. Loss of weight
   h. Restlessness, tremors, convulsions
   i. Diarrhea and vomiting
   j. Abdominal distension
   k. Skin rashes and/or skin lesions
   l. Hypothermia or hyperthermia

Analysis (see p. 387)

Planning, Implementation, and Evaluation

> **Goal:** Newborn will be free from undetected infection, will not experience complications or generalized sepsis.

Implementation
1. Treat immediately by administering antibiotics as ordered (e.g., penicillin, kanamycin, polymyxin); observe for side effects.
2. Prevent spread of infection by isolating septic newborns.
3. Monitor thermal environment.
4. Monitor body temperature (temperature rise is *not* an early sign of sepsis); in later stages, observe for severe hyperthermia or hypothermia.
5. Take daily weight.
6. Monitor I&O; observe for dehydration.
7. Provide adequate nutrition
8. Promote respiratory function.
9. Observe for central nervous system involvement (lethargy, apnea, seizures, tremors).

Evaluation
Newborn shows signs of decreasing infection (e.g., decreasing respirations, skin temperature between 36.1° C and 36.7° C); does not develop generalized sepsis.

☐ Neonatal Drug and Alcohol Addiction
General Information

1. Fetal alcohol syndrome
   a. Definition: a group of disorders characterized by teratogenesis as a result of chronic maternal alcoholism during pregnancy; high incidence in female newborns
   b. Associated problems
      1. intrauterine growth retardation; microcephaly
      2. ocular structural defects
      3. limb anomalies
      4. cardiovascular disturbances and anomalies (e.g., atrial and ventricular septal defects)
      5. mental retardation
      6. fine-motor dysfunction
      7. prematurity
      8. convulsions
2. Cocaine
   a. Exposure to the fetus during pregnancy may adversely affect the health and the growth and development of the neonate
   b. Associated problems
      1. congenital malformations

2. intrauterine growth retardation
3. prematurity
4. poorly organized infant state
5. decreased interactive behavior
6. irregular sleep behavior
7. increased risk of acute hypertension, cerebral artery injury/infarction, SIDS (not confirmed)

Nursing Process
Assessment (alcohol)

1. Signs and symptoms: onset according to time of last maternal use, type of combinations of drug taken, amount of drug taken, and length of addiction (onset of withdrawal generally occurs within 24 hours in alcohol addiction; can be up to 72 hours with some drugs)
   a. CNS signs
      1. restlessness
      2. jittery and hyperactive reflexes (e.g., constant sucking)
      3. high-pitched, shrill cry
      4. convulsions
   b. GI system signs
      1. feeds poorly
      2. vomiting
      3. diarrhea
      4. dehydration
   c. Respiratory system signs
      1. nasal stuffiness
      2. yawning and sneezing
      3. apnea
      4. tachypnea
      5. excessive secretions
2. Fluid-balance status

Assessment (cocaine)

1. Newborn urine testing can detect cocaine exposure within the preceding 6-9 days
2. Signs and symptoms vary with the degree of maternal substance abuse and time and dose of most recent exposure; may occur 4-5 days after birth
   a. CNS: tremulousness, irritability, muscular rigidity, increased startle response, disturbed sleep pattern
   b. GI: feeds poorly, vomiting, diarrhea, dehydration
   c. Cardiorespiratory: elevated respiratory and heart rate
   d. Fluid balance

Analysis (see p. 387)
Planning, Implementation, and Evaluation

> **Goal:** Newborn will remain free from injury; will have symptoms associated with withdrawal or seizures; parents will understand the need for follow-up care.

Implementation

1. Reduce stimuli in environment and minimize handling.
2. Protect from injury (swaddle newborn in snug-fitting blanket).
3. Promote bonding/attachment.
4. Ensure newborn receives required fluid and caloric intake; use pacifier between feeding.
5. Feed on demand; give small amounts at frequent intervals.
6. Use pacifier between feedings.
7. Administer IV therapy as ordered.
8. Position on side to avoid aspiration.
9. Measure I&O; watch for signs of dehydration resulting from vomiting, loose stools, poor feeding.
10. Weigh frequently.
11. Give skin care with special attention to body folds; expose to air.
12. Protect skin from injury (mittens on hands, sheepskin on crib, pads on sides of crib).
13. Give medications as ordered.
    a. Phenobarbital (6 mg/kg/day, IM or 2 mg po qid)
    b. Paregoric (2-4 gtt/kg orally q4-6h; dose may increase to 20-30 gtt/kg q4-6h)
14. Maintain patent airway if seizure occurs.
15. Maintain adequate warmth.
16. Document accurately.
17. Teach parents the importance of long-term follow-up health care.
18. See also *Substance Use Disorders*, p. 72, and reprints, pp. 106 and 414.

Evaluation

Newborn is comfortable and free from seizures, complications of withdrawal; has homeostasis restored; parents have an appointment with physician or clinic for follow-up care.

☐ Acquired Immunodeficiency Syndrome (AIDS)
General Information

1. Definition: a disase that affects the immune system (T cells) and renders one unable to fight disease or infection. High mortality rate in the first 3 years of life; no known cure. Currently 50% of infants born to HIV-positive women will be infected.
2. Modes of transmission to newborn
   a. Transplacental
   b. Through breast milk
   c. Contact with body fluids

Nursing Process
Assessment

1. Often small-for-gestational-age (SGA)
2. Hepatosplenomegaly
3. Neurological abnormalities (e.g., microcephaly)

4. Prominent, boxlike forehead
5. Increased distance between inner canthi; flattened nasal bridge
6. Recurrent infections (e.g., interstitial pneumonia)
7. Evidence of Epstein-Barr viral infection

Analysis (see p. 387)
Planning, Implementation, and Evaluation

> **Goal:** The newborn will be isolated from others to prevent the spread of the disease; will be free from complications of AIDS; parents will understand need for referral and follow-up care.

Implementation
1. Assess infants of mothers at risk (e.g., IV drug users, prostitutes, positive HIV test) for signs and symptoms of AIDS.
2. Promote bonding/attachment.
3. Maintain blood and body secretion precautions.
4. Educate parents about disease process, transmission, current treatment, follow-up care.
5. Provide emotional support to family.

Evaluation
Newborn is free from complications; parents keep follow-up care appointments.

☐ Birth Injuries/Congenital Anomalies
General Information
1. Birth injuries
   a. Definition: physical trauma to the newborn resulting from the birth process
   b. Predisposing factors: large-for-gestational-age newborn, dystocia
   c. Common types of injuries
      1. brachial plexus injuries
      2. cephalhematomas
      3. fractures
      4. intracranial hemorrhage
2. Congenital anomalies
   a. Definition: a variety of defects or disorders, which may be evident or concealed at birth; the physical and developmental consequences will vary with selected problem(s)
   b. Incidence: 6 in 1000 total births
   c. Predisposing factors
      1. past personal or family history of congenital anomalies, genetic factors (e.g., chromosomal aberrations)
      2. exposure to toxic agents, viruses, or drugs during pregnancy
      3. genetic-environmental interaction

Nursing Process
Assessment
1. Birth injuries

   a. Decreased mobility of arm, abnormal positioning (brachial-plexus injuries)
   b. Swelling of head caused by rupture of the blood vessels between a cranial bone and the periosteum (cephalhematoma)
   c. Swelling, irritability associated with pain, decrease mobility of affected extremity, abnormal positioning at rest (fractures)
   d. Respiratory irregularities with cyanosis, reduced responsiveness, high-pitched cry, tense fontanel, or convulsions (intracranial hemorrhage resulting from hypoxia and hypovolemia seen mainly in premature infants)
2. Congenital anomalies
   a. Antepartum/intrapartum high-risk factors, including maternal history of
      1. chronic alcoholism or drug addition
      2. family members born with congenital defects
      3. exposure to toxic agents in environment
      4. infections (e.g., TORCH)
      5. high-altitude resident
   b. Hydramnios: associated with
      1. neurological defects such as hydrocephalus, anencephalus, and spina bifida
      2. gastrointestinal malformation such as esophageal atresia, cleft palate, pyloric stenosis
      3. Down syndrome
      4. congenital heart disease
      5. maternal diabetes
      6. prematurity
   c. Oligohydramnios, associated with anomalies of the renal system

Analysis (see p. 387)
Planning, Implementation, and Evaluation

> **Goal 1:** Newborn will not develop undetected complications of birth injury.

Implementation
1. Assess for asymmetrical movements by placing newborn on back and observing movements of arms and legs.
2. Screen all LGA newborns for birth injuries; listen for high-pitched, weak cry; observe muscle tone (poor), hypertonicity, hyperactivity, flaccidity.
3. Palpate fontanels for bulging, tenseness.
4. Observe pupillary response.
5. Position head higher than hips (for intracranial hemorrhage); minimal handling; provide warmth; maintain adequate nutrition.
6. Implement specific treatment, which varies with nature and extent of insult.
7. Document observations.

Evaluation
Newborn receives early treatment of birth injury; is

free from long-term sequelae (e.g., mental retardation) when possible.

> **Goal 2:** Newborn will have anomalies recognized and treated early; will be free from complications; will maintain homeostasis; parents will understand need for referral.

Implementation

1. Screen for apparent and hidden congenital anomalies (often done upon admission to nursery).
2. Implement appropriate therapeutic measures (interdisciplinary health care team approach essential).
3. Refer family for care and genetic counseling.

Evaluation

Newborn adapts successfully to extrauterine life; receives appropriate treatment for defect; parents have an appointment for appropriate referral.

☐ Parental Reaction to a Sick, Disabled, or Malformed Newborn
General Information

1. The grief and mourning process initiated by birth (parents grieve over the loss of normality in their newborn)
2. Stages of grief and mourning (refer to *Loss and Death and Dying*, p. 26)
   a. First stage
      1. initial sadness
      2. guilt feelings ("What did I do to cause this? What happened?")
      3. shock over reality of situation
      4. denial
      5. general anger at situation; overprotectiveness of the newborn
      6. neglect of other family members
      7. isolation/loneliness (increases after mother's discharge from hospital)
   b. Second stage: developing awareness of reality of situation
   c. Restitution: coming to terms with situation

Nursing Process
Assessment
1. Stage of grief and mourning
2. Parental behavior: adaptive or maladaptive
Analysis (see p. 387)
Planning, Implementation, and Evaluation

> **Goal:** Parents will accept support in their grief over the ill, disabled, or malformed newborn.

Implementation

1. Allow parents to express grief (may be shown as anger, denial, depression, or crying); be supportive.
2. Modify hospital policies when possible to allow early contact with newborn and frequent visitation; encourage parents to see newborn, to touch and hold newborn in neonatal intensive care unit.
3. Point out normal characteristics of their newborn to parents.
4. Encourage parental participation in care (e.g., providing breast milk, bathing, and feeding).
5. Recognize signs of maladaptive responses.
   a. Possibility of abuse or neglect
   b. Overwhelming guilt
6. Expect repeated periods of sadness.
7. Provide simple explanations for procedures.
8. Refer parents to social worker for follow-up while newborn is in hospital, according to family need.
9. Encourage parents who are unable to visit to call nursery for progress reports.
10. Refer to public health nurse (official agency or visiting nurse) for health supervision upon discharge of newborn.
11. Plan for follow-up or institutionalization as necessary.

Evaluation

Parents grieve for their newborn's condition; express feelings of sadness and anger; allow nursing staff, family, and friends to support them.

BIBLIOGRAPHY
Women's Health

Bobak, I., Jensen, M., & Zalar, M. (1989). *Maternity and gynecologic care.* (4th ed.) St. Louis: Mosby–Year Book.

Hirsch, A., & Hirsch, S. (1989). The effect of infertility on marriage and self-esteem. *Journal of Obstetric, Gynecologic, and Neonatal Nursing, 18,* 13-20.

Louchs, A. (1989). A comparison of satisfaction with types of diaphragms among women in a college population. *Journal of Obstetric, Gynecologic, and Neonatal Nursing, 18,* 194-206.

Olson, R., & Mitchell, R. (1989). Self-confidence as a critical factor in breast self-examination. *Journal of Obstetric, Gynecologic, and Neonatal Nursing, 18,* 476-481.

Williams, S. (1989). *Nutrition and diet therapy.* St. Louis: Mosby–Year Book.

Antepartal Care

Aaronson, L., & Macnee, B. (1989). Tobacco, alcohol, and caffeine use during pregnancy. *Journal of Obstetric, Gynecologic, and Neonatal Nursing, 18,* 279-287.

Benoit, J. (1988). Sexually transmitted diseases in pregnancy. *Nursing Clinics of North America, 23,* 937-946.

Bernstein, J. (1990). Parenting after infertility. *Journal of Perinatal and Neonatal Nursing, 4,* 11-23.

Catado, C., & Whitney, E. (1986). *Nutrition and diet therapy.* St. Paul, MN: West Publishing.

Conner, G., & Denson, F. (1990). Expectant fathers' response to pregnancy. *Journal of Perinatal and Neonatal Nursing, 4,* 33-42.

Cunningham, F., MacDonald, P., & Gant, N. (1989). *Williams' obstetrics* (18th ed.). Norwalk, CT: Appleton & Lange.

Hytten, F. (1990). Nutrition regulation in pregnancy. *Midwifery, 6,* 93-98.

Jensen, M., Bobak, I., & Zalar, M. (1989). *Maternity and gynecologic care* (4th ed.). St. Louis: Mosby–Year Book.

Lopez, E. (1989). Prenatal diagnosis by ultrasound. *Journal of Perinatal and Neonatal Nursing, 2,* 34-42.

Moore, M. (1989). Recurrent teen pregnancy. *MCN: The American Journal of Maternal Child Nursing, 14*, 104-108.

Myhre, C., Richards, T., & Johnson, J. (1989). Maternal alphafeto-protein screening. *Journal of Perinatal and Neonatal Nursing, 2*, 13-20.

Olds, S., London, M., & Ladewig, P. (1990). *Maternal-newborn nursing* (3rd ed.). Menlo Park, CA: Addison-Wesley.

Reeder, S., & Martin, L. (1987). *Maternity nursing*. Philadelphia: Lippincott.

Shannon, D. (1987). HELLP syndrome: A severe consequence of pregnancy-induced hypertension. *Journal of Obstetric, Gynecologic, and Neonatal Nursing, 16*, 395-402.

Thomson, E., & Cordero, J. (1989). The new teratogens: Accutane and other vitamin A analogs. *MCN: The American Journal of Maternal Child Nursing, 14*, 244-248.

Intrapartal Care

Bobak, I., Jensen, M., & Zalar, M. (1989). *Maternity and gynecologic care* (4th ed.). St. Louis: Mosby–Year Book.

Clark, J., Queener, S., & Karb, V. (1990). *Pharmacologic basis of nursing practice*. St. Louis: Mosby–Year Book.

Gill, P., Smith, M., & McGregor, C. (1989). Terbutaline by pump to prevent recurrent preterm labor. *MCN: The American Journal of Maternal Child Nursing, 14*, 163-167.

Givens, S. (1988). Update on tocolytic therapy in the treatment of preterm labor. *Journal of Perinatal and Neonatal nursing, 2*, 21-32.

Johnson, F. (1989). Assessment and education to prevent preterm labor. *MCN: The American Journal of Maternal Child Nursing, 14*, 157-162.

Korbort, L. (1989). Are universal precautions changing the "nurture" of obstetric nursing? *American Journal of Nursing, 89*, 1609-10.

Roberts, J. (1989). Managing fetal bradycardia during second stage of labor. *MCN: The American Journal of Maternal Child Nursing, 14*, 394-398.

Postpartal Care

Bucknell, S., & Sikorki, K. (1989). Putting patient controlled analgesia to the test. *MCN: The American Journal of Maternal Child Nursing, 14*, 37-40.

Nice, F. (1989). Can a breastfeeding mother take medication without harming her infant? *MCN: The American Journal of Maternal Child Nursing, 14*, 27-31.

Newborn Care

Bobak, I., & Jensen, M. (1991). *Essential of maternity nursing* (3rd ed.). St. Louis: Mosby–Year Book.

Bobak, I., Jensen, M., & Zalar, M. (1989). *Maternity and gynecologic care* (4th ed.). St. Louis: Mosby–Year Book.

Brazelton, T. (1973). *Neonatal behavioral assessment scale*. Philadelphia: Lippincott.

Driscoll, J. (1990). Maternal parenthood and the grief process. *Journal of Perinatal and Neonatal Nursing, 4*, 1-10.

Lund, M. (1990). Perspectives on newborn male circumcision. *Neonatal Network, 9*, 7-10.

Novi, K., Nacion, K., & Abromson, R. (1988). Early discharge with home follow-up: Impact on low income mothers and infants. *Journal of Obstetric, Gynecologic and Neonatal Nursing, 17*, 133-141.

*Null, S. (1989). Nursing care to ease parents' grief. *MCN: The American Journal of Maternal Child Nursing, 14*, 84-89.

Weibley, T. (1989). Inside the incubator. *MCN: The American Journal of Maternal Child Nursing, 14*, 96-100.

Whaley, L., & Wong, D. (1991). *Nursing care of infants and children* (4th ed.). St. Louis: Mosby–Year Book.

*Wilkerson, N. (1988). A comprehensive look at hyperbilirubinemia. *MCN: The American Journal of Maternal Child Nursing, 13*, 360-364.

*See reprint section.

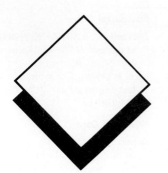

Reprints

Nursing Care of the Childbearing Family

Postpartum Depression as a Family Problem

Reprinted from MCN: The American Journal of Maternal Child Nursing, March/April 1989

We know little about the cause of postpartum depression, but we can assume the entire family is involved.

LOUISE K. MARTELL

Postpartum depression is more serious and longer lasting than the transitory depression commonly referred to as "maternity blues." It is less serious, however, than "postpartum psychosis," which is characterized by extremely altered perceptions of reality. Postpartum depression may begin within the first weeks after delivery and persist for months. Women feel inadequate and unable to cope. They do not enjoy life, tend to withdraw, and may complain of fatigue. Because many women with this problem are not diagnosed or seen by mental health professionals, its incidence is unclear. Various studies, however, estimate that postpartum depression affects 3 percent to 27 percent of all childbearing women (1).

According to systems theory, anything that affects one family member will also have an impact on others in the family. Life changes create stress or strain on each member's usual coping strategies, and often difficulties arise in interpersonal relationships. In addition, unrealistic perceptions may develop about the parent role. Understanding the impact of postpartum depression on family members can guide nurses in assessing depressed women and their families and in intervening in their behalf.

LOUISE K. MARTELL, R.N., M.N., is an assistant professor of family nursing at The Oregon Health Sciences University, Portland. She is currently a doctoral candidate of human development and family studies at Oregon State University, Corvallis.

Assessment of mothers for postpartum depression and subsequent intervention require careful listening, observation, and planning. (See Identifying and Managing Postpartum Stress.) Transition to parenthood is a stressful time, as various demands are made on the family to adapt to a new situation (2,3). Sleep is disturbed, and the family's usual daily activities are disrupted. Families may be further stressed by illness or hospitalization, the loss of a job, or inadequate resources for a new baby. Loss of the mother's income may impose

---

Identifying and Managing Postpartum Stress

Nursing Diagnosis
Ineffective family coping

Assessment
Isolation from usual support systems
Increased absence of family members from home
Energy levels lower than expected
Inappropriate expressions of anger, including family violence
Decreased functioning for usual everyday tasks
Financial burdens and worries
Sleep deprivation and extreme fatigue

Interventions
Help family work out strategies for increasing contact with usual support systems
Refer to community supports for new parents
Encourage family members to have times together for mutually enjoyable activities
Have family set priorities for everyday tasks and work out a plan for sharing them
Refer for financial counseling or encourage family to work through payment plans with health care provider and hospital
Teach about appropriate ways to express anger, such as vigorous exercise
Encourage verbal expression of grief, depression, and disappointment
Make appropriate referrals if abuse occurs
Help family arrange for uninterrupted sleep for affected members

additional financial worry. Loss may indeed be a prominent theme of postpartum depression; the mother has lost her usual energy levels, and the family has, in turn, lost an optimally functioning member.

When postpartum depression occurs, stressors are magnified. To cope, the family may express anger in nonfunctional ways, such as hitting children or speaking abusively. Such expressions have profound effects, as illustrated by a British community health nurse and sufferer of postpartum depression. She described her feelings: "The shouting and slapping which I inflicted on my daughter as my depression went untreated left her a sad and pathetic little girl" (4).

Isolation is another important factor in postpartum depression; but whether isolation causes or results from depression has not been determined. It is reported that social support can buffer the transition to parenting (5). Yet, childbearing families are often preoccupied and, thus, separated from family and friends. Seen in that light, isolation may precede postpartum depression.

Depressed persons tend to withdraw from social contact, because they are less energetic and have feelings of worthlessness. In turn, family and friends tend to decrease their interactions with the depressed person because the relationship is not sustained by the usual give-and-take. The mother's isolation can thus be exacerbated by postpartum depression. Family members may find that when they withdraw from each other, they compound the problem and withdraw from other supports too.

When family members do seek support outside the family system, their openness may have a positive impact, or it may have a negative effect.

Positively, opportunities for support are increased; negatively, if individuals seek all their support outside the family, other family members may find themselves more isolated than before.

Impact on Parenting

Mounting evidence shows that depressed mothers have different styles of interacting with their infants than nondepressed mothers (1). (See Identifying and Managing Alterations in the Parenting Role.) In one study, interactions were viewed of 12 depressed mothers and 12 who were not depressed as they played with their infants who were between the ages of three and five months (6). The behaviors of both groups, viewed during a 10-minute videotape, differed significantly. The infants of the depressed women were drowsier, displayed less relaxed physical activity, had less contented facial expressions, and were fussier. The depressed mothers played fewer games, showed tenser facial expressions, were less active, and had fewer contingent responses.

This purely descriptive study did not explain the behaviors; however, the findings do point to the possible dynamics of depressed mother-infant relationships. For example, some babies may have temperaments that make it difficult for mothers, especially when depressed, to respond to their infants with positive feelings and playfulness. Another possible dynamic is that infants develop the depressed style of their mothers.

Attitudes about parenting may also differ between depressed and nondepressed women (6,8). (See Identifying and Managing Unrealistic Perceptions of Parenting.) In the study described above, the depressed mothers had more controlling and

---

Identifying and Managing Alterations in Parenting Role

Nursing Diagnosis
  Alteration in parenting: actual and/or potential

Assessment
Interaction with infant characterized by low level of energy, somberness, tension, lack of enjoyment
Behavior problems in other children, such as tantrums that are inappropriate for age and separation anxiety
Signs of neglect and abuse

Interventions
Demonstrate enjoyable ways to interact with infant
Teach about expectations for age-appropriate behavior, behavior management, and care of infant and other children
Teach how to recognize tension and ways to relax
Refer when necessary for child behavior, neglect, or abuse

Identifying and Managing Unrealistic Perceptions of Parenting

Nursing Diagnosis
  Disturbance in role performance: parenting

Assessment
Attitudes about parenting include desire for high control and punitiveness
Locus of control tends to be external
Perceived capabilities for parenting are poor
Little satisfaction and enjoyment with motherhood

Interventions
Encourage mother to problem solve and make decisions about her own children
Expose to role models who have good child management skills and enjoy parenthood
Discuss individuality of children and parent's inability to have total control
Reward positive parenting efforts
Encourage parents and children to share activities that are mutually enjoyable

more punitive attitudes toward childrearing (6). Although the two groups of mothers did not differ in their knowledge of developmental landmarks among children, the depressed women were more anxious and had less internalized loci of control. The researchers speculated that depressed women's perceptions of themselves, their infants, and childrearing might lead to the depressed style of parenting.

In another study of parental attitudes, depressed women tended to use more punishment and were more irritable than nondepressed mothers (7). And, in another, depressed women rated themselves as less capable mothers and stated that they frequently disliked their mother role (8). Furthermore, in published case studies, dysfunctional parenting by postpartally depressed women is also a common theme (4,9,10). Questions arise about what influence this depression will have on children as they grow older. Furthermore, how postpartum depression affects older children in the family is not known and needs investigation. It is reasonable to hypothesize, however, that depression does have an impact.

Precisely how depression and parenting attitudes are associated is not known either (7). Possibly, depression precedes mothers' use of punishment, which results in children's behavioral problems. Or, perhaps, children's problems, such as being a "difficult" baby, precede depression. Whatever the case, parenting attitudes are different for postpartally depressed women, and their depression and subsequent parenting may have deleterious effects on their children.

Changes in Relationship with Partner

Postpartum depression affects many aspects of the partner relationship. (See Identifying and Managing Alterations in the Relationship with Partner.) Communication is impaired because depressed women tend to withdraw. In addition, the decreased libido commonly associated with depression may be confounded by postpartum fatigue and dyspareunia. Consequently, intimacy diminishes, and the couple may lose the opportunity for sexual expression of support for each other during their transition to parenthood.

Dissatisfaction with marriage is a recurring theme in writings about postpartum depression (4,9,10). Whether depression creates marital tension or marital tension exacerbates depression has not been determined (7,8).

Changes in men's lives and in their expectations of their partners are also recurring themes in descriptions of postpartum depression (4,9,10). Men may find that the demands of motherhood draw their partners away from them; postpartum depression may erode the situation even more. Housework does not get done, babies become more fussy, and women can become unattractive and run down by fatigue. As a result, tension between partners can escalate.

Scapegoating is one possible outcome of increasing tension (9). Either partner may blame the other for the less than ideal situation. Worse yet, the baby may be perceived as the source of their problems. Scapegoating is crippling, because it keeps the family from functional coping mechanisms, such as seeking counseling or treatment for the depression. Furthermore, labeling individuals, especially children, can impede their development.

Nursing Implications

The entire family of the postpartally depressed woman is at risk for dysfunction. Inadequate parenting, child behavioral problems for both the new infant and older children in the family, and marital discord are but a few examples of dysfunction. Although postpartum depression has an impact on the entire family, the family unit is rarely seen for care. A depressed mother may be seen during a postpartum examination, a disturbed infant during a well-baby check-up, and a withdrawn father for an occupational health physical. Assessing the extent of depression is, therefore, difficult. Nurses, however, can have an impact on the health of the entire family even though nursing assessment, diagnoses, and interventions are

---

Identifying and Managing Alterations in Relationship with Partner

Nursing Diagnosis
Alteration in marital role

Assessment
Level of intimacy and libido tend to be low
Life changes related to infant care, maternal depression
Unmet expectations about baby, parenting, partner's role performance
Scapegoating or inappropriate blaming for difficulties
Decreased family communications
Inappropriate expression of anger toward partner

Interventions
Discuss realistic expectations for the family situation, physical aspects of maternal recovery, and the demands of infant care
Encourage members to communicate honestly and directly without blaming, accusing, etc.
Clarify misconceptions about etiology and effects of postpartum depression
Discuss postpartum sexuality in terms of physical changes, the impact of fatigue, depression, and demands of infant care
Encourage partners to express love, concern, and tenderness toward each other in a variety of ways
Refer to counselor for extremely dysfunctional communication, hostility toward each other, or other signs of marital distress

directed toward the mother; health promotion and education, illness prevention, and emotional support are provided for the entire family. Collaboration among health care providers is often helpful.

Often during pregnancy, before postpartum depression occurs, women are in contact with nurses. Families who are vulnerable to postpartum depression can be identified at that time. Such families include those stressed by loss, limited support systems, financial burdens, or unexpected pregnancy complications. Also, families with rigid expectations about parenting or with marital discord may have more difficulties than others if postpartum depression occurs. After vulnerability is identified, the nurse can begin appropriate preventive measures.

In the early postpartum period, nurses have unique opportunities to observe mothers and infants together. Whether their behaviors provoke or result from postpartum depression is not important. What is important is taking an active role in promoting the best possible relationship between an infant and the mother. Nurses need to recognize babies who are not easy for parents to attach to; those babies might stimulate parent reactions that do not promote optimal development. Similarly, nurses must recognize parents' actions that do not stimulate infants to respond. Showing mothers ways to derive pleasure from interacting with their infants may offset some of the negative impact of postpartum depression (11).

The impact on families of postpartum depression can only be conjectured from our understanding of family systems, of case studies, and of depressed parents in general. This limited information, however, is enough to indicate that postpartum depression has a profound, negative impact on all family members. Interventions must address the depression and family functioning.

REFERENCES

1. AFFONSO, D. D., AND DOMINO, G. Postpartum depression: a review. *Birth* 11:231–235, Winter 1984.
2. COX, M. J. Progress and continued challenges in understanding the transition to parenthood. *J.Fam.Issues* 6:395–408, 1985.
3. COWAN, C. P., AND OTHERS. Transition to parenthood: his, her, and theirs. *J.Fam.Issues* 6:451–481, 1985.
4. HABGOOD, J. Postnatal depression. Exposing the blues and treating them. *Comm.Outlook* 14:4–11, Aug. 1985.
5. CRONENWETT, L. R. Network structure, social support, and psychological outcomes of pregnancy. *Nurs.Res.* 34:93–99, Mar.–Apr. 1985.
6. FIELD, T., AND OTHERS. Pregnancy problems, postpartum depression, and early mother-infant interactions. *Dev.Psychol.* 21:1152–1156, Nov. 1985.
7. GHODSIAN, M., AND OTHERS. A longitudinal study of maternal depression and child behavior problems. *J.Child Psychol. Psychiatry* 25:91–109, Jan. 1984.
8. BROMET, E. J., AND CORNELY, P. J. Correlates of depression in mothers of young children. *J.Am.Acad.Child Psychiatry* 23:335–342, May 1984.
9. CIARAMITARO, B. *Help for Depressed Mothers*, ed. by L. Meyer. Edmonds, WA, The Charles Franklin Press WA, 1982.
10. ARIZMENDI, T. G., AND AFFONSO, D. D. Research on postpartum depression: a critique. *Birth* 11:237–245, 1984.
11. SNYDER, C., AND OTHERS. New findings about mothers' antenatal expectations and their relationship to infant development. *MCN* 4:354–357, Nov.–Dec. 1979.

Type I Diabetes and Pregnancy

...are we hearing women's concerns?

Effective collaboration between the health care team and a pregnant woman with diabetes is based on thorough, sensitive discussions about the plan of care.

BY ELLEN W. LEFF/MARGARET P. GAGNE/SANDRA C. JEFFERIS

Reprinted from MCN: The American Journal of Maternal Child Nursing, March/April 1991

Even when women with high-risk pregnancies have frequent and intensive contact with the health care system, they may not have important needs identified. This unanticipated finding emerged from an analysis of data gathered during interviews with women who had type I diabetes (1). The women were asked about their pregnancy experiences as part of a larger study of diabetes and breast-feeding.* The responses revealed a depth of emotional experience and personal hardship that was surprising to researchers who had cared for some of the women during antepartum hospitalizations. The women de-scribed needs that were not fully understood by health care professionals in spite of their frequent contact with women. For some women, the unmet needs interfered with blood glucose control and may have adversely affected pregnancy outcomes. For others, the unmet needs resulted in increased stress for themselves and for their families.

Much theoretical and anecdotal literature has been written that explores the impact of high-risk and diabetic pregnancies that have on women and their part-

* The research described in this article was supported by a grant from the American Nurses Foundation, Inc.

ELLEN W. LEFF, B.S.N., *is the head nurse in the maternity/newborn nursery at the Medical Center Hospital of Vermont in Burlington;* MARGARET P. GAGNE, B.S.N., *is a lecturer in the School of Nursing at the University of Vermont, Burlington; and* SANDRA C. JEFFERIS, B.S.N., *is a staff nurse at the Medical Center Hospital of Vermont.*

ners. Several authors have described how the completion of the normal developmental tasks of pregnancy may be threatened by a woman's experience of being high risk. (See Bibliography.)

Researchers have begun to explore the effects of stress and social support on the women with high-risk pregnancy. For example, both life stress during the previous year and inadequate emotional support were significantly related to emotional disequilibrium in high-risk pregnancy (2). Ultimately, life stress and emotional disequilibrium were associated with complications of pregnancy, delivery, and infant condition. Tangible social support, however, such as someone to help during an emergency or illness, lessened the adverse effects of stress during pregnancy. In another study that compared high- and low-risk pregnancies, researchers found that women with high-risk pregnancies experienced greater negative life-events stress and greater depression and anxiety. But, women with high-risk pregnancies also received greater support (3). Moreover, a study of the effects of high-risk pregnancy on women with low incomes showed they had higher blood levels of epinephrine, which suggested increased physiologic stress (4).

In a study of pregnant women with insulin-dependent diabetes, high levels of psychosocial stress were associated with increased blood glucose levels (5). In yet another investigation, a majority of women with type I diabetes felt that amniocentesis, blood tests, and the diabetic diet were stressful (6). Another researcher, however, stated that while each woman with diabetes responds to her pregnancy in a unique way, childbearing may be an important way for these women to prove their self-worth, their femininity, and their ability to produce a normal child (7).

Confronting Unanswered Questions

Previous research on diabetes and pregnancy left unanswered questions, because the stressors had been identified by the investigators, not by the subjects. Moreover, the studies did not examine the perceived importance that the stressful experiences had for the women themselves. Thus, the purpose of our study was to describe from a woman's point of view, the experience of pregnancy complicated by diabetes, including the positive and negative aspects.

In this article, we emphasize the clinical issues that were raised by our findings and the resulting changes we made in practice. As indicated earlier, they were serendipitous findings of a study on diabetes and breast-feeding. The original study was descriptive and qualitative. The convenience sample consisted of 22 women who had had type I diabetes diagnosed prior to pregnancy. All subjects were white, and all but two were married when their infants were born. Their ages ranged from 18 to 38 years, and they lived in rural and urban areas of the northeastern United States. Gestational age of the infants ranged from 28.5 weeks to 42 weeks (average

36.8), and newborn weights ranged from 650 grams to 4,904 grams (average 3,119).

The Goals of Pregnancy

Traditionally, explicit discussions about the goals of a care plan often do not occur between pregnant women and their health care providers. Ideally, goals must be discussed early in pregnancy in order to identify and agree upon the priorities of ongoing care. We found as a result of interviews done during the study that we had to reconsider our nursing goals for these women and how the goals might be better achieved. Based on the interview data as well as our personal experiences providing nursing care for pregnant women with type I diabetes, we identified three major nursing goals in working with these women: first, the birth of a healthy baby; second, positive maternal feelings about meeting the challenges of diabetes and pregnancy; and third, increased maternal motivation and capability to control diabetes.

A healthy baby is the most obvious desired outcome of any pregnancy. When a pregnant woman has type I diabetes, her pregnancy is considered by the health care system to be at high risk. A great deal of effort is focused on maintaining proper blood glucose levels in the mother; satisfactory levels prevent complications that would adversely affect the baby's health.

A second goal — that a woman feel positively about meeting the challenges of diabetes and pregnancy — was not often found by the authors to be a priority of physicians and nurses caring for these women. The women who were interviewed, however, described strong feelings of success or failure about how well they managed their diabetes. One woman described her positive experience: "When I was pregnant, that's the best control I've ever been in in my entire life." Another woman had decided against future pregnancies because, as she said, "It takes too much out of me...I don't think I could face it again after having...two miserable pregnancies. I think that if I found out I was pregnant, I would go hang myself or something; I just couldn't do it."

The third goal is to help a woman increase her motivation and capability in controlling diabetes for the rest of her life. Health care professionals consider this a desirable goal, but not a high priority goal. For several women, however, that outcome was of considerable importance. One woman stated, "Even if I had known everything...about watching my sugar before I was married and had kids, I probably wouldn't have been very careful about it; whereas, now I'm much more careful...I think they (my family) need me."

To achieve these outcomes requires the cooperation of the woman and her health care team: the patient is responsible for managing control of the diabetes through blood glucose testing, insulin administration, diet, and exercise; the health care team is responsible for providing routine antepartal care as well as special health status monitoring and information and support

---

Pregnancy with Type I Diabetes

The following paragraphs include information as it might be presented to a pregnant woman with type I diabetes.

General Considerations

- Your pregnancy is labeled "high risk" because poor blood sugar control increases the risks of birth defects, stillbirth, or of having an excessively large baby. The newborn of a mother with diabetes may have problems with low blood sugar or jaundice.

- Prenatal care is very important to help prevent complications. You will have frequent check-ups and more tests than a woman without diabetes. You can expect more blood tests and perhaps some 24-hour urine collections. Some tests use ultrasound (harmless high frequency sound waves) to examine the baby. A fetal monitor may be used to observe how the baby's heart rate responds to the baby's movements or to the contractions of your uterus. Near the end of your pregnancy, an amniocentesis may be done to see whether the baby's lungs are ready to function normally. All tests will be explained to you.

- The chances are excellent that you will have a healthy baby if you take good care of yourself during pregnancy. A healthy pregnancy and a healthy baby depend in part on your ability to follow your doctor's instructions about blood sugar testing, insulin, diet, and exercise. Compared with your diabetic care before you were pregnant, more of your time and effort will be required now. Moreover, your care will be more expensive. If you do not understand or have difficulty following the instructions, discuss the situation with your doctor, nurse, dietitian, or social worker.

- Like all pregnant women, you will notice many physical and emotional changes. Your health care team wants to help you understand and adjust, so discuss your discomforts, concerns, fears, and questions with them.

Changes in Diabetic Care

- Your goal will be to maintain blood sugar levels close to the levels of a pregnant woman who does not have diabetes: 60 mg to 90 mg/dl before meals and less than 120 mg/dl two hours after meals. Blood sugar level may be especially difficult to control early in pregnancy; pregnancy causes your body to produce hormones that affect blood sugar (1).

- Your insulin needs will increase as pregnancy progresses, as the placenta produces more hormones that interfere with the effect of insulin. You may need more injections each day, and larger amounts and different types of insulin.

- You will probably need to test your blood sugar more often to find out if your insulin doses are adequate. Because your blood sugar level may be too high or too low at certain times of the day, frequent testing will be helpful to you in detecting those times.

- A dietitian will help you plan your pregnancy diet. Following the plan is important: You will need to eat snacks, including one at bedtime, in addition to three well balanced meals each day.

- Regular daily exercise and sleep patterns may be needed to help you keep your blood glucose under control. Discuss with your doctor what types of exercise are best for you.

- Your symptoms of low blood sugar may change, and you may not notice an insulin reaction in its early stage. Because the reaction occurs suddenly, a special bracelet must be worn or a card carried to identify you as a person with diabetes. Also, always have hard candy, sugar cubes, or glucose tablets with you. Treat low blood sugar immediately.

1. JOVANOVIC-PETERSON, L. AND OTHERS. *Diabetes and Pregnancy: What to Expect.* American Diabetes Association, 1989.

---

for diabetic management. This interdependent system is intended to prevent and resolve problems in pregnancy. The subjects interviewed, however, indicated that the system can fail in several ways. For example, disagreements or misunderstandings can occur in defining the health problem, determining the health care objectives, formulating a plan to achieve the objectives, implementing the plan, and monitoring results.

Reacting to "High Risk"

A pregnant woman who has had diabetes for years often does not easily comprehend why her pregnancy is at increased risk. As one woman described the situation, "I had no idea why they were so excited about my being pregnant...and I didn't get much of an explanation." This misunderstanding of the high-risk nature of the pregnancy may contribute to decreased motivation to follow a strict diabetic regimen throughout pregnancy. It is important, therefore, that the woman understand the effects that pregnancy will have on her diabetes and the effects that diabetes will have on pregnancy (see Pregnancy with Type I Diabetes).

While some of the women calmly accepted the high-risk designation and the need for special care during pregnancy, others responded with anxiety, fear, denial, or anger. These feelings were rarely spontaneously shared with nurses or physicians, but sometimes they affected a woman's ability to achieve the desired outcomes. For example, one woman described worrying about her baby throughout the entire pregnancy. She was afraid the baby would have missing arms or legs, be blind, or have diabetes. She stated, "I was always worried there was going to be something wrong because I had so many things wrong with me."

Her fears might have been alleviated by discussions with her nurse or physician. Perhaps she would have been reassured by information about the small likelihood of congenital malformations or inherited diabetes. She could have been told that her chances of having a healthy baby were excellent if she maintained good blood glucose control. By emphasizing the normal and healthy aspects of this woman's pregnancy, a nurse might have been able to alleviate some of the stress.

Another woman described her denial of risk during an unwanted pregnancy: "I think I could have watched [my blood sugar] more carefully...but I didn't really want to." This woman needed professional counseling to help her cope with marital problems and accept her pregnancy and diabetes. For her, as for other women, unresolved emotional conflicts that are related to having a chronic disease resurfaced in pregnancy. With professional assistance, she might have been able to take advantage of opportunities for personal growth and for learning new ways of coping.

Yet another woman's anger about her pregnancy's high-risk designation and its treatment prompted her to strive to normalize her pregnancy and childbirth experience. She resented "being treated as ill" even though her diabetic control was excellent. The resentment interfered with her relationships with health care professionals, and she did not come to terms with the high-risk designation until her third pregnancy. The problem might have been resolved sooner if it had been discussed frankly. This woman was capable of making more decisions regarding her care during pregnancy, and she wanted to. But, she also needed support in continuing to work through her grief associated with having a chronic disease.

Understanding Objectives

A major objective for the women who were interviewed was to maintain their blood glucose levels close to those of pregnant women without diabetes.

Although this objective was the same for each of the women, their understanding and acceptance of it varied considerably. At one extreme was the woman who constantly strove for perfection in diabetic control. Her attempt to overreach the goal led to unnecessary frustration and guilt: "I was just really burned out from having put so much into the pregnancy." At the other extreme was the woman who began her pregnancy by setting her sights much lower: "They wanted me to get to like 90 to 100 [mg/dl] at the beginning but there was no way...I run like 250 or a little bit higher."

Determining objectives may have been complicated because few of the women indicated an understanding of the effect of pregnancy on diabetic control. Moreover, some of the women did not know the possible adverse consequences of poor control, while others lived in constant fear of complications. The possible consequence of both over- and under-reaching is poor emotional or physical health. For that reason it is important that the nurse discuss how diabetes and pregnancy can interact to affect the health of mother and baby. Why the goals for blood glucose levels are lower during pregnancy needs to be explained.

Working to Achieve Objectives

When a woman with diabetes becomes pregnant, far-reaching lifestyle changes are often recommended by her physician: the frequency of blood glucose testing is increased; insulin type, dose, and frequency of injection may be changed; a strict diet with several snacks is followed; and a consistent daily pattern of activities is desirable. Although many of the women did not fully understand the complexities of the diabetic regimen, and many had great difficulty complying, they rarely questioned the need to make the prescribed changes.

The women's acceptance of a plan of care was probably facilitated by the health care team's creative, flexible approach in planning lifestyle changes. The women appreciated the opportunity to discuss the changes with the health care team, to participate in decision-making regarding insulin doses and to accommodate the plan as much as possible in their schedules and lifestyles.

A nursing database may help nurses to work with pregnant women with diabetes in developing an individualized plan of self-care. Information about the woman's usual blood sugar testing routine and insulin doses, her knowledge of diabetic control, and her daily schedule of activities is needed to accommodate necessary changes with a minimum of disruption for the woman and her family. Also, appropriate patient education can be planned that recognizes and builds upon her current level of knowledge.

Maintaining acceptable blood glucose levels is the responsibility of the pregnant woman. Most of the women who were interviewed felt their control of diabetes during pregnancy was good or the best they had ever achieved; however, great time and energy were often invested. The self-care regimen was stressful because it had to be followed every day. As one subject stated, "You live and breathe diabetes!"

The motivation to meet the regimen requirements was often based on fear: "If anything was wrong with [the baby], I know I would have blamed it on something I had done one day by not doing the best with my diabetes." For some women, knowledge and fears about the possible adverse effects of diabetes on the baby may be positive motivators, but for others, they may interfere with a positive adjustment to pregnancy. If a woman is able to openly discuss her fears with a nurse, the nurse can dispel misconceptions and confirm the actual risks. Professional counseling may be needed for a woman whose guilt and fear interfere with maintaining the diabetic care plan.

Another way that nurses can provide support for a woman maintaining the diabetic regimen is by asking more specifically about the woman's feelings and concerns about her pregnancy. Listening to and accepting those feelings may be helpful. Some women feel reassured to hear that their feelings of stress and anger are normal responses. It is encouraging for some women to have the nurse affirm that the baby benefits from efforts to maintain strict glucose control and that the care regimen may be relaxed after pregnancy.

Monitoring blood glucose levels was done during frequent clinic visits, by testing blood, and by making telephone calls to the women's homes or work. The women were aware that their antepartal care was much more involved than that of their friends and relatives, and they responded in a variety of ways: some were reassured, others were stressed or irritated. One woman said, "It felt like I was specimen number 236."

Women varied in their individual need for monitoring and support, and their need sometimes changed as pregnancy progressed. Increased stress due to social problems, such as marital difficulties or relocation to a new community, may increase a woman's need for contact, assistance, and support. On the other hand, when diabetic control is well maintained, the woman may feel more competent, trusted, and in control if monitoring is less intense; she may be encouraged to initiate contact with the health care team when she feels that it is necessary.

The women who were interviewed also expressed a need for normal pregnancy care. They had concerns about morning sickness, fatigue, depression, and preparation for labor and delivery; these concerns were often not addressed. It is important for nurses caring for women with high-risk pregnancies to educate and counsel them regarding normal pregnancy discomforts and events, to offer childbirth preparation, and to discuss with them the experiences common to all pregnant women.

The Challenge

In order to promote the physical and emotional health of the pregnant woman with type I diabetes, nursing care must be based on careful assessment. As circumstances change throughout pregnancy, assessment needs to be repeated.

A woman often does not volunteer information regarding her feelings and concerns, especially if she has negative feelings about her care. Moreover, both patient and nurse may be unaware of the woman's misunderstandings or conflicts regarding pregnancy risks, appropriate blood glucose levels, the lifestyle changes necesary to maintain control, the effectiveness of self-care routines, or how the health care team will monitor and support the woman as she implements the plan.

The nurse may inquire about the woman's feelings regarding these aspects of her care. Adequate time for discussion and listening, and mutual trust and respect between nurse and patient are required for a thorough assessment. An acknowledgment of both positive and negative feelings is necessary to improve a woman's understanding and motivation to maintain appropriate diabetic control. This sharing will help the woman prevent or diminish unnecessary guilt, anxiety, and anger, and thus promote positive feelings about meeting the challenge of her pregnancy.

Pregnancy presents a formidable challenge to a woman with type I diabetes, because to a large degree a successful outcome depends upon her ability to manage her diabetes. For some women with diabetes, pregnancy, childbirth, and breast-feeding are important expressions of their desire to live as full a life as possible. Health care professionals can provide care that is sensitive to and built upon individual needs and that is offered in the context of a collaborative relationship. In that way, the goals of pregnancy are more likely to be achieved by a woman with diabetes.

REFERENCES

1. GAGNE, M. P., AND OTHERS. *Diabetes and Breastfeeding: an Exploratory Approach.*(Report submitted for publication to the American Nurses Foundation.)
2. NORBECK, J. S., AND TILDEN, V. P. Life stress, social support, and emotional disequilibrium in complications of pregnancy: a prospective, multivariate study. *J.Health Soc.Behav.* 24:30–46, Mar. 1983.
3. MERCER, R.T., AND FERKETICH, S.L. Stress and social support as predictors of anxiety and depression during pregnancy. *Adv.Nurs.Sci.* 10:26–39, Jan. 1988.
4. KEMP, V.H., AND HATMAKER, D.D. Stress and social support in high-risk pregnancy.*Res.Nurs.Health* 12:331–336, Oct. 1989.
5. BARGLOW, P., AND OTHERS. Psychosocial childbearing stress and metabolic control in pregnant diabetics.*J.Nerv.Ment.Dis.* 173:615–620, Oct. 1985.
6. ZIGROSSI, S. T., AND RIGA-ZIEGLER, M. The stress of medical management on pregnant diabetics.*MCN* 11:320–323, Sept.-Oct. 1986.
7. PAPATHEODOROU, N. H. Diabetes and pregnancy: a psychosocial perspective. IN *Management of the Diabetic Pregnancy*, ed. by B. S. Nuwayhid and others. New York, Elsevier Science Publishing Co., 1987, pp. 136–167.

BIBLIOGRAPHY

FURLONG-LIND, R., AND BECK-BLACK, R. Psychosocial implications, family planning, and emotional support. IN *Diabetes Mellitus in Pregnancy: Principles and Practice*, ed. by E.A. Reece and D.R. Coustan. New York, Churchill Livingtone, 1988.
GALLOWAY, K.G. The uncertainty and stress of high-risk pregnancy. *MCN*, 1:294–299, Sept.-Oct. 1976.
KEMP, V.H., AND PAGE, C.K. The psychosocial impact of a high-risk pregnancy on the family. *J.Obstet.Gynecol.Neonatal Nsg.* 15:232–236, May-June 1986.
PENTICUFF, J.H. Psychologic implications of high-risk pregnancy. *Nurs.Clin.North Amer.* 17:69–78, March 1982.
SCHROEDER-ZWELLING, E., AND HOCK, R. Maternal anxiety and sensitive mothering behavior in diabetic and nondiabetic women. *Res.Nurs.Health* 9:249–255, Sept. 1986.
SNYDER, D.J. The high-risk mother viewed in relation to a holistic model of the childbearing experience. *J.Obstet.Gynecol.Neonatal Nsg.* 8:164–170, May-June 1979.
WEIL, S.G. The unspoken needs of families during high-risk pregnancies. *AJN* 81:2047–2049, Nov. 1981.

Nursing Care To Ease Parents' Grief

Reprinted from MCN: The American Journal of Maternal Child Nursing, March/April 1989

One hospital's program of nursing care for grieving parents has much to offer nurses in emergency room, home care, and other health care settings.

SALLY NULL

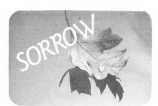

Candlelight and roses. That phrase is often heard in connection with the labor and delivery department at Stanford University Hospital (SUH). And for most parents, a trip to Stanford to deliver a baby ends in a celebration of life, complete with steak and champagne, compliments of the hospital.

However, there is another group of parents who come to Stanford who are not so fortunate. In 1987, labor and delivery reported 27 (.7 percent) stillbirths and 83 (2.7 percent) neonatal deaths. Because SUH is a tertiary hospital and receives mothers with high-risk pregnancies from all over central California, these percentages are probably higher than those at community hospitals.

These figures do not, however, reflect spontaneous abortions that occur at home or in SUH's emergency room, nor do they include ectopic pregnancies, which are treated on a surgical unit. According to Rana Limbo and Sara Wheeler, "Each year of over half a million babies born alive, some 30,000 babies are stillborn. Miscarriage occurs in 15 to 20 percent of pregnancies" (1).

Whether a miscarriage is suffered at home or in the emergency room, or a fetal demise, stillbirth, or neonatal death occurs in labor and delivery, the grief the parents experience is as painful to them as is grief for any lost loved one. For some, it feels even more wrenching because the death may have been unexpected or seems particularly unfair. One father recalled, "We did everything right: good prenatal care, prepared childbirth with no drugs, and we had a beautiful baby who died. No one ever told us this could happen. It's been over a year and I still don't feel the world is safe."

In addition to the parental grief that nurses confront, they must also contend with their own feelings. They can be overwhelmed by parents' grief. Or they may feel unsure about assisting grieving parents with their loss and with the decisions that need to be made after an infant's death.

In 1982, Charmaine Thomas and Rita Rodriguez, two SUH nurses, realized that some sort of plan to facilitate parents' progress through the grief process needed to be instituted. The Grief and Loss Committee, the means toward this end, was formed for several purposes: continuity of patient care, nurse credibility, and staff training.

How the Committee Operates

The Grief and Loss Committee is now comprised of nurses from SUH's labor and delivery and postpartum units; originally, only labor and delivery unit nurses participated. (Intensive care unit nurses have formed their own Grief and Loss Committee as well.) The committee's primary goal is to have a nurse visit parents as soon as they have heard their baby is going to die or has died. Committee members are represented on all shifts and work weekends, so they are available to grieving parents at all times. Several are grief counselors certified by Resolve Through Sharing.* Not all unit nurses are members of the committee. In fact, SUH labor and delivery nurses may ask not to be assigned to care for grieving mothers if they feel unprepared emotionally. Other nurses, who are willing to care for grieving mothers but are inexperienced, call on committee members for help with unfamiliar or daunting tasks.

Regardless of whether the nurse treating a particular mother and her family is a committee member, the standards of care remain constant. Most important, the nurse assures the parents that they are not alone. She also conveys to them the Grief and Loss Committee's philosophy: that the

SALLY NULL, R.N., B.S.N., is staff nurse IV, Stanford University Hospital, Stanford, California. She rotates among the perinatal units and is a member of the Grief and Loss Committee. She thanks Rana Limbo and Sara Wheeler of Resolve Through Sharing for their assistance in the establishment of the Grief and Loss Committee and for providing support materials, including the leaf design that appears above. For reprints of this article, see the classified section.

*Resolve Through Sharing is a support program for grieving parents. For information and materials, contact the group c/o Lutheran Hospital, 1910 South Ave., La Crosse, WI 54601; 608-785-0503.

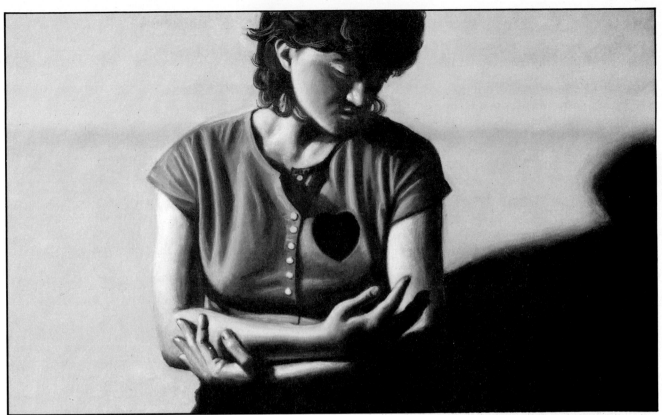

No matter how short the infant's life, parents will have formed attachments to the baby and will, therefore, mourn their loss.

grief and loss the parents are experiencing is very real; no matter how short the infant's life, parents will have formed attachments to the baby. "The best care we can give you is not to protect you from pain but to support you through it," accurately summarizes the committee's approach (2).

When the nurse visits the parents, she also conveys her acknowledgement of their loss by expressing her sympathy. And, while she recognizes that each family has unique needs, she offers them the value of her experience dealing with other grieving parents. Founding Grief and Loss Committee member Rita Rodriguez says she prefaces suggestions by saying, "I know this is a lot of information at one time, and I really don't know what you are feeling now. But this is what other families have found helpful. . . ."

In addition, she notes that for some newly grieving parents, any amount of information is an overload. Nurses working with these parents present one decision or one bit of information to them at a time, allowing plenty of time in between. Nurses working with these parents also make a point of assuring them that they may take their time making decisions and may change their minds.

Achieving Continuity of Care

One of the first tasks the Grief and Loss Committee tackled was to update the procedure manual. The new manual includes sample copies of all the forms it will be necessary to fill out, such as the birth certificate, death certificate, autopsy or genetic work-up consent, and disposition of remains instructions. Nurses are guided by step-by-step directions through the intricacies of the paperwork. Suggestions of what to say and do to effectively support the grieving family are included in the manual as well.

The Grief and Loss Committee also compiled a two-part packet of materials used by the nurse and the family. In the nurse's section are the forms the nurse may need and a picture card provided by Resolve Through Sharing. The card is placed outside the door to the mother's room so all axillary hospital personnel will be aware of the situation and act accordingly.

Also in the nurse's section is a checklist of forms to be completed, communications that need to be made, keepsakes parents may want, etc. The original of the checklist (see the sample) stays in the mother's file; one copy stays in the labor and delivery department; the second copy is sent to the unit to which the mother is transferred after delivery. The checklist is a valuable tool that helps nurses ensure continuity and completeness of patient care and documents nursing's role in that care.

The parents' section of the packet is given to them as soon as possible by their nurse. It includes:

• a booklet, "When Hello Means Goodbye; A Guide for Parents Whose Child Dies Before Birth, at Birth or Shortly After Birth" (2);

• a letter from the Grief and Loss Committee expressing its sympathy and offering assistance;

- a handout on dealing with engorgement after infant loss;
- a flyer from a local mortuary that offers free burial or cremation for the infant;
- a list of suggestions on dealing with grief;
- a list of local support groups;
- a memento card on which the baby's name, weight, length, footprints, parents' names, and date and location of birth are recorded; and
- an evaluation form of the labor and delivery unit care they received for parents to complete and return.

Caring for the Grieving Family

The information packet is a tangible way for nurses to show their support. Many fathers cling to the packet and involve themselves in the decisions they must make. This may represent their effort to regain control over a world that has been turned upside down for them. Giving the information packet to parents immediately after the death of their infant helps them take advantage of the many choices available to them at SUH.

Parents of a baby who is dying or has died are encouraged to hold their baby. They may want to provide whatever care their dying baby may need, such as feeding, diapering, or dressing, or may wish to unwrap their dead infant to see the baby's body. Often, parents are reluctant to hold or see a baby who has died or feel fearful of the experience. Yet, "seeing and holding the baby helps the parents face the reality of what has happened and begin the normal mourning process" (3). As a result of nurses' and physicians' support, many dying babies at SUH spend their last moments in their mothers' arms. Even parents who were initially reluctant to hold their baby usually comment, "I wish I had held my baby longer."

Pictures of the baby are another service nurses offer to parents. Photographs are taken of the baby clothed and unclothed in a basket lined with pastel-colored cloth. If the parents do not want the photographs, they are stored in the mother's chart. That way, they are still available in case the parents change their minds, which often happens. Or, parents may prefer keepsakes such as the baby's ID band, the blanket the baby was wrapped in, the completed crib card, hand and footprints, and/or a lock of hair, all of which nurses collect.

Naming the baby and baptizing or blessing the baby are other possibilities extended to parents. They can opt to have the baby baptized or blessed by a nurse, the SUH chaplain, or a religious official of their selection. If the baby is baptized, the seashell used is given to the parents.

Nurses also act as liaisons between the family and medical staff, social workers, and the chaplain. They offer to make contacts with other caregivers, answer questions, or provide services, such as checking on autopsy results, that family members require.

Adapted and reprinted with the permission of Stanford University Hospital, Stanford, CA.

If the family has chosen to have an autopsy performed, preliminary autopsy results, including reports of gross anomalies and the condition of the cord and placenta are usually available within 24 hours. Results are phoned to the physician, who is responsible for informing the parents. The family's nurse makes herself available to the parents to answer questions that invariably come up. Complete written autopsy results, including genetic findings, are discussed at the mother's postpartum checkup four to six weeks later. Couples may then be referred for genetic counseling, if appropriate.

Another nursing function, if the baby has not yet been born, is to physically and emotionally support the mother as she undergoes tests and procedures. Typically, the family's stress and denial levels are so high at this point that the already unfamiliar medical world becomes incomprehensible. One mother, told point-blank that her 36-week-old fetus was dead, asked five times in the next hour if the baby was okay.

Once the baby is born and the mother has recovered, she is encouraged to go to the maternity unit. Because the maternity unit is a family-centered

---

How To Deal With Grief: Suggestions For Parents

---

1. Resume old and new relationships both as a couple and by yourself.

2. *Nutrition:*
   A. Eat a balanced diet that includes milk, meat, vegetables, fruit, and whole grains.
   B. Avoid junk foods.

3. *Fluid Intake:*
   A. Drink eight glasses of liquids per day (juice, water, caffeine-free soda).
   B. Avoid caffeine and alcohol; they cause dehydration, headaches, and low back pain. Alcohol also depresses body function and natural emotional expression.

4. Eliminate tobacco. It depletes your body of vitamins, increases the acid level in your stomach, decreases circulation, and can cause palpitations.

5. Have a physical examination about four months after your loss; while you are grieving, your body is at risk for life-threatening disease.

6. Exercise daily; biking, walking, jogging, aerobics, and stretching exercises are all good choices.

7. *Rest:*
   A. Resume your normal sleep pattern as soon as possible.
   B. Avoid increased work activity.
   C. Make sure to rest even if you cannot sleep.

8. *Writing:*
   A. Keep a diary or journal of your thoughts or memories; keep mementos.
   B. Write letters, notes, and/or poems to or about your baby.

9. *Reading:*
   A. Read books, articles, and poems that help you understand your grief and find comfort so you do not feel so alone.
   B. Avoid "scare" literature and technical medical publications.

10. *Changes and decisions:*
    A. Don't move, change jobs, or alter relationships; wait 24 months then decide.
    B. Avoid long trips; your coping mechanisms are decreased.
    C. Don't put away the baby's clothes until you feel ready.
    D. Don't let others make decisions for you.
    E. Don't become pregnant until after the first anniversary of your loss.

11. Admit to yourself and family when you need help; it'll lessen your pain and loneliness.

12. Accept the help of others. Ask people to do specific things for you, such as bringing you food, keeping you company, or caring for living children.

13. Accept the support others offer; allow family and friends to share your grief.

14. Talk to your family and friends about the baby and share your feelings.

15. Request help or support from clergy to help you renew your faith and hope.

16. Join a support group. Couples who have "been there" already can give support, help, and hope.

Excerpted from a May 1983 lecture given by Glen W. Davidson, Ph.D., author of *Understanding Mourning* (Minneapolis, Augsburg Publishing House, 1984). Used with permission.

---

rest. For women who are mourning, these may be overwhelming activities. After studying mourners' grief reactions, one psychiatrist noted, "insomnia and loss of appetite were almost universal" (4). The mother's sleep is often punctuated with nightmares.

Fathers, Grandparents, and Siblings

At times, fathers may feel overlooked or may ignore their own grief in order to be strong for their partners. They may not feel able to cry or talk about their feelings as easily as their partners. This difference in coping styles, which may continue throughout the mourning process, may be misinterpreted if it is not discussed. Nurses encourage parents to keep the lines of communication between them open.

Grandparents may suffer doubly. Not only have they lost a grandchild, but they also see their own children in pain that they cannot prevent. In an effort to ease the grief, grandparents may attempt to smooth the situation over by encouraging the couple to get on with life and forget about the baby. In this case, nurses encourage grandparents to support the couple's open expression of grief.

Siblings are often bewildered and overwhelmed by the loss of "their baby." Young children miss their parents and may be frightened by the hospital setting. They often ask difficult questions such as, "Why did our baby die?" Many think they are somehow responsible for the baby's death. Nurses can help the family reassure the children or can talk with the children themselves.

An open visitation policy and a private room enables family members to congregate and support each other. A cot is supplied so the father can spend the night. Grandparents and siblings are allowed to hold the baby and, if the parents consent, take pictures. It is not uncommon for family members to turn to the nurse for guidance or to ask questions regarding the baby's death. In response, nurses offer support and information and make referrals, as necessary.

Postdischarge Reactions

Once the mother goes home and the funeral is over and friends and family members have gone on with their lives, the newly bereaved mother may begin to feel an overwhelming sense of loneliness. She may feel completely isolated and believe that no one else understands what she is going through. The numbness that helped shield the parents from the depth of their tragedy begins to wear off, intensifying their grief (5).

After the initial shock wears off, many parents next experience denial. They may deny the baby's importance since it "never really lived." Some women express their denial by continuing to feel the baby kick even after delivery, or hear their baby cry in the night. Along with denial often

care unit, nurses there are better able to assist not only the grieving mother, but the father, the grandparents, and siblings as well. The mother is also given the option of going to another unit.

During the postpartum period, the mother will experience the same discomforts as any newly delivered woman. When her milk comes in on the third or fourth day, a well-fitted bra, cold packs, pain medication, and minimal hand expression will relieve engorgement. Bromocriptine mesylate (Parlodel) is occasionally prescribed to help curtail lactation. Care in relation to lochia, hemorrhoids, and episiotomies is the same for a grieving mother as for any postpartal woman.

In addition, it is very important for mothers to eat well-balanced meals, walk, and get plenty of comes bargaining, especially if the baby's death, although imminent, has not yet occurred. "If my baby is alive," promise many women, "I will be the best mother in the whole world. . . ."

Anger, another stage of the grieving process, soon surfaces, leading many mothers to resent other mothers and their babies. A mother's anger may be directed at the father of the baby, the physician, the staff, God, and/or the world in general. A mother's sense of the unfairness is only intensified when well-meaning people say, "It was God's will" or "You can have another."

Guilt is also a major theme in many parents' mourning. Mothers are plagued with "If only" thoughts. If only I had gone to the doctor sooner . . . or If only I hadn't had that glass of wine. . . . They may also feel as if they've failed because their bodies and genes didn't produce a healthy child. If the pregnancy was unplanned or unwanted, parents' guilt may be compounded.

Customarily, the mourning period takes approximately one year; it may however, last as long as two years. Throughout the mourning period, most parents are overcome by feelings of sadness and emptiness. Their love for the child began before the baby was born; along with the infant's death die their dreams of tomorrow. All their fantasies of party dresses and baseball games now become bitter symbols of what will not be.

The emotions and reactions that characterize parental grief—shock, denial, bargaining, anger, sadness, loneliness, disorganization, acceptance—do not necessarily come in an orderly progression (5). The seemingly endless despair and conflicting emotions may make some women feel as if they are going crazy or that time has lost its meaning. Time weighs heavily on mourners as days go by, and even the simplest tasks seem too much to accomplish.

For some couples, intimacy is a source of comfort; for others it is a painful reminder that the last life they started ended in death. Some couples immediately begin another pregnancy, a reaction termed replacement child syndrome, without letting the emotional wounds from the previous pregnancy heal.

Relatives, friends, and acquaintances are often uncomfortable when the topic of the infant's death and surrounding events comes up. They change the subject or urge the parents to forget about it. Such avoidance of the issue can pervade every corner of the family's life, becoming a breeding ground for "continued sadness, anger, depression, and occasional bouts of madness" (6).

As a way to monitor the parents' progress through their grief, a week after the mother is discharged, her nurse or a nurse from the Grief and Loss Committee makes a follow-up call. The nurse making the call uses the labor and delivery unit's copy of the checklist for reference. During the follow-up call, parents are urged to keep the lines of communication between them and among other family members open and to talk about the pain. Remembering and talking about the baby makes the baby more real for parents and helps validate the infant's life, however short, as an important part of their lives.

Couples are reminded that every parent has a different timetable for grieving; therefore, the partners' reactions may often be out of sync. Writing their feelings down and reading books about how other parents have felt and coped with their loss may help as well. The nurse making the call often recommends participation in a support group for grieving parents to help ease their loneliness. Professional help is advised for parents who feel suicidal or whose relationship seems to be deteriorating.

Ensuring That Staff Is Well-Trained

As part of its goal of providing quality care to grieving parents, the Grief and Loss Committee also initiated staff training efforts. Initially, the committee's inservice coordinator rented a movie, *Some Babies Die*, for SUH staff members to see. (*Some Babies Die* is produced and directed by Martyn Langdon Doron, Langdon Films, Australia.) Now, members of the Grief and Loss Committee periodically distribute copies of the grief packet, offer inservices, and show *Some Babies Die* to nurses in the emergency room, maternity department, and intensive care nursery, and to doctors. That way, personnel other than labor and delivery and postpartum unit staff are well-prepared to help women who suffer spontaneous abortions or ectopic pregnancies.

In addition, a library of books on grief and neonatal death (see the reference list) was compiled and is kept in labor and delivery. The books are lent out to staff and parents to assist them with specific problems such as explaining a fetal demise to a sibling. And, in order to help nurses deal with their own grief and anxiety, one of SUH's nursing consultants periodically leads group discussions on the topic.

The Fruits of Evaluation

The Grief and Loss Committee evaluates its work in two ways. The first is through the postdischarge follow-up phone call. Mothers often voice their regrets or suggestions at this time. In addition, the Grief and Loss Committee judges its success by the many donations it has received from grateful families; these are acknowledged by a certificate of appreciation. The most poignant source of feedback, however, is letters from parents. Some recent comments include:

All of you have our sincere thanks for helping us through these very difficult times. The sadness is very overwhelming. But our moments with our daughter and our keepsakes of her will always be precious.

The compassion and kindness of all the nurses/ staff who dealt with me during the preparation for the actual birth was one of the best things about SUH. I feel that the way I was treated at the hospital helped me handle things better emotionally.

We especially appreciated that everyone respected our son's brief life and still made him a person. My husband particularly appreciated that they cared and acknowledged that this was his loss as well as mine.

I have wonderful memories of holding our precious and beautiful daughter for the first and last time. Because of your support and explicit guidance from the beginning, I was able to participate in all the preparations for our daughter's burial.

Some may question the validity of the nurse's role as advisor to grieving parents. Susan Borg and Judith Lasker wrote: "It is in [hospital staff members'] power, through their reactions and the quality of care they provide, to control the enormous difference between a tragedy that is bearable and one made worse by insensitivity, error, or inattention to need" (7). With support and counseling, parents can reach the final stage of the grief process, acceptance of the death of their baby, and recover from the experience.

REFERENCES

1. LIMBO, R. K., AND WHEELER, S. R. *When a Baby Dies: A Handbook for Healing and Helping.* La Crosse, WI, La Crosse Lutheran Hospital/Gunderson Clinic, Ltd., 1986.
2. SCHWIEBERT, P. T., AND KIRK, P. *When Hello Means Goodbye: A Guide for Parents Whose Child Dies Before Birth, At Birth or Shortly After Birth.* rev. 2nd ed. Portland, OR, Perinatal Loss, 1985, p. 24.
3. BORG, S. O., AND LASKER, J. *When Pregnancy Fails: Families Coping with Miscarriage, Stillbirth, and Infant Death.* Boston, MA, Beacon Press, 1985, p. 54.
4. _____ . p. 18.
5. ILSE, S. *Empty Arms: Coping after Miscarriage, Stillbirth and Infant Deathcarriage, Stillbirth or Neonatal Death.* Long Lake, MN, Wintergreen Press, 1985.
6. DEFRAIN, J., AND OTHERS. *Stillborn: The Invisible Death.* Lexington, MA, Lexington Books, 1986, p. 2.
7. Borg, *op. cit.,* p. 124.

BIBLIOGRAPHY

MANNING, D. *Don't Take My Grief Away: What to Do When You Lose a Loved One.* Springfield, IL, Human Services Press, 1979.
SCHWIEBERT, P. T., AND KIRK, P. *Still to Be Born.* Portland, OR, Perinatal Loss, 1986.

The Dangers Of Prenatal Cocaine Use

Reprinted from MCN: The American Journal of Maternal Child Nursing, May/June 1988

Because of the dramatic effects cocaine can have on both mother and fetus, prevention, early detection, and intervention are essential.

JUDY SMITH

On several different occasions, Beth, a 24-year-old, middle-class, married woman, had snorted small amounts of cocaine. She had used cocaine when she was with close friends, while alone with her husband, and a few times by herself. She was convinced that she could take it or leave it at will; addiction, she was sure, was not a problem for her.

When she found out she was six weeks pregnant, she discontinued her cocaine use entirely, and her pregnancy progressed without any observable problems. She used cocaine once at about 28 weeks' gestation without any complications.

At 34 weeks' gestation, she snorted an unspecified quantity of cocaine at 8:00 P.M. Shortly afterward, she felt strong contractions begin. She was admitted to the labor unit at 9:15 P.M. with contractions every 2 to 3 minutes and fetal tachycardia. Tocolysis was attempted with magnesium sulfate per protocol. An hour later, late decelerations appeared on the fetal monitor and Beth was quickly prepared for a cesarean birth. She delivered a viable, 4-pound 10-ounce girl with Apgars of 5 and 7 and no noticeable congenital anomalies.

Beth typifies the difficulties the health care system confronts when coping with cocaine abuse during pregnancy. There has been a marked increase in cocaine use in the United States during the past few years and cocaine has become more socially acceptable and more widely available to both the affluent and the poor of the nation. Thousands of women from middle and upper socioeconomic classes are addicted to what many see as the glamour drug of the 1980s.

Approximately 20 million people in the United States have used cocaine on one occasion, and 5 million use it regularly (1). The National Institute on Drug Abuse reports that among street drugs, U.S. high school students favor cocaine second only to marijuana (2). There is a lack of national data on maternal cocaine abuse, but indications that the problem is growing are unmistakable. One New York City hospital recently reported that 10 percent of all newborns born there had a positive urine screen for cocaine (1).

In addition to the physiologic dangers cocaine use during pregnancy produces, it also raises difficult legal and ethical questions. How do we balance the rights of the mother with the rights of her unborn child? Should the mother be held legally accountable for endangering her fetus, or are both the mother and the baby considered victims of a disease? Was the mother aware of the harmful effects cocaine can have on a growing fetus? Was she in need of preconceptional education? If a mother is identified as a cocaine user, should her infant be sent home with her to a potentially drug-using environment?

The legal obligations and responsibilities of caregivers are equally clouded. Does the caregiver have a legal responsibility to the fetus to report the mother's cocaine use? What impact will the caregiver's report have on the issues of patient confidentiality and the mother's right to privacy?

Lately, the national trend is to protect child welfare, health, and safety through enforcement of the child abuse and neglect reporting laws rather than to maintain maternal confidentiality (3). Keeping this trend in mind when determining legal obligation and responsibility to report suspected child abuse or neglect resulting from perinatal use of illicit drugs can be beneficial.

Pharmacology of Prenatal Cocaine Use

The rapidly growing number of cocaine-affected pregnancies has caught health care providers by surprise. Data related to the effects of cocaine on the developing fetus are now appearing in the literature and represent intense, ongoing investigation of cocaine's cause and effect relationships.

There are many common misconceptions about cocaine use (see Cocaine Misconceptions). For pregnant women, the most profound misconception is that the placenta protects the unborn baby from toxic substances taken during pregnancy.

JUDY E. SMITH, R.N.P., M.N., is a certified ob/gyn nurse practitioner and an associate professor of maternal-child nursing at California State University, Long Beach, California. For reprints of this article, see the classified section.

EFFECTS OF MATERNAL COCAINE USE ON MOTHERS AND FETUSES/BABIES

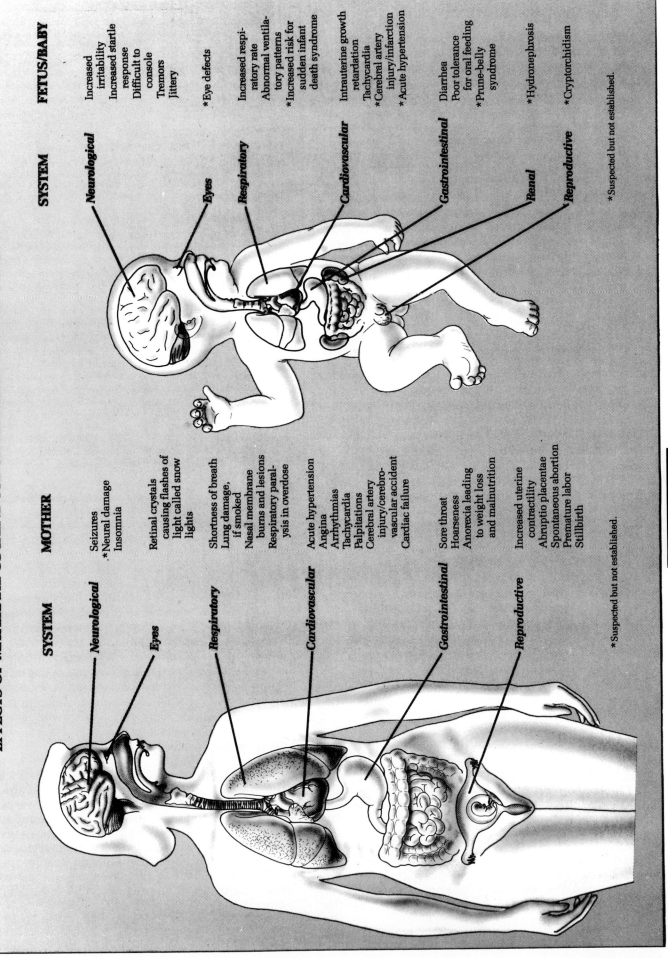

MOTHER

SYSTEM	MOTHER
Neurological	Seizures *Neural damage Insomnia
Eyes	Retinal crystals causing flashes of light called snow lights
Respiratory	Shortness of breath Lung damage, if smoked Nasal membrane burns and lesions Respiratory paralysis in overdose
Cardiovascular	Acute hypertension Angina Arrhythmias Tachycardia Palpitations Cerebral artery injury/cerebrovascular accident Cardiac failure
Gastrointestinal	Sore throat Hoarseness Anorexia leading to weight loss and malnutrition
Reproductive	Increased uterine contractility Abruptio placentae Spontaneous abortion Premature labor Stillbirth

*Suspected but not established.

FETUS/BABY

SYSTEM	FETUS/BABY
Neurological	Increased irritability Increased startle response Difficult to console Tremors Jittery
Eyes	*Eye defects
Respiratory	Increased respiratory rate Abnormal ventilatory patterns *Increased risk for sudden infant death syndrome
Cardiovascular	Intrauterine growth retardation Tachycardia *Cerebral artery injury/infarction *Acute hypertension
Gastrointestinal	Diarrhea Poor tolerance for oral feeding *Prune-belly syndrome
Renal	*Hydronephrosis
Reproductive	*Cryptorchidism

*Suspected but not established.

Many drugs freely cross the placenta. Drugs such as cocaine that act upon the central nervous system are often lipophilic and of relatively low molecular weight, characteristics that make it easier for the substance to cross the placenta and the fetal blood-brain barrier (1).

Animal studies documenting the pharmacologic effects of cocaine on physiology are consistent in their findings (see Effects of Maternal Cocaine Use on Mothers and Fetuses/Babies). Cocaine stimulates the central nervous system much as amphetamines do. It has a half-life in plasma of about one hour following administration, making it a stimulant of short duration. Additionally, cocaine stimulates the peripheral nervous system and prevents norepinephrine reuptake at the nerve terminals (4). The result is a high circulating level of norepinephrine, which causes vasoconstriction, tachycardia, acute hypertension, and uterine contractions. In pregnancy, placental vasoconstriction results, restricting blood flow to the fetus (1).

There has also been a recent and dramatic increase in the use of alkaloidal cocaine, better known as crack. Crack is often smoked because it vaporizes at relatively low temperatures. As it is absorbed by the pulmonary vasculature, it produces a rapid euphoria, which diminishes in 30 minutes. Crack is used repeatedly to regain the euphoric state, a pattern that can lead to high levels of fetal exposure in pregnant women (5).

Pregnancy Complications

Women who use cocaine during pregnancy are more likely than nonusers to have spontaneous first-trimester abortions, a finding consistent with the implication of placental vasoconstriction induced by cocaine use (1). The incidence of abruptio placentae, usually occurring within an hour of cocaine administration, is higher than in the nonusing population (1,5,7). This finding is attributed to the acute hypertension caused by cocaine and the well-established relationship between hypertension and abruptio placentae.

Third trimester use of cocaine by pregnant women has been reported to induce a sudden onset of uterine contractions, fetal tachycardia, and excessive fetal activity within hours or even minutes of ingestion (1,6). The premature labor and abnormal fetal heart rate patterns experienced by Beth are not unusual.

In the general population, cocaine has been associated with palpitations, angina, and arrythmias. Even small amounts of cocaine found in sensitive individuals have been linked to deaths resulting from cardiac failure (8). For pregnant women, cocaine-induced tachycardia further strains the already overworked maternal heart.

The teratogenic effect of cocaine on the developing fetus is relatively unknown at this time. Cocaine's profound impact on cardiovascular

---

COCAINE MISCONCEPTIONS

Cocaine is a harmless drug. The cocaine epidemic and all the talk about the hazards of using the drug are scare tactics and media hype. Cocaine is one of the most insidious drugs on the illicit market today. It can exacerbate psychiatric problems and cause severe physical problems, even death. Its use has wrecked innumerable families and careers. In some cities, cocaine deaths are becoming more common than heroin deaths.

Even if cocaine is harmful, it harms only the user. Cocaine abuse can hurt not only its users, but those around them—families, friends, co-workers, employers, employees. Treating drug abuse drives up health care costs, which affects everyone. Cocaine is the most expensive drug dependence to treat, perhaps because relapses and retreatment are common. The annual cost of cocaine abuse to American society is estimated at $25–$35 billion.

Cocaine is nonaddictive. Cocaine is the most powerful psychological reinforcer of any of the illicit drugs, allowing for profound dependence. The biochemical mechanisms of cocaine dependence are not understood and why some casual users become addicted while others don't is unclear.

Cocaine is only habit-forming if it is smoked or injected. Although the most serious dependencies are generally found among those who freebase (smoke cocaine) or use the drug intravenously, a significant number of people in treatment for cocaine-related problems have only inhaled it.

People who only use the drug once a week, or once a month, don't become dependent on it. Dependency and abuse can't be thought of only in terms of frequency. Some people who use cocaine once a month do so in binges during which they may ingest huge quantities. Any use at all, but particularly daily or binge use, puts a person at risk for addiction.

Based on "Cocaine Use In America," *Prevention Networks*, National Institute on Drug Abuse. (DHHS publ. No. ADM 86-1433) Washington, D.C., U.S. Government Printing Office, Apr. 1986.

---

function can potentially place the exposed fetus in jeopardy for both short- and long-term adverse effects (5). There have been only isolated reports and small-sample pilot studies that suggest cocaine might be responsible for congenital anomalies. One infant studied by Ira Chasnoff exhibited cryptorchidism, prune-belly syndrome, and hydronephrosis that may have been associated with maternal cocaine use (6). The effects of cocaine as a human teratogen must be studied more extensively before conclusions can be derived.

Effects on the Newborn

The consequences of cocaine exposure to the fetus are ambiguous. Unlike opiate-exposed neonates, cocaine-exposed infants do not seem to experience the classic neonatal abstinence syndrome. Infants born to mothers who have used cocaine during pregnancy tend to be shorter, lower in birthweight, and have smaller head circumferences as compared to infants of women who were drug-free during pregnancy (1).

Cocaine-exposed infants may show mild to

moderate tremulousness and increased irritability, muscular rigidity, and startle response. They are difficult to console and state lability is pronounced (5,6). In addition, elevated respiratory and heart rates, poor tolerance for oral feedings, diarrhea, and disturbed sleep patterns have been linked to cocaine exposure in utero (9,10). Newborns exhibiting these symptoms are evaluated for cocaine exposure in utero (see the section on postpartum care).

Maternal prenatal cocaine use also places the infant at potentially increased risk for sudden infant death syndrome (SIDS). Abnormal sleeping ventilatory patterns implicated in SIDS have been reported in cocaine-exposed neonates (10). The rate of SIDS in cocaine-exposed neonates may be as high as 15 percent, more than three times the rate in heroin-exposed neonates (1).

Perinatal cerebral infarction in infants exposed to cocaine just prior to birth has also been reported (1,11). The finding of perinatal cerebral infarction in cocaine-exposed neonates tends to parallel reports of acute cerebral and myocardial infarction in young adults shortly after cocaine use (1).

Caring for Cocaine Users

Planning appropriate nursing interventions for cocaine using women can be a difficult and intricate task. Assessment can be exceptionally complex due to the lack of clear physical signs that indicate cocaine use. Cocaine addiction can be concealed by demeanors from shy and secretive to outgoing and witty. Consequently, nurses may find it difficult to identify the cocaine abusing woman.

Prevention, undoubtedly, is the most effective and ideal nursing intervention. Many women, like Beth, are unaware of the potential dangers inherent in cocaine use. The key to any successful prevention effort is getting accurate information to those at greatest risk.

A substantial proportion of cocaine users are young, well-paid, well-educated, upwardly mobile professionals in their 20s and 30s (2). Anne, a 32-year-old advertising executive, visited her private obstetrician-gynecologist for a preconceptional consultation and evaluation. The office nurse asked her about any history of cocaine use, which Anne immediately denied. The nurse used a well-planned, nonjudgmental, natural-appearing pause at this point. Anne qualified her answer with, "Well, very, very rarely and not enough to cause any harm or alarm." The pause gave Anne a moment to think about the question. The nurse's nonjudgmental manner and nonthreatening attitude invited Anne's honest disclosure, paving the way for preconceptional education about the dangers of cocaine use in pregnancy.

Young professionals tend to be fairly sophisticated. Many grew up in the 1960s and early 1970s, when scare-tactic approaches to prevention destroyed the credibility of the information presented. For this reason, nurses must make special efforts to deliver information straightforwardly and unemotionally (2). The nurse in Anne's obstetrician-gynecologist's office gave Anne factual information about cocaine use and corrected her misconceptions (1).

Prevention efforts targeted to the teenaged population require a different approach than those designed for adult professionals. Teenagers are not apt to perceive health hazards as real and immediate dangers. Effective interventions for teens center around dispelling the popular idea that cocaine use is normal, acceptable, and that everybody uses drugs. Pairing the well-documented health hazards of cocaine use with those of amphetamines or heroin, which have been more widely studied and publicized, allows nurses to draw on teenagers' background knowledge to construct meaningful parallels. Enlisting the aid of teen peers to impart information to teen groups enhances the effectiveness of prevention efforts and can be accomplished cost effectively via a videotaped presentation shown in a clinic waiting room.

Educational efforts must rely on current preliminary data and will need to be updated as new information becomes available. Widespread knowledge is the best means to the long-term end—prevention.

Early detection of cocaine use in pregnancy complemented by appropriate intervention and follow-up affords the best outcome for both mother and infant. In order to identify maternal cocaine use, the nurse must be tactfully inquisitive. During the initial contact, assessing the woman's mood, attention to personal grooming, and affect may provide subtle or overt clues to the possibility of cocaine or other substance use.

As the nurse compiles a nursing and medical history, the ideal opportunity for questioning substance abuse presents itself. Standard history forms include questions about smoking practices, alcohol use, and over-the-counter drug use. Altering the form to guide the questioning toward ascertainment of illicit drug use is a simple task (see Drug Use Assessment).

Selecting nonjudgmental, sensitively-constructed questions and delivering them at the same speed and in the same tone of voice and matter-of-fact manner as nonsensitive questions maximize the likelihood that the woman will answer truthfully. A woman is more likely to respond honestly if the nurse has conveyed that she will not react with shock, accusations, or a guilt-laden lecture. The development of trust and rapport are prerequisites for helping substance-abusing pregnant women confront their drug problems.

Identifying cocaine use during pregnancy can be concurrently challenging and frustrating. Often the woman will deny that she uses cocaine and fails to realize how she has incorporated the drug into her life. The woman may believe she has control over her cocaine use. Showing her the connection between cocaine use and related health problems may enable her to more realistically face the impact of cocaine use on her pregnancy. Counseling, education, and careful prenatal health care management can help forestall continued maternal cocaine use, limiting adverse fetal effects from cocaine exposure and reducing the risk of related maternal complications (1).

Ellen, a 28-year-old woman pregnant with her second child, came to the clinic for her first prenatal visit at 21 weeks' gestation. She was underweight, appeared quite nervous, and was in a hurry to leave. Ellen denied use of any drugs or alcohol. She was referred to the clinic's nutritionist as intervention for her inadequate weight gain. She missed her next prenatal appointment.

At her next visit, Ellen still hadn't gained any weight, and complained of her heart racing at times, of having headaches, and of having insomnia. The nurse suspected drug use and used the fact that Ellen hadn't followed nutritional guidelines to build a trusting, nonjudgmental rapport. She then sensitively asked her about drug use.

Ellen admitted that she had used cocaine but had stopped when she suspected she was pregnant. As the nurse related her concerns about cocaine use in pregnancy in general terms, Ellen interjected that her current use of cocaine was quite regular. She appeared to be relieved at having revealed the problem. Her nurse identified the short-term goals of Ellen's care: correcting Ellen's nutritional deficit and helping her give up her use of cocaine.

The nurse referred Ellen to a local cocaine treatment program; her prenatal care continued to be provided at the clinic. She began to follow her nutrition program and gained adequate weight during the remainder of the pregnancy. At the clinic, Ellen received a great deal of support and encouragement for her weight gain, for her continued involvement in the treatment program, and for abstaining from cocaine. She gave birth to a normal appearing, 40-week gestation boy weighing 7 pounds 4 ounces; his Apgars were 9 and 9. Ellen continued to attend her treatment program's support group and abstained from cocaine use even after she delivered a healthy son.

Recognizing intrapartum cocaine effects is as difficult as antepartum detection. Many signs are subtle and can appear unrelated. Fetal tachycardia, excessive fetal activity, and a sudden onset of unusually strong uterine contractions at the beginning of labor alert the nurse to inquire about recent cocaine use. Fetal meconium passage and a precipitous labor and delivery can also be related to use of cocaine (1).

Toxicologic urine screening will detect cocaine

DRUG USE ASSESSMENT

Drug History	No	Yes	Type	Amount	Frequency of Use	Last Time Used	How Taken	Comments
A. Alcohol								
B. Nicotine								
C. Medications								
Vitamins								
Laxatives								
Antacids								
Cold Remedies								
Caffeine								
Aspirin								
Pain Relievers								
Sleeping Aids								
Sedatives								
Tranquilizers								
Marijuana								
Cocaine								
Heroin								
Hallucinogens								
D. Drug Allergies								

ingestion within the past 24 hours. Cocaine reaches the brain and neurons of the sympathetic nervous system in 3 minutes when it is inhaled, in 15 seconds when it is injected, and in 7 seconds when it is smoked. In the latter, it is rapidly metabolized by the liver, which makes it difficult to screen anything other than current use (2). Toxicologic blood screening also renders information regarding the quantity of cocaine in the blood.

The goal when treating a woman in labor who has recently ingested cocaine is to stabilize both mother and fetus. Placing the patient in a lateral recumbent position and administering oxygen via face mask may improve fetal oxygenation and bradycardia. Monitoring of the fetus and of maternal blood pressure and pulse provides valuable, continuous, assessment data. Seizure precautions and neurologic assessments are critical if the woman is in a transient, acute, cocaine-induced hypertensive episode. Assessment of respiratory rate and rhythm will enable the nurse to detect respiratory impairment and paralysis associated with cocaine overdose (2). Given the short half-life of cocaine in plasma, maternal stabilization usually occurs within an hour.

After the mother and fetus are stable, the mother must be carefully observed for the signs of abruptio placentae: headache, constant abdominal pain, and excessive vaginal bleeding. The potential for catastrophic abruptio placentae is high and must be anticipated.

Postpartum Care

Cocaine use by a pregnant woman may go unnoticed during prenatal and intrapartum care. Detection may first occur during the assessment of the infant in the nursery. If a nurse suspects neonatal cocaine exposure, she must initiate both treatment of the infant and maternal psychosocial interventions without delay.

Toxicologic urine screening will detect neonatal cocaine exposure within the past six to nine days. Most drugs persist longer in fetuses and newborns than they do in adults because immature neonatal livers take longer to metabolize the drug. Fetuses and infants have a relative deficiency of plasma cholinesterases, the enzymes that break down cocaine. Cocaine and cocaine metabolites can persist in the newborn's urine for several days after delivery (13).

If the neonate is being breast-fed and begins to demonstrate signs of cocaine exposure, evaluate the mother for current cocaine use. Cocaine can be transferred from mother to infant through breast milk (2).

The mother whose cocaine use has gone undetected until after delivery must be postpartally evaluated to determine the degree of her substance abuse. The mother's nurse does this by eliciting from the mother information about the magnitude of her drug use, whether her significant others use drugs, her treatment history, and her expectations for future cocaine use. With this information, nurses can plan appropriate interventions, including health education about cocaine use, referral to a local treatment program, and arranging close follow-up care that ensures a safe environment for the baby (12). In all cases, an approach individualized for each woman's situation is most likely to succeed.

Follow-up discussion with Beth after the birth of her daughter revealed that she was unaware of the risks she had imposed on her unborn baby and herself by using cocaine during her pregnancy. She explained her beliefs about the drug, saying that although cocaine use is illegal, she had thought her use of the drug was safe because she only inhaled small amounts. She had thought of her cocaine use as recreational because she had only taken the drug occasionally, usually in social settings. Many people across the nation share her view that small, recreational use of cocaine is harmless (8).

Beth had discontinued her cocaine use when she discovered she was pregnant because she wanted a healthy baby and knew she shouldn't take any kind of drug unless it was prescribed for her. Later in the pregnancy, on the two occasions when she used cocaine, Beth said that she had been influenced and pressured by her friends to try just a small amount. Because she had no adverse effects at 28 weeks' gestation, she had thought it would be safe to use cocaine again. Throughout the discussion, Beth cried, expressed a great deal of guilt and regret, and reached out for someone to help her cope with her overwhelming feelings.

Beth's nurses chose crisis intervention for her care plan because of Beth's overwhelming feelings of guilt and regret regarding the premature birth of her daughter. After coping with the immediate crisis, Beth was able to concentrate on learning about cocaine use. Once she became aware of the harmful effects of cocaine, she was able to discontinue further use of the drug. She was discharged from the hospital with written material about cocaine and a resource telephone number.

Who's At Risk?

The magnitude of the maternal cocaine abuse problem is just beginning to surface. Attempts to organize approaches to meet this new challenge are now emerging. One is a national drug treatment referral hotline (800-662-HELP), which was established so that people can call for information about treatment facilities within their communities. No one, regardless of their competence or success in other areas of life, is immune from the dangers of cocaine.

REFERENCES

1. CHASNOFF, I. J. Perinatal effects of cocaine. *Contemp.OB/GYN* 29:163–179, May 1987.
2. NATIONAL INSTITUTE ON DRUG ABUSE. Cocaine use in America. IN *Prevention Networks.* (DHHS Publ. No. ADM 86-1433) Washington, D.C., U.S. Government Printing Office, Apr. 1986, pp. 1–14.
3. CHASNOFF, I. J., ED. *Drug Use In Pregnancy.* Norwell, MA, MTP Press Ltd., 1986, pp. 147–155.
4. HOLLAND, D. J. Cocaine use and toxicity. *JEN* 8:166–169, July–Aug. 1982.
5. LeBLANC, P. E., AND OTHERS. Effects of intrauterine exposure to alkaloidal cocaine. *Am.J.Dis.Child.* 141:937–938, Sept. 1987.
6. CHASNOFF, I. J., AND OTHERS. Cocaine use in pregnancy. *N.Engl.J.Med.* 313:666–669, Sept. 12, 1985.
7. ACKER, D., AND OTHERS. Abruptio placentae associated with cocaine use. *Am.J.Obstet.Gynecol.* 146:220–221, May 15, 1983.
8. NATIONAL INSTITUTE ON DRUG ABUSE. *Cocaine Addiction.* (DHHS Publ. No. ADM 85-1427) Washington, D.C., U.S. Government Printing Office, 1985.
9. NEWALD, J. Cocaine infants: a new arrival at hospitals' steps? *Hospitals* 60:96, Apr. 5, 1986.
10. WARD, S. L., AND OTHERS. Abnormal sleeping ventilatory patterns in infants of substance-abusing mothers. *Am.J.Dis.Child.* 140:1015–1020, Oct. 1986.
11. CHASNOFF, I. J., AND OTHERS. Perinatal cerebral infarction and maternal cocaine use. *J.Pediatr.* 108:456–459, Mar. 1986.
12. CHYCHULA, N. M. Screening for substance abuse in a primary care setting. *Nurse Pract.* 9:15–24, July 1984.
13. CHASNOFF, I. J. Cocaine and pregnancy. *Childbirth Educator* 37–42, Winter 1986–1987.

A Comprehensive Look At Hyperbilirubinemia

Reprinted from MCN: The American Journal of Maternal Child Nursing, September/October 1988

Jaundice, although common, is not well-understood. This article, the first of two, explains its development, relevant research, and preventive measures.

NORMA NEAHR WILKERSON

Hyperbilirubinemia, although common among normal infants, is poorly understood and of uncertain clinical significance. Approximately 80 percent of all newborns become clinically jaundiced (1). Fifty percent of full-term newborns become visibly jaundiced in the first week of life (2). This article, the first of two, describes the natural history of neonatal jaundice in healthy, full-term infants, provides an overview of current literature on hyperbilirubinemia, distinguishes the various etiologic categories, and discusses preventive measures. The second article, to be published in MCN's January–February issue, describes methods of treating hyperbilirubinemia.

How Bilirubin Metabolizes

Bilirubin metabolism is a function of both the liver and the intestinal tract. Infants are born with relative polycythemia, a surplus of red blood cells. The excess compensates for the relative hypoxia of intrauterine life. As fetal red blood cells mature, die, and are catabolyzed, bilirubin, a breakdown product, is formed. One molecule of hemoglobin produces four molecules of bilirubin (1). In utero, the mother's hepatic and intestinal function clear the fetus's blood of excess bilirubin.

In normal, full-term infants, excess red blood cells deteriorate in neonatal circulation, causing a rise in serum bilirubin to between 3 and 5 mg/dl. The bilirubin molecules, which are insoluble in water, then bind to albumin, a carrier protein, for transport through the bloodstream to the liver (see

NORMA NEAHR WILKERSON, R.N., Ph.D., is associate professor of nursing, University of Wyoming School of Nursing, Laramie, Wyoming. This article is based on the presentation she made at the 1987 second national MCN Convention. For reprints, see the classified section.

Bilirubin Metabolism). Hepatocytes, with the assistance of a ligand, are able to conjugate (attach) albumin-bound bilirubin molecules with molecules of glucuronide, a product of liver glycogen. Conjugated bilirubin is water soluble and can thus be cleared from the bloodstream.

Conjugated bilirubin is excreted from the liver into bile. Via the gallbladder, it passes into the intestine. Meconium, which has accumulated in the fetus's bowel, is loaded with bilirubin. After birth, when the sterile fetal bowel is colonized with normal flora, bacterial enzymes convert bilirubin into urobilinogen, most of which is eliminated from the body when the infant defecates. If stool remains in the newborn's bowel for a prolonged period of time, bilirubin is reabsorbed by the bloodstream and must then be recirculated.

There are many opportunities for neonatal bilirubin metabolism to be disrupted in otherwise healthy, full-term infants. Such disruption causes hyperbilirubinemia. Prenatal or intrapartum hypoxia, associated with increased fetal blood volume, increased fetal-placental blood volume, and increased neonatal blood volume can ultimately result in increased bilirubin production (see Proposed Pathogenesis of Polycythemia). Delayed cord clamping at birth can also cause a large placental transfusion, predisposing the newborn to polycythemia and hyperbilirubinemia as well (3). Normal, full-term infants who experience bruising, hematomas, or trauma from long, difficult, or forcep deliveries are at risk for increased and more rapid breakdown of red blood cells, leading to elevated bilirubin levels. Or, increased bilirubin can result if the mother has been mildy sensitized to Rh, A, or B antigens and has produced antibodies that break down fetal/neonatal red blood cells into bilirubin products.

In addition, the immaturity of a newborn's liver inhibits the physiology of bilirubin transport. Because a newborn's bowel is sterile, the lack of normal bacterial enzymes can interrupt bilirubin excretion, resulting in reabsorption.

Relating Bilirubin to Jaundice

Thus, some degree of physiologic jaundice (PJ) is a normal finding as the infant matures. Visible jaundice occurs as insoluble bilirubin, at serum levels greater than 5 mg/dl, is deposited in fatty, subcutaneous tissue. Sclera, mucous membranes, and urine can also become yellow in color as hyperbilirubinemia progresses. But what does jaundice actually indicate?

Researchers first began to investigate hyperbilirubinemia in the 1950s by studying the importance of conjugated and unconjugated bilirubin, abnormalities of bilirubin excretion, and Rh isoimmunization (4). Studies supported the association between high serum bilirubin levels (unconjugated hyperbilirubinemia) and kernicterus in infants with hemolytic disease. Kernicterus rarely occurs with serum bilirubin levels less than 20 mg/dl, yet controversy over the potential neurological deficits that can occur with serum bilirubin levels less than 20 mg/dl persists (5).

Barbara Foerder retrospectively studied 175 children who had been normal, full-term infants (6). She found no differences in development, as measured by Brazelton and Bayley scales at 3 months, 10 months, and 24 months of age, between infants who were jaundiced as newborns (serum bilirubin levels of less than 20 mg/dl) and those who were not.

How Is Breast-Feeding Involved?

In the 1960s, researchers documented reports of breast-fed infants with prolonged jaundice (7–9). As the infants described in these reports had elevated serum bilirubin levels that continued for longer than normal periods of time, the syndrome was dubbed breast milk jaundice (BMJ) and received much attention. The condition was described as unconjugated hyperbilirubinemia in otherwise healthy, breast-feeding infants. The diagnosis is usually made after the infant's first two weeks of life. If the mother continues to breast-feed, BMJ can last for as long as four months.

Early theorists associated BMJ with pregnane-3 alpha, 20 beta-diol, a maternal steroid present in breast milk of mothers whose infants had BMJ (10,11). The steroid inhibits glucuronide formation. Later studies suggested that breast milk's glucuronide inhibiting property is related to elevated lipase activity in the milk (12). Breast milk in which lipase activity is abnormally high develops abnormally elevated concentrations of free fatty acids, which then inhibit glucuronyl transferase, the enzyme that allows unconjugated bilirubin to attach to glucuronide. The normal newborn's limited ability to absorb and digest fat may also affect bilirubin metabolism (13–15).

Most recently, researchers have arrived at another hypothesis. BMJ develops, they propose, because increased presence of beta-glucuronidase in breast milk leads to increased neonatal intestinal absorption of bilirubin; increased levels of beta-glucuronidase were found in the feces of breast-fed infants (15,16). Breast-fed infants, as

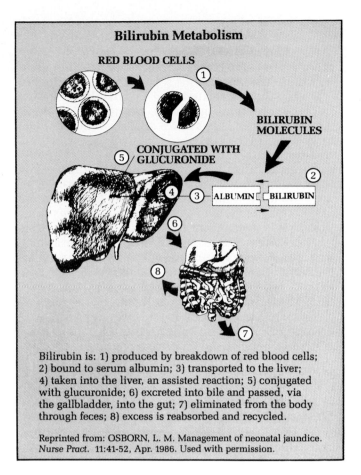

Bilirubin Metabolism

Bilirubin is: 1) produced by breakdown of red blood cells; 2) bound to serum albumin; 3) transported to the liver; 4) taken into the liver, an assisted reaction; 5) conjugated with glucuronide; 6) excreted into bile and passed, via the gallbladder, into the gut; 7) eliminated from the body through feces; 8) excess is reabsorbed and recycled.

Reprinted from: OSBORN, L. M. Management of neonatal jaundice. *Nurse Pract.* 11:41-52, Apr. 1986. Used with permission.

compared to formula-fed newborns, have more acidic feces, less output of stool, and have distinctive intestinal bacterial flora, all of which may account for the differences in fecal beta-glucuronidase activity and bilirubin levels between breast-fed and formula-fed newborns.

The rate at which the newborn evacuates stool directly relates to the amount of bilirubin reabsorbed. Frequent sucking shortens gut transit time and promotes greater output of stool. Studies to compare frequency of feeding with bilirubin levels in breast-fed and formula-fed infants are now being designed (17).

There is a difference, however, between BMJ and breast-feeding associated jaundice (BFAJ). Jaundice that presents within the first few days of life has been documented to occur with greater frequency in breast-fed infants than in formula-fed infants. This form of hyperbilirubinemia is not *caused* by breast milk, but may be correlated with the infant's success at breast-feeding. Lucy Osborne's research correlates BFAJ with lighter weight and poor weight recovery (1). She speculates that "the increased weight loss reflects the quality of nursing. Infants with good functional nursing stimulate an early adequate milk supply. Those who are not breast-feeding well may suffer a relative caloric deprivation, which can then lead to decreased hepatic clearance of bilirubin and subsequent indirect hyperbilirubinemia" (18).

Her findings can be compared with those of Manoel DeCarvalho (17). He demonstrated that feeding frequency and serum bilirubin levels were reliably correlated ($r = -.361$). Infants who nursed more than eight times per day had average serum bilirubin levels of 6.5 mg/dl as compared to an average of 9.3 mg/dl for babies who breast-fed less frequently.

Their findings are consistent with those of a population study of 498 full-term, appropriate for gestational age infants conducted by J. E. Clarkson and colleagues (19). They found that infants who first passed meconium less than 12 hours following delivery were less jaundiced than those who first passed meconium more than 12 hours after delivery. Babies who by four days of age had gained weight tended to be much less jaundiced than those who had lost more than 5 percent of their birth weight in their first four days of life.

Living at a high altitude is another factor associated with increased incidence of neonatal hyperbilirubinemia (20). In a retrospective study of all infants born during a 14-month period in Leadville, Colorado (elevation 3,100 meters), the incidence of hyperbilirubinemia (total serum bilirubin levels greater than 12 mg/dl) was more than twice that of infants born in Denver (elevation 1,600 meters); the incidence was four times that of infants born at sea level.

Jaundice Related to Obstetric Interventions

The incidence of physiologic jaundice not associated with pathophysiologic factors seems to have increased through the 1970s and 1980s. Four specific obstetric interventions are associated with the higher incidence: labor induction, epidural anesthesia, the use of intravenous fluids during labor, and delayed or limited feeding during the infant's first 24 hours of life (21).

Findings of studies investigating the use of oxytocin and prostaglandin for induction of labor are inconsistent. One multifactorial survey of 981 infants reports that elevated bilirubin levels occurred reliably more often when medium or high doses of oxytocin had been used during labor (22). In addition, artificial rupture of membranes and use of oxytocin to induce labor were associated with increased bilirubin levels. When oxytocin was used only to enhance labor (augmentation), it was not found to be related (23).

However, in J. E. Clarkson's population study, the effects of artificial membrane rupture, epidurals, and oxytocin for induction were not found to be significantly related to hyperbilirubinemia in the newborn (19). A Danish prospective study failed to substantiate relationships between hyperbilirubinemia and induction after premature rupture of membranes (N = 250), artificial membrane rupture (N = 270), or induction with oxytocin without amniotomy (N = 219) (24).

N. B. Knepp and colleagues investigated another intervention. They observed elevated bilirubin levels in infants of mothers receiving intravenous 5 percent dextrose (25). The researchers hypothesized a relationship between hydration and increased fetal insulin production. A study of 51 Jamaican women who received no intravenous fluids and 43 who received fluids in varying amounts yielded similar results (26). Serum bilirubin levels were above 10 mg/dl in 15 percent of the infants whose mothers received intravenous fluids; levels above 10 mg/dl were recorded in 4 percent of infants of mothers who did not.

Because well-controlled studies that eliminate potential maternal, fetal, or neonatal complications that increase the incidence of infant jaundice are difficult to design, the influence of obstetric interventions on time of the newborn's first feeding, the quality of the infant's suckling, the frequency of feedings, and gut transit time is difficult to measure. Further efforts to investigate the various hypotheses related to neonatal hyperbilirubinemia are necessary. It is vital to determine whether hospital routines, management, and structured interactions between mother and infant are related to the physiology of hyperbilirubinemia in breast-fed infants.

Applying Research to Practice

Given the well-documented relationships between normal neonatal physiology, infant feeding practices, and hyperbilirubinemia, it is obvious that rigid feeding schedules contribute to increased neonatal jaundice. Instead, mothers need to be encouraged to breast-feed their infants as soon after birth as possible and as frequently as possible thereafter. Based on the literature and my

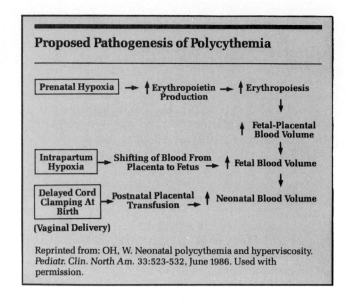

Proposed Pathogenesis of Polycythemia

Reprinted from: OH, W. Neonatal polycythemia and hyperviscosity. *Pediatr. Clin. North Am.* 33:523-532, June 1986. Used with permission.

Variables and Prevention of Nonpathologically-Induced Hyperbilirubinemia

Relevant Variables	Physiologic Jaundice (PJ)	Breast Milk Jaundice (BMJ)	Breast-Feeding Associated Jaundice (BFAJ)
Incidence	20 percent of all neonates have bilirubin levels of 5.0 mg/dl.	1–2 percent of breast-fed neonates have bilirubin levels of 15–25 mg/dl.	10 percent of breast-fed infants have bilirubin levels of 9.0–19.0 mg/dl.
Appearance of Jaundice	Usually in the second to third day of life.	After first week of life when physiologic jaundice is waning.	Usually in second to third day of life.
Clinical Progression	Bilirubin peaks at 5–10 mg/dl by third to fifth day of life; decreases to below 2 mg/dl by day seven. Rate of accumulation below 5 mg/dl/24 hours.	Bilirubin peaks at 10–15 days of life. Infants may remain jaundiced for weeks, rarely months. Diagnosis confirmed if level drops with cessation of breast-feeding for 24–48 hours. Levels usually rise slowly, but not to previous level with resumption of breast-feeding.	Bilirubin peaks by second to third day of life. Rate of accumulation below 5 mg/dl/24 hours. Typically, breast-feeding is not well-established. Bilirubin level may go as high as 15–19 mg/dl.
Etiology and Associated Factors	Excess of fetal red blood cells in neonatal circulation. Load can be increased by perinatal hypoxia, trauma, or passage of maternal serum antibodies to Rh, A, or B antigens during transition from fetal to neonatal circulation after birth. Mean peak serum conjugated bilirubin levels increase at higher elevations and in Chinese, Japanese, Korean, and American Indian populations.	Controversy still exists over cause. Current explanations are: increase in intestinal absorption of bilirubin due to beta-glucuronidase (present in feces of breast-fed infants); and less frequent stooling of breast-fed infants.	Smaller, less vigorous infants who do not nurse well. Caloric deprivation then leads to decreased hepatic transport and clearance of bilirubin. Poor intake of milk is the cause, not factors related to breast milk.
Primary Prevention	All neonates experience some degree of hyperbilirubinemia. It can be exacerbated by delayed passage of meconium, limited caloric intake, and higher elevations. Identify infants at risk, increase feedings, and decrease gut transit time.	Breast-fed infants should be monitored. If history of BMJ in previous sibling, promote early, frequent feedings and exposure to sunlight, and provide parental anticipatory guidance.	Infants at risk require early and frequent feedings. If breast-feeding is not well-established in first 24 hours, caloric supplementation may be useful.
Secondary Prevention	Increased feedings, exposure to sunlight, phototherapy if bilirubin approaches 18–20 mg/dl.	Interrupt nursing for 24–48 hours to confirm diagnosis. Follow-up required to support and reestablish breast-feeding.	Increase feedings to provide calories; phototherapy may be instituted if levels approach 18–20 mg/dl.
Tertiary Prevention	Usually no complications if infant is monitored and treated to keep level below 20 mg/dl. Risk of kernicterus increases as levels rise above 18–20 mg/dl.	Usually self-limiting and benign. No reported cases of kernicterus caused by BMJ.	Same as tertiary prevention of physiologic jaundice.

clinical experience, I recommend a two-hour interval between feedings during the first week, particularly if the infant's bilirubin level is rising. Frequent breast-feeding sessions that begin soon after birth stimulate maternal milk productivity, stimulate the infant's intestinal motility, and can help keep bilirubin levels low.

I also recommend rooming-in in order to keep mother and infant in close proximity. Mothers can be encouraged to nurse their infants whenever the infants begin to awaken, root, and suck on their fists, early signs of the stimulus to feed. If the infant is offered the breast at this time, rather than after crying has begun, breast-feeding sessions are more likely to be successful and mutually beneficial. Studies that investigate these variables in relation to nipple soreness have shown that limiting suckling time is not a proven technique for preventing or treating sore nipples (27–29).

Mothers can also be encouraged to expose their infants to natural sunlight. Feeding and caring for the infant in front of a window and giving the infant sun baths in warm daylight are primary prevention strategies. On the other hand, parents must be warned to avoid exposing the infant to excessive amounts of sun. With the trend toward early discharge, the need for outpatient monitoring of jaundiced infants cannot be overlooked.

When to Begin Treatment

Even if an otherwise healthy infant's serum indirect bilirubin concentration rises, the mother can continue breast-feeding. Generally, a healthy full-term infant with a bilirubin level greater than 12 mg/dl is examined to exclude pathophysiologic conditions such as blood incompatibilities, hypothyroidism, inherited glucuronyl transferase deficiency, or biliary atresia. Whether the infant is experiencing normal physiologic jaundice or breast milk jaundice, treatment (phototherapy) is not required unless serum bilirubin nears 12–15 mg/dl by the second day of life or reaches 15–18 mg/dl thereafter. Kernicterus has never been reported in an infant with BMJ (30).

Some caregivers accept 15–16 mg/dl as the level at which to initiate phototherapy. However, Barbara Foerder's findings support a higher cutoff (6). She found no significant differences in developmental outcomes between hyperbilirubinemic infants (levels ranged from 5 to 19 mg/dl) and controls. Furthermore, she found that hyperbilirubinemic children who were breast-fed scored better than formula-fed hyperbilirubinemics at 3, 10, and 24 months, findings that also support continuation of breast-feeding for hyperbilirubinemic infants. If the infant's serum bilirubin level approaches 20 mg/dl, diagnosis of BMJ must be made. If the mother stops breast-feeding for 24 to 48 hours and the infant's serum bilirubin level decreases, the diagnosis of BMJ is confirmed and no further tests are required (5). Interrupting breast-feeding if the infant's serum bilirubin level is below 15–16 mg/dl may unnecessarily impede breast-feeding.

Mothers who must interrupt breast-feeding in order to confirm BMJ diagnosis need supervision and support from nursing staff with well-prepared lactation skills. Nurses can teach these mothers to pump their breasts in order to maintain their milk supply until they resume breast-feeding. Nurses can also minimize stress mothers may feel if they believe that they have caused their infants to become ill. Discussions in which the mother can express her fears and concerns will alleviate some maternal stress. Assuring parents that their infant's jaundice is transitional also reduces parental distress.

Infants who must remain hospitalized for phototherapy and their parents require special intervention. (Specifics about phototherapy, its mechanism of action, side effects, and use at home are discussed in my second article on hyperbilirubinemia, to be published in the January–February *MCN*. Transcutaneous bilirubinometry and exchange transfusions are covered as well.) These infants will benefit from frequent contact with their parents and must be accessible to parents for feeding, holding, and comforting. Nurses can also teach parents to care for their infant even while the infant is receiving phototherapy.

However, it is important to remember that physiologic jaundice and breast milk jaundice have no long-term harmful effects if properly monitored and judiciously treated. Aggressive, early treatment with phototherapy or substitution of formula for breast milk is not generally justified for healthy, full-term infants diagnosed with physiologic hyperbilirubinemia (31).

──────── REFERENCES ────────

1. OSBORN, L. M. Management of neonatal jaundice. *Nurse Pract.* 11:41–52, Apr. 1986.
2. MAISELS, M. J. Jaundice in the newborn. *Pediatr.Rev.* 3:305–319, 1982.
3. OH, W. Neonatal polycythemia and hyperviscosity. *Pediatr.Clin.North Am.* 33:523–532, June 1986.
4. KIVLAHAN, C., AND JAMES, E. J. The natural history of neonatal jaundice. *Pediatrics* 74:364–370, Sept. 1984.
5. MAISELS, M. J. Hyperbilirubinemia. IN *Current Therapy in Neonatal Perinatal Medicine 1984-1985*, ed. by N. M. Nelson. St. Louis, C. V. Mosby Co., 1985.
6. FOERDER, B. A. Neonatal jaundice: effects on development to age two years. *Commun.Nurs.Res.* 20:38, 1987.
7. NEWMAN, A. J., AND GROSS, S. Hyperbilirubinemia in breast-fed infants. *Pediatrics* 32:995–1001, Dec. 1963.
8. ARIAS, I. M., AND OTHERS. Prolonged neonatal unconjugated hyperbilirubinemia associated with breast feeding and a steroid, pregnane-3 (alpha), 20 (beta)-diol, in maternal milk that inhibits glucuronide formation in vitro. *J.Clin. Invest.* 43:2037–2047, Nov. 1964.
9. STIEHM, E. R., AND RYAN, J. Breast milk jaundice. Report of eight cases and effect of breast feeding on incidence and severity of unexplained hyperbilirubinemia. *Am.J.Dis.Child.* 109:212–216, Mar. 1965.
10. BROOTEN, D., AND OTHERS. Breast-milk jaundice. *JOGNN* 14:220–223, May–June 1985.
11. ARIAS, I. M., AND OTHERS. Neonatal conjugated hyperbilirubinemia associated with breastfeeding and a factor in milk that inhibits glucuronide formation in vitro. *J.Clin.Invest.* 42:913–918, June 1963.
12. HARGREAVES, T. Effect of fatty acids on bilirubin conjugation. *Arch.Dis.Child.* 48:446–449, June 1973.
13. DEANGELIS, C., AND OTHERS. Breast milk jaundice. *Wis.Med.J.* 79:40–42, Feb. 1980.
14. POLAND, R. L. Breast-milk jaundice. *J.Pediatr.* 999:86–88, July 1981.
15. DeCARVALHO, M. D., AND OTHERS. Fecal bilirubin excretion and serum bilirubin concentrations in breast-fed and bottle-fed infants. *J.Pediatr.* 107:786–790, Nov. 1985.
16. GOURLEY, G. R., AND AREND, R. A. Beta-glucuronidase and hyperbilirubinaemia in breast-fed and formula-fed babies. *Lancet* 22:644–646, Mar. 1986.
17. DeCARVALHO, M. D., AND OTHERS. Frequency of breastfeeding and serum bilirubin concentration. *Am.J.Dis.Child.* 136:737-738, Aug. 1982.
18. OSBORN, L. M. Op. cit., p. 49.
19. CLARKSON, J. E., AND OTHERS. Jaundice in full term healthy neonates—a population study. *Aust.Paediatr.J.* 20:303–308, Nov. 1984.
20. MOORE, L. G., AND OTHERS. Increased incidence of neonatal hyperbilirubinemia at 3,100 m in Colorado. *Am.J.Dis.Child.* 138:157–161, Feb. 1984.
21. COGAN, R., AND HINZ, R. The etiology of "physiological" neonatal jaundice: the role of interventions. *ICEA Review* 7(1):1–7, 1983.
22. JEFFARIES, M. J. A multifactorial survey of neonatal jaundice. *Br.J.Obstet.Gynaecol.* 84:452–455, June 1977.
23. CHEW, W. C., AND SWANN, I. L. Influence of simultaneous low amniotomy and oxytocin infusion and other maternal factors on neonatal jaundice: a prospective study. *Br.Med.J.* 1:72–73, Jan. 8, 1977.
24. LANGE, A. P., AND OTHERS. Neonatal jaundice after labour induced or stimulated by prostaglandin E2 or oxytocin. *Lancet* 1:991–994, May 1982.
25. KNEPP, N. B., AND OTHERS. Fetal and neonatal hazards of maternal hydration with 5% dextrose before cesarean section. *Lancet* 1:1150–1152, 1982.
26. SINGHI, S., AND OTHERS. Hazards of maternal hydration with 5% dextrose. *Lancet* 2:335–336, Aug. 7, 1982.
27. DeCARVALHO, M. D., AND OTHERS. Does the duration and the frequency of early breastfeeding affect nipple pain? *Birth* 11:81–84, Summer 1984.
28. L'ESPERANCE, C., AND FRANTZ, K. Time limitation for early breastfeeding. *JOGNN* 14:114–118, Mar.–Apr. 1985.
29. BOROVIES, D. L. Assessing and managing pain in breast-feeding mothers. *MCN* 9:272–276, July–Aug. 1984.
30. LASCARI, A. D. "Early" breast-feeding jaundice: clinical significance. *J.Pediatr.* 108:156–158, Jan. 1986.
31. PALUDETTO, R., AND OTHERS. Moderate hyperbilirubinemia does not influence the behavior of jaundiced infants. *Biol.Neonate* 50:43–47, July 1986.

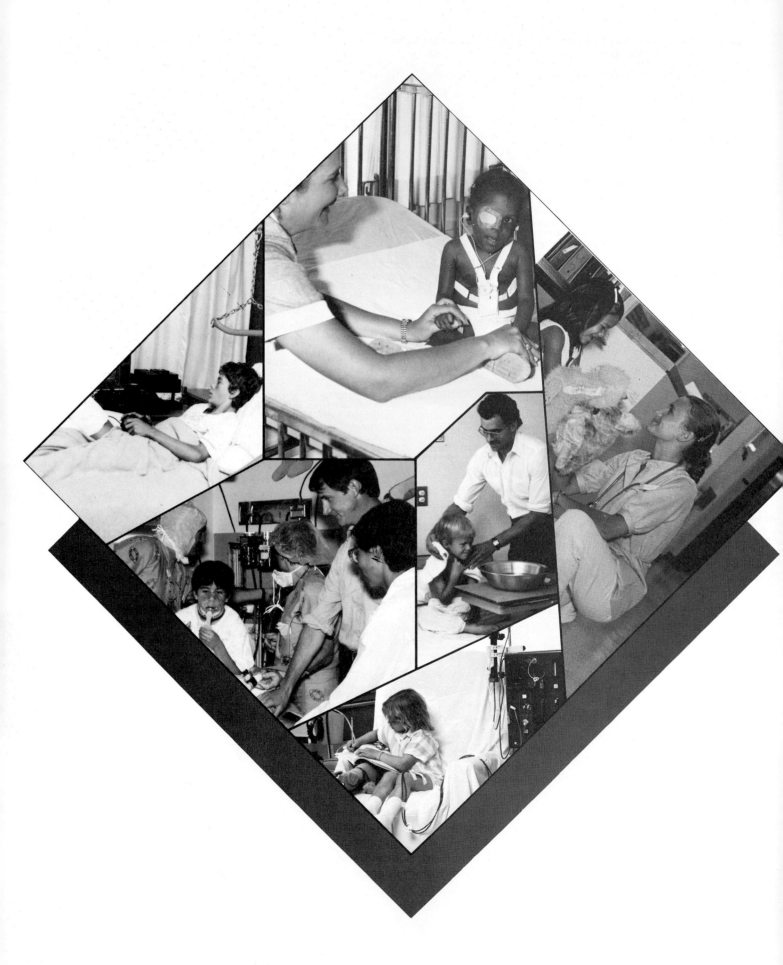

Nursing Care of
the Child

Coordinator

Susan Colvert Droske, MN, RN

Contributors

Karen S. Bernardy, MSN, RNC
Alice Copp Franz, MA, RN
Judith K. Leavitt, MEd, RN
Mariann C. Lovell, MS, RN
Michele A. Michael, PhD, RN
Maribeth L. Moran, MSN, RN
Bernadette Mazurek Vulcan, MSN, RNC,
PNP

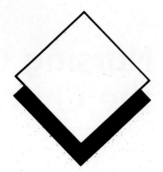

The Healthy Child

GENERAL CONCEPTS
Infant (1 month to 1 year)

1. Normal growth and development
   a. Psychosocial development—Erikson: trust vs. mistrust (see Table 2-1, p. 15)
      1. trust: infant's needs are met consistently, resulting in feelings of physical comfort and emotional security; learns to love and be loved
      2. depends on the quality of the relationship between the primary caregiver and infant
   b. Physical growth and development
      1. physical growth should follow standard growth curves
      2. length: 50% increase by 1 year (grows from average 20 inches at birth to 30 inches at 1 year)
      3. weight
         a. gains about 1½ pounds per month during the first 6 months; ¾ pounds per month the second 6 months
         b. doubles at 5-6 months
         c. triples by 1 year (18-25 pounds at 1 year)
      4. head circumference greater than chest circumference until age 2
      5. vital signs (see Table 5-1)
         a. pulse 80-150/min; average 100/min
         b. respirations 20-50/min
      6. developmental characteristics
         a. cephalocaudal (head to tail): gross motor skills
            ◆ 5 months: turns over, no head lag when in sitting position
            ◆ 6 months: sits alone with hands held forward for support
            ◆ 8 months: sits steadily without support, pulls to a standing position
            ◆ 9 months: able to "crawl," able to regain balance when sitting
            ◆ 1 year: stands upright, able to "cruise" about a room by holding onto objects; may take first "solo" steps
         b. proximal to distal (central axis of body outward) and general to specific (differentiate): fine motor skills
            ◆ 3-4 months: arm control; supports upper body weight; scoops objects with hands
            ◆ 6 months: transfers objects from one hand to the other
            ◆ 10 months: pincer (thumb and index finger) grasp
         c. fontanels
            ◆ anterior: closes at 12-18 months
            ◆ posterior: closes at 2 months (may be closed at birth)
         d. teeth: development begins in utero
            ◆ 4-8 months: central mandibular incisors
            ◆ 1 year: 8 teeth (average)
   c. Cognitive development—Piaget: sensorimotor stage (birth to 2 years)
      1. 1 month: reflexive
      2. 1-4 months
         a. visually follows objects 180°
         b. recognizes familiar faces and objects
         c. turns head to locate sounds
         d. discovers parts of own body (hands, feet)
      3. 4-8 months: beginning object permanence
         a. searches for objects that have fallen
         b. imitates expressions and gestures of others
         c. smiles at self in mirror (mirror-image play)
         d. begins development of depth and space
      4. 9-12 months: searches for hidden objects
   d. Socialization
      1. 1 month: differentiates between face and object
      2. 2 months: social smile
      3. 4 months: recognizes primary caregiver
      4. 7-8 months: shy with strangers
      5. 9-10 months: separation anxiety
   e. Vocalization (language development)
      1. 2 months: differentiated cry
      2. 3 months: squeals with pleasure
      3. 5 months: simple vocal sounds (ooh, aah), turns to voice

Table 5-1 Vital sign ranges in children (averages)

Pulse*	1 month-1 year	80-150/beats/min
	1-5 years	80-120/beats/min
	5-10 years	70-110/beats/min
	10-16 years	60-100/beats/min
Respiration*	1 month-1 year	20-50/min
	1-5 years	20-40/min
	5-10 years	18-30/min
	10-16 years	14-26/min
Blood pressure	1 month-1 year	80/50 mm Hg
	1-5 years	90/60 mm Hg
	5-10 years	100-110/60-70 mm Hg
	10-16 years	110-120/70-80 mm Hg

*Lower numbers in range represent values with child asleep.

Table 5-2 Average daily caloric needs of infants and children*

Age	Calories
Birth-6 months	53 × weight in pounds = kcal/day (400-800 kcal/day)
6 months-1 year	48 × weight in pounds = kcal/day (800-1200 kcal/day)
1-3 years	1300 kcal/day
4-6 years	1700 kcal/day
7-10 years	2400 kcal/day
11-16 years	
Boys	2700 kcal/day
Girls	2200 kcal/day

From the Food and Nutrition Board of the National Research Council, National Academy of Sciences.
*These daily averages may vary considerably for an individual child, depending on the child's activity level, length (height), and body build.

4. 6 months: begins to imitate sounds
5. 9 months: first word (dada, baba); says "dada," "mama" specifically
6. 12 months: two words besides mama and dada; uses gesture language (e.g., "up" [points] or "bye" [waves])

   f. Play (solitary)
1. purposes: to stimulate sensorimotor development
2. toys
   a. simple, easily handled
   b. safe; no sharp points or small removable parts
   c. stimulating
   d. washable
   e. nonlead paint
3. types of toys
   a. mobiles (black-and-white or bright colors)
   b. rattles, musical toys
   c. squeeze toys, sponge toys
   d. activity box for crib or playpen
   e. balls, blocks

   f. pots and pans (9-10 months)
4. games: peek-a-boo and patty-cake

2. Nutrition
   a. Caloric needs: approximately 400 (newborn) to 1200 (1-year-old) kcal/day (see Table 5-2 for recommended averages); actual caloric requirements depend on baby's activity and rate of growth.
   b. Introduction of solid foods
1. when to start solids: variety of opinions; some evidence that early feeding of solids is linked to food allergies and overweight
2. does not need solids first 4-6 months
   a. salivary enzymes and intestinal antibodies to aid digestion not present until 4-6 months
   b. extrusion reflex lasts until 3-4 months
   c. chewing movements begin at 6-7 months
3. introduce foods one at a time; continue 3 or 4 days before introducing another
4. give small quantities (start with 1 tsp)
   c. Types of foods: each introduced one at a time; wait 2-3 days before adding another
1. cooked cereals are introduced first at 4-6

months; rice cereal is preferable (high iron content, easily digested, less likely to cause allergic reaction)

2. strained/cooked vegetables are introduced next at 6-7 months (before fruits, which have lower iron content)

3. strained/mashed fruits are introduced at 7-8 months (bananas are preferable first fruit)

4. ground/pureed meats are introduced at 8-9 months, egg yolks at 10 months (delay egg whites until 12 months)

5. chewable and finger foods are introduced when teething begins (6-9 months): zwieback, toast, crackers

6. avoid nuts, raisins, popcorn, gum, candy, hot dogs (can be aspirated)

d. Self-feeding: at 6 months infant begins handling spoon, finger foods; by 1 year, most infants are able to use a spoon well; weaning—ready for introduction of a cup at 6-8 months, should be weaned gradually from breast or bottle; offer juice in a cup; drink independently from a cup at 1 year (may still want bottle or breast for security)

e. Food allergies (a common health problem in infancy)

1. common foods causing allergic responses include
   a. milk
   b. foods containing wheat, corn, or soy (protein gluten)
   c. egg white (albumin)
   d. chocolate
   e. citrus foods

2. indications of hypersensitivity to food
   a. urticaria
   b. abdominal pain, vomiting, and diarrhea
   c. respiratory symptoms

3. diagnosis
   a. singular addition of food
   b. food diary or history
   c. skin testing not useful (because of immature immune system)

4. treatment
   a. removal of causative food
   b. change to soy formula (if milk allergy)
   c. elimination diet

3. Sleep
   a. Most infants have nocturnal sleep pattern by 3 months
   b. 6 months: sleep through night
   c. 8-9 months: two naps during day, sleep 10-12 hours at night
   d. Anticipatory guidance for parents
      1. each infant's sleep patterns are unique
      2. best indicators of adequate sleep are normal activity during waking hours and normal physical growth

Table 5-3   Recommended immunization schedule

Age	Immunization
2 months	Diphtheria-pertussis-tetanus (DPT) no. 1; Trivalent oral poliovirus (TOPV) no. 1; haemophilus influenzae b conjugate vaccine (HbCV)
4 months	DPT no. 2, TOPV no. 2, HbCV
6 months	DPT no. 3, TOPV no. 3 (optional in United States), HbCV
12 months	Tuberculin test (may be done at 15-month visit)
15 months	Measles-mumps-rubella (MMR), DPT no. 4, TOPV no. 4, HbCV
4-6 years	DPT no. 5, TOPV no. 5
14-16 years	Tetanus and diphtheria toxoids (adult type)—Td; repeat every 10 years

Primary immunization for children not immunized in first year of life	
Age	**Immunization**

UNDER 7 YEARS

First visit	DPT no. 1, TOPV no. 1, MMR, HbCV (if older than 15 months)
Interval after first visit	
2 months	DPT no. 2, TOPV no. 2
4 months	DPT no. 3
10-16 months	DPT no. 4, TOPV no. 3
Preschool (4-6 years)	DPT no. 5, TOPV no. 4

7 YEARS AND OVER

First visit	Td no. 1, TOPV no. 1, MMR
Interval after first visit	
2 months	Td no. 2, TOPV no. 2
8-14 months	Td no. 3, TOPV no. 3
10 years later	Td; repeat every 10 years

3. sleeping arrangements are influenced by family's cultural beliefs and customs

4. Health care
   a. Immunizations
      1. see Table 5-3 for recommended schedule of the American Academy of Pediatrics
      2. contraindications
         a. febrile illness
         b. previous severe reaction to toxoid
         c. presence of skin rash
         d. malignancy
         e. pregnancy
         f. poor immunological response
         g. administration of gamma globulin, plasma, or blood in previous 6-8 weeks
         h. give measles vaccine only after Tb test has been found to be negative (Tb fulminates in presence of measles virus)

3. common side effects
   a. mild fever
   b. malaise
   c. soreness and swelling at injection site (DPT)
   d. mild rash (measles, rubella)
4. advise parents of possible side effects; use of acetaminophen for fever (aspirin is contraindicated because of possible link between viral illness, aspirin, and Reye's syndrome)

b. Accident prevention: accidents are the second leading cause of death in this age group
1. aspiration/suffocation
   a. avoid propping bottles
   b. keep small objects out of reach
   c. check toys for small parts or sharp edges
   d. close pins when changing diaper
   e. keep plastic bags away
2. falls
   a. never leave on elevated surface unattended
   b. keep crib rails up
3. auto accident: use infant car seats (crash tested, rear facing)
4. burns: check water temperature before immersing infant; keep hot substances away from infant (cigarette ashes, coffee, etc.); check temperature of foods/formulas; expose to sun gradually

Toddler (1-3 years)

1. Normal growth and development
   a. Psychosocial development—Erikson: autonomy vs. shame and doubt
   1. all activities move toward independence; expands independence by exploring evironment and extending its limits
   2. verbally negative ("No!") even when agreeable to request
   b. Physical growth and development
   1. vital signs: pulse and respirations decrease, blood pressure increases with increasing size and age (see Table 5-1)
   2. teeth: all 20 deciduous present by 2½-3 years
   3. general appearance: potbellied, exaggerated lumbar curve, wide-based gait
   4. practices and increases muscle coordination and physical abilities
      a. climbs; goes up steps, cannot get down, and won't accept help
      b. jumps in place
      c. pushes and pulls toys
      d. scribbles spontaneously
      e. builds a tower of cubes
      f. 18-24 months: learns to undress self
      g. 24-36 months: able to undress self with minimal help

   c. Cognitive development—Piaget: sensorimotor and preconceptual stages
   1. 13-18 months
      a. very curious
      b. identifies geometric shapes
      c. opens doors and drawers
      d. points to body parts
      e. puts objects into holes, smaller objects into each other
   2. 19-24 months
      a. egocentric thinking and behavior
      b. beginning sense of time; waits in response to "just a minute"
   3. 24-36 months
      a. beginning magical thinking
      b. understands prepositions (e.g., over, under, behind, up)
      c. animism (attributes lifelike characteristics to inanimate objects)
      d. understanding of cause-and-effect relationships is determined by proximity of two events; therefore, should be disciplined immediately
      e. increasing attention span
   d. Socialization
   1. 15 months
      a. resistant to sitting in laps
      b. wants to move independently
   2. 18 months to 2½ years: imitates parent behaviors (e.g., housework)
   3. dawdling and ritualistic behavior
   4. temper tantrums may be used to assert independence and gain control, especially when desires are thwarted
   5. may be attached to transitional objects, such as a favorite blanket or stuffed animal
   6. territorial: possessive of own toys and body
   e. Vocalization
   1. understands simple commands
   2. 18 months: 20 words, names 1 body part
   3. 2 years: makes simple two- or three-word sentences; uses pronouns, plurals; knows full name
   f. Play (parallel)
   1. purposes: to help child make transition from solitary to cooperative play, to stimulate motor development
   2. child will play beside, not with another child
   3. types of toys
      a. cars and trucks
      b. push-pull toys
      c. blocks, building toys, balls
      d. telephone
      e. stuffed toys and dolls
      f. large crayons, coloring and hardboard books
      g. clay, finger paints

h. wood puzzles

4. games: likes to throw and retrieve objects, prefers "rough and tumble" play

2. Nutrition and dental care
   a. Growth slows, appetite smaller; "physiological anorexia" (may eat a great deal one day and little the next); needs an average of 1300 calories/day (see Table 5-2)
      1. ritualistic food preferences
      2. likes finger foods (crackers, celery, carrot sticks)
      3. drinks from cup
      4. self-feeds by 18 months
      5. prone to iron-deficiency anemia, especially if milk intake is high
   b. Anticipatory guidance for parents
      1. serve small portions
      2. recommended daily milk intake 24-32 oz
      3. do not give bottle as a substitute for solid foods; give solids before or with milk
      4. do not use food as a reward
      5. recognize ritualistic needs (e.g., same dishes, utensils, chair)
      6. do not force child to eat
   c. Dental care guidelines
      1. brush and floss twice daily with help from parents
      2. first visit to dentist as soon as all primary teeth have erupted (2½-3 years)
      3. use fluoridated water or oral fluoride supplement (0.25-0.5 mg/day)
      4. limit concentrated sweets
      5. do not allow child to take a bottle containing juice or milk to bed since "bottle mouth caries" may result

3. Elimination: toileting practices
   a. Learning bowel and bladder control is one of the major tasks of toddlerhood and is dependent on physiological and cognitive factors
   b. Myelinization of nerve tracts occurs around 15-18 months of age (physiological readiness)
   c. Toddler uses toileting activities to control self and others
   d. Independent toileting depends on
      1. physiological readiness
      2. ability to verbally communicate need to defecate or urinate
      3. ability to get to toilet and manage clothing
      4. psychological readiness (desire to please)
   e. Ages
      1. 18 months: bowel control
      2. 2-3 years: daytime bladder control
      3. 3-4 years: nighttime bladder control

4. Limit setting and discipline help child learn self-control and socially appropriate behavior; promote security

   a. Enforcement of limits should be consistent and firm
   b. Discipline should occur immediately after wrongdoing
   c. Positive approach is best
   d. Disapprove of the behavior, *not* the child
   e. Types of discipline
      1. redirecting child's attention
      2. ignoring the behavior (often very difficult)
      3. time-out
      4. reasoning and reprimanding, loss of privileges (for older children; not effective with toddlers)
      5. corporal punishment (controversial)

5. Accident prevention: accidents are leading cause of death from 1-15 years of age
   a. Falls
      1. Motor development is far ahead of judgment and perceptions
      2. climbs over side rails; change to regular bed
      3. climbs stairs; use safety gates
      4. supervise at playgrounds
   b. Poisonous ingestions (leading cause of injury and death); keep poisons and sharp objects locked up and out of reach
   c. Supervise when near cars; use car safety seats; never leave unattended in car
   d. Burns: cover electrical outlets; do not leave unattended in bathtub, near hot stove, fireplace, etc.; teach child what "hot" means
   e. Drowning: supervise near water (e.g., bathtub, toilet, pools, lakes)

Preschooler (3-6 years)

1. Normal growth and development
   a. Psychosocial development—Erikson: initiative vs. guilt
      1. learns how to do things, derives satisfaction from activities
      2. needs exposure to variety of experiences and play materials
      3. imitates role models
      4. imaginative
         a. reality vs. fantasy blurred
         b. may have imaginary friends
      5. exaggerated fears (e.g., fear of mutilation, monsters)
   b. Physical growth and development
      1. body contours change: thinner and taller
      2. blood pressure 100/60 mm Hg
      3. motor skills: better control of fine and gross ones; posture more erect
         a. uses scissors and simple tools
         b. draws a person
            ◆ 4 years: three parts
            ◆ 5 years: six or seven parts
         c. rides a tricycle or "big wheel"

d. skips and hops, throws and catches a ball well (5 years)

e. walks downstairs as well as upstairs alternating feet on steps

f. dresses self completely

c. Cognitive development—Piaget: preconceptual and intuitive thought stages

1. increased sense of time and space (tomorrow, afternoon, next week)

2. less egocentric

3. perception dominates reasoning

4. centration

a. thinks of one idea at a time

b. unable to think of all parts in terms of a whole

c. conclusions based on immediate visual perceptions

5. increased ability to think without acting out; anticipates events

d. Socialization

1. beginning social awareness

2. capable of sharing; begins to have "best friends"

3. may be physically aggressive

4. boasts and tattles

5. learns appropriate social manners

6. separates easily from mother

e. Vocalization

1. 3-year-old: constantly asks "how" and "why" questions; vocabulary of 300-900 words

2. 5-year-old: uses sentences of adult length

3. knows colors, numbers, and alphabet

4. understands analogies ("If fire is hot, ice is [cold]")

5. stuttering (dysfluency) is fairly common among toddlers and preschoolers; normal variation of language development; parents should ignore stuttering so child does not become anxious; persistent stuttering beyond age 5 may require speech therapy

f. Play (cooperative)

1. purpose: to help child learn to share and to play in small groups, to learn simple games and rules, language concepts, and social roles

2. play may be dramatic, imitative, or creative; expresses self through play

3. types of toys

a. housekeeping toys

b. playground equipment

c. wagons

d. tricycles: "big wheels"

e. dress-up clothes

f. materials for cutting, pasting, and painting

g. simple jigsaw puzzles

h. picture books

i. dolls

j. TV (controversial but a contemporary reality)

2. Nutrition: a slow-growth period; needs an average of 1700 calories/day (see Table 5-2)

a. Appetite remains decreased; has definite food preferences; less picky

b. Self-feeding: 4-year-old uses fork, can use knife to spread; able to get snacks for self

c. Sets the table; learns table manners

d. Able to pour from a pitcher

3. Sleep

a. Sleep problems are most common in this age group

b. Requires 9-12 hours each night

c. May or may not take one nap during day

d. May have fears of the dark, or may awaken with nightmares

e. Guidelines for caregivers

1. provide quiet time before bedtime

2. use a nightlight

3. adhere to a consistent bedtime pattern

4. Sexuality

a. Knows sex differences by 3 years

b. Imitates masculine or feminine behaviors; gender identity well established by 6 years

c. Sexual curiosity and exploration

1. masturbation is normal; especially common in preschoolers, may increase in frequency when child is under stress

2. curious about anatomical differences and seeks to "investigate" them

d. Guidelines for caregivers

1. assess what child already knows when child asks a question

2. answer questions simply, honestly, and matter-of-factly (avoid detailed explanations), using correct terminology

3. masturbation: redirect child's attention without punishing or verbally reprimanding; teach child that touching genitals is not appropriate in public

5. Accident prevention

a. Motor vehicle accidents (leading cause of injury and death)

1. street safety: teach to wait at curb until told to cross; avoid riding cycles near street or driveways

2. wear seat belt

b. Drownings: teach to swim; supervise near pools, lakes, etc.

c. Burns: teach not to play with matches or lights; supervise near fireplace; teach how to escape from burning home

d. General safety: teach not to talk to strangers; child should know own name, address, telephone number, and how to seek help if lost

School Age (6-12 years)

1. Normal growth and development
   a. Psychosocial development—Erikson: industry vs. inferiority
      1. develops a sense of competency and esteem academically, physically, and socially
      2. school phobias may occur as a result of increased competition, desire to succeed, fear of failure
      3. desire for accomplishment so strong that young school-age child may try to change rules of game to win
      4. gains competence in mastering new skills and tasks; assumes more responsibilities
      5. desires to get along socially; more responsive to peers
      6. still needs reassurance and support from family and trusted adults
   b. Physical growth and development
      1. growth is slow and regular (1-2 inches gain in height per year, 3-6 lb weight gain per year), prepubertal females are usually taller than males
      2. motor skills: increases strength and physical ability, refines coordination
         a. 6 years: jumps, skips, hops well; ties shoelaces easily, prints
         b. 7 years: vision fully developed, can read regular-size print; can swim and ride a bicycle
         c. 8 years: writes rather than prints; increased smoothness and speed
         d. 9 years: fully developed hand-eye coordination; individual capabilities/talents emerge
         e. 10 years: increased strength, stamina, coordination
         f. 11 years: awkward; nervous energy (drumming fingers, etc.)
   c. Cognitive development—Piaget: concrete operations stage (7-11 years)
      1. decentering: can consider more than one characteristic at a time; leads to ability to emphathize and sympathize
      2. reversibility: able to imagine a process in reverse
      3. conservation: able to conserve (mentally retain) physical properties of matter even when form is changed
      4. able to classify objects and verbalize concepts involved in doing so
      5. reasons logically; reasoning dominates perception
      6. able to think through a situation and anticipate the consequences; may then alter course of action

   d. Socialization
      1. prefers friends to family; life is centered around school and friends
      2. relationships with peers and adults other than parents of increasing importance
      3. increasing social sensitivity
      4. more cooperative; improved manners
      5. school phobia: difficulty coping with the academic or social demands of school may result in psychosomatic complaints (stomachache, headache) and refusal to attend school; best managed by rewarding school attendance, withdrawing privileges and attention for school avoidance
      6. by 10 years enjoys privacy (e.g., own room, box that locks)
   e. Vocalization
      1. curious about meaning of different words; rapidly expanding vocabulary
      2. likes name-calling, word games (e.g., rhymes)
      3. develops a sense of humor; giggles and laughs a great deal; silly
      4. knows clock and calendar time
   f. Play (cooperative, team, rule-governed, same sex together)
      1. purposes: to learn to bargain, cooperate and compromise; to develop logical reasoning abilities; to increase social skills
      2. types of toys; entertainment
         a. play figures, trains, model kits
         b. games, jigsaw puzzles, magic tricks
         c. books: joke and comic books, storybooks, adventure, mystery
         d. TV, Nintendo, tapes, radio
         e. riding a bicycle
         f. organized activities (sports, scouting, music and dancing lessons, camping, slumber parties)
   g. "Collecting" age: stamps, cards, rocks, etc.
2. Nutrition and dental health
   a. Appetite increases; needs an average of 2400 calories/day (see Table 5-2); breakfast is important for school performance
   b. More influenced by mass media; more likely to eat junk food because of increased time away from home
   c. Nutrition education
      1. teach basic four food groups
      2. teach basic cooking skills, meal planning
      3. nutritious snacks
   d. Dental health
      1. loss of deciduous teeth (begins at 5-7 years of age); eruption of permanent ones, including first and second molars
      2. many school-age children will wear braces
         a. good oral hygiene is important

   b. reassure permanent teeth will appear
3. dental caries are a major health problem
   a. caused by poor nutrition, influence of TV advertising contributing to increased intake of carbohydrates and concentrated sweets, inadequate dental hygiene
   b. prevention: good brushing and flossing techniques, regular dental checkups, fluoridated water, good nutrition

3. Accident prevention
  a. Accepts increasing responsibility for own safety; safety education is essential
  b. Motor vehicle accidents
    1. teach how to cross street
    2. bike safety
    3. use car safety belts
  c. Drowning
    1. learn to swim
    2. teach water safety
  d. Burns
    1. teach safety around fires (e.g., fireplaces, camp fires) and safe use of candles and matches
    2. teach not to play with explosives or guns
  e. Sports injuries: teach about appropriate protective equipment

Adolescent (12-20 years)

1. Normal growth and development
  a. Psychosocial development—Erikson: identity vs. identity diffusion
    1. "Who am I?"
    2. "What do I want to do with my life?"
    3. has many changes in body image
    4. experiences mood swings; vacillates between maturity and childlike behavior
    5. continually reassesses values and beliefs
    6. begins to consider career possibilities
    7. gains independence from parents
  b. Physical growth and development: puberty (average onset in males occurs 2 years later than in females)
    1. males: development of secondary sex characteristics
     a. increase in size of genitalia
     b. swelling of breasts
     c. growth of pubic, axillary, facial, and chest hair
     d. voice changes
     e. increase in shoulder breadth
     f. production of spermatozoa; nocturnal emissions
    2. females: development of secondary sex characteristics
     a. increase in transverse diameter of pelvis
     b. development of breasts
     c. change in vaginal secretions

     d. growth of pubic and axillary hair
     e. menstruation: 12 years (average)
    3. both sexes
     a. acne
     b. perspiration
     c. blushing
     d. rapid increase in height and weight
     e. fatigue (since heart and lungs grow at slower rate)
  c. Cognitive development—Piaget: formal operations (11 years and older); attained at different ages and depends on formal education, experience, cultural background
    1. abstract thinking
    2. forms hypotheses, analytical thinking
    3. can consider more than two categories at same time
    4. generalizes findings
    5. thinks about thinking; philosophical; concerned with social and moral issues
  d. Socialization
    1. with adults
     a. may resent authority
     b. wishes to be different from parents: may ridicule them
     c. has need for parent figures
     d. develops crushes on adults outside the family, "hero worship"
    2. with peers
     a. overidentifies with group: same dress, same ethical codes
     b. has close friendships with members of same sex
     c. develops heterosexual relationships, sexual experimentation (may be sexually active)
  e. Recreation, leisure activity: expanding variety
    1. parties, dances
    2. Nintendo, television, movies, and music (radio, tapes)
    3. telephone conversations, daydreaming
    4. sports, games, hobbies
    5. reading and writing
    6. part-time jobs (especially babysitting) to earn extra money
  f. Sexual activity
    1. 50% of adolescents have engaged in sexual activity
    2. educate about birth control methods, pregnancy, sexually transmitted disease, and safe sex

2. Nutrition
  a. Appetite increases with rapid growth; puberty changes nutritional requirements; needs basic four food groups
  b. Caloric needs vary with activity level, sex, and body build (see Table 5-2)

1. girls need approximately 2200 calories/day
2. boys need an average of 2700 calories/day

c. Increased need for protein, calcium, iron, and zinc

d. Sports activity may increase nutritional requirements

e. Eating habits are easily influenced by peer group
    1. intake of junk food
    2. fad diets and dieting: can lead to health problems, including anorexia nervosa, bulimia
    3. overeating or inactivity: may result in obesity

3. Accident prevention
    a. Motor vehicle accidents: enroll in driver-training programs, wear seat belts
    b. Drownings: teach water safety, first aid, CPR
    c. Sports injuries: educate for prevention
    d. Alcohol and drug abuse: education
    e. Suicide: be alert for signs of depression

Application of the Nursing Process to the Healthy Child

Assessment

1. Health history
    a. General health status: incidence of illnesses in past year, visits to health provider, immunization history, current medications
    b. Developmental history: parents' health status, mother's obstetrical history with this child, child's neonatal history, achievement of developmental milestones, self-care abilities, behavior, and temperament
    c. Parents' perceptions and concerns
    d. Parents' knowledge of development, child care, safety, nutrition, etc.
    e. Child's home and school environments: safety, appropriate stimulation, barriers to development
    f. Nutrition: daily food and fluid intake, child's preferences and dislikes, self-feeding abilities, special needs (cultural/religious practices, allergies), eating patterns
    g. Dental care: number of teeth, tooth eruption (discomfort, management), daily oral hygiene, self-brushing and flossing, fluoride (water or daily supplement), dental visits
    h. Elimination: daily routine, toilet trained or diapers, problems (e.g., diarrhea, constipation, enuresis; how managed)
    i. Activity/sleep: exercise and activity patterns; sleep habits: sleep environment, daily total, special needs, problems
    j. Sexuality: gender knowledge and identity, sexual curiosity and exploration, sexual knowledge, primary and secondary sex characteristics; adolescent: knowledge, sexual activity, contraception, pregnancy, sexually transmitted disease

2. Clinical appraisal

a. Development
    1. observation of age-appropriate developmental behavior and abilities
    2. administration of developmental screening tools when indicated to screen for delays (e.g., Denver Developmental Screening Test [a screening tool to detect developmental problems in four areas: personal-social, fine motor–adaptive, language, and gross motor; *not* an intelligence test; does not predict future developmental potential])
    3. home environment: visit to appraise for support of or barriers to development

b. General physical appraisal
    1. growth: length, weight, head circumference; percentiles on standard growth curves
    2. vital signs: annual BP screening over age 3 (especially in high-risk children) (see Table 5-1)
    3. general health: skin, activity, attention span, ability to communicate, etc.
    4. vision/hearing screening
        a. vision testing
            ◆ binocularity tests for strabismus; if strabismus is not detected and corrected by age 6 years, amblyopia (dimness of vision, even blindness) may result
                • corneal light reflex test
                • cover test
            ◆ visual acuity tests; Snellen E (preschoolers or illiterate children) or Snellen alphabet chart
            ◆ head tilting or squinting may indicate visual impairment
            ◆ ophthalmoscopic exam
            ◆ referral criteria
                • 3 years: vision in one or both eyes 20/50 or worse
                • 4-6 years: vision in one or both eyes 20/40 or worse
                • 7 years and older: vision in one or both eyes 20/30 or worse
                • children with one-line or more difference between both eyes (example: 20/30 in left eye, 20/40 in right)
                • abnormal findings from cover test or corneal light reflex test
        b. hearing testing
            ◆ otoscopic exam
            ◆ conduction tests
                • Rinne test (comparison of bone and air conduction)
                • Weber's test (bone conduction)
            ◆ pure tone audiometry (audiogram) to test for conductive or sensorineural hearing impairments

Analysis

1. Safe, effective care environment
   a. High risk for injury
   b. Sensory-perceptual alteration: visual, auditory, kinesthetic, tactile, olfactory
   c. Knowledge deficit
2. Physiological integrity
   a. High risk for activity intolerance
   b. Altered nutrition: high risk for less/more than body requirements
   c. Fatigue
3. Psychosocial integrity
   a. Decisional conflict
   b. Altered role performance
   c. Body image disturbance, self-esteem disturbance
4. Health promotion/maintenance
   a. Ineffective family coping: high risk for growth
   b. Altered growth and development
   c. Health-seeking behaviors

General Nursing Planning, Implementation, and Evaluation

Goal 1: Child will achieve optimum development.

Implementation

1. Provide information to parents on normal growth and development.
   a. What to expect (skills, behavior)
   b. Age-appropriate play activities and materials
   c. Ways to stimulate development
2. Discuss child-rearing methods and styles, limit setting, and ways to cope with child-rearing problems.
3. Administer screening tools during well-child visits to detect developmental delays (e.g., language, speech, gross and fine motor skills, social, self-help).
4. Refer for further evaluation or to early intervention services if developmental delay detected.

Evaluation

Child grows and develops within expected range; is free from delays in development; parents cope effectively with child-rearing concerns and problems.

Goal 2: Child will experience a safe environment and will be free from accidental injury.

Implementation

1. Provide anticipatory guidance to parents concerning age-related safety hazards and ways to prevent accidental injury (safety proofing the home, auto safety restraints, swimming and bicycling safety, safe toys, driver education).

Evaluation

Child is free from accidental injury.

Goal 3: Child will receive optimal nutrition and dental care.

Implementation

1. Provide teaching and counseling to parents concerning child's nutritional requirements, feeding techniques, dental hygiene, tooth eruption, food allergies, and feeding abilities.

Evaluation

Child's physical growth follows growth curve; child receives daily nutritional requirements (calories, protein, carbohydrates, fats, vitamins/minerals); feeds self in accordance with developmental abilities; receives appropriate dental hygiene and care and is free from dental caries; child's food allergies are detected and diet is adjusted as needed.

Goal 4: Child will get adequate rest and sleep.

Implementation

1. Provide anticipatory guidance to parents concerning child's sleep needs, patterns of sleep in childhood, and ways to cope with sleep problems.

Evaluation

Child gets amount of sleep required for optimal growth and development; parents cope with child's sleep problems.

Goal 5: Child will develop healthy sexuality.

Implementation

1. Provide anticipatory guidance to parents concerning child's developing sexuality.
   a. What to expect (questions, behaviors)
   b. How to answer child's questions matter-of-factly, honestly, accurately
2. Teach child about sex and sexuality appropriate to child's age and expressed interest.

Evaluation

Child develops gender-appropriate sexual identity and healthy sexuality.

Goal 6: Child will be free from preventable communicable diseases.

Implementation

1. Reinforce to parents the importance of childhood immunizations.
2. Administer immunizations according to recommended schedule.

Evaluation

Child receives immunizations according to recommended schedule; is free from preventable communicable diseases.

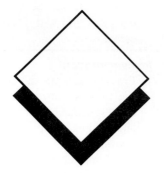

The Ill and Hospitalized Child

GENERAL CONCEPTS
Overview

1. Hospitalization and illness are stressful for children
   a. Difficulty changing routines
   b. Limited coping mechanisms
   c. Reason for hospitalization is often less significant than consequences (e.g., separation from familiar persons and surroundings, painful procedures, restricted mobility)
2. Major stressors for the child
   a. Separation
   b. Loss of control
   c. Body injury
   d. Pain
   e. Immobility
3. Factors that affect responses to illness and hospitalization
   a. Developmental level (see below, "Developmental Responses to Hospitalization")
   b. Past experiences, especially with hospitalization and surgery
   c. Level of anxiety: child and parents
   d. Relationship between parents and child
   e. Nature and seriousness of illness or injury; circumstances of hospitalization
   f. Family background: education, culture, support systems
4. Developmental responses to hospitalization
   a. Infant
      1. separation: before attachment (under 4-6 months) not as significant; older infant's response is significant with crying, rage, protest; stranger anxiety
      2. loss of control
         a. expects that crying will bring immediate response from caregiver (changed, fed, held); may interfere with development of trust
         b. in hospital
            ◆ immediate response may not occur
            ◆ need may be met by unfamiliar person
            ◆ unable to express needs or understand explanations
      3. immobility: restrictions and restraints interfere with activity and sucking (see Table 5-4)
      4. pain: procedures cause discomfort; responds by crying and withdrawal
   b. Toddler
      1. separation
         a. fear of unknown and abandonment
         b. separation anxiety is similar to grief; so encourage protest behaviors as healthy response
            ◆ protest: cries loudly, rejects attentions of nurses, wants parent
            ◆ despair: monotonous cries, state of mourning, "settling in"
            ◆ denial: renewed interest in surroundings; seems adjusted to loss, but actually repressing feelings for parent
         c. disruption in routines (eating, sleep, toileting) decreases security and control
         d. regression: attempts to seek comfort by returning to earlier, dependent behaviors
            ◆ clinging, whining
            ◆ wetting
            ◆ wanting bottle, pacifier
      2. loss of control: special concern because major task is to gain autonomy
      3. body injury: fears intrusive procedures (e.g., rectal temperature, injections) and reacts intensely
      4. immobility: cannot freely explore environment; may interfere with motor, language development
      5. pain: becomes emotionally distraught and physically resistant to painful procedures
   c. Preschooler
      1. body injury/body integrity
         a. confusion between reality and fantasy
         b. casts and bandages are particular problems, since child is not assured that all body parts

Table 5-4 Commonly used pediatric restraints

Type	Indications	Precautions
Jacket	In crib (alternative to crib net) In high chair To maintain horizontal position in crib	Tie in back. Secure ties underneath crib or high chair.
Crib net	To prevent infant or toddler from climbing over side rails	Avoid nets with tears or large gaps. Tie to bedsprings, not to crib sides.
Crib cover	To prevent toddler from climbing out of crib	Ensure that all latches are locked.
Mummy	For infant or small toddler needing short-term restraint venipuncture gavage feedings eye, ear, nose, and throat exams	Keep top of mummy sheet level with shoulder. Maintain arms and legs in anatomical position. Expose needed extremity only.
Clove hitch or commercial ties	For arm or leg restraints to limit motion for venipunctures	Observe for adequacy of circulation. Place pad under restraint. Tie ends to crib springs. Remove q2h for ROM exercise.
Elbow	To prevent touching of head or face scalp vein infusions after repair of cleft lip, palate	Use pad with stiff material. Use pins or ties to prevent slippage. Remove one at a time q2h for ROM exercise.

that were there before are there now; much worry over body integrity

2. loss of control: their active imagination may lead to exaggeration or misinterpretations of hospital experiences; fears and fantasies may get the best of them
3. separation
   a. may view as punishment for something thought or done
   b. more subtle responses than toddler (quiet crying, sleep problems, loss of appetite)
4. pain
   a. recognizes cues that signal an impending painful experience
   b. able to anticipate pain: may try to escape, may become physically combative
5. immobility: prevents mastery of fears; preschooler often feels helpless
d. School-age child
   1. separation
      a. from family and friends
      b. easier than other age groups because of cognitive level and better time concept
   2. fear of loss of control
      a. through immobility
      b. enforced dependence
      c. fear of injury and death; death anxiety peaks
      d. does not want others to see loss of control (e.g., crying), tries to appear brave
   3. pain: responses are influenced by cultural variables; usually uses passive coping strategies (lies rigidly still, shuts eyes, clenches teeth and fists)

4. immobility: affects sense of physical achievement and need for competition
e. Adolescent: loss of control/enforced dependence when the need is to move toward own identity and independence

Application of the Nursing Process to the Ill and Hospitalized Child

Assessment
1. Child's development level and major fear associated with age group
   a. Infant: separation
   b. Toddler: separation, intrusive procedures
   c. Preschooler: body mutilation, pain
   d. School age: loss of control, separation from peers
   e. Adolescent: change in body image and self-identity, loss of esteem
2. Child's perceptions/understanding of illness and hospitalization
3. Family responses to child's hospitalization
   a. Parents may react with denial, disbelief, guilt, fear, anxiety, frustration, and depression
   b. Alterations in family routines and life-style
   c. Parents' coping mechanisms
      1. support systems for parents (e.g., friends, extended family members)
      2. financial resources
      3. family's ability to cope with the child's illness
      4. ability to express reaction to child's illness
4. Child's response to pain: unable to express verbally; often results in underuse of pain-relief methods
   a. Through observation
      1. verbally: younger child often uses incorrect

words (e.g., "bad," "funny," "hot"); older child often reluctant to complain because of fear of "shots"

2. behaviorally: pulling at area (ear), irritable, loss of appetite, lying or moving in unusual position
3. physiologically: vomiting, change in vital signs, flushed skin, increased sleep time, sleep disruptions

   b. Asking child to rate the pain (e.g., using happy/unhappy faces, or scale of 0-10)

Analysis

1. Safe, effective care environment
   a. High risk for infection
   b. High risk for injury
   c. Sensory-perceptual alteration
2. Physiological integrity
   a. Ineffective airway clearance/high risk for aspiration
   b. Pain
   c. Fluid volume deficit
3. Psychological integrity
   a. Ineffective individual coping
   b. Anxiety/fear
   c. Body image disturbance
4. Health promotion/maintenance
   a. Altered growth and development
   b. Knowledge deficit
   c. Altered family processes

Planning, Implementation, and Evaluation

> **Goal 1:** Child will be prepared psychologically for hospitalization.

Implementation

1. Encourage preadmission preparation.
   a. *Before 2 years:* explanation is ineffective; allow to take favorite toy and objects
   b. *2-7 years:* usually tell child ahead in days equal to years of age (e.g., 2 years = 2 days ahead, 6 years = 6 days ahead)
   c. *Over 7 years:* tell child when parent knows (use judgment)
2. Orient child and family to surroundings.
3. Anticipate and alleviate age-related needs and fears.
   To develop trust in infant
   a. Arrange for rooming-in.
   b. Ensure consistency of caregiver.
   c. Provide security objects (e.g., toy, blanket).
   d. Make routine patterns as similar as possible to home.
   e. Hold, cuddle, stroke.
   To help toddler maintain control
   f. Use familiar words (e.g., child's word for toileting).

   g. Ask parents to leave familiar objects with child (e.g., toy, blanket).
   h. Encourage rooming-in and parental participation in care.
   i. Accept regressive needs but avoid promoting them (e.g., don't put toilet-trained child back in diapers).
   j. Provide explanations immediately before any procedure with use of simple, concrete words.
   k. Use time orientation in relation to familiar activities (e.g., "after naptime").
   l. Prepare parents to recognize and accept regressive behavior following discharge.
   m. Maintain limit setting to provide consistency for child.
   n. Don't offer choices when there are none.
To help preschooler relieve body-mutilation anxiety
   o. Allow child to wear underwear.
   p. Provide reassurance regarding invasive procedures.
   q. Encourage play that incorporates equipment and treatments.
   r. Concept of time is related to routine activities (e.g., when you wake up, after lunch).
   s. Allow some choices to promote feelings of control and mastery (choice of fluids, play activities).
To help school-age child maintain a degree of control
   t. Provide explanations of illness and treatment with pictures, simple anatomical diagrams, dolls (call them models or teaching models with older child), books, or step-by-step illustrations.
   u. Maintain educational level during long-term hospitalization to help meet need for accomplishment.
      1. homework; contact with own schoolteacher
      2. in-hospital teacher
   v. Allow to participate in planning care by choosing food, times for bath or treatments.
To help adolescent maintain esteem and identity
   w. Maintain peer contacts.
      1. visiting should be open to adolescents
      2. place in adolescent unit or room
   x. Encourage participation in decision making regarding own body.

4. Provide *honest* explanations, information, and support.
   a. Determine level of understanding based on cognitive development and preexisting knowledge.
   b. Use age-appropriate language, terminology, and timing before instruction.
5. Foster a sense of safety and security.
   a. Encourage rooming-in, security objects for younger children.
   b. Determine child's routine, rituals, and nickname.
   c. Implement age-appropriate safety measures (e.g.,

bubble top [covered] cribs, raised crib rails [see Table 5-4]).

Evaluation

Child maintains developmental level; expresses feelings/desires about hospital (e.g., wants to go home); maintains attachments (family, favorite objects, friends).

Goal 2: Parents will feel in control.

Implementation

1. Allow and encourage parents to participate in child's care; provide 24-hour open visiting and rooming-in facilities.
2. Foster family relationships between ill child for family members; include siblings.
3. Provide support; help family identify persons or community resources who can help.
4. Provide information about child's illness, treatment, and care at rate that parents are able to cope with and accept.

Evaluation

Parent's express satisfaction with caregivers and information provided; child and parents maintain/regain supportive relationships.

Goal 3: Child undergoing hospital procedures and surgery will be prepared.

Implementation

1. Refer to "Perioperative Period," p. 117.
2. Measure child's height and weight (used for calculating medications and IV fluids).
3. Explain procedure, recovery room, and postoperative care to child (appropriate for age) and to parents.
   a. Use concrete words and visual aids.
   b. Use neutral words (e.g., "fixed" instead of "cut").
   c. Emphasize body part involved and any change in function.

   d. Use drawings and storytelling to evaluate child's understanding.
   e. Take child and parent to see equipment and rooms if possible.

Day of surgery

4. Keep NPO (shorter duration for a child compared with an adult).
5. Check for loose teeth and inform anesthesiologist of findings.
6. Allow favorite toy to accompany child to OR.
7. Encourage parents to remain with child as long as possible.
8. Clothe child for OR: diaper for non–toilet-trained child; permit older child to wear underwear under hospital gown, if possible.
9. Administer preoperative medications as ordered; oral or parenteral form is influenced by type, amount, age, and accessibility; see Tables 5-5 and 5-6.

Evaluation

Child and family understand rationale for NPO and comply; child is prepared correctly for surgery; child and family correctly verbalize understanding of postoperative care.

Goal 4: Postoperatively, child will maintain adequate pulmonary ventilation and circulation, fluid and electrolyte balance.

Implementation

1. Turn, position, and get child to cough at least q2h.
2. Allow some crying in infants to achieve deep breathing.
3. Use inspirometer, straw games with older child to ensure deep breathing.
4. Monitor IV closely.
   a. If microdrip (60 gtt/ml used), gtt/min = ml/hr
   b. Check for fluid overload (pulmonary rales)

Table 5-5 Medication and temperature guide

Age group	Usual form of oral medication	Available injection sites	Usual route for temperature
Infant	L	VL	A R
Toddler	L P (crush)	VL	A R
Preschooler	L P (crush or chew)	VL VG GM D for all immunizations except DPT (give deep IM)	A R O (older child)
School-age child	L P	VL VG GM D	O A
Adolescent	L P C	VL VG GM D	O A
	P–pills L–liquid C–capsules	VL–vastus lateralis GM–gluteus medius CG–ventrogluteal D–deltoid	O–oral A–axillary R–rectal

Table 5-6   Medication administration for young children

Age	Developmental considerations	Nursing implications
1-3 months	Strong sucking reflex	Allow sucking for oral medications (e.g., nipples, syringes).
	Extrusion reflex	Give medications in small amounts to allow for swallowing.
		Keep head upright.
		Place liquid in center or side of mouth, toward back.
	Reaches randomly	Control child's hands when giving oral medications.
	Whole body reacts to painful stimuli	Use own body to control infant's arms and legs for parenteral medications.
3-12 months	Extrusion reflex disappears	Use medicine cup and syringe rather than spoon.
	Drinks from cup	Offer physical comforting more than verbal.
	Can finger-feed	
	Can spit out medication	
12-30 months	Development of large motor skills	Never leave medications where child can reach or throw.
	Can spit out medications or clamp jaw shut	May need two adults to give injections (one to restrain).
	Can use medicine cup	
	Auditory canal is not straight	Give ear drops by pulling pinna down and back.
	Autonomy vs. shame/doubt	Be honest about taste/pain; use distractions.
	Ritualistic	Be firm, ignore resistive behavior.
	Takes pride in tasks	Give choices when possible.
2½-3½ years	Has eating likes and dislikes	Disguise medicinal taste.
	Little sense of time	Use chewable medications.
	Tries to coerce, manipulate	Use concrete and immediate rewards (e.g., stickers, badges).
	Has fantasies	
	Body boundaries are unclear	Give choices when possible, but do not offer if there are none.
		Be consistent.
		Give simple explanations; assure medicine is not for a punishment.
		Use Band-Aids for covering injection sites.
3½-6 years	Develops proficiency at tasks	Allow child to handle equipment (e.g., syringes).
	Refining senses	Will be unable to disguise tastes and smells.
	Has loose teeth	Consider teeth when deciding route.
	Can make decisions	Allow choice about route, if possible.
	Has a sense of time	Allow participation in choice of administration time when possible (e.g., before or after meals).
	Takes pride in accomplishment	
	Developing a conscience	Explain in simple terms reason for medications.
	Fears mutilation, punishment	Avoid prolonged reasoning.
	May master pill swallowing	Use simple command by trusted adult that medication is to be given.
		Allow control when possible.
		Praise after medication is given.

Table 5-7   Estimating pediatric drug doses

Pediatric medication dosages may be estimated using *body surface area (BSA):* most reliable method; must plot child's height and weight on a nomogram (available in reference texts)

$$\frac{\text{Body surface area of child (m}^2)}{1.7 \text{ (m}^2)} \times \text{Adult dose} = \text{Estimated pediatric dose}$$

Example: Child's BSA is 0.34; usual adult dose is 500 mg. What is the child's estimated dosage?

$$\frac{0.34}{1.7} \times 500 \text{ mg} = 100 \text{ mg}$$

5. Exercise restrained limbs q2h; fasten restraint ties to crib or bed.
6. Monitor hydration status.
   a. Keep accurate I&O.
   b. Check urine specific gravity.

Evaluation

Child has adequate ventilation and circulation, normal color, and no evidence of cyanosis or fluid volume deficit or overload.

Goal 5: Child will be free from pain.

Implementation

1. Be alert to nonverbal messages in a very young child or child who may fear injections and not wish to communicate discomfort.
2. Medicate for nausea and pain as ordered (analgesics such as acetaminophen are often used).
3. Determine correct medication dosage (see Table 5-7).
4. Assess for response to medications.

Evaluation

Child experiences minimal pain.

Goal 6: Child will use diversionary activity and play to cope with the stress of hospitalization.

Implementation

1. Refer to *"Healthy Child,"* p. 428
2. Help child participate in nursing activities (e.g., tea party for fluid intake, inspirometer for deep breathing, bean bags for range of motion).
3. Use drawings, storytelling, or puppets to help child express feelings about illness.
4. Allow child to use syringes, needles with supervision.

Evaluation

Child expresses fears and feelings during play; adapts to hospital routine with minimal distress.

Goal 7: Child and family will receive appropriate discharge teaching.

Implementation

1. Provide oral and written instructions regarding
   a. Activities and restrictions
   b. Diet
   c. Procedures
   d. Medications: schedule, administration, storage, side effects
2. Teach parents procedures that must be performed at home.
3. Contact appropriate outside resources as needed (e.g., homebound teacher, Visiting Nurse Association).

Evaluation

Child (as appropriate) and parent describe medical regimen that must be carried on at home (e.g., medications, diet, restrictions); demonstrate how to do procedures or give medications; know how to obtain refills and arrange for follow-up appointments.

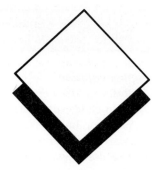

Sensation, Perception, and Protection

GENERAL CONCEPTS
Overview/Physiology

1. Immunological differences in children
   a. Newborn receives passive immunity from mother for most major childhood communicable diseases (assuming mother is immune)
   b. The young infant's immune system is not fully developed; therefore, the infant is more prone to infectious disease
   c. The eustachian tube in infants and young toddlers is shorter and straighter than in older children and adults, leading to increased risk of middle-ear infections
   d. Increasing exposure of preschoolers and school-age children to infectious disease and the immaturity of their immune system leads to increased incidence of infections
2. Integumentary (skin) differences in children
   a. The skin is less thick during infancy
   b. The epidermis is fragile and more prone to irritation
   c. The infant's skin is more sensitive to changes in temperature (especially extremes of heat and cold) and is more susceptible to invasion by bacteria and other infectious organisms
3. Neurological differences in children
   a. The greatest neurological changes occur during the first year of life
   b. The brain reaches 75% of adult size by age 2, 90% by age 4
   c. Cortical development is usually complete by age 4
   d. Primitive neonatal reflexes disappear as higher centers of the brain take over; most neonatal reflexes disappear or diminish by 3-4 months of age; their persistence may indicate a neurological problem

Application of the Nursing Process to the Child with a Sensory Problem
Assessment
1. Nursing history

   a. Frequent earaches or sore throats, persistent nosebleeds, sinus problems, or allergies
   b. Eye crosses, deviates outward or inward, tears excessively; history of other vision problems
   c. Parental concerns about child's vision or hearing
2. Clinical appraisal
   a. Otoscopic exam, ear pain or "fullness," and hearing loss
   b. Ophthalmoscopic exam, head tilting or squinting
   c. Hypertrophy of tonsils, sore throat
3. Diagnostic tests
   a. Vision and hearing testing (refer to "The Healthy Child," p. 436)

Analysis
1. Safe, effective care environment
   a. Sensory-perceptual alteration: visual, auditory, tactile
   b. High risk for injury
   c. High risk for infection
2. Physiological integrity
   a. Pain
   b. Actual/high risk for impaired skin integrity
3. Psychosocial integrity
   a. Body image disturbance
   b. Anxiety
4. Health promotion/maintenance
   a. Knowledge deficit
   b. Self-care deficit
   c. Altered growth and development

Nursing Planning, Implementation, and Evaluation
(refer to Selected Health Problems)

SELECTED HEALTH PROBLEMS: INTERFERENCE WITH SENSATION
☐ Otitis Media
General Information

1. Definition: middle-ear infection; two types:
   a. *Serous otitis media:* nonpurulent effusion of middle ear
   b. *Suppurative otitis media (acute or chronic):* ac-

444

cumulation of viral or bacterial purulent exudate in middle ear
2. Cause
   a. Serous: unknown, but there appears to be a relationship with allergies
   b. Suppurative: pneumococci, *H. influenzae*, streptococci
3. Incidence: one of the most common illnesses of infancy and early childhood
4. Medical treatment
   a. Diagnosis
      1. otoscopic exam
         a. inflamed, bulging tympanic membrane (acute) or dull gray membrane (serous)
         b. no visible landmarks or light reflex
      2. tympanometry (measures air pressure in auditory canal): decreased membrane mobility
   b. Antibiotic therapy: ampicillin (may cause diarrhea; given q6h) or amoxicilline (more expensive but fewer side effects; given TID) 10-14 days
   c. Surgical intervention: incision of membrane (myringotomy) and insertion of myringotomy tubes in cases of recurrent chronic otitis media; adenoidectomy

Nursing Process

Assessment
1. *Suppurative otitis*
   a. Pain (infants may pull or hold ears)
   b. Irritability
   c. High fever
   d. Lymphadenopathy
   e. Purulent discharge (indicates rupture of membrane)
   f. Nasal congestion, cough
   g. Anorexia, vomiting
   h. Diarrhea
2. *Serous otitis*
   a. Ear "fullness"
   b. Popping sensation when swallowing
   c. Conductive hearing loss

Analysis (see p. 444)
Planning, Implementation, and Evaluation

> **Goal 1:** Child will be free from infecting organism and recurrence of infection.

Implementation
1. Teach parents to administer antibiotics as prescribed.
2. Educate parents concerning importance of adhering to medication regimen for full course of therapy.
3. Clean drainage from ear with cotton balls and water.

Evaluation
Child shows no signs or symptoms of continuing infection (e.g., pulling at ears, fever); no discharge from ears; disease does not recur.

> **Goal 2:** Child will receive comfort measures and be free from pain and fever.

Implementation
1. Monitor body temperature.
2. Teach parents to administer antipyretic analgesics (acetaminophen or aspirin).
3. Control fever with tepid baths or sponging.
4. Avoid foods that require chewing.
5. Apply external heat (warm water bottle or heating pad).

Evaluation
Child is free from pain, able to play and sleep comfortably; child's temperature returns to normal.

> **Goal 3:** Child will have no permanent hearing impairment.

Implementation
1. Monitor for signs of hearing loss (decreased attention and responsiveness).
2. Conduct audiometry screening at routine intervals.
3. Refer child to appropriate resources if results are abnormal.

Evaluation
Child has normal hearing.

> **Goal 4:** Child and family will receive appropriate information concerning home care following a myringotomy and insertion of tubes.

Implementation
1. Tell parents to expect some drainage from the ear for several days postoperatively; obvious bleeding is not normal, so the physician should be notified.
2. Keep ear dry; avoid activities that require submerging the head in water (e.g., swimming).
3. Before bathing, place cotton balls in the external canal to keep the ear dry (some physicians recommend dipping them in petroleum jelly first); ear plugs are also available.
4. Advise parents to notify physician if the child develops fever, headache, or nausea/vomiting (meningitis).
5. Check the ears periodically in case the tubes become dislodged (they normally remain in approximately 6 months and then fall out spontaneously).

Evaluation
Child has uneventful recovery; family implements home care without problems or complications.

☐ Tonsillectomy and Adenoidectomy
General Information

1. Definition: surgical excision of the tonsils and adenoids; usually done after 3 years of age because of the danger of excessive bleeding and tonsillar regrowth

2. Indications for surgery: controversy exists regarding the value of surgery; most widely accepted reasons are chronic tonsillitis (most common cause is beta-streptococci, group A), airway obstruction, and chronic otitis media

Nursing Process

Assessment

1. Airway obstruction: noisy or increased respiration; restless/change in behavior; diaphoretic; pale/cyanotic
2. Active infection: fever, sore throat, enlarged lymph nodes; elevated WBCs
3. Bleeding disorders: bleeding and coagulation time: PT, PTT
4. Preoperative anxiety: child and family's knowledge concerning surgery

Analysis (see p. 444)

Planning, Implementation, and Evaluation

> **Goal 1:** Preoperatively, the child and family will be prepared psychologically for hospitalization and surgery (refer to "The Ill and Hospitalized Child," Goal 1, p. 440)

> **Goal 2:** Postoperatively, the child will remain free from excessive bleeding or hemorrhage; maintain a patent airway.

Implementation

1. Position child on side with knee on upper side flexed until alert and recovered from surgery.
2. Monitor vital signs frequently.
3. Observe for excessive swallowing, vomiting of fresh blood, restlessness, frequent clearing of throat.
4. Inspect surgical site for signs of oozing.
5. Discourage child from coughing, sneezing, crying, and sucking on straw (puts tension on suture line).
6. Employ comfort measures.
   a. Ice collar to promote vasoconstriction and reduce pain
   b. Analgesics prn (avoid aspirin)
   c. Nonirritating, cool liquids (ice chips, Popsicles, Jell-O); avoid milk products
   d. Mouth care (no gargling or toothbrush)

Evaluation

Child maintains patent airway free from hemorrhage; experiences minimal pain and discomfort.

> **Goal 3:** Child or family will receive appropriate information concerning home care.

Implementation

1. Observe for delayed hemorrhage (5-10 days postoperatively) caused by infection or tissue sloughing during healing process.

2. Limit child's activities for 1-2 weeks.
3. Provide daily rest periods.
4. Keep child away from anyone with an active infection (e.g., URI).
5. Provide nonirritating foods to child for 1-2 weeks; not hot, citrus, spicy, or rough foods; encourage clear liquids.
6. Have child refrain from coughing, clearing throat, or gargling (sore throat usually lasts 7-10 days).

Evaluation

Child's surgical site heals without complications; child resumes normal diet and activities 1-2 weeks postoperatively.

☐ Strabismus

General Information

1. Definition: neuromuscular defect of the eye that can cause visual impairment, either diplopia (double vision) or amblyopia (suppression of vision in one eye)
2. Incidence: normal in young infants; considered abnormal after 4 months of age, requiring evaluation and treatment
3. Medial treatment (done before age 6 to preserve or restore vision in affected eye)
   a. Eye muscle exercises (orthoptics)
   b. Corrective lenses
   c. Patching unaffected eye to strengthen muscles of affected eye
   d. Surgical correction

Nursing Process

Assessment

1. Eye crosses or deviates outward; may be unilateral or bilateral
2. Squinting; head tilting
3. Cover test: unaffected eye is covered while child focuses on an object, cover is removed, affected eye deviates
4. Corneal light reflex test: shine penlight on bridge of child's nose while child fixates on a distant object, light reflects from a different point on each pupil, indicating an imbalance

Analysis (see p. 444)

Planning, Implementation, and Evaluation

> **Goal 1:** Child and parents will implement treatment plan (exercises, patching, or corrective lenses).

Implementation

1. Teach child and parents how to carry out prescribed treatment measures.
2. Emphasize importance of adhering to treatment plan.

Evaluation

Child cooperates with and adheres to corrective measures; has vision restored; experiences no worsening of visual impairment.

Goal 2: Child will be prepared for eye surgery; complications will be prevented.

Implementation

1. Assist child in becoming familiar with postoperative environment (e.g., call light, bedside table).
2. Minimize changes in child's postoperative environment.
3. Speak to child in normal voice tones; identify self and purpose *before* proceeding with care.
4. Maintain eye patches or shields as prescribed.
5. Keep bed's side rails up; pad as necessary.
6. Teach child to avoid straining, coughing, sudden movement, rubbing eyes (use elbow restraints if necessary).
7. Observe and report ocular redness, discharge, itching, or pain.
8. Instill eye ointments or drops as prescribed (inner to outer canthus).
9. Provide auditory and tactile play activities (music, reading to child, story tapes, favorite attachment objects).

Evaluation

Child's eye heals without injury or infection; child cooperates with care and maintains age-apppropriate play activities.

Application of the Nursing Process to the Child with an Interference with Protection: Communicable Disease

Assessment

1. Nursing history
   a. Immunization history
   b. History of exposure to disease
   c. Previous communicable disease, how treated
   d. Signs and symptoms of current illness
      1. alterations in skin sensation
      2. skin lesions
      3. pain or tenderness
      4. itching
      5. fever
2. Clinical appraisal
   a. Skin lesions: size, color, distribution (general, localized), configuration (single, clustered, diffuse, linear), type of lesion (macule, papule, vesicle, pustule, crust)
   b. Description of infestation (lice, scabies, ringworm, pinworms)
3. Diagnostic tests
   a. Microscopic exam of lesions
   b. Culture of organism

Analysis

1. Safe, effective care environment
   a. High risk for poisoning
   b. High risk for infection
2. Physiological integrity
   a. Pain
   b. Fluid volume deficit
   c. Impaired skin integrity
3. Psychosocial integrity
   a. Body image disturbance
   b. Social isolation
   c. Anxiety
4. Health promotion/maintenance
   a. Knowledge deficit
   b. Self-care deficit
   c. Altered health maintenance

General Nursing Planning, Implementation, and Evaluation

Goal: Child will be free from communicable disease (infection, infestation) and will not spread communicable diseases to others.

Implementation

1. Ensure that child's immunizations remain up-to-date.
2. Explain prescribed treatment to parents and child, and encourage them to comply with therapy.
3. Prevent child's exposure to others during communicable period.
4. Identify contacts who also may require treatment.

Evaluation

Child is free from communicable disease; does not transmit disease to others.

SELECTED HEALTH PROBLEMS: COMMUNICABLE DISEASES, SKIN PROBLEMS, INFESTATIONS

☐ Communicable Diseases

General Information

1. Definition: a disease caused by a specific agent or its toxic products, transmitted by direct contact or indirectly through contaminated articles; the incidence of communicable disease has significantly decreased with availability and widespread use of immunizations
2. Types of immunity
   a. Active: antibodies formed by body as a result of having had the disease or through immunization
   b. Passive: introduction of antibodies formed outside the body, such as by placental transfer, breast milk, or gamma globulin injection
3. Medical treatment
   a. Prevent through immunization (refer to Table 5-3)
   b. Antibiotic therapy for scarlet fever (penicillin/erythromycin), Rocky Mountain Spotted Fever (tetracycline/chloramphenicol), and Lyme disease (doxycycline/tetracycline)
   c. Rubella titer before pregnancy or during first trimester

Nursing Process

Assessment

1. Prodromal period

a. Malaise
b. Anorexia
c. Coryza
d. Sore throat
e. Fever
f. Lymphadenopathy
g. Headache
2. Specific characteristics
   a. *Chickenpox (varicella zoster):* rash begins as macule, progresses to papule and vesicle that breaks open and crusts over; all stages present in varying degrees at same time; rash begins on trunk and spreads to extremities and face; intense pruritus; child communicable until all lesions crusted
   b. *Mumps (parotitis):* after puberty, sterility in males is major complication; encephalitis is frequent complication of mumps for any age group
   c. *German measles (rubella):* greatest concern is teratogenic effect on fetus during first trimester of pregnancy; rubella titer on women of childbearing age highly recommended
   d. *Rocky Mountain Spotted Fever (RMSF):* transmitted by ticks; found primarily along Atlantic coast and Rocky Mountain region; high fever and rash beginning on ankles, wrists, soles of feet; may see edema and CNS problems; methods for tick removal include withdrawing tick by turning counterclockwise with tweezers or pulling gently at 45° angle
   e. *Lyme disease:* transmitted by deer ticks throughout the continental United States; most common in late spring and early summer; spreading red-pink ringlike rash develops around tick bite 3-4 weeks after exposure accompanied by flulike symptoms—fever, fatigue, myalgias, nausea; if untreated, child may develop arthralgias, synovitis, neuropathy, and dysrhythmias 6 weeks to 3 years after exposure
   f. *Roseola (exanthema subitum):* seen in children age 6 months to 2 years; high fever for 3-4 days; temperature returns to normal with onset of rosy-pink, macular rash; rash fades with pressure and lasts 1-2 days; febrile convulsions
   g. *Scarlet fever:* caused by beta-hemolytic streptococcus group A; high fever, strawberry tongue, and red pinpoint rash, especially in skin folds; rheumatic fever or acute glomerulonephritis may follow
   h. *Reye's syndrome:* while not communicable, is a serious complication that may occur after a viral infection (e.g., chickenpox, flu); child appears to have recovered from viral infection and then usually begins to vomit; may see changes in LOC: increased intracranial pressure (ICP) and seizures; increased risk in children who received aspirin during viral illness; acetaminophen is drug of choice for this reason

Analysis (see p. 447)
Planning, Implementation, and Evaluation

> **Goal 1:** Child will be prepared for isolation, will not spread disease.

Implementation
1. Explain reason for isolation to child and parents.
2. Provide age-appropriate play.
   a. Diversion
   b. Plan time to play with child
   c. TV in room (except if photophobic)
3. Accept expressions of fear, anger, restlessness, boredom.
4. If child is hospitalized, use appropriate isolation procedures (see Table 5-8).
5. Discontinue isolation as soon as period of communicability is over.
Evaluation
   Child accepts restrictions of isolation (stays in room); engages in age-appropriate activities; other cases of disease do not occur.

> **Goal 2:** Child will be free from complications and long-term sequelae.

Implementation
1. Observe and report signs of encephalitis: headache, bizarre behavior changes, seizures, fever, muscle weakness.
2. Observe and report signs of vision or hearing loss.
3. Observe and report signs of respiratory or cardiac complications: pneumonia, laryngotracheitis, otitis media, rheumatic fever.
4. Observe and report signs of orchitis (mumps).
Evaluation
   Child is free from complications and long-term sequelae (e.g., neurological disability, sensory impairment, sterility, or cardiac damage).

> **Goal 3:** Child will ingest adequate food and fluids to meet nutritional needs.

Implementation
1. Avoid rough or acidic foods; offer bland foods.
2. Use colorful glasses, straws, or liquids to enhance appetite.
3. Offer favorite foods and fluids (ice cream, pudding, gelatin).
4. Advance from liquids to regular diet as tolerated.
Evaluation
   Child ingests adequate daily intake; is free from dehydration; eats a soft diet of sufficient caloric content.

> **Goal 4:** Child will experience minimal discomfort.

Table 5-8 Types of isolation

Mode of transmission	Isolation	Nursing responsibilities
Direct contact; airborne (droplets)	Strict	Private room Hand washing Gown, gloves, and mask Double-bag linen and trash Sterilize all reusable equipment Lab specimen precautions
Airborne (droplets)	Respiratory	Private room Hand washing Mask Double-bag respiratory trash Lab specimen precautions
Direct/indirect contact with feces	Enteric	Private room Hand washing Gowns and gloves when in contact with feces or materials contaminated with feces Double-bag contaminated articles Lab specimen precautions
Direct/indirect contact with purulent material or drainage from infected body sites	Drainage/secretions precautions	Hand washing Gown and gloves when in contact with contaminated linen, dressings, etc. Double-bag linen/trash
Direct/indirect contact with infected blood or body fluids	Universal precautions	Hand washing Gowns and gloves when in contact with body fluids, soiled linens, clothes, dressings, etc. Protective eyewear when splashing of body fluids can be expected Double-bag contaminated articles Avoid needle-stick injuries Dispose of used needles correctly Keep emergency ventilation devices at bedside if indicated Health care personnel with open skin lesions should avoid all direct client care
	Severely compromised client (reverse)	Private room with positive pressure airflow Hand washing Gowns, gloves, and mask Sterilize linen, clothing, etc.

Implementation

1. Give antipyretics for fever or discomfort (dose: 1 grain for every year of age up to 10 years qh4 prn); do not give aspirin. Tylenol dose is 5-10 mg/kg.
2. Place on bed rest until fever subsides.
3. Change bed linen and clothing daily.
4. Provide humidifer as needed.
5. Use tepid baths to relieve fever and itching; keep skin clean; observe for signs of secondary skin infection.
6. Apply calamine lotion for itching (wash off completely once a day to prevent maceration of skin); administer antihistamines or antipruritic medications.
7. Keep fingernails short and clean; apply mittens if needed.
8. Dim lights if photophobia is present.
9. Use warm compresses or irrigations of saline to eyes (measles).

10. Local applications of heat or cold to relieve parotid discomfort (mumps).

Evaluation

Child rests and sleeps comfortably; has only minimal fever and itching.

☐ Sexually Transmitted Diseases (STDs) General Information

1. Definition: a communicable disease transmitted by direct genital contact or sexual activity; STDs are the most prevalent communicable diseases in the United States; majority of cases occur in adolescents and young adults; some STDs are contracted by newborns (*Candida* [thrush], herpes, gonorrheal conjunctivitis); STDs in infants and children usually indicate sexual abuse and should be investigated
2. Cause (see Table 5-9)
3. Medical treatment (see Table 5-9)

Table 5-9 Sexually transmitted diseases

Causative agent	Incidence	Assessment	Medical treatment
Gonorrhea *Neisseria gonor-rheae*	Most commonly reported communicable disease	Males: dysuria, frequency, purulent urethral discharge Females: purulent vaginal discharge; 60% asymptomatic Diagnosis: by Gram stain or culture (Thayer-Martin medium) Complications if untreated: prostatitis and epididymitis in males; pelvic inflammatory disease, infertility, and arthritis in females	Penicillin or other antibiotics Probenecid may be given to delay excretion of penicillin
Herpes *Herpesvirus hominus* type 2	300,000-500,000 new cases each year	Active lesions: painful vesicular lesions that ulcerate Signs and symptoms of systemic illness: fever, headache, and/or general adenopathy Diagnosis: isolation of virus in tissue culture; demonstration of multinucleated giant cells on microscopic exam	Viscous lidocaine to ease pain Keep lesions clean and dry apply cornstarch use warm air blower wear loose clothing Females: dysuria may be eased by voiding in warm water Acyclovir (Zovirax) may decrease duration of the initial or subsequent episodes, but doesn't prevent recurrences
Syphillis *Treponema palidum*	Third most commonly reported communicable disease	Primary (3 weeks after exposure): classic chancre (painless, red, eroded lesions with indurated border at point of entry) Secondary (1-3 months after exposure): cutaneous, nonpruritic, diffuse lesions on face, trunk, and/or extremities Tertiary (10-30 years after exposure): cardiac and neurological destruction Diagnosis: positive darkfield slide of organism; VDRL, RPR, or FTA	Penicillin
Trichomoniasis *Trichomonas vaginalis*	May be the most frequently acquired sexually transmitted disease in the United States	Symptoms range from none to frothy, greenish-grey vaginal discharge Diagnosis: microscopic identification of motile protozoan	Metronidazole (Flagyl)
Candidiasis *Candida albicans*	Overall incidence in United States is unknown	Erythematous, edematous, pruritic vulva Thick, white, "cottage-cheese"-like discharge	Nystatin (Mycostatin) vaginal suppositories or cream; if this fails, clotrimazole 1% (Lotrimin)
Scabies *Sarcoptes scabiei*	Epidemic in United States	Intense, nocturnal genital itching Diagnosis: microscopic examination of shave excision lesion	1% gamma benzene hexachloride lotion (Kwell) A-200 Pyrinate, RID in children under 5

Table 5-9 Sexually transmitted diseases—cont'd

Causative agent	Incidence	Assessment	Medical treatment
Chlamydia *Chlamydia tra- chomatis*	More prevalent than gonor-rhea Affects approxi-mately 3 mil-lion Americans a year	Major cause of nongonococcal ure-thritis in men (frequency, dysuria) Accounts for 20%-30% of all pelvic inflammatory diseases May be transmitted to the newborn during delivery and result in con-junctivitis and pneumonia Many women are asymptomatic; others may complain of fre-quency, dysuria, urgency, abnor-mal vaginal discharge, even bleeding Diagnosis: identification of organ-ism through culture	Tetracycline/erythromycin; should take medication at least 7-10 days; sexual partners should also be treated
Acquired immu-nodeficiency syndrome (AIDS) *Human immu-nodeficiency vi-rus (HIV)*	Refer to p. 277		

Nursing Process

Assessment (see Table 5-9)
Analysis (see p. 447)
Planning, Implementation, and Evaluation

> **Goal 1:** Client will participate in treatment of STD; will not transmit the disease to others.

Implementation
1. Use a straightforward, nonjudgmental approach when taking nursing history.
2. Reassure client of confidentiality of information and exam.
3. Teach signs, symptoms, and transmission mode of STD.
4. Teach client to avoid sexual contact with partner while infected.
5. Provide clear, specific, written and oral explanations of medical treatment.
6. Counsel women of childbearing age concerning trans-mission of STD to newborn.
   a. Gonorrheal conjunctivitis (may cause blindness)
   b. Neonatal herpes infection (may cause blindness, deafness, mental retardation, or may be fatal)
   c. Congenital syphilis (passively transmitted through placenta)
   d. Oral candidiasis (thrush)
   e. Chlamydia conjunctivitis and pneumonia

7. Assist with identification and treatment of sexual con-tacts.
8. Report cases of gonorrhea, syphilis to health depart-ment.
9. Teach how to reduce risk of reinfection.

Evaluation
Client participates in treatment plan; is free from dis-ease recurrence; does not transmit disease to others.

> **Goal 2:** Client will resolve feelings of embarrass-ment, shame, guilt, and negative self-worth re-sulting from diagnosis.

Implementation
1. Treat with respect, dignity.
2. Ensure confidentiality.
3. Provide sexuality education to dispel myths and mis-information.
4. Encourage to express any feelings of shame, embar-rassment, guilt, loss of esteem.
5. Refer to self-help groups (herpes) in community as appropriate.

Evaluation
Client resolves negative feelings about diagnosis; uses support group (when appropriate); client's confidentiality is protected.

> **Goal 3:** Client will be aware of sexual practices that will reduce the chances of acquiring an STD.

Implementation
1. Avoid sex with individuals who have multiple partners.
2. Follow strict personal hygiene habits (e.g., bathing, diet).
3. Use only water-soluble lubricants.
4. Use condoms lubricated with nonoxynol-9.
5. Avoid douching before and after sex (increases the risk of infections because the body's normal defenses are reduced/destroyed).
6. Be aware of symptoms of STD (fever, weight loss, persistent diarrhea, enlarged lymph nodes, unusual discharge, dysuria, bruising).

Evaluation
   Client enjoys a healthy sex life; remains free from STD.

☐ Common Skin Problems and Infestations
General Information
1. Definition: inflammatory responses, bacterial infections, or insect infestation of the skin, hair, or scalp; common in preschoolers and school-age children whose close contact increases their susceptibility
2. Cause (see Table 5-10)
3. Medical treatment (see Table 5-10)

Nursing Process (see Table 5-10)
☐ Pinworms (Helminths)
General Information
1. Definition: parasitic infestation primarily of the intestinal tract; worms deposit eggs in anal area, causing severe itching; eggs attach to child's fingers, causing reinfection when fingers are put in mouth
2. Incidence: approximately half of all school-age children will have pinworms at some time
3. Medical treatment
   a. Stool for ova and parasites (not a reliable test for pinworms)
   b. Cellophane-tape test; child should be rechecked 2-3 times because of "false" negative findings; tape test should be done in early morning (i.e., 5 to 6 AM)
   c. Anthelmintic
      1. pyrvinium pamoate (Povan), single dose 5 mg/kg; stools turn red; tablets should not be chewed because they stain teeth
      2. piperazine citrate 65 mg/kg daily for 3 days; contraindicated in children with impaired renal/hepatic function or seizure disorders

Nursing Process
Assessment
1. Intense anal itching (worsens at night)/vaginitis
2. Enuresis
3. Irritability/restlessness
4. Night walking/insomnia

Analysis (see p. 447)
Planning, Implementation, and Evaluation

> **Goal:** Child will be free from infestation, will not reinfest self.

Implementation
1. Identify other family members and close contacts who may also need treatment.
2. Teach good hand washing and personal hygiene (after toileting and before eating).
3. Wear tight-fitting diapers or panties.
4. Change and launder underwear, pajamas, and bed linens daily.
5. Have child sleep alone.
6. Wear mitts or socks to prevent scratching.
7. Carry out proper disposal of feces.
8. Ensure that parents understand importance of carrying out these measures.

Evaluation
   Child is free from infestation; does not reinfest self or transmit infestation to others; parent establishes adequate sanitation.

Application of the Nursing Process to the Child with an Interference with Protection: Safety (See Selected Health Problems)

SELECTED HEALTH PROBLEMS RESULTING IN AN INTERFERENCE WITH PROTECTION: SAFETY
☐ Poisonous Ingestions
General Information
1. Definition: the swallowing of common nonnutritive materials that can cause health problems and/or poisoning; common ingested substances include lead, corrosives, hydrocarbons, aspirin, acetaminophen, and sedatives/hypnotics
2. Incidence: poisonous ingestions are fifth leading cause of death between 1 and 4 years of age; peak incidence is during toddler years
3. Cause: developmental curiosity; incorrect storage of potentially toxic substances
4. Aim of treatment is to remove ingested toxic substance from body or to neutralize its effects as quickly as possible
5. Vomiting, or use of an emetic, is contraindicated when
   a. Child is comatose, convulsing, or in severe shock (increases risk of apsiration)
   b. Substance is a hydrocarbon (aspiration may cause a chemical pneumonia)
   c. Substance is a corrosive (acid or alkali) (emesis may further damage or perforate esophageal mucosa); see Table 5-11 for general information, treatment, and assessment of specific ingestions

Table 5-10 Common skin problems and infestations

Cause	Assessment	Medical treatment	Plan/implementation
ACNE VULGARIS: SKIN LESIONS (COMEDOS) CAUSED BY INCREASED SEBACEOUS SECRETIONS DURING PUBERTY AND ADOLESCENCE; MORE THAN THREE FOURTHS OF ALL ADOLESCENTS ARE AFFECTED			
Corynebacterium acnes Dietary factors (chocolate, iodine) have not been substantiated Exacebated by menstruation, stress, oil-based cosmetics, and oral contraceptives	Sebum blocks skin pores, resulting in local inflammation Blackheads, papules, cysts, or nodules appear on face, back, chest, arms, and neck	Topical antibiotics. Tetracycline or prednisone for severe cases. Ultraviolet light. Isotretinoin (Accutane)	Teach adolescent to avoid picking or squeezing lesions (may cause infection and scarring). Encourage regular cleansing of skin, especially when sweaty (hot weather, after exercise). Avoid using caps, headbands. Recommend over-the-counter antiacne cleansers and cover creams (contain alcohol and benzoyl peroxide, a peeling and drying agent) to help keep skin dry. Encourage a healthy lifestyle: balanced diet, exercise, rest; minimize stress.
ATOPIC DERMATITIS (ECZEMA): ALLERGIC REACTION TO FOODS, ENVIRONMENTAL INHALANTS, AND POLLEN			
Unknown	Disease of remissions and exacerbations Lesions appear as papules, vesicles, and crusts; begin on cheeks and spread to face and flexor surfaces of body Intense itching that may lead to secondary skin infection Some consider eczema a precursor to asthma	Elimination diet. Topical steroids. Nonsoap preparations (Cetaphil). Wet soaks with Burow's solution. Antihistamines for itching.	Teach parents the importance of adhering to the diet. Teach administration of medications steroids may mask infections; may see rebound effect when ointment discontinued antihistamines may cause drowsiness Control itching by administering medications as ordered avoiding soap preparations keeping nails cut; covering hands with mittens; may need to use elbow restraints cotton clothing avoiding overheating exposure to ultraviolet light (irritates and dries the lesions) wet soaks with Burow's PRN (e.g., nap time)

Continued.

Table 5-10   Common skin problems and infestations—cont'd

Cause	Assessment	Medical treatment	Plan/implementation
IMPETIGO CONTAGIOSA: SUPERFICIAL BACTERIAL SKIN INFECTION			
Staphylococcus, strepto-coccus	Vesicles that rupture to form honey-colored crusts; erupt most often on face, axillae, and extremities; itches, highly contagious	Removal of crusts with Burow's solution. Topical bactericidal ointment (Neosporin). Penicillin in severe cases.	Teach child and parent how to soften and remove crusts, apply antibiotic ointment. Teach administration of oral antibiotics (penicillin/erythromycin). Prevent scratching by keeping nails clipped, using mitts or elbow restraints as necessary. Teach child to use own towels and washcloths until lesions heal.
LICE (PEDICULOSIS): PARASITIC INFESTATION OF HEAD (PEDICULOSIS CAPITIS), BODY (PEDICULOSIS CORPORIS), OR PUBIC AREA (PEDICULOSIS PUBIS)			
Pediculus humanus	Ova (nits) on hair shafts Itching, skin excoriation Enlarged lymph nodes	Kwell (Lindane 1%) shampoo or lotion. (Not recommended for children younger than 5) A-200 Pyrinate, RID (Pyrethrin) and NIX (permethrin)	Teach parents how to apply prescribed shampoo or lotion; caution against Kwell overuse (neurotoxicity); should repeat treatment in 7-10 days. May need to cut long hair. Use fine-tooth comb dipped in vinegar to remove nits. Discard contaminated combs and brushes. Teach children not to exchange such personal items as towels, combs, brushes, and hats. Launder bed linens and towels. Use gamma benzene spray on upholstered furniture.

Nursing Process

Assessment (see Table 5-11)

Analysis (see p. 447)

Planning, Implementation, and Evaluation (for all ingestions)

> **Goal 1:** Child will receive emergency treatment for acute poisonous ingestion.

Implementation

1. Instruct parent to contact poison control center (provide telephone number) or take child to nearest emergency facility.

2. Instruct to induce vomiting (if appropriate) by stimulating gag reflex and giving syrup of ipecac; do not use salt water as an emetic.
3. Position child to avoid aspiration when vomiting; give physical support while child is vomiting.
4. Tell parent to keep original container label for determining antidote.
5. Analyze ingested substance and child's output.
   a. Bring in container and any remaining substance.
   b. Bring in any vomitus or urine output since ingestion.
6. Make appropriate referrals (e.g., social service).

Table 5-10 Common skin problems and infestations—cont'd

Cause	Assessment	Medical treatment	Plan/implementation
RINGWORM (TINEA): SUPERFICIAL FUNGAL INFECTION OF HEAD (TINEA CAPITIS), BODY (TINEA CORPORIS), "JOCK ITCH" (TINEA CRURIS), OR "ATHLETE'S FOOT" (TINEA PEDIS)			
Various fungi	Scaly, *Capitis* circumscribed patches Areas of patchy hair loss Itching Green concentric ring under Wood's light (ultraviolet) illumination Positive culture	Oral griseofulvin: 20 mg/kg/day for 7-14 days. Local antifungal preparations Whitfield's ointment tolnaftate (Tinactin)	Teach parents how to administer oral and local antifungal agents. Shampoo frequently using clean towels, combs, and brushes. Keep child's hair short. *Corporis and cruris* Avoid wearing nylon underwear and tight-fitting clothes. Keep affected areas clean and dry. Identify and treat source (often from household pets). *Pedis* Wear clean, light, cotton socks. Wear well-ventilated shoes. Apply topical antifungal powder containing tolinaftate. Avoid bare feet in public places (such as school gym) until infection has cleared.

Evaluation

   Parent institutes correct emergency care of child; child receives appropriate follow-up care.

Goal 2: Child will maintain adequate oxygenation.

Implementation

1. Monitor vital and neurological signs at least q15min until stable and as indicated.
2. Administer O_2 therapy as ordered.
3. Assess color of skin, nail beds, and mucous membranes.
4. Report difficulty breathing or swallowing immediately; may require a tracheotomy; keep laryngoscope, endotracheal tube, and tracheotomy tray at bedside.
5. Observe for seizure activity.
6. If breathing is labored, stay with child to reduce fear and anxiety.

Evaluation

   Child remains free from respiratory distress; maintains normal respiratory rate, color.

Goal 3: Child's ingestion will be recognized and treated early to prevent complications; child will be kept safe during treatment regimen.

Implementation

1. Institute seizure precautions.
2. Check vital signs frequently until stable; if temperature elevated, sponge with tepid water; may need to use cooling blanket; observe for febrile seizures.
3. If child is confused, provide safety measures as appropriate.
4. Record I&O accurately.
5. Monitor urine output (EDTA is potentially toxic to kidneys).
6. Prepare child for painful injections (EDTA and BAL); mix with local anesthetic (procaine hydrochloride); rotate injection sites.
7. Increase fluid intake to 1-2 times maintenance (aspirin).

Evaluation

   Child returns to normal activities with no residual effects; is free from acquired injuries.

Table 5-11 Commonly ingested poisonous substances

General information	Nursing assessment	Medical treatment
ASPIRIN (SALICYLATE POISONING)		

Most common cause of childhood poisoning
Toxic dose: 2 grains/kg of body weight
Lethal dose: 4 grains/kg
Effects: stimulates respiratory center, which leads to respiratory alkalosis; increases metabolism, leading to fever, metabolic acidosis (from high level of ketones)
	GI effects
	  vomiting
	  thirst
	CNS effects
	  hyperventilation
	  confusion, dizziness
	  staggered gait
	  coma
	Hematopoietic effects
	  bleeding tendencies
	Metabolic effects
	  sweating
	  hyponatremia
	  hypokalemia
	  dehydration
	  hypoglycema
		Induce vomiting with syrup of ipecac:
		  6-12 months of age: 10 ml (2 tsp) and as much water as possible.
		  over 1 year: 15 ml (1 tbsp) and 2-3 glasses of water.
		Gastric lavage.
		IV fluids, sodium bicarbonate (enhances excretion), electrolytes.
		Vitamin K for hypoprothrombinemia.
		Glucose for hypoglycemia.
		Diuretics: acetazolamide (Diamox).
		Dialysis when potentially lethal doses have been ingested.

ACETAMINOPHEN (TYLENOL)		

Toxic dose: uncertain, do not exceed recommended levels
Effects: cellular necrosis of the liver resulting in liver dysfunction and, in some cases, hepatic failure
	First stage (first 24 hours)
	  nausea
	  vomiting
	  sweating
	  pallor or cyanosis
	  weakness
	Second stage (24-48 hours)
	  SGOT, SGPT elevated
	  liver tenderness (RUQ)
	  prolonged prothrombin time
	Third stage (1 week)
	  liver necrosis
	  hepatic failure
	  possible death
		Induce vomiting or gastric lavage (see aspirin).
		Acetylcysteine (Mucomyst) as an antidote, given PO with fruit juice or cola, or via NG tube (offensive odor).
		IV fluids.
		Sodium-restricted, high-calorie, high-protein diet.

CORROSIVES (LYE, BLEACH, AMMONIA)		
Extent of damage depends on the causticity of the substance and the amount ingested	Grossly visible whitish burns of mouth and pharynx; color darkens as ulcerations form Edema Respiratory distress Difficulty swallowing Excess drooling Severe pain Shock	DO NOT INDUCE VOMITING; DO NOT LAVAGE Activated charcoal may be given. Dilute with small amounts of water. Tracheostomy if respiratory distress is severe. IV fluids while child is NPO. Analgesics, steroids, antibiotics, antacids. Possible gastrostomy. Possible esophageal dilatations to prevent strictures (or maintain patency of esophagus). Colon transplant if esophageal damage is severe (done when child is older).
HYDROCARBONS (GASOLINE, KEROSENE, TURPENTINE, MINERAL SEAL OIL)		
Immediate concern is aspiration, which can cause severe (or fatal) chemical pneumonitis Systemic effects from GI absorption of hydrocarbons are relatively mild	Burning sensation in mouth and throat Characteristic breath odor Nausea, anorexia, vomiting Lethargy Fever	DO NOT INDUCE VOMITING Supportive measures for respiratory effects, pneumonitis (O_2 antibiotics, IV fluids).

Table 5-11 Commonly ingested poisonous substances—cont'd

General information	Nursing assessment	Medical treatment
LEAD (CHRONIC POISONING)		

Approximately 4% of children under age 6 years have excessive lead levels in their blood; peak age is 2-3 years; black children have 6 times greater risk	Hematopoietic effects
	  anemia
	CNS effects
	  irritability
	  lethargy
	  hyperactivity
	  developmental delays
	  clumsiness
	  seizures
	  disorientation
	  coma, possible death
	GI effects
	  anorexia
	  nausea, vomiting
	  constipation
	  lead line along gums
	Skeletal effects
	  increased density of long
	    bones
	  lead lines in long bones
	Renal effects
	  glycosuria
	  proteinuria
	  possible acute or chronic renal
	    failure
		Remove child from lead source, hospitalize.
		Chelating agents: EDTA usually used in combination with BAL; given IM q4h for 5 days (causes lead to be deposited in bone and excreted via kidneys); monitor kidney function because EDTA is nephrotoxic; monitor calcium levels because EDTA enhances excretion of calcium.
		Calcium, phosphorus, and vitamin D aid lead excretion.
		Anticonvulsants for seizure control.
		Oral or IM iron for anemia.
		Follow-up lead levels to monitor progress (lead is excreted more slowly than it accumulates in the body).

Goal 4: Child will regain fluid and electrolyte balance.

Implementation

1. Observe and reports signs of respiratory alkalosis (deep and rapid breathing, lightheadedness, tetany, convulsions, and coma).
2. Observe and report signs of metabolic acidosis (deep breathing, shortness of breath, disorientation, coma).
3. Observe and report signs of metabolic alkalosis (depressed respirations, hypertonicity, and tetany).
4. Observe and report signs of hypokalemia: malaise, thirst, polyuria, cardiac dysrhythmias, decreased BP, thready pulse, depressed reflexes.
5. Observe and report signs of hypoglycemia-hyperglycemia.
6. Monitor vital signs frequently until stable.
7. Offer clear liquids in small amounts (if child is able to swallow); observe for nausea, ability to swallow.
8. Evaluate hydration status frequently.

Evaluation

Child is well hydrated without electrolyte imbalance.

Goal 5: Child will rest comfortably and be free from pain.

Implementation

1. Administer analgesics as ordered.
2. Soothe child with gentle touching and soft voice.
3. Encourage parental contact and involvement.
4. Provide opportunities for age-appropriate play.

Evaluation

Child rests and sleeps normally; is free from pain.

Goal 6: Parents will receive appropriate information to prevent or reduce recurrences.

Implementation

1. Provide anticipatory guidance concerning developmental issues and accidents.
2. Teach the essentials of prevention (childproofing environment).
   a. Do not place substances in unmarked containers.
   b. Keep harmful substances out of child's reach, in locked cabinets.
   c. Teach child that medication is not candy.
   d. Emphasize poisonous quality of abused over-the-counter drugs.
3. Provide appropriate supervision of the child.
4. Provide love and attention to the child.
5. Observe child for pica.
6. Obtain continued medical care as appropriate.

7. Support parents and child in dealing with feelings about ingestion (guilt and anger).

Evaluation

Parent modifies home environment to prevent recurrence of ingestion.

☐ Cocaine and Drug-Addicted Infants
General Information

1. Definition: physical dependence and addiction appearing at birth in neonates whose mothers use and abuse illicit drugs; common drugs include cocaine, crack, heroin, PCP, opiates, alcohol, and CNS depressants
2. Incidence: estimates indicate 7%-16% of women of childbearing years are addicted to drugs: 2%-3% are cocaine-dependent
3. Cause: many drugs freely cross the placental barrier and are incorporated into the fetal circulation; the fetus metabolizes these drugs differently, often resulting in delayed excretion
4. Pathophysiology: crack and cocaine cause hypertension, tachycardia, and vasoconstriction in mothers that may result in abruptio placentae and fetal hypoxia; chronic maternal blood flow restrictions can cause fetal anoxia, prematurity, intrauterine growth retardation, precipitous delivery, and fetal demise
5. Medical treatment
   a. Diagnosis: antepartal history of drug abuse; blood and urine testing of mother and neonate
   b. Treatment: life-sustaining measures include cardiac and respiratory support, social services and law enforcement assistance as needed

Nursing Process
Assessment

1. Antepartal history: maternal crack and cocaine or other drug use
2. Intrapartal history: abruptio placentae, meconium staining, prematurity, intrauterine growth retardation, microcephaly, positive blood and urine drug screens in mother or infant
3. Neonatal period: increased startle reflex, tremulousness, irritability, muscular rigidity, poor feeding patterns, ineffective suck-swallow coordination, and transient EEG abnormalities
4. Infancy and childhood: developmental delays, delayed language acquisition, increased incidence of SIDS, asymmetrical muscle development, and poor interactive capabilities

Analysis (see p. 447)
Planning, Implementation, and Evaluation

Goal 1: Child will experience love and physical contact without overstimulation.

Implementation

1. Decrease stimulation to child: lower lights, minimize sudden noises and movements, and remove from stimuli as much as possible.
2. Swaddle infant; hold closely and securely when providing care; use rhythmic movements (e.g., rocking, swaying).
3. Be observant and responsive to cues of overstimulation including gazing away, tremors, increased irritability.
4. Provide totally darkened, quiet environment if necessary.

Evaluation

Child responds appropriately to external stimuli; is able to form attachments to primary caretakers.

Goal 2: Child will maintain adequate nutrition.

Implementation

1. Wake for feedings if needed (infant may sleep 20-22 hours if allowed).
2. Provide small feedings in upright position.
3. Establish quiet environment, calm routine surrounding feedings.
4. Monitor height and weight.

Evaluation

Child follows growth curve for height and weight, participates in self-feeding as appropriate.

Goal 3: Child will achieve optimum level of growth and development.

Implementation

1. As negative reactions to environment decrease (by 3-4 months of age), provide appropriate developmental stimulation with specific attention to language skills.
2. Provide massage therapy.
3. Hold child with child's arms in midline position to aid in development of hand coordination.

Evaluation

Child achieves normal developmental milestones within first year of life.

Goal 4: Child, family, and caretaker will receive appropriate teaching and follow-up.

Implementation

1. Assess family's ability to safely care for infant at home.
2. Contact social service immediately after birth to arrange involvement of foster parents as needed.
3. Provide information to caretaker about infant's difficulty responding to environment.
4. Explain possible short- and long-term effects of prenatal drug exposure to families.

Evaluation

Family states effects of drug exposure; demonstrates ability to safely provide physical and emotional care for infant.

☐ Burns
General Information

1. Definition: tissue damage that results from thermal, chemical, electrical, or radioactive agents (see Table 5-12)
2. Incidence
   a. Third leading cause of accidental injury and death in children
   b. Over 50% of burns occur in children 5 years of age or younger
   c. Thermal burns are most common
3. Classification
   a. Percentage of body surface burned
      1. rule of nines (adults) (see Fig. 5-1)
      2. modified rule of nines (children) (see Fig. 5-1)
   b. Degree of damage (depth of burn injury)
      1. first degree: superficial partial thickness; pain, redness, no tissue or nerve damage, superficial epidermis affected
      2. second degree: deep-dermal partial thickness; pain, pale-to-red, edematous skin, vesicles, entire affected area of epidermis and varying amounts of dermis affected
      3. third degree: full thickness; painless; skin white, red, or black; edematous; bullae; nerves, epidermis, dermis destroyed; subcutaneous adipose tissue, fascia, muscle and bone may also be destroyed or damaged
4. Medical treatment (moderate to severe burns)
   a. Medical intervention
      1. immediate emergency care
         a. extinguish burn (teach children to "Stop, drop, and roll")

Table 5-12   Systemic responses to burn injury

Alterations in fluid volume	Altered capillary permeability results in shifts of water, protein, and electrolytes from the intravascular to interstitial spaces, which reduces the circulating blood volume
	The body adapts through vasoconstriction, tachycardia, and conservation of fluid volume by renal reabsorption. However, this is temporary, and unless the deficit is corrected, burn shock will result
	fluid losses continue for 3-4 days with major losses in the first 12 hours
	severe edema of burned tissue occurs with mild to moderate edema to the rest of the body; once fluid begins to shift back to intravascular spaces, diuresis occurs (within 48 hours), and the edema subsides
	sodium and potassium are exchanged with sodium entering the cell and potassium entering intravascular spaces; once diuresis occurs, potassium is excreted, child becomes hypokalemic, and replacement therapy is essential
	fluid volume deficit results in decreased renal blood flow, which impairs glomerular filtration; acute renal failure may develop if fluid replacement is not adequate
	hemolysis of RBCs may lead to anemia and renal tubular obstruction
Alterations in metabolism	Increased metabolic rate and oxygen consumption are the body's usual responses to major burns
	the stress of a burn injury causes
	glycogen breakdown leading to depletion of energy stores within 24 hours after burn, followed by gluconeogenesis (breakdown of protein stores)
	negative nitrogen balance (elevated BUN and urine urea nitrogen)
	increased blood glucose levels
	elevated aldosterone and antidiuretic hormone (ADH) levels
	metabolic acidosis (often compensated for by respiratory alkalosis)
Potential complications related to burn injury	The body's response to a burn is systemic in nature and carries the potential of affecting every system of the body
	respiratory problems: inhalation injury, aspiration, bacterial pneumonia, pulmonary edema
	wound infection (usually occurs within 3-5 days after burn; most often caused by gram-negative organisms, especially *Pseudomonas*)
	Curling's ulcer (gastric or duodenal stress ulcer)
	paralytic ileus (most common when burned surface is greater than 20%)
	arterial hypertension
	CNS disturbances: disorientation, personality changes, seizures (especially in burned children), coma

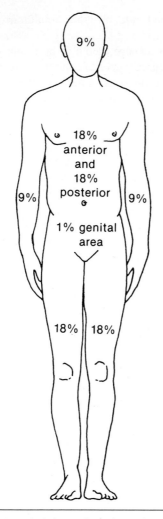

9%

18%
anterior
and
18%
posterior

9%   9%

1% genital
area

18%   18%

a) **Over 12 years:** Rule of Nines (see figure at left)

b) **Under 12 years:** Modified Rule of Nines

Head and neck	9% *plus* 1% for each year under age 12 years
Each arm	9%
Trunk	36%
Each leg	18% *minus* ½% for each year under age 12 years
Genital area	1%

Percentages include anterior and posterior aspects, except for genital area.

Fig. 5-1 Estimation of burn surface area. Percentages include anterior and posterior aspects, except for genital area.

b. slowly immerse burn injury in cool water if possible (relieves pain, inhibits edema formation, slows tissue damage)
c. do *not* use ice water, ice packs, or topical ointments
d. cover burn with clean cloth (e.g., clean bed sheet)
e. cover with blankets (uninvolved areas) if child is hypothermic
f. remove constrictive clothing and jewelry before swelling occurs
g. if child is alert and oriented, provide warm liquids
h. transport to nearest medical facility if burn is extensive

2. admission care
   a. establish airway (O₂, intubation if laryngeal edema is a risk)

b. *frequently* assess blood gases
c. initiate fluid and electrolyte therapy based on body weight and percent of surface area burned
   ◆ one-half of total estimated fluid requirements for the first 24 hours is usually replaced in the first 8 hours following the burn injury
   ◆ types of solutions used may vary
      • first 24 hours: crystalloid solutions, such as normal saline or Ringer's lactate
      • following diuresis, colloid solutions such as albumin or plasma
d. assess other injuries
e. insert urinary indwelling catheter for accurate assessment of urinary output
f. insert NG tube to prevent vomiting, abdom-

inal distension, or gastric aspiration

g. administer IV pain medication as ordered

h. administer antibiotics (penicillin or erythromycin) to prevent infection (broad-spectrum antibiotics are not used because of possibility of superimposed infections)

i. immunized with tetanus toxoid (according to recommended schedule)

3. care of burn wounds

a. initial therapy
- ◆ immersion in Hubbard tank with hypochlorite solution
- ◆ minor debridement; do not break vesicles
- ◆ hair removal next to burn area

b. open method: reverse isolation
- ◆ burn exposed to air; crust or eschar forms a protective barrier
- ◆ topical medication
  - • silver sulfadiazine (Silvadene): penetrates wound slowly; is soothing, causes no acid-base complications, keeps eschar soft; debridement easier; may also be used with closed method
  - • mafenide acetate (Sulfamylon): penetrates wound rapidly, is painful, causes mild acidosis; used when silver sulfadiazine is ineffective

c. closed method
- ◆ burn covered with nonadherent fine-mesh gauze and fluffed-gauze outer layer covered by stretch gauze bandages
- ◆ topical medication
  - • nitrofurazone (Furacin): acts by interfering with bacterial enzymes; most frequent problem is allergic contact dermatitis; may see superinfections
  - • silver nitrate: painless, bactericidal; liquid, must be kept moist; stains healthy skin and fabrics black

d. primary surgical excision: immediate surgical excision of burned tissue with grafting; reduces risk of infection; blood loss may be significant

e. debridement and hydrotherapy (Hubbard whirlpool tank): done regardless of the method of treatment used

f. grafting and reconstructive surgery: long-term treatment; to improve function and cosmetic appearance

Nursing Process

Assessment

1. Respiratory status: patency of airway (burns of head, neck, and chest areas predispose child to respiratory distress)

2. Extent and depth of burn; location of burn injury

3. Observe for early signs of shock (behavioral changes, tachycardia, alterations in BP, diminished output)

4. Presence of pain (frequently manifested as irritability, depression, hostility, or aggression)

5. Observe for signs of hemorrhage (decreased BP; rapid, thready pulse; diaphoresis; pallor; decreased body temperature)

6. Monitor laboratory findings
   a. Hematocrit, arterial blood gases
   b. Sodium, chloride, potassium, CO_2
   c. BUN, creatinine
   d. Serum protein
   e. Urine pH, specific gravity

7. Child and parents' emotional responses to burn injury

Analysis (see p. 447)

Planning, Implementation, and Evaluation

Goal 1: Child will maintain adequate oxygenation.

Implementation

1. Observe for respiratory distress (wheezing, rales, dyspnea, increased respiratory rate, nasal flaring, stridor, air hunger).

2. Monitor arterial blood gases.

3. Elevate burned extremities.

4. Assess arterial circulation in burned extremities qh.

5. Carefully monitor intubated child who is assisted by a respirator; humidified O_2 as ordered.

6. Use suction qh or prn.

7. Prevent aspiration: maintain patency of nasogastric tube.

8. Have child turn, cough, and deep-breathe; use inspirometer (to prevent hypostatic pneumonia); provide humidified air.

9. Check eschar on neck and chest for constriction; assist with escharotomy as needed.

Evaluation

Child is free from respiratory distress; has normal respiratory rate, pink color, adequate circulation (for age) in extremities.

Goal 2: Child will maintain adequate hydration and electrolyte balance.

Implementation

1. Monitor vital signs qh and as necessary; CVP line if appropriate.

2. Monitor I&O hourly (10-20 ml/hr for child under 2 years; 20-50 ml/hr for child over 2 years; 30-50 ml/hr for adult); check urine gravity and pH (may need to catheterize).

3. Observe for signs of hemorrhage (bleeding; decreased BP; decreased body temperature; rapid, thready pulse).

4. Observe for signs of dehydration (thirst, dry tongue, decreased urinary output, decreased BP, tachycardia, poor skin turgor).
5. Monitor IV therapy (NOTE: check for adequate urine output and serum K^+ level before adding potassium to IV).
6. Observe for signs of fluid overload (venous distension, increased BP, shortness of breath, rales, behavioral changes).
7. Observe for signs of electrolyte imbalance (e.g., abnormal lab results, cardiac dysrhythmias, tingling of fingers, abdominal cramps, convulsions, and spasms).

Evaluation

Child is free from shock, maintains adequate circulatory volume and electrolyte balance.

Goal 3: Child will be free from infection and have optimal wound healing.

Implementation

1. Maintain reverse (protective) isolation as ordered.
2. Administer antibiotics and tetanus prophylaxis as ordered.
3. Use sterile technique with wound care; handle wound carefully to prevent damage to healing tissues.
4. Keep wounds and surrounding areas shaved.
5. Encourage self-care to increase child's sense of control and autonomy; encourage child (when possible) to participate in dressing changes.
6. Observe for and report signs of wound infection (temperature elevation, redness at wound edge, purulent or green-grey drainage, offensive odor).
7. Observe for and report signs of systemic infection (increased body temperature, chills, tachycardia, hyperemia).
8. Observe for and report signs of respiratory infection (increased body temperature, signs of respiratory distress).

Evaluation

Child's wounds heal without complications; child assumes an active role in the wound care process.

Goal 4: Child will have minimal pain and discomfort.

Implementation

1. Administer analgesics as ordered (often given IV to ensure absorption); observe for response.
2. Medicate before painful procedures.
3. Use comfort measures (e.g., pillows).
4. Teach child to change focus to music, TV, friends; use imaging when appropriate.
5. Provide heat lamps, warmed blankets to assist with thermoregulation.

Evaluation

Child experiences no more than minimal pain or discomfort; develops coping strategies that reduce/modify painful experiences (e.g., dressing changes); maintains body temperature of 98° F-100° F.

Goal 5: Child will maintain adequate nutritional intake to prevent nitrogen loss and GI complications.

Implementation

1. Provide a high-protein, high-calorie diet; determine special likes and dislikes.
2. Weigh daily.
3. Offer small, frequent meals; encourage family to bring food from home.
4. Assess bowel sounds for possible paralytic ileus.
5. Observe for signs of Curling's ulcer (coffee-ground emesis, abdominal distension, anemia); usually occurs during the third and fourth weeks after the burn in children (first week after burn in adults).
6. Give supplemental vitamins and minerals (vitamins A, B, and C; iron and zinc), and antacids as ordered.

Evaluation

Child ingests therapeutic diet as ordered; is free from gastrointestinal complications; maintains weight.

Goal 6: Child will achieve functional use of burned area and successful cosmetic results.

Implementation

1. Protect graft site from injury; if grafted area is exposed, child may need to be immobilized.
2. When pockets of fluid accumulate under graft site, gently "roll" the fluid out at the graft edges with a sterile cotton-tipped swab.
3. Do not change dressing on donor site (prevents tearing of underlying delicate epithelium).
4. Observe for signs of infection at graft sites.
5. Minimize scar formation by maintaining affected areas in a functional position; use splints when appropriate.
6. Assist with range-of-motion (ROM) exercises as ordered.
7. Encourage ambulation when appropriate.
8. Encourage child's participation in self-care and activities of daily living.
9. Provide explanations to child and family for positioning requirements.

Evaluation

Child has full (or increasing) ROM of affected and unaffected joints; has no footdrop, contractures; graft sites heal without complications.

Goal 7: Child will verbalize concerns and feelings about altered body image.

Implementation

1. Assess child and parents' adjustment to altered body image (child's verbalizations and nonverbal behavior).
2. Spend time listening to concerns and feelings.
3. Use play therapy.
4. Offer preprocedure preparation according to age.
5. Use visual, auditory, and tactile simulation.
6. Use elastic bandages, camouflage clothes, and makeup to enhance appearance.
7. Refer to support groups.

Evaluation

Child talks about effect of burns on body; asks questions about what others will think of body; participates in activities appropriate for age and personal interest.

Goal 8: Child and family will receive appropriate information concerning home care of burns.

Implementation

1. Teach family how to change the burn dressing using clean technique; have family return demonstration; remember to adapt dressing change to family needs.
2. Instruct family to observe for signs of wound infection.
3. Review importance of vitamin C and protein in the healing process, and discuss ways to increase these nutrients in the child's diet.
4. Teach family appropriate care of a healed burn.
   a. Wash with mild soap and apply lubricating cream or jelly (nonperfumed).
   b. Avoid direct sun.
   c. Use medications prn for pruritus.
   d. Observe for signs of infection.
   e. Integrate ROM into daily routine.
5. Dicuss developmental aspects of disfiguring injures; include extended family, peers, school teachers, etc., in rehabilitation; return child to school as soon as possible.
6. Stress importance of self-care activities to strengthen sense of self.

Evaluation

Child's burns heal with minimal contractures; child participates in routine ADL; returns to school.

Application of the Nursing Process to the Child with Developmental or Neurological Disabilities

Assessment

Developmental and neurological disabilities include any serious, chronic disability caused by an impairment of physical or mental functioning, or both, that occurs in childhood, is likely to persist throughout life, and results in limitations in daily functioning; it may cause significant and permanent interruptions in the child's physical, emotional, and social growth and development; early detection and appropriate intervention are essential to promote optimum development; approximately 10% of all children and adolescents have some type of developmental disability

1. Nursing history
   a. Achievement of developmental milestones; child's self-care abilities
   b. Developmental delays: motor, language, social, cognitive (such as persistent head lag, failure to roll over, delayed speech, impaired social functioning)
   c. Perceptual problems: vision and hearing
   d. Perinatal history (refer to *Newborn Care,* p. 387)
   e. Family history: congenital anomalies, hereditary factors, infections
   f. Child's health history: illnesses, allergies, medications, immunizations
   g. Communication, memory, and attention problems; school performance
   h. Current health problem(s): signs and symptoms, medical treatment, home management, concerns or problems
   i. Parents and family's perception of health problem
      1. child's adaptation to disability
      2. family's ability to cope with loss of "perfect child" (refer to *Loss and Death and Dying,* p. 27)
      3. stressors: economic, marital, lack of time and energy
      4. threats to self-esteem and control
      5. overprotectiveness or rejection of child
2. Clinical appraisal
   a. General: level of consciousness, affect, attention span; head and circumferences, cranial sutures and fontanels; vital signs, including BP
   b. Persistent or absent neonatal reflexes
   c. Posture: persistent extension and flexion of extremities, scissoring, frog-leg position, opisthotonos
   d. Motor function: muscle size and tone; symmetrical, spontaneous movements of all extremities; involuntary movements such as tremors, spasticity, athetosis
   e. Developmental skills: assess for developmental progress (e.g., Denver Developmental Screening Test), gross and fine motor development, language, self-help skills (dressing, feeding, and toileting)
   f. Vision: infant's ability to focus on small objects;

vision screening tests for older children (refer to "Healthy Child," vision, hearing screening, p. 436)

   g. Hearing: startle reflex is a rough estimate of sound perception in infants; audiometry is unreliable with infants, toddlers, and mentally retarded children

3. Diagnostic tests (refer to *Nursing Care of the Adult*, diagnostic tests, p. 231)

Analysis

1. Safe, effective care environment

   a. High risk for injury

   b. Sensory-perceptual alteration: tactile and visual

   c. Impaired home maintenance management

2. Physiological integrity

   a. Impaired physical mobility

   b. Activity intolerance

   c. Altered nutrition: more/less than body requirements

3. Psychosocial integrity

   a. Anticipatory grieving

   b. Body image disturbance

   c. Altered thought processes

4. Health promotion/maintenance

   a. Altered growth and development

   b. Self-care deficit

   c. Altered family processes

General Nursing Planning, Implementation, and Evaluation

> **Goal 1:** Child will achieve optimum level of growth and development.

Implementation

1. Screen children at risk for developmental disabilities so that problems are detected and treated early to minimize developmental delays.

2. Keep child's activities in the mainstream as much as possible to promote self-sufficiency, adjustment, and mental development.

   a. Refer family to infant stimulation, developmental, and special education programs.

   b. Maintain open communication between family and all members of interdisciplinary team.

3. Treat child according to developmental (not chronological) age.

4. Provide guidance for learning acceptable social behaviors.

5. Identify parenting concerns and ways to handle them (e.g., consistent discipline; needs for nurturing are identical to any other child).

6. Include activities that enhance child's self-esteem and self-worth.

7. Provide a variety of stimuli; help child pay attention to distinct stimuli.

8. Break tasks into small components; use positive reinforcement (verbal praise, hugs, and stickers).

9. Provide visual and auditory cues and opportunities for practice (repetition enhances learning).

10. Teach self-care skills for activities of daily living (e.g., hygiene, feeding, and dressing).

   a. Allow child as much independence as possible, even if activities take longer (remember to stress that child is a family member, too).

   b. Acknowledge and positively reinforce parents' care of child and child's progress.

   c. Help parents provide a stimulating, healthful environment for the child (mainstreaming).

Evaluation

Child achieves and maintains optimum developmental potential; performs ADL as independently as possible; is maintained in a community setting.

> **Goal 2:** Adolescent or young adult will receive appropriate education regarding sexuality.

Implementation

1. Emphasize that adolescent may understand more than he or she can communicate.

2. Provide appropriate information concerning developmental changes, menstruation, or birth control.

3. Provide explanations at level adolescent can understand.

Evaluation

Adolescent or young adult verbalizes age-appropriate knowledge regarding sexuality.

> **Goal 3:** Parents and family members will express feelings about having a child with a developmental disability and their ability to cope.

Implementation

1. Allow parents and family members opportunities to express their grief; be supportive and anticipate repeated periods of sadness, anger; acknowledge that this is usually a lifetime process.

2. Help parents identify and reinforce child's capabilities and normal characteristics (this is *first* a child, and then a child with a disability).

3. Encourage family discussion and coping with changes that may occur in the family system as a result of caring for the child.

4. Refer the family to appropriate community resources.

Evaluation

Parents and family express feelings and concerns regarding child's limitations; develop realistic plans to care for the child at home; include child as a member of the family constellation; involve all family members in child's care; use appropriate community resources (e.g., parent-support groups, available programs).

> **Goal 4:** The family will remain cohesive and function at its optimal level.

Implementation

1. Identify families at risk for adapting poorly to disability and chronic illness.
   a. Recognize that certain family types (e.g., single-parent families, teen parents) may require more support and guidance in care of child.
   b. Consider the availability of extended-family members and their ability and willingness to participate in care of child.
2. Determine the family's perception of the child's disability and encourage realistic discussion about the child's capabilities and limitations.
3. Identify support systems within the family and community (e.g., home health care).
4. Encourage activities that enhance individual and family development for *all* family members.
5. Provide respite care to family when necessary.

Evaluation

Family discusses realistic perceptions about the child; uses available support systems; participates in activities outside the home.

SELECTED HEALTH PROBLEMS: DEVELOPMENTAL OR NEUROLOGICAL DISABILITIES

☐ Mental Retardation (MR)

General Information

1. Definition: below-average intellectual functioning that becomes apparent during childhood development and is associated with impairment in adaptive behavior; manifestations include impaired learning, inadequate social adjustment, and delayed or lowered potential capacity for achievement; see Table 5-13 for classification levels
2. Causes
   a. *Prenatal:* chromosomal and genetic variations (Down syndrome, PKU, Tay-Sachs), German measles or infection in mother during pregnancy, incompatible blood between mother and child (Rh or ABO), glandular disorders, toxic chemicals, nutritional deficiencies, excessive maternal drug or alcohol use
   b. *Perinatal:* birth injury such as anoxia or intracranial hemorrhage
   c. *Postnatal:* encephalitis, head trauma, glandular disturbances, inadequate developmental stimulation in early childhood, cardiac arrest, poisoning
3. Incidence: 3% of the U.S. population; 1 in 10 American families has an MR member; 70%-80% are in the borderline or mild (EMR) category (see Table 5-13); 20%-30% are moderately, severely, or profoundly retarded (the latter are most often cared for in residential institutions)

Nursing Process

Assessment
1. Developmental lags in motor and adaptive behaviors
2. Persistance of neonatal reflexes
3. Perceptual deficits
4. Level of functioning (see Table 5-13)

Analysis (see p. 464)

Planning, Implementation, and Evaluation (see General Nursing Plans, p. 464)

Table 5-13 Levels of retardation (classification system of American Association of Mental Deficiency)

Level	IQ range	Potential mental age	Rehabilitation potential
Level 0: Borderline	68-83	Close to normal	Usually capable of marriage, being *self-supporting* (probable low socioeconomic living standard).
Level 1: Mild or educable	52-67	8-12 years	Can usually be maintained in community. *Can work but needs supervision in financial affairs;* 4th- or 5th-grade academic possibilities (special classes for educable mentally retarded [EMR]) and vocational skills, but often has difficulty holding a job in a competitive market.
Level 2: Moderate	36-51	3-7 years	1st- to 3rd-grade academic potential (special classes for trainable mentally retarded [TMR]) or *vocational training in sheltered workshop in neighborhood job.*
Level 3: Severe	20-35	Toddler	*Minimal self-help skills* and independent behavior (toilet training, dressing self). School placement in handicapped or TMR program. Some are able to work in a sheltered workshop.
Level 4: Profound	Less than 20	Young infant	May require *total care;* may have CNS damage.

Goal: When hospitalized, the mentally retarded child will adapt to hospitalization, will maintain independence in ADL, will ingest adequate food and fluids.

Implementation
1. Adapt hospital routines to child's as much as possible.
2. Explain all procedures and treatments carefully, at level child can understand.
3. Maintain consistency to promote security within child's environment.
4. Encourage parent and family participation in care.
5. Assist with feeding as necessary; bring special cups and feeding utensils from home.
6. Be sure to follow through on what you tell child (e.g., if you say you will return at a certain time, be sure to do it).
7. Use positive reinforcement.

Evaluation
   Child accepts staff members' explanations and cooperates in care; feeds and dresses self; takes prescribed diet and fluids.

☐ Attention Deficit Disorder (ADD)
General Information
1. Definition: syndrome of behaviorally related problems that include inattention and impulsivity; *DSM-III-R* classification differentiates ADD with and without hyperactivity; previously known as minimal brain dysfunction or hyperkinesis
2. Causes: no definite pathophysiological basis has been determined; possible causes include neurotransmitter imbalances, lead poisoning, allergies, and genetic factors
3. Incidence: 5%-10% of school-age children, boys affected 4-6 times more frequently
4. Medical treatment
   a. Diagnosis: parent and teach report of behavior, objective home and classroom observation, psychological evaluation; results compared with *DMS-III-R* criteria
   b. Treatment
      1. behavioral management
      2. medication: methylphenidate (Ritalin)
         a. dosage: 0.3-1.0 mg/kg/day adjusted according to child's behavior
         b. side effects: anorexia, upper abdominal pain, insomnia, growth suppression, tachycardia
         c. nursing implications
            ◆ administer with or after meals to minimize appetite suppression
            ◆ do not administer after 4 PM to minimize insomnia

Nursing Process
Assessment
1. Distractability
2. Impulsiveness
3. Emotional lability
4. Low frustration tolerance
5. High incidence of learning disabilities
6. Hyperactivity (may or may not be present)
Analysis (see p. 464)
Planning, Implementation, and Evaluation

Goal: Child and parent will be prepared for home management.

Implementation
1. Help parents to
   a. Provide a very structured environment with regular routines.
   b. Establish clear, simple rules and firm limits.
   c. Prevent overstimulation and fatigue in the child.
   d. Provide daily rest or quiet times.
   e. Reward any partially successful efforts at self-control.
2. Teach parents and child administration, action, and side effects of medication.
3. Reinforce importance of regular, routine administration of medications.
4. Refer for family or individual counseling as necessary.
5. Encourage parents to work closely with school personnel to minimize impact of ADD on learning.

Evaluation
   Child continues to learn and progress in school; parents are satisfied with child's behavior pattern.

☐ Down Syndrome (Trisomy 21)
General Information
1. Definition: extra chromosome 21 (trisomy 21), resulting from a failure of the chromosome to split during gametogenesis; mental capacity varies from level 1 (educable) to level 3 (severely retarded); one of the most common causes of mental retardation
2. Cause: associated with increased maternal or paternal age
3. Incidence: 1 in 600-650 live births
4. Medical treatment: diagnosis is usually based on clinical manifestations; chromosome studies may be done

Nursing Process
Assessment
1. Physical manifestations
   a. Small, round head; flat nose; protruding tongue; high, arched palate
   b. Slanted eyelids, Brushfield's spots (speckles in iris)

c. Muscle hypotonia, hyperflexible joints

d. Simian crease, short fingers, clinodactyly

e. Congenital heart malformations in 40% of cases

f. Weak respiratory accessory muscles

g. Increased incidence of leukemia and GI anomalies

2. Mastery of development tasks
3. Intellectual functioning
4. Child's routine ADL

Analysis (see p. 464)

Planning, Implementation, and Evaluation

Goal 1: Child will be free from respiratory infection.

Implementation

1. Teach parents (and child as appropriate) preventive health measures.
   a. Prevent exposure to individuals with URIs.
   b. Encourage optimal nutrition, adequate rest.
   c. Keep immunizations up-to-date.
2. Obtain medical care at onset of infection (may need antibiotics).

Evaluation

Child has no more than 2 URIs each year.

Goal 2: Child will ingest adequate food and fluids and will experience minimal feeding difficulties.

Implementation

1. Teach parents appropriate feeding techniques.
   a. Use bulb syringe to clear nasal passages before feeding.
   b. Use a long-handled infant spoon (rubber-coated) to place food to side and back of mouth.
2. Reassure parents that infant's tongue thrust does not mean dislike of food.
3. When hospitalized or in school, encourage foods from home if child not ingesting adequate amounts.
4. Adjust caloric requirements based on child's size and activity level to prevent child from becoming overweight.
5. Provide high roughage and liberal fluids to prevent constipation.

Evaluation

Child's airway remains clear during feeding; child ingests food sufficient for growth; maintains weight within expected limits for height; remains free from constipation.

☐ Cerebral Palsy
General Information

1. Definition: nonprogressive muscular impairment resulting in abnormal muscle tone and uncoordination; spastic type most common (upper motor neuron in-

volvement), dyskinetic (athetoid) type second most common; may be mild to severe

2. Associated defects: mental retardation (may have normal or superior intelligence), seizures, minimal brain dysfunction; speech, hearing, oculomotor impairment
3. Incidence
   a. 25,000 babies with cerebral palsy born annually (5 per 1000 live births)
   b. Most common developmental disability of childhood
   c. Higher incidence in low-birth-weight babies or from birth with other complications, especially during the perinatal period, that result in cerebral anoxia
4. Medical treatment
   a. Braces, ambulation devices (crutches, walker)
   b. Surgical correction of extremity deformities (especially lengthening of heel cord to improve stability and function)
   c. Medications: muscle relaxants, anticonvulsants, tranquilizers

Nursing Process
Assessment

1. Spasticity
   a. Hypertonicity of muscles (continuous reflexive contraction of muscles leading to tightening and shortening)
   b. Persistence of neonatal reflexes
   c. Scissoring
   d. Poor posturing
   e. Delayed gross and fine motor development
   f. Uneven muscle tone
   g. Intellectual functioning may be impaired
2. Dyskinesis (athetosis)
   a. Continuous uncontrollable, wormlike movements of arms, legs, torso, face, and tongue
      1. intensified by stress
      2. absent during sleep
   b. Drooling
   c. Poor speech articulation

Analysis (see p. 464)

Planning, Implementation, and Evaluation

Goal 1: Child will ingest adequate nutrition.

Implementation

1. Provide adequate calories to meet additional energy demands of constant muscle activity (athetoid).
2. Feed slowly; provide calm, peaceful environment.
3. Modify feeding technique to deal with extrusion reflex.
4. Ensure adequate fluid intake.
5. Use special silverware and dishes as needed (e.g., padded spoon, nonskid dishes).

6. Teach importance of daily dental hygiene; routine dental care.

Evaluation

Child exhibits adequate growth; chews and swallows food adequately; is free from dental caries or gum problems.

> **Goal 2:** Child will develop maximum mobility and self-help skills.

Implementation

1. Teach parents appropriate stretching and range-of-motion exercises.
2. Teach use of braces or splints, special support chairs, or wheelchairs as needed.
3. Encourage participation in programs of physical and occupational therapy, speech therapy as needed.
4. Avoid movement that triggers abnormal reflexes.
5. Teach self-help skills, beginning with simplest ones first; teach only one skill at a time until it is learned.
6. Provide needed adaptive devices (special utensils, Velcro fastenings).

Evaluation

Child is free from contractures; demonstrates maximum mobility (with assistance as needed); participates in self-care tasks (e.g., feeds self, dresses self).

> **Goal 3:** Child will be free from skin breakdown.

Implementation

1. Reposition frequently and gently massage pressure points with lotion.

2. Check braces, splints for tightness and pressure; adjust as needed.
3. Use special equipment ("egg-crate" mattress, sheepskin).
4. Keep linens and clothes dry; if wet with urine or stool, change as soon as possible.

Evaluation

Child's skin is intact, free from pressure sores.

☐ Hydrocephalus
General Information

1. Definition: excessive accumulation of cerebrospinal fluid (CSF) within the ventricles of the brain; three common types
   a. Excess secretion of CSF
   b. Obstructive (noncommunicating): results from an obstruction in the ventricular pathway
   c. Communicating: results when the CSF is not absorbed from the subarachnoid space
2. Causes: developmental malformation (congenital), tumors, infections, head injury
3. Medical treatment
   a. Diagnosis: lumbar puncture, CAT scan (refer to *Nursing Care of the Adult*, Diagnostic tests, p. 231)
   b. Surgical insertion of shunt to bypass obstruction or drain excess fluid
      1. atrioventricular (AV) shunt: lateral ventricle to right atrium of heart
      2. ventriculoperitoneal (VP) shunt: lateral ventricle to peritoneal cavity
      3. one-way valves are used in both cases to

Table 5-14   Signs and symptoms of increased intracranial pressure in infants and children*

Causes	Hydrocephalus
	Intracranial tumors
	Cerebral trauma
	Meningitis, encephalitis
Manifestations (infants)	Bulging fontanels; wide suture lines
	High-pitched cry
	Vomiting, feeding difficulty (poor suck)
	Seizures
	Opisthotonos
	Rapid increase in head circumference (especially occipitofrontal diameter)
(older children)	Headache
	Nausea, vomiting
	Change in level of consciousness
	Papilledema
	Diplopia
	Motor dysfunction (grasp, gait)
	Behavior changes, irritability
	Change in vital signs (elevated systolic BP, wide pulse pressure, decreased pulse and respirations)
	Seizures

*Review *Nursing Care of the Adult*, p. 235, for content on head injury.

prevent backflow of blood or peritoneal secretions

c. Extraventricular drainage system
d. Rehospitalization is common for blocked or infected shunt, or for lengthening of shunt as child grows

Nursing Process

Assessment
1. For signs and symptoms of increased intracranial pressure to prevent or minimize brain damage (see Table 5-14)
2. Shiny scalp with dilated veins (congenital hydrocephalus)
3. Sunset eyes (congenital hydrocephalus)

Analysis (see p. 464)

Planning, Implementation, and Evaluation

> **Goal 1:** Child will maintain adequate nutrition and hydration.

Implementation
1. Offer small, frequent feedings; do not overfeed.
2. Burp often.
3. After feeding, position on side with head elevated.
4. Provide rest period after feedings.
5. Assess for dehydration.

Evaluation
Child demonstrates adequate growth; has elastic skin turgor, moist mucous membranes.

> **Goal 2:** Postoperatively, child will be free from complications.

Implementation
1. Measure head circumference daily.
2. Position on unoperative side relative to appearance of fontanel: if fontanel normal, elevate head; if fontanel depressed, position child flat in bed.
3. Observe for signs of redness, skin breakdown on scalp; use sheepskin or water mattress.
4. Turn at least q2h.
5. Do frequent neurological checks (LOC, PERRLA).
6. Observe for signs of infection.
7. *Pump shunt only with a physician's order*, to maintain patency (usually done when shunt valve is a bubble type).

Evaluation
Child's fontanels remain flat (no bulging or depression) with no further increase in head circumference; has no signs of infection or pneumonia (e.g., elevated temperature, increased pulse rate, reddened area around operative site); suffers no brain damage.

☐ Spina Bifida
General Information
1. Definition: congenital defect involving incomplete formation of vertebrae, often accompanied by herniation of parts of the central nervous system
   a. Meningocele: herniation of sac containing spinal fluid and meninges
   b. Meningomyelocele: herniated sac containing CSF, meninges and malformed portion of spinal cord and nerve roots (most serious type); sac may be covered by skin or a very thin, transparent tissue layer that tears easily and permits leakage of CSF
2. Motor and sensory impairment: relative to level and extent of defect; usually involves sensorimotor deficits of lower extremities, bowel and bladder dysfunction, associated orthopedic anomalies, and often hydrocephalus
3. Medical treatment
   a. Prenatal diagnosis: amniocentesis shows increased alpha-fetoprotein; done when mother has a history of having a child with a neural tube defect
   b. Surgical intervention to close defect within 24-48 hours to decrease chance of infection and minimize nerve damage

Nursing Process

Assessment
1. Condition of sac
2. Motor and sensory impairment: flaccid or spastic paralysis, response to painful stimuli, lower-extremity movement
3. Bladder and bowel function; dribbling of urine, leakage of stool
4. Associated orthopedic anomalies: clubfoot, congenital dislocated hip
5. Signs of infection (fever, irritability, lethargy)
6. Signs of increased intracranial pressure (see Table 5-14), increased head circumference (especially following surgery)

Analysis (see p. 464)

Planning, Implementation, and Evaluation

> **Goal 1:** Child will be free from rupture of sac and infection; postoperatively, incision will heal without complications.

Implementation
1. Position on side or prone.
2. Use Bradford frame.
3. Protect sac with sponge doughnut when holding infant.
4. Apply moist, sterile dressings as ordered.
5. Observe for leakage of CSF from sac.
6. Observe for signs of meningitis (e.g., fever, irritability, nuchal rigidity).

7. Meticulously cleanse diaper area to prevent contamination of sac or postoperative wound site with urine or stool; check incision frequently for signs of infection.
8. Postoperatively, observe for signs of hydrocephalus or shunt malfunction; daily head circumference; neurological checks.

Evaluation

Child is free from local or systemic infection (e.g., reddened skin around site, elevated temperature); has intact sac (preoperatively) has optimal wound healing postoperatively.

Goal 2: Child will maintain skin integrity (life-long goal).

Implementation
1. Observe for reddened areas, breaks in skin.
2. Change position frequently.
3. Use sheepskin or water mattress.
4. Massage pressure areas to promote circulation.
5. Teach self-help skills concerning skin care.

Evaluation

Child's skin is intact, free from reddened areas or pressure sores.

Goal 3: Child will experience love and physical contact.

Implementation
1. Talk to infant (use face-to-face position).
2. Touch and stroke child.
3. Encourage parents to caress, stroke, and talk to infant (cannot be held preoperatively or early postoperatively) to promote parent-infant attachment.

Evaluation

Child experiences physical and voice contact from staff and parents and family; parents caress and talk to infant.

Goal 4: Child will gain optimal bowel and bladder function (long-term goal).

Implementation
1. Empty bladder manually by applying gentle downward pressure (Credé method).
2. Provide diet with adequate fluids (those that acidify urine such as apple and cranberry juice) and fiber (as child grows older).
3. Teach parent (and child when older) to care for
   a. Intermittent catheterizations (self-catheterization)
   b. Indwelling Foley catheter
   c. Ileal conduit
4. Administer urinary antiseptics, stool softeners as prescribed.

Evaluation

Child has adequate urinary output and an established bowel routine; is free from urinary tract infection.

Goal 5: Child will develop minimal lower extremity deformity.

Implementation
1. Provide passive ROM exercises.
2. Keep hips abducted using blanket rolls.
3. Provide physical therapy; fitting with braces (usually long leg braces) and crutches for ambulation as child grows older.

Evaluation

Child maintains full ROM of joints; has no contractures of hip or lower extremity.

☐ Seizure Disorders
General Information

1. Definition: episode of uncontrolled electrical activity in the brain; neuronal discharges become excessive and irregular, resulting in loss of consciousness, convulsive body movements, or disturbances in sensations or behavior
2. Incidence: occur in 0.5% of all children; it has been estimated that 4%-6% of all children will experience one or more seizures by the time they reach adolescence
3. Cause: possible causes include infection, tumors, trauma, acid-base imbalances, epilepsy, allergies, anoxia, and hypoglycemia
4. *Epilepsy:* chronic brain dysfunction manifested by recurrent seizures; unknown etiology; higher incidence in children; may see *status epilepticus:* recurrent seizures occurring at such frequency that full consciousness is not regained between seizures.
5. Types of seizures and manifestation
   a. Generalized seizures
      1. *grand mal:* sudden loss of consciousness followed by tonic phase (stiffening of body) and clonic phase (jerky movements of trunk and extremities); periods of depressed or apneic breathing may occur; child may fall asleep after the seizure or be confused and irritable
      2. *petit mal* (absence seizures); child appears to be daydreaming; all verbal and motor behavior stops; may occur 10 or more times a day; usually lasts 10-30 seconds; child usually alert after the seizures; no memory episode
      3. *akinetic:* child experiences a sudden loss of body tone accompanied by loss of consciousness; lasts a few seconds; resumes ADL afterwards
      4. *infantile spasms:* similar to a startle reflex; involves jerking of the head and clonic move-

ments of the extremities; usually disappear by 2-3 years of age; may develop into more generalized seizures; usually accompanied by other problems (e.g., mental retardation)
b. Partial seizures
1. *Jacksonian:* twitching begins at distal end of extremity, eventually involving entire extremity and possibly entire side of body; no loss of consciousness; not commonly seen in children
2. *psychomotor:* characterized by altered state of consciousness (e.g., dreamlike); may chew, smack lips, mumble; lasts several minutes; child has no memory of behavior
c. Febrile seizures: transient disorder usually the result of an extracranial infection (e.g., otitis media); peak incidence between 6 months and 3 years of age; resemble grand mal seizures
d. Breath holding: usually benign; child begins to cry, holds breath, and experiences brief cyanosis with loss of consciousness; precipitating factors may be anger or frustration
6. Diagnosis: complete and accurate history and physical; thorough description of the seizure including onset, time of day, type of seizure, precipitating factors; EEG necessary for evaluating the seizure disorder
7. Medical treatment: anticonvulsants to elevate the child's excitability threshold and prevent seizures (refer to Table 5-15)

Table 5-15 Medications used to treat seizure disorders

Drug	Route	Side effects	Nursing implications
Carbamazepine (Tegretol)	PO	Drowsiness Ataxia Vertigo Anorexia Aplastic anemia	Periodic CBC and liver enzymes. Avoid excessive sunlight because of photophobia. Administer with food.
Clonazepam (Klonopin)	PO	Nausea and vomiting Rash Nystagmus Drowsiness Anemia	Monitor behavioral changes. Frequent respiratory assessment because bronchial secretions are increased.
Diazepam (Valium)	IV push over 1-2 min; may repeat q15min × 2	Drowsiness Dry mouth Constipation Anorexia	Used for status epilepticus. Only inject 5 mg/min. Monitor BP (hypotension) and respirations (respiratory depression). Do not dilute with IV solutions.
Ethosuximide (Zarontin)	PO	Drowsiness Ataxia Blurred vision Anorexia GI upset	Monitor liver and kidney function. Administer with food.
Phenobarbital	PO	Nausea and vomiting Drowsiness Rash Irritability Mild ataxia	Monitor BP and respiration during IV administration. Paradoxical reaction in children. Taper medication when discontinuing.
Phenytoin (Dilantin)	PO, IV	Gingival hypertrophy Dermatitis Ataxia Drowsiness Nystagmus Bone marrow suppression	Meticulous oral hygiene. Administer with food to reduce GI upset. Monitor liver enzymes.
Primidone (Mysoline)	PO	Nausea and vomiting Drowsiness Ataxia Headache Gum pain	Observe for folic acid deficiency. Taper medicine when discontinuing. Hemorrhage in newborns whose mothers are taking this medication.
Valproic acid (Depakene)	PO	GI upset Nausea and vomiting Drowsiness Leukopenia; thrombocytopenia	Administer with meals. Potentiates phenytoin/phenobarbital. Monitor liver enzymes. Periodic CBC, bleeding time.

Nursing Process

Assessment

1. History of seizure activity, recent episodes, management
   a. Preseizure behavior: aura, loss of consciousness
   b. Seizure activity: tonic/clonic phase; inappropriate behavior; fecal or urinary incontinence during the seizure
   c. Postseizure behavior: memory lapse, headache, instability, loss of consciousness, lethargy
2. Use of anticonvulsant medications, side effects

Analysis (see p. 464)

Planning, Implementation, and Evaluation

> **Goal 1:** Child will maintain adequate respiratory function and be free from injuries during a seizure (primary concern with status epilepticus).

Implementation

1. Gently lower the standing or sitting child to the floor (supine position).
2. Maintain a patent airway by hyperextending the neck and pulling the jaw slightly forward; turn the head to the side to facilitate drainage of mucus and saliva.
3. Have O_2 and suction available (if possible).
4. *Do not place anything in the child's mouth;* in the past it was believed that a padded tongue blade prevented the child from "swallowing" or biting tongue; simply turning the child's head to the side accomplishes the same effect and diminishes trauma.
5. Do not restrain child.
6. Remove any toys or dangerous objects that might injure the child during a seizure; pad side rails of bed if possible.
7. Loosen tight or restrictive clothing.
8. Observe the seizure carefully.
   a. Preseizure activity; aura, incontinence
   b. Seizure activity; include onset and initial focus of seizure, duration, change in respirations, progression of movement through body, and changes in neurological status
   c. Postseizure activity: duration, status, and behavior
9. Administer anticonvulsant medication as ordered.
10. Monitor blood gases.

Evaluation

Child has normal respiratory rate and pink color; is free from injuries; experiences cessation of seizure activity.

> **Goal 2:** Child and family will learn how to cope with the long-term problems associated with seizure disorders.

Implementation

1. Encourage good health practices including adequate sleep, good nutritional habits, and exercise.
2. Provide appropriate explanations concerning cause of seizure activity, actions of medications, importance of periodic reevaluation.
3. Teach the importance of adhering to medication routine, common side effects, importance of periodic blood and urine studies, behavior changes that may occur as a result of anticonvulsant medication.
4. Stress the importance of never discontinuing anticonvulsant medication abruptly.
5. Instruct family concerning care of child during a seizure.
6. Encourage child and family to discuss fears, anxieties concerning seizure disorder.
7. Inform child and family about situations that might precipitate seizure.
   a. Illness, fever, stress
   b. Occur more frequently during menses or as a result of alcohol ingestion
8. Ensure child wears a Medic Alert bracelet.
9. Provide information concerning vocational guidance and federal and state laws regarding limitations that might be imposed on the younger child or adolescent.
10. Provide information concerning support groups in the community.

Evaluation

Child functions independently regarding ADL; adheres to medical regimen; child and family discuss fears and anxieties concerning seizure disorder; become involved in support groups.

☐ Meningitis
General Information

1. Definition: a syndrome caused by inflammation of the meninges of the brain and spinal cord; two basic types
   a. *Bacterial: H. influenzae, Streptococcus pneumoniae,* or *Neisseria meningitidis* (meningococcus)
   b. *Aseptic:* viruses, parasites, fungi
2. Cause: may be preceded by otitis media, tonsillitis, or other URI
3. Incidence: occurs more often in boys; peak incidence is late infancy and toddlerhood; haemophilus influenza b conjugate vaccine (HbCV) will protect child from meningitis caused by *H. influenzae*
4. Characteristics
   a. Generally determined by age of child
      1. newborn presents with nonspecific symptoms such as poor sucking and feeding, apnea, weak cry, diarrhea, jaundice; tense anterior fontanel does not occur until late
      2. infant may present with fever, poor feeding,

nausea and vomiting, increased irritability, high-pitched cry, and seizures

3. child or adolescent shows classic signs of fever, headache, nuchal rigidity, seizures, altered sensorium, projectile vomiting

b. Petechial or purpural rash resulting from extravasation of RBCs usually seen in meningococcal meningitis

c. Long-term complications include bindness, deafness, mental retardation, hydrocephalus, cerebral palsy, and seizures

5. Medical treatment

a. Diagnosis: lumbar puncture to examine CSF; usual findings
1. elevated WBC
2. decreased glucose
3. elevated protein
4. positive results from culture

b. Medications
1. antibiotics (large doses given IV)
2. anticonvulsants
3. antipyretics

Nursing Process

Assessment

1. Neurological status (may see increased ICP [Table 5-14] secondary to cerebral edema resulting from inappropriate ADH secretion)

a. Neurological check (LOC, PERRLA, motor activity, vital signs)

b. Brudzinski's sign (pain on flexion of neck)

c. Kernig's sign (pain on knee extension while lifting knee from a supine position)

d. Opisthotonos

2. Meningeal irritation (e.g., high-pitched cry, nuchal rigidity, irritability)

3. Seizure activity (see p. 470)

4. Hydration (e.g., output, specific gravity, signs and symptoms of dehydration)

Analysis (see p. 464)

Planning, Implementation, and Evaluation

> **Goal 1:** Others will be free from infecting organism; disease will not spread.

Implementation

1. Place in strict isolation (for at least 24 hours after initiation of antibiotic therapy).

2. Teach parents and others isolation procedures.

3. Assist with lumbar puncture to determine causative organism.

4. Administer antibiotics as prescribed, observe side effects.

Evaluation

Disease does not spread to others; family adheres to isolation procedures.

> **Goal 2:** Child will remain free from neurological complications and long-term sequelae.

Implementation

1. Implement seizure and safety precautions (e.g., bed's side rails up [padded], oxygen and suction available).

2. Perform frequent neurological checks with vital signs.

3. Minimize environmental stimuli (lights, noise) and movement to lessen possibility of seizures.

4. Elevate head of bed slightly (to decrease intracranial pressure).

5. Administer anticonvulsants as ordered.

6. Monitor fluid intake to prevent dilutional hyponatremia (resulting from inappropriate ADH secretion).

7. Monitor for long-term sequelae: seizures, hydrocephalus, mental retardation, ataxia, hemiparesis, deafness.

8. Provide parental support and reassurance concerning recovery.

Evaluation

Child shows no signs of complications (e.g., seizure activity); resumes normal activities.

> **Goal 3:** Child will maintain adequate hydration and nutrition.

Implementation

1. Maintain NPO during acute phase of illness.

2. Administer IV fluids as ordered; restrain as needed to maintain infusion site.

3. Carefully monitor I&O to prevent fluid overload (can increase intracranial pressure), specific gravity, weight.

4. Advance diet as tolerated as child recovers.

Evaluation

Child is adequately hydrated; is free from signs of fluid overload; maintains weight.

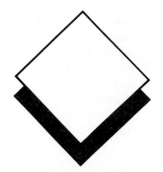

Oxygenation

GENERAL CONCEPTS
Overview/Physiology

1. Respiratory system (developmental differences)
   a. Chest configuration (AP diameter) changes from round to more flattened as child grows
   b. Steady increase in number and surface area of alveoli from birth to age 12; infants and young children have less alveolar surface for gas exchange
   c. Cricoid cartilage is at the level of the fourth cervical vertebra in infants and the fifth cervical vertebra in children (important when positioning children for resuscitation, intubation, or tracheostomy)
   d. Susceptible to respiratory obstruction and atelectasis because of narrow tracheal and bronchiolar pathways
   e. Susceptible to infections because of immature immune system and frequent contacts with infectious organisms
   f. In infancy, nasal passages are narrow and infants are obligatory nose breathers (important to remember when feeding infants—mucus accumulation and mucosal swelling may interfere with feeding)
   g. Diaphragmatic-abdominal breathing is normal at birth to age 5 years.
2. Cardiovascular system (developmental differences)
   a. Changes during transition from fetal to postnatal circulation
      1. lungs inflate, resulting in increased pressure in left side of heart
      2. foramen ovale closes
      3. ductus arteriosus closes
      4. obliteration of ductus venosus and umbilical vessels
   b. Blood pressure gradually increases, and pulse and respiratory rates gradually decrease as child grows
3. Hematological system (developmental differences)
   a. All components necessary for normal hematological functioning are present at birth except vitamin K, which is administered intramuscularly to the newborn (refer to *Nursing Care of the Childbearing Family,* p. 381); see Table 5-16 for normal values
   b. *All* bones are engaged in blood cell production until growth ceases in late adolescence

Application of the Nursing Process to the Child with Respiratory Problems

Assessment

1. Nursing history
   a. Any known breathing problems, respiratory allergies, activity intolerance (does child have problems keeping up with other children during play?), incidence of respiratory illnesses, medications, home management
   b. Environmental factors: dust, pollen, pets in home, or school environments; do parents or child smoke?
2. Clinical appraisal
   a. General appearance: color (pallor, cyanosis), respiratory effort (dyspnea, stridor, grunting, prolonged expirations), restlessness, irritability, fa-

Table 5-16 Hematology values in children

Hematocrit	35%-47%
Hemoglobin	10.5-16 g/dl
Red blood cell count (RBC)	3.9-5.1 million/mm³
White blood cell count (WBC)	5500-13,500/mm³ (between 2-13 years)
	5000-20,000/mm³ (under age 2)
Platelets	150,000-400,000/mm³
Arterial blood gases	
Po₂	83-108 mm Hg (65-80 mm Hg newborn)
Pco₂	35-45 mm Hg (27-40 mm Hg newborn)
pH	7.35-7.45 (7.27-7.47 newborn)

tigue, prostration, clubbing of fingers and toes
  b. Respiratory rate, depth, and character; presence of respiratory signs (cough: character, productive or nonproductive; rhinitis; retractions; nasal flaring)
  c. Fever
  d. Breath sounds: upper respiratory tract, all lobes of lungs; presence of wheezing, rales, or rhonchi
3. Diagnostic tests (refer to *Nursing Care of the Adult*, p. 125)

Analysis
1. Safe, effective care environment
  a. Knowledge deficit
  b. High risk for infection
2. Physiological integrity
  a. Ineffective breathing pattern
  b. Impaired gas exchange
  c. Ineffective airway clearance
3. Psychosocial integrity
  a. Anxiety
  b. Social isolation
4. Health promotion/maintenance
  a. Diversional activity deficit
  b. Altered growth and development

General Nursing Planning, Implementation, and Evaluation

Goal 1: Child will maintain adequate oxygenation and a patent airway.

Implementation
1. Monitor respiratory status.
  a. Vital signs (respirations, pulse, and temperature)
  b. Skin and nail-bed color, capillary refill, dyspnea, cough, nasal flaring, and retractions
  c. Adventitious lung sounds
  d. Use of sternal and thoracic muscles
  e. Behavioral changes (restlessness, irritability, or disruptions in patterns)
2. Be alert for signs of airway obstruction.
  a. Rapidly rising heart rate and increased respiratory rate; diaphoresis
  b. Restlessness, anxiety, or agitation (indicate hypoxia)
  c. Increased stridor, retractions
  d. Pallor or cyanosis
3. Position to ease respiratory effort (semi- to high-Fowler's); loosen clothing to allow maximum chest expansion.
4. Avoid sedatives that depress respirations and cough reflex (e.g., narcotics).
5. Keep endotracheal tubes, laryngoscope, and tracheostomy tray at bedside for emergency use.
6. Never leave child unattended if in respiratory distress (changes in condition can occur very rapidly).
7. Initiate CPR when necessary.

Infant (age 1 and younger)
  a. Position on back on a flat, firm surface (move child as a single unit).
  b. Clear airway of foreign matter and mucus.
  c. Open airway by placing head in a neutral position, lift chin (avoid overextension).
  d. Look, listen, and feel for breaths.
  e. Give 2 breaths of 1-1½ seconds each, mouth to mouth and nose.
  f. Check *brachial* pulse to assess circulation.
  g. Perform chest compressions if necessary.
     1. location: 1 finger-breadth below nipple line on sternum
     2. compress with 2 fingers ½-1 inch at a rate of 100 compressions a minute
     3. give 5 compressions to 1 breath
  h. Reassess after 10 cycles and every few minutes thereafter.

Child (age 1-8)
  i. Position on back on a flat, firm surface (move child as a single unit).
  j. Clear airway of foreign matter and mucus.
  k. Open airway and head tilt–chin lift maneuver (avoid overextension).
  l. Look, listen, and feel for breaths.
  m. Give two breaths of 1-1½ seconds each, mouth to mouth.
  n. Check *carotid* pulse to assess circulation.
  o. Perform chest compressions if necessary.
     1. location: 1 finger-breadth above costal-sternal notch in sternum
     2. compress lower sternum with heel of one hand 1-1½ inches at a rate of 80-100 compressions each minute
     3. give 5 compressions to 1 breath
  p. Reassess after 10 cycles and every few minutes thereafter.
8. Provide care for child with an endotracheal (ET) tube or tracheostomy.
  a. Perform ET tube/tracheostomy care and suctioning.
  b. Restrain child as needed.
  c. Provide reassurance to child and parents.
  d. Change position q2h.
  e. Anticipate needs since child cannot verbalize.
  f. Inform child of inability to speak.
  g. Devise alternate means of communication; reassure that voice will return when able to breathe normally again.

Evaluation
  Child maintains a patent airway; exhibits signs of adequate oxygenation (normal skin color, quiet breathing, alert and oriented, clear lung sounds).

Goal 2: Child will be free from respiratory distress.

Implementation

1. Provide care for child in mist tent with cool mist and O$_2$ as ordered (periodically analyze O$_2$ level).
   a. Plan care to minimize opening of tent.
   b. Tuck sides of tent tightly to prevent loss of O$_2$ and mist.
   c. Maintain ice chamber or cooling mechanism.
   d. Monitor tent-chamber temperature.
   e. Keep child as warm and dry as possible to prevent chilling (change clothing and bed linens frequently).
   f. Provide diversion and comfort measures to minimize child's fear and anxiety.
      1. reassure that child won't be left alone; encourage parent to stay with child
      2. provide favorite toy or object (no furry or mechanical toys)
2. Assist with chest percussion, vibration, and postural drainage as needed; position child so gravity facilitates drainage from specific lobes.

Evaluation

Child cooperates with mist tent therapy; is free from respiratory distress.

Goal 3: Child will be adequately hydrated.

Implementation

1. Provide humidified atmosphere to help loosen secretions.
2. Ensure adequate fluid intake.
   a. Withhold oral fluids until respiratory distress subsides.
   b. Monitor IV fluids to prevent dehydration or fluid overload.

Evaluation

Child has elastic skin turgor, normal urine output, adequate fluid intake; is free from signs of dehydration or fluid overload.

Goal 4: Child will conserve energy and remain physically comfortable.

Implementation

1. Administer sedatives (e.g., phenobarbital) as ordered (no narcotic sedatives, no cough suppressants).
2. Administer antipyretics, tepid sponge bath for fever.
3. Schedule treatments and nursing activities to allow uninterrupted periods for maximum rest and sleep.
4. Monitor child's response to care (feeding, chest physical therapy) to prevent tiring.
5. Provide quiet age-appropriate play activities.

Evaluation

Child conserves energy; cooperates with care and treatments; approximates normal rest and sleep patterns; engages in quiet play activities.

SELECTED HEALTH PROBLEMS RESULTING IN AN INTERFERENCE WITH RESPIRATION

☐ Sudden Infant Death Syndrome (SIDS), or "Crib Death"

General Information

1. Definition: sudden, unexpected death of an infant or young child, in which an adequate cause cannot be determined
2. Incidence: higher incidence in boys, infants with low birth weight, multiple births, lower socioeconomic status
3. Etiology: unknown; evidence supports theory of relationship between periodic apnea and chronic hypoxemia
4. Peak occurrence: winter or early spring; between ages 2 and 4 months

Nursing Process

Assessment

1. Parents' knowledge of SIDS
2. Availability of support systems (e.g., family, friends, SIDS organization, or mental health center)
3. Apnea monitoring of high-risk infants (premature infants, subsequent siblings) or "near-miss" infants
   a. Parents' knowledge of and adjustment to home apnea monitoring
   b. Infant's apnea patterns

Analysis (see p. 475)

Planning, Implementation and Evaluation

Goal 1: Parents will receive information and support to help them adjust to loss.

Implementation

1. Explain that they are not responsible for infant's death (parents feel guilty).
2. Provide information about SIDS.
3. Allow expression of feelings; provide support as parents cope with loss, grief, and mourning.
4. Refer to local SIDS organization or support group: Foundation for Sudden Infant Death.
5. Refer to other community supports (e.g., church or community mental health centers).

Evaluation

Parents ventilate feelings about loss of infant; have a referral for counseling.

Goal 2: Parents will maintain and cope with home apnea monitoring.

Implementation

1. Teach parents mechanics of home monitoring equipment.
2. Teach parents infant CPR.
3. Provide emotional support to parents.

4. Help parents identify and use resources for relief (e.g., qualified sitters).

Evaluation

Parents demonstrate ability to implement home monitoring, demonstrate correct infant CPR, adjust to home apnea monitoring.

☐ **Acute Spasmodic Laryngitis (Spasmodic Croup)**
☐ **Acute Epiglottitis**
☐ **Acute Laryngotracheobronchitis (LTB)**
☐ **Bronchiolitis** (refer to Table 5-17)
☐ **Bronchopulmonary Dysplasia**

General Information

1. Definition: an iatrogenic, chronic, obstructive pulmonary disease characterized by thickening of the alveolar walls and bronchiolar epithelium; most surviving infants recover by 1 year of age
2. Occurrence: primarily in low-birth-weight infants with insufficient levels of surfactant who have been mechanically ventilated with high concentrations of oxygen for prolonged periods of time
3. Medical treatment
   a. Oxygen and mechanical ventilation at lowest possible levels
   b. Medications: bronchodilators, diuretics (when

Table 5-17 Acute upper respiratory tract infections

	Acute spasmodic laryngitis (spasmodic croup)	Acute epiglottitis	Acute laryngotracheobronchitis (LTB)	Bronchiolitis
Definition	Acute spasm of larynx, resulting in partial upper airway obstruction	Severe inflammation of the epiglottis that progresses rapidly	Inflammation of larynx, to a lesser extent of trachea and bronchii, resulting in spasm and partial airway obstruction	Inflammation of the bronchioles with accumulation of mucus and exudate, resulting in lung hyperinflation, dyspnea, and cyanosis Lower airway disease
Peak age of occurrence	1- to 3-year-olds	3- to 8-year-olds	Infants and toddlers (most common form of croup)	2- to 12-month-olds (third leading cause of death in this age group)
Cause	Viral	Bacterial (usually H influenza, type B)	Usually viral, but may be bacterial	Viral (especially RSV*)
Assessment	Awakens with barklike, metallic cough Hoarseness Inspiratory stridor Usually occurs at night No fever May be preceded by URI Attack may recur for several nights	Sore throat Inflamed, cherry-red epiglottis Dysphagia, drooling Muffled voice Tripod posturing Suprasternal and substernal retractions High fever Restlessness Sudden onset, rapid progression	Preceded by URI Harsh, brassy cough Inspiratory stridor Substernal and suprasternal retractions, rales, and rhonchi Labored, prolonged expirations Low-grade fever	Paroxysmal cough Flaring nares Intercostal and subcostal retractions Rales with prolonged expirations, wheezing, grunting Diminished breath sounds, areas of consolidation Irritability, fatigue

Specific medications and treatment, additional nursing plan/ implementation (see also General Nursing Plans, p. 475)	Usually treated at home
	Teach emergency home care
	   steam inhalation
	   subemetic dose of ipecac
	   cool-mist humidifier
	Ensure adequate fluid intake (clear liquids)
	Prepare parents for possible recurrence for several nights
		Emergency hospitalization: intubation or tracheostomy
		IV antibiotics (ampicillin, chloramphenicol)
		Antipyretics
		Do not try to view child's throat (may precipitate laryngospasm and death)
		Be alert for signs of airway obstruction
			Hospitalization (intubation if needed)
			Racemic epinephrine in severe cases
			IV fluids until respiratory distress subsides
				Home care; hospitalization in severe cases
				Epinephrine or aminophylline in severe cases
				Percussion, vibration, and postural drainage
				If RSV, practice good handwashing

*Respiratory syncytial virus.

complicated by congestive heart failure), antibiotics for respiratory infection

Nursing Process

Assessment (refer also to "General Nursing Goal 2," p. 475)
1. Tachypnea
2. Cyanosis with feeding or crying
3. Signs of pulmonary hypertension and right-sided heart failure (e.g., fluid retention, rales, wheezing, and retractions)

Analysis (see p. 475)

Planning, Implementation, and Evaluation (see General Nursing Plans, p. 475)

☐ Bronchial Asthma (Reactive Airway Disease)
General Information

1. Definition: an obstructive, reversible condition of the trachea and bronchial tissues; a complex health problem that involves biochemical, immunological, endocrine, and psychological factors leading to

a. Edema of mucous membranes
b. Congestion of airways with tenacious mucus
c. Spasm of smooth muscle of bronchi and bronchioles causing narrowed airway and trapping of air in alveoli
2. Cause: believed to be an allergic hypersensitivity to foreign substances such as plant pollens, mold, dust, smoke, animal hair, or foods; other contributing factors are changes in environmental temperatures (especially cold air), emotional distress, fatigue, physical exertion, and infections
3. Medical treatment: acute asthma is a medical emergency
a. Drug therapy is directed toward relieving bronchial spasm, obstruction, and edema (see Table 5-18)
   1. bronchodilators
   2. corticosteroids
   3. no sedatives or cough suppressants
b. Supportive measures
   1. cool, humidified environment
   2. IV fluids to ensure adequate hydration

Table 5-18 Medications used to treat bronchial asthma*

Drug	Administration	Nursing responsibilities
BRONCHODILATORS		
Beta-adrenergic agents		
Epinephrine (Adrenalin)	Subcutaneously in 1:1000 aqueous solution Dose: 0.01 mg/kg	Short-acting smooth-muscle relaxant for acute attacks; doses may be repeated in 20 minutes for 3-4 doses. Discard if solution is discolored. Use tuberculin syringe for accuracy.
Albuterol (Proventil)	Oral and inhalation	Oral route recommended in young children. Lacks potency for acute attacks.
Methylxanthines		
Theophylline (Theo-Dur) Aminophylline	IV during acute attacks PO as maintenance regimen	Use IV pump to regulate. Monitor vital signs; observe for severe hypertension. Wide variation in rate of metabolism, but metabolized rapidly in children. Monitor blood levels. Therapeutic range between 10-20 μg/ml; toxicity >20μg/ml. Toxicity symptoms: irritability, restlessness, tachycardia, vomiting.
CORTICOSTEROIDS		
Hydrocortisone (Solu-Cortef) Prednisone Dexamethasone (Decadron)	IV Oral (shorter acting) Oral (longer acting)	Intravenous form used for status asthmaticus. Antiinflammatory, reduces allergic response, enhances smooth-muscle dilatation.
PROPHYLACTIC AGENT		
Cromolyn sodium (Aarane)	Inhalation	Prevents release of histamine. Used to prevent attacks.

*Refer to *Nursing Care of the Adult,* Tables 3-18 and 3-19 for additional drug information.

c. Status asthmaticus: continued severe respiratory distress in spite of medical intervention; child is in imminent danger of respiratory arrest and requires immediate hospitalization (to treat dehydration and acidosis and improve ventilation)
  1. NPO or sips of clear liquids
  2. IV fluids for hydration and medication administration
  3. sodium bicarbonate (IV) to correct acidosis
  4. humidified O_2
  5. mechanical ventilation in severe cases
  6. corticosteroids (hydrocortisone or methylprednisolone IV)
  7. aminophylline
  8. isoproterenol via intermittent positive pressure breathing

d. Long-term therapy includes removing the offending allergens, desensitization to allergens, normalization of respiratory function, and development of a personalized and effective therapeutic regimen

Nursing Process

Assessment
1. Prolonged expiratory wheezing
2. Hacking, paroxysmal, nonproductive coughing; cough then becomes rattling with thick, clear mucus
3. Deep-red lips; may progress to cyanosis
4. Anxious expression, restlessness
5. Child sits in upright position
6. Intercostal and suprasternal retractions (infants)
7. Coarse breath sounds
8. Shallow irregular respirations with sudden increase in rate and ineffective coughing may signal impending asphyxia (status asthmaticus)
9. Barrel chest and hunched shoulders (chronic asthma)

Analysis (see p. 475)

Planning, Implementation, and Evaluation

> **Goal 1:** Child will resume normal breathing pattern, will maintain a patent airway, and will liquefy and raise secretions.

Implementation
1. Monitor frequency, amount, and appearance of expectorated mucus.
2. Position in high-Fowler's or in a chair; administer O_2 to relieve cyanosis and anoxia (cyanosis appears in children with a Po_2 less than 55-65 mm Hg).
3. Teach child to use diaphragm rather than just lungs, to pull in and expel deep breaths of air when first feeling a tightening sensation in chest.
4. Administer prescribed medications, including nebulizers; know the action, dose ranges, side effects, and contraindications for all medications administered.

Evaluation
Child resumes normal breathing pattern (no wheezing, rales, or cyanosis), maintains patent airway, liquefies and raises excretions.

> **Goal 2:** Child will control anxiety during acute attacks.

Implementation
1. *Never* leave child alone during an acute attack; if parental anxiety is too high, it is better for child if someone who is calm and supportive stays with child; work with parent until parent can be a calming influence.
2. Hold child in an upright position and rock (as effective as bed rest if a relaxed, confident approach is used).
3. Reduce the level of nonproductive stimuli by keeping room quiet, with dimmed lighting; use touch, soft music, and controlled noise levels to induce relaxation and rest.
4. Teach child and parents panic control (i.e., teach to imagine how to stay calm [what works best] in stressful situations).

Evaluation
Child remains calm and copes with asthma attack.

> **Goal 3:** Child will avoid and/or eliminate allergens or precipitating factors in environment.

Implementation
1. Identify possible precipitating factors with child and family; teach child and parents to avoid stressful experiences, extremes of temperature, unnecessary fatigue, and exposure to infections.
2. Modify environment as indicated (no furry pets, damp dusting, nonallergic pillows and bedding, elimination of allergenic foods with diet, air filters).
3. Assist with immune therapy (hyposensitization for allergens such as dust, molds, and pollens).
4. Administer prophylactic antibiotics during periods of high susceptibility (e.g., winter, pollen or flu season).
5. Guide parents in planning a total program that promotes rest, moderate exercise, appropriate activities (swimming, baseball, skiing), balanced nutrition, controlled levels of emotional stress.
6. Remind and urge child and parents to see physician regularly and at the first indication of a respiratory infection or attack.
7. Refer family to psychological/mental health services when indicated.

Evaluation
Child and parents describe the importance of good nutrition and rest in preventing respiratory infections; identify situations or agents that precipitate an asthmatic

attack and conscientiously try to modify or avoid these; recognize signs of an impending attack (cough, wheezing, fever, nausea and vomiting, increased anxiety or tension) and the steps to take to minimize distress (position, rest, medications, fluids).

Application of the Nursing Process to the Child with Cardiovascular Dysfunction

Assessment

1. Nursing history
   a. Delayed growth patterns
   b. Frequent respiratory infections
   c. Activity intolerance, weakness, fatigue
   d. Anorexia, weight loss, fatigue during feedings
   e. Chest pain, dyspnea, pallor or cyanosis, clubbing of fingers and toes
   f. Medications: parental knowledge of side effects
   g. Family and obstetrical history
2. Clinical appraisal
   a. General appearance: pallor, cyanosis, clubbing of fingers and toes, cold extremities, mottling, edema, distended neck veins, and poor capillary refill
   b. Vital signs: apical pulse rate and character, presence of murmurs, gallops, friction rubs; blood pressure in upper and lower extremities; rate, depth, and character of respirations; rate, quality, and symmetry of peripheral pulses, especially of lower extremities
3. Diagnostic tests (refer to *Nursing Care of the Adult*, p. 125)
   a. Cardiac catheterization in infants and children: aids in diagnosis of congenital anomalies through direct visualization of chambers as well as abnormalities in oxygen saturation, pressure, and cardiac output; femoral artery or vein may be used for catheter insertion (see Table 5-19)
   b. Blood gas determination (see Table 5-16)
   c. Echocardiogram

Analysis

1. Safe, effective care environment
   a. High risk for infection
   b. Sensory-perceptual alteration
2. Physiological integrity
   a. Activity intolerance
   b. Decreased cardiac output
   c. Impaired gas exchange
3. Psychosocial integrity
   a. Anxiety
   b. Fear
4. Health promotion/maintenance
   a. Diversional activity deficit
   b. Ineffective family coping: compromised

General Nursing Planning, Implementation, and Evaluation

> **Goal 1:** Child will have adequate oxygenation and decreased work load of heart.

Implementation

1. Monitor vital signs frequently.
   a. Apical pulse 1 full minute while sleeping
   b. Peripheral pulses
   c. BP

Table 5-19 Cardiac catheterization in children: nursing considerations

Preprocedural	Postprocedural
Psychological preparation (see *Ill and Hospitalized Child* for developmental considerations)	Maintain bed rest with frequent checks on vital signs until stable.
Explain in simple terms what child will experience and what it will feel like (e.g., skin prep: "cold"; catheter insertion: "pressure"; injection of contrast medium: "warm all over" [do not use the word "dye"]; darkness of room, and sounds of "picture-taking"); do not explain too far in advance of procedure.	Do not take blood pressure in affected extremity.
Allow child to play with and manipulate equipment (e.g., gown and mask, syringes, sandbag).	Monitor skin color and warmth, especially distal to catheter insertion site.
Arrange for child and parent to visit catheterization room the day before to see the equipment and meet staff.	Palpate brachial or pedal pulses distal to catheter insertion for presence, strength, and symmetry.
Physical preparation	Observe operative site for bleeding, edema, and hematoma formation.
NPO 4-6 hr before the procedure (give 5% DW orally as prescribed 2-3 hr before the procedure for infants with cyanotic heart disease and polycythemia); use pacifier for infants.	Maintain sandbag or pressure dressing on operative site as ordered.
Obtain baseline vital signs, including brachial and pedal pulses.	Notify physician of any signs of complications (e.g., poor circulation, unstable vital signs, fever, and bleeding).
Administer preoperative medications as ordered (child is not anesthetized).	Apply direct pressure over site if bleeding occurs.

d. Respiratory status
e. Body temperature
f. Capillary refill

2. Schedule treatments and nursing care to prevent tiring and promote adequate rest and sleep.
3. Maintain bed rest as ordered.
4. Provide age-appropriate diversional activities to prevent boredom and help child maintain bed rest.
5. Avoid restrictive clothing and tight diapers.
6. Minimize crying and emotional distress (preoperatively).
   a. Encourage parent to room-in or visit frequently.
   b. Provide pacifier or favorite attachment object.
   c. Hold and cuddle child.
7. Relieve anoxic spells (cyanotic heart disease).
   a. Place child in knee-chest (squatting) position.
   b. Administer O_2 as ordered.
   c. Administer sedatives and analgesics as ordered.
8. Avoid extremes of environmental temperature.

Evaluation

Child is free from signs of respiratory or cardiac distress (e.g., no dyspnea, tachycardia); cooperates with bed rest, rests comfortably, plays quietly.

Goal 2: Child will be free from infections.

Implementation

1. Protect child from exposure to others with respiratory infections.
2. Immunize child according to recommended schedule (see Table 5-3).
3. Observe for signs of endocarditis (fever, malaise, anorexia) and pneumonitis (dyspnea, tachycardia, fever).
4. Teach child and parents importance of antibiotic prophylaxis (long-term therapy or short-term course for dental work, surgery, childbirth).

Evaluation

Child remains free from upper respiratory infections; is immunized on schedule; child and parents comply with antibiotic prophylaxis.

SELECTED HEALTH PROBLEMS RESULTING IN AN INTERFERENCE WITH CARDIAC FUNCTIONING

☐ Congenital Heart Disease

General Information

1. Hemodynamics: related to three principles
   a. Pressure gradients: blood flows from higher to lower; normally left side of heart is higher pressure
   b. Resistance: the higher the resistance the less the flow; normally the systemic circulation has higher resistance than pulmonary circulation; larger vessels have less resistance than smaller, narrow ones
   c. Quality of pumping action of heart effects the flow
2. Physical consequences of cardiac problems

a. Increased work load of the heart (causes changes in systolic and diastolic pressures)
b. Pulmonary hypertension (from increased pulmonary resistance)
c. Inadequate systemic output from recirculated blood flow
d. Cyanotic defects: no pure oxygenated blood in body, tissue hypoxia and hypoxemia, stimulates erythropoiesis, resulting in polycythemia

3. Cause: not known exactly; predisposing factors include
   a. Certain chromosome disorders (e.g., Down syndrome)
   b. Maternal and fetal infections (e.g., rubella in first trimester)
   c. Maternal alcoholism, undernutrition, diabetes, age over 40 years
4. Types of defects
   a. Acyanotic defects: blood flows from the arterial (left, oxygenated) side of the heart to the venous (right, deoxygenated) side; there is no mixing of unoxygenated blood with oxygenated blood in the systemic circulation (see Fig. 5-2)
      1. *atrial septal defect* (ASD)
         a. flow of blood is from left atrium to right atrium (normal flow resistance)
         b. increased blood flow to right side of heart
         c. treatment: surgical closure or patch graft of defect; 99% survival rate
      2. *ventricular septal defect* (VSD)
         a. most common cardiac defect
         b. flow of blood is from left ventricle (higher pressure) to right ventricle where oxygenated blood mixes with venous blood
         c. may cause right-ventricular hypertrophy and increased pulmonary-vascular resistance
         d. 50% close spontaneously within 1-3 years of age
         e. often associated with other cardiac defects (tetralogy of Fallot, transposition of great vessels, patent ductus arteriosus [PDA], pulmonic stenosis)
         f. infants with severe VSD may develop congestive heart failure and eventually right-to-left shunting
         g. treatment: surgical closure or patch graft of defect
         h. complications include conduction disturbances, CHF, or endocarditis
      3. *patent ductus arteriosus* (PDA)
         a. ductus arteriosus (normal in fetus) fails to close: some blood is shunted by higher pressure in aorta to pulmonary artery
         b. leads to recirculation through lungs and return to left atrium and ventricle; effect is increased work load on left side of heart

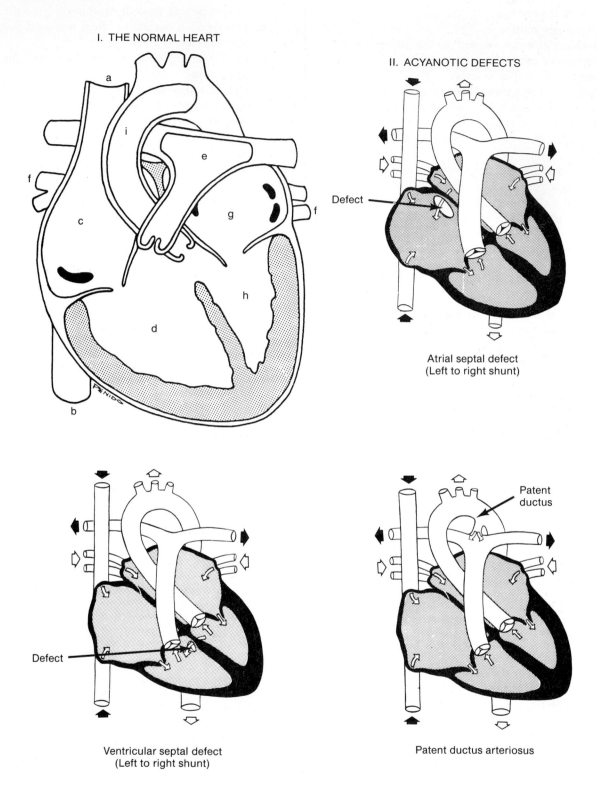

I. THE NORMAL HEART

II. ACYANOTIC DEFECTS

Defect

Atrial septal defect
(Left to right shunt)

Defect

Ventricular septal defect
(Left to right shunt)

Patent
ductus

Patent ductus arteriosus

Fig. 5-2 Normal and abnormal hearts. *a,* Superior vena cava; *b,* inferior vena cava; *c,* right atrium; *d,* right ventricle; *e,* pulmonary artery; *f,* pulmonary vein; *g,* left atrium; *h,* left ventricle; and *i,* aorta. (From *Nursing Inservice Aid #2, Congenital Heart Abnormalities Aid..* Columbus, OH: Ross Laboratories. Used with permission.)

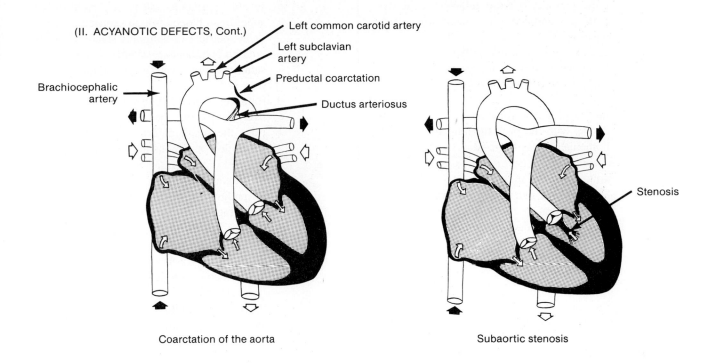

(II. ACYANOTIC DEFECTS, Cont.)

Left common carotid artery

Left subclavian artery

Brachiocephalic artery

Preductal coarctation

Ductus arteriosus

Stenosis

Coarctation of the aorta

Subaortic stenosis

III. CYANOTIC DEFECTS

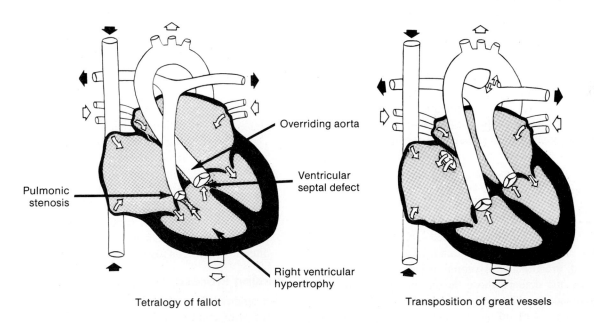

Overriding aorta

Ventricular septal defect

Pulmonic stenosis

Right ventricular hypertrophy

Tetralogy of fallot

Transposition of great vessels

Fig. 5-2, cont'd   For legend see opposite page.

and increased pulmonary congestion
c. pulse pressure is wide; left-ventricular hypertrophy and congestive heart failure may develop
d. characteristic machinery-like murmur
e. treatment: surgical ligation (closed-heart surgery) at 1-2 years of age; 99% survival rate
f. in very ill newborns, medical closure of the ductus with the prostaglandin inhibitor indomethacin may be tried
4. *coarctation of the aorta*
   a. a narrowing of the aorta
      ◆ preductal: narrowing proximal to ductus arteriosus
      ◆ postductal: distal to the ductus arteriosus
      ◆ effect is increased pressure proximal to defect and decreased pressure distal to defect
   b. blood pressure is higher in upper extremities
   c. bounding upper-extremity pulses, weak or absent femoral and popliteal pulses
   d. lower extremities may be cool, pale
   e. cramps (claudication)
   f. headaches, dizziness, epistaxis
   g. treatment: surgical resection and end-to-end anastomosis (or graft) at about age 4 (to allow for growth of aorta)
5. *pulmonic/aortic stenosis*
   a. pulmonic stenosis interferes with flow of blood from right ventricle to pulmonary artery
   b. aortic stenosis interferes with blood flow from left ventricle to aorta
   c. both pulmonic and aortic stenosis
      ◆ may be asymptomatic
      ◆ are usually of the valves
      ◆ increased resistance can cause right ventricular hypertrophy with pulmonary stenosis, left ventricular hypertrophy with aortic stenosis
      ◆ aortic stenosis may result in sudden death after strenuous exercise or activity because of increased sudden oxygen demand and resultant myocardial ischemia
   d. treatment: valvotomy or valve replacement
b. Cyanotic defects: those defects in which unoxygenated blood from right side of heart mixes with oxygenated blood on left side, causing the unoxygenated blood to be circulated through the systemic circulation (right-to-left shunt); results in cyanosis
   1. *tetralogy of Fallot*
      a. most common cyanotic heart defect in children

b. severe VSD
c. severe pulmonic stenosis: right-to-left shunting of blood through ventricular septal defect because of pulmonic stenosis and increased pulmonary resistance; results in desaturated blood entering systemic circulation
d. right ventricular hypertrophy
e. overriding aorta: because the aorta overrides the septal defect, much of the systemic flow is venous and therefore unoxygenated
f. treatment
   ◆ palliative surgical correction in infancy to increase pulmonary blood flow (Blalock-Taussig anastomosis of right or left subclavian artery and corresponding pulmonary artery)
   ◆ corrective surgical repair; closure of VSD (corrects overriding aorta) and pulmonary valvotomy or valve replacement
   ◆ palliative medical care: propranolol (Inderal) to decrease spasm
2. *transposition of the great vessels*
   a. the aorta arises out of the right ventricle so that venous blood enters directly into the systemic circulation, bypassing the lungs; the pulmonary artery arises out of the left ventricle and goes through the lungs; once the foramen ovale and ductus arteriosus close, the situation is incompatible with life (unless ASD or VSD is present)
   b. treatment
      ◆ palliative surgical correction to prevent CHF and reduce pulmonary vascular resistance
         • surgical creation of an ASD
         • balloon atrial septostomy during cardiac catheterization to enlarge existing ASD
         • pulmonary artery banding
      ◆ corrective surgical repair: creation of a new atrial septum that tunnels blood to the correct ventricle
5. Additional medical management: digoxin, potassium, diuretics (if in congestive heart failure), antibiotics

Nursing Process

Assessment

1. Infant or child with acyanotic heart defect
   a. Poor weight gain, small stature
   b. Increased incidence of respiratory infections
   c. Exercise intolerance
   d. Tachycardia, tachypnea, dyspnea
   e. *Not* cyanotic
2. Infant or child with cyanotic heart defect

a. Usually cyanotic at time of birth

b. Babies have difficulty eating because of inability to breathe and suck at same time

c. Delayed physical growth because of chronic hypoxia

d. Frequent and severe respiratory infections

e. Moderate to severe exercise intolerance

f. Chest pain that becomes severe with O_2 demand

g. Hypoxic spell may occur during periods of high O_2 demand (feeding, crying, or physical exertion during play)

    1. severe shortness of breath

    2. increased cyanosis and chest pain

    3. squats with arms thrown over knees, and knees on chest to relieve respiratory distress

h. Chronic hypoxia causes erythropoietin to be released from kidneys to stimulate bone marrow to produce more red blood cells; also causes clubbing of fingers and toes

    1. Hgb may rise 20-30 g or more with a hematocrit as high as 60%-80%

    2. increased RBC results in increased blood viscosity (polycythemia)

i. Polycythemia and sluggish circulation may cause cerebral thrombosis (stroke) and paralysis, sometimes occurring at a very young age

3. Preoperative assessment

a. Baseline vital signs, including apical pulse; existence and quality of peripheral pulses, especially of lower extremities; compare pulses

b. Educational needs of child and parents for preoperative teaching and postoperative experience

c. Laboratory values to assess potential problems

4. Postoperative assessment

a. Respiratory status, chest tubes, chest-tube drainage, breath sounds

b. Vital signs, including apical and femoral pulses, arterial and venous pressures, cardiac rhythm

c. Hydration status and output

d. Signs and symptoms of congestive heart failure

e. Color of skin, mucous membranes, nail beds, and earlobes

f. Level of discomfort and anxiety

g. Surgical incisions (suture line)

Analysis (see p. 480)

Planning, Implementation, and Evaluation

> **Goal 1:** Child will maintain adequate oxygenation and a patent airway.

Implementation

Preoperative and postoperative

1. Count respirations and apical pulse for 1 full minute.

2. Pin diapers loosely, use loose-fitting pajamas.

3. Feed slowly with frequent rest periods; burp frequently.

4. Position at 45° after feeding.

5. Suction nose and throat mucus if cough is inadequate.

6. Give O_2 as ordered and necessary.

7. Administer digoxin as prescribed.

    a. Give at regular intervals.

    b. Do not mix with other foods or fluids.

    c. Hold drug and notify physician if apical pulse rate is below 100 in infants, below 90 in toddlers, or below 70 in older children.

    d. Give 1 hour before or 2 hours after meals or feedings.

    e. Observe for signs of toxicity (bradycardia, nausea, anorexia, vomiting, disorientation).

8. Administer diuretics as prescribed.

    a. Monitor I&O closely.

    b. Ensure that fluid intake is within prescribed restrictions.

    c. Encourage high-potassium foods or administer prescribed potassium supplements.

Postoperative (palliative or corrective surgery)

9. Monitor constantly.

10. Take precautions in care of closed chest drainage (bottles below level of bed, no kinks in tubing, do *not* empty bottles, monitor fluid level and fluctuation in tube, character of drainage).

11. Avoid elevating foot of bed (causes intestines to put pressure on diaphragm).

12. Administer O_2 as ordered.

13. Establish and follow coughing routine; allow crying postoperatively in infant and young child to facilitate lung expansion; use inspirometer (incentive spirometry) with older children.

14. When child has recovered from anesthesia, elevate head of bed to reduce pressure on diaphragm.

15. Use nasogastric suction to reduce gastric distension.

16. Be alert to signs of CHF, hypovolemic shock, pneumonia, hemothorax (dyspnea), atelectasis (dyspnea, increased pulse), cerebral thrombosis.

Evaluation

Child has normal skin color, a patent airway, breathes freely; no signs of complications.

> **Goal 2:** Child will maintain adequate hydration and electrolyte balance.

Implementation

1. Encourage fluid intake within fluid restrictions for child; monitor I&O *very* accurately (be especially alert to thoracotomy drainage, fluid used to administer IV medications or flush CVP and arterial lines).

2. Monitor daily weights.

3. Check urine specific gravity and pH.

4. Be alert to early signs and symptoms of pulmonary edema, cardiac overload, and congestive heart failure (e.g., tachycardia, dyspnea, tachypnea, moist respi-

rations, rales, rhonchi, sweating [in infants], edema).

5. Be aware that dehydration with cyanotic heart disease increases blood viscosity and therefore risk of thrombosis.

6. Observe for signs of hypokalemia (altered lab values, cardiac dysrhythmias).

Evaluation

Child has adequate I&O; no signs or symptoms of fluid or electrolyte imbalance, stroke, or congestive heart failure.

> **Goal 3:** Child and parents will experience no more than moderate anxiety.

Implementation

1. Encourage child and parents to disclose their feelings about the surgery, hospitalization, and treatments (use projective techniques with child); answer their questions.

2. Prepare child and parents for treatments, surgical routine, and discharge; consider developmental age, environment, culture and ethnicity, timing needs, and ability to understand.

3. Help parents and others understand the importance of treating child as normally as possible (to provide for optimal emotional-social development and to avoid overprotecting and sheltering).

Evaluation

Child and parents describe realistic expectations about child's illness and hospitalization; establish and adhere to age-appropriate limits; demonstrate knowledge about procedures, medications.

> **Goal 4:** Child and parents will be adequately prepared for discharge and home care.

Implementation

1. Encourage and support parents in their attempts to allow child age-appropriate independence and responsibilities.

2. Teach parents safe administration of medications, side effects, signs of complications, when to seek medical attention.

3. Refer parents to community health nursing agency for home follow-up if indicated.

Evaluation

Child gradually assumes self-care responsibilities and age-appropriate independence; parents state signs of complications and when to seek attention; administer medications correctly.

☐ Rheumatic Fever and Rheumatic Heart Disease
General Information

1. Definition: an inflammatory disease caused by an immune response to group A beta-hemolytic strepto-coccal infection; affects collagen (connective) tissue such as heart, joints, central nervous system, and subcutaneous tissue

2. Occurrence: primarily affects school-age children; higher incidence in cold or humid climates, crowded living environments, and with strong family history of rheumatic fever

3. Medical treatment
   a. Antibiotics (penicillin or erythromycin)
      1. to eradicate any lingering infection
      2. for long-term prophylactic treatment
   b. Salicylates to control joint inflammation, fever, pain

Nursing Process

Assessment (revised Jones criteria [American Heart Association])

1. Major manifestations
   a. Carditis: mitral and aortic valves most commonly affected with symptoms of tachycardia, cardiomegaly, pericarditis, murmurs, congestive heart failure; carditis is the only manifestation that may cause permanent damage
   b. Painful migratory polyarthritis in large joints with manifestations of acute pain, warmth, redness, edema; permanent deformities do not follow
   c. Chorea (Saint Vitus' dance or Sydenham's chorea): purposeless, irregular movements of the extremities, muscular weakness, emotional lability, facial grimacing
      1. follows the acute febrile phase
      2. may last for months, but is self-limiting
      3. relieved by rest and sleep
   d. Erythema marginatum rheumaticum: macular rash with wavy, well-defined border on trunk
   e. Subcutaneous nodules: small, nontender swellings in groups over bony prominences

2. Minor manifestations
   a. Arthralgia
   b. Fever
   c. Nonspecific tests indicating inflammation
      1. elevated erythrocyte sedimentation rate (ESR)
      2. elevated C-reactive protein
      3. leukocytosis
   d. Anemia
   e. Prolonged PR and QT intervals on ECG

3. Other
   a. Positive throat culture
   b. Elevated antistreptolysin (ASO) titer (indicates a preceding streptococcal infection)

Planning, Implementation, and Evaluation
Analysis (see p. 480)

> **Goal 1:** Child will be free from pain and will rest comfortably.

Implementation

1. Administer salicylates as ordered.
2. Use cradles to keep bed linen off painful joints.
3. Position joints on pillows; handle gently.

Evaluation

Child does not complain of pain, rests and sleeps comfortably.

Goal 2: Child with chorea will be protected from injury.

Implementation

1. Use side rails and pad sides of bed.
2. Provide understanding and emotional support; reassure child and family that chorea will resolve spontaneously.
3. Provide with alternative means to do written work (e.g., typewriter, personal computer, oral reports).
4. Assist child in self-care to promote independence and positive self-concept.

Evaluation

Child ambulates without falling, does not sustain injury.

Goal 3: Child and family will be prepared for home care and long-term management.

Implementation

1. Emphasize importance of compliance with long-term antibiotic therapy for prevention of serious heart damage.
   a. Prepare child for injections of penicillin.
   b. Stress seriousness of recurrence and need to seek medical care for subsequent infections.
2. Plan for continuation of schoolwork, realistic career goals.
3. Refer to community health nurse for follow-up as needed.
4. Instruct parents to take vital signs, administer medications, ensure restrictions.

Evaluation

Child returns to full activity with no residual cardiac involvement.

Application of the Nursing Process to the Child with Hematological Problems

Assessment

1. Nursing history
   a. Dietary intake, especially dietary iron
   b. History of bleeding tendencies (easy bruising, gum bleeding, epistaxis), response to injury or trauma
   c. General symptoms: fatigue, irritability, anorexia, pain, or edema
   d. Recent stressful situations: exposure to temperature extremes, emotional stress
   e. Family history of hematological disorders
   f. Current treatment, home management, general health
2. Clinical appraisal
   a. General appearance: pallor, lethargy, bruising, physical growth (overweight or underweight for age)
   b. Vital signs: tachycardia, tachypnea, hypotension
3. Diagnostic tests (refer to *Nursing Care of the Adult*, p. 118)

Analysis

1. Safe, effective care environment
   a. High risk for injury
   b. High risk for infection
   c. Knowledge deficit
2. Physiological integrity
   a. Impaired gas exchange
   b. Fatigue
   c. Altered cerebral tissue perfusion
3. Psychosocial integrity
   a. Anxiety
   b. Altered role performance
   c. Body image disturbance
4. Health promotion/maintenance
   a. Ineffective family coping: compromised
   b. Diversional activity deficit
   c. Altered growth and development

General Nursing Planning, Implementation, and Evaluation

Goal 1: Child will be free from pain.

Implementation

1. Administer prescribed analgesics (no aspirin).
2. Handle and move child gently.
3. Provide bed rest with covers off affected areas.
4. Provide age-appropriate diversional activities.

Evaluation

Child is free from pain; rests comfortably.

Goal 2: Child will conserve energy.

Implementation

1. Schedule nursing care and treatment to prevent tiring and to provide uninterrupted periods of rest.
2. Provide quiet age-appropriate play activities.
3. Counsel parents concerning plan for activity and rest at home.

Evaluation

Child engages in activities of daily living without tiring, has age-appropriate rest and sleep periods.

SELECTED HEALTH PROBLEMS RESULTING IN AN INTERFERENCE WITH FORMED ELEMENTS OF THE BLOOD

☐ Iron-Deficiency Anemia

General Information

1. Definition: a decrease in the number of erythrocytes and/or a decreased Hgb level: less than 10 g/dl
2. Occurrence: most common nutritional disorder in United States, resulting in reduced oxygen-carrying capacity of blood; most common childhood anemia
   a. Primarily in children 6-24 months of age who have a diet low in iron
   b. In premature infants (inadequate iron stores)
   c. In adolescent girls, with increased growth and menstruation
   d. In adolescent boys, with androgen-related increase in hemoglobin concentration
3. Cause: impaired production of red blood cells, resulting from deficient iron stores
   a. Inadequate dietary intake
   b. Impaired absorption
   c. Blood loss
   d. Excessive demand (prematurity, puberty, or pregnancy)
4. Medical treatment
   a. Oral iron supplements (ferrous iron), 10-15 mg/day for 3 months
   b. Parenteral iron therapy (iron dextran [Imferon]) IM or IV
   c. Blood transfusions with packed red cells (if Hgb is less than 4 g/dl)

Nursing Process

Assessment
1. Nutritional history (daily intake)
2. Pallor (porcelain-like skin)
3. Poor muscle development
4. May be overweight ("milk baby")
5. Exercise intolerance, lethargy
6. Susceptible to infection

Analysis (see p. 487)

Planning, Implementation, and Evaluation

Goal: Child will ingest diet and medications to maintain adequate Hgb level.

Implementation
1. Explain the necessity for a proper diet to parents.
   a. Provide adequate sources of iron, and teach parent and child what they are.
   b. For infants, give iron-fortified formula and cereal and iron supplements.
   c. For older children, give foods high in iron (e.g., meat, vegetables, and fruit).
   d. Give solids before milk.
2. Teach parents correct administration of oral iron preparations as ordered.
   a. Give ferrous sulfate (Fer-In-Sol) in 3 divided doses/day, between meals with citrus juice.
   b. Continue for 4-6 weeks after red blood cell count returns to normal.
   c. Liquid iron temporarily stains teeth (use straw or dropper to back of mouth; brush child's teeth).
   d. Oral iron causes stools to become dark-green.
3. If oral preparations ineffective, administer parenteral iron as prescribed using IM Z-track method: painful and stains subcutaneous tissue; do not use deltoid; no more than 1 ml per site; use air bubble, don't massage over injection site, avoid tight clothing over injection site.
4. Limit milk intake to 1 q/day or less.

Evaluation
Child takes diet and medications as ordered; child's Hgb level returns to normal.

☐ Sickle Cell Anemia

General Information

1. Definition: autosomal recessive defect (see Fig. 5-3) found primarily in blacks, resulting in production of abnormal hemoglobin (hemoglobin S) and characterized by intermittent episodes of crisis
2. Occurrence 1:600 black Americans
   a. Sickle cell trait: heterozygous form (carrier); 1 in 12 black persons is a carrier
   b. Sickle-cell disease: homozygous form (has the disease); may have vasoocclusive crisis; painful, acute occurrence usually precipitated by decreased O_2 tension, which causes cells to become viscous and assume a sickle shape, obstruct blood vessels, and cause tissue ischemia, infarction, and necrosis
3. Cause: defective form of hemoglobin (hemoglobin S), inherited by autosomal-recessive genetic transmission
4. Medical treatment: symptomatic treatment of crisis
   a. Bed rest to decrease O_2 expenditure
   b. Adequate hydration: oral and IV fluids to increase blood volume and mobilize sickled cells
   c. Electrolyte replacement (hypoxia causes metabolic acidosis)
   d. Relief of pain
      1. acetaminophen
      2. codeine
      3. meperidine (Demerol)
      4. may use client-controlled analgesia
   e. Blood transfusions, for severe drop in hemoglobin (aplastic crisis)
   f. O_2 for severe hypoxia (on a short-term basis)
   g. Antibiotics to treat concurrent infection

A. Autosomal dominant diseases

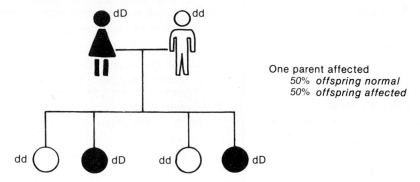

One parent affected
50% *offspring normal*
50% *offspring affected*

Key: d = normal gene; D = abnormal, *dominant* gene

Examples: Huntington's disease, osteogenesis imperfecta, neurofibromatosis

B. Autosomal recessive diseases

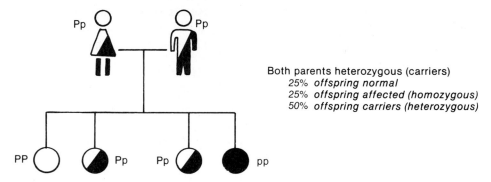

Both parents heterozygous (carriers)
25% *offspring normal*
25% *offspring affected (homozygous)*
50% *offspring carriers (heterozygous)*

Key: P = normal gene; p = abnormal, *recessive* gene

Examples: phenylketonuria, cystic fibrosis, sickle cell disease, galactosemia, Tay-Sachs disease, thalassemia

C. Sex-linked recessive diseases (X-linked)

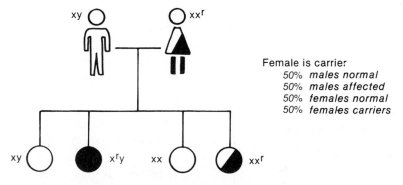

Female is carrier
50% *males normal*
50% *males affected*
50% *females normal*
50% *females carriers*

Key: xy = normal *male* sex chromosome pattern; xx = normal *female* sex chromosome pattern; r = sex-linked *recessive* gene

Examples: hemophilia, color blindness, agammaglobulinemia, G6PD deficiency, X-linked Duchenne's muscular dystrophy

Fig. 5-3 Common modes of genetic transmission.

Nursing Process
Assessment
1. Parents with sickle cell trait
2. Signs and symptoms (depend on organ involved); not evident until after 6 months of age
   a. Chronic hemolytic anemia
   b. Frequent infections, related to decreased ability of spleen to filter bacteria
   c. Organ deterioration (spleen, liver, kidney, heart, or CNS)
   d. Chronic pain: joints, abdomen, back
   e. Bone deterioration (osteoporosis, skeletal deformities) from increase in marrow
3. Manifestations of vasoocclusive crisis
   a. Severe abdominal pain: caused by organ hypoxia
   b. Hand-foot syndrome: swelling of hands and feet
   c. Fever: resulting from dehydration or possible concurrent infection
   d. Arthralgia

Analysis (see p. 487)
Planning, Implementation, and Evaluation

> **Goal 1:** Child's episodes of vasoocclusive crisis will be prevented or minimized.

Implementation
1. Teach crisis-prevention methods to child and parent.
   a. Avoid situations resulting in decreased O_2 concentration such as high altitudes, constrictive clothing, extreme physical exertion, and exposure to cold.
   b. Avoid emotional distress.
   c. Maintain adequate hydration (child should receive at least *minimum* daily fluid requirement).
   d. Protect from infection.
      1. prevent exposure to persons with infections
      2. promote adequate nutrition
      3. obtain medical care at onset of infection (may need antibiotics)
      4. keep immunizations current

Evaluation
Parent and child adhere to plan for crisis prevention; child's crisis episodes are minimized.

> **Goal 2:** Child will receive appropriate supportive care during crisis.

Implementation
1. Relieve pain.
   a. Administer analgesics.
   b. Handle gently.
   c. Use heating pad on painful areas.
2. Monitor hydration and electrolyte status.
   a. Monitor I&O; offer liquids frequently.
   b. Regulate IV fluids, blood transfusion.
   c. Observe for fluid or electrolyte imbalance.

3. Assess for signs of infection; protect from exposure to infectious sources during crisis.

Evaluation
Child is relieved of pain during crisis; has no elevated temperature; has elastic skin turgor, moist mucous membranes, adequate fluid intake.

> **Goal 3:** Parent and child at risk will receive screening and genetic counseling.

Implementation
1. Teach parent about screening and diagnostic techniques.
   a. Nonspecific screening tests for trait or disease: Sickledex
   b. Specific identification of trait and disease: Hgb electrophoresis ("protein fingerprinting") used if screening tests are positive
2. Give information on available genetic counseling.

Evaluation
Parents receive screening and genetic counseling as indicated; demonstrate knowledge of transmission and implications for subsequent pregnancies.

☐ Hemophilia
General Information
1. Definition, occurrence, and cause: hereditary coagulation defect, usually transmitted to affected male by female carrier through sex-linked recessive gene (see Fig. 5-3), resulting in prolonged clotting time; most common type is hemophilia A-factor VIII deficiency; severity of the deficiency varies from mild to severe; at risk for acquired immunodeficiency syndrome (AIDS) from contaminated bood products (see Table 5-9)
2. Medical treatment
   a. Replacement of factor VIII: transfusion of plasma, factor VIII concentrate, or cryoprecipitate to prevent bleeding episodes
   b. Additional treatment measures for more severe bleeding episodes
      1. immediate administration of factor VIII to control bleeding
      2. bed rest with covers off affected area to relieve pain; temporary immobilization of affected joints in a slightly flexed position with casts, splints, or traction
      3. physical therapy to prevent contractures, beginning 48 hours after bleeding stops
      4. pain relief with sedatives or narcotics

Nursing Process
Assessment
1. Infant
   a. Umbilical-cord hemorrhage
   b. Hemorrhage following circumcision

c. Family history of hemophilia
2. Any age
   a. Hemarthrosis (bleeding into a joint space) is the most frequent site of bleeding; may result in crippling bony deformities
   b. Epistaxis
   c. Spontaneous hematuria
   d. Hemorrhage following tooth extraction or minor falls and cuts
3. Diagnostic laboratory tests: only tests that measure clotting factors (e.g., PTT) are abnormal; platelet function tests (e.g., bleeding time) are normal

Analysis (see p. 487)

Planning, Implementation, and Evaluation

> **Goal 1:** Parent and child will receive education to *prevent* bleeding, provide safety measures; will know how to treat minor bleeding episodes.

Implementation

1. Prepare parents and child for home care and administration of factor VIII (where available).
   a. Teach about the disease.
   b. Teach venipuncture procedure and how to monitor the tranfusion.
   c. Provide regular follow-up (family must be sufficiently motivated and stable to maintain a home-care program).
2. Teach local treatment measures for minor bleeding episodes.
   a. Apply direct pressure to site (10-15 minutes).
   b. Apply ice pack.
   c. Immobilize and elevate affected part.
3. Teach safe administration of medication.
   a. Give orally if possible.
   b. Avoid injections; if necessary, after injection apply pressure until bleeding stops.
4. Avoid medications that increase bleeding (aspirin, phenacetin, phenothiazines, indomethacin [Indocin]).
5. Institute dental precautions: soft toothbrush, Water Pik, good dental hygiene to avoid extractions.
6. Encourage appropriate toys, games, and sports.
   a. Soft toys for infants

   b. Quiet activities (e.g., reading, swimming)
   c. Avoid body-contact sports
   d. Careful handling of sharp objects
   e. Use of electric shavers (not razors)
7. Use protective devices for young child: padded crib, playpen, side rails, protective padding and helmet for toddler.
8. Teach to avoid overweight (causes strain on affected joints).
9. Teach to wear Medic Alert identification.
10. Inform appropriate school personnel.
11. Avoid stressful situations (they increase susceptibility to bleeding).
12. Seek emergency medical treatment in cases of uncontrolled bleeding.

Evaluation

Parent and child demonstrate ability to correctly manage home administration of factor VIII; state medication precautions, activities to avoid, and those that are permitted; parent provides appropriate protective devices at home; adequately cares for minor bleeding episodes (e.g., local pressure, ice pack); school personnel and friends are informed about child's condition and necessary restrictions or appropriate action during a bleeding episode.

> **Goal 2:** Child and parents will receive emotional support.

Implementation

1. Encourage realistic career goals.
2. Allow child and family to discuss feelings and concerns about bleeding tendency and treatment, subsequent absences from school, reactions to peers, and parental protectiveness.
3. Encourage independence while maintaining safety.
4. Urge testing for HIV status.
5. Refer to the local chapter of the National Hemophilia Foundation.

Evaluation

Child seeks independence within reasonable limits; asks questions about reactions of school friends; adolescent seeks out appropriate job opportunities.

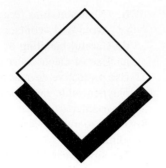

Nutrition and Metabolism

GENERAL CONCEPTS
Overview/Physiology

1. Fluid balance (developmental differences)
   a. Greater proportion of body water, especially in extracellular space, until 2 years of age (increases vulnerability to changes in body water)
   b. Three times greater water-turnover rate per unit of body weight in infants because of
      1. higher metabolic rate
      2. faster respiratory rate
      3. functional immaturity of kidneys that impairs ability to conserve water (increases infant's susceptibility to fluid volume deficit)
   c. Greater skin surface area in proportion to body weight (increases susceptibility to insensible water loss)
   d. Greater gastrointestinal surface area (leads to greater fluid loss from diarrhea)
2. Calculation of daily fluid requirements for infants and children
   a. Average daily fluid requirements are calculated according to child's weight in kilograms
      1. 100 ml/kg for the first 10 kg
      2. 50 ml/kg for the next 10 kg
      3. 20 ml/kg for each additional kg
   b. Example of calculation for a 25-kg child
      1000 ml (100 ml × 10 kg)
      500 ml (50 ml × 10 kg)
      <u>100</u> ml (20 ml × 5 kg)
   Total 1600 ml per day
3. Digestive system (developmental differences)
   a. High rate or peristalsis (increases susceptibility to diarrhea)
   b. Immature cardiac sphincter that relaxes easily (predisposes to gastroesophageal reflux)
   c. Low production of intestinal antibodies until 6-7 months of age (increases susceptibility to infection)
   d. Increased permeability of intestines to whole proteins such as those found in cow's milk (increases susceptibility to allergies)
   e. Decreased levels of lactase in intestinal mucosa (predisposes to lactose intolerance and subsequent diarrhea)
   f. Immature liver (leads to an inability to conjugate water-soluble bilirubin in the newborn, resulting in physiological jaundice; results in difficulties with drug metabolism)
4. Endocrine system (developmental differences)
   a. Functionally immature
   b. Blood glucose levels fluctuate (predisposes to hypoglycemia)
   c. Hormonal feedback mechanisms are not fully operational (leads to less ability to tolerate stresses and metabolic demands of illness)

Application of the Nursing Process to the Child with Problems of Nutrition and Metabolism

Assessment

1. Nursing history
   a. Dietary-intake history: type, amount, frequency, and tolerance
   b. Vomiting or diarrhea: onset, severity, duration, description, precipitating factors, and home management
   c. Infant/child behavior: irritability, lethargy, and change in disposition
   d. Other signs and symptoms of illness such as fever, respiratory infection, and abdominal pain
   e. Frequency and amount of voiding
   f. History of exposure to illness in family or community
   g. Family history of hereditary disorders: cystic fibrosis, phenylketonuria, diabetes mellitus, cleft lip and palate, or lactose intolerance
2. Clinical appraisal
   a. General appearance: color, cry, behavior
   b. Physical growth (refer to *Healthy Child*, p. 428)
   c. Vital signs, presence of fever

d. Nutrition and hydration status, including signs of dehydration
   1. milk dehydration: weight loss of up to 5%
      a. dry mucous membranes
      b. poor tear production
      c. decreased urine output with increased specific gravity (>1.030)
      d. pallor
      e. pulse normal or slightly increased
      f. normal blood pressure
   2. moderate hydration: weight loss between 5%-9%
      a. very dry mucous membranes
      b. poor skin turgor
      c. pale to gray skin color
      d. oliguria (<1 ml/kg/hr)
      e. tachycardia
      f. slight increase in BP
   3. severe dehydration: weight loss between 10%-15%
      a. parched mucous membranes
      b. very poor skin turgor
      c. marked oliguria
      d. gray to mottled skin color
      e. severe tachycardia
      f. decreased blood pressure
      g. sunken eyes and fontanel
      h. tetany and convulsions (late sign of electrolyte imbalance)
   4. laboratory findings: elevated hematocrit and BUN
3. Diagnostic tests (refer to *Nursing Care of the Adult*, p. 160)

Analysis
1. Safe, effective care environment
   a. High risk for infection
   b. High risk for injury
2. Physiological integrity
   a. Fluid volume deficit
   b. Altered nutrition: less than body requirements
   c. High risk for aspiration
   d. High risk for impaired skin integrity
3. Psychosocial integrity
   a. Anxiety
   b. Self-esteem/body image disturbance
   c. Fear
4. Health promotion/maintenance
   a. Altered family processes
   b. Altered growth and development
   c. Knowledge deficit

General Nursing Planning, Implementation, and Evaluation

Goal: Child will maintain fluid and electrolyte balance.

Implementation
1. Monitor for signs of electrolyte imbalance (refer to *Nursing Care of the Adult*, p. 191).
2. Administer fluids (PO, IV) as prescribed; usually includes sodium chloride and potassium replacement.
   a. Use infusion pump to maintain accurate rate.
   b. Restrain child as necessary to protect infusion site.
   c. Observe infusion site for infiltration or redness, and report promptly.
3. Provide pacifier if infant is NPO.
4. Administer electrolytes as prescribed (give potassium only when urinary output is adequate [i.e., 1-2 ml/kg/hr]).
5. Carefully monitor and record I&O (weigh diapers, indicate urine and stool output separately if possible).
6. Monitor response to therapy (improved skin color and turgor, moist mucous membranes, stable vital signs, urine output within normal limits, urine specific gravity within normal limits [e.g., 1.005-1.030]).
7. Weigh child daily before breakfast or every shift on same scale.
8. Administer antiemetics as ordered.
9. Gradually return to diet for age as tolerated.

Evaluation

Child regains and maintains fluid and electrolyte balance; shows no signs of dehydration or electrolyte or acid-base imbalance; returns to usual diet without recurrence of vomiting or diarrhea.

SELECTED HEALTH PROBLEMS RESULTING IN AN INTERFERENCE WITH NUTRITION AND METABOLISM

☐ Vomiting and Diarrhea

General Information

1. Although vomiting and diarrhea are usually symptoms of other underlying problems or diseases, they are often the primary diagnosis in infants because fluid and electrolyte imbalance can develop rapidly and become critical in a few hours
2. Occurrence: these are very common health problems in infancy; younger infants and children who are debilitated, and those who are exposed to unsanitary environmental conditions, are at greater risk of developing diarrhea
3. Causes
   a. Vomiting
      1. gastrointestinal infection
      2. allergy to formula, food, medications
      3. emotional upsets
      4. GI obstruction
      5. toxin ingestion
      6. increased intracranial pressure
      7. overfeeding
      8. diabetic ketoacidosis
      9. migraine headaches
      10. appendicitis

11. other infections (e.g., otitis media, meningitis, respiratory and urinary tract infections)
   b. Diarrhea (may be acute or chronic)
      1. infection
         a. viruses (e.g., rotavirus [self-limiting])
         b. parasites (e.g., Giardia)
         c. enteropathogenic organisms such as *Shigella, Salmonella, E. coli, Campylobacter*
      2. diet: formula or food allergy, high sugar or fat content, high bulk, overfeeding
      3. emotional upsets
      4. prolonged use of antibiotics (may destroy normal flora)
      5. intestinal malabsorption
      6. inflammatory bowel disease
      7. extraintestinal: hepatic, pancreatic, thyroid disorders
      8. ingestion of heavy metals such as lead and mercury
      9. parenteral infections
4. Medical treatment: depends on severity of symptoms and degree of dehydration
   a. Medical intervention
      1. bowel rest; IV and/or oral fluid and electrolyte replacement therapy (type and amount determined on basis of child's age and hydration status)
      2. antibiotic therapy for bacterial diarrhea
      3. antiemetics, usually by rectal suppository
      4. gradual reintroduction of solid foods
      5. diagnosis and treatment of extraintestinal cause
   b. Surgical intervention for GI obstruction

Nursing Process
Assessment
1. Feeding technique and formula preparation (amount, type, formula reconstitution, position of infant, and burping)
2. Type of vomiting and/or diarrhea
   a. Vomiting
      1. *forceful* vomiting: evacuation of stomach contents; usually caused by overdistension from formula or air
      2. *projectile* vomiting: stomach contents propelled 2-3 feet from infant; indicates GI obstruction or increased intracranial pressure
      3. *regurgitation:* "spitting up" milk after feeding; smells sour; usually associated with rumination or gastroesophageal reflux
   b. Diarrhea
      1. *mild:* weight loss of 5% or less; stools are loose, runny, usually brown and brownish-yellow
      2. *severe:* explosive, green, watery stools, 10-12/day; weight loss 10% or more

3. Character of vomitus or stool (ACCT)
   a. *A*mount: measure or estimate
   b. *C*olor/*C*onsistency
      1. vomitus
         a. undigested food, uncurdled milk
         b. sour milk curds
         c. bile stained (indicates lower GI tract obstruction)
         d. blood tinged or coffee ground
      2. diarrhea
         a. color (brown, green, yellow)
         b. consistency (bulky, watery, runny, mucoid, bloody, seedy, or pasty)
   c. *T*ime
      1. frequency
      2. precedents (feeding, stimulants, emotional upsets)
4. Diagnostic tests
   a. Stool pH and stool glucose with Clinitest
   b. Stool blood with guaiac or Hemoccult
   c. Stool sample for bacteria culture, ova, and parasites
5. Associated symptoms: anorexia, nausea, cramping, abdominal pain, fever, headache
6. Signs of dehydration
7. Change in acid-base balance
   a. Vomiting causes loss of HCl, which results in metabolic alkalosis
      1. compensation: kidneys conserve Na^+ and K^+, excrete HCO_3^-
      2. lab findings: urine pH greater than 7; serum pH greater than 7.45
   b. Diarrhea causes loss of HCO_3^-, which results in metabolic acidosis
      1. compensation: respiratory hyperventilation (deep, rapid respirations)
      2. lab findings: urine pH less than 6; serum pH less than 7.35

Analysis (see p. 493)
Planning, Implementation, and Evaluation

> **Goal 1:** Child's close contacts will be free from signs of infection.

Implementation
1. Obtain stool culture to determine infecting organism.
2. Isolate infant; use good hand-washing technique; dispose of excreta and contaminated laundry appropriately.
3. Teach parents protective measures.
4. Administer antibiotics as ordered, observe for side effects.

Evaluation
Individuals involved with care of child (and other children in close proximity) show no signs of spread of infection.

Goal 2: Child (with diarrhea) will maintain skin integrity.

Implementation

1. Cleanse perineum and buttocks well after each stool.
2. Expose to heat lamp or air (buttocks must be free of ointment before exposing to heat lamp).
3. Apply ointment to protect skin.
4. Take axillary temperatures to avoid stimulating peristalsis.

Evaluation

Child is free from skin breakdown; heals excoriated areas.

Goal 3: Child will maintain comfort and safety.

Implementation

1. Position to prevent aspiration (on side or abdomen, or in infant seat).
2. Give mouth care after vomiting and while NPO.
3. If infant is NPO, offer pacifier to meet sucking needs.
4. Change soiled clothing and linen immediately.
5. Exercise restrained limbs.

Evaluation

Child is free from aspiration; rests and sleeps comfortably.

Goal 4: Child will resume diet for age without recurrence of vomiting or diarrhea.

Implementation

1. Begin clear liquids such as noncarbonated soft drinks, Gatorade, and half-strength flavored gelatin; use oral rehydration solutions (e.g., Pedialyte, Lytren) for infants and young children
2. Give liquids at room temperature (cold liquids stimulate bowel activity).
3. If vomiting, offer frequent, small amounts (5-15 ml depending on child's age) every 20 minutes; increase the amount and intervals between feedings slowly.
4. For diarrhea, offer large amounts of clear liquids at infrequent intervals.
5. Discourage use of Popsicles and Kool-Aid as sole source of fluid replacement since they lack electrolytes.
6. Limit apple juice.
7. Discourage use of homemade electrolyte solutions.
8. If infant is breastfeeding, continue and supplement with clear liquids.
9. Add other liquids and solids gradually as tolerated.
10. Encourage bananas, applesauce, strained carrots, rice cereal, and toast for child with diarrhea.
11. Discourage foods with high fat content.
12. Add milk products last because temporary lactose intolerance is common after diarrhea.
13. Switch to soy formula for 1-3 weeks if necessary.

Evaluation

Child tolerates diet for age without recurrence of diarrhea or vomiting; gains or maintains present weight.

☐ Nonorganic Failure to Thrive
General Information

1. Definition: A syndrome used to describe infants and children who fail to gain weight as a result of psychosocial factors such as environmental deprivation; usually results from a disrupted relationship between child and primary caregiver
2. Medical treatment
   a. Comprehensive diagnostic testing to rule out organic failure to thrive, which results from physical causes (e.g., malabsorption syndrome, gastroesophageal reflux, cystic fibrosis, genitourinary or cardiac defects, and neurological or endocrine disorders)
   b. Criteria used for diagnosis
      1. absence of organic disease
      2. weight below the 5th percentile with subsequent weight gain when nurtured
      3. developmental lags that improve with stimulation
      4. improvement in clinical signs of deprivation when nurtured
      5. disruption in psychosocial environment

Nursing Process
Assessment

1. Infant
   a. Growth retardation: height and weight below 5th percentile
   b. Developmental delay: social, motor, language, or cognitive
   c. Flat affect, withdrawn
   d. Feeding and elimination disorders
   e. Absence of stranger anxiety
   f. Avoids eye-to-eye contact
   g. Visually scans the environment
   h. Posture stiff or floppy
   i. Difficulty in feeding or eating (e.g., poor suck, anorexia, vomiting, rumination)
   j. Slow in smiling or socially responding to others
2. Parent
   a. Handles infant only when necessary
   b. Does not talk to, play with, or cuddle infant
   c. Bothered by infant's sounds and smells
   d. Holds infant away from body, no eye contact with infant
   e. Responds inappropriately and inconsistently to infant's cues
   f. Refers to infant as "bad" and "unloving"

Analysis (see p. 493)
Planning, Implementation, and Evaluation

Goal 1: Infant will show evidence of weight gain.

Implementation

1. Calculate caloric requirements based on infant's weight: 115 kcal/kg/day for the first year of life.
2. Suggest dietary consultant.
3. Monitor I&O; describe frequency and precipitating events of any vomiting.
4. Obtain daily weights before breakfast on same scale, and weekly length and head circumferences.
5. Observe feeding patterns.
6. Observe parent-infant interactions around feeding.

Evaluation

Infant shows steady weight gain, ingests and retains appropriate amount of nutrients necessary to meet caloric requirements.

Goal 2: Infant will show progression in development while hospitalized.

Implementation

1. Use primary caregivers.
2. Hold, cuddle, talk to infant lovingly with reassurance to model for caregivers.
3. Monitor infant's response to care.
4. Provide age-appropriate developmental and sensory stimulation.

Evaluation

Infant responds appropriately to developmental stimulation and nurturing; maintains eye contact, smiles; allows self to be held closely; demonstrates interest in environment.

Goal 3: Parents will show positive interaction with infant.

Implementation

1. Welcome parents when visiting.
2. Encourage parent participation in care, teaching as appropriate.
3. Use anticipatory guidance regarding infant's capabilities, physical care, emotional needs (demonstrate by example).
4. Encourage parents to express feelings about infant and their parenting.
5. Urge parents to talk to infant; point out positive responses.
6. Identify stressors in family; refer to social services and family counseling as appropriate.
7. Praise parents' involvement with child.
8. Determine progress in parent-child relationship.
9. Maintain a nonjudgmental attitude.

Evaluation

Parents provide some care to infant; hold, cuddle, and talk to infant; express feelings about infant.

Goal 4: Parents will participate in follow-up care after discharge.

Implementation

1. Assess home environment.
2. Refer to community resources (e.g., public health nurse, parent support group) as needed.
3. Refer to agencies that can provide family counseling, financial assistance (e.g., WIC).
4. Review infant's regimen with parents (nutrition, elimination, stimulation, etc).
5. Arrange for return visit for infant to physician/clinic.
6. Review developmental milestones and age-appropriate stimulation.

Evaluation

Parent keeps all appointments, including those with community resources and groups; infant continues weight gain and developmental progress.

☐ Pyloric Stenosis
General Information

1. Definition and occurrence: narrowing of the pylorus caused by hypertrophy of circular muscle fibers; more commonly affects firstborn white males, 2 weeks to 3 months of age
2. Medical treatment
   a. Medical intervention
      1. barium swallow to confirm diagnosis
      2. IV fluids to hydrate and correct metabolic alkalosis
      3. nasogastric tube to decompress stomach
   b. Surgical intervention: Fredet-Ramstedt procedure (pylorotomy); hypertrophied muscle is *split down to but not through* submucosa, permitting pylorus to expand (if mucosa is cut, gastric contents will leak into peritoneum, causing peritonitis)

Nursing Process
Assessment

1. Vomiting: amount, color, consistency, and time
2. Classic signs
   a. Projectile vomiting (not bile stained since obstruction is above the duodenum)
   b. Palpable, olive-size mass (usually in RUQ)
   c. Observable left-to-right gastric peristaltic waves
3. Metabolic alkalosis, caused by loss of HCl and K^+
4. Signs and symptoms of food and fluid loss
   a. Hunger after feeding
   b. Weight loss, or failure to gain weight
   c. Dehydration
   d. Scanty, concentrated urine
   e. Progressive constipation

Analysis (see p. 493)
Planning, Implementation, and Evaluation

Goal 1: Preoperatively, infant will regain and maintain fluid and electrolyte balance.

Implementation

1. Assess vital signs frequently.
2. Assess signs of dehydration.
3. Offer pacifier while NPO.
4. Follow correct principles of IV fluid and electrolyte administration.
5. Carefully monitor I&O and urine specific gravity.
6. Weigh infant daily or every shift if condition warrants.
7. Maintain nasogastric decompression as ordered.

Evaluation

Infant regains and maintains fluid and electrolyte balance; is free from signs of dehydration and metabolic alkalosis.

Goal 2: Postoperatively, infant will be free from vomiting and will ingest adequate nutrition.

Implementation

1. Initiate glucose water or electrolyte solutions 4-6 hours postoperatively and gradually advance to full-strength formula during second postoperative day.
2. Give small, frequent feedings; feed slowly.
3. Burp infant after every ½ oz; position on right side in semi-Fowler's position after feeding.
4. Teach parent how to feed child; supervise as needed.
5. Handle gently and minimally after feeding.
6. Offer pacifier during period of restricted feeding.
7. Keep accurate I&O.

Evaluation

Infant ingests adequate caloric and fluid intake; has no vomiting, no signs of dehydration; gains or maintains present weight.

Goal 3: Postoperatively, infant will be free from infection.

Implementation

1. Observe operative site routinely for any drainage or signs of inflammation.
2. Perform incision care and dressing change as ordered.
3. Assess for signs of peritonitis (e.g., abdominal distension, fever, rigid abdomen, increased irritability, tachycardia, decreased or absent bowel sounds, or rapid thoracic breathing).

Evaluation

Infant remains afebrile, has soft abdomen, exhibits no signs of discomfort.

☐ Celiac Disease (Gluten Enteropathy)
General Information

1. Definition: a disease of unknown etiology characterized by the permanent inability to tolerate gluten (one of the proteins found in wheat, rye, oats, and barley)
2. Occurrence: 21 in 100,000 live births; second leading cause of malabsorption in children; positive familial tendency
3. Pathophysiology: the ingestion of gluten results in the inability to fully digest gliadin (a fraction of gluten); subsequently, there is an accumulation of the amino acid glutamine, which is toxic to the mucosal cells of the small intestine; this may lead to malabsorption of the following nutrients, causing various complications
   a. Fats: steatorrhea, malnutrition
   b. Proteins and carbohydrates: peripheral edema
   c. Vitamin D and calcium: osteomalacia, osteoporosis
   d. Vitamin K: bleeding
   e. Iron, folic acid, and vitamin B_{12}: anemia
4. Medical treatment
   a. Diagnosis
      1. positive fecal fat
      2. decreases in serum protein, prothrombin, folic acid, vitamin B_{12}, calcium
      3. anemia
      4. x-rays to determine bone age
      5. sweat test (to rule out cystic fibrosis)
      6. improvement of clinical signs and symptoms after withdrawal of gluten from diet
      7. bowel studies
      8. peroral jejunal biopsy (diagnosis is confirmed when atrophic changes are seen in the mucosal wall)
   b. Dietary management
      1. gluten-free diet (corn and rice are substituted for wheat, rye, oats, and barley)
      2. supplemental calories, vitamins, iron, and calcium
      3. parenteral alimentation if malnourished
   c. Management during celiac crisis (acute episode of profuse, watery diarrhea and vomiting that frequently leads to severe dehydration and metabolic acidosis; usually precipitated by gastrointestinal infection, dietary sources of gluten, and anticholinergic drugs)
      1. IV fluids and electrolytes
      2. albumin infusions (to prevent shock)
      3. nasogastric decompression
      4. corticosteroids (to decrease bowel inflammation)

Nursing Process
Assessment

1. Clinical manifestations (highly variable)
   a. Chronic diarrhea (usually begins late in the first year of life after gluten-containing foods have been introduced)
   b. Failure to thrive
   c. Irritability

d. Anorexia
e. Vomiting
f. Abdominal pain and distension
g. Excessive appetite
h. Rectal prolapse
i. Peripheral edema
j. Clubbing of fingers
k. Wasting of muscles
l. Excessive bruising
2. In celiac crisis
    a. Severe pale, bulky, foul-smelling stools
    b. Vomiting
    c. Signs of shock and metabolic acidosis
    d. Dependent edema

Analysis (see p. 493)
Planning, Implementation, and Evaluation

> **Goal 1:** Child will remain free from injury during intestinal biopsy.

Implementation
1. Prepare child and family for diagnostic procedure.
2. Assess bleeding times and platelet count.
3. Administer vitamin K prophylactically as ordered.
4. Assess frequently, following procedure for shock (early signs: tachycardia and signs of peripheral vasoconstriction; late signs: hypotension).

Evaluation
Child tolerates intestinal biopsy well, recovers free from signs of hemorrhage.

> **Goal 2:** Child will adhere to nutritional management.

Implementation
1. Assess family's understanding of disease process and need for gluten-free diet.
2. Educate family regarding gluten-free foods; show parents how to read food labels (gluten is often listed as hydrolyzed vegetable protein or cereal fillers).
3. Encourage balanced diet (offer foods high in calories and protein such as pudding and milkshakes); consult dietitian to help in meal planning.
4. Reinforce to family the need for lifelong dietary adherence.

Evaluation
Parents list elements of a gluten-free diet; child ingests only gluten-free, balanced meals.

> **Goal 3:** Child will remain free from fluid and electrolyte imbalance during celiac crisis.

Implementation
1. Monitor vital signs frequently.
2. Assess for signs of shock and metabolic acidosis.
3. Keep accurate I&O.
4. Weigh child daily on same scale.
5. Maintain nasogastric decompression as ordered.
6. Administer corticosteroids, albumin, IV fluids, and electrolytes as ordered.
7. Test all stools and nasogastric drainage for occult blood.
8. Educate family regarding precipitating factors of celiac crisis.

Evaluation
Child recovers from celiac crisis free from complications; achieves homeostasis.

☐ Cleft Lip and Palate
General Information

1. Definition
    a. *Cleft lip:* incomplete fusion of facial process; may be small notch in the upper lip (incomplete) or extend to nasal septum and dental ridge (complete); may be unilateral or bilateral
    b. *Cleft palate:* fissures in soft and/or hard palate and alveolar (dental) ridge; may be midline, unilateral, or bilateral
2. Occurrence
    a. Cleft lip (with or without cleft palate): 1:1000 live births; higher in males, whites, and Asians
    b. Cleft palate: 1:2500, higher in females
3. Cause: often unknown, multifactorial inheritance, chromosomal abnormalities, maternal alcohol or drug ingestion, prenatal infection
4. Surgical treatment: cleft *lip* is usually repaired (by Z-plasty surgical technique) within the first 3 months of life if the infant is demonstrating steady weight gain and is free from infection; early correction is important for nutrition and cosmetic purposes; cleft *palate* repair is usually delayed until 12-18 months of age to allow for bone growth and changes in contour of palate

Nursing Process
Assessment
1. Infant's ability to suck and and swallow (will depend on type and extent of defect)
2. Nutritional status
3. Parents' reaction to birth of an infant with a facial defect

Analysis (see p. 493)
Planning, Implementation, and Evaluation

> **Goal 1:** Preoperatively, child will maintain adequate nutrition and will not aspirate fluids.

Implementation
1. Feed slowly in upright position; use one of the following
    a. Soft nipple with large or cross-cut opening

b. Asepto syringe (bulb syringe with rubber catheter tubing attached)

c. Cup for older infant with cleft palate

2. For palate cleft infants with be careful not to place nipple inside cleft.

3. Burp frequently.

4. Rinse mouth with water after feedings to keep lip/palate cleansed.

5. Teach parents how to feed and burp infant.

6. Teach parents use and care of palate prosthesis.

Evaluation

Child ingests adequate fluids and calories; is free from aspiration and lip/palate infections.

Goal 2: Postoperatively, child will maintain a patent airway.

Implementation

1. Observe for respiratory distress; assist in respiratory effort by positioning child to facilitate breathing; aspirate oral secretions *gently* from the sides of the mouth.

2. Cleft palate: place in mist tent.

3. Position infant to provide for drainage of mucus and to prevent trauma to suture lines.

a. Cleft lip repair: on side or in infant seat

b. Cleft palate repair: on side or abdomen

4. Keep oxygen and suction equipment at bedside; suction only if assessment reveals signs of airway obstruction.

Evaluation

Child has patent airway and adequate oxygenation; has no signs of respiratory distress.

Goal 3: Postoperatively, child will be free from trauma and infection of suture lines.

Implementation

1. Monitor vital signs including temperature every 4 hours.

2. Minimize crying by holding and soothing infant as needed do not use pacifiers.

3. Put elbow restraints on child; remove *one at a time* q2h for ROM exercises.

4. Position as stated above.

5. Maintain Logan bar (a metal-wire arch) on upper lip to decrease tension o suture line.

6. Cleanse suture lines after feeding with sterile swabs and solution (usually diluted hydrogen peroxide) as ordered to limit crusting and inflammation

a. For cleft lip repair: *roll* applicator without rubbing

b. For cleft palate repair: rinse mouth with sterile water after feeding

7. Apply antibiotic ointment to lip suture line as prescribed.

8. Encourage parents to stay with infant and participate in care.

Evaluation

Child has healing of suture lines without trauma and scarring associated with infection.

Goal 4: Postoperatively, child will ingest adequate nutrition.

Implementation

1. Feed with medicine dropper, Asepto syringe (cleft lip), or cup (cleft palate); *no sucking,* straws, or spoons to prevent trauma to suture line.

2. For children with cleft palate repair, give soft diet high in calories and protein (encourage milkshakes and pudding); avoid hard foods such as toast or cookies.

Evaluation

Child takes food and fluids (appropriate for age); is free from choking or aspiration.

Goal 5: Child and parents will be referred for ongoing, long-term intervention and promotion of optimum development.

Implementation

1. Teach parents signs of otitis media (fever, turning head to side, pulling at ear, discharge from ear, pain, or crying); encourage parents to seek medical treatment for upper respiratory infections.

2. Refer for regular evaluation of child's hearing, speech, and dental development.

3. Help parents to express feelings and concerns about defect and surgery.

4. Refer parents to community resources.

a. Parent groups; local and state cleft-palate associations

b. Crippled Children's Services or social services

Evaluation

Parents list early signs of ear infections and when to seek treatment; child has no permanent hearing loss; has age-appropriate language development, intelligible speech, and normal tooth alignment; parents and child receive community support (emotional, financial, and social).

☐ Congenital Hypothyroidism
General Information

1. Definition: congenital condition in which the fetal thyroid fails to develop, resulting in inadequate levels of T_4 and other thyroid hormones in the fetus and newborn; also called cretinism; early diagnosis is essential to prevent mental retardation

2. Incidence: one of the most common endocrine problems of childhood; 1 in every 4500 live births; twice as common in females and in males; higher incidence in Down syndrome
3. Pathophysiology: thyroid hormones have a stimulating effect on metabolic rate, heart production, cardiac output, and growth of almost all tissues; lack of these hormones specifically affects brain, bone, and muscle growth in infants
4. Diagnosis
   a. Elevated serum TSH and decreased T_4 levels in early days of life; screening is mandatory in most state
   b. Decreased uptake of radioactive iodine by thyroid after oral administration of isotope
5. Causes
   a. Hypoplasia or aplasia of thyroid gland
   b. Pituitary dysfunction
   c. Unresponsiveness of tissue to existing thyroid hormones
   d. Autoimmune destruction of the thyroid (juvenile hypothyroidism)
6. Medical treatment: thyroid replacement as soon as diagnosis is suspected
   a. Levothyroxine (Synthroid), 0.006 mg/kg/day or desiccated thyroid (Proloid), 4 mg/kg/day; adjusted according to clinical symptoms and T_4 level
      1. doses in children usually *higher* than adult doses
      2. given as a single dose in morning
      3. replacement is a lifelong necessity
   b. Side effects of excessive dosage: dyspnea, tachycardia, fever, irritability, tremors, diarrhea, weight loss, and sleep disturbance

Nursing Process

Assessment
1. Prolonged gestation and high birth weight
2. Puffy face with coarse features
3. Wide fontanels and sutures
4. Flattened nasal bridge
5. Low anterior hairline
6. Described as "good, quiet baby"
7. Hoarse, weak cry
8. Lethargy and excessive sleeping, resulting in poor feeding
9. Poor abdominal muscle tone; constipation
10. Weak reflexes
11. Large, protruding tongue
12. Cold, mottled skin (hypothermia: 95° F or less)
13. Delayed cognitive and motor development
14. Delayed physical growth
15. Prolonged physiological jaundice
16. Delayed passage of meconium
17. Respiratory distress
18. See also "Hypothyroidism," p. 178

Analysis (see p. 493)
Planning, Implementation, and Evaluation

Goal 1: Child's condition will be identified at the earliest possible stage.

Implementation
1. Screen all children before discharge from the hospital or within first week of life.
2. Be alert to earliest clinical manifestations and parental comments (e.g., "She is such a good baby, she hardly ever cries").
3. Educate and support parents during diagnostic tests.
Evaluation
Infant if diagnosed within first several weeks of life; replacement therapy begins.

Goal 2: Child will experience normal growth and development.

Implementation
1. Provide information to family about condition.
2. Encourage expression of concerns about child's behavior and development.
3. If diagnosis is delayed, explore possible guilt feelings and discuss probability of mental retardation.
4. Teach parents about medication administration, side effects, need for lifelong administration.
   a. Do not change brands without physician knowledge since hormone content varies.
   b. Store in dry, dark place.
   c. Measure pulse daily before administration (indication of drug effectiveness).
   d. Teach importance of regular, consistent administration of medication.
   e. If a dose is missed, give twice the dose the next day.
   f. Look for signs of overdose (e.g., dyspnea, fever, diaphoresis, irritability, and rapid pulse).
5. Teach parents how to measure pulse rate; consult physician if pulse is above normal range (see Table 5-1).
6. Monitor child's growth and development periodically.
7. Refer family to community support groups if needed.
Evaluation
Child is alert, active; grows normally; development continues within normal range; parents and child assume self-care responsibilities.

☐ Insulin-Dependent Diabetes Mellitus (IDD: Type I)
General Information

1. Definition: metabolic disease of unknown inheritance mechanism that results in insulin deficiency because of reduction in pancreatic islet cell mass or destruction of islets and consequent alterations of carbohydrate, fat, and protein metabolism; also results in long-term

Table 5-20 Comparison of Type I (insulin-dependent) and Type II (non–insulin-dependent) diabetes mellitus

	Type I	Type II
CHARACTERISTICS		
Age of onset	Usually less than 20 years (peaks: 5-7 years; puberty)	Usually over 35 years
Type of onset	Abrupt	Gradual
Nutritional status	Underweight	Overweight
Symptoms	Polydipsia, polyuria, polyphagia	May be none
Remission	Yes (honeymoon period)	No
Plasma insulin	Absent	Usually decreased
MANAGEMENT		
Medication	Insulin only	Oral hypoglycemics frequently used
Meal planning	Free or exchange	Exchange
Self-monitoring	Blood glucose monitoring preferred; when testing urine, use Clinitest; first-voided specimen acceptable	Blood glucose monitoring preferred; when testing urine use Tes-Tape or Clinitest on second voided specimen
Hypoglycemia	Oral sugars and glucagon (for severe reactions)	Oral sugars only

alterations in vascular, nervous, renal, and ocular systems; damage to other organ systems may be related to degree of control of diabetes (see Table 5-20 for comparison with adult-onset diabetes)

2. Theories of etiology
   a. Viral infection (e.g., mumps, coxsackievirus): stress of the illness may decrease glucose tolerance and precipitate onset of IDD
   b. Genetic inheritance
   c. Autoimmune disease child produces antibodies that destroy the islet cells of the pancrease)
3. Pathophysiology: refer to "Diabetes mellitus," p. 183
4. Medical treatment
   a. Medication
      1. insulin therapy: human insulin usually recommended because of limited antigenicity, decreased dosage, increased solubility, and increased absorption
         a. dosage: 0.5-1.0 U/kg/day (usually in 2 divided doses)
         b. refer to Table 3-34, p. 184
      2. oral hypoglycemics: not used with children
   b. Meal plan: more flexible nutrition options than with adults; most commonly used are free (no concentrated sweets, exchange, and basic four food groups (usually three meals and three snacks a day); prudent fat intake
5. Modifying factors
   a. Puberty
      1. onset complicates control by increasing insulin demands (growth is stimulated by gonadal steroids, which antagonize isulin action; larger doses of insulin usually needed)
      2. asociated growth significantly increases caloric needs

   b. Exercise
      1. reduces insulin requirements because glucose is catabolized without insulin during muscular activity
      2. increases risk of insulin shock if an extra snack is not provided before vigorous exercise
   c. Illness and emotional disturbance
      1. lessens ability to use glucose
      2. may increase insulin requirements because of decreased activity
   d. Alcohol and drug usage (common problem in adolescents)
      1. alcohol suppresses gluconeogenesis, which may recipitate hypoglycemia
      2. stimulant drugs (e.g., cocaine and amphetamines) increase metabolism and decrease appetite, which may results in hypoglycemia

Nursing Process

Assessment
1. Initial
   a. Polydipsia, polyphagia, polyuria (bedwetting): classic signs
   b. Weight loss
   c. Irritability, fatigue
   d. Abdominal discomfort
   e. May be mistaken for influenza, gastroenteritis
   f. Frequent infections, slow-to-heal skin injuries
2. Often characterized by remission or honeymoon period
   a. Common in children with IDD
   b. Decreased amounts of insulin required
   c. Occurs once, lasting a few weeks up to a year
3. Diabetic ketoacidosis (DKA): polydipsia, polyphagia,

polyuria, dehydration with possible hypovolemic shock, nausea and vomiting, acetone breath, Kussmaul's respiration, flushed dry skin (children with DKA for the first time often show signs of abdominal pain and rigidity, which may mimic appendicitis); refer to Table 3-36

4. Hypoglycemia: irritability, trembling; apprehension; headache; hunger, blurred vision; mental confusion; sweating, pallor seizures (more likely in infants and children); temper tantrums (common in toddlers)

Analysis (see p. 493)

Planning, Implementation, and Evaluation

> **Goal:** Child and parents will be prepared for home management.

Implementation

1. Teach blood glucose monitoring (preferred self-monitoring method).
   a. Finger-stick technique
   b. Importance of exact timing
   c. Variation among different products (use same product for consistency and accuracy)
   d. Importance of checking expiration dates
   e. Four measurements per day (before each meal and bedtime snack)
   f. Interpretation of results
   g. Importance of record keeping
2. Contact community resources for financial assistance as needed for blood glucose monitoring at home.
   a. Medicaid coverage in some states
   b. Local diabetes association
   c. Rentals available
   d. Private insurance
3. Demonstrate urine testing for glucose and acetone (to be done if blood glucose level is greater than 240 mg); 2- to 5-drop Clinitest preferred; first-voided specimens used because of difficulty in obtaining second-voided specimens in children.
4. Teach insulin administration.
   a. Knowledge of medication
   b. Proper mixing
   c. Injection technique
   d. Rotation of sites
   e. Use of insulin pump when indicated
5. Involve dietitian with nutrition planning; adjust meal plans for activity and growth with periodic reassessment at least every 6 months.
6. Teach management of hyperglycemia.
   a. Recognition of early signs and symptoms
   b. Importance of good control
   c. Food, activity, and insulin adjustment to improve control
7. Teach management of hypoglycemia: ingest a rapidly absorbed glucose-containing food or liquid,

such as 4 oz of orange juice, 2 teaspoonfuls of honey, 5-6 Life Savers (chewed); for the unconscious child with a severe reaction, squeeze glucose gel or cake frosting between the child's cheek and gums and administer glucagon subcutaneously (raises blood glucose level by stimulating the release of glucose from glycogen stores in the liver).

8. Demonstrate foot care: same as adult except bare feet acceptable.
9. Prepare parents for developmental concerns with respect to management.
   a. For toddlers and preschoolers
      1. inform parents of major concerns (finger sticks and injections threaten body integrity; fears of loss of control and autonomy)
      2. encourage parents to offer choices when possible
      3. prepare parents for finicky eating habits and assist in meal planning
      4. teach parents how to recognize hypoglycemia and hyperglycemia
      5. encourage parents to involve child in creative play to allow expression of fears and emotions
   b. For school-age children
      1. inform school, teacher, and peers about symptoms/treatment
      2. arrange for child to participate in gym classes and sports, adjusting medication as needed
      3. anticipate nutrition needs of lunches, parties, and holidays
      4. feelings of being different
   c. For adolescents
      1. discuss feelings and concerns about future: career, marriage, and pregnancy
      2. acting-out behaviors (anticipate and prevent)
      3. onset of puberty, changes in body image
      4. discuss the effects of drugs, alcohol, and birth control pills on blood glucose levels
10. Teach self-management as appropriate.
    a. At 6 to 8 years: assisting with urine tests, injections, diet selection, and blood glucose measurement
    b. At 8 to 9 years: physical readiness; teach to do urine tests, injections, and blood glucose monitoring
    c. At 12 to 13 years and beyond: cognitive readiness; teach meal planning, how to maintain food, activity, and insulin balance
11. Develop an exercise program that allows for optimal growth and development.
12. Advise child and parents of need to obtain and wear medical-alert identification.

Evaluation

Child and parents incorporate necessary skills to daily routine; child does not have recurrent episodes of ketoacidosis or hypoglycemia; continues normal growth and development.

☐ Cystic Fibrosis (CF)
General Information

1. Definition: an inherited multisystem disorder characterized by widespread dysfunction of the exocrine glands (those whose secretions reach an epithelial surface, either directly or through a duct)
2. Cause and occurrence: autosomal recessive disorder (both parents are carriers: see Fig. 5-3); most common genetic defect in white children; approximately 1 in 2000 live births; 1 in 20 persons estimated to be a carrier
3. Pathophysiology: abnormal secretion of thick tenacious mucus by the exocrine glands causes obstruction and results in varying degress of pathology
   a. *Pulmonary effects:* depressed respiratory-cilia cells result in increased infection, bronchiole obstruction, and eventually pulmonary fibrosis; child ultimately develops chronic obstructive pulmonary disease; may progress to cor pulmonale; death can occur from respiratory infection or heart failure
   b. *Pancrease effects:* pancreatic fibrosis and eventual decrease of digestive enzymes (lipase, amylase, and trypsin) resulting in severe malnutrition and failure to thrive; steatorrhea: fatty, bulky, foul-smelling stools that float because of undigested fat cells; also can affect pancreatic endocrine functions, resulting in hyperglycemia, glucosuria, and ultimately requiring insulin replacement (occurs late in the disease process)
   c. *Salivary effects:* fibrosis and enlargement of glands caused by thickened secretions; elevated sodium and chloride in saliva
   d. *Sweat gland effects:* elevated sodium and chloride in sweat
   e. *Reproductive effects*
      1. males: inability to produce sperm; the semen is thickened and tenacious; it plugs the ducts in the testes, resulting in fibrosis; males are generally sterile but not impotent
      2. females: difficult to conceive because cervical plug cannot be penetrated by normal sperm
   f. *Hepatic effects:* bile secreted by the liver to emulsify fat in the duodenum is thickened (inspissated) and may plug liver ductules, resulting in biliary cirrhosis and jaundice; can lead to esophageal varices; (in newborn and infant, condition may be misdiagnosed as biliary atresia)
4. Medical treatment
   a. Diagnostic testing
      1. prenatal diagosis: DNA analysis of chorionic villi samples; DNA or enzyme analysis of amniotic fluid samples
      2. postnatal diagnosis: pilocarpine electrophoresis (sweat chloride test)
         a. normal sweat chloride values: less than 40 mEq/L
         b. suggestive of CF: 40-60 mEq/L
         c. diagnostic of CF: greater than 60 mEq/L
   b. Medication
      1. pancreatic enzymes by mouth (Pancrease, Cotazym-S: preparations that resist destruction by stomach acids)
      2. fat-soluble vitamins A, D, E, and K in water-miscible form
      3. "high-dose" antibiotics for respiratory infections: penicillins and aminoglycosides (ticarcillin, piperacillin, tobramycin); NOTE: with aminoglycoside therapy, toxic effects include renal toxicity and ototoxicity
      4. stool softeners, when necessary, for constipation
      5. NaCl tablets added to diet in hot weather, during febrile illness, or strenuous activity; liberal dietary salt encouraged
      6. oral iron supplements
   c. Oxygen therapy, aerosols, nebulizers, bronchodilators
   d. Percussion, postural drainage, and breathing exercises
   e. Sweat chloride testing or gene-marker studies of other family members along with genetic counseling

Nursing Process
Assessment
1. Effects of mucous gland involvement
   a. Dry, paroxysmal cough
   b. Wheezing
   c. Barrel-shaped chest as child grows older
   d. Cyanosis and clubbing of child's fingers and toes as a result of hypoxia from chronic pulmonary disease
   e. Thick, mucoid, tenacious pulmonary secretions expectorated following chest physical therapy
   f. Since GI tract has a mucoid lining, newborn is at risk of meconium ileus (failure to pass meconium; impacted meconium causes bowel obstruction); older children are also at risk of bowel obstruction caused by fecal impactions
2. Effects of pancreatic involvement
   a. Abdominal distension
   b. Ravenous appetite
   c. Small stature
   d. Delayed puberty
   e. Decreased subcutaneous tissue
   f. Pale, transparent skin
   g. Easy fatigability
   h. Malaise
   i. Fatty, bulky, foul-smelling stools
   j. Rectal prolapse
3. Child tastes "salty" when kissed
Analysis (see p. 493)

Planning, Implementation, and Evaluation

> **Goal 1:** Child will maintain effective airway clearance and remain free from pulmonary complications.

Implementation

1. Teach parents how to administer nebulizer treatment with prescribed solution and carry out percussion and postural drainage at least twice daily, including on arising and at bedtime; discourage treatments immediately before or after meals.
   a. Percussion and postural drainage are carreid out before and after nebulizer treatment.
   b. Nebulizer solution usually contains beonchodilators and saline; mucolytics rarely used.
2. Teach child and family correct administration of medications (antibiotics, bronchodilators, expectorants).
3. Teach child breathing exercises (done after postural drainage).
4. Encourage child to engage in physical activities (e.g., swimming, gymnastics, or baseball).
5. Teach child and family general health measures to prevent respiratory infections (e.g, immunizations on time avoid crowds and people with URIs, prevent chilling, no smoking in the home, provide proper nutrition).
6. Observe and record sputum amount, color, and consistency.
7. Review social implications of sputum by age.
   a. 2-year-olds and under cannot expectorate.
   b. *Socially unacceptable for older children to spit, especially for teenage with beginning sexual identity and relationships.*
   c. Review with older children how to take care of bad breath.
   d. If tetracycline given, warn that it stains teeth.

Evaluation

Child and parents implement daily pulmonary therapies; child is free from respiratory infections or they are detected and treated early and vigorously; maintains optimal ventilation.

> **Goal 2:** Child will maintain adequate nutritional and electrolyte intake.

Implementation

1. Give pancreatic enzymes as ordered.
   a. Dosage; individualized
   b. Side effects nausea, vomiting, and gastric irritation
   c. Just before meals to assist digestion
   d. Do not crush enteric-coated preparations
   e. Capsules may be opened and sprinkled on food
   f. Mix with pureed fruit for infants; older children can swallow capsules
   g. Antacid may be prescribed concurrently
   h. Monitor I&O, appetite, quality of stools, and weight
2. Encourage intake of balanced nutrition high in protein and carbohydrate (use supplements such as Carnation Instant Breakfast or Sustacal); give snacks with high food value preceded by appropriate amounts of enzymes (these children have additional protein and caloric requirements); fats should be unsaturated.
3. Administer water-miscible vitamins daily.
4. Encourage child to assume responsibility for healthy food selection.

Evaluation

Child's nutritonal intake is adequate to meet growth needs.

> **Goal 3:** Child and parents will learn to cope with the chronicity of cystic fibrosis.

Implementation

1. Encourage and permit child and parents to express their feelings regarding diagnosis and its effects, and prognosis.
2. Discourage parents from overprotecting child and interfering with normal developmental processes.
3. Provide ongoing support and teaching as disease progresses.
4. Encourage hcild to assume age-appropriate responsiblity for care to increase feelings of control.
5. Provide positive reinforcement to enhance child's self-esteem.
6. Plan exercise program that allows for optimal growth and development.
7. Refer for genetic counseling: essential for persons wtih CF and all family members.
8. Support family in decision to seek genetic counseling.
9. Refer to community supoprt groups and Cystic Fibrosis Foundation.

Evaluation

Child and parents verbalize their feelings about the disease; show adaptive behaviors; and seek genetic counseling and community support groups.

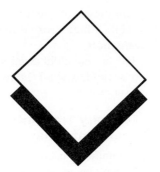

Elimination

GENERAL CONCEPTS
Overview/Physiology

1. Urinary elimination
   a. Kidney development is not complete until approximately 1 year of age
   b. Immature functioning of nephrons; poor filtration and absorption during first year of life; ability to concentrate urine increases gradually during first year of life
   c. Urinary bladder is an abdominal organ during infancy; as pelvic shape changes, the bladder gradually settles and becomes a pelvic organ
   d. Average daily urine output
      1. newborn: 150-300 ml
      2. infant: 400-500 ml
      3. 1-6 years: 500-700 ml
      4. 6-15 years: 700-1400 ml
2. Bowel elimination
   a. Large and small intestines serve as the major organs for detoxification during infancy while the liver and kidneys are maturing
   b. Development of digestive processes is complete by the early toddler years
3. Voluntary control of elimination
   a. Myelinization of the spinal cord is complete by 18-24 months of age, resulting in capacity for voluntary control of urinary and anal sphincters
   b. Bladder capacity increases (greater in girls than in boys) as voluntary control is achieved

Application of the Nursing Process to the Child with Elimination Problems
Assessment

1. Nursing history
   a. Voiding patterns: day and night; frequency; color, clarity, and estimated amount of urine output; recent changes or problems (e.g., nocturia, urgency, dysuria, or infections)
   b. Bowel elimination patterns: frequency, consistency, and color; recent changes or problems (e.g., diarrhea, constipation, or abdominal cramping)

   c. Alterations in elimination: neurogenic bowel and bladder, ostomy, enuresis, encopresis; problem management; medications (e.g., urinary antiseptics, laxatives, antidiarrheal drugs)
2. Clinical appraisal
   a. Observation of urine and stool
   b. Palpation and auscultation of abdomen and bladder (normally nonpalpable), including bowel sounds (all quadrants)
3. Diagnostic tests (refer to *Nursing Care of the Adult*, p. 194)

Analysis

1. Safe, effective care environment
   a. High risk for infection
   b. High risk for impaired skin integrity
2. Physiological integrity
   a. Activity intolerance
   b. High risk for fluid volume deficit/excess
   c. Constipation
   d. Altered patterns of urinary elimination
   e. Altered tissue perfusion
3. Psychosocial integrity
   a. Body image disturbance
4. Health promotion/maintenance
   a. Altered family processes
   b. Knowledge deficit

General Nursing Planning, Implementation, and Evaluation (see Selected Health Problems)

SELECTED HEALTH PROBLEMS RESULTING IN AN INTERFERENCE WITH URINARY OR BOWEL ELIMINATION

☐ Hypospadias
General Information

1. Definition: congenital abnormality in which urethral opening is located behind the glans penis or lies on the ventral surface of penis; frequently associated with chordee, which results in a downward curve of penis
2. Medical treatment
   a. Surgical intervention to provide normal function

and appearance (usually two or three surgeries)
1. urethroplasty: skin grafting to extend urethra and surgically construct a new urinary meatus
2. surgical release of chordee
   b. Circumcision is contraindicated, since foreskin may be needed for reconstructive surgery

Nursing Process
Assessment

1. Abnormal placement of urethral meatus
2. Abnormal urine stream
3. Associated problems
   a. Chordee
   b. Undescended testes

Analysis (see p. 505)

Planning, Implementation, and Evaluation

> **Goal 1:** Child will maintain integrity of surgical repair.

Implementation

1. Check pressure dressing for evidence of bleeding and to ensure intact dressing.
2. Monitor function of urinary diversion apparatus (permits urine to bypass the operative site).
   a. Foley catheter
   b. Suprapubic tube
   c. Perineal urethrotomy
3. Check for adequate circulation to tip of penis.
4. Observe for difficulties following catheter removal.
   a. Inability to void
   b. Painful voiding (dysuria)
   c. Urinary tract infection
   d. Hematuria
   e. Frequency
5. Prevent trauma to surgical site.

Evaluation

Child voids normally; maintains dry and intact surgical dressing and site.

> **Goal 2:** Parents and child will experience minimal mutilation fears; will cope with altered body image.

Implementation

1. Identify defect in infancy to allow complete surgical repair before 5-6 years of age (preferred age: 6-18 months).
2. Encourage child to express mutilation fears through play before surgery.
3. Reinforce that surgery is to repair anomaly child was born with and is not punishment for sex play or masturbation.
4. Prepare parents and child for appearance after surgery.
5. Encourage child to examine surgical site after repair to minimize castration anxiety.

6. Encourage expression of parental concerns about child's future sexual functioning.

Evaluation

Parents and child discuss surgical outcome in positive terms; child expresses, through play, appropriate reasons for surgery.

☐ Urinary Tract Infection
General Information

1. Definition: bacteriuria with or without signs and symptoms of inflammation of the urinary bladder or kidneys, resulting in risk of renal damage; *E. coli* most common infecting organism
2. Incidence: 1%-2% of the childhood population; girls have a 10-30 times greater risk than boys because of short female urethra close to vagina and anus (5% of girls have a urinary tract infection by age 18); peak age is 2-6 years
3. Predisposing factors
   a. Poor perineal hygiene, prolonged use of a single diaper (especially disposable diapers)
   b. Tight-fitting clothing (e.g., blue jeans)
   c. Ureteral reflux caused by congenital malposition of ureters
   d. Concurrent vaginitis or pinworms
   e. Neurogenic bladder
   f. Concentrated and alkaline urine
4. Medical treatment
   a. Antibiotic therapy: usually ampicillin, cefaclor (Ceclor), amoxicillin, or sulfonamides (e.g., Bactrim, Septra) for short, intensive treatment, 10-14 days
   b. Longer-term urinary antiseptic therapy: nitrofurantoin (Furadantin) or methenamine mandelate (Mandelamine) to maintain sterility of urine
   c. Surgical correction of congenital malposition of ureters (ureteral reimplantation) to correct reflux

Nursing Process
Assessment

1. Frequency, urgency, dysuria, dribbling, enuresis
2. Foul-smelling urine
3. Lower abdominal pain
4. Nausea, poor feeding, lethargy
5. Fever, chills, flank pain (all usually indicate an acute infection of the upper urinary tract)

Analysis (see p. 505)

Planning, Implementation, and Evaluation

> **Goal 1:** Child's urinary tract infection will be detected and treated early.

Implementation

1. Ensure that child receives annual routine urinalysis (especially girls, ages 2-6 years).
2. Provide age-appropriate preparation of child for in-

trusive diagnostic tests (usually done under general anesthesia).

3. Emphasize importance of full course of antibiotic therapy and continuing antiseptics even when child has no signs of infection.
4. Emphasize necessity of follow-up urine culture after antibiotic therapy completed.

Evaluation

Child is free from urinary tract infection; has no recurrence.

> **Goal 2:** Child and parents will be knowledgeable about prevention of urinary tract infection.

Implementation

1. Teach good hygiene measures.
   a. Wipe front to back.
   b. Avoid bubble baths.
   c. Wear loose-fitting clothing and cotton panties.
2. Caution child not to "hold" urine, but to void as soon as urge is felt.
3. Teach child to empty bladder completely with each voiding.
4. Advise an increase in daily fluid intake, especially fluids that acidify urine (e.g., apple and cranberry juice).

Evaluation

Child is free from urinary tract infection; uses appropriate hygiene measures; empties bladder with each voiding; child's daily fluid intake is adequate.

☐ Vesicoureteral Reflux (VUR)
General Information

1. Definition: retrograde flow of bladder urine into the ureters; increases the chance for infection
2. Causes
   a. Primary; results from congenitally abnormal insertion of the ureters into the bladder
   b. Secondary: occurs as a result of infection or a neurogenic bladder
3. Peak age: 46% of infants younger than 23 months with urinary tract infections and 9% of children 24-60 months of age with urinary tract infections exhibit VUR
4. Medical treatment
   a. Continuous, low-dose antibiotic therapy (nitrofurantoin and trimethoprim-sulfamethoxazole)
   b. Frequent urine cultures
   c. Surgical intervention (ureteral reimplantation is the procedure of choice)

Nursing Process
Assessment

1. Reflux of urine into kidneys
2. Chronic urinary tract infections
3. Associated problems

Analysis (see p. 505)
Planning, Implementation, and Evaluation

> **Goal 1:** Child will be free from infection.

Implementation

1. Monitor vital signs.
2. Encourage fluid intake.
3. Monitor urine cultures.

Evaluation

Child is afebrile, has no complaints of dysuria.

> **Goal 2:** Child will maintain integrity of surgical repair.

Implementation

1. Check dressing for intactness and evidence of bleeding.
2. Monitor function of urinary diversion apparatus (suprapubic catheter and left and right ureteral catheters or stent).
3. Monitor separate outputs from each catheter (suprapubic catheter will contain gross blood immediately following surgery).
4. Check bed, cradle, and 4-point restraints if used to prevent trauma.
5. Hydrate with IV or oral fluids.
6. Administer postoperative antibiotics as ordered.
7. Observe for difficulties following catheter removal (removed separately beginning 5-10 days postoperatively).

Evaluation

The child has clean, dry wound; maintains patency of suprapubic catheter.

> **Goal 3:** Child will not retain urine.

Implementation

1. Encourage child to void in a continuous stream and to empty bladder completely.
2. Observe and record amount, color, and frequency of each voided specimen.

Evaluation

Child empties bladder completely with each void.

> **Goal 4:** Child and parents will understand methods to prevent problems.

Implementation

1. Teach child and family correct administration of antibiotics.
2. Teach regarding general health measures to prevent urinary tract infections. (e.g., no bubble baths, empty bladder completely).

Evaluation

Child and parents list and follow measures to prevent further infections.

☐ Nephritis
General Information

1. Definition: acute glomerulonephritis (AGN) is an immune complex disease that occurs as a reaction to the group-A beta-hemolytic *Streptococcus;* it causes inflammation and transient damage to the glomerulus; there is a latent period of 10-14 days between the streptococcal infection and the onset of symptoms (see Table 5-21)
2. Incidence: peak age is 6-7 years; history of URI, scarlet fever, or impetigo 1-3 weeks before the onset of symptoms; two times higher incidence in boys
3. Medical treatment
   a. Bed rest until hypertension and hematuria subside
   b. Medication
      1. antibiotics (penicillin) to eradicate streptococcal infection (indicated by an elevated antistreptolysin-O [ASO] titer)
      2. antihypertensives and diuretics to control BP (diuretics are of limited value since they do not reach the distal tubules)
      3. digitalis (with congestive heart failure)
      4. anticonvulsants (with hypertensive encephalopathy)
   c. Diet
      1. fluid restriction for cardiac failure or anuria
      2. moderate sodium restriction
      3. low potassium until urine output is normal
      4. regular protein

Nursing Process
Assessment
1. Moderate edema
2. Elevated BP
3. Moderate proteinuria (rarely seen)
4. Gross hematuria

5. Elevated serum K^+
6. Mild hypoproteinemia
7. Elevated urine specific gravity
8. ASO titer

Analysis (see p. 505)
Planning, Implementation, and Evaluation

> **Goal 1:** Child will be free from infection and hematuria.

Implementation
1. Monitor temperature.
2. Keep child away from infected persons.
3. Administer antibiotics as ordered.
4. Teach parents administration, action, and side effects of medications.
5. Record frequency of urinary output; test each voided specimen for occult blood.
6. Measure I&O.
7. Restrict fluids if anuria is present.

Evaluation
Child has vital signs and lab values within normal ranges; has normal urine output.

> **Goal 2:** Child will regain and maintain good nutrition within dietary limitations.

Implementation
1. Offer regular diet or low-protein and low-sodium diet if ordered.
2. Offer small, frequent, attractive meals.
3. Restrict fluids if anuria is present.
4. Restrict high-potassium foods during oliguria.

Evaluation
Child ingests a diet adequate for age.

Table 5-21 Comparison of nephrosis and nephritis

	Nephrosis	Nephritis/inflammatory
GENERAL INFORMATION	*Chronic* condition	*Acute* condition
	Unknown cause	Caused by antigen-antibody response to group-A beta-hemolytic streptococci
PEAK AGE	2-3 years (toddler)	6 years (school-age)
MEDICATIONS	Prednisone	Antibiotic therapy; possibly antihypertensives and diuretics
DIET	High potassium	Low potassium until urine output normal
ASSESSMENT		
Edema	Massive	Moderate, usually facial and periorbital
Blood pressure	Normal	Elevated
Proteinuria	Massive	Moderate
Hematuria	Microscopic	Gross
Serum K^+	Normal	Elevated
Hypoproteinemia	Marked	Mild
Hyperlipidemia	Present	Absent

Goal 3: Child will maintain normal tissue perfusion.

Implementation
1. Monitor vital signs, especially BP.
2. Monitor urinary output.
3. Observe skin color.
4. Assess changes in edema by weighing daily.
5. Monitor arterial pulses.
6. Administer antihypertensives as ordered.
7. Keep environment calm.

Evaluation
Child is free from renal failure or cardiac decompensation; maintains BP within normal range.

Goal 4: Child and family will be prepared for home care.

Implementation
1. Let family verbalize concerns.
2. Refer to support groups as necessary.
3. Teach the family about
   a. Urine testing
   b. Side effects of drugs
   c. Diet therapies
4. Plan follow-up care.
5. Obtain throat cultures of each family member to check for streptococcal infections.

Evaluation
Child and family accurately describe discharge instructions in their own words.

☐ Nephrosis
General Information
1. Definition: a chronic condition characterized by glomerular membrane permeability to proteins, especially albumin; also called nephrotic syndrome (see Table 5-21)
2. Causes
   a. Idiopathic (80% of cases)
   b. Congenital
   c. Drug toxicity
   d. Sequelae of various diseases
3. Peak age: 2-5 years; 60% of those affected are boys
4. Medical treatment
   a. Activity as tolerated unless edematous, then bed rest
   b. Medication
      1. prednisone to reduce proteinuria and edema, to induce remission, to produce diuresis
         a. dosage is 2 mg/kg/day until urine is free from protein
         b. side effects: immunosuppression, potassium loss, gastric ulcer, hypertension, growth failure, and Cushing's syndrome
      c. nursing implications
         ◆ taper dose gradually to avoid adrenal insufficiency
         ◆ administer with meals or milk to minimize gastric irritation
         ◆ monitor fluid balance
         ◆ protect from infection
      2. antibiotics to decrease risk of infection
      3. IV salt-poor albumin during acute phase
   c. Diet
      1. fluid and sodium restriction if edema present
      2. high protein, high potassium

Nursing Process
Assessment
1. Insidious weight gain
2. Severe edema
   a. Periorbital, facial
   b. Generalized: feet, scrotal/labial, ascites
3. Respiratory difficulty because of pleural effusion
4. Oliguria, increased urine specific gravity
5. Massive proteinuria
6. Marked hypoproteinemia
7. Hyperlipidemia
8. Irritability
9. Increased susceptibility to infection
10. Anorexia
11. Diarrhea

Analysis (see p. 505)
Planning, Implementation, and Evaluation

Goal 1: Child will be free from infection and skin breakdown.

Implementation
1. Monitor vital signs and lab values.
2. Keep child away from infected persons.
3. Administer antibiotics as ordered.
4. Give medications by mouth if possible.
5. Teach parents administration, action, and side effects of medications.
6. Give good skin care.
7. Support edematous organs (if needed, support scrotum with pillows or a rolled towel).
8. Change body position often.
9. Cleanse edematous eyelids with saline wipes.
10. Place in a semi-Fowler's position to facilitate breathing.
11. Handle gently with any movement.

Evaluation
Child has intact skin; has normal vital signs, lab values.

Goal 2: Child will conserve energy and play quiet activities suitable for age.

Implementation
1. Balance rest and activities; maintain bed rest with edema.
2. Provide quiet activities for age.
3. Observe for fatigue.
4. Explain reasons for bed rest.

Evaluation
Child tolerates play activities without fatigue.

Goal 3: Child will maintain fluid balance.

Implementation
1. Measure I&O; weigh diapers.
2. Weigh and measure abdominal girth daily.
3. Assess changes in edema each shift.
4. Limit fluids if necessary.

Evaluation
Child has no generalized edema or increased abdominal girth; maintains urine output, balanced I&O.

Goal 4: Child will maintain nutritional intake.

Implementation
1. Offer high-protein, high-carbohydrate, high-potassium diet.
2. Restrict sodium intake if edematous.
3. Serve small, frequent, attractive meals.

Evaluation
Child eats an adequate diet for age (within dietary restrictions).

Goal 5: Child will accept body changes.

Implementation
1. Provide feedback to child about body changes; reassure as needed.
2. Encourage child to verbalize feelings about body changes.
3. Teach child that changes are caused by medications and will diminish when medications are discontinued.

Evaluation
Child expresses feeling about body changes, capitalizes on positive aspects of self, looks forward to discontinuing medications.

Goal 6: Child and family will be prepared for home care.

Implementation
1. Let family verbalize concerns.
2. Refer to support groups as needed.
3. Teach about
   a. Urine testing
   b. Side effects of drugs
   c. Prevention of infection
   d. Diet therapies

4. Maintain follow-up contact with the family.

Evaluation
Child and family describe discharge instructions correctly.

☐ Lower GI Tract Obstruction
General Information

1. Definitions
   a. *Intussusception:* telescoping of one portion of intestine into another, usually involving ileocecal valve, resulting in obstruction of blood supply with ischemia and death of telescoped portion; one of the most common causes of intestinal obstruction in infancy; most cases occur in previously healthy children under 2 years of age; three times more common in boys; higher incidence in children with cystic fibrosis and celiac disease
   b. *Hirschsprung's disease* (aganglionic megacolon): congenital absence of parasympathetic ganglia of distal colon and rectum, resulting in inadequate peristalsis; stool and flatus accumulate in colon proximal to defect, causing dilatation and hypertrophy of bowel; usually diagnosed in neonatal period or early infancy; four times more common in boys; higher incidence in children with Down syndrome
2. Medical treatment
   a. *Intussusception*
      1. hydrostatic reduction with barium enema before bowel becomes necrotic
      2. surgical intervention (resection and anastommosis) if bowel necrosis has occurred
   b. *Hirschsprung's disease*
      1. barium enema to aid diagnosis
      2. rectal biopsy to confirm absence of ganglion cells
      3. resection of aganglionic portion of bowel, temporary colostomy of sigmoid or transverse colon to rest bowel and restore nutritional balance; abdominal-perineal pull-through anastomosis at approximately 1 year of age

Nursing Process
Assessment

1. *Intussusception:* acute, recurrent, episodic, severe, colicky, abdominal pain; "currant jelly" stools containing blood and mucus, caused by bowel gangrene (occurs about 12 hours after onset of abdominal pain); palpable sausage-shaped mass in right upper quadrant
2. *Hirschsprung's disease*
   a. Delayed passage of meconium in newborn; failure to thrive
   b. Chronic constipation
   c. Ribbonlike, foul-smelling stools
   d. Breath has foul odor

e. Severe abdominal distension with shortness of breath
f. At risk for enterocolitis, which increases risk of fatality
3. Both
   a. Bile-stained vomiting (the obstruction is below ampulla of Vater, which empties bile into duodenum)
   b. Abdominal distension

Analysis (see p. 505)
Planning, Implementation, and Evaluation

Goal 1: Child will maintain adequate hydration and nutrition and regain normal elimination.

Implementation
1. Give IV fluids as ordered; hyperalimentation may be ordered for infants with Hirschsprung's disease.
2. Usually keep NPO; give mouth care, pacifier.
3. Keep accurate I&O; measure and record drainage (NG, colostomy); irrigate NG tube as ordered.
4. Assess bowel sounds frequently.
5. Take axillary temperature only.
6. Gradually reintroduce feedings and return to normal diet postoperatively after NG tube has been removed and bowel sounds have returned.

Evaluation
Child is adequately hydrated (elastic skin turgor, moist mucous membranes, etc.), has adequate caloric intake; returns to normal diet without complications (e.g., vomiting); is free from abdominal distension and establishes normal bowel elimination postoperatively.

Goal 2: Child with colostomy/ileostomy will have intact, functioning stoma without irritation or infection.

Implementation
1. Refer to "Mechanical Obstruction of the Colon," p. 223.
2. Instruct child and parent about stoma care.
   a. Diaper only may be used in infants with sigmoid colostomy.
   b. Select appliance that fits child's size, activity level, and development.
   c. Use hypoallergenic supplies, as children's skin tends to be more sensitive.
   d. Encourage self-care
      1. by 6-7 years, child should be able to remove an reapply pouch with assistance
      2. by 10-11 years, child should be able to assume all responsibility
3. Inspect stoma daily for redness, irritation, or breakdown.
4. Do not submerge colostomy in bath water.
5. Refer parents to local ostomy association for assistance and support.

Evaluation
Child has healthy, functioning stoma; becomes involved in developmentally appropriate self-care.

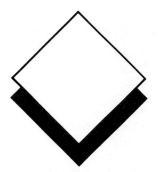

Mobility

GENERAL CONCEPTS
Overview/Physiology

1. Skeletal maturation
   a. Accurate "bone age" is determined by x-ray of ossification centers
   b. Correlates closely with other measures of physiological maturity (e.g., onset of menarche) rather than with height or chronological age
   c. Complete when epiphysis fuses completely with diaphysis, usually 18-21 years of age (earlier in girls than boys)
2. Differences in children's skeletal system compared with the adults'
   a. Thick periosteum: stronger, more active osteogenic potential
   b. More plastic (pliable) bone: more porous, allows bending and buckling; this flexibility diffuses and absorbs a significant amount of the force of impact
   c. Rapid healing: decreases as child gets older (younger bones can be remolded more easily)
   d. Stiffness is unusual, even after lengthy immobilization

Application of the Nursing Process to the Child with an Interference with Mobility

Assessment
1. Nursing injury
   a. Development of motor skills; delays, recent changes or interferences
   b. Signs and symptoms of current health problem; pain, altered structure or mobility
2. Clinical appraisal
   a. Muscle strength and symmetry
   b. Balance, gait, and posture
   c. Range of motion
   d. Obvious structural deformities or functional deficits
3. Radiological tests of affected body part (refer to *Nursing Care of the Adult*, p. 256)

Analysis
1. Safe, effective care environment
   a. High risk for injury
   b. Knowledge deficit
   c. High risk for infection
2. Physiological integrity
   a. High risk for aspiration
   b. Impaired physical mobility
   c. High risk for altered peripheral tissue perfusion
3. Psychosocial integrity
   a. Body image disturbance
   b. Social isolation
   c. Altered role performance
4. Health promotion/maintenance
   a. Altered growth and development
   b. Diversional activity deficit
   c. Bathing/hygiene self-care deficit

General Nursing Planning, Implementation, and Evaluation

Goal 1: Child's deformity will be detected and treated early.

Implementation
1. Screen child for skeletal deformity.
   a. In newborn period for congenital clubfoot and congenital hip dysplasia
   b. During preadolescence and adolescence for scoliosis
2. Refer child with possible deformity for immediate treatment.
3. Teach child and parents the importance of adhering to prescribed treatment plan to minimize or prevent serious, permanent deformity.
4. Stress importance of continued follow-up care to prevent recurrence.

Evaluation
Child's deformity is detected at an early age; parents initiate recommended treatment plan.

Goal 2: Child will maintain correct alignment of the affected body part during the period of treatment.

Implementation

1. Teach child and parents prescribed exercises, application of splints or brace, and cast care.
2. Provide care for child in traction (see Table 5-22, Fig. 5-4).
   a. Maintain traction apparatus (elastic bandages, splints, rings, ropes, pulleys, and weights).
   b. Do not allow weights to rest on floor or bed.
   c. Maintain correct body alignment (emphasis on shoulder, hip, and leg alignment).
   d. Elevate head or foot of bed as needed to provide correct pull and countertraction.
   e. Assess skin color, sensation, and movement of extremity every hour for the first 48 hours, then every 4 hours.
3. Provide care for child in cast (see *Nursing Care of the Adult*, p. 259).
   a. "Petal" cast edges of plaster cast (protects cast and skin); use waterproof adhesive tape petals (see Fig. 5-5).
   b. Protect cast from being soiled with urine or stool (position child with buttocks lower than shoulders during toileting).
   c. Use Bradford frame for smaller children.
   d. Provide toys too large to fit down cast.
   e. Stay with child during mealtimes.
   f. Observe for signs of impaired circulation and infection (fever, lethargy, foul odor), do *not* rely on child to verbalize discomfort; change position frequently; do *not* use abduction-stabilizer bar on hip spica as a handle for turning child.

Evaluation

Child maintains correct alignment of affected body part; has permanent deformity prevented; parents provide appropriate care to child in cast, splint, or brace.

> **Goal 3:** Child's skin integrity will be maintained during period of immobilization.

Implementation

1. Assess for areas of skin breakdown.
2. Change position frequently or encourage movement within limitations imposed by traction, cast, or brace to relieve pressure.
3. Check pin sites (skeletal traction) for bleeding, redness, edema, and infection.
4. Provide pin care as needed.
5. Monitor circulation of affected extremities (normal skin color, blanches easily, warm to touch; able to wiggle fingers and toes; peripheral pulses present).
6. Give meticulous skin care to areas near edges of cast or in contact with brace or traction apparatus.

Evaluation

Child's skin integrity is maintained; circulation is maintained; child is free from skin breakdown or infection.

> **Goal 4:** Child's developmental progress will be maintained during immobilization (brace, cast, or traction).

Implementation

1. Provide age-appropriate stimulation and activity.

Table 5-22   Types of traction

	General
Skin traction	Direct pull to skin surface and indirect pull to skeletal structures by means of adhesive strips or elastic bandage.
Skeletal traction	Direct pull to skeletal structures by means of pin, wire, or tongs inserted into bone distal to fracture.
	Specific
Bryant's traction	Unidirectional, lower-extremity skin traction with child's hips flexed at 90° angle, knees extended, and legs and buttocks suspended.
Buck's extension	Skin traction to lower extremity with hips and legs extended. Used mostly when short-term traction is needed.
Russell traction	Two-directional, lower-extremity skin traction with padded knee sling; immobilizes hip and knee in flexed position. One pull line is longitudinal; the other is perpendicular to leg. Traction pull is twice the amount of weight applied.
Balance suspension with Thomas ring splint and Pearson attachment	Two-directional, skin or skeletal traction that suspends leg with hip slightly flexed; Thomas ring circles uppermost portion of the thigh while Pearson attachment supports lower part of leg. Alignment is maintained even when child lifts off bed.
Halo-femoral traction	Metal rings (halo) are attached to the skull and pins are inserted into distal femur also. Progressive traction is applied upward to the halo and downward to the distal end of the femur, increasing weights twice daily until alignment is achieved.

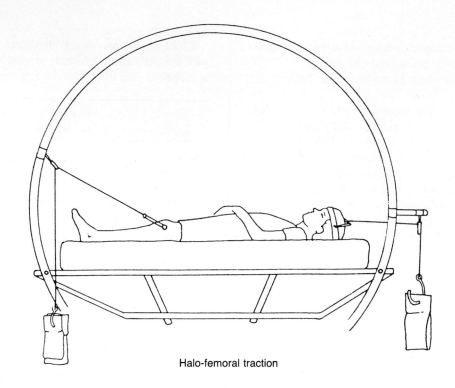

Halo-femoral traction

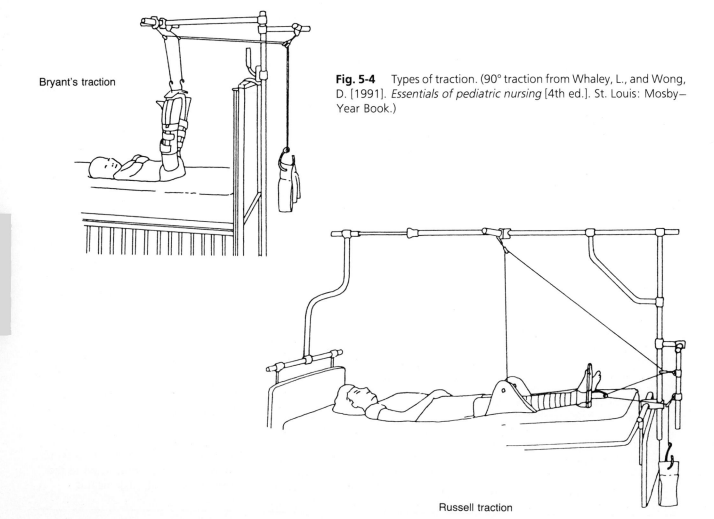

Bryant's traction

Fig. 5-4 Types of traction. (90° traction from Whaley, L., and Wong, D. [1991]. *Essentials of pediatric nursing* [4th ed.]. St. Louis: Mosby—Year Book.)

Russell traction

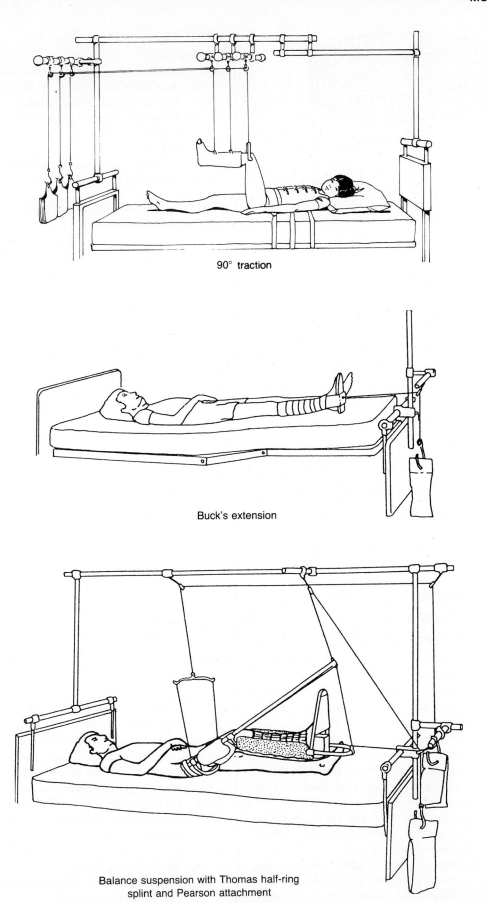

90° traction

Buck's extension

Balance suspension with Thomas half-ring
splint and Pearson attachment

Fig. 5-4, cont'd Types of traction

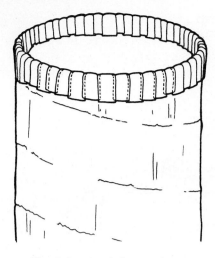

Fig. 5-5 Petaled cast edges.

2. Encourage child to participate in own daily care and maintain control as much as possible.
3. Provide for child to maintain educational progress while immobilized (hospital teacher, homebound teacher, daily contact with regular teacher).
4. Arrange for and encourage interaction with peers, siblings if child is hospitalized or confined to home.

Evaluation

Child maintains developmental and educational progress while immobilized; has no developmental delays; participates in own care.

SELECTED HEALTH PROBLEMS RESULTING IN AN INTERFERENCE WITH MOBILITY

☐ Congenital Clubfoot

General Information

1. Definition; congenital skeletal deformity of the foot; the most common type is talipes equinovarus (95% of cases), characterized by inversion and plantar flexion (directed inward and downward) of foot; may be unilateral or bilateral
2. Incidence
   a. Boys are affected twice as often as girls are
   b. Unilateral is slightly more common than bilateral
   c. Frequency: 1:1000 in general population
3. Medical treatment
   a. Early correction: successive casts until foot is manipulated into an overcorrected position, followed by Denis Browne splint to maintain correction
   b. Later correction in older child or for recurrent clubfoot: surgical intervention (tendon transfer, arthrodesis) followed by casting, corrective shoes

Nursing Process

Assessment

1. Differentiate true clubfoot from positional deformity
   a. True clubfoot cannot be passively manipulated into an overcorrected position
   b. Positional deformity can be passively corrected or overcorrected

Analysis (see p. 512)

Planning, Implementation, and Evaluation (see General Nursing Plans, p. 512)

☐ Congenital Hip Dysplasia

General Information

1. Definitions
   a. *Subluxation:* head of femur is partially displaced but remains in contact with acetabulum
   b. *Complete dislocation of hip:* head of femur is completely displaced
2. Incidence
   a. 70% are female
   b. Unilateral twice as common as bilateral
   c. Frequency: 1 in 500
   d. Incidence increases with breech delivery and among siblings of affected children
3. Medical treatment
   a. Very mild cases: triple diapering can be useful
   b. Newborn to 6 months: keep hips flexed and adducted with the Pavlik harness (most common) or the Ilfeld or Frejka splints worn continuously for 2 to 3 months
   c. Older infants and young children: may require traction (Bryant's or Russell) or hip spica cast
   d. Older children: may require traction, open reduction, and casting
   e. If treatment is not completed in childhood, total hip replacement may be done in young adulthood

Nursing Process

Assessment

1. *Infant*
   a. Limited abduction of affected hip
   b. Wide perineum
   c. Shortening of leg on affected side (Galeazzi's sign, Allis' sign)
   d. Asymmetry of thigh and gluteal folds
   e. Positive Ortolani's sign: clicking when leg abducted, caused by femoral head slipping over acetabulum (infant under 4 weeks of age)
   f. Barlow's sign: hand placed over knee, adduct leg past midline; abnormal movement is positive response
2. *Older child*
   a. Trendelenburg's sign: when child stands on affected leg, pelvis tilts downward on unaffected side instead of upward

b. Limp on affected side

c. Flattening of buttock on affected side

Analysis (see p. 512)

Planning, Implementation, and Evaluation (see General Nursing Plans, p. 512)

☐ Legg-Calvé-Perthes Disease
General Information

1. Definition: self-limiting avascular necrosis of the femoral head; if untreated, the head becomes flattened and deformed, resulting in permanent disability
2. Incidence
   a. Onset usually between 3 and 11 years of age
   b. Four times more common in boys
   c. Usually unilateral; 15% bilateral
   d. Possible familial tendency
3. Medical treatment: the earlier the age of onset, the better the results of treatment
   a. Bed rest and skin traction to the limb during the painful initial period
   b. Some weight bearing allowed after resolution of the initial stage of the disease; use of abduction braces, casts, or hip sling
   c. Full weight bearing if no new dense areas develop in femoral head in 2 months
   d. Surgical osteotomy of femur done if medical management is ineffective

Nursing Process
Assessment
1. Hip, groin, or thigh pain (insidious onset)
2. Referred knee pain
3. Limp; stiffness
4. Limited motion—abduction and internal rotation
5. Atrophy of thigh muscles from disuse

Analysis (see p. 512)

Planning, Implementation, and Evaluation (see General Nursing Plans, p. 512)

☐ Scoliosis
General Information

1. Definition: lateral curvature of the spine, which results in structural and functional alterations in spine, chest, and pelvis
2. Incidence
   a. 15% of children between ages 10-21 are affected
   b. Eight times more common in adolescent females
   c. 70% of cases are idiopathic (i.e., without apparent cause)
3. Medical treatment
   a. Nonsurgical management techniques
      1. bracing and exercise; 2 basic types of braces used:
         a. Boston brace (most common) is underarm brace used for lumbar curves; made of molded plastic

      b. Milwaukee brace (older, but still in use) is an individually adapted steel-and-leather brace extending from chin to pelvis
      2. electrical stimulation: stimulation plates placed next to spine cause muscles to contract, straightening the spine; worn at night
   b. Surgical management techniques (curves greater than 40°)
      1. Harrington instrumentation: metal rods implanted to hold vertebrae and bone fragments for permanent fusion
      2. Luque segmental instrumentation: flexible L-shaped metal rod fixed by wires to spinous processes. NOTE: child can get up and walk within a few days, and no postoperative immobilization is necessary
      3. Dwyer instrumentation: cable through cannulated screws that are fixed to each vertebra
      4. Cotrel-Dubousset procedure: bilateral segmental fixation using two knurled rods and multiple hooks

Nursing Process
Assessment
1. Spinal curve may be obvious
2. Elevated shoulder or hip
3. Structural asymmetry (scapulae, waist, hips, shoulders, breasts)
4. Rib hump apparent when child bends at waist

Analysis (see p. 512)

Planning, Implementation, and Evaluation

> **Goal:** Adolescent and family will adjust to lengthy treatment regimen.

Implementation
1. Allow adolescent and parents to express feelings and concerns about long-term bracing or casting (6 months to 3 years for medical intervention).
2. Help adolescent cope with altered body image.
   a. Emphasize and enhance positive attributes (hair, makeup).
   b. Help with selection of attractive camouflage clothing.
   c. Encourage involvement in appropriate activities (choir, school clubs, etc.).
3. Demonstrate alternative ways of getting in and out of bed, dressing, etc.
4. Advise standing at drafting table or easel for homework.
5. Teach application and removal of brace (must wear 23 hr/day; remove for 1 hour for hygiene or swimming).
6. Teach adolescent to wear T-shirt under brace.
7. Check for loosening of the brace; tighten the brace as necessary.

8. Keep brace clean: wash plastic with soap and water, clean leather with saddle soap.
9. Provide for needs of adolescent following surgical intervention (spinal fusion).
   a. Keep bed flat; log-roll q2h.
   b. Assess circulatory and neurological status in legs and feet.
   c. Administer analgesics for pain.
   d. Monitor incision sites for bleeding and signs of infection.
   e. Monitor respiratory status.
   f. Cough and deep-breathe; use incentive inspirometry.

Evaluation

Child with scoliosis copes with treatment regimen and altered body image; recovers from surgery free from complications; is free from permanent disability.

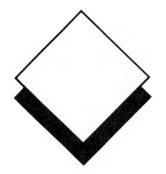

Cellular Aberration (Childhood Cancer)

General Concepts (see also *Nursing Care of the Adult,* p. 267)

Overview/Physiology

1. Cancer is the leading cause of death from disease between the ages of 3 and 15
   a. Leukemias and lymphomas account for more than 40% of childhood malignancies
   b. Brain tumors account for 20% of childhood cancers
   c. Embryonal tumors (e.g., Wilms' tumor and neuroblastoma) and sarcomas account for another 20% of childhood malignancies
   d. The survival rate for childhood cancer has dramatically increased in the last two decades, especially for acute lymphocytic leukemia
2. Differences in childhood cancers as compared with adult cancers
   a. Higher incidence of embryonal tumors
   b. Occur more frequently in rapidly growing tissues, such as bone marrow
   c. Higher rate of metastasis
3. Medical treatment
   a. Surgery: excision of all or part of solid tumors; may only be palliative if cancer has metastasized; most successful with localized and encapsulated tumors
   b. Chemotherapy: administration of antineoplastic drugs
      1. classification
         a. cell-cycle specific: destroys cells in specific phases of cell division
            ◆ most effective for rapidly growing cells
            ◆ least toxic
            ◆ examples: cytosine arabinoside, methotrexate
         b. cell-cycle nonspecific: destroys cells at any phase
            ◆ most effective for slow-growing, solid tumors
            ◆ examples: alkylating agents, hormones, antibiotics, nitrosoureas

   c. cytotoxic action (see Table 5-23 for specific drugs)
      ◆ alkylating agents: alkyl group; replaces hydrogen atom, causing cell to die
      ◆ antimetabolites: similar to essential elements needed for cell growth, but in altered form; prevent synthesis of DNA or RNA
      ◆ plant alkaloids: stop cell growth in metaphase
      ◆ antitumor antibiotics: interfere with cell division by reacting with DNA and RNA
      ◆ hormones, adrenocorticosteroids: depress mitosis of lymphoid cells; androgens and estrogens are used for breast and prostatic cancers, probably affecting growth regulation
      ◆ miscellaneous agents: enzymes, such as L-asparaginase, hydroxyurea, nitrosoureas; metals such as cisplatin
      2. combination chemotherapy: two or more drugs used simultaneously; each drug has a different effect on cell growth; increases effectiveness, decreases resistance of cancer cells to drugs
   c. Irradiation: frequently used in childhood cancers as an adjunct to surgery and/or chemotherapy; may be curative or palliative

Application of the Nursing Process to the Child with Cancer

Assessment

1. Nursing history (see *Nursing Care of the Adult,* p. 268)
2. Clinical appraisal: physical findings will vary according to the type of cancer
3. Diagnostic tests: same as for adult except that bone marrow aspiration is usually performed on the posterior iliac crest

Analysis

1. Safe, effective care environment

Table 5-23 Commonly used chemotherapeutic agents

Drug	Uses	Side effects	Specific nursing concerns
ALKYLATING AGENTS			
	Hodgkin's and other lymphomas Leukemias Neuroblastomas Retinoblastomas Multiple myeloma	Nausea and vomiting, occurring 2-6 hours after administration and lasting up to 48 hours Bone marrow depression Alopecia	
Cyclophosphamide (Cytoxan)			Chemical cystitis may result; force fluids, report burning or hematuria.
Mechlorethamine (nitrogen mustard, Mustargen)			Use immediately after reconstitution. Avoid vapors in eyes; if solution comes into contact with skin, flush with liberal amounts of water. Ensure IV is in place to prevent necrosis and sloughing.
Chlorambucil (Leukeran)			Side effects occur slowly and with high doses.
Cisplatin			Toxic to kidneys and ears; can cause anaphylaxis. Hydrate well before and during treatment with IVs and mannitol. Monitor renal function and audiograms.
ANTIMETABOLITES			
	Acute lymphocytic leukemia; acute myelocytic leukemia; brain tumors; ovarian, breast, prostatic, testicular cancers	Mild to moderate nausea and vomiting Bone marrow depression Stomatitis Dermatitis Photosensitivity	
5-Fluorouracil (5-FU, Adrucil)			Chronic nausea and vomiting with prolonged use. Check oral mucosa. If stomatitis and diarrhea are severe, stop drug.
Methotrexate (MTX)			Toxic to liver and kidney; avoid aspirin, sulfonamides, and tetracycline while on drug. Avoid vitamins containing folic acid. Leucovorin used as an antidote for high doses ("leucovorin rescue"). When outdoors, use sun screen.
6 Mercaptopurine (6-MP)	Give allopurinol concurrently to inhibit uric acid production from cell destruction, thus increasing drug's potency.		
Cytosine arabinoside (ara-C, Cytosar-U)			Crosses blood-brain barrier; may be hepatotoxic; monitor liver function.

Table 5-23 Commonly used chemotherapeutic agents—cont'd

Drug	Uses	Side effects	Specific nursing concerns
PLANT ALKALOIDS			
	Acute lymphocytic leukemia, Hodgkin's disease, Wilms' tumor, sarcomas, breast cancer, testicular cancer	Minimal nausea and vomiting Alopecia Neurotoxicity	
Vincristine (Oncovin)			Monitor for neurotoxicity: reflexes, weakness, parasthesias, jaw pain, constipation. Check IV placement to prevent cellulitis.
Vinblastine (Velban)			Headaches; less neurotoxic than vincristine.
ANTITUMOR ANTIBIOTICS			
	Sarcomas; neuroblastomas; head and neck tumors; testicular, ovarian, breast cancer	Severe nausea and vomiting Stomatitis Diarrhea Bone marrow depression Photosensitivity	
Dactinomycin (cosmegen)			Used for Wilms' tumor; enhances effects of radiation (also increases toxicity). Extravasation can cause necrosis; maintain patent IV.
Doxorubicin hydrochloride (Adriamycin)			Monitor for cardiac dysrhythmias (cardiotoxicity is irreversible). Caution that urine turns red.
HORMONES			
Adrenocorticosteroids Prednisone Dexamethasone (Decadron)	Leukemia, Hodgkin's disease, breast cancer, lymphomas, multiple myeloma, cerebral edema caused by brain metastasis	See Table 3-33	See Table 3-33
Androgens Testosterone (Oreton) Fluoxymesterone (Halotestin)	Breast cancer in postmenopausal women	Fluid retention Nausea Masculinization	Give low-sodium diet; provide psychological support for masculinization effects.
Estrogens Diethylstilbestrol (DES) Ethinyl estradiol (Estinyl)	Prostatic cancer, breast cancer that is estrogen-receptor-positive in postmenopausal women	Fluid retention Feminization Gynecomastia in males	Give low-sodium diet; provide psychological support to males experiencing feminization.
Antiestrogens Tamoxifen (Nolvadex)	Breast cancer; prostatic cancer	Hot flashes Generally mild nausea	
MISCELLANEOUS AGENTS			
Enzymes L-asparaginase	Leukemias, Hodgkin's disease	Severe nausea and vomiting; fever Liver dysfunction Anaphylaxis	Monitor BUN and serum ammonia levels. Observe for allergic reaction (have epinephrine 1:1000 at bedside).

a. High risk for infection
b. High risk for injury
c. Impaired home maintenance management
2. Physiological integrity
   a. Pain
   b. Diarrhea, constipation
   c. Fluid volume deficit
3. Psychosocial integrity
   a. Fear
   b. Social isolation
   c. Ineffective individual coping
4. Health promotion/maintenance
   a. Knowledge deficit
   b. Altered parenting
   c. Altered growth and development

General Nursing Planning, Implementation, and Evaluation

Goal 1: Child and family will be prepared for diagnostic tests.

Implementation
1. Provide age-appropriate explanation of procedure (what will happen, what it will feel like, what child is expected to do).
2. Give parents option of staying with child during procedure so they can provide needed emotional support to child.
3. Hold child firmly during procedure to facilitate needle insertion (e.g., bone marrow aspiration, lumbar puncture).
4. Reassure child throughout procedure.
5. After the procedure, provide child opportunities to express feelings (verbally, through therapeutic play).
6. Provide positive feedback to child concerning child's cooperation during the procedure.

Evaluation
Child copes with diagnostic procedures; cooperates with procedure; expresses feelings during and after procedure.

Goal 2: Child and family will be prepared for surgery (refer to "Ill and Hospitalized Child," p. 438).

Goal 3: Child and family will be prepared for chemotherapy.

Implementation
1. Explain benefits of chemotherapy, using terms the child and family can understand.
2. Reinforce physician's explanation of types of chemotherapy child will receive.
3. Explain side effects that may occur and identify measures that will help lessen side effects.

a. Nausea and vomiting: administer antiemetics before chemotherapy; ensure adequate hydration
b. Diarrhea: administer antispasmodics, adjust diet; monitor perianal skin condition
c. Anorexia: monitor weight; provide soft diet; small, frequent feedings; favorite foods and liquids; give choices
d. Stomatitis (see Goal 6)
e. Alopecia: provide wig, scarf, or hat as desired; reassure that hair will grow back
f. Fatigue: provide frequent rest periods, encourage quiet activities

Evaluation
Child and family list side effects; implement measures that minimize these effects and promote/enhance child's comfort.

Goal 4: Child and family will be prepared for radiation therapy.

Implementation
1. Reinforce reasons for and benefits of radiation.
2. Prepare for and manage side effects of radiation therapy.
   a. Nausea and vomiting: administer prescribed antiemetics as needed, bland diet, clear liquids
   b. Peeling skin: meticulous skin care; avoid direct exposure to sun; do not wash off skin markings (dark purple lines that define area to be irradiated)
   c. Risk of fracture: explain to child and family why child should avoid weight bearing; help plan to meet child's need for mobility through alternative means, such as crutches or stimulating activities while on bed rest
   d. Delays in physical development: discuss possible outcomes with parents and child (as appropriate) such as pathological fractures, spinal deformities, growth retardation, sterility, delayed appearance of secondary sex characteristics, chromosomal damage

Evaluation
Child and family state reasons for radiation and knowledge of side effects that may occur.

Goal 5: Child will be free from infection.

Implementation
1. Maintain reverse isolation, or private room with strict hand washing if child is severely immunosuppressed.
2. Prevent contact with anyone with infection.
3. Have child rinse mouth regularly before meals, after meals, and q4h (removes debris as a source for growth of bacteria and fungi).
4. Administer antibiotics and observe for side effects.
5. Take measures to prevent skin breakdown.
6. Do not give immunizations until child's immune response is adequate.

7. Permit return to school when WBCs approach normal level (2000/mm^3).

Evaluation

Child remains free from infection; maintains skin integrity; child and family correctly assess immune response, risk factors, and modify life-style appropriately.

Goal 6: Child will receive care for ulcerations of mouth and rectal area.

Implementation

1. Provide meticulous oral hygiene before and after meals.
2. Offer mouthwash frequently; apply local anesthetic (viscous lidocaine [Xylocaine]) prn.
3. Encourage fluids, nonirritating foods (soft foods, cool drinks).
4. Avoid rectal temperatures and suppositories.
5. Encourage sitz baths; offer pericare after voiding or BM.
6. Expose ulcerated anal area to air and heat.

Evaluation

Child is free from increased ulceration; experiences healing of lesions in mouth and rectum.

Goal 7: Child will ingest foods and fluids to meet nutritional needs.

Implementation

1. Rinse mouth before child eats.
2. Offer small, frequent meals.
3. Provide soft foods; permit favorite foods child tolerates.
4. Use nutritional supplements.

Evaluation

Child maintains appropriate nutrition and hydration status to meet developmental needs.

Goal 8: Child's pain will be relieved and comfort promoted.

Implementation

1. Administer nonnarcotic and narcotic analgesics as needed.
2. Maintain comfortable body position, turning at least q2h and PRN.
3. Teach child to focus on TV, music, or friends when having pain.
4. Provide soothing skin care.

Evaluation

Child experiences relief of pain; child and family verbally identify and use available comfort measures.

Goal 9: Child's growth and development will be fostered throughout the course of illness and treatment.

Implementation

1. Refer to "Healthy Child," p. 428 for developmental needs appropriate to child's age.
2. Encourage child to participate in self-care to the extent possible.
3. Provide opportunities for child to exercise some control over daily routine (food choices, selection of play activities).
4. Maintain child's educational progress as much as possible.
5. Maintain child's contact with siblings and friends (through visiting, telephone calls, letters).

Evaluation

Child is free from significant developmental or educational delays; demonstrates age-appropriate skills and behaviors.

Goal 10: Child and family cope with the stresses of living with cancer and its treatment.

Implementation

1. Encourage parents and family to continue to provide care of child as much as desired and possible.
2. Encourage expressions of fear, feelings, and concerns about cancer and its treatment.
3. Refer to parent-support groups (Candlelighters, Compassionate Friends).
4. Assess child's understanding of diagnosis and prognosis (see Table 5-24).
5. Help child express feelings through play and art.

Table 5-24 Child's concept of death

INFANTS AND TODDLERS

React more to pain and to parents' responses and behaviors than to probability of death; cannot verbalize their understanding; only understand "alive," not "dead"; may persist in ritualistic activities.

PRESCHOOL

Death is a kind of sleep, temporary; believe their own illness is punishment; fear painful procedures and being separated from parents.

SCHOOL AGE

6-7 years old: personify death, such as God, devil, "bogeyman"; fear the mutilation of death.

9-10 years old: similar to adult concept; understand death is eventually inevitable and irreversible; fear the unknown about death; need concrete explanations and a chance to share their fears and gain some control.

ADOLESCENTS

Have the most difficulty coping with death; have adult cognitive understanding, but death is a threat to their identity; fear the physical changes of terminal illness.

6. Encourage family to treat child as normally as possible (i.e., age-appropriate limit setting and enforcement, avoid excessive gifts or privileges).
7. If child's condition becomes terminal, support family as they prepare for child's death; refer for home or hospice care, as appropriate and desired by family.

Evaluation

Child and family cope with child's illness and treatment; parents participate in community support groups as desired, express their fears and feelings about child's illness and prognosis.

SELECTED HEALTH PROBLEMS RESULTING FROM CELLULAR ABERRATION

☐ Leukemia

General Information

1. Definition: malignant neoplasm of unknown etiology that involves blood-forming organs and is characterized by abnormal overproduction of immature forms of any of the leukocytes; interferes with normal blood cell production, resulting in decreased erythrocytes, decreased platelets
   a. Types
      1. lymphocytic: predominance of stem cells, lymphoblasts, usually known as acute lymphocytic leukemia (ALL); 80% of childhood leukemias are of this type
      2. myelogenous: predominance of monocytes and immature granulocytes (more common in adults); 10%-20% of childhood leukemias are myelogenous
   b. Pathophysiology: leukemic cells proliferate and deprive normal blood cells of nutrients needed for metabolism
      1. anemia results from decreased red blood cell production, blood loss
      2. immunosuppression occurs from large numbers of *immature* white blood cells or profound neutropenia
      3. hemorrhage results from thrombocytopenia
      4. leukemic invasion of other organ systems occurs (extramedullary disease)
         a. liver
         b. spleen
         c. lymph nodes
         d. CNS
         e. kidneys
         f. lungs
         g. gonads
      5. hyperuricemia may result after the start of chemotherapy when large numbers of cells are rapidly destroyed
2. Incidence
   a. Most common childhood cancer
   b. Peak age of onset is 2-5 years; more frequent in males
   c. 50% of children with ALL who are treated in major research centers live 5 years or longer
3. Medical treatment
   a. Diagnostic measures
      1. bone marrow aspiration
      2. lumbar puncture
      3. frequent blood counts
   b. Chemotherapy—three phases
      1. remission induction: to reduce leukemia-cell population and attain remission, usually with corticosteroids and vincristine
      2. consolidation (sanctuary): usually begun after remission is achieved; may be done along with induction; prophylactic treatment of the CNS, usually with intrathecal use of methotrexate
      3. maintenance course: to maintain remission, usually with combination drugs
   c. Additional therapies
      1. radiation: irradiate cranium and spine as prophylaxis against CNS involvement
      2. bone marrow transplantation
4. Prognosis: disease is characterized by remissions and exacerbations; outlook varies according to type of cell involved, response to treatment, age at diagnosis, initial WBC, and extent of involvement

Nursing Process

Assessment

1. Bleeding tendencies
   a. Petechiae often the first sign, as a result of low platelet count
   b. Hemorrhage (nosebleeds, gingival bleeding; intracranial hemorrhage in advanced disease)
2. Anemia: fatigue, pallor
3. Neutropenia: immunosuppression leads to secondary infection and fever, since cells are not capable of normal phagocytosis
4. Pain
   a. Abdomen: resulting from enlarged liver, spleen, lymph nodes, and other organs from cell infiltration
   b. Bones and joints
5. Anorexia and weight loss; ulcers of mucous membranes of GI tract
6. Vomiting and increased intracranial pressure from CNS involvement
7. Impaired kidney function
8. Emotional reaction, coping skills of parents, siblings, child, and significant extended-family members
9. Developmental and educational needs of child

Analysis (see p. 519)

Planning, Implementation, and Evaluation

Goal 1: Child will be free from hemorrhage.

Implementation
1. Observe for epistaxis, gingival bleeding.
2. Handle gently.
3. Inspect skin and mucous membranes daily.
4. Keep lips and nostrils clean and lubricated.
5. Pad bed/crib to avoid trauma.

6. Monitor blood work.
Evaluation
   Child is free from bruises and bleeding; has early signs of hemorrhage detected and reported.

Goal 2: Child will receive transfusions properly and safely.

Table 5-25   Common solid-tumor cancers in children

Definition	Assessment	Medical treatment	Nursing planning/implementation
BRAIN TUMORS			
Neoplasms in the cranium; most brain tumors in children are *infratentorial* (below the tentorium cerebelli), thus affecting the cerebellum and brain stem, making them less operable	Signs of increased ICP: see Table 5-14	Surgical excision to extent possible Irradiation Chemotherapy: methotrexate, vincristine	Perform frequent neurological checks. Institute seizure precautions. Postoperative care 　Observe cranial dressing for drainage and record. 　Reinforce but DO NOT CHANGE cranial dressing. 　Position flat or on side with neck slightly extended. 　Monitor fluid intake (IV, PO) carefully to prevent overload. 　Avoid analgesics and sedatives that cause CNS depression. 　Avoid coughing, straining, jarring movements.
NEUROBLASTOMA			
Malignant, embryonic abdominal tumor; most common in infancy	Abdominal mass that crosses midline Lymphadenopathy Urinary frequency or retention (pressure from tumor) Urine catecholamines (elevated)	Surgical excision and staging (to determine extent of other treatment and prognosis) Irradiation Chemotherapy	See General Nursing Plans, p. 522.
WILMS' TUMOR			
Malignant, embryonic tumor of kidney, usually encapsulated until late stages; 90% survival rate if detected while encapsulated; peak age of occurrence—3 years; more common in boys; increased incidence in siblings or twin; usually unilateral	Palpable abdominal mass Abdominal distension Hypertension (excess renin secretion)	IV push Nephrectomy and adrenalectomy, staging (to determine treatment and prognosis) Irradiation Chemotherapy: actinomycin D, vincristine	Handle carefully; DO NOT PALPATE ABDOMEN. Monitor kidney function (e.g., I&O, urine specific gravity, BP).
OSTEOGENIC SARCOMA			
Primary bone tumor, usually affecting distal femur or proximal tibia; most common in adolescent males	Pain Localized swelling Limp or limited ROM	Amputation (above the knee or total hip disarticulation) Prophylactic lung irradiation Chemotherapy: doxorubicin, cisplatin, methotrexate with leucovorin rescue	Postoperative stump care (see *Nursing Care of the Adult*, p. 261). Support coping response in adjusting to loss of body part.

Implementation

1. Administer blood products properly.
   a. Take baseline vital signs before transfusion.
   b. Check label with RN before transfusion for name, blood type, RH, hospital number, and physician's name.
   c. Flush tubing with isotonic saline solution (hemolysis can occur if dextrose is in line).
   d. Administer blood at room temperature within 4 hours of refrigeration.
   e. Administer transfusion slowly to determine possible transfusion reaction, to prevent circulatory overload, and to protect small veins.
   f. Stay with child for first 15 minutes; have parent or other adult stay with young child throughout transfusion.
   g. Take vital signs q15 min for first hour.
   h. Do not give IV medications while blood is infusing.
   i. Use blood filter.
2. Monitor intravenous transfusions.
   a. Whole blood/packed cells (cannot be continuously maintained on tranfusions since preservative in whole blood functions as anticoagulant)
   b. Platelets last 1-3 days; do not need to crossmatch for blood group or type, but doing so decreases chance of immunization to another platelet group; spontaneous hemorrhage can occur at platelet levels below 20,000/mm^3
   c. Leukocytes last 2-3 days; need compatible donors; febrile responses (with moderate to severe chills) are common; give antihistamines or antipyretics as ordered
3. Observe for complications and reactions to blood transfusions.
   a. Chills
   b. Fever (give antipyretic PRN)
   c. Headache
   d. Apprehension (give sedatives PRN)
   e. Pain in back, legs, or chest
   f. Hypotension (give IV fluids, vasopressors)
   g. Dyspnea (give O$_2$, bronchodilator [epinephrine] as ordered)
   h. Urticaria (give antihistamines PRN)
4. Promptly manage a transfusion reaction.
   a. Stop the transfusion of blood.
   b. Monitor vital signs.
   c. Do not leave child alone.
   d. Run IV fluids to maintain patency of the IV line.
   e. Notify physician.
   f. Return untransfused blood to blood bank.

Evaluation

Child receives correct transfusion, is free from preventable complications (e.g., hemolysis); early signs of reaction (e.g., rash) are detected, and transfusion reaction is managed properly.

☐ **Solid Tumors**
General Information (see Table 5-25)
Nursing Process (see Table 5-25)

BIBLIOGRAPHY

General

Foster, R. Hunsberger, M., & Anderson, J. (1989). *Family-centered nursing care of children.* Philadelphia: Saunders.

Mott, S., James, S., & Sperhac, A. (1990). *Nursing care of children and families* (2nd ed.). Redwood City, CA: Addison-Wesley.

Scipien, G.M., et al. (1990). *Pediatric nursing care.* St. Louis: Mosby–Year Book.

Servonsky, J., & Opas, S. (1987). *Nursing management of children.* Boston: Jones and Bartlett.

Whaley, L., & Wong, D. (1991). *Nursing care of infants and children* (4th ed.). St. Louis: Mosby–Year Book.

Healthy child

Castiglia, P., & Petrini, M. (1985). Selecting a developmental screening tool. *Pediatric Nursing, 11*(1), 8-17.

Dickey, S. (1987). *A guide to the nursing of children.* Baltimore: Williams and Wilkins.

Lee, J., & Fowler, M. (1986). Merely child's play? Developmental work and playthings. *Journal of Pediatric Nursing, 1*, 260-270.

Pipes, P. (1989). *Nutrition in infancy and childhood* (4th ed.). St. Louis: Mosby–Year Book.

Report of the Committee on Infectious Diseases (21st ed.) (1988). American Academy of Pediatrics.

Rimar, J. (1986). Haemophilus influenzae type b polysaccharide. *MCN: American Journal of Maternal Child Nursing, 11*, 8-17.

Scipien, G.M., et al. (1990). *Pediatric nursing care.* St. Louis: Mosby–Year Book.

Servonsky, J., & Opas, S. (1987). *Nursing management of children.* Boston: Jones and Bartlett.

Whaley, L., & Wong, D. (1991). *Nursing care of infants and children* (4th ed.). St. Louis: Mosby–Year Book.

Wishon, O., & Kinnick, V. (1986). Helping infants overcome the problem of obesity. *MCN: American Journal of Maternal Child Nursing, 11*, 118-121.

The ill and hospitalized child

Gordin, P. (1990). Assessing and managing agitation in a critically ill infant. *MCN: American Journal of Maternal Child Nursing, 15*, 26-32.

Jackson, P.L., & Vessey, J.A. (1991). *Primary care of the child with a chronic condition.* St. Louis: Mosby–Year Book.

Landier, W., Barrell, M., & Styffe, E. (1987). How to administer blood components to children. *MCN: American Journal of Maternal Child Nursing, 12*, 178-184.

O'Brien, S., & Konsler, G. (1988). Alleviating children's postoperative pain. *MCN: American Journal of Maternal Child Nursing, 13*, 183-186.

*Reynolds, E., & Ramenofsky, M. (1988). The emotional impact of trauma on toddlers. *MCN: American Journal of Maternal Child Nursing, 13*, 106-109.

Rimar, J. (1987). Guidelines for the IV administration of medications used in pediatrics. *MCN: American Journal of Maternal Child Nursing, 12*, 322-340.

*Rimar, J. (1988). Recognizing shock syndromes in infants and chil-

*See reprint section.
†Highly recommended.

dren. *MCN: American Journal of Maternal Child Nursing, 13,* 32-37.

Ruddy-Wallace, M. (1987). Temperament: Assessing individual differences in hospitalized children. *Journal of Pediatric Nursing, 2,* 30-36.

Rushton, C. (1986). Promoting normal growth and development in the hospital environment. *Neonatal Network, 4,* 21-30.

Zweig, C. (1986). Reducing stress when a child is admitted to the hospital. *MCN: American Journal of Maternal Child Nursing, 11*(1), 24-26.

Sensation, perception, and protection

Dyer, C., & Roberts, D. (1990). Thermal trauma. *The Nursing Clinics of North America, 25*(1), 85-117.

Ellis, J. (1988). Using pain scales to prevent undermedication. *MCN: The American Journal of Maternal Child Nursing, 13,* 180-182.

Engle, N. (1989). AZT for children with AIDS. *MCN: American Journal of Maternal/Child Nursing, 14*(2), 121.

Hurley, A., & Whelan E. (1988). Cognitive development and children's perception of pain. *Pediatric Nursing, 14,* 21-24.

Lewis, K., Bennett, B., & Schmeder, N. (1989). The care of infants menaced by cocaine abuse. *MCN: American Journal of Maternal Child Nursing, 14*(5), 324-329.

Mott, S., James, S., & Sperhac, A. (1990). *Nursing care of children and families* (2nd ed.). Redwood City, CA: Addison-Wesley.

Paparone, P. (1990). The summer scourge of Lyme disease. *American Journal of Nursing, 90*(6), 44-47.

Parks, B., & Smith, D. (1989) Treatment of head lice and scabies infestations in children. *Pediatric Nursing, 15*(5), 522-524.

Scheinblum, S., & Hammond, M. (1990). The treatment of children with shunt infections: Extraventricular drainage system care. *Pediatric Nursing, 16*(2), 139-143.

Scipien, G.M., et al. (1990). *Pediatric Nursing Care.* St. Louis: Mosby–Year Book.

Servonsky, J., & Opas, S. (1987). *Nursing management of children.* Boston: Jones & Bartlett.

Thomson, E., & Cordero, J. (1989). The new teratogens: Accutane and other vitamin-A analogs. *MCN: American Journal of Maternal Child Nursing, 14*(4), 244-248.

†Ward-Wimmer, D. (1988). Nursing care of children with HIV infection. *The Nursing Clinics of North America, 23*(4), 719-729.

Williams, A. (1989). Nursing management of the child with AIDS. *Pediatric Nursing, 15*(3), 259-261.

Oxygenation

Agamalian, B. (1986). Pediatric cardiac catheterization. *Journal of Pediatric Nursing 1*(2), 73-79.

Foster, R., Hunsberger, M., & Anderson, J. (1989). *Family-centered nursing care of children.* Philadelphia: Saunders.

Higgins, S., & Kashani, I. (1986). The cyanotic child: Heart defects and parental learning needs. *MCN: American Journal of Maternal Child Nursing, 11*(4), 258-262.

Mott, S., James, S., & Sperhac, A. (1990). *Nursing care of children and families* (2nd ed.). Redwood City, CA: Addison-Wesley.

Nederhand, K.C. (1989). Respiratory syncytial virus: A nursing perspective. *Pediatric Nursing, 15*(4) 342-345.

Servonsky, J., & Opas, S. (1987). *Nursing management of children.* Boston: Jones & Bartlett.

Smith, J. (1988). Big differences in little people. *American Journal of Nursing, 88*(4), 458-462.

Swoiskin, S. (1986). Sudden infant death: Nursing care for the survivors. *Journal of Pediatric Nursing,1*(1), 33-39.

Zahr, L.K. (1989). Assessment and management of the child with asthma. *Pediatric Nursing, 15*(2), 109-114.

Nutrition and metabolism

Bishop, W.P., & Ulshen, M.H. (1988). Bacterial gastroenteritis. *Pediatric Clinics of North America, 35*(1), 69-87.

Brink, S.J. (1988). Pediatric, adolescent, and young-adult nutrition

issues in IDDM. *Diabetes Care, 11,* 192-199.

Dibble, S.L., & Savedra, M.C. (1988). Cystic fibrosis in adolescence: A new challenge. *Pediatric Nursing, 14* (4), 299-303.

Foster, R., Hunsberger, M., & Anderson, J. (1989). *Family-centered nursing care of children.* Philadelphia: Saunders.

Gavin, J.R. III. (1988). Diabetes and exercise. *American Journal of Nursing, 88,* 178-180.

Hodges, L., & Parker, J. (1987). Concerns of parents with diabetic children. *Pediatric Nursing, 13*(1), 22-24, 68.

Lipman, T.H. (1988). What causes diabetes? *MCN: American Journal of Maternal Child Nursing, 13*(1), 40-43.

Lipman, T.H., Difazio, D.A., Meers, R.A., & Thompson, R.L. (1989). A developmental approach to diabetes in children: Birth through preschool. *MCN: American Journal of Maternal Child Nursing, 14*(4), 255-259.

Lipman, T.H., Difazio, D.A., Meers, R.A., & Thompson, R.L. (1989). A developmental approach to diabetes in children: School age–adolescence. *MCN: American Journal of Maternal Child Nursing, 14*(5), 330-332.

Meyer, P.A. (1988). Parental adaptation to cystic fibrosis. *Journal of Pediatric Health Care, 2*(1), 20-28.

Stullenbarger, B., et al. (1987). Family adaptation to cystic fibrosis. *Pediatric Nursing, 13*(1), 29-31.

Tucker, J.A., & Sussman-Karten, K. (1987). Treating acute diarrhea and dehydration with an oral rehydration solution. *Pediatric Nursing, 13*(3), 169-174.

Vaughan, V., & Behrman, R. (1987). *Nelson's textbook of pediatrics* (13th ed.). Philadelphia: Saunders.

Wells, P.W., & Meghdadpour, S. (1988). Research yields new clues to cystic fibrosis. *MCN: American Journal of Maternal Child Nursing, 13*(3), 187-190.

Yoos, L. (1987). Chronic childhood illnesses: Developmental issues. *Pediatric Nursing, 13*(1), 25-28.

Elimination

Foster, R., Hunsberger, M., & Anderson, J. (1989). *Family-centered nursing care of children.* Philadelphia: Saunders.

James, S., Mott, S. (1988). *Child health nursing: Essential care of children and families.* Menlo Park, CA: Addison-Wesley.

Marlow, D., & Redding, B. (1988). *Textbook of pediatric nursing* (6th ed.). Philadelphia: Harcourt-Brace-Jovanovich.

Servonsky, J., & Opas, S. (1987). *Nursing management of children.* Boston: Jones and Bartlett.

Sperhac, A. M. (1989). Abdominal pain in pediatric patients: Assessment and management update. *Journal of Emergency Nursing,* 93-100.

Wilson, D., (1989). Urinary tract infections in the pediatric patient. *Nurse Practitioner 14*(38), 41-42.

Cellular aberration

Austin, J. (1990). Assessment of coping mechanisms used by parents and children with chronic illness. *MCN: American Journal of Maternal Child Nursing, 15,* 98-102.

Hockenberry, M.J., & Coody, D.K. (1986). *Pediatric oncology and hematology.* St. Louis: Mosby–Year Book.

Hockenberry, M.J., Coody, D.K., & Bennett, B. (1990). Childhood cancers. *Pediatric Nursing, 16,* 239-245.

Krulik, T. (1988). *The child and family facing life threatening illness.* Philadelphia: Lippincott.

Lilley, L. (1990). Side effects associated with pediatric chemotherapy: Management and patient education issues. *Pediatric Nursing, 16,* 252-272.

Marcoux, C., Fisher, S., & Wong, D. (1990). Central venous access devices in children. *Pediatric Nursing, 16,* 123-133.

Meehan, J. (1989). Pain control in the terminally ill child at home. *Issues in Comprehensive Pediatric Nursing, 12,* 187-197.

Young, J., Eslinger, P., & Galloway, M. (1989). Radiation treatment for the child with cancer. *Issues in Comprehensive Pediatric Nursing, 12,* 159-169.

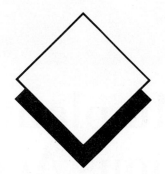

Reprints

Nursing Care of the Child

An Implantable Venous Access Device for Children

Children who require repeated intravenous therapy now have the option of having a venous access device implanted — a mechanism that can remain in place for two to three years.

BY KIMBERLY A. KANDT

Reprinted from MCN: The American Journal of Maternal Child Nursing, March/April 1988

The implantable venous access device (IVAD) is a system that delivers blood and blood products, drugs, and intravenous fluids to children for whom regular vascular access is necessary. The system, used for children only during the past few years, facilitates peripheral venipuncture, which is time-consuming, stressful, and painful. It is recommended for children who require daily, weekly, or monthly intravenous therapy; for example, children with oncologic problems, AIDS, thalassemia, sickle cell anemia, cystic fibrosis, or any chronic illness that requires intravascular therapy. In addition, children who need frequent hyperalimentation and lipid administration are candidates. Blood sampling, too, can be done.

The implantable device has two parts, the port, or chamber, and the catheter, which are connected. The port-reservoir is a stainless steel or hard plastic chamber measuring approximately 1 to 1-1/2 inches. The top is a rubber disk. To implant the chamber requires approximately an hour. The surgical procedure begins with an incision in the upper chest. A short subcutaneous tunnel is then made, through which the catheter enters a vessel and continues to a bony, stabilizing pocket — usually the bony prominence under the clavicle. That pocket stabilizes the reservoir. The port is secured in place, and the incision closed. The position is confirmed by fluoroscopy or chest x-ray. Externally, the IVAD is visible only as a small bump under the skin on the chest (1).

KIMBERLY A. KANDT, R.N., B.S.N., is the assistant unit manager of pediatrics at the University Medical Center of Southern Nevada. Certified as a chemotherapy nurse, the author assists in both inpatient and outpatient therapy programs. She would like to recognize Tara Brascia, her mentor in maternal/child nursing, for her encouragement, support, and expertise.

The port costs from $250 to $350. Three systems are commonly used: Infuse-A-Port (from Infusaid in Norwood, Massachusetts), Port-A-Cath (Pharmacia, in Piscataway, New Jersey), and Hickman Subcutaneous Port (Davol-Bond, Cranston, Rhode Island). Maintaining an implantable device costs less than maintaining a percutaneous catheter, because irrigations are less frequent and no dressing changes required. The only significant cost is that of a special needle (Huber-noncoring, 90-degree angle). It is attached to the extension tubing (1).

The Pros and Cons

Because many factors must be considered before the IVAD is implemented, the nurse's guidance will help a child and family choose the most suitable system. The table Criteria Used to Select Venous Access System presents guidelines for decision making.

The advantages of the implantable venous access device extend to both the child and parent or other caregiver. One advantage is that the device is easily palpable and can be used immediately after it is inserted. In addition, the IVAD can be punctured up to 2,000 times before replacement is necessary. Infection is also less likely than when using the percutaneous catheter.

Cosmetic changes are few, and when the system is not being used, a child's activity is not limited — an especially important factor for both adolescents and toddlers. A child may also shower or bathe with no difficulty. Finally, no daily care is required when the catheter is not being used. Maintaining it entails flushing every 28 days. The implanted device needs to be changed every two to three years. (When it is finally removed, a surgical procedure is performed.)

The biggest disadvantage of the IVAD is that a needle puncture is required with each access, unless continuous intravenous therapy is required. The pain associated with the puncture may cause some children to prefer a percutaneous catheter. During the first two weeks after surgery, more pain is experienced with the puncture due to tenderness and edema. Stabilizing the system for punctures may be diffi-

cult. Care must be taken to prevent extravasation due to leakage of fluids or medications, or accidental dislodgment of the needle. The IVAD can be used for only one infusion at a time; if multiple infusions are needed, a system that uses a multilumened catheter may be a better choice. Although dual IVADs are on the market, none has been designed that is small enough to be used for pediatric care.

Nursing Management

Routine care and discharge planning and teaching are among the responsibilities of the nursing staff. Routine injections, flushes, infusions, needle changes, and dressing changes are important in caring for the system. Hospital policies and procedures may vary but general guidelines facilitate consistency in care. They are part of the nurse's orientation to her responsibilities on the pediatric unit.

Specific guidelines are also used for inserting and withdrawing the Huber needle when accessing the device. (See Accessing the Implanted Device.)

The drawing and infusing of blood require special care. When drawing blood through the device, at least 3 cc of blood (the capacity of the extension tubing and the port) must be discarded before blood can be used for studies in order to ensure accurate tests. It is not recommended that blood be drawn from the implantable venous access device for coagulation or pharmacologic studies, because residual heparin or drug in the portal may affect test results. Instead, blood may be aspirated through a syringe or a vacuum adapter attached directly to the tube used to aspirate blood; the system is flushed immediately after this procedure according to the protocol established by the institution.

When using the implantable venous access device for the transfusion of blood or blood products, close observation is necessary to detect intraluminal clot formation with resultant catheter occlusion. During an infusion of blood, a positive pressure pump must be used along with a saline flush. Heparinized saline is used after the transfusion. Hyperalimentation also requires the use of heparin.

The implantable device has few disadvantages and many advantages when used for children. To circumvent those disadvantages and to carry out routine strategies effectively, a careful plan of care must be devised. (See Nursing Care Plan for a Child with an Implantable Venous Access Device.)

Complications

Complications may occur in children even with meticulous aseptic use of the port. Problems that are encountered in children include venous thrombosis, extravasation, and/or infection.

Venous Thrombosis

The most common complication appears to be venous thrombosis. A clot can develop around the catheter in either the subclavian or the superior vena cava, and may go undetected until symptoms devel-

---

Criteria Used to Select Venous Access System

1. The cognitive and psychosocial developmental levels of the child.
2. The child's physical condition (type and severity of illness), diagnosis, and ability to cope with the system.
3. The parents' or significant others' understanding and reaction to the system.
4. The child's skills level related to catheter care versus IVAD care.
5. Understanding the necessity of the device, why it is needed, what it does.
6. Financial status, ability to pay for supplies.
7. Home environment, availability of support system.
8. Parent and child preference.
9. Type of therapy, types of medications to be infused, time projected for catheter usefulness.

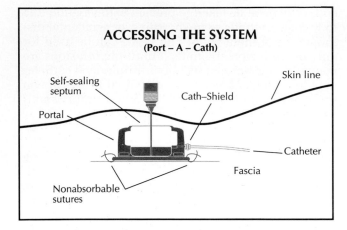

ACCESSING THE SYSTEM
(Port – A – Cath)

Self-sealing septum
Skin line
Portal
Cath–Shield
Catheter
Fascia
Nonabsorbable sutures

op. Symptoms may include the presence of pain in the neck, arm, and/or shoulder on the ipsilateral side of the catheter insertion site. Supraclavicular and neck swelling, as well as swelling of the face can occur. Thrombosis is diagnosed by x-raying the catheter, using dye to observe configuration and flow. If a catheter is partially blocked, aspiration with saline may help to clear the tubing. In addition, the needle is replaced. If the clot remains, a physician may order streptokinase or urokinase to dissolve the clot.

Extravasation

Inadvertent dislodgment of the needle from the port, catheter migration, or the catheter's becoming disconnected from inside the portal system may cause extravasation. If the child experiences chest pain, shortness of breath, or coolness in the chest, the physician is called. The catheter is not flushed; what has been infused must be identified, because certain drugs, such as Dilantin, calcium, or certain chemotherapy, may cause untoward effects outside venous access.

Infection

The incidence of infection among children with an IVAD is lower than among those with indwelling catheters; some indwelling catheter use has resulted in infection rates as high as 80 percent; local cellulitis has also been reported. The rate of infection among IVAD users has been documented as low as 5 percent (2). In addition to the nurse's observing for signs of infection, teaching observation skills to the child's parent is also essential. The site must be inspected for redness, swelling, and other indications of induration. If the child has a fever, both peripheral and central blood are obtained for culture. The culture will identify systemic infection. Localized infection is treated with oral antibiotics and/or antibiotic ointment at the site of infection. The device may need to be removed.

Although complications may occur, the advantages of the IVAD are many for a child who must cope with chronic illness. As familiarity with the device increases, the IVAD may become the answer to less traumatic therapy and to fewer complications.

Accessing the Implanted Device

1. Explain the procedure to the child and parents. Information is presented appropriately for the child's growth and development.

2. Assemble equipment. Prime the tubing that is attached to the 22-gauge Huber needle with bacteriostatic saline. Have a syringe of normal saline flush and heparinized saline ready.

3. Position the child either supine or sitting. Locate the site of the port by trapping it between two fingers of the nondominant hand so that the device cannot slip and move. Feel for the septum — a small rubber disc found at the center of the port — where the needle is inserted.

4. Wash hands and put on sterile gloves. Occasionally, a physician may order 0.1 to 0.15 cc of 2 percent lidocaine injected subcutaneously to "numb" the area prepared for injection.

5. Prepare skin according to hospital policy for sterile procedure; for example, povidone-iodine/alcohol solution. Let the area dry.

6. Again, feel the port and trap it with the two fingers , as described. Grip the port securely, and palpate the disk for injection.

7. Hold the needle perpendicularly to the septum and push it firmly through the skin and septum until it makes contact with the bottom of the portal chamber. The needle may still not look totally inserted because of the size of the child. When the bottom is reached, the catheter is checked for placement. Once the septum is punctured, the needle is not tilted or rocked; these actions may cause fluid leakage, extravasation, and damage to the septum. The needle is secured when it hits the bottom of the septum, and blood flow is checked. Three other factors are also checked: positive blood return on aspiration; the ability to prime solution; and that no sign of subcutaneous tissue infiltration is present after infusion of priming solution and flush.

8. Flush the system with heparinized saline. To avoid reflux, maintain a positive pressure when flushing. Clamp the tubing as the flush is finished.

9. Huber needles, when fitted with the proper "hep-lock" adapter, may be left in place for 7 days before they need to be changed. If, because of the child's size, the needle does not appear totally implanted, a 2x2 gauze dressing is arranged on each side of the needle to secure it, thereby preventing manipulation or dislodgment. An occlusive dressing is then applied to the catheter and needle site. A piece of tape can be used to coil the tubing before the dressing is applied to secure the system. A stopcock type of extension set also helps to decrease manipulation. Dressings should be changed at the same time the needle is changed (every 7 days); sterile technique must be used, but no mask is necessary. If the patient is allergic to tape, a sterile dressing and foam dressing may be used. Some institutions require the use of povidone or antibiotic ointment on the site before the dressings are applied.

10. When removing the needle, a positive pressure is maintained while simultaneously withdrawing the needle. Press firmly with two fingers.

11. Cleanse the site and apply a light dressing or band-aid.

12. Record the procedure and note observations on the nursing chart.

Nursing Care Plan for a Child with an Implantable Venous Access Device

Nursing diagnosis: Anxiety related to insertion of the catheter

Rationale — Child and parents may have questions about the insertion procedure and care of the catheter after it is inserted. Providing information can promote their feelings of control and thus decrease anxiety.

Goal — For child and parents to verbalize decreased anxiety about catheter insertion and care.

Intervention (preoperative) — Assess level of knowledge and elicit statement of fears and concerns from the child and family. Encourage questions and provide information. Provide visual aids that are appropriate for the child's level of growth and development. Familiarize the child with his room and the usual preoperative and postoperative routines.

Outcomes — Child and parents can explain the insertion procedure and care; they demonstrate a decreased level of anxiety.

Nursing diagnosis: Potential for alteration in cardiac output related to hemorrhage, injury-related catheter migration, misplacement, occlusion, and disconnection that results in air embolism or thrombosis

Rationale — Air embolism and hemorrhage may result if the catheter becomes disconnected; catheter may become occluded by clot formation if not properly irrigated after use or drawing of blood; extravasation of fluids may occur if catheter is misplaced.

Goals — For the child to be free of complications; for the catheter to be patent.

Intervention — Observe for signs of migration and dislodgment: edema of the arm, neck pain, jugular venous distention, confusion, pallor, and lightheadedness. Use dressings for 24 hours after use of the system. Monitor intake and output. Observe for difficulty irrigating or infusing fluids, for edema, subcutaneous fluid along the tunnel, or leakage around the catheter. Irrigate the catheter with flushes, as ordered.

Outcomes — Child has no hemorrhaging, thrombosis, or air embolism. Blood flows easily through the catheter prior to irrigation. The catheter is irrigated easily.

Nursing diagnosis: Child's and parent's knowledge deficit related to catheter/system maintenance and to use of the system on discharge due to lack of recall, cognitive limitations, and lack of interest in learning

Rationale — Child and parents must have sufficient knowledge to manage independently the care of the system at home. Planned instruction and the child's and/or parent's return demonstrations will assist learning.

Goal — For the parent to demonstrate care of the system and to state signs of complications.

Intervention — Begin teaching preoperatively. Stress signs of infection and complications. Teach what to do in emergencies, such as a needle becoming dislodged. Monitor the learning process, reinforcing and demonstrating so that return demonstrations of all aspects of care can be given. Refer family to social service, public health, or other agencies if applicable.

Outcomes — Parent and child can state signs of complications and what to do if complications occur, can demonstrate care of the system, and can carry out aspects of care.

Nursing diagnosis: Potential for infection related to entry of Huber needle into the port, altered skin integrity at needle site, or body's rejection of the IVAD

Rationale — Introduction of any foreign object into the body increases the risk of infection and presents the potential for rejection. Signs and symptoms of impending sepsis include fever or chills; signs of localized site infection may be drainage, inflammation, redness.

Goal — For the patient to remain free of infection systemically and at port site; 72-hour blood culture and sensitivity tests are negative.

Intervention — Know hospital policy regarding dressing and needle changes. Use aseptic technique when cleaning the site and inserting needle. With each dressing change, inspect the site for signs of infection. When no dressing is used, be aware of signs of minor temperature elevations or vital sign changes.

If port is being used, the dressing can be protected and the patient may shower or bathe, keeping the dressing dry.

For a continuous infusion, change needle and tubing, redress site every week or according to hospital policy. At least every 4 hours, monitor for signs of sepsis, such as fever, increased heart and respiratory rates, and decreased blood pressure. If physician orders antibiotics, monitor for therapeutic or toxic effects.

Nursing diagnosis: Potential for injury related to infiltration of toxic drugs/copious fluids

Rationale — Some drugs are caustic and may cause severe tissue damage if infiltration occurs. Subsequently, tissue necrosis may occur, necessitating skin grafts.

Goal — For the child to experience safe administration of fluids and drugs — tubing remains patent and no infiltration occurs.

Intervention — Monitor entrance site for signs of infiltration, such as pain, burning, no blood return, edema; have written policy available for nursing staff regarding intake and output management.

Adapted from GREENBERG, C. *Nursing Care Planning Guides for Children*. Baltimore, MD, Williams & Wilkins, 1987. Used with permission.

REFERENCES
1. WAINSTOCK, J. Making a choice: the vein access method you prefer.*Oncol.Nurs.Forum* 14:79–82, Jan.-Feb. 1987.
2. *PORT-A-Cath; Implantable Access System* (Professional Nursing Pamphlet). St. Paul, MN, Pharmacia Deltec, Inc., 1989, pp. 35-39.

BIBLIOGRAPHY
ABBOTT, P., AND SCHLACHT, K. Pediatric IV's: a special challenge. *Can.Nurse* 80:24–26, Nov. 1984.

GREENBERG, C. *Nursing Care Planning Guides for Children*.Baltimore, MD: Williams & Wilkins, 1987.
GULLATTE, M. Managing an implanted infusion device.*RN* 52:44–49, Jan. 1989.
HARRIS, L.C., AND OTHERS. Implantable infusion devices in the pediatric patient: a viable alternative. *J.Pediatr. Nurs.* 2:174–183, June 1987.
MOORE, C., AND OTHERS. Nursing care and management of venous access ports.*Oncol.Nurs.Forum* 13:35–39, May-Jun. 1986.

Shock In Infants And Children: Assessment And Treatment

Reprinted from MCN: The American Journal of Maternal Child Nursing, March/April 1988

As a youngster progresses through the phases of shock, his nurse must be ready to adjust care accordingly.

JOAN M. RIMAR

Because of the evolving nature of shock, nursing assessment and treatment of the various stages is a demanding, ongoing process. Signs and symptoms appear and disappear, and treatment is initiated, modified, or discontinued throughout the course of the illness. (Types of shock, their stages, and their symptoms were discussed in "Recognizing Shock Syndromes In Infants And Children," MCN, January/February 1988.) A child's ability to survive this fast-paced series of actions and reactions depends heavily on the services and skills of an astute, vigilant nurse.

Shock symptoms are caused by circulatory dysfunction and tissue oxygen and tissue nutrient deficits. Physical findings (temperature, skin color, etc.) and hemodynamic indices (blood pressure, central venous pressure, etc.) reflect the consequences of perfusion impairment on organ function and the child's general condition. Laboratory tests quantify the damage suffered.

Clinical Assessment

Impairment of peripheral circulation can be assessed by examination of the temperature, color, pulse, and capillary refill of the child's extremities. Normally, a child's extremities are warm and pink, with strong, equal pulses and brisk capillary refill. The child in shock, however, presents with cool and clammy skin, mottled or gray extremi-

JOAN M. RIMAR, R.N., M.S.N., *is head nurse of the infant-toddler ward at Yale–New Haven Hospital in New Haven, Connecticut. To order reprints of this article, see the classified section.*

ties, diminished pulses, and sluggish capillary refill, abnormalities primarily resulting from decreased cardiac output (CO) and increased systemic vascular resistance (SVR). However, septic shock, which in its early stage is associated with normal or increased CO, causes different initial signs and symptoms. Septic shock patients have warm and dry skin (they are often febrile) and they are well-perfused. They often look good despite the fact that they suffer from a life-threatening condition.

The circulatory dysfunction and depleted vascular volume characteristic of most shock syndromes are reflected in low blood pressure (BP), central venous pressure (CVP), and pulmonary capillary wedge pressure (PCWP)/left atrial pressure (LAP). Compensatory tachycardia can also occur and is often the first indicator of circulatory impairment. Again, the exception is septic shock. In the early stages of septic shock, and in cardiogenic shock, the CVP and PCWP/LAP are often normal or elevated.

Signs of dehydration also accompany these signs of hypovolemic shock. Skin turgor is poor, and the skin may remain "tented" when pinched. Mucous membranes are often dry, the fontanelle may be sunken, and daily weight may decrease.

Signs and symptoms of cerebral perfusion dysfunction are often subtle in the early stages of shock. The child's sensorium may be clouded, his response to stimuli may be poor, and he may be anxious, irritable, or lethargic. Infants frequently exhibit a weak cry and poor suck. As shock progresses, somnolence advances to obtundation.

In addition, arrhythmias, which impair cardiac function, are not uncommon in the presence of electrolyte imbalance, metabolic acidosis, and hypoxemia. All of these can occur in shock.

Even with normal or increased cardiac output, the child in shock may suffer myocardial injury. The reasons for the infarctions sustained by some patients in shock are not clear. Indications of damage to the heart muscle include S-T segment elevation on electrocardiogram (EKG) and abnormal cardiac enzyme values (creatine kinase-myocardial enzyme, or CK-MB) (1).

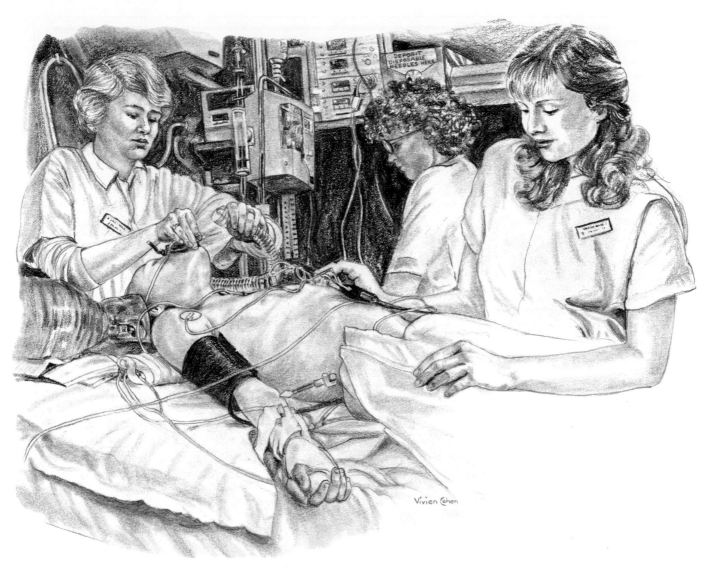

Because changes occur rapidly in shock and the effects of therapy must be evaluated quickly, continuous monitoring is an essential part of the treatment of an infant or child in shock.

Urine output is an extremely important measurement when assessing infants and children in shock. Particularly in hypovolemic patients, output may decrease long before other signs of impaired tissue perfusion become evident. In general, urine output decreases when renal blood flow drops, and increases as flow increases. Renal blood flow, in turn, is dependent on cardiac output. Sudden drops in renal blood flow or pressure cause urine output to decrease and urine specific gravity to rise. Low urine output is <0.5–1.0 ml/kg/hour in infants and children and <1.0–2.0 ml/kg/hour in neonates. But, if the fall in renal blood pressure or flow is gradual, changes in urine output may appear slowly. In some patients with sepsis, urine output may initially be normal or increased, despite the relative hypovolemia associated with the condition (2).

Laboratory Evaluation

Laboratory tests are obtained as soon as possible after a child presents in shock. Further tests are acquired as dictated by the child's clinical condition. They are necessary in order to monitor a variety of potentially lethal conditions and irregularities that may be encountered in shock patients. Metabolic acidosis, hypoglycemia, electrolyte and coagulation abnormalities, infection, and renal failure are a few of these conditions.

Tests commonly obtained include: arterial and mixed venous blood gases; blood lactate; serum electrolytes, osmolality and glucose; coagulation studies; complete blood count with differential; creatinine and blood urea nitrogen; blood cultures; urinalysis; and urine sodium and osmolality. If the cause of shock is unclear, the possibility

Cardiovascular Drugs Used in the Treatment of Pediatric Shock

Drug	Usual Intravenous Dose	Comments
Isoproterenol	0.05–1.5 mcg/kg per min	Increases strength and rate of cardiac contraction. Dilates peripheral vessels. May increase myocardial work and oxygen consumption. May include arrhythmias.
Epinephrine	0.05–0.5 mcg/kg per min	At low doeses, increases strength and rate of cardiac contraction to moderate degree and causes systemic vascular resistance (SVR) to decrease slightly at low doses. At high doses, causes marked increase in strength and rate of cardiac contraction and severe vasoconstriction of peripheral vasculature (increased SVR). As epinephrine may decrease renal blood flow significantly, monitor urine output.
Dopamine	1–20 mcg/kg per min (higher doses may be used)	Effects vary with dose: low dose response primarily dopaminergic; mid-range cause moderate increase in heart rate and contractility; high doses (10–20 mcg/kg min) vasoconstriction predominates. May cause arrhythmias.
Dobutamine	2–15 mcg/kg per min (higher doses may be used)	Increases strength of cardiac contraction but causes minimal change in heart rate. On occasion, causes tachycardia and hypertension.
Amrinone	0.75 mg/kg initially; 5–10 mcg/kg per min (adult dose recommendation)	Increases strength of cardiac contraction and relaxes vascular smooth muscle, causing decreased afterload and preload. Clinical studies regarding use in children are ongoing.
Nitroprusside	0.5–10 mcg/kg per min	Dilates peripheral arteries and veins. May produce severe hypotension. Do not use in boluses. Immediate onset and short duration (2–4 sec) of action. Protect from light.
Phentolamine	1–20 mcg/kg per min	Dilates peripheral arteries and, to a lesser extent, veins. Also causes cardiac stimulation. May cause marked hypotension, tachycardia, and arrhythmias.
Hydralazine	0.1–0.5 mg/kg per dose every 3–6 hr	Primarily vasodilates peripheral arteries. Also maintains or increases renal and cerebral blood flow. May cause tachycardia.
Tolazoline	1–2 mg/kg initially; 1–2 mg/kg per hr	Decreases peripheral resistance and increases venous capacitance. Causes cardiac stimulation. Reduces pulmonary arterial pressure and resistance.

that it may be due to a drug overdose must be considered. Accordingly, blood and urine are screened, especially for barbiturates and major tranquilizers. Sequential chest x-rays will aid in the diagnosis of some complications of shock (pulmonary edema, for example) and facilitate evaluation of corresponding treatment.

Initial Treatment

Children in shock are often significantly hypotensive, obtunded, and require resuscitation. Immediate therapeutic goals at this time include establishment of a patent airway and maintenance of respiration and circulation while the underlying problem is assessed. Endotracheal intubation and mechanical ventilation with 100 percent oxygen is usually indicated. The heightened susceptibility of newborns to oxygen toxicity (particularly retrolental fibroplasia) must always be considered when determining inspired oxygen concentration for infants.

Emergency medications and fluids are given as soon as administration routes are available. The following routes (in the order of their desirability) are used for drug administration: central venous; peripheral venous/intraosseous (anterior tibial bone marrow); endotracheal; and intracardiac (3). Fluid boluses may be infused via any of the venous routes.

Two central lines (or one multilumen catheter) constitute optimal intravenous (IV) access. One of the central venous lines is used for pressure measurement and the other for infusion of drugs into the central circulatory system close to their sites of action (3). Because some drugs cause tissue necrosis when they infiltrate at peripheral sites, central infusion is preferable. Peripheral IV lines are inserted as they are required.

Monitoring

Continuous monitoring is essential in treating shock patients. Changes occur rapidly, and the effects of therapy must be evaluated quickly.

Cardiac function is followed in several ways. The EKG displays cardiac rate and rhythm. The arterial line measures systemic BP, including diastolic pressure (which reflects SVR), and pulse pressure (related to stroke volume). It also provides a way to obtain arterial blood for calculating the arteriovenous oxygen difference ($avDo_2$). The CVP line quantifies right ventricular preload and, in most children without right ventricular outflow obstruction, left ventricular preload, too. If necessary, a pulmonary artery catheter is inserted to measure left ventricular filling pressure. Cardiac output can be measured directly by using the pulmonary artery catheter and indirectly with the $avDo_2$. An echocardiogram will gauge left ventricular contractility and help determine whether a pericardial effusion is present (4).

Renal function and, indirectly, cardiac function are followed by monitoring urine output. A urinary drainage catheter and collection system is necessary for output measurement.

In addition, pulse oximeters or transcutaneous oxygen and carbon dioxide monitors help monitor respiratory function in infants and children.

Fluid Management

Fluid replacement is generally accepted as the most important immediate therapeutic goal in shock. Early correction of the volume deficit is necessary to increase CO (by increasing preload) and to reestablish the even distribution of microcirculatory flow. It also prevents later complications of shock such as acute renal failure. Improvement in pressure, flow, oxygen delivery, and oxygen consumption indicate successful fluid therapy (5).

Controversy exists, however, as to whether colloid or crystalloid distribution is best suited to fluid resuscitation; the literature is replete with apparently contradictory studies (6). Colloid usually refers to albumin, but also includes other prepared plasma fractions, synthetic plasma substitutes, whole blood, red blood cells, and fresh-frozen plasma. Normal saline and Ringer's lactate are the isotonic, crystalloid (electrolyte) solutions used for acute volume replacement in shock (7). More than twice as much crystalloid as colloid is necessary to achieve the same degree of hemodynamic stability (8).

Proponents of colloid use claim that colloids are more effective than crystalloids in achieving optimum hemodynamic and oxygen transport goals. They also cite the importance of colloids for maintaining plasma colloid osmotic pressure and minimizing interstitial edema (9). Prevention of interstitial edema, particularly in the lung, is important because accumulation of interstitial fluid (i.e. pulmonary edema) leads to deterioration in gas exchange (8).

Those who advocate crystalloid infusion argue that a balanced salt solution is all that is necessary to restore and maintain effective extracellular fluid volume (6). They also affirm that colloid therapy increases the risk of pulmonary edema in some patients (10). In addition, colloid is expensive and extremely difficult to titrate, making the possibility of fluid overload much greater than when crystalloid is used. Underreplacement is more likely to occur with crystalloid therapy.

In most clinical situations, theoretical considerations give way to practical concerns. A variety of volume expanders are usually employed, depending upon their availability and the kinds of losses the child has suffered. In a life-threatening situation, a balanced salt solution is probably the ideal infusate; it can be infused rapidly and is immediately available. The amount and rate of infusion depend on the child's condition; 10 ml/kg of estimated body weight of Ringer's lactate solution infused over several minutes is a reasonable starting point. A second bolus of the same amount is infused if there is no improvement in blood pressure or perfusion (11). The child is evaluated between boluses for the presence of pulmonary edema (4). If there continues to be no improvement in the child's condition, impaired myocardial function must be considered.

Blood is administered as soon as possible in order to replace whole-blood loss and correct anemia. If there is evidence of continued bleeding or consumption of clotting factors, fresh-frozen plasma should be given as well.

Efforts to improve cardiac output and tissue perfusion by volume augmentation when treating children with cardiogenic or septic shock must be carefully monitored (12). The volume of fluid that may be safely administered is contingent on cardiac competence. Routine measurement of CVP, pulmonary artery pressure, and PCWP enable early detection of cardiac decompensation and pulmonary edema and therefore provide an important guide for volume replacement (13).

Pharmacologic Management

If fluid therapy fails to improve the child's condition, a drug to enhance cardiovascular performance (see Cardiovascular Drugs Used in the Treatment of Pediatric Shock) is administered. Increasing the *inotropy* (strength) and/or *chronotropy* (rate) of cardiac contraction by continuous infusion of intravenous catecholamines (sympathomimetic amines) is particularly well-suited to this task. The rapid onset, controllable dosage, and ultrashort half-life of catecholamines make them effective for treating shock (11).

Epinephrine, dopamine, isoproterenol, and dobutamine are the most frequently used exogenous catecholamines. In general, epinephrine is used when the child is in cardiopulmonary arrest or arrest is imminent; dopamine is used for children with diminished urine output; isoproterenol is used when the child has bradycardia or acidemia; and dobutamine is used when the child has high ventricular filling pressures or as a substitute for isoproterenol when the child has tachycardia (4,

14). Frequently, more than one catecholamine is given at a time; finding the right doses and combinations may take a while. Because catecholamines increase myocardial oxygen consumption, signs of myocardial hypoxia or ischemia such as S-T segment and T-wave changes on the EKG may become apparent during administration.

Sympathomimetic amines stimulate alpha, beta, and dopaminergic receptors throughout the body causing a variety of effects. (See Adrenergic Receptors and Functions for a discussion of physiologic responses.) Isoproterenol is a pure beta agonist that increases heart rate and cardiac contractility and causes dilatation of skeletal muscle beds and a fall in SVR. This vasodilatation often reduces venous return to the heart, decreasing preload and stroke volume; therefore, hypovolemia must be corrected before initiating isoproterenol infusion and the child's CVP is to be followed closely during therapy.

Adequate oxygenation must be ensured for children receiving isoproterenol. Additionally, the lowest effective dose is used because the drug can induce severe cardiac arrhythmias such as ventricular tachycardia and fibrillation in hypoxic children (11). Isoproterenol is valuable for children with bradycardia or acidosis due to poor perfusion from vasoconstriction (4).

Epinephrine acts on both alpha and beta receptor sites. Its most pronounced action is on the beta receptors of the heart, vascular, and other smooth muscle. The drug increases the heart rate, BP (mainly systolic), and strength of ventricular contractions. Total peripheral resistance may be decreased, increased, or unaffected by epinephrine administration, depending on the ratio of alpha to beta activity in different vascular areas; the vasodilator effect usually predominates (16). High doses can increase resistance in the kidney and decrease renal blood flow to such an extent that irreversible renal failure develops. Epinephrine may be particularly helpful in septic shock and anaphylaxis when SVR is abnormally low (11).

Dopamine activates alpha and beta receptors in a dose-dependent fashion. At low doses (2–4 mcg/kg/minute), it causes a decrease in SVR and splanchnic and renal vasodilatation; the dopaminergic effect on the kidney results in increased urine output. It stimulates $beta_1$ receptors at moderate doses (5–8 mcg/kg/minute), and exhibits a moderate positive inotropic effect. At high doses (> 10–15 mcg/kg/minute), dopamine is primarily an alpha agonist that causes renal vasoconstriction and increased SVR (11). Increased SVR will cause increased systemic afterload, which may diminish CO. When doses greater than 15 mcg/kg/minute are used, the child must be monitored for tachycardia, arrhythmias, and severe peripheral vasoconstriction.

Dobutamine, a synthetic catecholamine, is a $beta_1$ stimulant that increases cardiac contractility

---

Adrenergic Receptors and Functions

Receptor	Site Of Action	Response
Beta, (β_1)	Heart	cardioacceleration (sinoatrial and atrioventricular nodes), increased myocardial strength (atria and ventricles)
Beta$_2$ (β_2)	Peripheral vasculature: skeletal muscle	vasodilatation
	Lung	bronchodilatation
Alpha (α)	Heart: coronary circulation	vasoconstriction
	Lung	bronchoconstriction
	Peripheral vasculature: skin, mucosa, renal, splanchnic	vasoconstriction
Dopaminergic	Kidney	increased renal blood flow, increased urine output

Based on Crone, R.K., Acute circulatory failure in children, *Pediatr. Clin. North Am.* 27: 525–538, Aug. 1980 and Guyton, A. C., *Textbook of Medical Physiology*, 7th ed. Philadelphia, W. B. Saunders Co. 1986.

---

but causes only a slight increase in heart rate. The drug's opposing alpha and beta$_2$ effects on the peripheral vasculature minimize direct vascular activity, although SVR is usually decreased and minimal vasoconstriction is occasionally observed (16). Dobutamine has been found to be less effective in infants less than one year old than in older children (17).

Amrinone is a new, nonadrenergic, positive inotropic agent with vasodilator activity that is now undergoing research for use in children. Amrinone reduces afterload and preload by its direct relaxant effect on vascular smooth muscle. In children with depressed myocardial function, amrinone produces a prompt increase in CO (16).

Increased vascular resistance and consequent, increased ventricular afterload can result from activation of compensatory mechanisms and/or use of sympathomimetic agents in children who have shock. When an element of heart failure coexists with impeded ventricular outflow, the use of vasodilators, usually in combination with inotropic agents, is commonly indicated.

Vasodilators decrease ventricular afterload primarily by reducing impedance to left ventricular ejection (18). Afterload reduction may be accomplished with a direct vasodilator (nitroprusside sodium or hydralazine), a beta agonist (isoproterenol), or an alpha antagonist (phentolamine or tolazoline). All of these drugs, except hydralazine, are administered by continuous IV infusion. Hydralazine is given in single doses by slow intravenous push. Vasodilators can cause severe hypotension; hence, vasoconstricting agents, such as phenylephrine or norepinephrine, and fluid should be readily available (11).

Nitroprusside causes direct, balanced vasodilatation of peripheral veins and arteries. The subsequent fall in afterload and preload improves CO only when the effects of the drug that reduce outflow resistance predominate over the effects that reduce venous return (16). Filling pressures, therefore, must be at the upper limits of normal before nitroprusside infusion is begun (18). The dose range for the drug is 0.5–10 mcg/kg/minute for adults (19). However, manifestations of toxicity (headache, nausea, palpitations, hyperventilation, metabolic acidosis, and unexplained elevation of venous oxygen tension) have occurred at relatively low doses, leading some authors to suggest a maximum infusion rate of 4–8 mcg/kg/minute for adults and probably less for neonates and young children (20). Several precautions must be taken when the drug is administered: monitor serum levels of thiocyanate and cyanide, the toxic metabolites of nitroprusside; protect the 5 percent dextrose infusate containing the drug from light; and monitor BP continuously.

The alpha-adrenergic blocking agent phentolamine causes vasodilatation of peripheral veins and arteries. It dilates veins less effectively than does nitroprusside, resulting in a smaller reduction of left ventricular preload for a given reduction of afterload (18). Constraints to phentolamine use include its high cost and the large doses needed to maintain consistent vasodilatation.

Hydralazine exerts a peripheral vasodilating effect through direct relaxation of vascular smooth muscle, primarily arterial muscle, with little effect on venous beds. SVR decreases, but the change in filling pressure is minimal (16).

Tolazoline is a direct peripheral vasodilator with moderate alpha-adrenergic blocking activity. It decreases peripheral resistance, increases venous capacitance, and causes cardiac stimulation. In addition, tolazoline usually reduces pulmonary artery pressure and vascular resistance, which decreases right ventricular afterload and left ventricular preload. The use of epinephrine with large doses of tolazoline may cause epinephrine reversal, a further reduction of blood pressure that is followed by an exaggerated rebound (16).

Stimulation of peripheral $beta_2$ receptors by isoproterenol can enhance forward flow from the left ventricle by decreasing SVR. Other vasodilator drugs that are used occasionally in the treatment of shock include nitroglycerin, a potent venodilator that decreases preload, and captopril, an angiotensin-converting enzyme inhibitor that generally causes a decrease in both peripheral arterial pressure and resistance (16).

Other Pharmacologic Therapy

Acidosis depresses myocardial function, impairs ventilatory response, and renders sympathomimetic drugs ineffective. Therefore, when arterial blood pH is less than 7.20 and adequate ventilation has been established (i.e. the partial pressure of carbon dioxide is normal), correction with sodium bicarbonate is indicated (11). The initial dose is 1–2 mEq/kg given intravenously. Subsequent doses are titrated to the bicarbonate content of arterial blood.

Antibiotics are started as soon as possible if the etiology of shock is unknown or if infection is documented or suspected. Calcium replacement may be necessary because hypocalcemia occurs frequently in circulatory failure, especially after administration of large amounts of albumin, whole blood, or fresh-frozen plasma.

Recent evidence suggests that the release of endogenous opiate beta-endorphins during shock may contribute to hypotension. The opioid antagonist naloxone has been found to rapidly reverse hypotension secondary to endotoxin and blood loss in animals (22, 23). Naloxone has been used successfully in some children with septic shock who failed to respond to conventional therapy (24, 25). Further clinical trials are necessary, as response to naloxone therapy has been inconsistent and severe reactions may occur (26).

Similar variable results have been obtained with corticosteroid use in shock. In certain subgroups of septic shock patients, corticosteroids may improve short-term survival and instigate reversal of shock (27). Steroid administration is considered when adrenal insufficiency is suspected (4). Numerous other agents for the treatment of shock (particularly septic shock) are under investigation: endotoxin antiserum, anticomplement$_{5a}$ antibody, arachidonic acid inhibitors, fibronectin, toxic oxygen scavengers, and glucose-insulin-potassium (GIK) (28, 29).

Additional Therapies and Nutritional Support

The MAST (Military Anti-Shock Trousers) suit provides rapid redistribution of intravascular fluid. For children in hypovolemic shock, inflation of the suit quickly "autotransfuses" the upper circulatory system with blood compressed from the venous beds in the abdomen and legs. Circulation to the brain and heart are thus preserved. There is concern, however, that inflation of the abdominal compartment may impair ventilation and cause respiratory acidosis by limiting diaphragmatic excursion. The MAST suit is not used to treat cardiogenic shock because it increases left ventricular afterload (7, 30).

Extracorporeal membrane oxygenation (ECMO), left ventricular assist devices, and intra-aortic balloon pumps have been used to treat shock in children, but further clinical experience and evaluation of their efficacy and indications for use are needed. Plasmapheresis (removal of the child's blood, separation of plasma, and reinjection of the packed cells in fresh plasma) and continuous arteriovenous hemofiltration (CAVH) have also been used to successfully treat septic shock (31–33). However, too few patients have received these treatments for their use to be recommended at this time.

Critically ill infants and children are particularly prone to malnutrition because of the nature and duration of their illnesses. Previously well-nourished infants and children will probably develop nutritional deficiencies after five to seven days of intensive care; infants and children who have been hospitalized for some time before the development of shock may already be malnourished (34). Parenteral or enteral nutritional support is initiated as soon as practical.

What Can Nurses Do?

The initial role of the nurse will vary depending on when in the course of shock she first encounters the child. In some cases, the nurse's primary role will be prevention of shock, particularly with children likely to develop septic shock. Septic shock may be avoided by reducing the potential for transmission and colonization of bacterial organisms by thorough handwashing, meticulous catheter and wound care, encouraging patients to do deep breathing exercises, and turning patients routinely (35). Nurses caring for infants and children at risk for sepsis must implement preventive measures immediately.

Prevention of shock is also possible for certain hospitalized infants and children with conditions that can lead to hypovolemia (vomiting and diarrhea, diabetes mellitus and insipidus, for example). Recording intake and output carefully, monitoring vital signs, and weighing patients frequently will enable the alert nurse to recognize deviations soon after they occur. She will then notify appropriate personnel.

The nurse's primary aim when treating the child with established shock is to increase tissue perfusion. Nursing care that facilitates this goal includes monitoring and interpreting indices that reflect circulatory adequacy, administering medical and nursing prescriptions for drugs and treatments, and monitoring and evaluating effects of interventions. Preventing complications and supporting the patient's family are other important aspects of good care.

Continuous assessment of cardiac, respiratory, neurologic, renal, hematologic, and integumenta-

---

Potential Nursing Diagnoses for the Child in Shock*

- Airway clearance, ineffective
- Gas exchange, impaired
- Tissue perfusion, alteration in: cerebral, cardiopulmonary, renal, gastrointestinal, peripheral
- Cardiac output, alteration in: decreased
- Fluid volume deficit, actual or potential
- Infection, potential for
- Nutrition, alterations in: less than body requirements
- Body temperature, potential alteration in
- Hyperthermia
- Tissue integrity, impaired
- Skin integrity, impairment of: actual or potential
- Urinary elimination, alteration in patterns
- Bowel elimination, alteration in: constipation or diarrhea
- Self-care deficit: feeding, bathing/hygiene, toileting
- Comfort, alteration in: pain
- Sleep pattern disturbance
- Mobility, impaired physical
- Communication, impaired verbal
- Fear
- Anxiety
- Knowledge deficit
- Coping, ineffective family: compromised
- Family processes, alteration in
- Grieving, anticipatory

*Diagnostic categories approved by the North American Nursing Diagnosis (NANDA) Seventh National Conference

---

ry function is essential. The importance and significance of information obtained from physical assessment, indwelling pressure lines, laboratory tests, and urinary drainage systems cannot be overemphasized. It is the nurse's responsibility to integrate and interpret this information to guide nursing care. She can also provide specific nursing interventions based on potential nursing diagnoses; see Potential Nursing Diagnoses for the Child in Shock.

Because the nurse is often the first person to encounter the data that may indicate an evolving problem, she may be the key to preventing the often lethal complications of shock. She ensures the minute to minute operation of equipment such as ventilators and medication infusions that will support system functions. It takes no more than an obstructed endotracheal tube or a kinked intravenous line to precipitate a crisis that will ultimately result in death.

The nurse can also play a valuable role by reducing the anxiety and fear that the infant or the child and his family will certainly experience. Hospital admission of almost any child causes strain, which is magnified when the child has a life-threatening condition (36). The strange environment, limitations on visiting, painful procedures, and the potential for death that accompany advanced shock are issues that must be addressed. The nurse must listen attentively and calmly to parents and explain policies, procedures, prognosis, and shock itself to them. Parents are to be encouraged to verbalize their questions, thoughts, and feelings and support personnel are to be involved.

For the child, relief from both physical and psychological pain through the use of potent analgesics such as intravenous morphine and antianxiety agents becomes important when comfort measures, distractions, etc., are unsuccessful or inappropriate. Family members can help themselves and the ill child by participating with him in active or passive play, as appropriate, and involving themselves in the activities of his daily life. They are never ushered from the bedside without good reason (37).

In these ways, a capable nurse can offset the extremely complicated and deadly progress of shock. Recognizing the child's condition early, diligently attending to the administration and evaluation of his treatment, and preventing the onset of common complications comprise a challenging and trying nursing role. Yet, the fulfillment of this role can decrease the degree of morbidity and increase the child's chance of survival, the most satisfactory outcome that can be achieved from the treatment of an infant or child in shock.

REFERENCES

1. McGRATH, R. B., AND REVTYAK, G. Secondary myocardial injury. *Crit.Care Med.* 12:1024–1026, Dec. 1984.
2. WILSON, R. F., ED. Shock. In *Critical Care Manual: Principles and Techniques of Critical Care.* Kalamazoo, MI, Upjohn Co., 1977, pp. C1–C42.
3. Standards and guidelines for cardiopulmonary resuscitation (CPR) and emergency cardiac care (ECC). *JAMA* 255:2905–2992, June 6, 1986.
4. VARGO, T. Shock. In *Life-threatening Episodes in Infants and Children: Cardiovascular Failure.* Kalamazoo, MI, Upjohn Co., 1984, pp. 5–10.
5. SHOEMAKER, W. C., AND HAUSER, C. J. Critique of crystalloid versus colloid therapy in shock and shock lung. *Crit.Care Med.* 7:117–124, Mar. 1979.
6. DODGE, C., AND GLASS, D. D. Crystalloid and colloid therapy. *Semin.Anesth.* 1:293–301, Dec. 1982.
7. SHINE, K. I., AND OTHERS. Aspects of the management of shock. *Ann.Intern.Med.* 93:723–734, Nov. 1980.
8. VIRGILIO, R. W., AND OTHERS. Balanced electrolyte solutions: experimental and clinical studies. *Crit.Care Med.* 7:98–106, Mar. 1979.
9. SHOEMAKER, W. C. Pathophysiology, monitoring, outcome prediction, and therapy of shock states. *Crit.Care Clin.* 3:307–357, Apr. 1987.
10. WEAVER, D. W., AND OTHERS. Pulmonary effects of albumin resuscitation for severe hypovolemic shock. *Arch.Surg.* 113:387–391, Apr. 1978.
11. CRONE, R. K. Acute circulatory failure in children. *Pediatr.Clin.North Am.* 27:525–538, Aug. 1980.
12. PERKIN, R. M., AND LEVIN, D. L. Shock in the pediatric patient: Part II: Therapy. *J.Pediatr.* 101:319–332, Sept. 1982.
13. WEIL, M. H., AND HENNING, R. J. New concepts in the diagnosis and fluid treatment of circulatory shock. *Anesth.Analg.* (Cleve) 58:124–132, Mar.–Apr. 1979.
14. CHERNOW, B., AND ROTH, B. L. Pharmacologic manipulation of the peripheral vasculature in shock: clinical and experimental approaches. *Circ.Shock* 18(2):141–155, 1986.
15. GUYTON, A. C. *Textbook of Medical Physiology.* 7th ed. Philadelphia, W. B. Saunders Co., 1986.
16. KASTRUP, E. K., AND OLAN, BERNIE, III, EDS. *Drugs Facts and Comparisons.* St. Louis, J. B. Lippincott Co., 1987.
17. PERKIN, R. M., AND OTHERS. Dobutamine: a hemodynamic evaluation in children with shock. *J.Pediatr.* 100:977–983, June 1982.
18. MASON, D. T. Afterload reduction and cardiac performance. Physiologic basis of systemic vasodilators as a new approach in treatment of congestive heart failure. *Am.J.Med.* 65:106–125, July 1978.
19. COLE, C. H., ED. *The Harriet Lane Handbook.* 10th ed. Chicago, Year Book Medical Publishers, 1984.
20. VESEY, C. J., AND COLE, P. V. Blood cyanide and thiocyanate concentrations produced by long-term therapy with sodium nitroprusside. *Br.J.Anaesth.* 57:148–155, Feb. 1985.
21. TRISSEL, L. A. *Handbook on Injectable Drugs.* 4th ed. Bethesda, MD, American Society of Hospital Pharmacists, 1986.
22. HOLADAY, J. W., AND FADEN, A. I. Naloxone reversal of endotoxin hypotension suggests a role of endorphins in shock. *Nature* 275:450–451, Oct. 5, 1978.
23. FADEN, A. I., AND HOLADAY, J. W. Opiate antagonists: a role in the treatment of hypovolemic shock. *Science* 205:317–318, July 20, 1979.
24. TIENGO, M. Naloxone in irreversible shock. (letter) *Lancet* 2:690, Sept. 27, 1980.
25. COCCHI, P., AND OTHERS. Naloxone in fulminant meningococcemia. (letter) *Pediatr.Infect.Dis.* 3:187, Mar.–Apr. 1984.
26. ROCK, P., AND OTHERS. Efficacy and safety of naloxone in septic shock. *Crit.Care Med.* 13:28–33, Jan. 1985.
27. SPRUNG, C. L., AND OTHERS. The effects of high dose corticosteroids in patients with septic shock. A prospective, controlled study. *N.Engl.J.Med.* 311:1137–1143, Nov. 1, 1984.
28. ZIMMERMAN, J. J., AND DIETRICH, K. A. Current perspectives on septic shock. *Pediatr.Clin.North Am.* 34:131–163, Feb. 1987.
29. BRONSVELD, W., AND OTHERS. Use of glucose-insulin-potassium (GIK) in human septic shock. *Crit.Care Med.* 13:566–570, July 1985.
30. CARTER, J. L., AND SMITH, B. L. Use of military antishock trousers: nursing implications. *Heart Lung* 11:422–425, Sept.–Oct. 1982.
31. SCHARFMAN, W. B., AND OTHERS. Plasmapheresis for meningococcemia with disseminated intravascular coagulation. (letter) *N.Engl.J.Med.* 300:1277–1278, May 31, 1979.
32. BJORVATN, B., AND OTHERS. Meningococcal septicaemia treated with combined plasmapheresis and leucapheresis or with blood exchange. *Br.Med.J.* 288:439–441, Feb. 11, 1984.
33. OSSENKOPPELE, G. J., AND OTHERS. Continuous arteriovenous hemofiltration as an adjunctive therapy for septic shock. *Crit.Care Med.* 13:102–104, Feb. 1985.
34. SEASHORE, J. H. Nutritional support of children in the intensive care unit. In *Topics in Pediatric Critical Care,* ed. by R. I. Markowitz and R. S. Baltimore. New Haven, CT, The Yale Journal of Biology and Medicine, 1984, pp. 111–134.
35. KEELY, B. R. Septic Shock. *Crit.Care Q.* 7:59–67, Mar. 1985.
36. LEWANDOWSKI, L. Psychosocial aspects of pediatric critical care. In *Nursing Care of the Critically Ill Child,* ed. by M. Hazinski. St. Louis, C. V. Mosby Co., 1984, p. 12.
37. RIMAR, J. M., AND OTHERS. Fulminant meningococcemia in children. *Heart Lung* 14:385–391, July 1985.

The Emotional Impact Of Trauma On Toddlers

Reprinted from MCN: The American Journal of Maternal Child Nursing, March/April 1988

Attending to toddlers' emotional needs is as critical to their overall well-being as treating their physical wounds.

ELLEN A. REYNOLDS/MAX L. RAMENOFSKY

Multiple trauma is a term that evokes images of sudden, intense injury, rapid transport, resuscitative efforts by a team of health care professionals, multiple procedures, and an extended hospital stay. For the injured toddler, this stressful event occurs at a time of developmental transition. The toddler is starting to move from passivity to autonomy, is beginning to view himself as an individual person separate from his mother, and is learning to communicate with the world through language and other symbols.

Erik Erikson indicated that life is not only a sequence of developmental transitions, but of accidental crises as well (1). When one of these accidental crises occurs at a crucial stage of development, the effects may be severe. Such is the case when a toddler is hospitalized for trauma.

Toddlers (children between the ages of one and three) are at greater risk for permanent emotional problems related to the experience of hospitalization than any other developmental group (2). One-to four-year-olds comprise 31 percent of all pediatric trauma admissions (3). Because of the critical need for rapid, thorough diagnosis and treatment, especially with multitrauma patients, caregivers often neglect to consider the overwhelming emotional impact that trauma has on the child.

ELLEN A. REYNOLDS, R.N., M.S.N., is pediatric trauma coordinator for the University of South Alabama Medical Center, Mobile, Alabama. She is a former staff nurse of the Emergency Medical Trauma Center, Children's Hospital National Medical Center, Washington, D.C. MAX L. RAMENOFSKY, M.D., is chief of the division of pediatric surgery, University of South Alabama Medical Center, chairman of the trauma committee of the American Pediatric Surgical Association, and co-principal investigator of the National Pediatric Trauma Registry, Department of Education Grant No. G008300042, Tufts-New England Medical Center and University of South Alabama. For reprints of this article, see the classified section.

The Parent-Child Relationship

The toddler is in the process of individuation. After a successful attachment to the parent during the first year, the child is able to use the parent as a secure base from which to come and go, enabling him to deal with stresses as they arise. The security in this relationship comes from the sense of reliable accessibility provided by the parent. The child is likely to display intense proximity-seeking behaviors when he is separated from the parent, tired, in pain, or perceives threat (4).

Even in the most family-centered pediatric trauma centers, children are separated from their parents for a great deal of this critical time. From the time the paramedics arrive on the scene until the child is transported to an intensive care unit (ICU), there is little opportunity for parents to be with their child. For the conscious toddler, the combined experience of pain, unfamiliar surroundings, multiple strangers performing procedures, and the rapid sequence of invasive events is overwhelming. The child's natural instinct is to seek his attachment figure . . . the parent.

But, during the initial period of treatment, the child's parents are also experiencing the crisis. The child's injury, in all likelihood, was sudden and unexpected. The child's survival may be questionable and his parents may be confronting their own feelings of guilt for allowing the child to get hurt. The stress can alter the parents' usual responses to the toddler, causing the child further distress. One study demonstrated that parents in an emergency room did not function effectively in the parenting role due to their own helplessness, regression, and anxiety (5). The parents' anxiety may be unconsciously transmitted to the child.

Because of the physical unavailability of the parents caused by resuscitation and stabilization efforts, and because the parents may not be able to be emotionally supportive, the child may perceive his parents as having abrogated their role as protectors by allowing strangers to perform painful procedures. The toddler may experience a loss of trust in his parents and may demonstrate this by temporarily rejecting them. Two-year-old Jackie was hit by a car and spent eight days in a pediatric intensive care unit. During this time she was on a ventilator and received pancuronium (Pavulon) with sedation. For two days after extubation, she refused to look at her mother and rejected all of her mother's overtures of affection. Calmed by a nurse's explanation of what was going through Jackie's mind, her mother was able to persist with her efforts to reassure Jackie. Jackie gradually became more responsive and had become her normal self a few days before she was discharged.

The Child's Developmental Phase

Cognitively, toddlers move through two sensorimotor stages and into the preconceptual stage within approximately two years of life. From 13 to 18 months, differentiation of self continues and memory begins to develop. By 18 to 24 months, egocentrism and magical thinking evolve. The rapid sequence of developmental events and the immaturity of his thought processes put the toddler at heightened risk for misinterpretation of treatment explanations, thus aggravating the emotional insult of the overall care.

For example, a toddler may interpret his hospitalization as a punishment for misbehavior, especially if he thinks his injury is the result of his own curiosity or exploration. Brief, simple explanations of procedures are easiest for toddlers to understand. A toddler cannot understand that a painful treatment will help him get better.

Following trauma, the toddler finds his expression of many of his newfound tasks and abilities restricted. A child who is just beginning to master verbal communication may suddenly find his skill thwarted by an endotracheal tube or tracheostomy. Restraints and traction may prevent him from dealing with the environment in his customary way. Generally, all aspects of autonomy have been taken away and the toddler finds himself again dependent on someone to feed, dress, and diaper him. In addition, body integrity may be of major concern to the toddler. Minor abrasions and lacerations may be more worrisome to him than is a less visible broken arm.

The Child's Past Experiences

Trauma is often the toddler's first introduction to the hospital. Well-child visits may have been the extent of the child's exposure to health care personnel. The most painful procedure he may have experienced may have been an immunization injection. While hospital tours and other types of preparation often help the older toddler cope with elective admission to a hospital, no such preparation precedes a traumatic admission. Therefore, the toddler has limited past experience on which he can draw to develop successful coping behaviors during hospitalization.

Extent of the Injury and Treatment

The severity of traumatic injuries runs the gamut from minor to life-threatening. Traumatic injuries tend to be painful and to require frequent diagnostic procedures for periodic reassessment. They also usually require some degree of immobilization, which in itself is stressful to a toddler.

A toddler who has suffered loss of consciousness prior to admission may be especially confused. Two-year-old Mia sustained a severe head injury and was comatose for several days. When she regained consciousness, she would stare out the window for long periods of time as if she was thinking. Finally, her mother asked her, "Mia, do you know why you are here?" Mia burst into tears and shook her head. Normal egocentrism and a tendency toward magical thinking, compounded by her coma, had made it difficult for her to understand what she'd been told and had made assessment of her comprehension difficult.

Invasive procedures, common elements of trauma care, are particularly threatening to the toddler. Blood drawing, tube insertions, and injections occur on a regular basis. Recollection of a painful event may cause anxiety over similar events. For example, the pain the toddler felt when a tourniquet was tightened may make him apprehensive about the inflation of a blood pres-

The toddler's tendency toward animism may lead the child to perceive machines as lifelike, frightening monsters.

sure cuff, a procedure that may not seem significantly different to the child. A toddler who sees a painful procedure performed on another child may become anxious about procedures to be performed on himself, due to his egocentrism.

In addition, because of the toddler's tendency toward animism, he may perceive machines and equipment as having lifelike qualities. The toddler may believe that he is about to be eaten by the computed tomography scanner or that alarms he hears are monsters trying to scare him.

The lengthy stay that trauma admission often entails causes stress for the toddler, too. Ritual and routine, so important in the toddler's life, are disrupted. Siblings may not be allowed to visit. Parents may not be able to room-in after the initial crisis is over, due to family and work responsibilities. As the child's immobility continues, his frustration will almost certainly increase.

Psychosocial Interventions

Equipped with knowledge of a toddler's developmental needs and the effects of hospitalization due to trauma, nurses can do a great deal to alleviate the child's resulting stress. First and foremost, parents must be included in the child's treatment and will need support throughout the hospitalization. Beginning with the initial resuscitation, parents of an injured child take on a new role. They will need information in order to successfully assume their new role and to cope accordingly. Questions regarding their child's injuries, treatment procedures and their outcomes, and prognostic indicators are uppermost in parents' minds and are to be answered as fully and truthfully as possible. From the time they enter the emergency room, through the completion of surgery, and until the child is released, they must be provided with frequent updates on their child's condition. As they become more comfortable in their new role, they will be better able to respond to their child's needs.

All toddlers need consistent parental presence (4,6,7). This need becomes even greater during stressful times such as hospitalization and is at its keenest during periods of highest stress such as when painful procedures are taking place. Preparing the parents by themselves ahead of time often enables them to work through their anxiety on their own, enabling them to provide greater support for the child. If possible, facilities should be made available to the parents so they can sleep in the hospital while their child is in the ICU.

With the multitude of disciplines involved in pediatric trauma care, every effort must be made to ensure a coordinated team approach. Often, this becomes the responsibility of the pediatric trauma coordinator or the child's primary nurse. She can see that duplication of special exams and tests is avoided and that specific hands-off times are scheduled and respected so that the toddler can

have uninterrupted rest periods. If a child life specialist is available, she is to be included in the child's care as soon as possible.

With the wide range of developmental tasks characteristic of toddlers, it will take special effort for the nurse to correctly assess the patient's individual developmental level. Careful observation and taking a thorough history from the parents are the best ways to accomplish this. Questions such as "Is the child using words to convey needs?" and "Does he take a bottle or use a cup?" help pinpoint the child's developmental level. Hospitalization is not the time to introduce new routines such as toilet training, but encouraging the child to maintain established routines can give him a sense of control and mastery within the hospital environment. The child's nurse must understand that some regression is normal and convey her knowledge to the parents; regressive behavior is met with understanding, not punishment.

Recognizing the child's particular body image concerns will also facilitate treatment. For example, most toddlers are comforted by the application of an adhesive strip after a procedure, but this is not always the case. Two-year-old Bobby cried hysterically after blood drawing was over and a Band-Aid was put on. Observing the procedure one day, his mother remarked that Bobby had always been fearful of Band-Aids, preferring to be able to see his wounds. Bobby's crying decreased dramatically when his nurse applied site pressure for a longer time and left the Band-Aid off.

Involving the Child

Traumatic injuries and associated procedures are often extremely painful. Young children rarely fake or imagine pain, but because of their limited ability to communicate verbally, the nurse may find it difficult to assess the amount of the child's pain. His facial expressions, whether he is guarding himself, and whether he is crying are clues that the child feels pain. Maintenance of consistent medication schedules during the acute stages of trauma helps prevent pain from becoming unmanageable. Proper positioning, which also minimizes pain, is especially important for toddlers with head injuries, for whom the use of medications may be limited.

Children being pharmacologically paralyzed require particularly careful attention. Their pain is not affected by the drugs that paralyze their muscles, but the signs and signals of their pain will be masked. In such situations, the child's nurse has to rely on physiologic indicators such as elevated blood pressure, tachycardia, and diaphoresis to determine if the current pain control interventions are effective. Remember, too, that the paralyzed child may well be aware of and extremely frightened by his inability to move and communicate. Be sure to explain, comfort, and reassure the child throughout the period of paralysis.

If the child is in traction or on bedrest, efforts must be made to counteract the effects of immobility. Often the bed—traction and all—can be wheeled to the playroom or outdoors. Throwing games give toddlers a sense of mobility and can help them vent frustration.

When describing a procedure to the child, try to relate it to his past experience. Tamika, a 20-month-old, was terrified of blood drawing. But, her mother explained that Tamika had been fascinated by the wheal raised during a recent tine test for tuberculosis and had asked, "Bubble? Bubble?" during subsequent visits to the pediatrician. The next time the phlebotomist drew blood, she prefaced the stick by saying, "It's going to feel just like making the bubble." Tamika cooperated and showed no further signs of fear. Always give the child lots of reassurance after any procedure.

The toddler needs as much control of and independence in his care as possible. The nurse can make sure that all choices the child is given are acceptable options. A child's need for control is frequently expressed through negativism in eating behavior, which is of special concern when trying to maintain the high caloric intake required following multiple trauma. The issue can be minimized by creative nursing interventions. Parents can be asked to bring the child his favorite foods from home. A trip to the hospital cafeteria for a meal with siblings may be arranged. Maximizing the child's oral intake is preferable, but if nasogastric or parenteral supplements are necessary, make sure the child understands that the tube isn't a punishment for his not eating enough.

The toddler's need for reassurance and TLC throughout his hospitalization cannot be overemphasized. If resuscitation is needed, the presence of a single nurse who provides comfort and explanations will often decrease the child's physical resistance and crying. Ideally, one primary and one associate nurse will be assigned to the child. Encouraging parents to be with, hold, and touch their child fosters another source of comfort and reassurance for the child.

Interventions with the Parents in Mind

Providing support to the child's parents during trauma care is essential to their ability to support their critically injured child. Some suggestions that will help nurses see parents through this critical period are:

Encourage parents to verbalize their concerns. A nurse's warm, responsive approach and honest reassurance without raising false hopes will enable parents to share their thoughts and work through their fears (8).

Continue to provide information on the child's condition and treatment. Involve the parents in decision making whenever possible, giving them control in a situation in which they may otherwise feel themselves to be relatively helpless.

Help the parents develop their participation in their child's care to a level that is comfortable for them. Because parents are often torn between their desire to be there for their child and their discomfort with hospital equipment, they may need to be taught how to touch or hold their child. The child's nurse can provide options such as, "Would you like to bathe your child or hold her hand while I bathe her?"

Provide a comfortable environment for parents. A bedside chair, a pillow and blanket for sleeping, and a coffee pot in the waiting room are small amenities that can make a big difference in parents' perceptions of hospital staff support.

Making Trauma Less Traumatic

Regardless of the quality of nursing care and participation of the parents, hospitalization for trauma is frightening to children. No amount of nursing care can undo the event that caused the trauma to occur. But sensitive, thorough nursing care can alleviate the physical and emotional stresses prompted by the injury and ensure not only a successful physical recovery, but a successful emotional one as well. Nurses can effectively minimize the consequences of trauma that can haunt a toddler. In some cases, they can even help the child come away from the experience with a positive sense of mastery and accomplishment.

REFERENCES

1. ERIKSON, E. H. *Childhood and Society.* New York, W. W. Norton and Co., 1964.
2. ROBERTSON, JAMES. *Young Children in Hospital.* New York, Basic Books, 1969.
3. NATIONAL PEDIATRIC TRAUMA REGISTRY, DEPARTMENT OF EDUCATION. *Annual Report.* Presented to the American Pediatric Surgical Association, meeting held in Toronto, Canada, May 1986.
4. BOWLBY, JOHN. *Attachment and Loss.* New York, Basic Books, Vol.1, 1969, p. 259. (2nd ed. in 1983)
5. ROSKIES, E., AND OTHERS. Emergency hospitalization of young children: some neglected psychological considerations. *Med.Care* 13:570–581, July 1975.
6. FREUD, ANNA, ED. The role of bodily illness in the mental life of children. *Psychoanalytic Study of the Child* 7:69–80, 1952.
7. RUTTER, MICHAEL. Attachment and the development of social relationships. In *Scientific Foundations of Developmental Psychiatry,* ed. by Michael Rutter. London, Heinemann Medical Books, 1980, (1987, text ed.)
8. CARNEVALE, F. A. Nursing the critically ill child: a responsive approach. *Focus Crit.Care* 12:10–13, Oct. 1985.

BIBLIOGRAPHY

BROOME, M. E. The child in pain: a model for assessment and intervention. *Crit.Care Q.* 8:47–55, June 1985.
ETZLER, C. A. Parents' reactions to pediatric critical care settings: a review of the literature. *Issues Compr.Pediatr.Nurs.* 7:319–331, June 1984.
LANNING, J. Pediatric trauma: emotional aspects. *AORN J.* 42:345–351, Sept. 1985.
LEWANDOWSKI, L. A. Psychosocial aspects of critical care. In *Nursing Care of the Critically Ill Child: American Association of Critical Care Nurses,* ed. by M. F. Hazinski. St. Louis, C. V. Mosby Co., 1984.
WOLTERMAN, M. C., AND MILLER, M. Caring for parents in crisis. *Nurs.Forum* 22(1):34–37, 1985.

A Button for Gastrostomy Feedings

Reprinted from MCN: The American Journal of Maternal Child Nursing, March/April 1988

A skin-level gastrostomy device addresses many of the problems of a gastrostomy tube. Whatever the disadvantages of this device, they are minimized by carefully preparing the child and parents.

KATHI C. HUDDLESTON/KAY L. PALMER

The gastrostomy tube, which has been used for more than 100 years, is for many the preferred method for long-term administration of enteral feedings to children with gastroesophageal anomalies, psychomotor retardation, or gastrointestinal disorders (1,2). Conventional gastrostomy tubes, however, cause numerous problems, particularly in children (3). Skin irritation, tube migration, and inadvertent removal are common difficulties.

Clinical practice indicates that children with gastrostomies often have additional physical problems that complicate gastrostomy feedings. For example. infants have small gastric capacities and high nutritional needs. With gastrostomy feedings, that small capacity is further limited by the balloon that is in the stomach; therefore, the volume of feeding necessary to meet the child's nutritional needs, often results in leakage of gastric contents (4). In addition, the incidence of gastroesophageal reflux, which is very common among infants, increases after placement of the gastrostomy tube. Moreover, many children who require gastrostomy feedings also have some degree of underlying pulmonary disease. Their increased respiratory effort often increases the incidence of aerophagia, or swallowing of air, which, in turn, increases the occurrence of gastroesophageal reflux. Gastroesophageal reflux has been directly related to life-threatening respiratory problems. (5,6).

Another physical concern is the length of the catheter in relation to the length of the infant or child; the long tube makes accidental dislodgment easier. Gastrostomy tubes also interfere with an infant's development (4,7). For example, younger infants develop upper torso and head control in the prone position, but often infants with gastrostomy tubes are not comfortable when prone. Similarly, infants attempting gross motor movements, such as pushing up on their arms or crawling, find that the long cumbersome tube prevents their moving.

Parents are also distressed by the catheter hanging from their infant's belly. Cosmetically, it reinforces that their child is different. This constant reminder of their child's impaired ability to eat can also affect bonding. Neighbors, friends, and extended family are often afraid to hold the child because of the tube.

The gastrostomy tube is familiar to a majority of nurses as the Foley, Malecot, and Mushroom catheters or the newer gastrostomy tubes such as the ones produced by Bard, Ross, or MIC. In the past few years, however, skin-level nonrefluxing devices—replacing the traditional gastrostomy tube—have been developed. (The original is The Button, developed by Bard Interventional Products (8). Ross developed the Stomate and Superior has the Gastroport. We—the authors—are experienced with The Button, but all skin-level nonrefluxing devices are similar in design.)

The gastrostomy button is a flexible silicone device with the intragastric portion resembling a mushroom or dePezzer catheter. The shaft varies from 1.5 cm to 3.7 cm and its diameter from 18 French to 28 French. The button is anchored by the internal mushroom dome and the external flat, short silicone wings. At the base of the shaft a one-way valve functions as an antireflux valve to prevent gastric contents from leaking. The button is designed to be used in an established gastrostomy tract, which was constructed by laparotomy, Stamm procedure and modifications, or percuta-

KATHI C. HUDDLESTON, R.N., M.S.N., *is a surgical clinical nurse specialist at Children's Hospital of the King's Daughters in Norfolk, Virginia.* KAY L. PALMER, R.N., M.S.N.,*is associate professor in the School of Nursing at Old Dominion University, Norfolk. Both authors are partners in a health consulting firm, Health Information System.*

neous gastrostomy (PEG) (9). (See Criteria for Successful Adaptation to the Gastrostomy Button).

At the time of the gastrostomy surgery the family is introduced to the available feeding devices. Clinical practice has demonstrated that some parents are more accepting of gastrostomy tube placement if they can look forward to the skin level feeding device two or three months following surgery. Parents have identified the button as much less threatening than the "long" tube.

Determining Size

Skin-level, nonrefluxing gastrostomy devices are not placed until the tract is completely healed—usually two or three months after surgery. It is imperative that the child have an 18- to 22-French catheter in place. If the stoma is not large enough to accommodate that size, a home health nurse or a knowledgeable parent may dilate the stoma by increasing the gastrostomy tube size by one each week. The size of the device used will depend on the size of the child and type of feeding.

For example, the 18-French button is suitable for formula feeding but will easily clog or have valve failure with blenderized, or thicker, feedings. Use of 18-French, therefore, is limited to the infant population.

A 28-French button is primarily used for older children or any child taking medications that may clog the button, such as Depakene, Klonopin, magnesium citrate, Carafate, pectin, or calcium supplements. It is important to note that a button size that is 4 French sizes larger than the gastrostomy tube can be used. A 24-French button is easily inserted into a stoma with a 20-French tube.

The most important factor that determines which size device to use is the length of the shaft. The majority of infants and children will need a length of 1.2 cm to 1.5 cm. The button is packaged according to its size and length. The package con-

tains a device to measure the stoma, a button, an obturator, a 60 cc syringe, a short bolus feeding tube, a continuous feeding tube with a 90-degree adaptor, and instructions for the parents about feedings. For professional education, Bard Interventional Products and Ross have produced a video that demonstrates button insertion.

Comfort Measures

Measures are taken to minimize the discomfort of insertion. One hour before the procedure, a dose of acetaminophen, given either orally or by gastrostomy, will assist in pain management. In addition, 20 to 30 minutes prior to insertion, a topical analgesic, such as 5 percent lidocaine ointment, may be applied to the skin. While the device is being inserted, the child is immobilized and comforted. Parents are told that if it is necessary during the 48 hours following the procedure, they may give acetaminophen in doses that are appropriate for the child's age.

After the Button Is Inserted

After the button is in place, it is rotated 360 degrees to ensure proper placement. The nurse also makes sure the antireflux valve is in the closed position by tapping the valve several times with the obturator or with the plunger of a 1 cc syringe. If the valve is open, drainage will persist from within the lumen. A sterile 2x2 gauze pad is slit and placed under the wings of the button so that the pad surrounds the button to absorb the minimal bleeding that is expected.

After button placement the child receives an initial feeding of sterile water to ensure that the device is properly placed (10). Accurate placement is indicated if the water flows in quickly by gravitational force. If feedings are to be given by family members, the sterile water feeding is at first done by them under the supervision of the nurse, who validates the correct feeding procedure. Parents are taught to tap the valve periodically, because when the child "burps," the valve may become wedged open in the lumen of the button. Prior to leaving the clinic or office, the parent is informed that some abdominal discomfort may be experienced for three to five days after the procedure. In addition, a circular area around the stoma may be slightly red and warm during that period. The parent is told to notify the physician if the child develops a fever; if redness tracks off beyond the circle around the stoma; or if the formula does not flow easily by gravity (10).

Nursing Care

Nursing care after gastrostomy button placement focuses on skin care, feeding technique, and family and caregiver teaching.

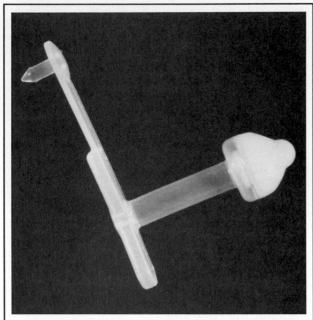

The gastrostomy button is a flexible silicone device; an intragastric portion resembles a mushroom.

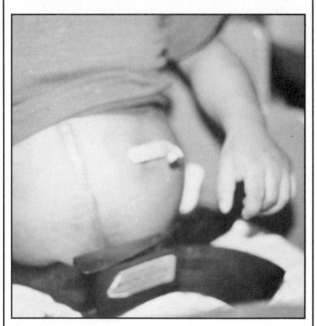

The skin around the gastrostomy button is one focus of nursing care; families are carefully instructed.

Skin care. Because the device is skin level, children are not as likely to play with it or pull it as they would a tube. The limited manipulation results in less skin irritation. Under the wings the skin may normally appear slightly red and moist, but to prevent skin breakdown the button is periodically rotated (11). If skin breakdown occurs under the wings as a result of the button pressing against the skin, the button is changed to one having a longer shaft. Daily cleansing with soap and

water around the stoma is also beneficial; bath time is a perfect time to do this (12). More frequent cleansing, however, may be necessary. Keeping the skin dry may be difficult if the button is in a fold of the skin. A clean piece of gauze cut like a tracheostomy dressing may be placed under the wings, although this is not usually necessary.

The skin around the stoma may appear erythematous and moist for the first seven to ten days after insertion of the button. Generally, routine skin care during this period is all that is required. Any time that the stoma appears larger than the button, that the skin is erythematous, or that drainage is a problem, skin breakdown is likely to occur. The early stage is treated with an adhesive powder to fill the area between the button and the skin (8). The powder protects the skin from any irritating effects by absorbing gastric acid.

If skin breakdown does occur, relatively easy remedies will aid healing. A stoma adhesive powder and a skin barrier, such as Duoderm, are usually sufficient. The powder is placed around the stoma. A 2x2 square of skin barrier with a small hole and a slit opening like a tracheostomy dressing is placed around the stoma under the wings of the gastrostomy button so that the shaft is touched by the skin barrier The skin barrier must be cut so that no skin around the button is left uncovered to collect gastric drainage. If skin irritation or breakdown does not respond to these measures or if drainage becomes excessive, the physician is notified.

Small amounts of fluid draining around the gastrostomy tube is not uncommon or harmful. Similar to the skin surrounding the anus or other body orifices, the stomal area has bacterial growth that does not require treatment (10). Culturing the drainage is therefore usually unnecessary. Slight overgrowth tissue, also considered normal, may be present. If the overgrowth tissue, however, becomes a concern due to the amount of drainage or stomal erosion, application of silver nitrate may be prescribed.

Feeding techniques. What equipment is used depends upon whether feeding is bolus or continuous. (See Equipment for Bolus Feedings, and Equipment for Continuous Feedings.) The feeding tube used for both techniques must be of the same size as the gastrostomy button. A 24-French button will require a 24-French feeding tube. The feeding tube is rinsed with hot water after each feeding. At least once a day the tube is washed with hot soapy water and then rinsed thoroughly (13,14). A clogged tube is disconnected from the button and flushed to remove the obstruction.

Research studies have shown that food occlusion is best treated with hot tap water irrigation if discovered early. But enzyme solutions may be required for occlusions that have remained in the tube for longer periods. Occlusions secondary to

---

**Equipment Required for Two Types
of Infant Feedings**

Bolus Feedings
(For feedings and medications that are less than 60 cc)

- Bolus feeding tube (short length tube)
- 60 cc catheter tip syringe
- Premeasured formula, fluid, or medicine
- Water

Continuous Feedings

- Continuous feeding tube with a right–angle connector
- Gravity feeding system, such as Flexiflow
- Premeasured formula, fluid, or medicine
- Water

---

medications have been successfully removed with hot tap water (15). If the tube becomes coated with formula, it is first flushed with hot water. Then, if the tube remains occluded, it is flushed with a soft drink or cranberry or pineapple juice. The effects of carbonated beverages, fruit juices, meat tenderizer, and Vivonase occlusions were compared, and no one better method was found (16).

Clinical experience indicates that a soft drink should be in the feeding tube for approximately one hour to enable the carbonation to loosen the formula. If a child is on fatty supplements or oil-based medicines and the tube becomes occluded, one teaspoon of meat tenderizer can be safely added to the eight-ounce soft drink soak to facilitate breakdown of residual fat in the tube (16). The button, itself, rarely becomes clogged.

A parent's hands must be washed before starting a feeding or handling equipment. The first step in the feeding process is to twist the button a full circle; the button is correctly positioned in the gastrostomy tract when it turns easily. If the gastrostomy button does not turn easily, the child is not given a feeding and the physician is contacted for further instructions.

If the button turns easily, a syringe or gravity feed system is attached to the clamped feeding tube, the tube purged with the fluid to be given, and then the tube is reclamped. Then, the feeding tube is attached to the button by holding one of the wings securely and pushing the end of the feeding tube into the button. While the wing is held in order to insert the tube, the child's abdomen is not pushed upon, because it may be tender, especially during the first seven to ten days after button insertion. In addition, extreme pressure on the button during insertion of the feeding tube may cause the button to be pushed into the stomach (11). After the feeding tube is attached, the clamp is slowly opened until the fluid begins to flow. If the fluid doesn't start to flow freely, the tube is milked. The flow is then regulated so that the feeding takes at least 20 minutes.

Following the feeding, the system is flushed. Water flushes are recorded as intake. A 5-cc flush for a child receiving two ounces every three hours would provide almost 10 percent of his intake. The feeding tube is removed by firmly grasping a wing of the button and withdrawing the tube. The attached plug, then, is firmly snapped into the lumen of the button.

The antireflux valve in a button necessitates decompression tubes to vent the stomach when a child is very uncomfortable from too much air or formula in his stomach. The tube is inserted for no longer than five to ten minutes, which is ample time to evacuate excess air or formula from the stomach. If used frequently or for prolonged periods, a decompression tube may prematurely weaken the button's valve. Decompression tube sizes are the same as button sizes.

The antireflux valve is below the fitting of the feeding tube connector. To vent, or "burp," the child is therefore not possible by removing the attached plug or connecting the feeding tube. A decompression tube must be used. If the child's abdomen is distended, the excessive pressure may push the antireflux valve up into the lumen of the button. If the valve becomes stuck in an open position, the button will drain stomach contents profusely from within the lumen of the button. Whenever drainage is reported, it is important to

---

The family is given a telephone number that they may call should help be necessary during the transition from gastrostomy tube to button.

---

ascertain whether the drainage is from around the button or from within its lumen. The only reasons for drainage from within the lumen is that the antireflux valve is stuck in the open position or that the valve has failed. The antireflux valve can be returned to a normal position by gently tapping the one-way valve through the lumen of the button back into the secure position, using the plunger of a 1 cc syringe.

Unlike the gastrostomy tube, the button will probably work well for nine months to a year. If, however, a child receives continuous or very frequent feedings, the valve may fail earlier.

Family teaching. Because the gastrostomy button is usually inserted in outpatient settings, opportunities for ideal teaching are often lacking. It is imperative that the family receive instruction about gastrostomy feedings and the button during visits prior to the time of insertion. They will need to handle the button and other feeding equipment. Any teaching at the time of insertion is done before the actual procedure, because afterwards, the family will need to comfort the crying child. Information for the family is written. Because of the differences between the button and the gastrostomy tube they had used before, the family will need a telephone number they may call concerning questions they have about the button.

The parent is instructed to keep an 18-French or 20-French catheter in the home so that a gastrostomy tube can be placed into the stoma should inadvertent removal of the button occur. Because the child has had a gastrostomy for at least three months, the parent is experienced in replacing the gastrostomy tube. The button, however, is reinserted only by a trained health professional.

Staff members from home health agencies who are involved in the care of a child with the button must receive information about the device. The interdisciplinary team who inserted the gastrostomy button may be resource persons for home health staff and the family.

The Pros and Cons

The disadvantages of the button have been identified by many practitioners: painful insertion procedure; high initial cost; higher cost for reinsertion (the cost of visiting a physician's office to have the button reinserted versus the cost of having a parent reinsert the gastrostomy tube); and premature valve failure. With a systematic approach, however, including the appropriate child selection, button selection, and child and family preparation, the disadvantages can be minimized. The button gives a family the semblance of a more normal life-style, but the advantages and disadvantages of the device, as well as the quality of life issues, must be researched to assess the full impact of this new technology.

REFERENCES

1. HAWS, E. B., AND OTHERS. Complications of tube gastrostomy in infants and children. *Ann.Surg.* 164:284–290, Aug. 1966.
2. HOLDER, T. M., AND OTHERS. Gastrostomy: its use and dangers in pediatric patients. *N.Engl.J.Med.* 286:1345–1347, June 22, 1972.
3. HUDDLESTON, K., AND OTHERS. MIC or Foley: comparing gastrostomy tubes. *MCN.* 14:20–23, Jan.-Feb. 1989.
4. PERRY, S. E., AND OTHERS. Gastrostomy and the neonate. *Am.J.Nurs.* 83:1030–1033, July 1983.
5. BEREZIN, S., AND OTHERS. Gastroesophageal reflux secondary to gastrostomy tube placement. *Am.J.Dis.Child.* 140:699–701, July 1986.
6. CYR, J. A., AND OTHERS. Nissen fundoplication for gastroesophageal reflux in infants. *J.Thorac.Cardiovasc.Surg.* 92:661–666, Oct. 1986.
7. WINK, D. M. The physical and emotional care of infants with gastrostomy tubes. *Issues Compr.Pediatr.Nurs.* 6:195–203, May-June 1983.
8. HUTH, M. M., AND O'BRIEN, M. E. The gastrostomy feeding button. *Pediatr.Nurs.* 13:241–245, July-Aug. 1987.
9. GAUDERER, M. W., AND OTHERS. The gastrostomy "button"—a simple, skin-level nonrefluxing device for long-term enteral feedings. *J.Pediatr.Surg.* 19:803–805, Dec. 1984.
10. GAUDERER, M. W., AND OTHERS. Gastrostomies: evolution, techniques, indications, and complications. *Chicago Year Book,* 1986.
11. BARD INTERVENTIONAL PRODUCTS. Gastrostomy feeding button. C. R. Bard, Inc. 68:1–3, 1986.
12. PAARLBERG, J., AND OTHERS. Gastrostomy tubes: practical guidelines for home care. *Pediatr.Nurs.* 11:99–102, Mar.–Apr. 1985.
13. ADAMS, M. M., AND WIRSCHING, R. G. Guidelines for planning home enteral feeding. *J.Am.Diet.Assoc.* 84:68–71, Jan. 1984.
14. GRUNOW, J., AND OTHERS. Contamination of enteral nutrition systems during prolonged intermittent use. *J.Parenter.Enteral.Nutr.* 13:23—25, Jan.-Feb. 1989.
15. BOMMARITO, A., AND OTHERS. A new approach to the management of obstructed enteral feeding tubes. *Nutr.Clin.Prac.* 4:111–114, June 1989.
16. MARCUARD, S., AND OTHERS. Clearing obstructed feeding tubes. *J.Parenter.Enteral.Nutr.* 13:81–83, 1989.

A Descriptive Study of Infants and Toddlers Exposed Prenatally to Substance Abuse

Reprinted from MCN: The American Journal of Maternal Child Nursing, March/April 1988

TERESA FREE/FAY RUSSELL
BRENDA MILLS/DONNA HATHAWAY

Investigating family patterns and interaction helped identify environmental deficits in families where children had been exposed prenatally to drugs.

Children affected by prenatal abuse of alcohol, illegal drugs, and drugs available at pharmacies or groceries are a growing concern of nurses. Professional literature describes maternal substance abuse and the damage evident in neonates at birth (1-3). Limited information, however, is available that reflects in-depth study of affected neonates as they progress to infancy and toddlerhood. (See *MCN*, Jan./Feb. 1989, pp. 44–46.)

Probably the most commonly used teratogenic substance is alcohol (1). Because the placenta affords no protection to the fetus from alcohol, the ethanol concentration in the mother's blood reaches the fetus essentially unaltered. The impact of alcohol on the fetus, however, may be greater than it is on the mother because of the higher ratio of fetal blood alcohol to body weight, and inefficient fetal liver and renal ethanol clearance. Alcohol and its first metabolite, acetaldehyde, probably impair nutrient and oxygen transport to the fetus, and thereby inhibit protein synthesis and cellular growth (2).

The most severe effect of maternal alcohol ingestion—fetal alcohol syndrome (FAS)—is characterized by cranial and midface dysmorphia, central nervous system dysfunction, and poor prenatal and postnatal growth (evident in weight, height, and head circumference, and organ systems development). The most characteristic dysmorphic facial features are short palpebral fissures; broad, low nasal bridge; short, upturned nose; and flattened philtrum and thin upper lip (2). Related features frequently include microcephaly with associated mental deficit, epicanthic folds, strabismus, ptosis, and micrognathia. Mothers who have more than five drinks daily or who go on binges risk having a baby with fetal alcohol syndrome. (The reported incidence is 1 to 3 per 1,000 live births in the United States, although it varies for different cities and population subgroups (2).)

Alcohol-related birth defects (ARBD) occur among more children than fetal alcohol syndrome does, although the actual incidence is unknown. Mothers who drink as few as two drinks per day significantly increase their chances of having a low-birth-weight, hypotonic infant who may have minor or major birth defects, such as facial, cardiac or renogenital aberrations (4,5). These infants also run the risk of central nervous system dysfunction. For example, borderline to moderate mental retardation and behavioral abnormalities, such as irritability among infants and hyperactivity among children, have been reported (5–7). The

TERESA FREE, R.N.C., Ph.D., *is assistant professor at the University of Tennessee, Memphis, College of Nursing.* FAY RUSSELL, R.N.C., M.N., *is associate professor also at the University's College of Nursing in Memphis, and chief of nursing at the University of Tennessee, Memphis, Boling Center for Developmental Disabilities.* BRENDA MILLS, R.N.C., M.S., *and* DONNA HATHAWAY, R.N., Ph.D.,*are both assistant professors at the University College of Nursing. Ms. Mills is also a pediatric clinical specialist at the University of Tennessee, Memphis, Boling Center for Developmental Disabilities.* This study was supported in part by USPHS MCJ 00090023 from the Bureau of Maternal and Child Health and Resources Development and by the University of Tennessee, Memphis, College of Nursing.

severity of physical abnormalities appears to predict the degree of intellectual handicap (8). The lower limits of how much a mother can drink without affecting her baby have not been established; therefore, total abstinence during pregnancy is currently recommended (2).

The Effects of Other Drugs

Much less is known about the exact effects of other drugs (9). The most common illegal drugs used by childbearing women in the United States probably are marijuana and cocaine (10). One quarter of Americans between the ages of 18 and 25 years have been estimated to smoke marijuana (11). Whether it crosses the placenta is debated (11,12). No malformations due to marijuana smoking during pregnancy have been reported, however-

er. Some studies do suggest associated fetal distress, neonatal tremors, startles, high-pitched crying, and low birth weight, but these findings are not confirmed (13-15). One study reported that the quality of the caregiving environment had greater effect on the infant's outcome than the prenatal use of marijuana (12).

Cocaine, on the other hand, has been associated with perinatal insults and congenital anomalies (10,16). Cocaine, like other central nervous system stimulants, is thought to cross the placenta and the fetal blood-brain barrier (10). The drug's physiological effects of maternal vasoconstriction, tachycardia, and acute hypertension cause restricted blood flow to the fetus, fetal tachycardia, and hyperactivity. Reports also associate cocaine with increased incidence of first trimester abortions, abruptio placentae, premature labor, intrauterine

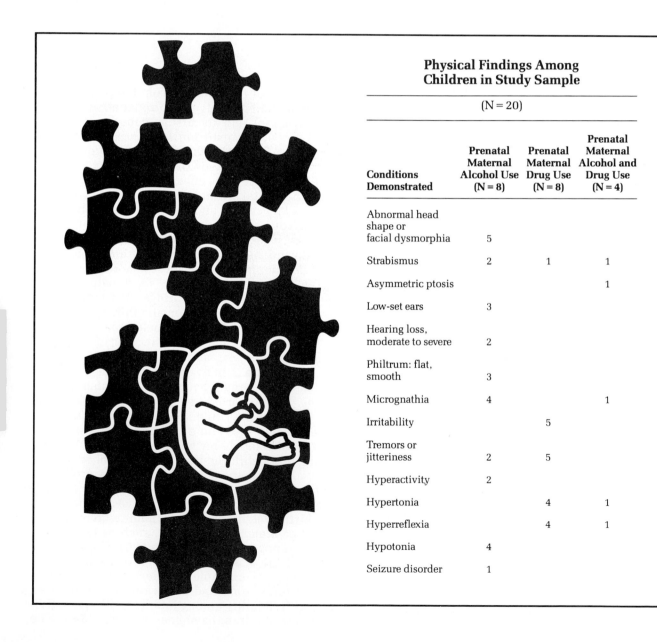

Physical Findings Among Children in Study Sample

(N = 20)

Conditions Demonstrated	Prenatal Maternal Alcohol Use (N = 8)	Prenatal Maternal Drug Use (N = 8)	Prenatal Maternal Alcohol and Drug Use (N = 4)
Abnormal head shape or facial dysmorphia	5		
Strabismus	2	1	1
Asymmetric ptosis			1
Low-set ears	3		
Hearing loss, moderate to severe	2		
Philtrum: flat, smooth	3		
Micrognathia	4		1
Irritability		5	
Tremors or jitteriness	2	5	
Hyperactivity	2		
Hypertonia		4	1
Hyperreflexia		4	1
Hypotonia	4		
Seizure disorder	1		

growth retardation, and fetal distress (10,16,17). For an infant, the physiologic and behavioral consequences of prenatal maternal cocaine use include irritability, tremulousness, jitteriness, seizures, abnormal respiratory rates and patterns, tachycardia, abnormal sleep patterns, feeding problems, diarrhea, and increased risk for sudden infant death syndrome (SIDS) and cerebral infarction (10,17). Moreover, the caregiver finds it difficult to console the infant. (See "The Care of Infants Menaced by Cocaine Abuse" by Keeta Lewis in MCN, Sept.–Oct. 1989.) The incidence of morbidity appears to be dose-related (17).

A Study Describing Affected Children

A descriptive pilot study was undertaken in a University-Affiliated Early Intervention Program to determine the characteristics of a representative sample of infants and toddlers who had been exposed as fetuses to substance abuse. In addition, we wanted to identify the health and developmental status of these children, and determine who the caregivers were and the quality of care they provided. In this way, the interactive environment was investigated. Twenty children and their caregivers from 15 families were included in the study. (See How the Study Was Conducted.) The findings of the study may be limited due to the use of a small, nonrandom, convenience sample and cross-sectional measurement of outcomes rather than a longitudinal design. In addition, although the prematurity and low birth weight may have been caused by substance abuse, the two factors confound the developmental effects.

What We Discovered

The growth measures among children in the 20 families studied confirmed literature reports that many children exposed prenatally to alcohol and/or drugs fail to grow normally (2,10). Three children were born (to alcoholic mothers) with clinical microcephaly. Six of the children were below the fifth percentile for both weight and height, one was below the fifth percentile for weight only, and one was below the fifth percentile for height only. Of the nine children born prematurely, five were below the fifth percentile for weight for their corrected age at the time of the study and five were below the fifth percentile for height.

Among the children studied, the incidence of

How the Study Was Conducted

Twenty infants and toddlers with their caregivers from 15 families participated in an exploratory-descriptive study. These children had measurable levels of alcohol or drugs in their urine or blood at the time of birth or were identified by confirmed history of prenatal substance abuse. Only 11 of the caregivers were the biological mothers; the other nine were maternal grandmothers (five) and maternal aunts (four), because the mothers had neglected or abandoned their child, or because they were incarcerated. All but one child was black and all but two families were from the lower socioeconomic group. Thirteen children were less than 1 year old, five were between 1 and 2 years, and two were between 2 and 3 years. Mean maternal age was 29.6 years, and mean educational grade level for mothers and caregivers was 11.6.

Home visits were made to each child to assess the home environment and the interaction between child and caregiver (see Description of Assessment Tools). Using established measures—the Home Observation for Measurement of the Environment (HOME) and the Nursing Child Assessment Training (NCAT) feeding and teaching scales—we compared the subscale scores of the children whose primary caregiver was their biological mother with those children whose primary caregiver was a relative other than the mother. (The biological mother had abused drugs during pregnancy; none of the relatives who were caregivers had abused drugs.) Study investigators were certified in the use of the HOME and NCAT scales.

In addition to assessing the home environment, a health history and physical assessment and a developmental screening test were used to measure the characteristics, health, and developmental status of the children. Growth and developmental data were collected at the early intervention program site.

According to MCN's guidelines for authors, this study is a systematic clinical investigation. The authors used a standardized process to collect data that document practice. Systematic clinical investigation can, among other approaches, examine responses to practice; lead to definitions of a research question; apply knowledge from clinical and/or research literature to practice; or analyze the conceptual connections between practice and theory.

Relationship of Substance Abuse to Infant Status

	Developmental Screening		Birth Weight		Gestation	
	Normal	Abnormal	More than 2,500 grams	Less than 2,500 grams	Term	Less than 37 weeks
Alcohol	4	4	2	6	3	5
Other drugs	6	2	6	2	6	2
Alcohol and drugs	3	1	2	2	2	2
	13	7	10	10	11	9

developmental delay was 35 percent, much higher than in the general population, where the incidence is generally thought to be 3 to 5 percent. Greatest lags were in language and other cognitive skills, a pattern that usually occurs with mentally retarded children. The table Physical Findings Among Children in Study Sample includes a list of all the physical abnormalities that were evident. (See also Relationship of Abused Substances to Developmental Status, Birth Weight, and Prematurity.) The environments of those children living with their biologic mothers (n=11) were compared with those of the children living with other relatives (n=9). A statistically significant difference was found on only one subscale of the HOME: maternal involvement with child. The mothers' mean score was 2.73, while the other caregivers' mean was 4.44; p was less than 0.5. This difference, however, was not significant on the total HOME score.

It is noteworthy that not more differences were found in child interactions with the mothers who were using alcohol or drugs and with the family caregivers who did not abuse substances in the pilot study. This suggests that the family members who take care of infants relinquished by substance-abusing mothers are as much in need of emotional support and information about infant care as are the mothers.

Interestingly, no significant statistical differences were found between mothers and other caregivers when the NCAT feeding scale was administered. Similarly, when the teaching scale was administered to all 20 children and caregivers, no significant differences were found between mothers and other family members.

The particularly low mean of the HOME scale total for all 20 children (28.9) indicates that the caregiver relatives and substance-abusing mothers failed to provide an environment for promoting the child's cognitive development. Another comparison of HOME scores was made between the drug-exposed children who were developmentally normal and those who were not. This

---

Description of Assessment Tools

The Caldwell Home Scale and the NCAT Feeding and Teaching Scales were used to measure the interactive environment. The Home Observation for Measurement of the Environment (HOME) Inventory Scale for Families of Infants and Toddlers measures the availability of caregiver and developmental stimulation for the child under 3 years (1). Items assess (a) frequency and consistency of adult contact with the child; (b) satisfaction of basic physical needs, including health and safety; (c) emotional environment; (d) provision of appropriate amounts and timing of sensory and developmental stimulation; (e) physical, verbal, and emotional responsivity of the environment to the child; (f) avoidance of restrictions on exploratory and motor behaviors; (g) availability of appropriate play materials; and (h) parental investment of concern and activity to foster developmental achievement.

A nurse visits the home while the child is awake to observe the child's interaction with the primary caregiver. The nurse also asks the caregiver to recount the activities of a typical day for the child and asks to see the child's toys. The nurse scores the HOME's 45 items on a binary system of Yes or No. Tool development demonstrated that Cronbach alpha coefficients of the six subscales were 0.49–0.78. Total scale internal consistency using the Kuder-Richardson 20 formula was 0.89 (1).

The Nursing Child Assessment Training (NCAT) Feeding Scale and Teaching Scale (2) measure the quality of caregiver/infant interaction. Both scales were developed to assess (a) how the caregiver sets up the environment to make it conducive for interaction, such as positioning the infant, the food, the teaching materials, and herself; (b) the degree of infant and caregiver attentiveness and distractibility; (c) the visual, auditory, and tactile stimulation of the infant and response to it; (d) the emotional warmth of the caregiver and response to the infant; (e) the degree of give and take in the interaction; and (f) the flexibility of the caregiver and responsiveness to the infant's cues of readiness or satiation (3). The teaching scale also focuses on the mother's use of such strategies as demonstration, reinforcement of attempts, timing, and physical guidance. Both scales have six subscales; four describe caregiver interaction behaviors and two, infant interaction behaviors.

Kathryn Barnard, R.N., Ph.D., found that items within each subscale of the feeding and teaching scales were positively correlated, indicating unidimensional constructs and internal consistency (4). When corresponding subscales of the two scales were combined, correlations were much lower, indicating that the scales measure different information. The feeding situation is a familiar, practiced one, and the teaching situation is more structured and may be more novel.

REFERENCES

1. CALDWELL, B. M., AND BRADLEY, R. H. Home Observation for Measurement of the Environment. Little Rock, AR: Caldwell and Bradley, 1978.
2. BARNARD, K. E., AND EYRES, S. J. Child Health Assessment, Part 2: The First Year of Life (DHEW Publication No. HRA 79-25). Hyattsville, MD, US Department of Health, Education, and Welfare, June, 1979.
3. EYRES, S. J., BARNARD, K. E., AND GRAY, C. A. Child Health Assessment, Part 3: 2–4 Years. Seattle, WA, School of Nursing, University of Washington, 1979.
4. BARNARD, K. E. Nursing Child Assessment Satellite Training: Instructor's Learning Resource Manual. Seattle, WA, the Author, 1978.

comparison demonstrated statistically significant differences on two subscales but not on the total HOME scale. The developmentally delayed group had lower scores on organization of the environment (p less than .01) and on opportunities for variety in their daily stimulation (p less than .01). From this study, it appears that a mother's prenatal substance abuse and the quality of the home environment both affect a child's development.

Families and Their Needs.

The families who participated in the study were motivated to obtain special health and developmental evaluations and intervention for their children. The social workers in the university-affiliated program surveyed the study mothers and family member caregivers regarding family needs. A majority wanted information regarding teaching their child, growth and development, behavior management, and community resources, but stated they were not interested in knowing more about how to play or talk with the child. All families reported that primary health care was available to them.

Most of those surveyed wanted assertiveness training but were not interested in a GED class. Several indicated that talking with other mothers or caregivers would be helpful, and most wanted more time for themselves. Only one saw the need to talk regularly with a counselor. Day care and transportation were the community services most frequently needed.

All the families studied appeared to need counseling and intermittent respite from the children. The caregivers in families where drugs were a problem especially wanted information on how drugs affect users and how to help their family member who was using substances. All caregivers required more time for themselves and information on the growth and developmental needs of their children.

The social workers reported a combination of three or more of the following risk factors for family dysfunctioning occurring among 14 of 15 families: single parent; low socioeconomic status; guardianship of child—not natural parent; continued use of alcohol and/or drugs; or problematic relationships between family members. In making their determination, the social workers utilized psychosocial risk factors that were identified during their professional experience or that appeared in the professional literature (18,19).

How Great the Need

Because of the multifaceted nature of these families' problems, everything from crisis management to group sessions to referrals to an interdisciplinary team is needed. To describe in-depth the health care given to these families through our own University-Affiliated Facility is beyond the scope of this article. But, many services, including emotional support, are required for caregivers—parents and family members—to help them cope with the teratogenic effects of prenatal substance abuse and to help them provide an environment that will assist these children and themselves to develop to their full potential.

REFERENCES

1. STREISSGUTH, A. P., AND LADUE, R. A. Psychological and behavioral effects in children prenatally exposed to alcohol. *Alcohol Health Res. World* 10:6–12, Fall 1985.
2. PETRAKIS, P. L. *Alcohol and Birth Defects: The Fetal Alcohol Syndrome and Related Disorders* (DHHS Publ. No. (ADM) 87-1531). Rockville, MD: U.S. Department of Health and Human Services, 1987.
3. DOBERCZAK, T. M., AND OTHERS. Impact of maternal drug dependency on birth weight and head circumference of offspring. *Am.J.Dis.Child.* 141:1163–1167, Nov. 1987.
4. SMITH, D. W. The fetal alcohol syndrome. *Hosp.Pract.* 14:121–128, Oct. 1979.
5. McCARTHY, P. A. Fetal alcohol syndrome and other alcohol-related birth defects. *Nurse Pract.* 8:33–37, Jan. 1983.
6. STEPHENS, C. J. The fetal alcohol syndrome: cause for concern. *MCN* 6:251–256, July–Aug. 1981.
7. ERB, L., AND ANDRESEN, B. D. Hyperactivity: a possible consequence of maternal alcohol consumption. *Pediatr.Nurs.* 7:30–33, 51 July–Aug. 1981.
8. STREISSGUTH, A. P., AND OTHERS. Natural history of the fetal alcohol syndrome: a 10-year follow-up of eleven patients. *Lancet* 2:85–92, July 13, 1985.
9. DAY, N. L., AND OTHERS. Measurement of substance use during pregnancy: methodological issues. *Natl.Inst.Drug Abuse, Res. Monogr. Ser.* 59:36–47, 1985.
10. SMITH, J. E. The dangers of prenatal cocaine use. *MCN* 13:174–179, May–June 1988.
11. ABEL, E. L. Effects of prenatal exposure to cannabinoids. *Natl.Inst. Drug Abuse Res. Monogr. Ser.* 59:20–35, 1985.
12. HAYES, J. S., AND OTHERS. Newborn outcomes with maternal marijuana use in Jamaican women. *Pediatr.Nurs.* 14:107–110, Mar.–Apr. 1988.
13. TENNES, K., AND OTHERS. Marijuana: prenatal and postnatal exposure in the human. *Natl.Inst.Drug Abuse Res.Monogr.Ser.* 59:48–60, 1985.
14. FRIED, P. A. Postnatal consequences of maternal marijuana use. *Natl.Inst.Drug Abuse Res.Monogr.Ser.* 59:61–72, 1985.
15. HINGSON, R., AND OTHERS. Effects of maternal drinking and marijuana use on fetal growth and development. *Pediatrics* 70:539–546, Oct. 1982.
16. CHASNOFF, I. J., AND OTHERS. Cocaine use in pregnancy. *N.Engl.J.Med.* 313:666–669, Sept. 12, 1985.
17. ORO, A. S., AND DIXON, S. D. Perinatal cocaine and methamphetamine exposure: maternal and neonatal correlates. *J.Pediatr.* 111:571–577, Oct. 1987.
18. HEINS, M., AND SEIDEN, A. M. Parenting and the pediatrician. *Am.J.Dis.Child.* 141:1188–1192, Nov. 1987.
19. HOWARD, B. Single parenting in America. *Early Childh. Update* 5:1, Winter 1989.

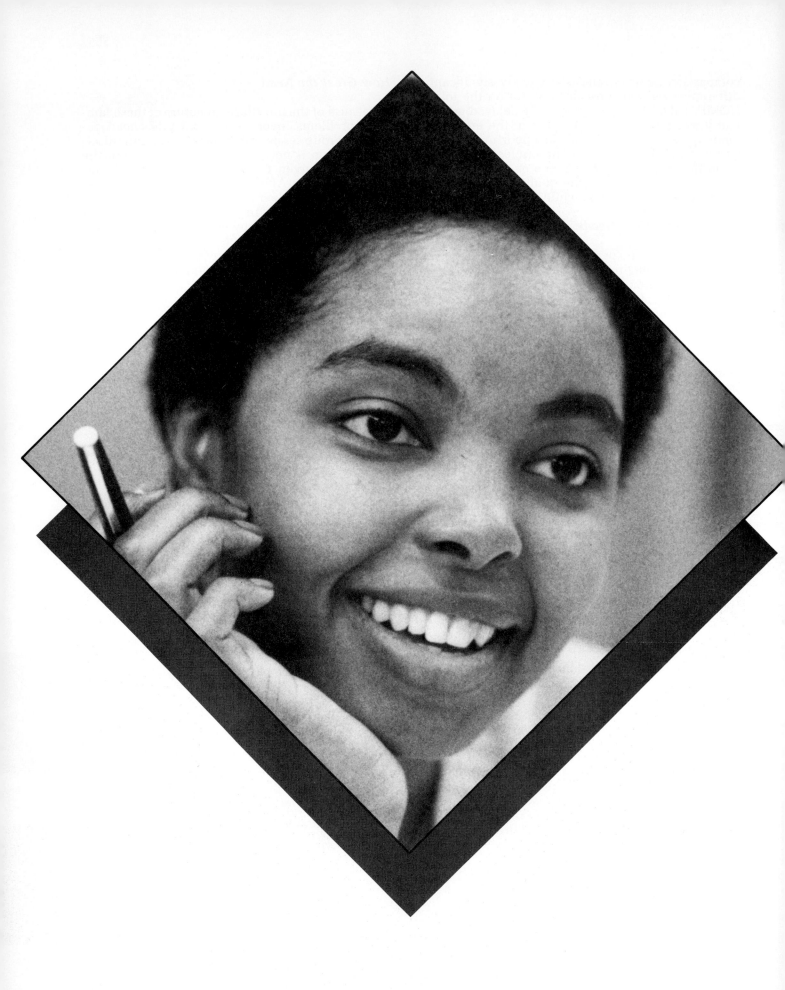

Questions and Answers

The questions and answers in this section have been organized to simulate the NCLEX-RN exam.

The 374 questions have been divided into four sections of 93 or 94 questions each. Each section tests your nursing knowledge regarding care of the adult, the child, the childbearing family, and the client with psychosocial problems.

INSTRUCTIONS FOR TAKING THE TEST

1. Review the information in Section One: Preparing for the NCLEX-RN.
2. Time yourself, allowing 1½ hours per section.
3. Read each question carefully, and select *one* best answer to each question.
4. Do not leave questions blank, since you will not be penalized for random answers on the NCLEX-RN.
5. Score your exam using the answer key. Count any questions left unanswered as incorrect. A score of 75% (70 questions) or more correct answers per section is roughly equivalent to a passing grade.
6. Review the questions you answered incorrectly and restudy that specific material.

At the end of each answers and rationales section, you will find information regarding the assignment of each question into the section of this book covering the content, nursing process, and client need categories. These decisions were made after consultation with the section coordinators and the National Council of State Boards of Nursing. You may use this information to determine if your incorrect answers reflect a weakness in a particular area. Remember, however, that NCLEX-RN is testing your abilities *to apply the steps of the nursing process*, not your ability to assign a category to an individual question.

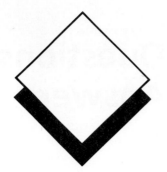

Sample Test Questions: Part One

The community health nurse makes a home visit to the Stephens family. Mona Stephens is a single mother with a 2½-year-old daughter, Vanessa, and a 3-week-old son, Burton. The family lives on public assistance and receives food stamps. Burton's formula is supplied by the WIC program.

1. The nurse would best initiate the visit with which remark?
   - ☐ 1. "You look tired. Are you getting enough sleep?"
   - ☐ 2. "Vanessa seems to like her new brother."
   - ☐ 3. "Tell me what a typical day is like for you."
   - ☐ 4. "Are you having any trouble meeting your expenses?"

2. Ms. Stephens tells the nurse she is concerned about Burton's "throwing up; he does it every time he eats." What would be the nurse's best first response to further clarify this potential problem?
   - ☐ 1. "About how much does he throw up each time, and what does it look like?"
   - ☐ 2. "Are you burping him after every ounce?"
   - ☐ 3. "Perhaps you aren't diluting his formula correctly. Let's check."
   - ☐ 4. "Is he taking formula with iron?"

3. After ascertaining that Burton is experiencing normal newborn regurgitation, the nurse reassures his mother that newborns often experience this problem based on what knowledge?
   - ☐ 1. The newborn's stomach capacity is small.
   - ☐ 2. It takes some time for the newborn to adjust to the formula's richness.
   - ☐ 3. The lining of the newborn's stomach is easily irritated.
   - ☐ 4. The cardiac sphincter between the esophagus and stomach is not fully matured.

4. The nurse has just finished talking with Ms. Stephens about accident prevention. Which of the following statements by the mother suggests that the nurse's teaching was *not* effective?
   - ☐ 1. "I can simply close the door to the bathroom and basement in order to keep Vanessa out."

   - ☐ 2. "It's very important that my daughter not think of medicine as candy."
   - ☐ 3. "I've put the poison control center phone number by all the phones in the house."
   - ☐ 4. "You know, no matter how hard I try I just can't monitor everything she does."

5. The nurse makes a follow-up visit in 3 months. Which finding presents the greatest cause for concern?
   - ☐ 1. Burton is taking 28 ounces of formula daily and 2 tbsp of cereal and pureed fruit twice daily.
   - ☐ 2. Vanessa wets the bed 2 or 3 times a week.
   - ☐ 3. Ms. Stephens says she is "always exhausted."
   - ☐ 4. The only toys in the home are makeshift ones, such as shoe boxes, tissue paper, and pots and pans.

6. The nurse assesses Burton's development at this visit. He should be exhibiting which of the following behaviors?
   - ☐ 1. Bears some weight on his legs.
   - ☐ 2. Imitates speech sounds.
   - ☐ 3. Sits with minimal support.
   - ☐ 4. Uses a thumb-finger grasp.

Margaret Dunneden is a 40-year-old businesswoman who was admitted to the psychiatric unit 2 days ago for severe depression.

7. Mrs. Dunneden says to the nurse, "I'm terrible. I don't deserve to live." Which of the following responses by the nurse would be most appropriate?
   - ☐ 1. "Yes, it has occurred to us that you have that opinion of yourself."
   - ☐ 2. "If you continue to talk this way, I can't listen to you any more."
   - ☐ 3. "What has led you to think that you don't deserve to live?"
   - ☐ 4. "I don't think you're terrible. Don't you think you're liked here?"

8. When the nurse tells Mrs. Dunneden that he will be meeting with her for regular interviews, she says,

"Why would you want to do that?" What would be the most therapeutic response?

- ☐ 1. "I think you're worth the time and effort."
- ☐ 2. "I have been assigned as your therapist."
- ☐ 3. "You need to talk about your feelings."
- ☐ 4. "You can't get better without help."

9. In planning Mrs. Dunneden's care, which of the following objectives is *first* priority?

- ☐ 1. Promotion of self-esteem.
- ☐ 2. Establishment of the nurse-client relationship.
- ☐ 3. Promotion of expression of feelings.
- ☐ 4. Protection from suicidal gestures.

10. Mrs. Dunneden tells the nurse she has just received a promotion and is in line for another significant advance in her company if she does as well in the new position as she did in the last. How is this information most likely related to her depression?

- ☐ 1. Success can sometimes result in a depression.
- ☐ 2. Depression includes grandiose delusions.
- ☐ 3. This will help validate that she is not worthless.
- ☐ 4. The promotion will give her a goal.

11. One day, the nurse notices Mrs. Dunneden sitting alone in the television lounge; and although the TV is on, she is not watching it. Which of the following would be the most therapeutic way to open a conversation with her?

- ☐ 1. "What are you feeling?"
- ☐ 2. "Do you like TV?"
- ☐ 3. "Tell me how you're doing today."
- ☐ 4. "You're not watching TV."

12. Instead of responding verbally, Mrs. Dunneden gets up and walks away. Which of the following is the most therapeutic thing for the nurse to do?

- ☐ 1. Let her go.
- ☐ 2. Follow her and encourage her to talk.
- ☐ 3. Follow her and confront her avoidance behavior.
- ☐ 4. Send another staff person to check on her.

13. One of the staff members reports that Mrs. Dunneden has been eating very little at meals. Which of the following is the most likely explanation of this behavior?

- ☐ 1. It is a common side effect of antidepressants.
- ☐ 2. The hospital food is probably unfamiliar to her.
- ☐ 3. She is trying to get attention from the staff.
- ☐ 4. It is part of her psychiatric problems.

14. Mrs. Dunneden begins to respond to her antidepressant trazodone hydrochloride (Desyrel), and will continue to take it after she is discharged. Which of the following is the correct information to give her about her medication?

- ☐ 1. It may be addicting and should be stopped as soon as she can tolerate being without it.
- ☐ 2. Dizziness can be minimzed by not taking the drug on an empty stomach.
- ☐ 3. The drug may cause hypertension, and she should monitor her blood pressure.

- ☐ 4. She should avoid foods such as aged cheeses and yogurt and products made with yeast, beer, and wine.

15. Mrs. Dunneden has become very involved in activities on the unit. She is talking to other clients and making plans to see all her family. She tells the nurse, "I know everything will work out now." The nurse's most appropriate response would be

- ☐ 1. "Are you making plans to harm yourself?"
- ☐ 2. "I'm concerned that you are taking on too much too fast."
- ☐ 3. "What is it that you are doing now?"
- ☐ 4. "I'm glad to see that you've become interested in activities and people again."

16. Which of the following statements about suicide is accurate?

- ☐ 1. Suicide is the leading cause of death in this country among all groups and among adolescents.
- ☐ 2. Depressed persons attempt suicide as an expression of anger.
- ☐ 3. Hospitalized persons rarely attempt suicide.
- ☐ 4. A person who talks about suicide will not attempt it.

17. When would the nurse best begin preparing for the termination of the relationship with Mrs. Dunneden?

- ☐ 1. At the first meeting.
- ☐ 2. During the working phase.
- ☐ 3. After rapport has been established.
- ☐ 4. When her discharge date is set.

18. A few days before Mrs. Dunneden's scheduled discharge, the nurse finds her crying alone in her room. She says, "I just don't know if I'll be able to make it." What is the most therapeutic response?

- ☐ 1. "You're worried that you'll get depressed again."
- ☐ 2. "You won't be able to 'make' what?"
- ☐ 3. "You wouldn't be leaving if you couldn't make it."
- ☐ 4. "Everyone feels that way sometimes."

19. What is the most likely explanation for Mrs. Dunneden's behavior?

- ☐ 1. She is not ready for discharge.
- ☐ 2. She has become overly dependent on the hospital.
- ☐ 3. She is having a common reaction to discharge.
- ☐ 4. She needs to know the nurse still cares about her.

Alda Clark is a 75-year-old widow who maintains her own residence. While cleaning the snow off her walk, she slips and falls.

20. The nurse notices that Mrs. Clark is unable to move her left leg. The first priority is to

- ☐ 1. Extend her leg into a normal position.
- ☐ 2. Try to reduce the fracture.
- ☐ 3. Elevate the extremity.
- ☐ 4. Treat her as if a fracture has occurred.

21. The nurse suspects that Mrs. Clark fractured her left hip because of which of the following manifestations?
    □ 1. Edema around the site.
    □ 2. Internal rotation of the left hip.
    □ 3. Abduction of the left hip.
    □ 4. Shortened right leg.

22. Preparation of Mrs. Clark's skin before applying Buck's extension traction should include which of the following?
    □ 1. Surgical preparation of the area where pins will be inserted.
    □ 2. Close shaving of the leg with a safety razor.
    □ 3. Washing and drying of the skin.
    □ 4. Application of talc to area.

23. The diagnosis of extracapsular fracture of the left hip requiring internal fixation is made. The plan of care in the postoperative course includes which of the following?
    □ 1. Sedation to reduce Mrs. Clark's pain.
    □ 2. Early ambulation with weight bearing on the left leg to prevent muscle atrophy.
    □ 3. Provisions for "log-rolling" Mrs. Clark.
    □ 4. Maintaining adduction of the left hip to prevent dislocation of the prosthesis.

24. Mrs. Clark has had osteoarthritis for years. She takes 600 mg of aspirin q4h to relieve the pain. Side effects of aspirin are indicated by which of the following signs?
    □ 1. Urinary retention.
    □ 2. Bradycardia.
    □ 3. Tinnitus.
    □ 4. Diplopia.

25. Mrs. Clark expresses concern over her impending discharge. What would be the most effective intervention for Mrs. Clark?
    □ 1. Ask her what concerns her.
    □ 2. Discuss the possibility of placing her in a nursing home.
    □ 3. Teach her about hazards in her environment.
    □ 4. Have the social worker make a visit to Mrs. Clark's home.

Phillip Witten is employed as the manager of a real estate business. Subsequent to increasing pressures at work, hurried and irregular meals, and an unhappy home and family environment, Mr. Witten developed a duodenal ulcer.

26. Which of the following may be a manifestation of a duodenal ulcer?
    □ 1. Pain relieved by food ingestion.
    □ 2. Pain ½ hour after meals.
    □ 3. Vomiting.
    □ 4. Hematemesis.

27. Mr. Witten was placed on a bland diet regimen. Foods permitted on this diet include which of the following?
    □ 1. Creamed soup and pureed squash.
    □ 2. Potato chips and whole wheat bread.
    □ 3. Sponge cake and fried chicken.
    □ 4. Bran muffins and unsalted butter.

28. Anticholinergic drugs are useful in managing gastrointestinal problems such as Mr. Witten's duodenal ulcer. Which is their major action?
    □ 1. Increase gastric motility.
    □ 2. Reduce production of gastric secretions.
    □ 3. Neutralize hydrochloric acid in the stomach.
    □ 4. Absorb excess gastric secretions.

29. Mr. Witten has an order for antacids q2h. At 2 AM when the night nurse goes to his room to give him the antacid, he is asleep. What action is most appropriate?
    □ 1. Wake him and give the medication.
    □ 2. Let him sleep, but wake him at 4 AM and give him a double dose of medicine.
    □ 3. Let him sleep until he wakes up, and then resume the antacid q2h.
    □ 4. Wake him, but give him a double dose of medicine in order to avoid waking him at 4 AM

30. Mr. Witten requires surgical intervention and has a gastric resection. Postoperative nursing interventions include connecting his Salem sump tube to low, continuous wall suction. If he starts to regurgitate, which action should the nurse take?
    □ 1. Irrigate the tube with normal saline.
    □ 2. Notify the physician.
    □ 3. Switch the Gomco suction to a low setting.
    □ 4. Reposition the tube.

31. After Mr. Witten's abdominal surgery, the nurse must be particularly conscientious in encouraging him to cough and deep-breathe hourly for which of the following reasons?
    □ 1. Marked changes in intrathoracic pressure will stimulate gastric drainage.
    □ 2. The high, abdominal incision will lead to shallow breathing to avoid pain.
    □ 3. The phrenic nerve has been permanently damaged during the surgical procedure.
    □ 4. Deep-breathing will prevent postoperative vomiting and intestinal distension.

32. The nurse should be aware of potential complications after a total gastrectomy. For example, 2 months postoperatively, Mr. Witten sought help for complaints of dizziness, sweating, and tachycardia, which occurred 30 minutes after he ate. He also had lost 10 pounds. Symptoms were probably due to which of the following?
    □ 1. Pernicious anemia.
    □ 2. Dumping syndrome.
    □ 3. Recurrence of the ulcer at the incision.
    □ 4. Pyloric stenosis.

Mark Parker, 3 years old, has Down syndrome. During a routine clinic visit, Mrs. Parker tells the nurse that her husband is being transferred to another city. She is very concerned about the effect this move will have on Mark.

33. Which of the following suggestions should receive the highest priority when discussing the move with Mrs. Parker?
    - ☐ 1. Adhere to Mark's daily routine as much as possible during and after the move.
    - ☐ 2. Include Mark in all the family discussions concerning the move.
    - ☐ 3. Have Mark stay with relatives until the move is complete.
    - ☐ 4. Enroll Mark in a special day-care program as soon as possible.

34. Mrs. Parker is also concerned about Mark's weight. "He is so much smaller than other children his age." The nurse's response should be based on the knowledge that
    - ☐ 1. Mark needs more fluids and calories than the average 3-year-old.
    - ☐ 2. The height and weight of children with Down syndrome is usually below chronological norms.
    - ☐ 3. Mrs. Parker should discuss this concern with Mark's pediatrician.
    - ☐ 4. Mark's growth will "catch up" in a few years.

35. Which of the following childhood problems poses the most serious threat to Mark's health?
    - ☐ 1. Conjunctivitis.
    - ☐ 2. Milk allergy.
    - ☐ 3. Chickenpox.
    - ☐ 4. Bronchitis.

36. A comprehensive preschool stimulation program has been planned for Mark according to his abilities. The primary goal of this program is which of the following?
    - ☐ 1. Mark will improve his muscle tone.
    - ☐ 2. Mark will achieve an optimal developmental level.
    - ☐ 3. Mark's family will be involved in his care.
    - ☐ 4. Mark will be ready to enter first grade at age 6.

37. Which of the following actions is likely to have the greatest impact on Mark's learning outcomes during the preschool stimulation program?
    - ☐ 1. Giving Mark's parents written instructions explaining the learning activities.
    - ☐ 2. Observing Mark's parents carrying out Mark's learning plan.
    - ☐ 3. Explaining the activities to Mark while they are being performed to increase his understanding.
    - ☐ 4. Praising Mark for his accomplishments and cooperation with the learning activities.

Thirteen-year-old Darren has hemophilia, and he has recently been diagnosed with acquired immunodeficiency syndrome (AIDS) resulting from contaminated blood products. Darren is currently free from infectious disease.

38. Darren has been hospitalized for hemarthrosis of his left elbow. He is complaining of severe elbow pain. In addition to placing Darren on bed rest, the nurse should
    - ☐ 1. Apply a heating pad to Darren's left elbow.
    - ☐ 2. Give Darren aspirin gr x PO.
    - ☐ 3. Gently perform passive range-of-motion exercises to Darren's left elbow.
    - ☐ 4. Elevate and immobilize Darren's left elbow in a flexed position.

39. The nurse plans to obtain a nursing history from Darren and his mother. No direct body contact with Darren will be necessary during this time. Since Darren has AIDS, the nurse should take which precautions?
    - ☐ 1. Wear a mask only.
    - ☐ 2. Wear a mask and gown.
    - ☐ 3. Wear a mask, gown, and gloves.
    - ☐ 4. No special precautions are needed.

40. A nursing student on Darren's unit tells the nurse she has a cousin with hemophilia and wants to know how the disease is inherited. The nurse explains that a female is usually the carrier of the disease, and when she marries a male who is free of the disease, the risk to their offspring for each pregnancy is what?
    - ☐ 1. All female children will be carriers of hemophilia.
    - ☐ 2. All male children will have the disease.
    - ☐ 3. Half the male children will have hemophilia.
    - ☐ 4. Half the female children will have hemophilia.

41. While Darren is on bed rest, which activity should the nurse *not* include as part of Darren's nursing care plan?
    - ☐ 1. Reading the daily newspaper.
    - ☐ 2. Playing Nerf basketball with his older brother.
    - ☐ 3. Watching his favorite football team on television.
    - ☐ 4. Playing chess with his father.

Ann Cooper, age 28, was referred to the infertility clinic after 6 years of unsuccessful attempts to conceive. She and her husband, Tim, wish to exhaust all possibilities before applying to a community adoption agency.

42. After taking a complete health history from both partners, the nurse prepares them for further assessments. Which of the following fertility tests are generally suggested at the time of the initial visit?
    - ☐ 1. Testicular biopsy and culdoscopy.
    - ☐ 2. Laparoscopy and hormonal studies.
    - ☐ 3. Huhner test and thyroid screening.
    - ☐ 4. Semen analysis and cervical mucus observation.

43. After several months of consultation, the cause of infertility still has not been established. Mr. Cooper expresses his frustration that so little specific information has been given. Which of the following statements by the nurse is most appropriate?
   □ 1. "I know you want a family, but these tests take time."
   □ 2. "Your doctor is a very competent infertility specialist."
   □ 3. "It is hard when you don't know which one of you is at fault."
   □ 4. "Feeling frustration is understandable; let's discuss it."

44. The physician completes all tests and finds no physical reason for the inability of Mrs. Cooper to conceive. He prescribes the drug clomiphene citrate (Clomid) and will continue with hormonal studies. The couple should be aware that a side effect of this therapy may be
   □ 1. Uterine fibroids.
   □ 2. Multiple gestation.
   □ 3. Hypertension.
   □ 4. Transitory depression.

45. Several months after initiating Clomid therapy, the couple visit the clinic for confirmation of pregnancy. The physician estimates that Mrs. Cooper is approximately 8 weeks pregnant, and the couple is delighted. In setting a goal for antepartal care, which of the following is a priorty?
   □ 1. Mother will adhere to regular clinic visit schedule.
   □ 2. Father will participate in each prenatal class.
   □ 3. Couple will practice exercises each day.
   □ 4. Mother will rest for 30 minutes daily.

46. In the tenth week of pregnancy, Mrs. Cooper experiences scant vaginal bleeding for several days. Urine HCG levels remain elevated, and the physician believes that there is no imminent risk of abortion. As the couple prepare to return home, which of the following must be included in teaching?
   □ 1. "Please call if you experience abdominal pain or cramping."
   □ 2. "Notify the doctor if you are nauseated or if you vomit."
   □ 3. "If you are very tired, please let us know."
   □ 4. "Report any signs of urinary frequency."

47. An ultrasound examination is scheduled at the next visit, in the twelfth week of pregnancy. What is the chief purpose of this test?
   □ 1. Measure biparietal diameters.
   □ 2. Identify potential problems.
   □ 3. Confirm fetal viability.
   □ 4. Assess placental function.

48. The pregnancy advances without complications, and Mrs. Cooper keeps all clinic appointments faithfully. After an examination at 32 weeks gestation, she discusses her concerns and discomforts. Mrs. Cooper reports occasional nightmares about labor and delivery. The nurse listens to her feelings and understands that this experience
   □ 1. Is common with a history of infertility.
   □ 2. Is unique to a primigravida.
   □ 3. May indicate deep psychological problems.
   □ 4. Is quite usual in the third trimester.

49. The Coopers plan on a birthing-room delivery. Their Lamaze classes include an orientation to the unit and a tour of the nursery, in addition to the usual content and practice sessions. Which of the following statements following delivery indicates that the couple learned from the classes?
   □ 1. Breathing and relaxation techniques were used effectively.
   □ 2. Early mother-father-infant bonding was initiated.
   □ 3. No analgesics were requested during the first stage of labor.
   □ 4. Father remained supportive throughout the labor and delivery.

50. A 7-pound daughter was put to breast within an hour of birth. The nursing student asks the benefit of early nursing. The staff nurse explains that the chief reason for early breastfeeding is to
   □ 1. Enhance closeness to the newborn.
   □ 2. Promote uterine contraction.
   □ 3. Meet the nutritional needs of the infant.
   □ 4. Stimulate meconium passage.

51. On the infant's admission to the newborn nursery, a gestational assessment is performed. Which of the following observations indicates that the newborn is probably full term?
   □ 1. Apgar scores of 9 and 10 at 1 and 5 minutes.
   □ 2. Good reflex responses.
   □ 3. Many sole creases present.
   □ 4. Birth weight at 50th percentile.

52. While assessing the Cooper infant, the nurse notes that the newborn sneezes frequently and appears to be a nose breather. What is the correct analysis of these data?
   □ 1. There may be a respiratory problem.
   □ 2. Further assessment is indicated.
   □ 3. The environment may be cold.
   □ 4. These are normal responses.

53. The infant looks directly at her mother while breast-feeding and seems to react to the voices of both parents. Mr. Cooper asks the nurse if their daughter can see and hear. Which of the following responses is most accurate?
   □ 1. "We think that the newborn can see light and hear loud sounds."
   □ 2. "Research has shown that close-up vision and hearing are present."
   □ 3. "The newborn only appears to respond to sensory stimuli."
   □ 4. "It is impossible to determine this in the first days of life."

54. During the first 2 days of rooming-in, Mrs. Cooper is taught many aspects of newborn care. On the day of discharge, she is observed feeding and handling the baby. Which of the following actions best indicates that Mrs. Cooper has learned safe handling of her daughter?
   - [ ] 1. The infant is placed on her right side after the feeding.
   - [ ] 2. Breastfeeding is managed comfortably and effectively.
   - [ ] 3. The diaper area is cleansed after passage of a stool.
   - [ ] 4. The mother handles the baby gently while dressing her.

55. The father asks you about laboratory charges for PKU screening, and questions the need for the test. The nurse understands that PKU testing is valuable because
   - [ ] 1. It identifies newborns with chromosomal abnormalities.
   - [ ] 2. Routine screening tests meet state laws.
   - [ ] 3. A rare metabolic disorder can be detected.
   - [ ] 4. Autoimmune adaptation is evaluated.

Judy Rogers is a 25-year-old, type I insulin-dependent diabetic. She works as a bookkeeper and has a young son. She has maintained fairly good diabetic control until recently and is now being admitted for reevaluation. Her insulin routine has been 22 units of NPH plus 5 units of regular insulin daily. She takes her insulin each morning at 7 o'clock.

56. Which piece of subjective data obtained on the nurse's admission assessment indicates a potentially serious problem with Mrs. Rogers' self-care management?
   - [ ] 1. "I'm not getting as much sleep as I used to. Tommy seems to wake up at least once every night."
   - [ ] 2. "I've been promoted at work, but the new job has more responsibility."
   - [ ] 3. "I can't seem to find the time for morning urine tests anymore."
   - [ ] 4. "I'm careful about never skipping meals, but I frequently have to eat breakfast at our 10 A.M. coffee break."

57. Since Mrs. Rogers takes NPH insulin, the nurse reinforces her knowledge of a proper diet by testing her understanding of the importance of snacks at which time of day?
   - [ ] 1. Midmorning.
   - [ ] 2. Midafternoon.
   - [ ] 3. Early evening.
   - [ ] 4. Bedtime.

58. Mrs. Rogers administers her insulin in two injections. What is the most accurate evaluation of this routine?
   - [ ] 1. This is the only safe method because NPH should never be mixed with any other form of insulin.
   - [ ] 2. This is the preferred method because it prevents mistakes in dosage.
   - [ ] 3. There are no real advantages or disadvantages to administering the insulin in one or two injections.
   - [ ] 4. Accurately mixing the two insulins in one injection means that injection sites can be used less frequently.

59. Which statement indicates that Mrs. Rogers rotates injection sites appropriately?
   - [ ] 1. "I use each site only once a month."
   - [ ] 2. "I can give myself my insulin with either hand."
   - [ ] 3. "I alternate daily between sites on my thighs and upper arms.
   - [ ] 4. "I can use sites on my arms, thighs, stomach, and buttocks for injections."

Two-month-old Evan Martin was born with a unilateral complete cleft lip. It is twelve hours after surgical repair of the lip. His mother is staying in his hospital room.

60. Evan is acting fussy and starts to cry softly. The nurse should
   - [ ] 1. Encourage Evan's mother to hold and rock him.
   - [ ] 2. Give Evan his pacifier and rub his back.
   - [ ] 3. Sedate Evan with 2.5 mg of diphenhydramine hydrochloride (Benadryl) elixir.
   - [ ] 4. Allow Evan to cry to facilitate lung inflation.

61. Evan's oral feedings of 4 to 6 ounces of infant formula every 4 or 5 hours are to be resumed. The nurse should teach Mrs. Martin to feed Evan using what method?
   - [ ] 1. A bottle with a soft nipple.
   - [ ] 2. A small paper cup.
   - [ ] 3. A syringe with catheter tubing.
   - [ ] 4. Nasogastric gavage.

62. While feeding Evan, Mrs. Martin asks the nurse, "Why do you think this happened to Evan?" The nurse should reply
   - [ ] 1. "Cleft lip probably runs in your family."
   - [ ] 2. "Sometimes it's hard to know why these things happen."
   - [ ] 3. "Did you have any infections or take any drugs while you were pregnant?"
   - [ ] 4. "What thoughts do you have about why it happened?"

63. Evans is seen for follow-up in the pediatric clinic 3 weeks after his surgery. What is the most crucial indicator of successful treatment of Evan's defect?
   - [ ] 1. Evan's suture line is clean and well healed.
   - [ ] 2. Evan's parents say they are "thrilled with how he looks now."
   - [ ] 3. Evan is making cooing and babbling sounds.
   - [ ] 4. Evan is now sleeping through the night.

Oscar Brown, age 37, has had a cough and fatigue for several weeks. A sputum culture is positive for *Mycobacterium tuberculosis*.

64. Which of the following best prevents the transfer of the tuberculosis organism?
□ 1. Having Mr. Brown cover his nose and mouth with double-ply tissue when he coughs or sneezes.
□ 2. Instructing Mr. Brown's family in effective hand washing.
□ 3. Having Mr. Brown's laundry disinfected after use.
□ 4. Having Mr. Brown's dishes sterilized after use.

65. Mr. Brown and his family ask many questions when first told about his diagnosis of active tuberculosis (e.g., "How did this happen? What can we do? What will happen?"). The nurse's best response might be which of the following?
□ 1. "Mr. Brown probably contracted tuberculosis from another person with tuberculosis."
□ 2. "Mr. Brown will be given medication and be treated at home."
□ 3. "You need not be concerned; tuberculosis is curable."
□ 4. "You seem very worried about the tuberculosis. What concerns you most?"

66. The definitive test for the diagnosis of tuberculosis is
□ 1. A positive PPD skin test.
□ 2. A positive sputum culture.
□ 3. Abnormal findings on chest x-ray.
□ 4. Abnormal results of a pulmonary function test.

67. Screening a population for tuberculosis with tuberculin skin testing is an example of
□ 1. Primary health promotion.
□ 2. Secondary health promotion.
□ 3. Tertiary health promotion.
□ 4. Primary prevention.

Harry Collins, a 39-year-old draftsman for a small engineering firm, came to the mental health center at the insistence of his wife. In his leisure time, Mr. Collins designs household gadgets. Mr. Collins has the persistent belief that someone is attempting to steal his designs. His attempts to prevent this are interfering with his marital relationship and with other social relationships. He has installed an elaborate alarm system in their home and spends hours finding places to hide his designs. He refuses to attend social functions because "someone will steal his ideas." Other than self-imposed isolation from his co-workers, he has no difficulties at work. He completes his work on time and is respected by colleagues as a hard worker.

68. Mr. Collins' symptoms are delusions of
□ 1. Grandeur.
□ 2. Persecution.
□ 3. Reference.
□ 4. Religiosity.

69. The nurse who takes Mr. Collins' admission history understands that his delusion is related to
□ 1. A desire for attention.
□ 2. Anger at his employer.
□ 3. Fear of losing control.
□ 4. Low self-esteem.

70. Mr. Collins is given a diagnosis of chronic paranoia. Based on this, the nurse would expect Mr. Collins to have
□ 1. Hallucinations.
□ 2. Hostility.
□ 3. Impaired intellectual functioning.
□ 4. Poor reality testing in all areas.

71. Which of the following problems is also true of Mr. Collins?
□ 1. Attention-getting behavior related to mistrust of others.
□ 2. Decreased intellectual functioning.
□ 3. Impaired marital relationship caused by suspiciousness.
□ 4. Paranoia.

72. Initial plans for Mr. Collins would best include
□ 1. Allowing Mr. Collins to initiate relationships and activities.
□ 2. A one-to-one relationship initiated by the nurse.
□ 3. Participation in a competitive sport.
□ 4. Participation in an occupational-therapy group.

73. Mr. Collins attends his first group-therapy session the second day of hospitalization. He leaves in the middle of the session and tells his nurse, "They don't know what they're doing in there. They're all crazy. I won't go to those meetings." The nurse's most appropriate action would be to
□ 1. Develop a one-to-one relationship with Mr. Collins before he begins group therapy again.
□ 2. Explain the benefits of group therapy in helping Mr. Collins overcome his delusions.
□ 3. Insist that Mr. Collins return to the group session immediately.
□ 4. Tell Mr. Collins that he is excluded today but must return to group therapy tomorrow.

74. All of the following nursing actions will be important in developing a one-to-one relationship with Mr. Collins *except*
□ 1. Accurate and honest communications.
□ 2. Clearly stated mutual expectations.
□ 3. Confrontation regarding delusions.
□ 4. Consistency in keeping appointments.

75. Mr. Collins has been hospitalized for a week. He still talks at length about the measures he can take to protect his designs. The nurse's most appropriate action is to
□ 1. Involve Mr. Collins in an activity on the unit.
□ 2. Listen attentively and encourage further discussion.
□ 3. Tell Mr. Collins his plans are unnecessary.
□ 4. Tell Mr. Collins she is aware of his actions.

76. Which of the following is the best indicator that Mr. Collins is improving?
☐ 1. He attends occupational therapy.
☐ 2. He attends to his personal hygiene and grooming.
☐ 3. He freely discusses his attempt to protect his designs.
☐ 4. He discusses feelings of anxiety with the nurse.

Sixteen-month-old Mi Lin Ngyen and her family moved to the United States from Southeast Asia 1 month ago. Mi Lin and her parents visit the pediatric clinic for the first time.

77. Which of the following is *least* important for the nurse to consider when initiating interaction with Mi Lin?
☐ 1. Developmental level.
☐ 2. Racial heritage.
☐ 3. Cultural experiences.
☐ 4. Inability to comprehend English.

78. To gain Mi Lin's trust and cooperation, the nurse should first
☐ 1. Offer Mi Lin a toy to play with.
☐ 2. Pick Mi Lin up and hug her warmly.
☐ 3. Use a puppet to "talk" to Mi Lin.
☐ 4. Establish a positive interaction with Mi Lin's parents.

79. The nurse measures Mi Lin's length and weight and finds she is below the 5th percentile for both. A nutritional history reveals Mi Lin's caloric and nutrient intake is consistent with recommended guidelines. Which of the following interpretations is most valid?
☐ 1. Growth norms are based on American children, who tend to be larger on the average.
☐ 2. Mi Lin's parents may not have been truthful concerning her intake.
☐ 3. A hormone deficiency may be causing a growth lag.
☐ 4. Mi Lin may not be getting adequate activity and exercise.

80. When preparing to administer Mi Lin's DTP booster, the nurse should
☐ 1. Allow Mi Lin to play with a syringe for a few minutes.
☐ 2. Talk in a soothing tone to Mi Lin while her mother holds her firmly in her lap, and proceed quickly.
☐ 3. Explain to Mi Lin that she must "get a shot so you won't get sick."
☐ 4. Secure the assistance of at least one other nurse to help restrain Mi Lin.

Kathy Smith, 5 years old, has been admitted with a diagnosis of noncommunicating hydrocephalus secondary to postmeningitis adhesions.

81. What was probably the earliest manifestation of increased intracranial pressure that Kathy exhibited?

☐ 1. Early morning headache.
☐ 2. Clumsy gait.
☐ 3. Projectile vomiting.
☐ 4. Papilledema.

82. Following insertion of a ventriculoperitoneal shunt, the nurse should plan for Kathy to be placed in what position?
☐ 1. Semi-Fowler's on the operative side.
☐ 2. Semi-Fowler's on the unoperative side.
☐ 3. Flat on the operative side.
☐ 4. Flat on the unoperative side.

83. Postoperatively, which of the following findings is the most reliable indicator of a change in Kathy's intracranial pressure.
☐ 1. Change in sensorium.
☐ 2. Tachycardia.
☐ 3. Nausea and vomiting.
☐ 4. Pulmonary rales.

84. The physician has ordered Kathy's shunt to be pumped four times every shift. When preparing Kathy for this procedure, the nurse should
☐ 1. Explain to Kathy how it will feel when the shunt is pumped.
☐ 2. Tell Kathy why the shunt has to be pumped.
☐ 3. Remind Kathy to be brave so she will get well soon.
☐ 4. Ask Kathy to close her eyes and relax so it will be over quickly.

Julio Cortez, age 47, is admitted from the ER with severe substernal chest pain. A diagnosis of acute myocardial infarction is made. He is in severe pain and is cold, clammy, and dyspneic.

85. All of the following interventions are important. Which should be done first?
☐ 1. Administer oxygen.
☐ 2. Place in semi-Fowler's position.
☐ 3. Institute complete bed rest.
☐ 4. Administer morphine by slow IV push.

86. Mr. Cortez is started on heparin therapy. The nurse should tell Mr. Cortez he is receiving heparin to
☐ 1. Thin his blood.
☐ 2. Slow the clotting of his blood.
☐ 3. Stop his blood from clotting.
☐ 4. Dissolve the clot in his heart.

87. Mr. Cortez begins to have blood in his stool and has episodes of epistaxis. In view of this development, which drug should the nurse have available?
☐ 1. Vitamin C (ascorbic acid).
☐ 2. Vitamin K (AquaMEPHYTON).
☐ 3. Protamine sulfate.
☐ 4. Calcium chloride.

88. Mr. Cortez suffers congestive heart failure and is given digitalis. Which of the following indicates a toxic effect of digitalis?

☐ 1. Hypokalemia.
☐ 2. Tachycardia.
☐ 3. Nausea and vomiting.
☐ 4. Gynecomastia.

89. With left-sided congestive heart failure, which of the following symptoms is most expected?
☐ 1. Nocturnal dyspnea.
☐ 2. Sacral edema.
☐ 3. Oliguria.
☐ 4. Anorexia.

90. Mr. Cortez is advised to eliminate foods high in cholesterol from his diet. This means he should avoid eggs and
☐ 1. Liver.
☐ 2. Yogurt.
☐ 3. Chicken.
☐ 4. Corn oil.

Three-year-old Nicole Lyon's mother brings her to the emergency room because Nicole ate "half a bottle of my acetaminophen tablets 15 minutes ago."

91. The nurse ascertains that the bottle originally contained 100 tablets. The nurse's first action should be what?

☐ 1. Have Nicole drink an 8-ounce glass of milk.
☐ 2. Give Nicole 30 ml of syrup of ipecac followed by a glass of water.
☐ 3. Insert a nasogastric tube and administer activated charcoal.
☐ 4. Obtain a brief history of events leading up to the ingestion from Mrs. Lyon.

92. Nicole is admitted to the pediatric unit for observation. Which laboratory findings should the nurse monitor most closely for changes in Nicole's health status?
☐ 1. Hemoglobin and hematocrit.
☐ 2. White-blood-cell count and differential.
☐ 3. Blood gases (PO_2, PCO_2, and pH).
☐ 4. Serum transaminase levels (SCOT and SGPT).

93. Nicole is receiving acetylcysteine (Mucomyst) as an antidote to the acetaminophen. To make the drug more palatable for Nicole to drink, the nurse should mix the drug with what fluid?
☐ 1. Water.
☐ 2. Orange juice.
☐ 3. Milk.
☐ 4. Flavored milkshake.

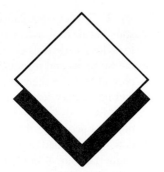

Correct Answers and Rationales: Part One

KEY TO ABBREVIATIONS

KEY TO ABBREVIATIONS
Section of the Review Book

P = Psychosocial and Mental Health Problems
    I = Introduction
    T = Therapeutic Use of Self
    L = Loss and Death and Dying
    A = Anxious Behavior
    C = Confused Behavior
    E = Elated-Depressive Behavior
    SM = Socially Maladaptive Behavior
    SS = Suspicious Behavior
    W = Withdrawn Behavior
    SU = Substance Use Disorders
A = Adult
    H = Healthy Adult
    S = Surgery
    O = Oxygenation
    NM = Nutrition and Metabolism
    E = Elimination
    SP = Sensation and Perception
    M = Mobility
    CA = Cellular Aberration
CBF = Childbearing Family
    W = Women's Health Care
    A = Antepartal Care
    I = Intrapartal Care
    P = Postpartal Care
    N = Newborn Care
C = Child
    H = Healthy Child
    I = Ill and Hospitalized Child
    SPP = Sensation, Perception, Protection
    O = Oxygenation
    NM = Nutrition and Metabolism
    E = Elimination
    M = Mobility
    CA = Cellular Aberration

Nursing Process Category

AS = Assessment
AN = Analysis
PL = Planning
IM = Implementation
EV = Evaluation

Client Need Category

E = Safe, Effective Care Environment
PS = Physiological Integrity
PC = Psychosocial Integrity
H = Health Promotion/Maintenance

1. no. 3. This opening statement allows the nurse to gain an overall perspective of family functioning, yet is specific enough to focus the response (as opposed to, "Tell me how you are doing"). The other choices focus narrowly on one aspect, which might be appropriate as the visit proceeds, but are haphazard initial questions. Also, two of them (no. 1 and no. 4) require only a "yes" or "no" response and thus do not encourage disclosure by the client. P-T, AS, PC

2. no. 1. The nurse's first response should be to clarify and validate the problem by gathering additional information. Option no. 2 might be asked as the nurse proceeds to narrow the scope of the cause. no. 3 is likely to make the parent feel defensive, and no. 4 is irrelevant, since research does not implicate iron as a cause of regurgitation or vomiting. C-H, AS, E

3. no. 4. The young infant's cardiac sphincter is not yet fully matured and as a result often relaxes, allowing regurgitation of stomach contents. Although the newborn's stomach capacity is small, it is not the size per se, but the weak cardiac sphincter that precipitates spitting up. There is no scientific basis to support options no. 2 or no. 3. CBF-N, AN, PS

4. no. 1. Usually by 2 years, the toddler can turn knobs and open doors; simply closing the door is not enough; the door should be locked and all harmful substances placed in a locked cabinet. Parents need to be told that medicine should not be treated as candy, the Poison Control Center number should be easily accessible and no matter how hard they try, they cannot watch their children all the time. Accidents will happen. C-H, EV, H

5. no. 3. Although tiredness is a common complaint of mothers of small children, Ms. Stephens' feeling "exhausted" may indicate anemia or poor coping. This needs to be further investigated. Although Burton does not need solids at his age, his caloric intake is within recommended ranges. Bed-wetting is not considered unusual in children of Vanessa's age, and she may still be adjusting to her new brother. The homemade toys provide appropriate developmental stimulation for Ms. Stephens' children. C-H, AN, H

6. no. 1. Burton should be bearing some weight on his legs when held upright. Inability to do so may indicate a neuromotor delay. The other skills are too advanced for Burton's age. C-H, AS, H

7. no. 3. This is the only response that recognizes and acknowledges the client's perception of her situation and that encourages her to explore it with the nurse. This response is therapeutic and conveys respect for the client's point of view and a desire to help her learn to cope with her problems. It promotes a relationship of trust. Option no. 1 is slightly sarcastic and no. 2 makes a listening relationship contingent on the client's behavior. Option no. 4 contradicts the client's ideas. P-T, IM, PC

8. no. 3. This option focuses on the client's needs without challenging the client. No. 1 reassures a client of his/her worth, but does not provide information necessary to set tone for nurse-client relationship. No. 2 presents factual information but does not focus on client needs or the purpose of nurse-client relationship. No. 4 challenges the client and does not focus on needs. P-T, IM, PC

9. no. 4. 50%-80% of all suicides are committed by depressed persons. Mrs. Dunneden is a high suicide risk; she has already expressed that she doesn't desire to live anymore and may, therefore, have a plan. Although options no. 1, no. 2, and no. 3 are good objectives of care, they are not the first priority at this time. P-T, PL, PC

10. no. 1. Success can cause depression in some persons because of a fear of failure, which will lead to a loss of self-esteem. The promotion will increase stress and responsibility. Option no. 2 is not correct because there is no indication of delusions, and no. 3 may lead to argument over worth. P-E, AN, PC

11. no. 3. Encourage the client to talk by using general, open-ended question. Option no. 1 is too vague and no. 4 does not encourage the client to talk. The TV is not the concern. P-T, IM, PC

12. no. 2. Stay with her to demonstrate caring. Encourage her to talk, but do not push or confront her. Options no. 1 and no. 4 may be interpreted by the client as a lack of caring. In this initial, early phase, confrontation might be destructive to the relationship. P-T, IM, PC

13. no. 4. Anorexia is a common occurrence in depressed clients, but it is not a common side effect of antidepressants. Hospital food usually meets client needs. There has been no indication that she desires staff attention. P-E, AN, PC

14. no. 2. The most common side effect of trazodone hydrochloride (Desyrel) is dizziness. Antidepressants are not addicting. No. 3 and no. 4 are common for MAO inhibitors. P-E, IM, H

15. no. 3. Further assessment is necessary to determine if the client is suicidal or is making realistic plans and taking positive steps to become reinvolved with her environment. no. 1 is a possibility, however, more information is necessary before asking this direct question. no. 2 and no. 4 do not encourage further exploration of the client's actions and feelings and cut off communication about plans for self. P-E, IM, PC

16. no. 2. Suicide is an act of self-punishment, of anger directed toward the self. The suicidal person is depressed, feels guilty, condemns self, and directs anger inward. Suicide is not the leading cause of death in all persons. Hospitalized clients and those who talk of suicide are vulnerable. P-E, AN, PC

17. no. 1. Preparing for termination begins with the inception of the therapeutic relationship. Introduction of termination at any of the other times listed would disrupt the complete process of the relationship. P-T, PL, E

18. no. 1. Reflection will encourage the client to discuss her fears. Option no. 2 is too direct and does not acknowledge underlying concerns. No. 3 minimizes fear and closes off exploration of feelings and planning coping methods upon discharge. No. 4 fails to recognize client as an individual and is an attempt at unrealistic reassurance. P-T, IM, PC

19. no. 3. Clients often become anxious near discharge and reexperience symptoms they may not have shown for some time. There has been no data given to indicate that she is not ready for discharge or that she is overly dependent. Crying is unlikely to

be directly related to the nurses caring for her. P-A, AN, E

20. no. 4. The diagnosis has not been confirmed; you only suspect a fractured hip. Never attempt to reduce a fracture, or extend or elevate the extremity. You may cause more damage. A-M, AN, PS

21. no. 3. Fractured hips are indicated by abduction of the affected extremity and movement away from the main axis of the body. There is also external rotation of the hip, and the leg is shortened. It is difficult to assess edema at this point. A-M, AS, PS

22. no. 3. Washing and drying of the skin aids in securing the traction. Buck's traction does not involve the insertion of pins. Healthy skin (i.e., without abrasions) tolerates skin traction well. C-M, IM, E

23. no. 3. When the client is moved, she needs to be "log-rolled" with abductor splint or pillows between her legs. Abduction of the affected leg is to be maintained at all times. Sedation does not relieve pain. Early ambulation is advocated; however, no weight bearing is allowed on the operated side. A-M, PL, PS

24. no. 3. Doses of aspirin sufficient to relieve pain may cause tinnitus. The other side effects listed are not characteristic of aspirin. A-S, AS, PS

25. no. 1. Additional information is needed from Mrs. Clark regarding her concerns. The other choices *may* be appropriate, but clarification regarding the clients' concerns is needed first. P-T, IM, PO

26. no. 1. Manifestations of a duodenal ulcer include: pain relieved by food ingestion, pain occurring 1-4 hours after eating, and melena. Vomiting and hematemesis are characteristic of gastric ulcers. A-NM, AS, PS

27. no. 1. All fried foods and whole grains are prohibited on a bland diet. A-NM, AN, E

28. no. 2. Anticholinergic drugs block the effect of acetylcholine at receptor sites, thereby reducing the production of gastric secretions. A-NM, AS, PS

29. no. 1. Antacids are given to coat the ulcer to protect it from irritation. To be effective, they must be given on time. A-NM, IM, PS

30. no. 2. Irrigation is contraindicated after gastric surgery, unless ordered, to avoid trauma to the surgical site. Salem sumps are repositioned after gastric surgery *only* by the physician. Repositioning can cause disruption of the suture line. Gomco suction is contraindicated because it is intermittent suction; to be effective, the Salem tube requires continuous suction. A-NM, EV, PS

31. no. 2. After abdominal surgery, the client is at greatest risk for pulmonary complications. Therefore, encourage him to take deep breaths at least hourly. The other statements listed are not true. A-S, AN, PS

32. no. 2. These are signs and symptoms of late dumping syndrome. Rapid emptying of the stomach contents into the intestine ultimately leads to a hypoglycemic reaction that causes the symptoms. A-NM, EV, PS

33. no. 1. Maintaining consistency in Mark's environment is the single most effective way to promote a sense of security and continuity during the move. no. 2 is unrealistic in view of Mark's age and limitations. no. 3 and no. 4 may increase Mark's fear by adding more change in his life. C-I, PL, PC

34. no. 2. Children with Down syndrome are smaller than healthy children the same age and will continue to be as they grow older. No data suggests that Mark's fluid and caloric intake is inadequate. Referring this mother's concern to the pediatrician is inappropriate since it is within the scope of nursing practice. C-SPP, AN, H

35. no. 4. Respiratory infections are common in children with Down syndrome and account for high morbidity. The hypotonicity of the chest and abdominal muscles is a major predisposing factor to respiratory infections. C-SPP, AN, H

36. no. 2. The priority goal of caring for a child with any form of retardation is to promote optimal development. Options no. 1 and no. 3 are important goals, but are not as crucial as the broader goal of maximizing development. No. 4 may be unrealistic because of the mental retardation that accompanies Down syndrome. C-SPP, PL, H

37. no. 4. While all the options are necessary in a comprehensive preschool stimulation program, motivating the child to want to learn is the critical factor. This is best accomplished through praising the child's accomplishments. This option is also helpful in promoting self-esteem. C-SPP, EV, H

38. no. 4. During a bleeding episode involving a joint, the joint should be elevated and immobilized in a flexed position to minimize further bleeding and decrease pain. Heat will cause vasodilation and aggravate the bleeding episode. Ice packs, which promote vasoconstriction, should be applied to the elbow instead. Aspirin is contraindicated for the child with hemophilia because it interferes with platelet function. Range-of-motion exercises may cause further trauma to the joint during a bleeding episode. C-O, AN-E

39. no. 4. AIDS is transmitted in body secretions such as urine, stools, blood, and saliva. As long as the nurse does not have direct body contact with Darren, no special precautions are needed. C-SPP, IM, E

40. no. 3. When a female carrier of hemophilia has children fathered by a male who is free of the disease, the risk to their offspring (*with each pregnancy*) is as follows: half the males will have hemophilia (XrY), half the males will be normal

(XY), half the females will be carriers of the hemophilia gene (XrX), and half the females will be normal (XX). C-O, AS, PS

41. no. 2. Playing Nerf basketball would be contraindicated for Darren because it would require him to move his elbow, which should remain immobilized while he is on bed rest to prevent further bleeding. The other activities are age appropriate and acceptable for his treatment plan. C-H, IM, E

42. no. 4. While the other tests may be performed later, they are involved or invasive. Semen analysis is a simple assessment. Cervical mucus consistency changes during the menstrual cycle and gives clues to ovulation. CBF-W, IM, PC

43. no. 4. This response indicates understanding of common feelings about infertility and is considered therapeutic communication, as it encourages further discussion. While options no. 1 and no. 2 are true, neither is helpful to the father. Option no. 3 blocks communication by introducing the concept of blame. P-T, IM, PC

44. no. 2. Clomiphine citrate (Clomid), a drug frequently prescribed to correct infertility, increases the risk of ovarian cysts and multiple births. None of the other choices is correct. CBF, W, IM, E

45. no. 1. The priority goal for any pregnant client is compliance with regular prenatal care. CBF-A, PL, H

46. no. 1. If the client experiences contractions, cramping, or more bleeding, she may be experiencing a miscarriage. The other symptoms listed are common in the first trimester and need not be reported. CBF-A, IM, PS

47. no. 3. At this time in pregnancy, when the client has a history of bleeding, the test is performed to confirm fetal viability. Biparietal diameters are a useful assessment between 18 and 24 weeks' gestation. Neither option no. 2 nor no. 4 is accurate. CBF-A, AS, PS

48. no. 4. These fears and dreams are common, especially in the last trimester. There is no higher incidence with infertility or in a first pregnancy. CBF-A, AN, PC

49. no. 1. The focus of Lamaze classes is the practice of breathing, relaxation, and conditioned responses for use during labor. While it is positive that bonding and support were noted, these are not criteria for evaluation of learning. Requests for analgesics during labor do not influence successful delivery outcome of Lamaze couples. CBF-A, EV, PC

50. no. 1. While uterine contractions are stimulated by lactation, the major reason for initiating nursing soon after delivery is to promote closeness. Nutritional needs are minimal at this time. Breastfeeding has no specific effect on meconium passage, which normally occurs within the first 24 hours. CBF-P, IM, H

51. no. 3. This is the only assessment that refers to gestational age. Apgar scores measure immediate adaptations to extrauterine life; birth weight is not necessarily related to length of gestation; reflexes may be good in some infants who were born before term. CBF-N, AN, PS

52. no. 4. These are normal responses. BF-N, AN, PS

53. no. 2. Studies indicate that sensory development at birth is quite good. This response is more specific than option no. 1. CBF-N, IM, H

54. no. 1. A newborn should be positioned on the abdomen or right side after feeding to prevent aspiration of milk or mucus. The other behaviors are appropriate, but do not evaluate *safe* care. CBF-N, EV, E

55. no. 3. While state laws do require PKU screening, the most appropriate response gives the major purpose of the test. The PKU test is specific for one inherited metabolic disorder rather than for vague chromosomal abnormalities. CBF-N, AS, H

56. no. 4. This is a potentially serious problem because she takes her insulin at 7 AM but does not eat until 10 AM. Regular insulin's onset is 1 hour, and it peaks in 2-4 hours. A-NM, AS, E

57. no. 2. Peak action for NPH is 8-12 hours after administration. Since she takes her insulin at 7 AM, the NPH peak action will be from 3 to 7 PM. If she eats a snack between 3 and 4 PM, she will cover the beginning peak time of the NPH. A-NM, AN, H

58. no. 4. NPH and regular insulin may be mixed. Accurately and consistently drawing up insulin, whether mixed or not, is the key to preventing mistakes in dosage. There is no need for two injections, and this gives the client more sites for rotation, decreasing the incidence of lipohypertrophy. A-NM, EV, E

59. no. 1. No injection site should be used more than once a month. While the other statements are all correct to some degree, this statement tells you the exact, correct information. A-NM, EV, E

60. no. 1. Sucking and crying are contraindicated postoperatively in infants who have had a cleft lip repair because of potential damage to the repair. Sedation with diphenydramine hydrochloride (Benadryl) is indicated only if Evan becomes very restless or agitated and is unable to be calmed by other measures such as holding, stroking, or rocking. Allowing Evan's mother to hold and rock him also involves her directly in his care and thus increases her sense of control. C-NM, IM, E

61. no. 3. A syringe fitted with soft catheter tubing will allow Evan's mother to feed him adequate amounts of formula to the side and back of his mouth and prevent Evan from sucking, which may injure the lip repair. Evan should not be allowed to suck from a nipple in the postoperative period

because of possible damage created by tension on the suture line. Evan is too young to be able to drink from a cup; additionally, placement of the cup to his lips may stimulate his suck reflex or directly irritate the suture line. There is no reason to institute nasogastric feedings when a less invasive method, effective in providing adequate nutrition, is available. C-NM, IM, E

62. no. 4. This reply allows the nurse to ascertain what Mrs. Martin believes to be the cause of Evan's defect, and what specific concerns or unanswered questions about the cause she may have. The nurse can then further validate the mother's concerns before responding with information or appropriate supportive comments. Although cleft lip is known to be transmitted multifactorially, thus increasing the possiblity of occurrence in families with a history of defect, option no. 1 has not been validated and is not responsive to the mother's concern. Option no. 2 ignores Mrs. Martin's feelings in the situation. Teratogens, such as viruses or drugs, may also cause cleft lip, but option no. 3 is worded as a closed question and does not address the mother's question. C-NM, IM, PC

63. no. 1. The goal of surgical repair of cleft lip is to achieve primary closure of the defect to ensure adequate nutrition through normal sucking and to minimize scarring for cosmetic reasons. A clean, well-healed suture line indicates that Evan has the capacity to suck and that he will have minimal scarring. Although it is important for the parent-infant relationship that Evan's parents are pleased with the repair, Evan's physiological needs are more crucial when evaluating treatment outcomes. Options no. 3 and no. 4 illustrate typical development progress for a 3-month-old and do not provide direct evidence of goal achievement. C-NM, EV, H

64. no. 1. Tuberculosis is an airborne disease transmitted by droplet nuclei. The client should cover his nose and mouth with double-ply tissues when he coughs or sneezes; his bare hand will not stop the droplets. Proper hand washing removes the tubercle bacilli from the hands but eliminating droplet transmission best prevents the transfer of the disease. No special laundry or dishwashing techniques are needed. A-O, IM, E

65. no. 4. The multiple questions suggest anxiety and fear. No. 4 encourages Mr. Brown and his family to express their feelings. The other options, while factually correct, will probably not allay anxiety and imply that the nurse knows what is bothering Mr. Brown and his family. P-A, IM, H

66. no. 2. A positive sputum culture for acid-fast bacilli confirms the diagnosis of active tuberculosis. A positive PPD indicates exposure to the tubercle bacillus, but not necessarily the presence of active disease. Abnormal findings on a chest x-ray or pulmonary function tests are not definitive for a diagnosis of tuberculosis. Skin testing, chest x-ray, and pulmonary function tests must all be confirmed by a positive sputum culture. A-O, AN, H

67. no. 2. The goal of tuberculin skin testing is the early diagnosis and treatment of tuberculosis, (i.e., secondary health promotion). Primary health promotion and primary prevention aim at preventing the occurrence of a disease. Tertiary health promotion aims at preventing the complications of a disease. A-H, AS, H

68. no. 2. Delusions of persecution are defined as false beliefs that oneself has been singled out for harassment. Delusions in this situation do not relate to ideas of superiority (no. 1), or focus on the self (no. 3) or on religious ideation (no. 4). P-W, AN, PC

69. no. 4. Content of the delusion serves to build up the person's self-esteem. Insufficient data are given to support the other choices. Delusions of persecution are not usually attributed to the behavior patterns described in options no. 1, no. 2, and no. 3. P-SS, AN, PC

70. no. 2. Persons with paranoid ideation have underlying hostility. There is no evidence of hallucinations. Intellectual functioning appears intact. Reality testing remains intact in paranoid clients except for the area related to the delusion. P-SS, AS, PC

71. no. 3. Mr. Collins has marital problems because of his behavior. There is no evidence that his behavior is attention seeking and his intellectual functioning is not disturbed. Paranoia is a medical diagnosis, not a nursing diagnosis. P-SS, AS, PC

72. no. 2. Interventions would begin with one-to-one activities. Socialization is increased gradually. The client will need assistance in developing a relationship. Participation in demanding group activities may seem threatening. P-SS, PL, E

73. no. 1. Involve the suspicious client in group activity and relationships gradually. Begin by developing a one-to-one relationship; involve others slowly. Options no. 2, no. 3, and no. 4 do not allow for this gradual involvement. P-SS, IM, PC

74. no. 3. Do not argue with the client about delusions. Consistency and clarity will enhance development of trust and are crucial in developing a relationship. P-T, IM, PC

75. no. 1. Maintain a focus on reality without demeaning the client or becoming involved in arguments. Options no. 2 and no. 3 may lead to an argument. Option no. 4 shows a condescending attitude by the nurse and is not therapeutic. P-SS, IM, PC

76. no. 4. The goal for a suspicious client is to recognize and express the anxiety that causes the de-

lusion. No disruption of work or self-care abilities has been indicated. Discussion of delusions would indicate no change. P-SS, EV, PC

77. no. 2. Although Mi Lin's racial heritage is an important factor to consider when assessing growth and physical health status, it has little bearing on how the nurse would approach Mi Lin in a clinical situation, wheras the other factors listed are essential in guiding the nurse's interaction with Mi Lin. C-H, AS, PC

78. no. 4. At this age, it is best to allow the child to make the first move. Establishing interaction with Mi Lin's parents gives Mi Lin time to size up the nurse and see that her parents demonstrate trust in the nurse. The other nursing actions may be perceived by Mi Lin as direct threats because of her language barrier and developmental level. C-H, IM, PS

79. no. 1. Asian children are shorter and weigh less, on the average, than American children, on whom growth norms are usually based. Even though the graphs have been revised recently to be more representative of children from varying backgrounds, the nurse should always consider the child's family heritage when evaluating variances from normal. No information has been provided to support any of the other options. C-H, AN, PC

80. no. 2. It is best to have a parent assist with holding the child during a briefly painful procedure, such as an immunization, if possible. Proceeding quickly is the desirable approach with a child this age for a procedure that will be over quickly. Prolonged explanations only increase the child's anxiety and, in Mi Lin's case, would not be understood because she does not speak English. She may be given the needleless syringe to play with *following* the injection. C-I, IM, PC

81. no. 1. Early morning headaches are frequently the earliest sign of increased intracranial pressure. The other manifestations are later signs of increased ICP. C-SPP, AS, PS

82. no. 4. Positioning the client flat on the unoperative side will prevent pressure on the shunt valve and allow for gradual drainage of the spinal fluid. The other positions would place additional pressure on the shunt. C-SPP, PL, E

83. no. 1. The primary indicator of changing intracranial pressure is a change in sensorium or level of consciousness. C-SPP, EV, PS

84. no. 1. Six-year-olds are in the preoperational stage of cognitive development and are most concerned about what sensations they will feel when facing an unfamiliar experience. Kathy would have difficulty understanding why the shunt must be pumped and, in any event, why is not as important as what or how. Options no. 3 and no. 4 do not actively involve Kathy in the experience or give her any sense of control and will probably increase her fear and lessen her cooperation. C-I, IM, PC

85. no. 4. Relief of pain is the priority goal for a client with a myocardial infarction. All the interventions may be carried out, but relief of pain is first. A-O, IM, PS

86. no. 2. Anticoagulant therapy is used to prolong, not prevent, clotting. Anticoagulants have no thrombolytic (clot-dissolving) action. "Blood thinner" is a term commonly used by lay persons for anticoagulants, but actually anticoagulants have no effect on hemoconcentration. A-O, IM, PS

87. no. 3. Protamine sulfate is the antidote for heparin. Vitamin K is the antidote for *oral* anticoagulants. Neither vitamin C nor calcium chloride acts as an antidote against anticoagulant drugs. A-O, AN, E

88. no. 3. Digitalis toxicity is manifested by gastrointestinal upset. Bradycardia, not tachycardia, is a side effect that may or may not indicate toxicity. Hypokalemia potentiates the effects of digitalis, but is not a toxic effect. Gynecomastia is an uncommon side effect. A-O, AS, PS

89. no. 1. Left-sided congestive heart failure causes pulmonary congestion and symptoms. Oliguria, although present in both right-sided and left-sided congestive heart failure, is primarily a symptom of right-sided failure. Sacral edema and anorexia occur with right-sided congestive heart failure. A-O, AS, PS

90. no. 1. Organ meats are high in cholesterol. Chicken and yogurt are low in cholesterol. Vegetable oils such as corn oil have no cholesterol. A-O, AN, H

91. no. 2. Use of syrup of ipecac in age-appropriate dosage is the safest, most effective emergency treatment of accidental ingestion of all substances *except* hydrocarbons or caustics. The priority goal is to empty the potentially toxic acetaminophen from the stomach. Having the child drink milk may cause more rapid absorption of the tablets. Gastric lavage with administration of activated charcoal should be carried out *after* gastric emptying. Option no. 4 would waste valuable time and allow greater amounts of the acetaminophen to be absorbed. The history may be obtained during or immediately following administration of the syrup of ipecac. C-SPP, IM, E

92. no. 4. Acetaminophen is potentially toxic to the liver. Serum transaminase (SGOT and SGPT) levels should be closely monitored every 24 hours for 3 to 5 days following the ingestion to detect hepatic damage. Acetaminophen toxicity is not reflected by any of the other laboratory findings listed. C-SPP, AN, PS

93. no. 2. Orange juice will help disguise the taste of acetylcysteine (Mucomyst), whereas water will not. Milk products may interfere with the absorption of the Mucomyst and are, therefore, not recommended. C-SPP, IM, E

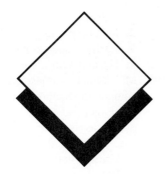

Sample Test Questions: Part Two

Josephine Harrod has been admitted to the hospital with hepatitis A.

94. Which of the following precautions is *inappropriate* to include in Mrs. Harrod's care?
    ☐ 1. Stool and needle isolation.
    ☐ 2. Special care of linens and food.
    ☐ 3. Use of a gown and gloves during client contact.
    ☐ 4. Reverse isolation.

95. Several months following her hospitalization for hepatitis, Mrs. Harrod reentered the hospital with complaints indicative of cholecystitis and cholelithiasis. Because she has an existing jaundice, which of the following tests should be performed before surgery?
    ☐ 1. Lee-White clotting time.
    ☐ 2. Bleeding time.
    ☐ 3. Prothrombin time.
    ☐ 4. Circulation time.

96. For which postoperative complication is Mrs. Harrod at risk after gallbladder surgery?
    ☐ 1. Atelectasis.
    ☐ 2. Pneumonia.
    ☐ 3. Hemorrhage.
    ☐ 4. Thrombophlebitis.

97. Following surgery, Mrs. Harrod has a nasogastric tube in place with an order to irrigate it as needed. What is the rationale for postoperatively irrigating a client's nasogastric tube?
    ☐ 1. To remove secretions from the stomach.
    ☐ 2. To decrease abdominal distension.
    ☐ 3. To minimize bleeding.
    ☐ 4. To maintain patency of the tube.

Barbara Tilson developed insulin-dependent diabetes at age 11. She is now 21; diet and insulin were balanced during this, her first pregnancy. A healthy 10-pound girl is delivered in the birthing room at 38 weeks' gestation.

98. When caring for Baby Girl Tilson in the delivery room, what is the priority nursing action?
    ☐ 1. Ensure proper identification.
    ☐ 2. Establish a warm environment.
    ☐ 3. Maintain a patent airway.
    ☐ 4. Facilitate parental bonding.

99. Considering the maternal history, which of the following goals is critical during the first hours of newborn care?
    ☐ 1. Hydration will be adequate.
    ☐ 2. Temperature will be maintained in the normal range.
    ☐ 3. Nutrition will be maintained.
    ☐ 4. Blood glucose will remain normal.

100. Mother and newborn will be sent home in 48 hours. Both appear to be adapting to breastfeeding. In preparing Mrs. Tilson for discharge the nurse includes infant-care teaching. Which of the following indicates the nurse understands the needs of the newborn with a diabetic mother?
    ☐ 1. "Observe the baby after feedings since asphyxia is a common problem."
    ☐ 2. "Watch the baby for signs of hypoglycemia in the first few weeks."
    ☐ 3. "Visit the pediatrician regularly throughout childhood because diabetes is hereditary."
    ☐ 4. "Supplement breastfeeding with skim milk to control weight."

101. The nurse reviews diabetic teaching with Mrs. Tilson, including manifestations of hypoglycemia. It is suggested that she immediately drink orange juice if she experiences
    ☐ 1. Nausea and vomiting and flushed dry skin.
    ☐ 2. Increased temperature, pulse, and perspiration.
    ☐ 3. Polyuria, thirst, and dry skin.
    ☐ 4. Hunger, dizziness, and clammy skin.

102. At the postpartum check-up, diabetic teaching is reinforced, with emphasis on hygiene and foot care. Which of the following practices indicates that further teaching is needed?
    □ 1. Nails are trimmed straight across.
    □ 2. Shoes fit well and give support.
    □ 3. Feet are bathed and inspected daily.
    □ 4. Hot Epsom salt soaks are used for painful corns.

103. Diet management for the breastfeeding diabetic focuses on an increase in
    □ 1. Saturated fats, vitamin C, and fibers.
    □ 2. Potassium, protein, and iodine.
    □ 3. Fluids, simple sugars, and iron.
    □ 4. Calcium, protein, and complex carbohydrates.

Allen Spinet, 23 years old, was injured in an automobile accident.

104. Of the following sequences, which would be the most appropriate in the minutes immediately following trauma?
    □ 1. Control the hemorrhage; establish an open airway; stabilize the fractured vertebrae; splint the fractured leg.
    □ 2. Establish an open airway; control the hemorrhage; stabilize the fractured vertebrae; splint the fractured leg.
    □ 3. Establish an open airway; stabilize the fractured vertebrae; control the hemorrhage; splint the fractured leg.
    □ 4. Establish an open airway; control the hemorrhage; splint the fractured leg; stabilize the fractured vertebrae.

105. Which is the most important intervention in treating hemorrhage?
    □ 1. Allay apprehension.
    □ 2. Give oral fluids.
    □ 3. Prevent chilling, but do not overheat.
    □ 4. Restore blood volume.

106. Shock causes which of the following?
    □ 1. A Po_2 greater than 80 mm Hg.
    □ 2. A pH less than 7.34.
    □ 3. A Pco_2 less than 45 mm Hg.
    □ 4. A decrease in capillary permeability.

107. If cardiopulmonary resuscitation were performed on Mr. Spinet by two persons, which of the following ratios of cardiac compression to pulmonary ventilation would be used?
    □ 1. 1:1.
    □ 2. 5:1.
    □ 3. 15:2.
    □ 4. 20:2.

108. Effective cardiopulmonary resuscitation would be best indicated by which sign?
    □ 1. Palpable carotid pulse.
    □ 2. Dilated pupils.
    □ 3. Easily blanched nail beds.
    □ 4. Normal skin color.

109. Mr. Spinet is conscious and is bleeding from a compound fracture of the right leg. The adequacy of his general tissue perfusion can be determined by the assessment of all of the following except one. Which of the following is *incorrect?*
    □ 1. Urinary output.
    □ 2. Blood pressure.
    □ 3. Level of consciousness.
    □ 4. Skin color.

110. Mr. Spinet has been admitted to the ICU. He has a mean blood pressure of 90. He is on nitroprusside drip and an epinephrine drip with orders to keep blood pressure at a mean of 80. What is the most appropriate action?
    □ 1. Decrease nitroprusside.
    □ 2. Increase nitroprusside.
    □ 3. Decrease epinephrine.
    □ 4. Increase epinephrine.

111. What is the primary objective of therapy for Mr. Spinet's shock?
    □ 1. Maintain adequate blood pressure.
    □ 2. Improve tissue perfusion.
    □ 3. Maintain adequate vascular tone.
    □ 4. Improve kidney function.

112. Mr. Spinet's injuries include a skull fracture. One of the goals of care for him is to observe for increasing intracranial pressure. Increased intracranial pressure would be indicated by which signs?
    □ 1. Increased pulse rate and increased blood pressure.
    □ 2. Increased pulse rate and decreased blood pressure.
    □ 3. Decreased pulse rate and increased blood pressure.
    □ 4. Decreased pulse rate and decreased blood pressure.

113. In addition, which of the following would best indicate increased intracranial pressure?
    □ 1. BP change from 110/80 mm Hg to 140/50 mm Hg.
    □ 2. Pulse change from 78/min to 92/min.
    □ 3. Respirations change from 16/min to 26/min.
    □ 4. Change in level of consciousness from stupor to drowsy and restless.

Herb Leva, 68 years old, is admitted to a long-term care facility with a diagnosis of idiopathic parkinsonism.

114. Mr. Leva is likely to have which one of the following manifestations?

- ☐ 1. Resting (intentional) tremors.
- ☐ 2. Hyperkinesia.
- ☐ 3. Propulsive gait.
- ☐ 4. Loss of sensation in both feet.

115. Upon admission, the nurse notes that Mr. Leva has been taking the medication levodopa. The nurse knows that one side effect of this drug that should be monitored and included in the care plan is
- ☐ 1. Hypertension.
- ☐ 2. Increased appetite.
- ☐ 3. Euphoria.
- ☐ 4. Orthostatic hypotension.

116. The physician orders a screening test to assess Mr. Leva for glaucoma. That test is a(n)
- ☐ 1. Myringotomy.
- ☐ 2. Fundoscopy.
- ☐ 3. Tonometry.
- ☐ 4. Iridectomy.

John David Jankowski, 14 months old, is scheduled for palliative surgery for tetralogy of Fallot. His mother is staying in his hospital room until he is taken to surgery.

117. When reviewing John David's preoperative lab reports, the nurse should be most concerned about which value?
- ☐ 1. White-blood-cell count $14,000/mm^3$.
- ☐ 2. Hematocrit 52%.
- ☐ 3. Serum pH 7.33.
- ☐ 4. Platelets $220,000/mm^3$.

118. The surgeon plans to anastomose John David's left subclavian artery to his pulmonary artery. Mrs. Jankowski asks the nurse to explain the reason for this temporary palliative surgery. The nurse should reply
- ☐ 1. "The surgery will increase the amount of blood that flows through John David's lungs so that his body gets more oxygen."
- ☐ 2. "This procedure will change the direction of blood flow in his heart so his skin color will be less blue."
- ☐ 3. "The pressure on the heart chamber that pumps blood to the body will be relieved."
- ☐ 4. "The surgery will allow John David to grow and develop like a normal child."

119. Which activity would be most appropriate for John David preoperatively?
- ☐ 1. A play stethoscope.
- ☐ 2. A push-pull toy.
- ☐ 3. A shape sorter.
- ☐ 4. A toy trumpet.

120. John David is playing beside his mother's chair when he starts to investigate the contents of her purse. When Mrs. Jankowski takes her purse away

from him, John David begins to cry, then screams, stomps his feet, and starts to gasp. Which action should the nurse take?
- ☐ 1. Allow Mrs. Jankowski to handle the situation.
- ☐ 2. Distract John David with one of his favorite toys.
- ☐ 3. Advise Mrs. Janowski to "be as easy as possible on him" until after surgery.
- ☐ 4. Hold John David in a squatting position.

Janice Carter is in the thirty-seventh week of pregnancy. Her husband calls the physician to report that his wife awakened in the middle of the night, lying in a pool of bright-red blood.

121. The onset of third-trimester painless bleeding is usually a sign of potential
- ☐ 1. Abruptio placentae.
- ☐ 2. Placenta previa.
- ☐ 3. Incomplete abortion.
- ☐ 4. Ectopic pregnancy.

122. Mrs. Carter is admitted to the labor room. Which of the following is contraindicated during the admission assessment?
- ☐ 1. Vaginal examination.
- ☐ 2. X-ray pelvimetry.
- ☐ 3. Type and crossmatch.
- ☐ 4. Perineal prep.

123. Mrs. Carter is worried about her condition, and about her 2-year-old twins at home. Mr. Carter asks the nurse if he should remain with Mrs. Carter or return home to check on the children and their teenaged sitter. Which response indicates an understanding of their feelings at this time?
- ☐ 1. "You would feel more secure if you checked on your family."
- ☐ 2. "Your wife is well cared for here. You may go home for a while."
- ☐ 3. "You really belong here now. Call home and check on the children."
- ☐ 4. "Why not ask your wife what she feels would be best for her?"

124. An ultrasound confirms that the placenta totally covers the cervical os. Mrs. Carter is prepared for a cesarean birth. In addition to providing emotional support, preparation for the client includes all *except*
- ☐ 1. Type and crossmatch.
- ☐ 2. Insertion of Foley catheter.
- ☐ 3. Skin prep and shave.
- ☐ 4. Tap-water enema.

125. Mrs. Carter will receive a spinal anesthetic. As she signs the consent forms, she asks about the possibility of postanesthesia headaches. An appropriate response is

1. "Headaches rarely occur and are usually mild."
2. "Medication is available to counteract headaches and is given as needed."
3. "If there is an allergy to the agent used, headaches may occur."
4. "This problem may be prevented by keeping the bed flat."

126. A client having a spinal anesthetic is at most risk for which of the following complications?
1. Respiratory paralysis.
2. Permanent motor dysfunction.
3. Paralytic ileus.
4. Hypotension.

127. An IV of 1000 ml of 5% dextrose in saline with 10 units of oxytocin (Pitocin) is ordered. The solution is to infuse in 6 hours. Drop factor is 10. At what rate should the IV infuse?
1. 2.7 drops per minute.
2. 3.7 drops per minute.
3. 27 drops per minute.
4. 37 drops per minute.

128. In evaluating Mrs. Carter's response to oxytocin (Pitocin), which observation indicates a potential problem?
1. Fundus is firmly contracted.
2. Urinary output is 20/ml/hr.
3. IV is infusing well.
4. Slight cramps are reported.

Loretta Neter, a 22-year-old woman, is admitted to an inpatient psychiatric unit. Paralysis developed in her right arm, for which no physical cause can be found. The admitting diagnosis is conversion reaction.

129. Miss Neter is using which of the following defense mechanisms?
1. Reaction formation and projection.
2. Suppression and compensation.
3. Isolation and undoing.
4. Repression and displacement.

130. Miss Neter tends to focus on her paralysis in her interactions with others by asking for help, even for things she can do herself, and by talking about how she feels about having a paralyzed arm. Which of the following interventions would be most appropriate when dealing with this dynamic?
1. Allow the client to discuss her symptoms to help relieve her anxiety.
2. Encourage the client to get involved in activities on the unit and to discuss other topics.
3. Insist that the client not discuss her paralysis or receive help from others to force her to learn new ways of handling anxiety.
4. Insist she discuss her physical symptoms with the nurses and the physician only, not with friends and family.

131. One day Miss Neter says to the nurse, "I suppose you think I'm faking my paralysis." Which of the following would be the best nursing response?
1. "Yes, I think you could move your arm if you chose to do so."
2. "I think you know that there is no physical cause for your paralysis."
3. "I believe you are currently unable to move your arm, regardless of the cause."
4. "I believe your paralysis is physical and that you may have been misdiagnosed."

132. Miss Neter's comment is most likely a result of which of the following explanations?
1. She is having auditory hallucinations.
2. She is having paranoid delusions.
3. She is seeking reassurance.
4. She is lonely.

Three-month-old Pedro Cruz is seen in the pediatric clinic for well baby care. During this visit, the physician diagnoses congenital hypothyroidism.

133. When explaining the diagnosis to Mr. and Mrs. Cruz, the nurse should describe which findings as characteristic of congenital hypothyroidism?
1. Hyperirritability and prominent nasal bridge.
2. Tachycardia and small oral cavity.
3. Constant hunger and runny stools.
4. Inactivity and mottled skin.

134. Pedro is placed on levothyroxine (Synthroid), 25 μg per day. The nurse should provide which instruction to Pedro's parents?
1. The medication should be given until symptoms subside, then gradually discontinued.
2. Pedro can be expected to lose some weight as he adjusts to the medication.
3. The medication should be administered as a single morning dose.
4. Constipation may develop, indicating toxicity.

Janie Olivera, age 5, has just been diagnosed with acute lymphoblastic leukemia. She has been admitted to the pediatric unit for induction chemotherapy.

135. In assessing the Oliveras' response to Janie's diagnosis, the nurse should initially expect which parental reaction?
1. Expressing feelings of guilt and remorse.
2. Hoping that the diagnosis is wrong.
3. Making frequent demands on the staff.
4. Asking about unconventional types of treatment.

136. Which of the following behaviors would best indicate to the nurse that Janie is adequately prepared for bone marrow aspiration? Janie

□ 1. Explains that her healthy blood cells are sick and need special medicine.

□ 2. Tells her mom that she like her nurse and wants to play after the test.

□ 3. Willingly allows the nurse to take her to the treatment room.

□ 4. Tells her dolls that she has to have a needle in her hip to test her blood.

137. A chemotherapeutic regimen of vincristine and prednisone has been initiated for Janie. The nurse should report which of the following reactions to the physician?

□ 1. Petechiae appear on Janie's chest and face.

□ 2. Janie vomits two times after breakfast.

□ 3. Janie complains of tingling in her fingers and toes.

□ 4. Janie develops small ulcerations on her lips.

138. Janie is receiving a unit of packed cells intravenously. Which intravenous solution would be appropriate to use to flush the tubing before initiating the transfusion?

□ 1. Lactated Ringer's solution.

□ 2. 5% dextrose in water.

□ 3. 5% dextrose in one-fourth normal saline.

□ 4. Hyperalimentation solution.

139. Janie is also receiving radiation therapy. Mr. Olivera says he has heard that there are serious side effects, and asks the nurse what these are. Which one of the following is *not* a side effect of radiation therapy?

□ 1. Delays in physical development.

□ 2. Susceptibility to bone fractures.

□ 3. Early onset of secondary sex characteristics.

□ 4. Possible damage to chromosomes.

140. Janie is crying softly and says she is "hurting." Janie's pulse rate is elevated. Which of the following protocols would be most effective when administering Janie's pain medication?

□ 1. Give when she becomes restless and is unable to sleep.

□ 2. Give on a preventive schedule after assessing her pain responses.

□ 3. Give whether Janie or her parents request it be given.

□ 4. Give every 3 to 4 hours around the clock.

141. Mrs. Olivera tells the nurse that Janie is supposed to receive a DPT and TOPV booster before she starts kindergarten this year, and asks when she should take Janie to the health department to receive these. Which response by the nurse is accurate?

□ 1. "We can give it before she leaves the hospital."

□ 2. "Wait until a week or so before she starts school."

□ 3. "When her white-blood-cell count returns to a normal level."

□ 4. "Because of her diagnosis, Janie won't ever be able to be immunized again."

Olivia Carnelli, age 76, is scheduled for a right modified mastectomy tomorrow.

142. Preoperatively, the nurse would discuss postoperative

□ 1. Skin grafting.

□ 2. *Peau d'orange* skin changes.

□ 3. Treatment of intraductal edema.

□ 4. Use of a HemoVac.

143. During a discussion with Mrs. Carnelli about the surgical skin prep she will receive, the nurse notices that Mrs. Carnelli seems close to tears. What would be the nurse's most appropriate response?

□ 1. "I'll stop this discussion for a while."

□ 2. "You must pay close attention to what I'm saying."

□ 3. "You seem close to tears, can you tell me what you're feeling?"

□ 4. Continue on with the explanation.

144. When Mrs. Carnelli returns from surgery, she is monitored for signs and symptoms of hemorrhage. In addition to assessing her vital signs, the nurse should

□ 1. Ask her if her back feels wet.

□ 2. Assess her level of consciousness.

□ 3. Observe the amount of drainage in the HemoVac.

□ 4. Visually check under her back for drainage.

145. Which of the following plans would be most likely to meet Mrs. Carnelli's learning needs for discharge planning?

□ 1. Provide written materials for her to read during the day.

□ 2. Offer brief, frequent one-to-one sessions.

□ 3. Teach her during a single session, taking a sufficient amount of time to provide complete factual material.

□ 4. Have her join a group session with peers; use charts, several speakers, and handouts.

146. The nurse discusses ways of minimizing lymphedema with Mrs. Carnelli. Which of the following statements indicates a need for more teaching?

□ 1. "I'll avoid any constriction around my arm."

□ 2. "I'll make sure I drink plenty of fluids."

□ 3. "I'll sleep with my arm elevated on pillows."

□ 4. "I'll keep my right arm elevated as much as possible during the day."

147. Before Mrs. Carnelli is discharged, the nurse would expect her to
    ☐ 1. Be able to explain incision care.
    ☐ 2. Have adapted to her altered body image.
    ☐ 3. Have completed the grieving process.
    ☐ 4. Have received an order for a Jobst pressure machine.

Mrs. Keller brings her son, Jermaine, who just turned 5, to the pediatrician's office for a complete health appraisal before he enters kindergarten next month.

148. The nurse should focus part of the assessment on Jermaine's achievement of psychosocial tasks. At this age, Jermaine should be trying to accomplish a sense of
    ☐ 1. Autonomy.
    ☐ 2. Identity.
    ☐ 3. Mastery.
    ☐ 4. Initiative.

149. The nurse evaluates Jermaine's readiness to attend kindergarten. Jermaine should be able to
    ☐ 1. Tie his shoelaces.
    ☐ 2. Count to 20.
    ☐ 3. Tell time on a clock.
    ☐ 4. Print his name.

150. Part of the assessment of Jermaine includes vision screening using the Snellen E chart to test for visual acuity. Jermaine's results are 20/30 vision in both eyes. Which action should the nurse take?
    ☐ 1. Rescreen Jermaine immediately.
    ☐ 2. Rescreen Jermaine in 2 weeks.
    ☐ 3. Refer Jermaine to an opthalmologist for a complete eye exam.
    ☐ 4. Explain to Jermaine and his mother that his vision is normal.

151. While conducting vision screening, the nurse should also screen Jermaine for
    ☐ 1. Strabismus.
    ☐ 2. Diplopia.
    ☐ 3. Papilledema.
    ☐ 4. Pupil reactivity.

152. Jermaine's height is at the 50th percentile. His weight is at the 90th percentile. A nutritional history reveals that Jermaine's diet is very high in carbohydrates and fats. The nurse helps Jermaine's mother develop a plan to ensure that Jermaine gets the nutrients he needs without overeating. This diet should provide Jermaine with approximately how many calories per day?
    ☐ 1. 1200.
    ☐ 2. 1700.
    ☐ 3. 2400.
    ☐ 4. 2800.

153. Treatment of Jermaine's overweight would best include
    ☐ 1. A planned program of activity and exercise.
    ☐ 2. A daily appetite suppressant.
    ☐ 3. Large doses of supplemental vitamins.
    ☐ 4. Withholding all sweets.

154. Jermaine returns for a follow-up visit in 6 months. Which of the following best indicates Jermaine is progressing satisfactorily with his nutritional plan?
    ☐ 1. Jermaine has lost 5 pounds.
    ☐ 2. Jermaine's daily intake has been 300 calories less than recommended.
    ☐ 3. Jermaine's weight is now in the 75th percentile.
    ☐ 4. Jermaine has stopped craving junk food.

Gloria Rock, age 31, gravida 5, para 4, has just delivered her fifth son following a 2-hour labor. The baby weighs 9 pounds 10 ounces.

155. Based on the data given, a potential problem for Mrs. Rock is
    ☐ 1. Thrombophlebitis.
    ☐ 2. Postpartal hemorrhage.
    ☐ 3. Puerperal infection.
    ☐ 4. Urinary retention.

156. One day postpartum, Mrs. Rock complains that excessive perspiring kept her awake at night. She is worried that there is a problem. An appropriate response is
    ☐ 1. "IV fluids administered during labor sometimes cause sweating."
    ☐ 2. "Maybe you drank too much fluid during the day."
    ☐ 3. "Fluids that were retained during pregnancy are normally lost."
    ☐ 4. "You may be experiencing signs of infection."

157. Mrs. Rock comments, "I hope this is our last baby because we can't afford any more." The nurse's best response would be
    ☐ 1. "Discuss this with your physician at your postpartum check-up."
    ☐ 2. "You need not worry until you quit breastfeeding."
    ☐ 3. "Let's talk about birth-control methods."
    ☐ 4. "Perhaps the social worker can help you."

158. Mrs. Rock goes home from the hospital and returns to the clinic for measurement of a diaphragm. The nurse explains to Mrs. Rock that this type of contraception is effective only if the device is used properly. The teaching has been effective if Mrs. Rock reports
    ☐ 1. Using K-Y jelly as a lubricant.
    ☐ 2. Removing the device 6 hours after coitus.
    ☐ 3. Storing it in a jar of alcohol.
    ☐ 4. Wearing the diaphragm for 1-2 days.

Otis O'Shea, age 28, is admitted to the hospital after becoming embroiled in an argument with the police during a routine traffic check. His admitting diagnosis is paranoid schizophrenia.

159. As the nurse is orienting Mr. O'Shea to the unit, he states, "They can't arrest me; I'm J. Paul Getty, and I don't have to fool with inconsequential people like the police." Which of the following would be the best initial response?

- ☐ 1. "Can't arrest you?"
- ☐ 2. "What made you so angry, Mr. O'Shea?"
- ☐ 3. "This is your room, Mr. O'Shea."
- ☐ 4. "Your record indicates your name is Otis O'Shea."

160. The defense mechanism being used by Mr. O'Shea is which of the following?

- ☐ 1. Denial.
- ☐ 2. Fantasy.
- ☐ 3. Introjection.
- ☐ 4. Projection.

161. The physician leaves orders for Mr. O'Shea to have halperidol (Haldol), 75 mg qid. Which of the following would be the most appropriate action for the nurse to take?

- ☐ 1. Call the physician; the dose is too low.
- ☐ 2. Call the physician; the dose is too high.
- ☐ 3. Call the physician; haloperidol is not effective for paranoid schizophrenia.
- ☐ 4. Administer the drug; the medication and dose are appropriate.

162. Shortly after admission, Mr. O'Shea is seen ordering the other clients around. What action should the nurse best take?

- ☐ 1. Confront him with his behavior on a one-to-one basis.
- ☐ 2. Encourage other clients to confront him in a group meeting.
- ☐ 3. Seclude him.
- ☐ 4. Spend more time with him on a one-to-one basis.

163. Shortly after breakfast one morning the nurse hears Mr. O'Shea talking loudly and notes that he is beginning to pace in the hall. What would be the best initial action for the nurse to take?

- ☐ 1. Tell him, "Let's have a cup of coffee and talk about what's making you angry."
- ☐ 2. Offer him a PRN medication for agitation.
- ☐ 3. Suggest that he use the punching bag.
- ☐ 4. Isolate him before he hurts someone on the unit.

164. Mr. O'Shea has not had a bowel movement for 6 days. This is most likely related to which of the following?

- ☐ 1. His decreased activity level.
- ☐ 2. Lack of fiber in his diet.
- ☐ 3. A side effect of haloperidol (Haldol).
- ☐ 4. Constriction of the bowel as a result of tension.

165. Mr. O'Shea has a great deal of difficulty making decisions. This is most likely the result of which of the following?

- ☐ 1. Autism.
- ☐ 2. Mixed feelings.
- ☐ 3. Ambivalence.
- ☐ 4. Apathy.

166. When Mr. O'Shea's behavior becomes more appropriate, the nurse decides to include him in the preparation for the next unit party. Which of the following would be the most appropriate activity for him?

- ☐ 1. Assign him to the entertainment committee.
- ☐ 2. Ask him to take charge of making the coffee and seeing that the pot is kept filled.
- ☐ 3. Put him in charge of the clean-up committee.
- ☐ 4. Ask him to arrange for the pizza to be delivered.

167. Mr. O'Shea has an erratic employment history and is at present unemployed. He is planning to secure a job before discharge. What nursing action would be the most useful?

- ☐ 1. Help him read the want ads.
- ☐ 2. Role-play the job interview with him.
- ☐ 3. Refer him for vocational testing.
- ☐ 4. Encourage him to write a resume.

Thirteen-year-old Tim McMichael is brought to the emergency department by his camp leader. During a summer overnight youth camp-out, Tim's kerosene lamp overturned and ignited his sleeping bag. Tim's shirt sleeve caught fire when he tried to put out the fire. He has second-degree burns of his right hand and forearm.

168. Immediate care of the burn wound should include

- ☐ 1. Immersing Tim's hand and forearm in cool water.
- ☐ 2. Applying ice packs to the injury.
- ☐ 3. Pulling adherent charred clothing from the burn wounds.
- ☐ 4. Covering the burn with cortisone cream.

169. Tim's immunization history indicates that he has received all childhood immunizations according to the recommended schedule. At this time, tetanus prophylaxis for Tim should include

- ☐ 1. Tetanus toxoid.
- ☐ 2. Tetanus immune globulin.
- ☐ 3. Tetanus toxoid and tetanus immune globulin.
- ☐ 4. No additional protection.

170. After cleansing and debridement of the wound, the physician decides to apply silver sulfadiazine (Silvadene) and cover the wound with a bulky gauze dressing. The primary advantage of the closed method used to treat Tim's burn is that it

- ☐ 1. Protects the wound from further injury.
- ☐ 2. Minimizes fluid loss from the burn surface.

☐ 3. Alleviates pain caused by exposure of the wound to air.

☐ 4. Prevents contractures of the hand and wrist.

171. Tim's parents come to take him home. The nurse is teaching them how to change his dressing. Which discharge instruction should the nurse include in the teaching plan?

☐ 1. The silver sulfadiazine cream will be painful when first applied to the burn.

☐ 2. Tim should return to the laboratory each day to have his blood pH monitored.

☐ 3. Old cream should be removed by soaking the wound in warm, soapy water.

☐ 4. The silver sulfadiazine cream may cause a change in color of adjacent healthy skin.

172. Which of the following foods should the nurse suggest Tim eat most often during the next several weeks?

☐ 1. Meats, citrus fruits, and milk.

☐ 2. Vegetables, cheese, and yogurt.

☐ 3. Breads, cereals, and pastas.

☐ 4. Milkshakes, salads, and soups.

173. Tim returns for follow-up. His wound is healing well. Which behavior indicates that Tim may be having difficulty coping with his burn injury?

☐ 1. Asks when he can begin playing football again.

☐ 2. Says he is not interested in girls.

☐ 3. Refuses to wear short-sleeve shirts.

☐ 4. Is quiet and nontalkative during the office visit.

174. The nurse observes that Tim has mild acne, and that the lesions are especially noticeable on his forehead and chin. When asked if he would like some suggestions to help clear up the lesions, Tim nods. The nurse should suggest that Tim

☐ 1. Use a commercial sunlamp for 5 minutes daily.

☐ 2. Wear an absorbent headband during exercise or hot weather.

☐ 3. Purchase an over-the-counter product that contains benzoyl peroxide.

☐ 4. Avoid chocolate, fried foods, and iodized salt.

Jeff Tate, 34 years old, complains to the health clinic of urinary burning, frequency, and urgency; hematuria; fever and chills. Lab tests on a clean-catch urine sample reveal RBCs and WBCs (too many to count), numerous hyaline casts, and bacteria greater than 100,000/ml. A physical exam reveals extreme costovertebral angle (CVA) tenderness. Mr. Tate is diagnosed as having pyelonephritis, and he is admitted to the hospital.

175. The most important blood test of kidney filtration ordered for Mr. Tate would be

☐ 1. Glucose.

☐ 2. Electrolytes.

☐ 3. Creatinine.

☐ 4. BUN.

176. An intravenous pyelogram (IVP) is ordered for Mr. Tate. Which of the following would be the most important for the nurse to do the night before the IVP?

☐ 1. Give a cathartic and enemas to cleanse the bowel.

☐ 2. Instruct the client to be NPO after midnight.

☐ 3. Identify by history any client allergies to medicine or foods.

☐ 4. Teach the client that x-rays will be taken at multiple intervals.

177. Mr. Tate is placed on a regimen of a sulfonamide antibiotic (Bactrim). As a nurse, you know which of the following to be true concerning this drug?

☐ 1. It is metabolized by the liver and excreted through the bile.

☐ 2. It produces a false-negative glucose on urine tests.

☐ 3. It is more soluble in acidic urine.

☐ 4. It can crystalize in the urine if fluid intake is insufficient.

178. Upon Mr. Tate's discharge, the physician wants him to maintain his urine in a more acidic state by eating an acid-ash diet. Which of the following foods would you teach the client can be unrestricted in his diet?

☐ 1. Milk.

☐ 2. Carrots.

☐ 3. Grape Nuts cereal.

☐ 4. Dried apricots.

179. Which of the following interventions would be a priority in discharge teaching for Mr. Tate?

☐ 1. Drink at least 3-4 L of fluid/day.

☐ 2. Take sitz baths 3-4 times/day for urethral burning.

☐ 3. Void immediately after sexual intercourse.

☐ 4. Avoid exposure to persons with upper respiratory infections.

180. After 3 weeks, Mr. Tate returns to the ER with severe, sharp, deep lumbar pain radiating to his right side. A repeat IVP reveals a kidney stone in the right ureter at the bifurcation of the iliac vessel. Upon his admission to the hospital, which of the following goals would take initial priority in this client's nursing care?

☐ 1. Client will decrease risk of future kidney stones.

☐ 2. Client will be prepared for possible urinary tract surgery.

☐ 3. Client will be free from discomfort of kidney stones.

☐ 4. Client will have fluid intake of 3-5 L/day.

Carol Clay, gravida 1, para 0, is being admitted to the hospital in labor. She has had regular prenatal care, attended prenatal classes with her husband, and had an uncomplicated pregnancy.

181. Which of the following observations would be the most reliable guide to assess Mrs. Clay's progress in labor?

☐ 1. Contractions that are getting more intense.

☐ 2. Breathing that is becoming more rapid.

☐ 3. Progressive dilatation of the cervix.

☐ 4. Increased vaginal discharge (or rupture of membranes).

182. Mrs. Clay ambulates with her husband. Which of the following would warrant bed rest or further evaluation of her condition?

☐ 1. Contractions that are intense and last 60 seconds.

☐ 2. Progressive sacral discomfort during contractions.

☐ 3. Rapid, shallow respirations during contractions.

☐ 4. A desire to defecate at the peak of contractions.

183. Mrs. Clay's blood pressure is monitored every 2 hours. Blood pressure is recorded in between contractions because

☐ 1. Assessing during contractions gives erratic readings.

☐ 2. Monitoring blood pressure during contractions is inaccurate.

☐ 3. Taking blood pressure during contractions distracts the client from breathing patterns.

☐ 4. Maintaining the arm in position during contractions is difficult for the client.

184. In early labor, the fetal heart tones (FHT) are auscultated at regular intervals. The most appropriate time to listen to FHT is

☐ 1. During contractions.

☐ 2. Between contractions.

☐ 3. Soon after contractions.

☐ 4. During and soon after contractions.

Virginia Ryan calls the adolescent mental health clinic worried about her 16-year-old daughter, Kathleen. She tells the nurse that Kathleen is obsessed about dieting and exercising even though she seems healthy and has not lost any weight.

185. Mrs. Ryan says her daughter eats very well but spends more and more time in the bathroom after meals. Kathleen denies anything is troubling her. The nurse's initial response to Mrs. Ryan would be

☐ 1. "She's a typical teenager, gobbling her food and then shutting herself off in a room."

☐ 2. "It sounds as if Kathleen is anorexic."

☐ 3. "Are you worried Kathleen may have an eating disorder?"

☐ 4. "Let's figure out if she's depressed."

186. Kathleen's symptoms suggest she is

☐ 1. Depressed.

☐ 2. Anorexic.

☐ 3. A chemical abuser.

☐ 4. Bulimic.

187. Mrs. Ryan brings Kathleen into the emergency room the next day because Kathleen has admitted to her she has been abusing laxatives and diet pills. The first goal of treatment will be to

☐ 1. Help Kathleen develop insight into her behavior.

☐ 2. Promote Kathleen's acceptance of herself and her body.

☐ 3. Promote adequate nutritional intake and retention of food.

☐ 4. Help her develop realistic expectations for dieting and exercising.

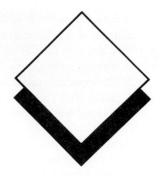

Correct Answers and Rationales: Part Two

94. no. 4. The hepatitis A virus is spread by way of contact with oral and respiratory secretions, feces, and serum from an infected person. A-NM, IM, PS

95. no. 3. Jaundice is a sign of obstructive disease (i.e., obstruction of the bile duct, possibly from a gallstone). Prothrombin, a protein produced by the liver, is used in the clotting of blood. Its production depends on adequate intake and absorption of vitamin K. Obstruction of the bile flow may impair absorption. Prolonged prothrombin time may lead to hemorrhage. The Lee-White clotting time is a relatively insensitive test for coagulation; bleeding time only measures the initial phase of hemostasis. A-NM, IM, PS

96. no. 1. Because of the high incision and upper abdominal pain, the postoperative client resists coughing and deep-breathing and is likely to develop atelectasis. A-S, AN, PS

97. no. 4. Irrigation maintains the patency of the tube, which will also accomplish options no. 1 and no. 2. A-NM, AN, PS

98. no. 3. Although all are appropriate interventions, the priority is to establish and maintain a patent airway. CBF-I, IM, E

99. no. 4. The plan is based on an understanding that in the first hours after delivery, excess insulin may lead to hypoglycemia. Brain damage will result if low blood glucose is not corrected. Glucose level is assessed frequently. If low, early feeding is essential. Hydration is not critical in the first hours of life. All newborns need an environment that conserves body temperature. CBF-N, PL, E

100. no. 3. The teaching for this mother must include emphasis on regular pediatric care, considering the possibility of inherited tendency to diabetes. Asphyxia is a potential problem for a diabetic's newborn in the immediate delivery process. Skim milk is never suggested for a newborn. Risk of hypoglycemia passes after initial adaptation to feedings. CBF-N, EV, H

101. no. 4. The release of epinephrine in response to an abnormal drop in blood glucose level results in dizziness and trembling. Hunger is characteristic of hypoglycemia. The other symptoms are manifestations of acidosis or infection. A-NM, IM, E

102. no. 4. Evaluation of the care of the feet indicates that the client needs further teaching if hot Epsom salt soaks are being used. This solution is drying and could burn the feet. Daily washing of the feet prevents skin breakdown. A-NM, EV, E

103. no. 4. Protein and calcium are needed to meet lactation needs. Complex carbohydrates provide fiber and enhance blood-glucose control. Saturated fats should be reduced for diabetics. Increased potassium is not recommended, as it may be a factor in hypoglycemia. Simple sugars may lead to blood-glucose imbalance. CBF-P, IM, PS

104. no. 2. An open airway is the first priority following trauma. Control of hemorrhage is second. Stabilization of the fractured vertebrae takes precedence over splinting of the leg. A-O, PL, PS

105. no. 4. Primary intervention with hemorrhage includes measures to stop bleeding and restore blood volume in order to prevent irreversible shock. The other interventions are appropriate but of secondary importance. A-O, IM, PS

106. no. 2. Shock causes metabolic acidosis (a pH less than 7.34). Tissue metabolism continues so that large amounts of acid are emptied and accumulate in the stagnant blood. With progressive tissue hypoxia, anaerobic metabolism produces nonvolatile lactic acid, which further increases the acidosis. Shock also produces hypoxia (Po_2 less then 80 mm Hg); hypercapnia (Pco_2 greater than 45 mm Hg); and an increase in capillary permeability. A-O, AN, PS

107. no. 2. According to the American Heart Association, the two-rescuer CPR compression-ventilation ratio is 5:1 with a 1- to 1½-second pause for ventilation. The recommended compression-ventilation ratio for one-rescuer CPR is 15:2. The compression rate for either one- or two-rescuer CPR is 80-100 per minute. Compression-ventilation ratios of 1:1 or 20:2 are not recommended. A-O, IM, PS

108. no. 1. A palpable carotid pulse would be the best indicator of adequate sternal compression. It is a better indicator of effective CPR than skin color. Easily blanched nail beds and dilated pupils indicate inadequate perfusion. Some emergency drugs alter pupil reaction (e.g., atropine). A-O, EV, PS

109. no. 4. Alterations in skin color may result from changes in vasomotor tone yet give little indication of perfusion of the vital organs. Options no. 1, no. 2, and no. 3 are reliable indicators of vital tissue perfusion. A-O, AS, PS

110. no. 3. Doing either no. 2 or no. 3 would bring the BP down; but since vasoconstriction causes other problems, the nurse would want to decrease the epinephrine rather than increase the nitroprusside. Options no. 1 and no. 4 would cause BP to rise further. A-O, IM, PS

111. no. 2. All are goals of treatment, but tissue perfusion must be improved to prevent irreversible damage and death of tissues. If tissue perfusion improves, the other goals will be accompanied secondarily. A-O, PL, PS

112. no. 3. Cerebral pressure rises as a result of tissue injury, edema, and hypoxia. BP increases in response to the hypoxic stimulation of the vasomotor center. Pulse rate slows as blood pressure increases. A-SP, AS, PS

113. no. 1. A widening pulse pressure is characteristic of increasing intracranial pressure; also, pulse rate decreases, respirations decrease, and level of consciousness decreases. A-SP, AS, PS

114. no. 3. With bradykinesia (not hyperkinesia) and muscle rigidity, the older adult is unable to lift his feet; hence, he shuffles and propels forward with such momentum that he often is unable to control body movement. Parkinsonian clients manifest nonintentional or resting tremors. Option no. 4 is not a manifestation of parkinsonism. A-SP, AS, PS

115. no. 4. This is a common side effect of this drug. Rather than euphoria, the client often becomes depressed as a second common side effect. Option no. 2 is incorrect. Most parkinsonian clients have a decreased appetite. A-SP, AN, PC

116. no. 3. A myringotomy is an opening into the tympanic membrane. Fundoscopy is a procedure to observe the tissue in the cavity of a body of any organ (e.g., the eye or uterus). An iridectomy is the removal of the iris of the eye. A-SP, AS, H

117. no. 2. The child with cyanotic heart disease is prone to polycythemia (an increase in circulating red blood cells), which leads to a rise in hematocrit. Normal hematocrit values for a child are 32%-47%.

All other values are within normal limits. C-O, AN, PS

118. no. 1. The purpose of palliative surgery for the child with tetralogy of Fallot is to increase the pulmonary blood flow, which increases the amount of oxygenated blood to the tissues. The procedure will not affect the intracardiac shunting of blood from right to left or provide enough oxygen to his tissues to allow for normal development. In tetralogy of Fallot, the pressure is increased in the right ventricle (not the left) because of the pulmonary stenosis. C-O, IM, PS

119. no. 3. The shape sorter is age appropriate (toddlers are interested in how things fit together, such as how different shapes fit into their respective slots) and is a quiet activity. A priority goal preoperatively is to minimize the work load of the heart. The push-pull toy and the toy trumpet will increase the oxygen demands and, therefore, the cardiac work load. A play stethoscope is too advanced for John David (it is an appropriate toy for a pre-schooler). C-H, IM, H

120. no. 4. Gasping indicates that John David is at risk for having an anoxic spell and should be placed in a knee-chest (squatting) position to increase the blood flow to his heart, lungs, and brain. Although options no. 1 and no. 2 are appropriate responses for handling a toddler's temper tantrums, in this instance, John David's physiological needs take priority over his developmental needs. Encouraging Mrs. Jankowski to set few limits is not in John David's best interests developmentally. C-O, IM, E

121. no. 2. Low implantation of the placenta causes painless bleeding in the third trimester. Abruptio placentae often is accompanied by pain or tenderness. Ectopic pregnancy and abortion occur earlier in pregnancy. CBF-A, AN, PS

122. no. 1. A vaginal examination is contraindicated for this client, because it might stimulate contractions and increase the risk of placental delivery. The other options if ordered may be safely done. CBF-A, IM, E

123. no. 4. Since the mother is worried, her feelings should be considered. The nurse appropriately suggests shared decision making. CBF-I, IM, PC

124. no. 4. All of these are part of preparation for cesarean birth except an enema, which could stimulate contractions and cause bleeding. CBF-I, IM, E

125. no. 4. The bed will be kept flat for 8-12 hours after use of spinal anesthetic to minimize the possibility of headaches. Although it is true that medication is available, the chief focus of teaching is on position. CBF-P, IM, H

126. no. 4. Spinal anesthesia results in vasodilation and pooling of blood with a resultant decrease in effective circulatory volume. Respiratory paralysis could occur if the anesthetic is given improperly, but it is not a potential complication. The anesthetic agent is injected below the level of the spinal cord, so spinal cord injury is not a complication. Paralytic ileus is a complication of surgery but is due to factors other than spinal anesthesia. A-S, AN, PS

127. no. 3. With a drop factor of 10 drops/ml, the desired rate is 27 drops/min. CBF-I, IM, PS

128. no. 2. Oxytocin (Pitocin) has an antidiuretic effect in addition to stimulating contractions and causing cramps. Urinary output must be carefully monitored. Less than 30-50 ml/hr is cause for concern and should be reported. The medication may be discontinued. CBF-I, EV, PS

129. no. 4. She is repressing conflicting feelings that she unconsciously believes she cannot handle and displaces the resulting anxiety into the physical symptom of paralysis. In this way, her focus is on the paralysis. As a result, she is relieved of the need to deal with the original conflict. Suppression is a conscious mechanism; and if she were using suppression, she would consciously know that her paralysis was an emotional response, and it would be within her conscious control. Reaction formation expresses feelings opposite those being experienced. Projection ascribes to another person or object the unacceptable thoughts and feelings. Compensation is substituting an unattainable goal for another to make up for a real or imagined inadequacy. Isolation is blocking the feelings associated with an unpleasant, threatening situation or thought. Undoing cancels the effect of another response just made. P-A, AN, PC

130. no. 2. It is important to encourage her to give up the symptom by not focusing on it. However, since the symptom is a method she uses to relieve anxiety, staff members need to help her find new ways of relieving anxiety before she will give up her present method of relieving it. However, one cannot force a person to learn new ways of handling anxiety that comes out of the unconscious. Since her symptoms unconsciously control the anxiety, discussion alone would not relieve the symptoms. It is inappropriate to focus on physical symptoms since they are of unconscious origin. P-A, IM, PC

131. no. 3. This is the response that demonstrates the nurse's understanding of the pain the symptom is causing the client and its reality to her. Options no. 1 and no. 2 contradict the client's behavior. Option no. 4 would promote doubt in competence of staff and is untrue. P-A, IM, PC

132. no. 3. The client is seeking reassurance about the origin of her symptoms. This client is not psychotic, and loneliness, though painful, does not cause the dramatic, unconscious behavior and symptoms described. P-A, AN, PC

133. no. 4. The infant with congenital hypothyroidism is inactive (often described as a good, quiet baby) and undemanding. The disease is also characterized by mottling of the skin, constipation, a large protruding tongue, and a flattened nasal bridge. C-NM, AS, PS

134. no. 3. Thyroid replacement should be given as a single morning dose throughout the child's lifetime. Diarrhea, tachycardia, and weight loss indicate toxicity. C-NM, IM, E

135. no. 2. The initial response to diagnosis of a life-threatening illness is shock, disbelief, and hope that "it's not real." Frequent demands and feelings of guilt and remorse characterize later stages of the grieving process. Asking about unconventional treatments should alert the nurse to be concerned that the parents may not understand the meaning of the diagnosis. P-L, AN, PC

136. no. 4. Option no. 1 indicates some understanding of the disease, but not the bone marrow procedure. No. 2 and no. 3 reflect adaptation to hospitalization. No. 4 indicates that Janie comprehends what will happen to her during the procedure. C-I, EV, PC

137. no. 3. Petechiae result from the leukemic process. Vomiting and stomatitis are expected side effects of chemotherapy. Vincristine causes neurotoxic responses, such as numbness and tingling, jaw pain, and constipation, which should be reported because they may indicate toxicity. C-CA, AN, E

138. no. 1. When administering blood products, only saline solutions or solutions that don't contain any dextrose or glucose should be used. Dextrose and glucose solutions (hyperalimentation solutions contain hypertonic glucose concentrations) will cause hemolysis of the blood cells. C-CA, IM, PS

139. no. 3. Radiation therapy may cause delayed onset of puberty, delays in physical growth, pathological bone fractures, and chromosomal damage because of its effects on normal cells. C-CA, AN, PS

140. no. 2. Pain control is best achieved on a preventive schedule after assessing the period that a particular dosage is effective for the child and the child's general pain responses. This prevents fluctuation in pain threshold levels. Waiting until the child becomes restless and unable to sleep will lessen the effectiveness of analgesics when given. Pain medications should not be given more often than every 3 to 4 hours, but giving them that often around the clock may not be necessary for a particular child. C-I, IM, E

141. no. 3. Immunosuppression is a contraindication for giving immunizations. Immunizing a child who is immunosuppressed can lead to overwhelming infection and death. As soon as the child's white blood cell count is normal, the DPT and TOPV boosters may be given since the child's immune system can respond normally. C-CA, IM, E

142. no. 4. Postoperatively, Mrs. Carnelli will probably have a HemoVac in place. Skin grafting is associated with the more extensive Halsted radical mastectomy. *Peau d'orange* change in skin is a preoperative assessment parameter, noted on breast self-examination. A-CA, IM, PS

143. no. 3. Acknowledging what the client is feeling encourages verbalization about the feeling. No. 1 avoids an opportunity for further discussion. No. 2 is too demanding and does not acknowledge what the client is feeling. No. 4 avoids even observation of the client's feelings. P-I, IM, PC

144. no. 4. Drainage is drawn to the back of the dressing by gravity. Unless her back is checked for drainage, Mrs. Carnelli may hemorrhage significantly without it being detected. Alterations in level of consciousness are associated with decreased oxygenation resulting from a number of factors. She would have to lose a significant amount of blood before her state of consciousness would be altered. A-CA, IM, E

145. no. 2. This best allows the nurse to assess understanding of material and provides an opportunity to adapt to the client's concentration span. Option no. 1 is not best with this age group since those in this group may have trouble with written content or may not be motivated to read. No. 3 and no. 4 may overtax the client and do not allow feelings about the surgery and diagnosis to be expressed. Option no. 4 is more appropriate with 20- to 30-year-olds. A-H, IM, H

146. no. 2. The client should decrease her intake of sodium and liquids. This response indicates she needs additional teaching. A-CA, EV, PS

147. no. 1. Before discharge, Mrs. Carnelli should be able to explain incision care. Adapting to an altered body image takes weeks or months, as does the grieving process. The latter may even be delayed 2 or 3 months. A Jobst pressure machine is used only if other methods for preventing lymphedema are ineffective. A-CA, EV, E

148. no. 4. The psychosocial task at this age is accomplishing a sense of initiative. Autonomy is the toddler's major task, and identity is the adolescent's. Mastery is important throughout childhood but is most characteristic of the school-age child. C-H, AS, PC

149. no. 2. The average 5-year-old can count to 20, recite the alphabet, and recognize most colors. It is not until about age 6 that children can print their names. At age 7, children can tell clock time and tie their shoelaces. C-H, AS, H

150. no. 4. These results are normal; 20/20 or 20/30 vision is considered within normal limits at this age, because visual acuity may not be fully developed. C-H, AN, H

151. no. 1. Strabismus is a common health problem that must be detected early to prevent amblyopia. The other options are used to assess neurological status. C-H, AS, H

152. no. 2. Recommended caloric intake at this age is approximately 1700 calories/day. C-H, IM, H

153. no. 1. A carefully planned program of diet and exercise that meets the child's continued needs for growth is essential. Focus should be on slowing weight gain to allow height to catch up over a period of several months, rather than trying to have the child lose weight. Appetite suppressants are without merit in the treatment of childhood overweight and obesity. Large doses of vitamins are unnecessary if the child is eating a well-balanced diet, and they may actually be harmful to the child. Withholding all sweets is unrealistic and may lead to cheating. The child should be helped to change his eating habits with the recognition that an occasional sweet treat is acceptable. C-NM, PL, PS

154. no. 3. Because of the slowing of Jermaine's weight gain, his weight is now only one standard deviation from his height. Weight loss and caloric restriction are not desired outcomes. Jermaine may not be craving junk food, but this option doesn't give enough information to evaluate his progress (e.g., he may not be eating junk food, but his caloric intake may be as high as previously if he is substituting other foods). C-NM, EV, PS

155. no. 2. The uterine muscle may contract poorly as a result of overdistension from a large baby and several past pregnancies. Rapid labor may delay involution as well. While the other complications may occur, they are not specific in this case. CBF-P, AN, PS

156. no. 3. Fluid shifts during the postpartal period cause a normal diaphoresis and diuresis. Intake is related to urinary output, but options no. 1 and no. 2 are not accurate. While hormones dramatically affect adaptation after delivery, this symptom alone does not suggest infection. CBF-P, IM, H

157. no. 3. This is the best option and is an appropriate way to initiate teaching. Breastfeeding is not a means of contraception. Delaying a discussion until the check-up may lead to another pregnancy. CBF-P, IM, PC

158. no. 2. This describes the proper time for removal of a diaphragm. Spermicide, not K-Y jelly, should be used. Alcohol rapidly dries rubber and reduces

effectiveness. While a cervical sponge may be left in place for 1-2 days, a diaphragm should be removed 6 hours after intercourse. CBF-W, EV, H

159. no. 3. This response keeps the interaction reality oriented. No. 1 and no. 2 probe into the client's delusion. No. 4 may provoke an argument. P-W, IM, PC

160. no. 4. Projection is unconsciously attributing one's own unacceptable qualities and emotions to others. He is saying, "I'm not inconsequential. They are." No. 1, no. 2, and no. 3 are not found in this clinical situation. P-W, AN, PC

161. no. 2. The maximum therapeutic dose for haloperidol (Haldol) is 100 mg daily. P-W, IM, E

162. no. 4. The suspicious, hostile, or aggressive client should be worked with initially, and probably for an extended time, on a one-to-one basis. This will allow a trusting relationship to develop. No. 1 and no. 2 will provoke anger and hostility and will reinforce defenses. Option no. 3 isolates the client and may also reinforce defenses and perpetuate the delusional system. P-SS, IM, E

163. no. 1. Intervene while the client is still able to talk about feelings. Option no. 2 will not allow the client the opportunity to learn to deal with negative feelings. No. 3 also will not allow the client to learn verbal methods of dealing with anger. No. 4 is not justified by his behavior at this time. P-SS, IM, E

164. no. 3. Constipation is a side effect of haloperidol (Haldol). No. 1, no. 2, and no. 4 can cause constipation, but no data have been given to support them. P-W, AN, PS

165. no. 3. Ambivalence is the coexistence of two opposing feelings toward another person, object, or idea. Although the term "mixed feelings" is sometimes used, ambivalence is the proper term. Extreme withdrawal (autism) and low level of interest in or response to surroundings (apathy) have not been described. P-W, AN, PC

166. no. 2. Put the suspicious, hostile, aggressive client in charge of things, not people. Option no. 2 is the only response that meets that criterion. No. 1, no. 3, and no. 4 will subject this client to the stress of relating to people, especially in situations of authority. P-SS, IM, E

167. no. 2. This allows the client to practice verbally what he is going to say before he is in the actual situation (one that is likely to be stressful). Options no. 1, no. 3, and no. 4 may also be useful; but with Mr. O'Shea's employment history, vocational counseling, a resume, and the want ads are less likely to be useful than learning to deal with stressful situations. P-W, IM, H

168. no. 1. Emergency care of a burn wound such as this involves dousing or immersing the injury in cool water to prevent further thermal damage. Ice packs or ice water can cause further damage to the injured tissue and are contraindicated. Adherent clothing should never be pulled from a burn injury because of the possibility of damaging remaining tissue. Covering the burn with any kind of substance (cream, margarine, ointments) can trap heat and also cause further damage and increase the risk of infection. C-SPP, IM, E

169. no. 1. Because Tim's wound is not tetanus prone (i.e., does not involve muscle tissue, is not contaminated with saliva or excrement, and is less than 24 hours old) and he has received a full series of primary immunizations with his last booster less than 10 years ago (between 4 and 6 years of age) but more than 5 years ago, he needs tetanus toxoid (given in the form of Td). Tetanus immune globulin (passive immunity) is indicated only if the previous immunization history is unknown or uncertain or the burn wound is tetanus prone (i.e., burn wounds that involve muscle tissue or are highly contaminated). C-SPP, IM, H

170. no. 2. The major advantage of the closed method is to minimize fluid lost from the burn surface by applying gentle pressure to the burn wound. Use of silver sulfadiazine (Silvadene) will also reduce the possibility of wound infection. Although the dressing will protect the wound and reduce pain, these are not the primary reasons for using this method. Wrapping the wound will partially immobilize the hand and wrist and, therefore, may increase the possibility of contracture. C-SPP, IM, PS

171. no. 3. Removal of old cream is essential in keeping the wound clean and ensuring that newly applied cream is effective in reducing the chance of bacterial contamination. The wound should be cleansed with warm sudsy water (using a soap such as Ivory flakes or Dreft, *not* a detergent). Silver sulfadiazine (Silvadene) is not painful when applied and does not interfere with acid-base or electrolyte balance. Silver nitrate, not Silvadene, may cause skin discoloration when used to treat burn wounds. C-SPP, PL, E

172. no. 1. The burn-injured client needs large amounts of protein and vitamin C for wound healing. Meats and milk are high in protein, and citrus fruits are high in vitamin C. C-SPP, PL, PS

173. no. 3. Refusal to wear short-sleeve shirts in the summer indicates that Tim may be trying to hide his burn injury from himself and others and therefore may need help in coping with this body change. Asking about resumption of physical activity is a healthy sign. Many teenage boys this age are not yet interested in girls, and adolescents are often quiet and nontalkative in unfamiliar situations or with adults. P-L, EV, PC

174. no. 3. Acne is caused by sebum blocking skin pores and is most effectively treated by adequate daily cleansing, followed by application of anti-acne product that contains benzoyl peroxide, a peeling and drying agent. Use of a headband during exercise or hot weather can cause secretions to be retained, with further blockage of skin pores. There is no evidence that chocolate, iodine, or greasy foods contribute to acne. Use of ultraviolet light should be reserved for severe cases of acne and done under the supervision of a physician. C-SPP, PL, PS

175. no. 3. This is a specific measurement to determine kidney function, primarily glomerular filtration. Creatinine is produced at a constant rate; it is not reabsorbed and is only minimally secreted. BUN is less reliable because urea, after being filtered, is reabsorbed back into renal tubular cells. Additionally, urea production varies according to liver function and protein intake and breakdown. The test for serum glucose is used to screen for disorders of metabolism. Electrolyte studies are not specific to kidney filtration. A-E, PL, PS

176. no. 3. The dye used for an IVP is iodine based and can cause a severe allergic reaction (anaphylaxis) in sensitive individuals. Food allergies to shellfish can indicate an iodine allergy, because shellfish are high in iodine content. The other options should be done, but because of the possible danger to the client, the allergy history takes priority. A-E, EV, E

177. no. 4. Sulfonamides dissolve well in urine and are excreted unchanged in the urine; therefore they are excellent for treating urinary tract infections. However, if fluid intake is not sufficient, the drug can crystalize, resulting in renal toxicity. While on the drug regimen, intake should be sufficient to maintain a urine output of at least 1 L/day. Sulfonamides are metabolized by the liver and excreted through the kidneys, may produce a false-positive glucose on urine tests, and are more soluble in alkaline urine. A-E, AS, PS

178. no. 3. Whole grains are unrestricted in an acid-ash diet. Carrots and dried apricots are not allowed and only 1 pint of milk is allowed daily. A-NM, IM, H

179. no. 1. A high urine output helps flush out bacteria from the urinary tract and maintain a low urine osmolarity. Encourage clients to void every 2 to 3 hours during the day and 1 to 2 times during the night. Sitz baths are helpful during an acute episode but are not a priority of discharge planning. Voiding after intercourse is recommended for women who have repeated urinary tract infections. Avoidance of exposure to respiratory infections would be highly desirable if the client was showing signs and symptoms of renal failure. At this point, Mr. Tate is not in this category. A-E, IM, H

180. no. 3. All of these goals are worthwhile and will need to be met before discharge; however, because of the severity of the renal colic, option no. 3 must be the first priority. Only then can the client respond to teaching and begin taking increased fluids. Morphine may have to be given for the pain, depending upon the severity. IV fluids may have to be started to increase intake initially. A-E, PL, PS

181. no. 3. Cervical dilatation is the most reliable index of the progress of labor. Other options may or may not indicate true progress. No. 1 is possible with hypertonic dysfunction, no. 2 could be related to anxiety, and no. 4 can occur at any time and may not relate to progress. CBF-I, AS, PS

182. no. 4. This symptom is related to sacral pressure and progression into the second stage of labor. The other options do not warrant further evaluation as long as the client is comfortably ambulating. CBF-I, AS, E

183. no. 2. Blood pressure rises during contractions and, therefore, gives an inaccurate reading. Option no. 1 is incorrect because erratic could mean increasing or decreasing. Options no. 3 and no. 4 may be true but they are not valid reasons. CBF-I, IM, E

184. no. 4. To assess for late decelerations, it is necessary to listen during and soon after contractions. Early fetal distress would be completely missed if option no. 2 were followed. CBF-I, AS, PS

185. no. 3. From the signs Mrs. Ryan describes, it is evident she suspects Kathleen has an eating problem. But the lack of weight loss does not seem to fit with what she knows, so she's not sure. Option no. 3 verbalizes the implied question Mrs. Ryan seems to be asking as well as gets to the point of her daughter having an eating disorder, which the symptoms support. Options no. 1 and no. 2 are wrong because Kathleen is showing typical symptoms of bulimia. Option no. 4 may be true, but the central problem is the eating disorder, bulimia. P-A, IM, PC

186. no. 4. Kathleen is showing the classic signs of bulimia, specifically the ones that differentiate it from anorexia (healthy appearance, normal weight, furtive trips to the bathroom after meals). Options no. 1, no. 2, and no. 3 are wrong for the symptoms presented. P-A, AN, PC

187. no. 3. Initially Kathleen will show some of the physical effects of long-term vomiting and use of laxatives. Options no. 1, no. 2, and no. 4 are also good objectives of care, but they are secondary to stabilizing her food retention and intake. P-A, PL, PC

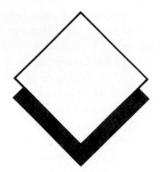

Sample Test Questions: Part Three

Carol Perez, 21 years old, is in acute renal failure following a large loss of blood from injuries she received in a car accident. Her 24-hour urine output is 275 ml. Her serum BUN is 90 mg/100 ml and her serum creatinine is 7.2 mg/dl.

188. During the oliguric phase of acute renal failure, which of the following would be an appropriate nursing intervention?
    □ 1. Increase dietary sodium and potassium.
    □ 2. Restrict fluid to 1500 ml daily.
    □ 3. Weigh client three times weekly.
    □ 4. Provide a low-protein, high-carbohydrate diet.
189. Mrs. Perez fails to respond to therapy to correct her acute renal failure. She goes into chronic renal failure with the prospect of having to start dialysis or have a kidney transplant. Which of the following indicators would you expect to see in Mrs. Perez as the renal failure becomes more severe?
    □ 1. Anemia.
    □ 2. Hypokalemia.
    □ 3. Diaphoresis.
    □ 4. Hypotension.
190. In planning Mrs. Perez's diet, which of the following food sources would be the best source of high biological-value protein?
    □ 1. Bananas.
    □ 2. Asparagus.
    □ 3. Eggs.
    □ 4. Mushrooms.
191. While waiting for a suitable transplant kidney to be identified, Mrs. Perez has to begin dialysis. An arteriovenous (AV) fistula is created for hemodialysis. As a nurse, you understand that one major complication you must observe for following an AV fistula is
    □ 1. Rejection of the Silastic cannula connecting the artery and vein.
    □ 2. Accidental dislodgment of the cannula with resulting hemorrhage.
    □ 3. Thrombosis of the artery and vein site.
    □ 4. Cardiac irritation caused by the cannula's insertion.

192. Nursing assessment of the access site to the AV fistula would best include
    □ 1. Taking blood pressures in the affected arm to monitor the presence of good circulation.
    □ 2. Making sure the color of the blood in the fistula is bright cranberry-red.
    □ 3. Checking skin temperatures and pulses proximal to the fistula to assess circulation.
    □ 4. Palpating the access site for a thrill to assess circulation.
193. While waiting for the AV-fistula site to mature for hemodialysis, Mrs. Perez is maintained using peritoneal dialysis. During peritoneal dialysis, the nurse notes a retention of 600 ml of dialysate fluid after draining the peritoneal cavity. The best initial response of the nurse would be to
    □ 1. Infuse an additional 1400 ml of fresh dialysate, and continue with dialysis.
    □ 2. Have the client turn from side to side to help localize fluid to promote drainage.
    □ 3. Check vital signs to assess whether a fluid overload is occurring.
    □ 4. Notify the physician of the fluid retention.
194. Today Mrs. Perez will undergo hemodialysis for the first time. Which of the following interventions, if implemented, would be most likely to help her avoid disequilibrium syndrome?
    □ 1. Withhold her antihypertensive medications.
    □ 2. Dialyze her for a short time.
    □ 3. Dialyze her in a sitting position.
    □ 4. Withhold protein from her diet.
195. While waiting for a compatible kidney for transplant, Mrs. Perez will be discharged home. Because of the distance of the hemodialysis center from her home, the physician decides to provide her with continuous ambulatory peritoneal dialysis (CAPD). When educating Mrs. Perez about CAPD, the top priority is to teach her
    □ 1. Sterile technique to help prevent peritonitis.
    □ 2. To maintain a more liberal protein diet.
    □ 3. To maintain a daily written record of blood pressure and weight.

4. To continue regular medical and nursing follow-up.

196. Mrs. Perez returns to the hospital for a kidney transplant. Which of the following interventions would do the most to help prevent transplant rejection?
   1. Transfusion of 4 units of typed and cross-matched blood.
   2. Administration of prophylactic antibiotics.
   3. Hemodialysis until the transplant begins to function.
   4. Administration of immunosuppressive drugs.

197. When Mrs. Perez has her kidney surgery, there is a high thoracic incision. The most appropriate outcome criterion to evaluate the status of the pulmonary system in this client would be
   1. Client is free from temperature elevation greater than 38.5° C.
   2. Client's breath sounds are clear.
   3. Client's PO_2 is greater than 60 mm Hg.
   4. Client shows no signs of cyanosis.

Chris and Jack O'Neal delayed childbearing for several years. After a year of planning, the O'Neals conceive. During her pregnancy, Mrs. O'Neal is carefully monitored because of a history of cardiac surgery as a child.

198. An internist follows her condition periodically during pregnancy and shares information with the obstetrician and primary nurse. The chief potential problem for this client during the third trimester is
   1. Premature delivery.
   2. Cardiac decompensation.
   3. Dehydration.
   4. Infection.

199. Mrs. O'Neal develops severe hypertension, experiences headaches, and is hospitalized. She is given IV magnesium sulfate to prevent convulsions. In evaluating the client's response to therapy, which effect is expected?
   1. Muscle cramps.
   2. Hyperreflexia.
   3. Polyuria.
   4. Central nervous system depression.

200. Mr. O'Neal stays with his wife all through labor. Which of the following statements made by him would best indicate that he understands his role during labor?
   1. "I should take my coffee break soon, as Chris will need me with her in transition."
   2. "I will be able to leave Chris around lunch time, as she will prefer the professional care as the pain gets intense."
   3. "My presence distracts her, and she tries to talk to me instead of resting between contractions."
   4. "Transition is a hard time and she is getting very irritable. I will take my break now and be back to help her to push."

201. Mrs. O'Neal's condition is stabilized, and she delivers an 8-lb son. The infant has an initial axillary temperature of 96° F. If the infant is cold stressed and is not warmed immediately, the nurse would initially observe
   1. Shivering.
   2. Cyanosis.
   3. Respiratory rate increase.
   4. Irritability.

202. Baby Boy O'Neal appears pink and active, but slight grunting on expiration is noted when he is scored using the Silverman-Anderson scale. What additional assessments are indicated?
   1. Heart rate.
   2. Chest movements.
   3. Blood gases.
   4. Color.

203. While performing a physical assessment of Baby Boy O'Neal, a swelling is observed on the side of the infant's head. This swelling is soft, does not pulsate or bulge when the infant cries, and does not cross suture lines. The parents ask about the mass. The problem is most likely
   1. Intracranial hemorrhage.
   2. Cephalhematoma.
   3. Caput succedaneum.
   4. Hydrocephalus.

204. Mrs. O'Neal holds her baby on the first day of rooming-in. Which of the following behaviors could indicate potential problems with early attachment?
   1. Mrs. O'Neal complains of episiotomy pain while sitting with her infant.
   2. She appears discouraged with early breastfeeding attempts.
   3. There is little attempt to touch or speak to the alert newborn.
   4. When the infant is quiet, Mrs. O'Neal often naps.

205. On her third postpartum day, Mrs. O'Neal is found crying and expresses inadequacy in meeting her baby's needs. The nursing student asks about this behavior. The nurse suggests that Mrs. O'Neal is probably experiencing.
   1. Postpartum blues.
   2. Normal taking-in behavior.
   3. Abnormal bonding.
   4. Early psychotic depression.

206. Two weeks have elapsed. Mrs. O'Neal is breast-feeding. What is a goal of care at this time?
   1. Mother will limit nursing to 20- to 30-minute periods.
   2. Parents will supplement feedings with bottle once daily.

☐ 3. Mother will reduce caloric intake to prepregnancy amount.

☐ 4. Couple will alternate night feedings.

Roger Caine, a 30-year-old insurance salesman, was awarded an expense-paid Caribbean cruise for his outstanding sales record. While on his trip, he became restless and overactive. He insisted on eating every meal at the captain's table. He danced until the wee hours and was up early, ready to go. He talked fast and behaved grandiosely. Upon his arrival in New York, he spent money excessively. He demanded a luxurious hotel suite and loudly berated the hotel manager because no luxurious hotel suite was available. Shortly thereafter, he was admitted to a hospital with a diagnosis of manic-depression. At the hospital, history taking revealed he had been hospitalized 2 years earlier for depression.

207. When it's time for lunch, Mr. Caine tells you he's too busy. He says he has an impending multimillion-dollar deal he has to negotiate, and he has people to call and see. The nurse's best response would be

☐ 1. "Visiting hours aren't until 4 PM, so you can't see anyone now."

☐ 2. "When you're finished, please come to the dining room to eat."

☐ 3. "Mr. Caine, you need to eat now. I'll go with you to help you."

☐ 4. "If you don't eat now, we'll need to put you in the seclusion room."

208. Which of the following actions must be *avoided* to ensure effective intervention with Mr. Caine's manipulative or demanding behavior?

☐ 1. Give a short, clear definition of limits that will be set.

☐ 2. Consistently enforce the limits that were set.

☐ 3. Allow some leeway when limits are violated.

☐ 4. Hold frequent staff conferences to ensure cohesiveness and consistency in carrying out the plan of care.

209. Which of the following should be considered first when planning Mr. Caine's physical care?

☐ 1. Mr. Caine will be overly concerned about cleanliness.

☐ 2. Mr. Caine is an adult who needs to be given autonomy in his care.

☐ 3. Mr. Caine needs more knowledge about his illness.

☐ 4. Mr. Caine may disregard his physical needs.

210. Mr. Caine is to be maintained on a regimen of lithium carbonate. What is the therapeutic blood level for lithium?

☐ 1. 0.8-2.6 mEq/L.

☐ 2. 0.8-1.5 mEq/L.

☐ 3. 1.6-2.4 mEq/L.

☐ 4. 2.9-3.2 mEq/L.

211. Mr. Caine should be observed for side effects of lithium. Which of the following is *not* an expected side effect?

☐ 1. Nausea and sluggish feeling.

☐ 2. Muscle weakness.

☐ 3. Thirst and polyuria.

☐ 4. Diffuse rash.

212. Mr. Caine has difficulty sleeping. He rarely sleeps more than 3 hours at a time. All of the following might alleviate his insomnia *except* one. Which one?

☐ 1. Provide an evening of quiet activity.

☐ 2. Give him a warm drink at bedtime.

☐ 3. Administer a sedative for sleep.

☐ 4. Encourage him to take a cool shower before retiring.

Antoinette Davis, a newborn, has a meningomyelocele. She is being transferred directly from the delivery room to a special care unit.

213. The nurse should place Antoinette in which position?

☐ 1. Semi-Fowler's.

☐ 2. Supine.

☐ 3. On her side.

☐ 4. Prone.

214. Mr. and Mrs. Davis have consented to surgical closure of Antoinette's defect. Before surgery, the defect should be

☐ 1. Covered with dry, sterile dressings.

☐ 2. Left open to the air.

☐ 3. Covered with sterile saline soaks.

☐ 4. Covered with gauze impregnated with petroleum jelly.

215. Twenty-four hours before surgery, Antoinette develops a fever. She is fussy, irritable, and refuses her formula. Which nursing measure should the nurse carry out first?

☐ 1. Examine the meningomyelocele sac.

☐ 2. Contact Antoinette's physician.

☐ 3. Place Antoinette in strict isolation.

☐ 4. Ask Mrs. Davis to feed Antoinette.

216. While caring for Antoinette postoperatively, which nursing action should receive the highest priority?

☐ 1. Maintain her legs in abduction.

☐ 2. Measure her head circumference daily.

☐ 3. Provide tactile and verbal stimulation.

☐ 4. Change her position frequently.

217. Antoinette is receiving ampicillin, 75 mg IV every 6 hours. When reconstituted with sterile saline, the vial contains 125 mg/1.2 ml. The nurse should administer what amount of the solution in the drip chamber?

☐ 1. 0.60 ml.

☐ 2. 0.72 ml.

☐ 3. 0.84 ml.

☐ 4. 1.00 ml.

218. The physician has also prescribed phenytoin (Dilantin) elixir, 20 mg PO BID, for Antoinette. The drug comes in a concentration of 30 mg/4 ml. The nurse should administer what amount?
- ☐ 1. 0.67 ml.
- ☐ 2. 1.5 ml.
- ☐ 3. 2.6 ml.
- ☐ 4. 3.0 ml.

219. Which potential problem presents the most serious threat to Antoinette's long-term management?
- ☐ 1. Flexion contractures of the hips.
- ☐ 2. Frequent colds.
- ☐ 3. Constipation.
- ☐ 4. Recurrent urinary tract infection.

Henry Duboff, a 50-year-old white man, awakes in the middle of the night with severe dyspnea, bilateral basilar rales, and expectoration of frothy, blood-tinged sputum. He is brought to the hospital by the paramedics in congestive heart failure complicated by pulmonary edema.

220. Dyspnea is a characteristic sign of left-sided congestive heart failure. This is primarily the result of which mechanism?
- ☐ 1. Accumulation of serous fluid in alveolar spaces.
- ☐ 2. Obstruction of bronchi by mucoid secretions.
- ☐ 3. Compression of lung tissue by a dilated heart.
- ☐ 4. Restriction of respiratory movement by ascites.

221. Edema caused by right-sided congestive heart failure tends to be which of the following?
- ☐ 1. Painful.
- ☐ 2. Dependent.
- ☐ 3. Periorbital.
- ☐ 4. Nonpitting.

222. What is the optimal bed position for the client with congestive heart failure?
- ☐ 1. Position of comfort, to relax the client.
- ☐ 2. Semirecumbent, to ease dyspnea and metabolic demands of the heart.
- ☐ 3. Sims, to decrease danger of pulmonary edema.
- ☐ 4. Dorsal recumbent, to decrease edema formation in the extremities.

223. Respirations of the client with congestive heart failure are usually of which kind?
- ☐ 1. Rapid and shallow.
- ☐ 2. Deep and stertorous.
- ☐ 3. Rapid and wheezing.
- ☐ 4. Biot's respirations.

224. How do rotating tourniquets relieve the symptoms of acute pulmonary edema?
- ☐ 1. Cause vasoconstriction.
- ☐ 2. Cause vasodilation.
- ☐ 3. Decrease the amount of circulating blood.
- ☐ 4. Increase the amount of circulating blood.

225. When tourniquets are applied to extremities to relieve the symptoms of pulmonary edema, one tourniquet should be rotated, in order, on a regular basis. How often are they rotated?
- ☐ 1. Every 5 minutes.
- ☐ 2. Every 10 minutes.
- ☐ 3. Every 15 minutes.
- ☐ 4. Every 20 minutes.

226. When Mr. Duboff is admitted to CCU, his ECG shows changes indicative of an anterior myocardial infarction. Which criteria should the nurse monitor to assess his cardiac status?
- ☐ 1. ECG changes, serum enzymes, and leg cramps.
- ☐ 2. Chest pain, ECG changes, and serum enzymes.
- ☐ 3. Chest pain, ECG changes, and serum creatinine.
- ☐ 4. ECG changes, serum electrolytes, and blood urea nitrogen.

227. Mr. Duboff continues to have ventricular dysrhythmias even though he is being treated with lidocaine (Xylocaine). On his second hospital day, he goes into a cardiac arrest. Which of these responses by the nurse would be appropriate initially?
- ☐ 1. Open his airway.
- ☐ 2. Start chest compression.
- ☐ 3. Check his carotid pulse.
- ☐ 4. Put him on a hard surface.

228. Mr. Duboff has been resuscitated with success and is transferred to the medical floor 4 days after the cardiac arrest. At this time, he is scheduled for a cardiac catheterization. The nurse emphasizes to him that during the procedure he will be
- ☐ 1. Heavily sedated and will not be able to move.
- ☐ 2. Under general anesthesia and unconscious.
- ☐ 3. Awake, not sedated, and asked to remain still.
- ☐ 4. Awake, mildly sedated, and asked to change his position.

229. The information gathered from the left cardiac catheterization will include all but one of the following. Which one is *incorrect*?
- ☐ 1. Patency of the coronary arteries.
- ☐ 2. Status of collateral circulation.
- ☐ 3. Patency of the pulmonary artery.
- ☐ 4. Perfusion of the myocardium.

230. After cardiac catheterization, in what position will Mr. Duboff be placed?
- ☐ 1. Supine with affected leg extended.
- ☐ 2. Supine with affected leg flexed.
- ☐ 3. Side lying with both legs flexed.
- ☐ 4. Any position he desires.

Jo Ellen Baxter, a 50-year-old with a diagnosis of chronic, undifferentiated schizophrenia, is hospitalized on a surgical unit for an appendectomy.

231. The day after surgery, Mrs. Baxter tells the nurse that she feels creatures eating away at her abdomen. What is the first thing the nurse needs to do?
    - ☐ 1. Request an increase in her phenothiazines to control the psychosis.
    - ☐ 2. Talk with her more often to help control her stress level.
    - ☐ 3. Assess for possible abdominal pains.
    - ☐ 4. Request an order for benztropine (Cogentin) to control her extrapyramidal symptoms.

232. The care needs of a chronic schizophrenic client are best reflected in which of the following statements?
    - ☐ 1. Have a different staff member care for her each day to avoid intimacy.
    - ☐ 2. Have one staff member care for her as much as possible to increase trust.
    - ☐ 3. Have one staff member care for her and remain with her the entire shift to increase intimacy and closeness.
    - ☐ 4. There is no need to be concerned about the assignment, since Mrs. Baxter will not know the difference.

233. Oral antibiotics are started. Mrs. Baxter has been taking her phenothiazines at home reliably for years. Which of the following is the most appropriate nursing intervention?
    - ☐ 1. Set up a plan to describe to Mrs. Baxter the cause of her problem, the effects on her body, and physiological changes caused by her disease.
    - ☐ 2. Tell her how often to take the medication and have her do it a few times while in the hospital.
    - ☐ 3. Insist that she not be discharged until the course of the medication has been given.
    - ☐ 4. Request a home health nurse to come into her home and give her the medication.

234. While you are talking to Mrs. Baxter one day, she tells you that the "creatures from Odum have just left my room." The creatures from Odum are probably which of the following?
    - ☐ 1. The result of an extrapyramidal reaction.
    - ☐ 2. A response to a phobic fear of being alone.
    - ☐ 3. A symbol from her autistic world.
    - ☐ 4. An example of flight of ideas.

235. Which of the following is the most appropriate nursing response to Mrs. Baxter's statement about the creatures from Odum?
    - ☐ 1. Acknowledge that the creatures have special meaning for Mrs. Baxter.
    - ☐ 2. Suggest a variety of interpretations of the creatures for Mrs. Baxter.

    - ☐ 3. Tell Mrs. Baxter to call you the next time she sees them.
    - ☐ 4. Tell her you don't like to talk about creatures.

Justine Turner, 10 years old, has had insulin-dependent diabetes mellitus (IDDM) since age 5. She is seen with her father in the diabetics' clinic for a routine follow-up.

236. Which statement made by Justine to the nurse indicates that Justine has achieved developmentally appropriate self-management of her diabetes?
    - ☐ 1. "My mom does my urine tests most of the time."
    - ☐ 2. "I give my injections, but Dad checks to be sure I do it right."
    - ☐ 3. "I'm not allowed to help with my finger sticks yet."
    - ☐ 4. "I decide what I want to eat and when."

237. Justine tells the nurse, "I'm on our school's soccer team now. We just started practice, and we sure do a lot of running." What changes in Justine's control of her diabetes should be expected as a result?
    - ☐ 1. Decreased insulin requirements.
    - ☐ 2. Increased insulin requirements.
    - ☐ 3. Decreased risk of insulin shock.
    - ☐ 4. Increased risk of ketoacidosis.

238. As Justine enters early adolescence, it is most important that the nurse prepare Justine and her family for which occurrence?
    - ☐ 1. A rapid gain in weight.
    - ☐ 2. Changes in diet and insulin requirements.
    - ☐ 3. The need to limit physical activity.
    - ☐ 4. A switch to oral hypoglycemics.

239. Two weeks later, Justine is admitted to the hospital in diabetic ketoacidosis. Which manifestation should the nurse expect to oberve?
    - ☐ 1. Seizures and trembling.
    - ☐ 2. Pallor and sweating.
    - ☐ 3. Vomiting and dry mucous membranes.
    - ☐ 4. Hunger and diplopia.

240. During the hospitalization, which of the following is most likely to be a major concern for Justine?
    - ☐ 1. Placement in unfamiliar surroundings.
    - ☐ 2. Fear of painful treatments.
    - ☐ 3. Absence from school and social activities.
    - ☐ 4. Worry over restricted mobility.

John Coates, 15 years old, was admitted to a psychiatric unit 2 weeks ago because his adolescence had been turbulent. His relationships with peers have been troubled. He goes to occupational therapy and becomes angry during the group activity.

241. When John returns to the unit, he says that the occupational therapists don't like him. John is probably experiencing which one of the following?

   □ 1. Trying to avoid OT because he is shy.

   □ 2. Feeling threatened by the group.

   □ 3. Feeling angry with a group member.

   □ 4. Being annoyed by the occupational therapists.

242. What is a more appropriate plan for John?

   □ 1. Require that he attend OT so that he will learn to adjust.

   □ 2. Tell him he cannot go to OT until he learns to act properly.

   □ 3. Put him in group therapy instead.

   □ 4. Have him work alone with an occupational therapist for awhile.

Eight-year-old Chad Fredricks is brought to the emergency room by his mother. He has multiple bruises over his entire body and a fractured right arm. His mother states he was playing with his wagon and fell on his right arm. The mother describes him as a "troublemaker and a bad kid." He is not crying and refuses to speak to the nurse or his mother. The nurse thinks that Chad may be a victim of child abuse.

243. All but one of the following reasons make the nurses suspicious. Which is the one *exception?*

   □ 1. The multiple bruises do not fit the description of the accident.

   □ 2. The mother identifies him as a bad child.

   □ 3. Chad does not turn to his mother for solace.

   □ 4. Chad, by playing with a wagon, shows regression or retarded development for an 8-year-old.

244. Mrs. Fredricks is advised that Chad will need to have his arm set and placed in a cast; then he will be hospitalized for further assessment and treatment. She is questioned about her methods of disciplining Chad. She responds angrily by saying, "Of course, I spank him. He's such a troublemaker; he does things purposely to upset me. He's so ungrateful. Sometimes I feel overwhelmed by it all, but I do not abuse him. I'm not overly violent. I hit him only when he asks for it." The nurse knows that Mrs. Fredricks is probably doing which of the following?

   □ 1. Lying to the hospital personnel to protect herself; she knows she's abusive.

   □ 2. Telling the truth, and it is someone else who hits the child.

   □ 3. Is not aware that her behavior is abusive.

   □ 4. Disciplining the child appropriately, since he seems to have a behavior problem.

245. The nurse realizes that the hospital has certain legal responsibilities in Chad's case. All of the following should be done *except* which one?

   □ 1. Document all bruises and cuts; include their placement and size.

   □ 2. Chart interaction patterns between Chad and his mother.

   □ 3. Document staff perceptions of the relationship between Chad and his mother.

   □ 4. Report to the state child-welfare agency.

246. The nurse needs to understand that parents who abuse their children

   □ 1. Frequently do not know or are unable to ask for help until after they have felt overwhelmed by problems.

   □ 2. Plan ahead as to when and how to abuse their children.

   □ 3. Rarely were abused themselves; so they do not recognize the problem until it is too late.

   □ 4. Usually are not concerned about their abusive actions.

247. After providing for physical care of the hospitalized abused child, the nurse needs to give priority to play activities that encourage the child to

   □ 1. Describe details of the traumatic events.

   □ 2. Maintain control over his feelings (e.g., games that are quiet or include many rules).

   □ 3. Be distracted from unpleasant experiences.

   □ 4. Share feelings of joy, anger, fear, or loneliness.

248. The nurse assigned to Chad recognizes her own negative feelings toward Mrs. Fredricks. The nurse's best action would be to

   □ 1. Continue to care for Chad and relate to the mother during visiting hours, and not share feelings with other staff, since they might be influenced by negativism.

   □ 2. Be open with the mother about feelings (e.g., saying, "I can help you more if I am honest with you.").

   □ 3. Ask other nurses to discuss the case over lunch to reduce guilt feelings about disliking the mother.

   □ 4. Discuss feelings with the head nurse, along with details of the care plan, asking for evaluation of the nursing care for the client and her mother, and discussing implications of reassignment to another case.

249. Best interventions to assist Mrs. Fredricks include which of the following?

   □ 1. Techniques to handle angry behavior before it goes out of control.

   □ 2. Encouragement that the problems of parents lessen as a child grows older.

   □ 3. Opportunities to discuss how child abuse started in the family.

   □ 4. Discussions on how parents can make children follow rules.

250. The nurse will know Mrs. Fredricks is responding to treatment when Mrs. Fredricks takes which of the following steps?

   □ 1. Decides to place Chad for adoption.

2. Begins to talk more realistically about Chad's mistakes.

3. Talks about her own frustrations and anxieties.

4. Realizes that her needs are secondary to Chad's.

251. Another good indicator of progress for both the child and the mother is which of the following?

1. Both sleep and eat well and carry out daily activities with no thoughts about past abusive behavior.

2. They rarely encounter frustrating conflicts.

3. When frustrated by Chad, Mrs. Fredricks uses one or two of the alternatives to physical punishment she has learned.

4. The mother has planned many separate activities for herself and Chad so they have much less time together.

Lan Yang, age 60, undergoes a total laryngectomy for cancer of the larynx. He returns from surgery with a laryngectomy tube and an NG tube.

252. In the immediate postoperative period, Mr. Yang requires both nasopharyngeal suctioning and suctioning through the laryngectomy tube. Which of the following should the nurse do when performing these procedures?

1. Use a clean suction setup each time.

2. Apply constant suction.

3. Suction the laryngectomy tube, then the nose.

4. Lubricate the catheter with a petroleum jelly.

253. The nasogastric tube is used to provide Mr. Yang with fluids and nutrients for approximately 10 days for which of the following reasons?

1. To prevent pain while swallowing.

2. To prevent contamination of the suture line.

3. To decrease need for swallowing.

4. To prevent aspiration.

254. When should Mr. Yang best start speech rehabilitation?

1. When he leaves the hospital.

2. When esophageal suture line is healed.

3. Three months after surgery.

4. When he regains all his strength.

A 28-year-old neighbor, Lucia Ortega, is in the second month of pregnancy and feels fairly well. While giving a history, she talks about her job in a small animal hospital, where she is a helper to the veterinarian. She plans to continue working during the pregnancy.

255. Which of the following tasks should the nurse suggest Mrs. Ortega assign to a high school student who helps part time?

1. Operating a computer to prepare weekly statements.

2. Preparing the surgical suite for minor procedures.

3. Handling rabies and distemper vaccines and syringes.

4. Administering antibiotic ear drops to small animals.

256. Mrs. Ortega takes home a small, abandoned kitten who appears to be in good condition. What teaching is most appropriate at this time?

1. "Realize that the kitten may be jealous of your infant."

2. "Ask your husband if he will care for the litter box."

3. "Check to see if you and your husband have any allergies."

4. "Be sure to keep the animal indoors at all times."

257. Several weeks later, Mrs. Ortega develops vague flulike symptoms. Which of the following statements by the client indicates she has learned what was taught at the early antepartal visits?

1. "I know I shouldn't take any over-the-counter remedies now."

2. "I feel so tired all the time; so I must need the rest."

3. "I urinate frequently, so I probably am drinking too many fluids."

4. "Between the morning sickness and the flu, I'll be happy to lose weight."

258. It is established that Mrs. Ortega's symptoms are caused by toxoplasmosis. As the pregnancy advances, the physician is concerned that fetal growth is not appropriate for gestation. Which of the following tests would best provide information about the development of the fetus?

1. Urine estriol.

2. Amniocentesis.

3. Ultrasound.

4. Nonstress test.

259. Suspicions are confirmed, and the couple is told that it appears the fetus suffers from intrauterine growth retardation. The physician spends much time with them, drawing sketches of the placenta and the fetus. As the nurse talks with them afterward, Mrs. Ortega begins to cry. "I don't think I can cope with a retarded baby." Which response is most appropriate?

1. "Perhaps you were not listening to the doctor's explanation."

2. "Are there other retarded children in either family?"

3. "There are many resources available to help you."

4. "Let's talk about what the doctor said to us all."

260. A 5-lb infant is delivered vaginally at 39 weeks' gestation. Apgar scores are 9 and 10 at 1 and 5 minutes. The newborn appears active, wide-eyed, and alert. There was slight meconium staining of the placenta and cord. What analysis is justified?

1. The baby may have suffered chronic hypoxia.

2. It appears that the baby's condition is normal.

3. Assessments indicate good adaptation.

4. This child may have been somewhat premature.

261. Although the Ortega infant appears to behave normally, it is observed that the child occasionally cries, then appears to quiet himself and fall asleep. What is the best explanation of this behavior?

1. The baby's needs have not been met.

2. This is normal, expected behavior.

3. The central nervous system may be immature.

4. The newborn is not able to deal with frustration.

262. Which of the following is most important in the discharge teaching plan for the Ortega infant?

1. Parents will keep pediatric clinic appointments.

2. Mother will feed the newborn every 2 to 3 hours.

3. Mother will weigh the child daily.

4. Father will participate in care daily.

The admission of Sam Levitt to a young-adult psychiatric unit was precipitated by his attempts to beat up his father. A history of episodic agitation and aggressive behavior for many months preceded this event.

263. The admitting nurse would best give priority attention to which one of the following areas?

1. The client's thoughts about being harmed by others.

2. His thoughts of harming other persons at a future time.

3. Thought patterns that are disconnected and unrelated.

4. Thoughts that describe false, fixed beliefs.

264. When the unit becomes especially active and noisy with visitors and newly admitted persons, Mr. Levitt is most likely to

1. Insist in a loud voice that a staff member escort him to the canteen immediately.

2. Retreat to his room for an extra nap.

3. Initiate a pool game with another client and play to win.

4. Engage a staff person in a heated discussion about client-government activities.

265. A priority nursing goal for Mr. Levitt on admission is to help him to

1. Discuss childhood situations in which he lashed out at persons, in order to increase his self-understanding.

2. Participate in a variety of physical activities in order to dissipate his destructive feelings.

3. Talk at length about his deep-seated anger in order to reduce the chance that he will strike out again.

4. Make plans to reapply for admission to the community college he had attended.

266. Mr. Levitt was found pacing, striking his fists in the air, and cursing another client named Mrs. Sanders. The nurse would best say

1. "Mr. Levitt, stop cursing at Mrs. Sanders. I will stay and help you control yourself."

2. "You must feel very angry. Maybe you should calm down."

3. "Mr. Levitt, Mrs. Sanders did nothing to upset you; so please stop threatening her."

4. "Mr. Levitt, calm down. You can get rid of all this energy in the gym this afternoon. Come and eat breakfast now."

267. When Mr. Levitt's father escorts his son to the unit following the son's first weekend pass from the inpatient setting, the nurse speaks to them together. The nurse's most important focus is

1. How both the father and son felt about the weekend.

2. What activities they did that were satisfying to both.

3. How frequently, if at all, Mr. Levitt lost control.

4. What events occurred that indicated progress in Mr. Levitt's ability to refrain from threatening behavior.

268. A long-term indicator of Mr. Levitt's progress will be his

1. Ability to move from verbal to physical activities when he senses increased anger.

2. Deliberate actions to engage in several community activities separate from his family.

3. Assuming responsibility to be punctual for all therapy sessions.

4. Willingness to admit that he has a bad temper and that he must do something about it.

When Edward Barden, a 37-year-old construction worker, is admitted to the nursing unit, he tells you that he has pain radiating down his right leg.

269. Which of the following is *not* appropriate to include in the assessment?

1. Activities that occur before the pain.

2. What relieves the pain.

3. How he carries out activities of daily living.

4. How he got to the hospital.

270. Mr. Braden is scheduled for a myelogram. Which of the following nursing care considerations is best included in the postprocedure care?

1. Keep the client in bed for 6-8 hours.

2. Allow the client to go to the bathroom as soon as he gets back to his room in order to excrete the dye.

3. Limit fluids.

4. Provide heavy sedation for his spinal headache.

271. The myelogram indicates that Mr. Barden has a ruptured intervertebral disk at L4-5 and is scheduled for a laminectomy. What does the nurse include in the preoperative teaching?

1. Postop "log-rolling."

2. Getting out of bed the third postoperative day.

3. Activities to be avoided after discharge.

4. Use of a turning frame.

272. In the immediate postoperative period, Mr. Barden complains of a severe headache, numbness and tingling in his feet. What is the nurse's first action?
   □ 1. Notify the physician at once.
   □ 2. Medicate him for the discomfort.
   □ 3. Explain that this is normal.
   □ 4. Compare this numbness and tingling with his preoperative neurologic assessment data.

Mrs. Jan Tiplady is seen in the obstetrical clinic to confirm a suspected pregnancy. Her history reveals that she has two children at home, both born at 40 weeks' gestation. She delivered a stillborn at 36 weeks' gestation.

273. Which of the following is a correct determination of Mrs. Tiplady's obstetrical statistics?
   □ 1. T3, P0, A0, L2.
   □ 2. T2, P1, A0, L2.
   □ 3. T2, P0, A1, L2.
   □ 4. T3, P0, A1, L2.
274. Upon assessment, these signs and symptoms are found to be present in Mrs. Tiplady. Which of the following is a correctly identified sign of pregnancy?
   □ 1. Amenorrhea: probable.
   □ 2. Chadwick's sign: probable.
   □ 3. Urine human chorionic gonadotropin (HCG): positive.
   □ 4. Nausea and vomiting: presumptive.
275. Blood is drawn on Mrs. Tiplady for hemoglobin and hematocrit. The results are compared with the CBC done 6 months before conception. Because of the normal physiological changes occurring during pregnancy, the nurse can expect to find
   □ 1. An increase in the hematocrit.
   □ 2. A decrease in the hematocrit.
   □ 3. An increase in the hemoglobin to meet the requirements of the fetus.
   □ 4. No change in the blood levels since the body will maintain homeostasis.
276. At a clinic visit in the tenth week, Mrs. Tiplady relates to the nurse that her pregnancy was planned. However, she finds herself questioning whether this was realistic, with two preschoolers at home. Which of the following responses by the nurse is most appropriate?
   □ 1. "Perhaps you should explore the possibility of terminating the pregnancy."
   □ 2. "It's normal to feel ambivalent. Let's talk about it."
   □ 3. "Once you feel the life within you, these feelings will subside."
   □ 4. "I can arrange an appointment for counseling if you wish."
277. Mrs. Tiplady reveals that she had experienced bladder infections with her past pregnancies. The nurse explains to the client that

   □ 1. Many women have a hereditary predisposition to bladder infection in pregnancy.
   □ 2. Pregnancy predisposes a woman to bladder infections because of dilatation of the ureters and decreased bladder tone.
   □ 3. Although bladder infections occur frequently in pregnancy, they are of little consequence.
   □ 4. Clients are generally placed on prophylactic antibiotics when such a history exists.
278. The nurse provides nutritional counseling for Mrs. Tiplady. Since the client does not like to drink milk, which of the following would best meet her need for calcium?
   □ 1. Nuts and sardines.
   □ 2. Yogurt and cheese.
   □ 3. Meat and leafy vegetables.
   □ 4. Custard and dried fruits.
279. In the sixteenth week, Mrs. Tiplady phones the clinic to report symptoms of frequency and burning when urinating. Which of the following statements indicates that she learned from the early discussion of bladder infection?
   □ 1. "I realize the frequency is due to pressure of the uterus on the bladder."
   □ 2. "I have noticed mild symptoms for the last 10 days."
   □ 3. "I called immediately. I understand this can be serious."
   □ 4. "I refilled my prescription for antibiotics from last year."

Carla Davis comes to the emergency room by herself and tells the admitting nurse that she has been raped.

280. Which of the following is the first action the nurse would take?
   □ 1. Determine Miss Davis' most immediate concern and needs.
   □ 2. Encourage Miss Davis to report the rape to the police.
   □ 3. Identify Miss Davis' support network and contact them.
   □ 4. Perform a vaginal examination.
281. Miss Davis tearfully tells the nurse, "It's all my fault. If I hadn't gone shopping this evening, it wouldn't have happened." The most appropriate response is
   □ 1. "Do you usually go shopping alone in the evening?"
   □ 2. "It is understandable that you feel very upset now; as time goes on you'll feel less uncomfortable about going out alone."
   □ 3. "It would be better to take someone with you in this neighborhood."
   □ 4. "You did not cause this to happen; the person who raped you is responsible."

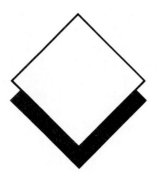

Correct Answers and Rationales: Part Three

188. no. 4. Nitrogenous waste products from protein metabolism result in an elevation of BUN; therefore a low-protein diet is needed. The protein given should be of high biological value (i.e., contain all essential amnio acids). A high-carbohydrate diet will help reverse gluconeogenesis. The client should be weighed daily. Intake is calculated on urine output plus 500-1000 ml of insensible water loss every 24 hours. Her potassium is already elevated; therefore the diet should be restrictive of potassium and may even require the administration of ion-exchange resins such as sodium polystyrene sulfonate (Kayexalate). A-E, IM, PS

189. no. 1. Anemia occurs in chronic renal disease because renal erythropoietin production is decreased and the bone marrow is depressed by the increasing uremia. Because of the decreased ability of the kidneys to excrete waste products and maintain normal fluid and electrolyte balance, hyperkalemia and hypertension develop. The stimulation of the renin-angiotensin mechanism also contributes to the hypertension. The skin becomes very dry because the sweat glands atrophy. A-E, AS, PS

190. no. 3. Milk, meats, fish, and eggs are considered the best sources of high biological-value protein. Some vegetables have all of the essential amino acids but are not consistently the best sources. In contrast, fruits are poor sources of high biological-value protein. A-E, PL, E

191. no. 3. An AV fistula is an *internal* access created by a side-to-side or end-to-end anastomosis of an adjacent vein and artery. This results in an enlarged vein because of the high pressure in the artery. The resulting vessel provides an easy access for venipuncture. Thrombosis at this site can be a major complication. Rejection does not occur, because no foreign material is involved. Dislodgment is not a problem, because the fistula is internal. (An AV *shunt* is external.) Cardiac irritation is a problem with subclavian catheters used for temporary access for hemodialysis. A-E, AS, PS

192. no. 4. The presence of a bruit and a thrill indicates good circulation. Skin temperatures and pulses should be assessed *distal* to the fistula. Blood pressure and venipunctures should never be done in the affected limb in order to help promote the longevity of the fistula. Since an AV fistula is *internal*, it is not possible to assess the color of the blood. A-E, AS, E

193. no. 2. Any fluid retention greater than 300 ml needs to be assessed before continuing with dialysis. Turning the client from side to side may help drain the remaining dialysate, thereby eliminating the need for contacting the physician. Vital signs must be monitored at frequent intervals throughout the dialysis. A-E, IM, PS

194. no. 2. Disequilibrium syndrome is believed by some to be caused by too rapid or excess fluid removal from the circulatory system. Dialysis for a short time (2 to 4 hours) and at a reduced rate of blood flow is effective in decreasing occurrence and severity. A-E, IM, E

195. no. 1. The most common recurring problem with peritoneal dialysis is peritonitis; therefore, education on proper techniques to help decrease its occurrence should take priority. All other listed interventions are also important and should be included in the teaching. A-E, IM, H

196. no. 4. The main defense against transplant rejection is immunosuppressive drugs (e.g., azathioprine [Imuran], prednisone). This therapy is begun before surgery and continues following surgery. It is important for the client not to discontinue this drug therapy unless instructed to do so by a physician, and then the reduction is done slowly over an extended time. Immunosuppressive drugs increase the client's susceptibility to infection. A-E, IM, E

197. no. 2. Atelectasis is the major pulmonary risk for this client. Clear breath sounds are the best indicator of an adequately functioning pulmonary system in the client. Temperature elevation is not an early sign of atelectasis and, if present, might signify many other problems. A lowering of the P_{O_2} may not occur early in atelectasis, and cyanosis is a very late sign of hypoxia. A-E, EV, PS

198. no. 2. This is a period of maximum cardiac output, and as a result, cardiac decompensation may occur. The other potential problems are not necessarily associated with cardiac disease. CBF-A, AN, PS

199. no. 4. Magnesium sulfate is a central nervous system depressant. The client must be closely observed for profound symptoms such as diminished respiratory rate. Muscle cramps indicate toxic effects of the drug; hyperstimulation of reflexes may indicate impending seizure. Anuria is sometimes observed in such a client. CBF-A, EV, E

200. no. 1. The most-needed time for the husband's presence is during transition. The other options show a lack of understanding of the client's needs during labor. CBF-I, EV, PC

201. no. 3. Cold stress increases metabolic efforts; respiratory distress can result. Cyanosis is a late change. A newborn does not shiver to maintain body temperature. CBF-N, AS, PS

202. no. 2. All are important assessments of respiratory function, but only breathing movements are scored as part of the Silverman-Andersen scale. CBF-N, AN, E

203. no. 2. Cephalhematoma is an effusion of blood between the bone and the periosteum. This problem resolves shortly after birth. Intracranial hemorrhage is a life-threatening occurrence. Hydrocephalus requires close monitoring and intervention. CBF-N, AS, H

204. no. 3. Talking to the infant in the first 24 hours is part of early bonding. Since this is the first day, she may need more time to get acquainted with the newborn. It is normal to feel discouraged with initial feeding; this is not likely to indicate attachment problems. CBF-P, AN, H

205. no. 1. Fatigue and hormone changes cause this behavior. If the behavior is prolonged beyond 6 weeks, there may be a serious psychological problem. The client is in the "taking hold" phase of adaptation. CBF-P, AN, PC

206. no. 1. Mastitis can occur 2 to 3 weeks after delivery as organisms enter through a traumatized nipple; thus, nursing periods should be limited and breasts alternated. In early breastfeeding, supplemental feedings should be infrequent. The nursing mother should not attempt weight reduction. CBF-P, PL, H

207. no. 3. When a person is in the manic phase of bipolar disorder he tends to disregard physical needs, and he needs clear, concise, firm, and explicit directions to meet these needs. Option no. 1 evades the issue of taking care of his physical

needs. Option no. 2 is too passive, and, left on his own, he won't come. Option no. 4 is too premature and punitive. P-E, IM, PC

208. no. 3. Manipulative and/or demanding behavior of the manic client is most effectively controlled by limit setting that is clearly spelled out to him, is fair, and is consistently enforced. Leeway when limits are violated may only increase pathological behavior. Since his behavior often provokes staff anger, staff-client arguments and rejection of the client are common. This reaffirms the client's feelings of rejection. It is important to note that only frequent staff conferences and staff planning can provide both a therapeutic plan of care for the client and support for the staff, which is essential if they are to give the needed care. P-E, IM, E

209. no. 4. A manic client often will disregard the basic needs of eating, sleeping, bowel/bladder control, etc., so nurses need to carefully monitor all physical needs. Options no. 1, no. 2, and no. 3 generally are not true during the acute phase of mania. P-E, AN, PC

210. no. 2. Lithium toxicity is closely related to serum lithium levels and can occur at doses close to therapeutic levels. Adverse reactions are seldom encountered at levels below maximum therapeutic levels, except in clients sensitive to lithium. P-E, AS, PS

211. no. 4. Options no. 1 through no. 3 are clinical signs of toxicity that must be detected and reported to the physician immediately. P-E, AS, PS

212. no. 4. This would stimulate the client, not sedate him. Activities that decrease stimuli may help counteract insomnia. Rest and sleep are vital for the manic client, because hyperactivity may lead to dangerous exhaustion. P-E, IM, E

213. no. 4. Antoinette must be kept in the prone position to reduce tension on and prevent trauma to the sac. The spine and semi-Fowler's position would place tension on the sac. The side-lying position is difficult to maintain in a newborn. C-SPP, IM, E

214. no. 3. Before surgical closure of the sac, it is important to prevent drying of the sac so the fragile tissue does not tear and allow cerebrospinal fluid to leak, increasing the risk of meningitis. Sterile saline soaks help to prevent drying. Dry, sterile dressings or leaving the sac open to the air is advocated only if surgery is to be delayed. Petroleum jelly gauze is contraindicated in either case. C-SPP, IM, E

215. no. 1. An elevated temperature accompanied by behavioral changes may be an early sign of infection. Any leak, abrasion, or tear of the meningomyelocele sac would further support the possibility of infection (e.g., meningitis). Assess the sac before notifying the physician. Isolation precautions

should be instituted to protect the other babies and would be appropriate once the sac has been assessed. While Mrs. Davis might help calm Antoinette, it is not appropriate until the nursing assessment is complete. C-SPP, AN, E

216. no. 2. While all of these nursing actions would be appropriate, measuring head circumference daily is essential. Hydrocephalus is a common complication of meningomyelocele. The primary sign of hydrocephalus in infants is head enlargement. Any change in the size of the infant's head can be assessed with daily measurements. C-SPP, IM, E

217. no. 2. The equation should be set up with 125 mg per 1.2 ml = 75 mg per X ml. Thus, 125X = 1.2 multiplied by 75, which becomes 125X = 90.90 divided by 125 = 0.72. Therefore, the nurse should administer 0.72 ml as the correct dose. C-I, IM, PS

218. no. 3. The equation is set up with 30 mg per 4 ml = 20 mg per X ml. Thus, 30X = 20 multiplied by 4, which becomes 30X = 80.80 divided by 30 = 2.6. Therefore, the nurse should administer 2.6 ml as the correct dose. C-I, IM, PS

219. no. 4. Renal problems present a major threat to the life of the child with spina bifida as well as to her self-image and willingness to become involved with activities and individuals outside the home. The other areas may become problematic but are generally not life threatening. C-SPP, AN, PS

220. no. 1. Left-sided congestive heart failure causes pulmonary circulatory congestion, which reduces the diffusion of O_2 and CO_2 across the alveolar membrane. The resultant hypoxia causes dyspnea. Options no. 2, no. 3, and no. 4 may be present with congestive heart failure, but they are not the primary cause of the dyspnea. A-O, AS, PS

221. no. 2. Because of gravity, dependent edema occurs in right-sided congestive heart failure. Cardiac failure edema is also painless and pitting. It does not involve the face. A-O, AS, PS

222. no. 2. The client with congestive heart failure can breathe with more ease in a Fowler's or semi-Fowler's position. Maximal lung expansion is permitted because there is full expansion of the rib cage and there is less upward pressure from the abdominal organs on the diaphragm. A-O, IM, PS

223. no. 1. Respirations in congestive heart failure are rapid and shallow because of the pulmonary circulatory congestion. Deep, stertorous, wheezing, or Biot's respirations are not characteristic of congestive heart failure. A-O, AS, PS

224. no. 3. Rotating tourniquets used in pulmonary edema decrease (not increase) venous return to the right side of the heart. The reduced blood volume decreases the pulmonary and circulatory congestion and pulmonary edema. Rotating tourniquets pro-

duce neither vasoconstriction nor vasodilatation. A-O, AS, PS

225. no. 3. Rotation every 15 minutes ensures that the venous return of a single extremity is occluded for no more than 45 minutes. Shorter or longer periods of venous occlusion are not recommended. A-O, IM, E

226. no. 2. Chest pain, ECG changes, and serum enzymes best indicate the status of a postmyocardial infarction client. All will show definite changes as the infarction process evolves. Leg cramps and changes in serum electrolytes, serum creatinine, and blood urea nitrogen are not indicators of cardiac status following an infarction. A-O, AS, PS

227. no. 1. The first step in a cardiac arrest is to ensure that the client has an open airway. The second priority is to establish breathing. The third priority is to establish cardiac function. A-O, IM, PS

228. no. 4. During a cardiac catheterization, the client may be asked to make verbal responses, change position, and cough and deep-breathe. In order to do this, the client will be only mildly sedated. A-O, IM, E

229. no. 3. A left-sided cardiac catheterization will show coronary artery patency and perfusion of the myocardium. A left-sided cardiac catheterization will not demonstrate any pathological condition in the right side of the heart or the pulmonary artery. A-O, AS, E

230. no. 1. During the left-sided cardiac catheterization, the catheter is introduced into the femoral artery of the leg. After catheterization, the client is cautioned to keep the affected leg extended (not flexed) to avoid any increase in pressure at the puncture site. A-O, PL, PS

231. no. 3. Chronic schizophrenics will sometimes incorporate pain into their delusional system. Option no. 1 may be needed, but only after assessment of the behavior is completed. Although talking is important, the abdominal pains take priority. The symptom described is not an extrapyramidal reaction. P-W, IM, E

232. no. 2. Sameness will increase trust in Mrs. Baxter, but intimacy will frighten her and cause her to withdraw more into herself. A wide variety of caretakers will only increase confusion and reduce trust. Option no. 3 has advantages, but may be overpowering to this client. P-W, IM, PC

233. no. 2. Lengthy explanations will be too confusing. Rather, tell and show her how to take the drugs and she will probably be as reliable with them as she has been with phenothiazines. It is better to return the client to her usual environment than to hold her in the hospital for the needs described. Reliable self-administration is better than forced dependency. P-W, IM, H

234. no. 3. The creatures are part of her hallucinatory world into which she withdraws at times. Hallucinations as described are not usually associated with extrapyramidal reactions, nor is hallucinatory activity viewed as phobic or as flight of ideas. P-W, AN, PC

235. no. 1. This statement acknowledges the importance of the hallucination for Mrs. Baxter without undermining her need for the symptom; it also does not indicate that the nurse regards the hallucination content as real. Interpretation is not usually a part of nursing practice. Option no. 3 supports her hallucination. Option no. 4 is not sensitive to the client's needs. P-W, IM, PC

236. no. 2. The 10-year-old should be involved in all aspects of managing her diabetes, but still requires supervision and support by an adult. Options no. 1 and no. 3 indicate overinvolvement of the parents, while option no. 4 indicates the parents are not providing adequate supervision. A 10-year-old is not yet capable of full self-management. C-I, EV, PC

237. no. 1. Exercise reduces insulin requirements since glucose can be used without insulin during periods of muscular activity. There is an increased risk of insulin shock if nutrition is not modified to reflect changes in caloric requirements during exercise. The risk of hyperglycemia is lowered as a result of exercise. C-NM, AN, PS

238. no. 2. The effect of changes in puberty on dietary and insulin management should be anticipated and discussed with the preadolescent and her family. Rapid weight gain is unexpected in adolescents with IDD, and they cannot be maintained on oral hypoglycemics at any point in their lives. Physical activity should be encouraged. C-NM, PL, PS

239. no. 3. Ketoacidosis is manifested by nausea, vomiting, acetone breath, flushing, dry skin and mucous membranes, and dehydration. The other manifestations are commonly seen with hypoglycemia. A-NM, AS, PS

240. no. 3. The school-age child is developmentally concerned with a sense of industry, which is accomplished through peer interactions and school activities. Fear of painful procedures characterizes preschoolers. The school-age child has little difficulty adjusting to new environments. Justine's activity should not be restricted; therefore, restricted mobility will not be a concern, C-I, AS, PC

241. no. 2. He is probably indicating his discomfort with the group. Perhaps projection is the main defense used in this situation. There is no evidence that John is shy nor that he is angry with any one group member; likewise, there is no evidence that the therapists annoy him. P-T, AN, PC

242. no. 4. He will have the benefit of OT without feeling threatened by the group. Requiring attendance may be useful in the future, but interpersonal group skills are best learned gradually. Withholding the OT experience will not facilitate his learning. Group therapy is entirely different from OT. P-T, PL, E

243. no. 4. Although a symptom of child abuse is that the child exhibits behavior not appropriate to age, playing with a wagon is appropriate for an 8-year-old. Options no. 1, no. 2, and no. 3 are classic behaviors found in abusive relationships. P-SM, AS, PC

244. no. 3. Some abusive parents do not see their behavior as inappropriate. They may have been abused as children and so raise their children as they were raised. None of the behaviors in no. 1, no. 2, and no. 4 are characteristics of abusive parent's actions. P-SM, AN, PC

245. no. 3. The nurse documents behaviors and factual information, which may become evidence. Ideas about what might have happened are not the hospital staff's responsibility to report. Accurate documentation and reporting is required and in the best interest of parent and child. P-SM, IM, E

246. no. 1. Complex, lifelong dynamics of being abused or unable to handle frustration leave the parent overwhelmed by problems. The parent loses control and the ability to change the behavior. Abuse is usually impulsive, not planned. Abusers are frequently the abused of past years. Usually the parent is concerned about actions, but out of control. P-SM, AN, PC

247. no. 4. Recovery for the abused child can be facilitated by the freedom to express emotion in a caring, safe environment. Although sharing details and gaining emotional control are important to the healing process, the expression of emotion is a priority if therapeutic interventions are to be successful. P-SM, PL, PC

248. no. 4. Negative feelings toward abusing parents are not uncommon, and the nurse can handle them professionally by discussing them with the head nurse. Carrying burdens alone does not promote mental health, but the mother should not be burdened with rejection. Staff discussions might be helpful, but violation of professional confidentiality is possible. A-SM, IM PC

249. no. 1. Effective control of anger is important in order to reduce abuse. Problems of child raising tend to increase with the child's age, the complexity of child abuse does not allow for finding a starting point, and focusing on making children follow rules usually reflects negative feelings and does not foster a positive environment. P-SM, IM, PC

250. no. 3. In discussing her own feelings, Mrs. Fredricks can learn how to control stress more effectively. Options no. 1, no. 2, and no. 4 are inappropriate because they focus on Chad rather than Mrs. Fredricks and the interaction. P-SM, EV, PC

251. no. 3. This indicates learning alternatives to anger and harmful punishment, which are significant aspects of nursing interventions for the abusive parents. No. 1 does not indicate changes in behavior patterns when frustrated or angry. No. 2 is a positive change, but, again, does not indicate constructive coping during frustration. No. 4 indicates avoidance rather than successful coping. P-SM, EV, PC

252. no. 3. The laryngectomy tube enters directly into the trachea; it should be suctioned first with sterile equipment. Sterile technique is used to prevent lower airway infections by the introduction of bacteria into the trachea. The nose requires clean technique and can be suctioned with the same catheter after the trachea is suctioned. Intermittent, not constant, suction is used. Only a sterile, water-soluble lubricant is used for the catheter. Oil-based lubricants, such as petroleum jelly, can cause pneumonia if aspirated into the lower airway. A-O, IM, E

253. no. 2. The NG tube is used primarily to prevent food and fluid from contaminating the pharyngeal and esophageal suture line during healing. Swallowing may also be reduced, but it is not the primary reason for the use of the NG tube. A-O, PL, E

254. no. 3. Speech rehabilitation can be started as soon as the esophageal suture line has healed. Time of healing is determined on an individual basis. A-O, IM, H

255. no. 3. This is a task that poses potential danger to a pregnant woman in the first trimester. There would appear to be no risks with the other tasks. CBF-A, AN, H

256. no. 2. There is danger in handling cat litter, so this is an essential aspect of teaching. CBF-A, IM, H

257. no. 1. This response indicates she has learned *essential* content of antepartal teaching. Rest is always important, but first-trimester fatigue is related to hormone changes. The pregnant woman should drink 6 to 8 glasses of fluids daily. Weight should be maintained in early pregnancy to provide for fetal growth. CBF-A, EV, H

258. no. 3. An ultrasound examination would provide information on the fetal development. Estriol and nonstress tests indicate placental-fetal well-being, while the amniocentesis may provide a variety of information, from genetic information to the extent of lung development. CBF-A, AS, PS

259. no. 4. This best meets the couple's needs. Apparently they have misunderstood the physician's explanation. Time to discuss feelings should be provided. CBF, IM, PC

260. no. 1. The signs indicate hypoxia. While the Apgar score is normal, the deprivation of nutrients and oxygen in utero causes retarded intrauterine growth. CBF-N, AN, PS

261. no. 2. The newborn has the ability to calm itself and go into a quiet sleep state. CBF-N, AN, PC

262. no. 1. Since the baby was exposed to infection and deprived of nutrients and oxygen during pregnancy, it is essential to monitor health and growth throughout infancy and childhood. Feeding frequently may depend on volume ingested. A weekly assessment of weight gain is sufficient. CBF-N, PL, H

263. no. 2. The nurse would give priority to collecting data relevant to the known history. The safety of others takes precedence over thought disorders described in options no. 3 and no. 4. Client's fears of being harmed can be worked with later. P-SM, AS, E

264. no. 1. The high-activity milieu may precipitate a sense of losing control in angry clients. Likewise, they rarely can give to others or sustain interaction. Seeking self-centered attention from staff might be viewed as a plea for help. It is the most likely action of this client under the circumstances. The desire for extra sleep is unlikely, as is initiation of interaction in a game requiring competition and concentration. It is also unlikely that he would be concerned with the world outside himself. P-SM, AS, PC

265. no. 2. Only after anger is constructively released can the client focus on specific feelings and self-understanding. Future plans, although important, cannot be realistically developed until anger is reduced. Retrospective understanding requires that present feelings be relieved *first*. P-SM, PL, PC

266. no. 1. To disrupt angry outbursts, get the client's attention by using his name. Give firm, simple directions. Stay with client in order to help him gain internal control. Options no. 2, no. 3, and no. 4 are examples of weakly stated interventions that delay action or do not provide structure. P-SM, IM, E

267. no. 4. It is important to learn about situations that the potentially violent person has handled well. This information can disclose strengths and give the nurse a chance to give positive reinforcement and assess the effects of hospitalization. The feelings in options no. 1 and no. 2 are of secondary importance to control of violent behavior. Option no. 3 does not focus exclusively on negative behavior. P-SM, PL, PC

268. no. 2. The ability to extend relationships beyond the family indicates developing security and independence. It also dilutes the intense family situations that often precipitate violence. Although the behaviors in options no. 1, no. 3, and no. 4 are positive, they do not suggest a high level of significant behavioral change. P-SM, EV, PC

269. no. 4. The mode of transportation to the hospital is not significant as part of the initial assessment. The other assessments listed are pertinent to the client's admitting complaint. A-M, AS, E

270. no. 1. Bed rest is necessary for 6 to 8 hours to prevent a spinal headache. Although the client may need to void, he cannot get out of bed. Fluids are to be encouraged for rehydration and replacement of cerebrospinal fluid and to minimize headache after the lumbar puncture. Only mild sedation is required for a spinal headache. If an oil-based dye was used, the head of the bed is elevated after the procedure to prevent the dye from coming into contact with the meninges and causing irritation. If a water-based dye was used, the bed may be kept flat. A-M, IM, E

271. no. 1. Postoperatively, the client is turned as a unit (i.e., log-rolled). A turning frame is used if the client has a fusion. The client will be out of bed on the first or second postoperative day. Activities to be avoided after discharge would be included in discharge instructions. A-M, IM, E

272. no. 4. Postoperative numbness and tingling should be compared to the client's preoperative neurological assessment data. If the client had no numbness and tingling preoperatively, or if numbness and tingling are more severe, the nurse notifies the physician. Sensory manifestations may be due to inflammatory changes and will be temporary. However, they always must be assessed. A-M, EV, E

273. no. 2. This item requires correct identification of terms used in a TPAL chart; analysis of data in the history leads to the only correct response. T = term births (two pregnancies carried to 40 weeks' gestation); P = premature births (the stillborn delivered at 36 weeks' gestation is considered a premature birth); A = abortion history (the client has no history of abortions, since all pregnancies extended beyond 20 weeks); L = number of living children (two living children). CBF-A, AS, H

274. no. 4. Morning sickness is correctly classified as a "presumptive sign." Amenorrhea and Chadwick's sign are also presumptive signs of pregnancy. Urine positive for HCG is a probable sign of pregnancy (95%-98%) accuracy). CBF-A, AN, PS

275. no. 2. There is an increase in both plasma and cells during pregnancy. However, the increase in plasma is greater than the increase in red blood cells. This results in a hemodilution of blood, causing a fall in the hematocrit. This is referred to as the normal physiological anemia of pregnancy. CBF-A, AS, PS

276. no. 2. Ambivalence is a normal psychological reaction during the first trimester. In communicating therapeutically, it is important to relate to the client that such feelings are frequently experienced. The nurse should allow the client to ventilate her feelings regarding this. The other options do not encourage the client to share feelings; rather, they immediately suggest an alternative or focus on long-term changes. CBF-A, IM, PC

277. no. 2. Increasing progesterone levels during pregnancy result in smooth-muscle relaxation, leading to dilatation of the ureters (especially the right ureter) and decreased bladder tone. Urinary stasis is thus created, contributing to bladder infections. Bladder infection during pregnancy can lead to serious complications for both mother and fetus. If an infection occurs, antibiotics may be prescribed. However, using such medication preventively is never suggested because of the teratogenic potential. CBF-A, IM, H

278. no. 2. Cheese and yogurt are both good substitutes for milk. Other sources of calcium include some fish, including sardines, ice cream, and dried beans. Although leafy vegetables and grains contain calcium, recent research indicates that it is poorly absorbed. CBF-A, IM, H

279. no. 3. This reflects an understanding of potential risks. Although bladder pressure causes frequency in the first and third trimesters, burning is never expected. Since the remaining options indicate delayed or self-treatment, they are incorrect. CBF-A, EV, E

280. no. 1. This is a nonjudgmental, empathetic intervention. It allows the client to begin to reestablish a sense of control that was lost when she was raped. No. 2 presents the nurse's viewpoint and can impede the client's independent decision making. No. 3 and no. 4 are important, but should be done when client is ready. P-SM, PL, PC

281. no. 4. Reinforce the responsibility of the rapist, not the victim. Recognize that victims feel guilt, but do not reinforce those guilt feelings. No. 1 does not acknowledge the client's feelings and may be interpreted by the client as reinforcement of them. No. 2 offers reassurance, but does not address guilt feelings. No. 3 would reinforce guilt feelings. P-SM, IM, PC

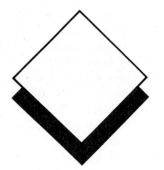

Sample Test Questions: Part Four

A new client, John Small, has been admitted to a 20-bed psychiatric unit of a university hospital. He was brought in by the police after getting in a fight and tearing up a bar. He is 6 feet 3 inches tall and weighs 275 pounds. At present, he is pacing in the unit recreation room, mumbling. His jaws are tight and his hands are clenched. Other clients are afraid of him and are trying to avoid him by going to their rooms.

282. Which of the following would the nurse best use initially in an attempt to prevent a crisis on the unit?
    ☐ 1. Keep the other clients away and observe Mr. Small's behavior until he calms down.
    ☐ 2. Place Mr. Small in seclusion immediately and then help him to verbally express his anger.
    ☐ 3. Approach Mr. Small on a one-to-one basis and offer him a PRN medication immediately.
    ☐ 4. Approach Mr. Small on a one-to-one basis, help him identify his anger, and offer him alternatives.

283. The milieu (environment) is a very important tool in working with an angry client. The environment may be therapeutic or nontherapeutic. Which of the following descriptions suggests an environment that would be most helpful in preventing a crisis for Mr. Small?
    ☐ 1. Large outside grounds, art activities, and a variety of places for Mr. Small to be alone.
    ☐ 2. Many programmed activities that encourage him to become involved in his own goals and treatment.
    ☐ 3. Setting firm, clear rules and limits.
    ☐ 4. Freedom for him to determine his own privileges.

284. Mr. Small continues to exhibit increasing signs of anxiety. He is shouting at and threatening the nurse and other clients. The nurse would take all of the following actions except
    ☐ 1. Offer Mr. Small a chance to dice the carrots for the salad being served at dinner.
    ☐ 2. Call a crisis team that could, if necessary, quickly subdue Mr. Small.

    ☐ 3. Prepare for Mr. Small a PRN medication and a seclusion room with restraints.
    ☐ 4. Keep the other clients away from Mr. Small.

285. Mr. Small continues to become more agitated, and he attempts to hit another client. The nurse decides that he needs to be placed in seclusion with full leather restraints. Which one of the following interventions would not be used when restraining a client?
    ☐ 1. Have an established team that can move as quickly as possible.
    ☐ 2. Remove the glasses and jewelry of staff and the client to prevent Mr. Small from destroying anything.
    ☐ 3. Identify for Mr. Small the positive behaviors the staff expects from him.
    ☐ 4. Use more staff and security guards whenever possible as members of the team.

286. Mr. Small has been out of seclusion for several hours. He is saying that his rights have been violated, and he demands to leave the hospital. The law includes several important provisions that apply to seclusion, restraints, and medication. Which one of the following statements would not apply in this situation?
    ☐ 1. Mr. Small can refuse to be placed in seclusion and restraints.
    ☐ 2. He can refuse to take his medication.
    ☐ 3. He can be retained in the hospital against his will if he is admitted by the state under an emergency or involuntary admission.
    ☐ 4. Mr. Small is entitled to legal counsel to discuss his future plans and concerns.

287. Mr. Small expresses concern about others knowing all about his "private life and behavior." Provisions have been made in the law to speak to his concerns. Which one of the following would not pertain to his concern?
    ☐ 1. Clients should have access to phones where others cannot hear conversations.
    ☐ 2. Information in clinical records should not be a part of the public record.

3. Information cannot be released without the client's consent.

4. Staff must include specific information in a separate document that is not part of the hospital record.

288. The timing of interventions for angry, aggressive behavior is best when the intervention occurs
    1. Before the initial anxiety is converted to aggressive behavior.
    2. After the aggressive act has occurred.
    3. During the aggressive act.
    4. After the initial anxiety.

Seven-month-old Maria Juarez has a congenitally dislocated right hip.

289. The nurse should expect to note which finding when assessing Maria?
    1. Easily abducted right hip.
    2. Lengthening of the right leg.
    3. Severe pain on hip movement.
    4. Widening of the perineum.

290. Maria has been fitted with a von Rosen splint. During a home visit to evaluate the effectiveness of teaching Maria's parents how to care for Maria during the treatment period, which outcome demonstrated by the parents indicates they understand the seriousness of Maria's defect?
    1. Her parents apply and remove the splint correctly.
    2. The Juarezes keep Maria in the splint at all times except when she is being bathed.
    3. Mr. and Mrs. Juarez change Maria's position at least every 2 hours.
    4. The parents provide age-appropriate sensorimotor activities and stimulation for Maria.

The labor-room nurse is monitoring the induction of labor for a primigravida, Mary Albert, who has failed to progress in labor over 24 hours.

291. In evaluating the action of the medication oxytocin (Pitocin), which of the following indicates an adverse effect?
    1. A contraction lasting over 120 seconds.
    2. A decrease in blood pressure.
    3. Urinary output of 100 ml per hour.
    4. Increasing intensity of contractions.

292. The induction stimulates regular contractions, and Mrs. Albert is now in active labor. She expresses concern about her ability to behave as she would wish during the remainder of labor. Which of these nursing interventions would be most supportive?
    1. Acknowledge that responses are often influenced by culture.
    2. Inform her that medication is available if she needs it.

3. Instruct the client in relaxation and breathing exercises.

4. Reassure her that she is accepted regardless of behavior.

293. Mrs. Albert delivers a 7-lb daughter. Thirty minutes after delivery, the fundus is firm, 1 in below the umbilicus; lochia is rubra; client complains of thirst; there are slight tremors of lower extremities. Analysis of these data suggests
    1. Impending shock.
    2. Circulatory overload.
    3. Subinvolution.
    4. Normal postpartum adaptation.

294. Two hours after delivery, Mrs. Albert complains of severe perineal pain. Which nursing action is a priority?
    1. Administer prescribed pain medication.
    2. Initiate sitz baths.
    3. Inspect the perineum.
    4. Teach perineal muscle exercises.

295. Which of the following nursing assessments suggests bladder distension 6 hours after delivery?
    1. Poor abdominal muscle tone.
    2. Increased lochia rubra with clots.
    3. hard, contracted uterus.
    4. Uterus soft to the right of midline.

Juanita Sanchez, age 78, has been living with her daughter since her husband's death 5 years ago. She has become increasingly forgetful and unable to care for herself. She wanders away from home frequently and is argumentative because of organic brain syndrome. The family has decided to place Mrs. Sanchez in a nursing home.

296. Based on the diagnosis of organic brain syndrome, nursing assessment of Mrs. Sanchez would most likely reveal which of the following intellectual changes?
    1. Decreased ability to handle anxiety.
    2. Disorientation to time and place.
    3. Emotional lability.
    4. Paranoid ideation.

297. Mrs. Sanchez becomes more confused after she has been admitted to the nursing home. Which of the following actions would be most helpful to decrease her confusion?
    1. Assist Mrs. Sanchez with all activities of daily living.
    2. Find out from the family what her usual daily routine is and follow it as closely as possible.
    3. Restrict visitors during the first 2 weeks so that she can adjust to the nursing home.
    4. Wait for the confusion to decrease as Mrs. Sanchez adjusts to her new environment.

298. Mrs. Sanchez's increased confusion is probably caused by
   ☐ 1. Anger at her daughter.
   ☐ 2. Decreased personal space.
   ☐ 3. Increased brain deterioration.
   ☐ 4. Unfamiliar surroundings.

299. Mrs. Sanchez frequently wanders from her room into other clients' rooms or out to the street. The most effective nursing intervention would be to
   ☐ 1. Accompany Mrs. Sanchez when she wanders and guide her to her room or the dayroom.
   ☐ 2. Ask Mrs. Sanchez to explain why she cannot remain in her room or public areas.
   ☐ 3. Confine Mrs. Sanchez to her room, because she gets lost too frequently.
   ☐ 4. Restrain Mrs. Sanchez in her chair; so she will not disturb others or become lost.

300. Mrs. Sanchez repeatedly attempts to leave the nursing home, stating, "My husband is waiting at home for me. I have to leave work now." The nurse's most appropriate response is
   ☐ 1. "He knows you're staying here tonight; come back in now."
   ☐ 2. "Mrs. Sanchez, you know you retired 13 years ago and your husband is dead."
   ☐ 3. "You can't leave now; you have to stay here."
   ☐ 4. "Your husband died 5 years ago, and you're in the nursing home now."

301. Mrs. Sanchez's daughter states that Mrs. Sanchez had lost 11 pounds in the past 3 months. Which of the following would be the most appropriate nursing intervention to ensure adequate nutrition?
   ☐ 1. Feed Mrs. Sanchez when she does not finish her meal.
   ☐ 2. Give Mrs. Sanchez six small feedings during the day.
   ☐ 3. Tell Mrs. Sanchez that she will be tube-fed if she does not eat.
   ☐ 4. Observe Mrs. Sanchez's eating, and weigh her before developing a plan.

302. Which of the following will be most effective in helping Mrs. Sanchez to maintain a reality orientation?
   ☐ 1. Call Mrs. Sanchez by name and identify yourself each time you enter her room.
   ☐ 2. Encourage Mrs. Sanchez to spend her time watching television in her room.
   ☐ 3. Plan a different schedule of activities every day to prevent boredom.
   ☐ 4. Rotate staff assignments so she will know each staff member.

303. Mrs. Sanchez is most likely to demonstrate which of the following?
   ☐ 1. Decreased attention span and ability to learn new things.
   ☐ 2. Equal recall of both recent and past events.

   ☐ 3. Increased ability to adapt to change in her environment.
   ☐ 4. Increased interest in hygiene and grooming.

304. The nurse notes that Mrs. Sanchez frequently confabulates when asked about her everyday activities. She does this in order to
   ☐ 1. Fill in memory gaps.
   ☐ 2. Get attention from the nurse.
   ☐ 3. Increase her attention span.
   ☐ 4. Prevent regression.

305. The night nurse reports that Mrs. Sanchez is very confused, is in and out of bed, and makes multiple requests for assistance throughout the night. Which of the following nursing actions would most effectively lessen her confusion?
   ☐ 1. Alter her bedtime routine to increase physical activity.
   ☐ 2. Give her a detailed explanation of her need for adequate rest.
   ☐ 3. Turn on night-lights in her bedroom and bathroom.
   ☐ 4. Give her a sedative to help her sleep.

306. Mrs. Sanchez has difficulty deciding what to wear in the morning. The most effective nursing intervention would be to
   ☐ 1. Give her as much time as she needs to make her own decision.
   ☐ 2. Help her select an outfit and get dressed.
   ☐ 3. Lay out her clothes each morning before she awakens.
   ☐ 4. Tell her she must hurry or she will miss breakfast.

307. Mrs. Sanchez tells her daughter not to visit since she does not care enough to let her own mother stay at home. The daughter tells the nurse, "I don't know what to do. Mother's so angry she doesn't want to see me. But I had to do something. We couldn't take care of her anymore." The nurse's most appropriate initial response would be
   ☐ 1. "Wait a few days and she'll get over this."
   ☐ 2. "She'll be OK once she gets settled here; don't worry."
   ☐ 3. "You feel guilty about leaving your mother here."
   ☐ 4. "This is a very difficult time for you and your mother."

308. The daughter asks if she should come back the next day to visit. The nurse's most appropriate response would be
   ☐ 1. "Come back tomorrow; your interest is important for your mother."
   ☐ 2. "Is there anyone else who could visit your mother?"
   ☐ 3. "Wait until your mother calls you to say she wants to see you."
   ☐ 4. "Your mother will be busy with the staff and clients. She won't miss you if you don't come."

309. An hour after her daughter leaves, Mrs. Sanchez tells the nurse, "I haven't seen my daughter in days. Something must be wrong." The nurse's most appropriate response would be
    □ 1. "Are you afraid she won't come back to visit you?"
    □ 2. "I'm sure you'll hear from her again soon."
    □ 3. "You're confused; she was here earlier tonight."
    □ 4. "Your daughter was here before dinner this evening."

310. Which of the following would be most helpful in providing ongoing care for Mrs. Sanchez?
    □ 1. Follow her usual routine as much as possible.
    □ 2. Involve her in all unit activities to decrease her loneliness.
    □ 3. Provide one-to-one teaching sessions to help her understand her limitations.
    □ 4. Adhere strictly to the unit's routine.

Eleven-year-old Gail is hospitalized with rheumatic fever with carditis and polyarthritis. She also has Sydenham's chorea.

311. Which of the following is true concerning rheumatic fever?
    □ 1. It is usually associated with glomerulonephritis.
    □ 2. Symptoms disappear shortly after the fever abates and the temperature returns to normal.
    □ 3. The child should resume normal activities as soon as she feels well.
    □ 4. It usually follows a streptococcal infection.

312. In planning nursing care, the nurse notes that Gail is on bed rest. What is the rationale for this?
    □ 1. To help the pain of the arthritis that accompanies the disease.
    □ 2. To minimize the effects of the carditis.
    □ 3. So other children will not see Gail's choreiform movements.
    □ 4. To help alleviate the febrile effects of the disease.

313. Which of the following is likely to be the major psychological stressor of Gail's illness and hospitalization?
    □ 1. Fear of painful procedures.
    □ 2. Separation from her family.
    □ 3. Activity restriction.
    □ 4. Worry about possible outcomes.

314. Which of the following children should the nurse select as Gail's roommate?
    □ 1. Seven-year-old Susan, who also has rheumatic fever.
    □ 2. Ten-year-old Amy with insulin-dependent diabetes.
    □ 3. Thirteen-year-old Sharon with sickle cell vasoocclusive crisis.
    □ 4. Twelve-year-old Evelyn with fever of unknown origin.

315. Which of the following activities is most appropriate for Gail?
    □ 1. Listening to records and the radio.
    □ 2. Watching television.
    □ 3. Playing Ping-Pong in the game room.
    □ 4. Crocheting a small afghan.

316. Gail's blood tests show the following results. Which is the most indicative of an improvement in her condition?
    □ 1. Positive C-reactive protein.
    □ 2. White blood cell count of 11,000.
    □ 3. Decreased erythrocyte sedimentation rate (ESR).
    □ 4. Elevated antistreptolysin O (ASO) titer.

317. Gail is readmitted to the hospital 2 months later for a cardiac catheterization. When preparing Gail for the procedure, the nurse should take into account which of the following?
    □ 1. Concrete explanations and experiences will be most meaningful.
    □ 2. Gail is likely to misinterpret the procedure as punishment for previous misbehavior.
    □ 3. Gail should be given a full verbal explanation of the procedure using correct medical terminology.
    □ 4. Gail should be allowed to make all decisions concerning her care.

Elizabeth Johnson, 21, delivered her first child this morning, after a long and difficult labor, with the fetus in posterior position.

318. Which of the following behaviors is common during this time of restoration and is characteristic of "taking-in"?
    □ 1. Showing an interest in newborn care.
    □ 2. Asking if "rooming-in" can begin immediately.
    □ 3. Talking constantly about the labor and delivery.
    □ 4. Experiencing mild transient feelings of depression.

319. In evaluating Mrs. Johnson's condition on the day after delivery, which finding suggests normal reproductive adaptation?
    □ 1. Fundus firm, 1 cm below the umbilicus.
    □ 2. Scant lochia serosa.
    □ 3. Moderate breast engorgement.
    □ 4. Perineal sutures healed.

320. On the third day after delivery, Mrs. Johnson complains of breast engorgement. Her 6-lb infant sucks briefly, then sleeps when put to breast. An appropriate plan is for the client to
    □ 1. Restrict intake of fluids until engorgement is relieved.
    □ 2. Use ice packs on breasts just before nursing.
    □ 3. Pump or express milk when the baby does not empty breasts.
    □ 4. Discontinue breastfeeding temporarily until the newborn is alert.

321. Mrs. Johnson asks if breastfeeding will change the shape of her breast. Which of the following is an appropriate response?
   □ 1. "Yes, the shape of your breast may be affected if the baby is allowed to nurse too vigorously."
   □ 2. "Breastfeeding does not affect the shape of the breast. However, wearing a proper breast support is important."
   □ 3. "If you breastfeed for more than 6 months, the shape of the breast will change."
   □ 4. "Breastfeeding may change the shape of the breast; however, this shouldn't be the most important consideration."

322. Before discharge, both Mr. and Mrs. Johnson attend several classes on infant care. Which statement by the new father indicates he has a realistic understanding of newborn behavior?
   □ 1. "I hope we can get him on a schedule of two naps and a full night's sleep."
   □ 2. "I don't want him to be spoiled, so he'll learn quickly not to cry for attention."
   □ 3. "If we can get him on a schedule for feedings, he'll nurse better."
   □ 4. "It looks like the next weeks will be mostly feeding, changing, and caring for baby."

323. At the postpartum clinic visit, Mrs. Johnson seems very discouraged about breastfeeding. She says, "Neither baby Tim nor I seem to be successful at this breastfeeding. Maybe it's because I am so small." The nurse's response to the mother is based on the understanding of which of the following?
   □ 1. Hormone levels may vary in individual women.
   □ 2. Desire to breastfeed affects milk production.
   □ 3. Primigravidas are usually apprehensive about feeding.
   □ 4. Breast size is not a factor in volume of milk produced.

Twenty-two-month-old Katie is admitted to the pediatric unit with acute laryngotracheobronchitis.

324. When a nursing history is taken, Katie's mother tells the nurse that Katie is toilet trained. Which additional information is the most important for the nurse to ascertain?
   □ 1. The age at which Katie began toilet training.
   □ 2. Katie's toilet habits and routine at home.
   □ 3. Katie's mother's understanding of the possibility of regression in Katie's toileting habits while she is hospitalized.
   □ 4. Katie's willingness to accept help from the nursing staff with her toileting needs.

325. Developmentally, Katie should exhibit which of the following behaviors?
   □ 1. Dress and undress herself without help.
   □ 2. Share her toys with other children.
   □ 3. Speak in 5- to 6-word sentences.

   □ 4. Feed herself well with a spoon.

326. Katie has an IV of 500 ml of 5% dextrose in 0.25% normal saline ordered to infuse over 8 hours. The nurse should set the microdrip regulator to infuse at a rate of how many drops per minute?
   □ 1. 21.
   □ 2. 30.
   □ 3. 63.
   □ 4. 125.

327. Katie is in a croup tent with compressed air. Nursing care of Katie should include which measure?
   □ 1. Explain to her why she must stay in the tent.
   □ 2. Restrict her fluid intake to no more than 32 oz a day.
   □ 3. Administer a cough suppressant to control her cough.
   □ 4. Change her wet bed linens frequently.

328. Chest percussion and postural drainage are prescribed four times a day for Katie. When should the nurse plan to carry out Katie's chest therapy?
   □ 1. Just before Katie eats and at bedtime.
   □ 2. Halfway between mealtimes and at bedtime.
   □ 3. Upon arising and 1 hour after meals.
   □ 4. During intervals between Katie's naps.

329. Following chest percussion and postural drainage, which finding indicates that the treatment has not been entirely effective?
   □ 1. Inspiratory stridor.
   □ 2. Rales and rhonchi.
   □ 3. Suprasternal retractions.
   □ 4. Harsh metallic cough.

330. Katie is hospitalized for 4 days. Katie's parents visit every evening but are unable to stay with her overnight. Which behavior is Katie most likely to demonstrate when separating from her parents?
   □ 1. Readily seeks comfort from the nurse.
   □ 2. Sucks her thumb, whines, and curls up in a corner of her crib.
   □ 3. Cries loudly and tries to cling to her parents.
   □ 4. Waves and blows them a kiss.

331. When planning care for the hospitalized toddler whose mother cannot room-in, which nursing action would be most appropriate?
   □ 1. Encourage the mother to leave an article of her clothing.
   □ 2. Assign the toddler a roommate close in age to keep him or her company.
   □ 3. Inform the mother that toddlers handle separation easily.
   □ 4. Suggest that mother limit visits to reduce the toddler's separation anxiety.

332. When Katie is discharged, which instruction to Katie's parents is not appropriate?
   □ 1. Katie may show some regression in her behavior for a few weeks.

☐ 2. Katie should not be separated from her parents for lengthy periods until she feels secure again.

☐ 3. Katie should be allowed to sleep with her parents for a few nights until she readjusts to being home.

☐ 4. Katie's parents should reinstate limits that were in effect before her hospitalization.

Stanley Brown, a 50-year-old man who has been a heavy smoker for the past 20 years, is admitted to the hospital with a diagnosis of emphysema with right-lower-lobe pneumonia. Upon his arrival at the medical floor, the nurse carries out the assessment, which is as follows: extremely dyspneic, ashen in color, perspiring profusely, very agitated, and coughing up large amounts of tenacious white sputum. Mr. Brown's orders include stat blood gases; O_2 at 2 L; aminophylline IV drip; sputum for culture and sensitivity; start ampicillin (Polycillin) 1 g after sputum is obtained.

333. All of the following information is provided by Mr. Brown. What probably precipitated his emphysema flare-up?

☐ 1. He wore a new cotton suit 2 days ago.

☐ 2. He smoked more cigarettes than usual 3 days ago.

☐ 3. He went bowling last week.

☐ 4. He has had a cold for the past week.

334. What is the expected action of aminophylline?

☐ 1. Increase the production of sputum.

☐ 2. Relax the bronchial muscle.

☐ 3. Promote sleep and relieve anxiety.

☐ 4. Liquefy tenacious sputum.

335. To detect a common side effect of aminophylline, the nurse should assess Mr. Brown for the possible development of which symptom?

☐ 1. Generalized dermatitis.

☐ 2. Hematuria.

☐ 3. Urinary retention.

☐ 4. Tachycardia.

336. Mr. Brown's blood-gas results demonstrate a pH of 7.37, Po_2 of 65 mm Hg, and a Pco_2 of 50 mm Hg. On the basis of this information, which statement is most justified?

☐ 1. Mr. Brown has acute respiratory insufficiency and needs to have his O_2 turned up to 8 L.

☐ 2. Mr. Brown has acute pulmonary failure and needs to be placed on a ventilator.

☐ 3. Mr. Brown has adapted to his high level of arterial CO_2 and is in chronic respiratory acidosis.

☐ 4. Mr. Brown demonstrates chronic respiratory acidosis and will soon display neurological changes.

337. Mr. Brown produces sputum, which is sent to the lab for culture and sensitivity. Then, IV ampicillin (Polycillin) is started. The nurse knows that this drug belongs to the penicillin family of antibiotics and that the pencillins, among all the antimicro-

bials, are most often responsible for which of the following?

☐ 1. Anaphylaxis.

☐ 2. Urinary retention.

☐ 3. Nausea and vomiting.

☐ 4. Gastric perforation.

338. Mr. Brown does not improve. On the third day after hospital admission, his temperature is 103.4° F (39.7° C), he has right-sided chest pain and decreased right-sided chest excursion. A portable chest x-ray reveals further extension of his pneumonia with a spontaneous pneumothroax. Mr. Brown is informed by Dr. Stone that a chest tube must be inserted immediately. To assist Mr. Brown in complying with this procedure, which of the following pieces of information does the nurse need to have in order to be of most help in answering his questions?

☐ 1. The pneumothorax is caused by disruption in the integrity of the pleura.

☐ 2. A rib has fractured and is causing changes in thoracic pressures.

☐ 3. Air has collected in the mediastinal space.

☐ 4. The pneumothorax is caused by the accumulation of pus in the lung tissue.

339. Mr. Brown asks the nurse how the chest tube will help him to breathe with greater ease. Which of the following responses by the nurse would be *incorrect*?

☐ 1. The chest tube will allow for the drainage of fluid and air from the pleural space.

☐ 2. The chest tube will aid in reestablishing positive pressure in the pleural space.

☐ 3. The chest tube will aid in reexpanding the lung.

☐ 4. The chest tube will aid in reestablishing negative pressure in the pleural space.

340. After the chest tube is inserted and connected to the Pleur-Evac, Mr. Brown wants to know why there are water "bubbles" in the water-seal container. Which of these responses by the nurse would be best?

☐ 1. "You should ask your doctor for more information."

☐ 2. "It indicates that the system is working correctly."

☐ 3. "Oh! Don't worry about it. I am taking good care of you."

☐ 4. "It indicates that your lung has not fully expanded."

341. Mr. Brown progresses well. After one week postoperatively, his chest tube is removed. Mr. Brown tells the nurse he realizes proper nutrition is very important for his future health, but he just does not have much of an appetite. Which of these responses by the nurse would be most helpful?

☐ 1. Eat three large meals a day that are high in carbohydrates.

    2. Eat three large meals a day that are high in protein.

    3. Eat six small meals a day that are high in carbohydrates.

    4. Eat six small meals a day that are high in protein.

342. When Mr. Brown is discharged, he and his wife are referred to the Visiting Nurse Association. Mr. Brown and his wife will more readily accept aid from this organization if which of the following is noted?

    1. The need they think they have for such help.

    2. The enthusiasm of the nurse who plans their care.

    3. The availability of the help.

    4. The willingness of Mrs. Brown to accept the help.

Following a car accident, Michael Lamaroux, a 34-year-old construction worker, is admitted to a medical-surgical unit for treatment of fractured femurs and a fractured right hip. He had been drinking and hit another car. Although Mr. Lamaroux's blood-alcohol level is high, he insists that he only had one beer. He is to have surgery for reduction of his fractured hip.

343. He tells his nurse that he is especially sensitive to pain and has used oxycadone (Percodan) for headaches in the past. What is the best initial statement the nurse can make?

    1. "Do you have any medications with you that were not prescribed by a physician?"

    2. "Be sure not to take any medications except what we give you for pain."

    3. "Have you ever felt like you needed medication to help you get through the day?"

    4. "I need you to make a verbal contract with me right now that you will not take any medication except what is ordered for you at this time. Other drugs may interfere with your anesthetic tomorrow."

344. In order for withdrawal symptoms to occur in a person with a substance use disorder, which of the following is *not* necessary?

    1. Physiological dependence.

    2. Marked tolerance.

    3. Diminished intake.

    4. Cessation of intake.

345. Which of the following ego-defense mechanisms is a top and continuing priority in dealing with alcoholic clients?

    1. Dependency.

    2. Denial.

    3. Paranoia.

    4. Projection.

346. Of all the following approaches to the treatment of alcoholism, which has been found to be the most effective to date?

    1. Membership in Alcoholics Anonymous.

    2. Family-systems approach.

    3. Treating the alcoholism as a chronic disease.

    4. Individual psychotherapy.

347. Following inpatient treatment for his fractures and for his substance abuse, Mr. Lamaroux agrees to involve himself in therapy. Which of the following would have the *least* influence on the structure of family-therapy sessions?

    1. Genetic factors and chronic disease effects of alcoholism.

    2. History of alcoholism in other family members and the previous generation.

    3. Overfunctioning and underfunctioning within the family.

    4. How closeness and distance are dealt with in the family.

348. Which of the following interventions would be the nurse's highest priority in the detoxification stage of alcoholism?

    1. Confront manipulative behavior designed to gain access to alcohol.

    2. Administer vitamin B supplements, knowing that alcoholism has resulted in a severe depletion.

    3. Report potassium level of 1.4 mEq/L.

    4. Provide ample opportunities to decrease social isolation and improve social skills.

349. As Mr. Lamaroux progresses in his treatment he remarks to the nurse, "I'm no good. My drinking has almost destroyed everything I value most." Which response from the nurse would be most helpful?

    1. "What did you do that was so bad?"

    2. "Yes, it's time you stopped drinking."

    3. "Have you been to this stage of treatment before?"

    4. "It sounds like you're feeling guilty about your drinking."

350. In revising the goals, the nurse writes, "Client will decrease drug-seeking, manipulative, and acting-out behaviors." Which of the following nursing orders is *not* appropriate for the updated care plan in light of Mr. Lamaroux's drug and alcohol problems?

    1. Set firm and consistent limits.

    2. Clearly define acceptable and unacceptable behavior.

    3. Hold a care conference to assure that entire staff adopt a consistent approach to client's behavior.

    4. Provide a high level of sympathy and empathy for his difficulties.

Sylvia Marlin, a 28-year-old newlywed, is admitted to the hospital with an enlarged thyroid gland.

351. In taking a nursing history, which of the following is considered a risk factor in the development of cancer of the thyroid?
☐ 1. A diet low in iodine.
☐ 2. A diet high in iodine.
☐ 3. A history of high doses of vitamin D.
☐ 4. A history of irradiation of the head or neck.

352. In carrying out an initial and daily assessment of a client with thyroid enlargement, the nurse will carefully observe for which of the following?
☐ 1. Difficulty in swallowing or breathing.
☐ 2. Excessive saliva production.
☐ 3. Muscle twitching.
☐ 4. Tingling around the lips.

353. In addition to having an enlarged thyroid gland, Mrs. Marlin has been experiencing symptoms suggestive of hyperthyroidism. What might these symptoms include?
☐ 1. Fatigue, weight gain, dry skin, and cold intolerance.
☐ 2. Decreased pulse rate, slurred speech, constipation, and cold intolerance.
☐ 3. Nervousness, weight loss, tachycardia, and heat intolerance.
☐ 4. Abdominal pain, diarrhea, fatty food intolerance, and heat intolerance.

354. Mrs. Marlin's laboratory workup will probably indicate which of the following?
☐ 1. Deficiency of serum T_3 and/or T_4.
☐ 2. Increased levels of serum T_3 and/or T_4.
☐ 3. Deficiency of serum TSH.
☐ 4. Increased levels of serum ACTH.

355. A serious form of hyperthyroidism results in a condition known as what?
☐ 1. Myxedema.
☐ 2. Cretinism.
☐ 3. Graves' disease.
☐ 4. Addison's disease.

356. Mrs. Marlin's hyperfunctioning thyroid results in exophthalmos. Nursing interventions specific for this problem should include which of the following?
☐ 1. Frequent mouth care using a soft toothbrush and normal saline mouthwash.
☐ 2. A private room with decreased environmental stimulation and light.
☐ 3. Lubricating eye drops and instructions to blink at regular intervals.
☐ 4. Frequent monitoring of vital signs and body temperature.

357. Mrs. Marlin's diagnosis workup includes a radioactive iodine (RAI) uptake. In preparing the client for this procedure, what should the nurse do?
☐ 1. Take a history of all recent medications and x-ray examinations.
☐ 2. Place the client on a low-sodium diet for 3 days before the test.
☐ 3. Prepare the client for isolation using radiation precautions.
☐ 4. Instruct the client in 24-hour urine collection techniques.

358. To inhibit thyroid hormone synthesis, Mrs. Marlin is given propylthiouracil (PTU). In reviewing this medication with her before discharge, the nurse would include all of the following *except* which one?
☐ 1. Report weight loss and increased pulse rate.
☐ 2. Report fever, sore throat, or rash.
☐ 3. Take the drug once daily at the same time each day.
☐ 4. Some weight gain is to be expected.

359. Antithyroid drug therapy has proved to be ineffective. Mrs. Marlin is readmitted to the hospital for thyroidectomy. Before the thyroidectomy, an iodine solution has been administered for several weeks in order to decrease the vascularity and size of the thyroid gland. When giving an iodine solution, the nurse should do which of the following?
☐ 1. Give the drug on an empty stomach to speed its rate of absorption.
☐ 2. Dilute the drug in fruit juice, milk, or water.
☐ 3. Avoid giving the drug with milk or antacids.
☐ 4. Avoid giving the drug at bedtime.

360. Before her surgery, Mrs. Marlin acquires coryza, stomatitis, and swollen salivary glands. What should the nurse do?
☐ 1. Put the client in protective isolation.
☐ 2. Isolate the client from other preoperative clients.
☐ 3. Evaluate the client's diet for excessive iodine intake.
☐ 4. Hold the iodine solution and report the client's symptoms.

361. Postoperative care of the client following thyroidectomy includes which of the following?
☐ 1. Keep the head of the bed flat to prevent neck flexion.
☐ 2. Avoid coughing and deep-breathing to prevent injury to the suture line.
☐ 3. Restrict ambulation until the suture line is healed.
☐ 4. Check the back of the neck and upper part of the back when assessing the dressing.

362. Following the thyroidectomy, the nurse frequently assesses the client's voice and ability to speak. What is the nurse trying to evaluate?
   □ 1. Changes in level of consciousness.
   □ 2. Recovery from anesthesia.
   □ 3. Injury to the parathyroid gland.
   □ 4. Spasm or edema of vocal chords.

363. Mrs. Marlin begins to experience respiratory distress. A check of the surgical dressing reveals it to be tight about her neck with a small amount of bloody drainage. What should the nurse do?
   □ 1. Administer oxygen at 2 L via nasal prongs.
   □ 2. Reinforce the dressing and notify the doctor.
   □ 3. Loosen the dressing and notify the doctor.
   □ 4. Place the client in low-Fowler's position and notify the doctor.

364. The nurse will instruct Mrs. Marlin to avoid which of the following activities for several weeks following a thyroidectomy?
   □ 1. Turning the head.
   □ 2. Sitting in a chair.
   □ 3. Brushing the teeth.
   □ 4. Side-lying position.

365. The nurse observes Mrs. Marlin for injury to the parathyroid gland as a result of her surgery. Which of the following indicates parathyroid damage?
   □ 1. Vague abdominal pain.
   □ 2. Nausea and vomiting.
   □ 3. Decreased serum calcium.
   □ 4. Decreased serum phosphorus.

366. Treatment of parathyroid hormone deficiency can be expected to include which of the following?
   □ 1. Thyroid preparations.
   □ 2. Digitalis.
   □ 3. Calcium gluconate.
   □ 4. High-phosphorus diet.

367. Following a total thyroidectomy, what should the nurse teach the client?
   □ 1. Take thyroid medication daily for the rest of life.
   □ 2. Thyroid medication will be prescribed for 1-2 years.
   □ 3. Restrict intake of seafood, iodized salt, and green vegetables.
   □ 4. Take iodine solution daily for the rest of life.

Seven-year-old Kenisha Collins had acute poststreptococcal nephritis.

368. The nurse makes a home visit to monitor Kenisha's response to treatment. Which of the following is necessary for the nurse to include when evaluating Kenisha?
   □ 1. Blood pressure measurement.
   □ 2. Auscultation of breath sounds.
   □ 3. Urine test for glucose and acetone.
   □ 4. Abdominal circumference measurements.

369. Which of Kenisha's meals reported by her mother indicates that Mrs. Collins does not fully understand Kenisha's dietary restrictions?
   □ 1. Fried chicken, mashed potatoes, green beans, and apple juice.
   □ 2. Broiled fish, macaroni salad, applesauce, and grape juice.
   □ 3. Scrambled eggs, bacon, muffin with jelly, and orange juice.
   □ 4. Grilled cheese sandwich, carrots, fruit cocktail, and milk.

370. Mrs. Collins asks the nurse if Kenisha will "probably end up on one of those kidney machines." The nurse's reply should be based on the knowledge that Kenisha will most likely
   □ 1. Return to normal renal functioning.
   □ 2. Develop acute renal failure, requiring dialysis.
   □ 3. Develop chronic renal failure, necessitating a kidney transplant.
   □ 4. Have numerous recurrences of the disease.

David James is a 31-year-old married man with two children. He is a devout Catholic. He has been diagnosed with leukemia, and the disease has been treated with drug therapy for 2½ years. Mr. James has been admitted to the hospital with pneumonia and has been placed in protective isolation.

371. Mr. James has told the nurses that he knows he is going to die, but that is all he has said about it. He talks about his disease in clinical terms to the nurses, never about his own experiences. One day he comments to his primary nurse, "I am so worried." The best response from the nurse is
   □ 1. "It must frighten you to know you are dying."
   □ 2. "It must make you very uncomfortable."
   □ 3. "Have you shared these feelings with your family?"
   □ 4. "Tell me exactly what things are worrying you."

372. Which of the following interventions would be most significant in helping Mr. James cope with this death?
   □ 1. Distract him by initiating conversation that does not deal with his disease.
   □ 2. Encourage him to reach out and spend more time with his wife and children.
   □ 3. Listen and allow Mr. James to reminisce about his life.
   □ 4. Help him spend most of his time sleeping.

373. Mr. James tells the nurse he does not want his wife and children to know that he is dying. What would be the most helpful response?

- ☐ 1. "They would not want you to upset yourself by worrying about them."
- ☐ 2. "You are concerned that they will be upset?"
- ☐ 3. "I think we should talk about something less stressful for you."
- ☐ 4. Sit quietly and say nothing.

374. Which of the following interventions is the most effective in helping Mrs. James and her two children deal with Mr. James's impending death?

- ☐ 1. Try to keep all of the family members at the same stage in the grieving process.
- ☐ 2. Encourage the family members to verbalize their anger, sadness, and guilt to the nurse.
- ☐ 3. Encourage the family members to spend as much time as possible at the hospital, even if they are just sitting in the waiting room.
- ☐ 4. Encourage the family members to cry, but not in the presence of Mr. James.

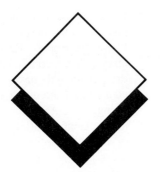

Correct Answers and Rationales: Part Four

282. no. 1. Many clients view a nurse entering "their space" as a threat, and Mr. Small is exhibiting signs of increased anxiety. His history indicates that he has used violent, aggressive behavior in response to increased anxiety. The nurse and the client do not have an established nurse-client relationship, and the nurse has not assessed his behavior and responses to others. Therefore, the nurse should reduce the environmental stimuli and assess his response to the decrease. Seclusion is a last resort to help clients to control behavior. The one-to-one attempt may be viewed as a violation of personal space, and behavioral distractions should be employed before medications if possible. Option no. 4 is not appropriate because at this stage of acting out, clients usually are unable to make decisions or identify anger. P-SM, IM, E

283. no. 3. Mr. Small is having difficulty maintaining self-control. Clear, firm limits will reduce his anxiety by providing a sense of control. Rules provide a sense of security until the client can provide his own controls. An expansive environment does not provide controls needed, and Mr. Small is not ready to develop his own treatment plan or determine his own needs. P-SM, IM, E

284. no. 1. The client is showing signs of escalating anxiety. He has a history of doing harm to others. The nurse needs to offer simple, limited, alternative behaviors without providing the client access to any weapons that could be used to do harm to himself or others. Nursing intervention with the angry client is best done with a team, and preparation for this client's care is in order for his protection. It is appropriate to help the client avoid altercations when possible. P-SM, IM, E

285. no. 3. When a client is placed in seclusion, communication should be kept simple and aimed at helping the client understand that the staff is assuming control until he can control his own behavior. When the staff is placing the client in restraints, his anxiety level will be raised and his hearing will become more selective. Expectations should be communicated at a time when the client's anxiety is lower. Options no. 1, no. 2, and no. 4 are all measures directed at staff and client safety. P-SM, IM, E

286. no. 1. Client's rights are addressed in state laws. State laws have statutes to include the conditions under which restraints can be used. Mr. Small's aggressive, violent behavior supports the need to protect others. Options no. 2, no. 3, and no. 4 all reflect state laws or client rights applicable in this situation. P-I, AN, PC

287. no. 4. The law does deal with the confidentiality concerns of clients. Limiting the documentation of staff is in violation of the portion of most state laws that indicates the record must contain specific data. Options no. 1, no. 2, and no. 3 address laws protecting client confidentiality. P-I, AN, PC

288. no. 1. Anger is cyclic. Once the client works out his anger and frustration in an aggressive act, he feels guilty and needs to justify and explain his behavior. While his anxiety is temporarily decreased, he experiences a decrease in self-esteem, which further increases the anxiety and can result in more acting-out behavior. The best intervention is to stop the anger cycle before it begins. Options no. 2, no. 3, and no. 4 reflect the later aspects of the anger cycle when intervention is more difficult. P-SM, IM, PC

289. no. 4. The findings of congenital dislocated hip include *limited abduction* of the affected hip, *shortening* of the leg on the affected side, and widening of the perineum caused by the head of the femur slipping out of the acetabulum. The infant rarely experiences pain in the affected hip. C-M, AS, PS

290. no. 2. All of these outcomes are desirable, but the parents' compliance with keeping Maria in her splint at all times except bath time is the most crucial indicator that they understand the possible consequences of not adhering to the treatment plan. C-M, EV, H

291. no. 1. If contractions exceed 90 seconds in duration, there is a danger of a ruptured uterus. Adverse blood pressure changes with oxytocin (Pitocin) are seen in hypertension. A desired effect is increased strength and frequency of contractions. CBF-I, AN, E

292. no. 4. Acceptance is needed in time of stress, as the woman seeks to maintain control. CBF-I, IM, E

293. no. 4. These are normal adaptations. CBF-P, AN, PS

294. no. 3. Such pain may be associated with the development of a hematoma. Assessment should precede intervention. Comfort measures may follow. CBF-P, PL, E

295. no. 4. A full bladder displaces the uterus and prevents contraction. Suggest that the client void and reassess fundus and lochia. CBF-P, AN, E

296. no. 2. This is the only symptom listed that is indicative of a problem with intellectual function. Options no. 1, no. 3, and no. 4 indicate changes in emotional functioning. P-C, AS, PC

297. no. 2. A familiar, established routine decreases confusion and the demands on the client's coping mechanisms. Efforts should be made to follow previous dependence. No. 3 would lead to increased feelings of isolation. Waiting will not lessen the confusion. P-C, IM, E

298. no. 4. Admission to a care facility often exacerbates symptoms because of the new environment. Although options no. 1, no. 2, and no. 3 are important considerations, it is unlikely that they "cause" the confusion as it is described in this situation. P-C, AN, PC

299. no. 1. Personal attention and assistance for client's safety will enhance feelings of security. Confinement and restraints increase feelings of hopelessness and inadequacy, which may lead to increased confusion. These clients will not be able to explain their behavior, and requests for such explanations may increase argumentativeness. P-C, IM, PC

300. no. 4. This provides reality orientation without degrading or arguing with the client. Inaccurate information confuses the client further. Option no. 2 does not tell the client where she is now and verbal constraints may confuse the client. P-C, IM, E

301. no. 2. Provide smaller meals that require less attention to complete. The other choices would decrease independence, threaten the client, or allow the problem to continue. P-C, IM, E

302. no. 1. Identify yourself to avoid misidentification and call the client by name to reinforce her sense of identity. Option no. 2 would decrease her interaction with others, possibly increasing confusion. Options no. 3 and no. 4 provide an inappropriate degree of stimulation. P-C, IM, PC

303. no. 1. Decreased ability to learn because of decreased attention span are characteristics of organic brain syndrome. Recent and remote memory changes are variable. As memory changes occur, the person will have more difficulty adapting to change and attending to usual activities of daily living. P-C, AS, PC

304. no. 1. Confabulation involves using old memories or inventing information to fill in memory gaps about present experiences. There is no evidence of a special need to gain attention. Confabulation does not increase attention span or prevent regression. P-C, AN, PC

305. no. 3. Avoiding shadows and darkness will help decrease her disorientation. Maintain her usual bedtime routine; alterations may only increase restlessness. These clients will not understand or remember explanations. Sedatives often increase activity and confusion in the elderly. P-C, IM, PC

306. no. 2. Provide assistance and direction with activities of daily living as needed. Giving her time will not increase her decisiveness or lessen confusion. Laying out her clothes makes the decision for her and decreases independence. Rushing her will increase confusion. P-C, IM, H

307. no. 4. Help family members to explore their feelings. Maintaining family contact is necessary for orientation and self-identity. Reassurance will not help family members deal with feelings or the situation. There is insufficient evidence to justify an inference of guilt. P-T, IM, PC

308. no. 1. Assist with feelings and client situations so family members will not withdraw from the client. Encourage regular visits. Options no. 2, no. 3, and no. 4 tend to separate family and client rather than enhance their feelings at this difficult time. P-C, IM, H

309. no. 4. Provide concrete information that reinforces reality without emphasizing the client's deficits. Probing for feelings increases confusion and argumentativeness in these clients. P-C, IM, PC

310. no. 1. Decreasing the number of adjustments needed in a new environment lessens confusion. Do not overstimulate or confront clients with deficits. Provide for individualization of care instead of rigid routines. P-C, PL, PC

311. no. 4. Two possible sequelae of a streptococcal infection are rheumatic fever and glomerulonephritis, but the two do not necessarily occur in conjunction with each other. C-O, AS, PS

312. no. 2. The major sequela of rheumatic fever is heart damage, particularly scarring of the mitral valve. Bed rest is recommended for the client with carditis to minimize metabolic needs and ease the work load of the heart. C-O, PL, E

313. no. 2. All are potential stressors, but the school-age child is especially vulnerable to the loss of

control that results from decreased and restricted mobility. Gail is old enough to understand and accept explanations of possible outcomes, reasons for hospitalization, and procedures such as venipuncture, but is likely to be easily frustrated by bed rest requirements. C-I, PL, PS

314. no. 2. Seven-year-old Susan is somewhat young to be the best choice, even though she has the same health problem. Because Gail has carditis, she should not be placed with Sharon; Gail had a recent streptococcal infection, and Sharon's condition may be aggravated by exposure to a potential source of infection. On the other hand, Evelyn has a fever, which may indicate a concurrent infection to which Gail should not be exposed. Amy is the best choice, because she is close enough in age, has no infectious condition, and, like Gail, has a chronic illness. C-O, PL, H

315. no. 4. Gail is on bed rest with bathroom privileges and cannot go to the playroom. Listening to records and watching television are passive activities. Crocheting requires minimal exertion, does not involve the large joints (which may be painful), and also fosters Gail's feelings of accomplishment. C-I, IM, E

316. no. 3. A decreasing ESR indicates a decrease in the body's inflammatory response. The WBC is slightly elevated; a positive C-reactive protein indicates continued inflammation; the elevated ASO titer indicates a recent streptococcal infection. C-O, EV, PS

317. no. 3. Gail is able to cognitively understand full explanations using correct terminology. Such explanations also consider her emotional needs and foster feelings of control. However, although she should be included in making decisions that affect her, she is not legally able to give consent for or refuse necessary care. Concrete thinking and misunderstanding of the causes of illness characterize the younger child. C-H, AN, PS

318. no. 3. There is a need during this phase to integrate the experience of delivery into reality. An interest in rooming-in and care usually follow in 2-3 days. CBF-P, AN, PC

319. no. 1. This indicates normal uterine involution. At this stage lochia should be rubra. Serosa is a sign that the cervix is blocked, probably by clots. Engorgement and healing do not occur this early. CBF-P, AS, PS

320. no. 3. Complete emptying of the breasts is important for the comfort of the mother. Engorgement is a normal physiological process. The newborn should be stimulated to suck. Restriction of fluids to less than 6-8 glasses daily is not appropriate. Ice packs may relieve discomfort between feedings but may reduce flow of milk as blood vessels and ducts constrict. CBF-P, PL, E

321. no. 2. The shape of the breast will not be changed by breastfeeding. The bra will prevent breakdown of breast musculature and provide comfort. CBF-P, IM, E

322. no. 4. The newborn sleeps more than 20 hours daily, nurses every 2 to 3 hours, urinates often, and has frequent stools. New parents will find their lives dramatically changed. The newborn will feed on demand in the first weeks, and parents cannot "schedule" naps or feedings. The father's comment on crying indicates a lack of understanding of the newborn's need to communicate and need for love. CBF-N, EV, H

323. no. 4. Breast size is not a factor in volume of milk produced. This mother needs support and teaching. CBF-P, IM, H

324. no. 2. Although all these pieces of information may be important and may be ascertained at some point during Katie's hospital stay, the nurse must know Katie's usual patterns in order to develop an appropriate care plan to meet Katie's toileting needs. C-I, AS, H

325. no. 4. Dressing without supervision, sharing with other children, and using complete sentences are characteristics of preschoolers, not toddlers. Katie should have learned to use a spoon well by 18 months of age. C-H, AS, H

326. no. 3. When a microdrip is used for an intravenous infusion, the number of milliliters per hour is equal to the number of drops per minute. Therefore, the nurse should divide the total amount of 500 ml by 8 hours to determine the amount per hour to be infused. This amount equals 63 ml per hour; therefore, the microdrip regulator should be set at 63 drops per minute. C-H, IM, E

327. no. 4. Bed linens should be changed frequently to prevent chilling and promote comfort. Cough suppressants are contraindicated, and children with croup need a liberal fluid intake because of the possibility of dehydration secondary to increased sensible fluid loss. Katie is too young to comprehend an explanation of why she must stay in the tent. C-O, IM, E

328. no. 1. Chest therapy in a child with a respiratory infection should be carried out just before mealtimes so the airway is cleared and Katie will be able to eat without tiring. Chest therapy should also be done at bedtime to facilitate sleep by helping Katie breathe more easily. Chest therapy after meals may cause Katie to vomit. Trying to schedule the treatment around Katie's nap times is inefficient and too unpredictable. C-O, PL, E

329. no. 2. Chest therapy is carried out to keep the lower airway passage clear and to facilitate drainage of lower airway secretions. Inspiratory stridor, suprasternal retractions, and a harsh metallic cough indicate upper airway involvement and are not used

to evaluate the effectiveness of chest percussion and drainage. The presence of rales and rhonchi indicates that the lower airway passages are still congested, and therefore the treatment has not been completely effective. C-O, EV, PS

330. no. 3. Protest behavior most characterizes the toddler's separation from parents. Despair or detachment behavior is unlikely to appear when hospitalization is short, especially when parents visit daily. C-I, AS, PS

331. no. 1. Of all the age groups, toddlers handle separation and hospitalization very poorly. If a mother cannot room-in, the next best thing is an article of clothing to remind the child of the mother. C-I, PL, PS

332. no. 3. Allowing Katie to sleep with her parents may increase Katie's insecurity and reinforces dependency (not autonomy), since this was not part of her routine before hospitalization. C-H, PL, PS

333. no. 4. Respiratory infections, such as flu or colds, are the most common cause of exacerbations in clients with emphysema (chronic obstructive pulmonary disease [COPD]). Health teaching for clients with COPD includes instructions on how to prevent respiratory infections and directions to seek early treatment of respiratory infections that do occur. A-O, AS, E

334. no. 2. Aminophylline has a beta-adrenergic effect that results in the relaxation of the bronchial muscle. Aminophylline has no mucolytic or sedative effects. A-O, AS, PS

335. no. 4. Tachycardia and palpitations are common side effects of aminophylline because it stimulates the cardiac muscle. Other side effects include GI upset, urinary frequency, nervousness, and insomnia. A-O, AS, PS

336. no. 3. A normal pH with elevated Pco_2 indicates chronic respiratory acidosis. Clients with chronic COPD adjust to the high level of arterial CO_2, and signs of neurological involvement are usually not present. Oxygen is always administered in low concentrations (1–2 L/min) in the presence of hypercapnia and hypoxia because of the danger of CO_2 narcosis and respiratory failure. A-O, AN, PS

337. no. 1. Among the antimicrobial drugs, penicillins are most often responsible for anaphylaxis because of their allergic properties. Persons known to be allergic to one penicillin preparation should not be given any form of the drug. A-O, AS, PS

338. no. 1. Disruption in the integrity of the pleura allows air from the lung to enter the pleural (not mediastinal) space. In this case, there is no rib involvement. A-O, AS, PS

339. no. 2. The primary purpose of a chest tube is to reestablish subatmospheric (negative) pressure in the pleural space by the removal of air and fluid.

This allows reexpansion of the lung. A-O, AS, E

340. no. 4. Correct information allays anxiety. Option no. 4 is the most accurate and is more specific than option no. 2. Options no. 1 and no. 3 do not answer the client's question. When the lung is fully expanded, the bubbling will cease. In a chest drainage system, connected to suction, continuous bubbling in the second bottle indicates normal functioning. A-O, AS, E

341. no. 3. Clients with emphysema may not be able to tolerate eating large meals; they might tolerate small, frequent meals better. Also, their need for carbohydrates is increased as a result of the increased energy expended for the work of breathing. A-O, IM, A

342. no. 1. The willingness to accept professional help depends upon the need as the client and family see it. All the other factors are important also, but first the client and family must want the service. P-T, AN, H

343. no. 3. This response encourages the client to discuss his feelings and can provide important clues to what is troubling him or what has been difficult for him. P-T, IM, E

344. no. 4. Even diminished intake can lead to withdrawal symptoms. Cessation is not a prerequisite to their occurrence. P-SU, AN, PC

345. no. 2. The alcoholic client's denial of problems is evidenced by recognition that something is wrong, but denying that medical, emotional, or social problems are related to the consumption of alcohol. No. 1 and no. 4 may be seen, but are not the priority for developing nursing care. Once the problem of denial is addressed, dependency and projection will decrease. No. 3, paranoia, is not a defense mechanism. P-SU, AN, PC

346. no. 1. The lowest rate of recidivism has been shown for those alcoholic clients who become involved with AA. Peer support and networking has more success than family or individual therapy or the chronic disease approach. Alcoholics Anonymous may be used in combination with these treatment approaches. P-SU, PL, PC

347. no. 1. Although genetic factors and chronic disease effects are important, options no. 2 through no. 4 are important areas to explore and focus upon in the family-therapy sessions. P-SU, AN, PC

348. no. 3. In the detoxification stage of alcoholism the body chemistry changes can be rapid and severe. Sodium-potassium level changes are especially vulnerable because of vomiting and fluid shifts. The heart, already burdened by the process of detoxification, is especially sensitive to low potassium levels. Option no. 1 is important, but not as dangerous a problem. No. 2 is true but is not an immediate concern. No. 4 is a priority at a later stage. P-SU, PL, PS

349. no. 4. The client needs to do his own evaluating as to his readiness to change direction. The nurse serves best by helping him to clarify his thoughts and feelings. No. 2 is judgmental and insensitive. The timing belongs to the client. No. 3 is inconsequential in light of the client's remarks. No. 1 might be appropriate, but no. 4 is geared more to the feeling level of the statement. P-SU, IM, PC

350. no. 4. Too much sympathy and empathy reinforces the client's view of himself as a victim of alcohol, drugs, or other people. The client will not accept responsibility for himself, nor will he be able to break through his denial, if a high level of sympathy and empathy is given. The client would then manipulate his nurse and avoid dealing with his problems. Options no. 1, no. 2, and no. 3 are critical to setting the stage for the client to work on his problems. The client needs to internalize limits. P-SU, IM, E

351. no. 4. Although a dietary deficiency of iodine may cause goiter and hypothyroidism, dietary iodine is not now considered a risk factor in the development of thyroid cancer. However, a history of irradiation of head, neck, or chest (e.g., for acne, enlarged thymus or tonsils, or Hodgkin's disease) is strongly associated with the development of thyroid cancer. High doses of vitamin D are used to treat hypoparathyroidism. A-NM, AS, PS

352. no. 1. An enlarged thyroid may encroach on organs in close proximity. Swallowing and breathing are usually the first functions to be affected. Muscle twitching and tingling around the lips would be the result of parathyroid involvement. A-NM, AS, PS

353. no. 3. Options no. 1 and no. 2 suggest hypofunction of the thyroid gland. The symptoms listed in option no. 4 are not, as a group, specific for thyroid dysfunction. A-NM, AS, PS

354. no. 2. Primary thyroid hyperactivity is characterized by elevations in serum triiodothyronine (T_3) and/or thyroxine (T_4). Secondary hyperthyroidism, caused by malfunction of the pituitary gland, is characterized by an overproduction of thyroid-stimulating hormone (TSH). Serum ACTH levels remain unaffected unless hyperpituitarism is involved. A-NM, AS, PS

355. no. 3. Graves' disease is hyperthyroidism accompanied by goiter and/or exophthalmos. It is thought to be autoimmune in nature because of the presence of long-acting thyroid stimulators (LATS) in the blood of many, but not all, affected persons. Myxedema is caused by hypofunction of the thyroid; cretinism is caused by congenital hypothyroidism. Addison's disease is caused by adrenocortical hypofunction. A-NM, AS, PS

356. no. 3. Exophthalmos is characterized by bulging eyes. To prevent drying of the overly exposed eyeballs, lubricating eye drops, such as methylcellulose drops, are frequently prescribed. In addition, self-lubrication and protection through regular blinking are encouraged. Although not specific to exophthalmos, both placement of clients in areas of low environmental stimuli in order to decrease adrenergic activity and frequent monitoring of vital signs for changes are considered important aspects of the nursing care plan. A-NM, IM, E

357. no. 1. Results of the test are affected by the client's intake of iodides (in medications or x-ray contrast media) and thyroid hormones. Proper interpretation of results requires this information be noted on laboratory slips. This test does not involve a 24-hour urine collection. Rather, the thyroid is scanned, and the amount of radioactivity is determined. The client is not placed in isolation. A-NM, PL, E

358. no. 3. Propylthiouracil should be taken every 8 hours to ensure adequate levels over a 24-hour period. Too low a dosage will be evidenced by a return of weight loss and rapid pulse rate. A serious side effect of this drug is agranulocytosis, evidenced by indications of infection (fever, sore throat, or rash). In returning to a euthyroid state, the client can be expected to regain previously lost weight. A-NM, IM, H

359. no. 2. To disguise the salty taste and to decrease gastric irritation, iodine solutions should be well diluted in a full glass of fruit juice, milk, or water and administered after meals and at bedtime. A-NM, IM, E

360. no. 4. These symptoms are indicative of iodine poisoning (iodism). The nurse's first action should be to discontinue iodine therapy and report the client's signs and symptoms to the physician. A secondary consideration is to explore additional sources of iodine in the diet (e.g., iodized salt, seafood, vegetables grown near the seaside). Isolation of the client is not required, and symptoms will subside with adjustment of iodine intake. A-NM, IM, E

361. no. 4. Hemorrhage is a serious complication following thyroidectomy. Because of gravity, drainage may not be visible along the suture line on the anterior neck dressing, but rather at the back of the neck and upper part of the back. The preferred position for the client after a thyroidectomy is semi-Fowler's with good neck support. Turning, coughing, and deep-breathing as well as early ambulation can be accomplished while the head and neck are supported in a neutral position. A-NM, IM, PS

362. no. 4. Increasing hoarseness after a thyroidectomy may indicate injury to the recurrent laryngeal nerve or swelling in the area of the glottis. Parathyroid injury will be evidenced by muscular tingling or twitching. A-NM, EV, PS

363. no. 3. Respiratory distress and a tightening neck dressing may indicate hemorrhage into tissues or increasing edema in the neck area. Loosening the dressing to prevent further tracheal compression should be the nurse's first action. Reinforcement of the dressing would only increase tracheal compression. High-Fowler's position alone will not decrease swelling; the dressing must also be loosened. A-NM, IM, PS

364. no. 1. Sitting in a chair, brushing the teeth, and lying on one's side may all be accomplished without the flexion, extension, or rotation of the neck that should be avoided in the early postoperative period because of the strain this places on the suture line. The client must be instructed to turn the whole body, not just the head during this time. A-NM, IM, H

365. no. 3. Injury to the parathyroid gland would be accompanied by decreased serum calcium, elevated serum phosphorus, painful muscle spasms, tingling around the lips, and numbness of the fingertips. A-NM, AS, PS

366. no. 3. The treatment of choice, both on an emergency and long-term basis, is the administration of calcium gluconate. Thyroid preparations have no influence on parathyroid functioning. Digitalis is a cardiotonic and requires normal levels of calcium to produce desired effects. Since phosphate levels increase in hypoparathyroid conditions, dietary phosphorus would be contraindicated. A-NM, PL, PS

367. no. 1. Following total removal of the thyroid gland, the client must take thyroid medication daily for the rest of life to supply the hormones essential for maintaining body metabolism. Since the thyroid hormones themselves are taken, dietary iodine is no longer needed to support their synthesis within the body. Dietary iodine need not be advised or restricted. A-NM, IM, H

368. no. 1. Elevated blood pressure is one of the primary manifestations of poststreptococcal nephritis and should be monitored on a regular basis. Return of the blood pressure to normal indicates the disease process is resolving. The edema associated with this disease affects the face and extremities, not the abdomen, so it is not necessary to measure abdominal girth. The urine should be checked for specific gravity, protein, and blood. Although assessment of breath sounds is an important part of evaluating general health status, it is not essential in this case. C-E, EV, PS

369. no. 3. The child with poststreptococcal nephritis needs a diet with normal protein, moderate sodium restriction, and low potassium. This meal is high in sodium (bacon) and high in potassium (orange juice) and therefore indicates the mother does not clearly understand the diet or the importance of the restrictions. C-E, AN, PS

370. no. 1. Fewer than one-quarter of the children with poststreptococcal nephritis develop chronic renal failure. Recurrences are very rare. With proper treatment, these children return to normal renal functioning within 3 to 4 weeks. C-E, EV, PS

371. no. 2. This response acknowledges empathy and encourages further expression of feeling. No. 1 is too confrontive, too fast. No. 3 cuts off communication of feelings between client and nurse. No. 4 is too demanding of information and cuts off spontaneous discussion of feelings by the client. P-L, IM, PC

372. no. 3. Terminally ill clients need to review their lives to explore the meaning their lives have had. No. 1 and no. 4 reinforces denial and nonacceptance of the inevitable. Withdrawal from relationships normally occurs among the terminally ill. P-L, IM, PC

373. no. 2. Verbalize implied feelings, give the client permission to discuss feelings, and help the client to work through the denial stage. Options no. 1 and no. 3 cut off communication. Silent support is important, but is not appropriate when the client is demonstrating a need to talk and is asking for information. P-L, IM, H

374. no. 2. Verbal expression of grief facilitates mourning. Option no. 1 is too controlling, does not permit individual needs of family members in dealing with their grief. No. 3 discourages family members from taking care of themselves and could hamper the family grieving process. No. 4 does not facilitate the family's communication about the grieving process. P-L, IM, PC

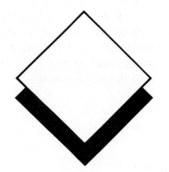

Appendix A

Approved Nursing Diagnoses from the North American Nursing Diagnosis Association, June 1990

Exchanging
Altered nutrition: more than body requirements
Altered nutrition: less than body requirements
Altered nutrition: high risk for more than body require-
  ments
High risk for infection
High risk for altered body temperature
Hypothermia
Hyperthermia
Ineffective thermoregulation
Dysreflexia
Constipation
Perceived constipation
Colonic constipation
Diarrhea
Bowel incontinence
Altered patterns of urinary elimination
Stress incontinence
Reflex incontinence
Urge incontinence
Functional incontinence
Total incontinence
Urinary retention
Altered tissue perfusion (specify type: renal, cerebral,
  cardiopulmonary, gastrointestinal, or peripheral)
Fluid volume excess
Fluid volume deficit (1)
Fluid volume deficit (2)
High risk for fluid volume deficit
Decreased cardiac output
Impaired gas exchange
Ineffective airway clearance
Ineffective breathing pattern
High risk for injury
High risk for suffocation
High risk for poisoning
High risk for trauma
High risk for aspiration
High risk for disuse syndrome

Altered protection
High risk for impaired skin integrity
Impaired skin integrity
Impaired tissue integrity
Altered oral mucous membrane
Communicating
Impaired verbal communication
Relating
Impaired social interaction
Social isolation
Altered role performance
Altered parenting
High risk for altered parenting
Sexual dysfunction
Altered family processes
Parental role conflict
Altered sexuality patterns
Valuing
Spiritual distress
Choosing
Ineffective individual coping
Impaired adjustment
Defensive coping
Ineffective denial
Ineffective family coping: disabling
Ineffective family coping: compromised
Family coping: potential for growth
Noncompliance
Decisional conflict
Health-seeking behaviors
Moving
Impaired physical mobility
Activity intolerance
Fatigue
High risk for activity intolerance
Sleep pattern disturbance
Diversional activity deficit
Impaired home maintenance management
Altered health maintenance

Feeding self-care deficit
Impaired swallowing
Ineffective breastfeeding
Effective breastfeeding
Bathing/hygiene self-care deficit
Dressing/grooming self-care deficit
Toileting self-care deficit
Altered growth and development

Perceiving
Body image disturbance
Self-esteem disturbance
Chronic low self-esteem
Situational low self-esteem
Personal identity disturbance
Sensory/perceptual alterations (specify) (visual, auditory, kinesthetic, gustatory, tactile, or olfactory)
Unilateral neglect

Hopelessness
Powerlessness

Knowing
Knowledge deficit
Altered thought processes

Feeling
Pain
Chronic pain
Dysfunctional grieving
Anticipatory grieving
High risk for violence: self-directed or directed at others
Post-trauma response
Rape-trauma syndrome
Rape-trauma syndrome: compound reaction
Rape-trauma syndrome: silent reaction
Anxiety
Fear

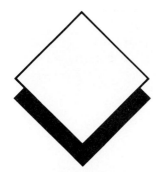

Appendix B

Common Laboratory Values—Adult*

	Conventional	SI units
HEMATOLOGICAL TESTS		
Hematocrit	Male: 42%-52%	0.42-0.52
	Female: 37%-47%	0.37-0.47
Hemoglobin	Male: 14-18 g/dl	8.1-11.2 mmol/L
	Female: 12-16 g/dl	7.4-9.9 mmol/L
Red blood cells	4.7-6.1 million/mm³	4.7-6.1 × 10¹²/L
White blood cells	5000-10,000/mm³	5-10 × 10⁹/L
Platelets	150,000-400,000/mm³	150-400 × 10⁹/L
Erythrocyte sedimentation rate	Male: 0-15 mm/hr	
	Female: 0-20 mm/hr	
Prothrombin time	11.0-12.5 seconds	11.0-12.5 seconds
Partial thromboplastin time	30-40 seconds	30-40 seconds
BLOOD CHEMISTRY TESTS		
Acid phosphatase†	0.10-0.63 U/ml	28-175 nmol/sec/L
Alkaline phosphatase†	30-85 ImU/ml	
Albumin	3.5-4.5 g/dl	35-55 g/L
ALT†	5-35 IU/L	5-35 U/L
Ammonia	15-110 μmol/dl	47-65 μmol/L
Amylase†	56-190 IU/L	25-125 U/L
AST†	5-40 IU/L	5-40 U/L
Bilirubin	Direct: 0.1-0.3 mg/dl	1.7-5.1 μmol/L
	Total: 0.1-1.0 mg/dl	5 ¹ ;7 μmol/L
Calcium	9.0-10.5 mg/dl	2.25-2.75 mmol/L
CO_2	23-30 mEq/L	21-30 mmol/L
Chloride	90-110 mEq/L	98-106 mmol/L
Cholesterol	150-250 mg/dl	3.90-6.50 mmol/L
Creatine phosphokinase†	5-75 mU/ml	12-80 U/L
Creatinine	0.7-1.5 mg/dl	<133 μmol/L
Globulin	2.3-3.4 g/dl	20-35 g/L

Modified from Pagana, K., & Pagana, T. (1990). *Diagnostic testing and nursing implications* (3rd ed.). St. Louis: Mosby—Year Book.

*Normal value ranges will vary from laboratory to laboratory.

†Enzyme value ranges may vary widely from laboratory to laboratory. Any actual client result must be compared with laboratory standards for accurate evaluation.

Continued.

	Conventional	SI units
BLOOD CHEMISTRY TESTS—cont'd		
Glucose	70-115 mg/dl	3.89-6.38 mmol/L
Iron	60-190 μg/dl	13-31 μmol/L
Iron-binding capacity	250-420 μg/dl	45-73 μmol/L
Lactic dehydrogenase†	90-200 ImU/ml	0.4-1.7 μmol/sec/L
Lipase†	Up to 1.5 U/ml	0-417 U/L
Lithium	0.8-1.4 mEq/L	
O_2 saturation	95%-100%	0.95-1.00
P_{CO_2}	35-45 mm Hg	
pH	7.35-7.45	7.35-7.45
P_{O_2}	80-100 mm Hg	
Potassium	3.5-5.0 mEq/L	3.5-5.0 mmol/L
Protein	6-8 g/dl	55-80 g/L
Sodium	136-145 mEq/L	136-145 mmol/L
Triglycerides	40-150 mg/dl	0.4-1.5 g/L
Urea nitrogen	5-20 mg/dl	3.6-7.1 mmol/L
Uric acid	Male: 2.1-8.5 mg/dl	0.15-0.48 mmol/L
	Female: 2.0-6.6 mg/dl	0.09-0.36 mmol/L
URINE TESTS		
pH	4.6-8.0	
Specific gravity	1.010-1.025	
Odor	Aromatic	
Color	Amber-yellow	
Turbidity	Clear	
Glucose	Negative	
Protein	<8 mg/dl	
Hemoglobin	Negative	
Acetone	Negative	

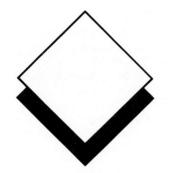

Appendix C
State and Territorial Boards of Nursing

Alabama

State Board of Nursing
Suite 203, 500 East Blvd.
Montgomery, Alabama 36117

Alaska

Alaska State Board of Nursing
Div. of Occupational Licensing
3601 C. Street, Frontier Bldg., Suite 722
Anchorage, Alaska 99503

Arizona

State Board of Nursing
5050 N. 19th Avenue, Suite 103
Phoenix, Arizona 85015

Arkansas

State Board of Nursing
Westmark Bldg., Suite 308
4120 W. Markham Street
Little Rock, Arkansas 72205

California

State Board of Registered Nursing
1030 13th Street, Suite 200
Sacramento, California 95814

Colorado

Colorado Board of Nursing
State Services Bldg., Room 132
1525 Sherman Street
Denver, Colorado 80203

Connecticut

Department of Health Services, Nurse Licensure
150 Washington Street
Hartford, Connecticut 06106

Delaware

State Board of Nursing
Margaret O'Neill Bldg., Third Floor
Federal and Court Streets
Dover, Delaware 19901

District of Columbia

Nurses Examining Board
614 H. Street, N.W., Room 923
Washington, D.C. 20001

Florida

State Board of Nursing
111 Coastline Drive East, Suite 504
Jacksonville, Florida 32202

Georgia

State Board of Nursing
166 Pryor Street, S.W., Suite 400
Atlanta, Georgia 30303

Guam

Guam Board of Nurse Examiners
P.O. Box 2816
Agana, Guam 96910

Hawaii

Board of Nursing
P.O. Box 3469
Honolulu, Hawaii 96801

Idaho

Board of Nursing
700 West State Street
Boise, Idaho 83720

Illinois

Department of Registration and Education
320 W. Washington Street
Springfield, Illinois 62786

Indiana

State Board of Nursing
Health Professions Bureau
1 American Square, Suite 1020
Indianapolis, Indiana 46282

Iowa

Board of Nursing
Executive Hills East
1223 E. Court
Des Moines, Iowa 50319

Kansas

Board of Nursing
503 Kansas Avenue, Suite 330
P.O. Box 1098
Topeka, Kansas 66601

Kentucky

Kentucky Board of Nursing
4010 Depont Circle, Suite 430
Louisville, Kentucky 40207

Louisiana

Board of Nursing
150 Baronne Street, Room 907
New Orleans, Louisiana 70112

Maine

Board of Nursing
295 Water Street
Augusta, Maine 04330

Maryland

Board of Examiners of Nurses
201 W. Preston Street
Baltimore, Maryland 21201

Massachusetts

Board of Registration in Nursing
100 Cambridge Street, Room 1519
Boston, Massachusetts 02202

Michigan

Board of Nursing
P.O. Box 30018
Lansing, Michigan 48909

Minnesota

Board of Nursing
2700 University Avenue W., #108
Minneapolis, Minnesota 55114

Mississippi

Board of Nursing
135 Bounds Street
Jackson, Mississippi 39206

Missouri

Board of Nursing
P.O. Box 656, 3523 N. Ten Mile Drive
Jefferson City, Missouri 65102

Montana

Montana Board of Nursing
1424 9th Avenue
Helena, Montana 59620-0407

Nebraska

Board of Nursing Department of Health
Bureau of Examining Boards
P.O. Box 95007
Lincoln, Nebraska 68509-5007

Nevada

Board of Nursing
1281 Terminal Way, Suite 116
Reno, Nevada 89502

New Hampshire

Board of Nursing Education and Registration
State Office Park South
101 Pleasant Street
Concord, New Hampshire 03301

New Jersey

New Jersey Board of Nursing
1100 Raymond Blvd., Room 319
Newark, New Jersey 07102

New Mexico

Board of Nursing
4125 Carlisle, N.E.
Albuquerque, New Mexico 87017

New York

State Board of Nursing
State Education Department
Cultural Education Center, Room 3013
Albany, New York 12230

North Carolina

Board of Nursing
P.O. Box 2129
Raleigh, North Carolina 27602

North Dakota

Board of Nursing
Kirkwood Office Tower, Suite 504
7th and Arbor Avenues
Bismarck, North Dakota 58501

Ohio

Board of Nursing Education & Registration
65 S. Front Street, Suite 509
Columbus, Ohio 43266-0316

Oklahoma

Board of Nurse Registration and Education
2915 Classen Blvd., Suite 524
Oklahoma City, Oklahoma 73106

Oregon

Oregon Board of Nursing
1400 S.W. 5th Avenue
Portland, Oregon 97201

Pennsylvania

Board of Nurse Examiners
P.O. Box 2649
Harrisburg, Pennsylvania 17105-2649

Puerto Rico

Accreditation & Development for Schools of Nursing
Council on Higher Education, University of Puerto Rico
Rio Piedras, Puerto Rico 00931

Rhode Island

Board of Nursing Education and Registration
Cannon Health Bldg.
75 Davis Street
Providence, Rhode Island 02908

South Carolina

Board of Nursing
1777 St. Julian Place, Suite 102
Columbia, South Carolina 29204

South Dakota

Board of Nursing
304 S. Phillips Ave., Suite 205
Sioux Falls, South Dakota 57102-0783

Tennessee

Tennessee Board of Nursing
283 Plus Park Blvd.
Nashville, Tennessee 37219-5407

Texas

Texas Board of Nurse Examiners
1300 E. Anderson Lane, Bldg. C, Suite 225
Austin, Texas 78752

Utah

Board of Nursing
Division of Professional Licensing
160 E. 300 South
Box 45802
Salt Lake City, Utah 84145

Vermont

Board of Nursing
26 Terrace Street
Montpelier, Vermont 05602-2198

Virgin Islands

Board of Nurse Examiners
Division of Professional Licensing
P.O. Box 7309
Charlotte Amalie
St. Thomas, Virgin Islands 00801

Virginia

State Board of Nursing
517 West Grace Street
P.O. Box 27708
Richmond, Virginia 23261

Washington

Board of Nursing
Division of Professional Licensing
P.O. Box 9649
Olympia, Washington 98504

West Virginia

Board of Examiners
922 Quarrier Street
Embleton Bldg., Suite 309
Charleston, West Virginia 25301

Wisconsin

Board of Nursing
1400 E. Washington Avenue
P.O. Box 8936
Madison, Wisconsin 53708

Wyoming

Board of Nursing
2301 Central Avenue, Barrett Bldg., 4th Floor
Cheyenne, Wyoming 82002

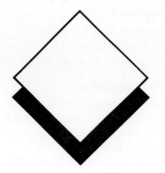

Canadian Provincial Registered Nurses Associations

Registrar

Alberta Association of Registered Nurses
10256 112th Street
Edmonton, Alberta T5K1M6

Registrar

Manitoba Association of Registered Nurses
647 Broadway Avenue
Winnipeg, Manitoba R3C0X2

Registrar

Registered Nurses Association of British Columbia
2855 Arbutus Street
Vancouver, British Columbia V6J3Y8

Registrar

New Brunswick Association of Registered Nurses
231 Saunders Street
Fredericton, New Brunswick E3B1N6

Registrar

Association of Registered Nurses of Newfoundland
A.R.N.N. House
55 Military Road
St. John's, Newfoundland A1C6A1

Registrar

Registered Nurses Association of Nova Scotia
6035 Coburt Road
Halifax, Nova Scotia B3H1Y8

Executive Director-Registrar

Association of Nurses of Prince Edward Island
41 Palmers Lane
Charlottetown, Prince Edward Island C1A5V7

Executive Director and Secretary

Order of Nurses of the Province of Quebec
4200 Dorchester Blvd. West
Montreal, Quebec H3Z1V4

Registrar

Saskatchewan Registered Nurses Association
2066 Retallack Street
Regina, Saskatchewan S4T2K2

Executive Director, Registrar

Northwest Territories Registered Nurses Association
P.O. Box 2757
Yellowknife, Northwest Territories X0E1H0

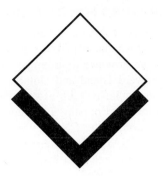

Appendix D

Information for Foreign Nurse Graduates Who Wish to Practice in the United States

Nursing practice in the United States is regulated by each state through its Nurse Practice Act and the State Board of Nursing (or State Board of Nurse Examiners). These licensing laws and appointed boards establish the qualifications for obtaining a license in the state and the grounds for denying a license to an applicant or suspending a nurse's license. Of particular significance is the board's role in defining the scope of nursing practice in a particular state. Qualifications for obtaining a license generally include:

◆ graduation from an accredited nursing education program
◆ a satisfactory score on the National Council Licensure Examination (NCLEX) or Canadian Nursing Association Testing Service (CNATS)
◆ submission of a completed application form with specified fee

Foreign nurse graduates must also obtain an H1 visa, which is a temporary working visa granted to individuals who are not seeking permanent residency in the United States. To obtain an H1 visa, a foreign nurse graduate must have a certificate issued by the U.S. Commission on Graduates of Foreign Nursing Schools (CGFNS). This requirement also applies to Canadian nurses who want to obtain a license in Indiana, Montana, South Dakota, and Washington state. The CGFNS certificate is awarded for successful scores on an examination. This multiple-

choice examination is intended to screen foreign nurse graduates and evaluate their understanding of written English and medical terminology, as well as their basic nursing knowledge. The CGFNS examination is given twice a year in sites throughout the world. To take this examination, the foreign nurse graduate must submit a completed application form and a filing fee 3 months before the examination is held (i.e., January 1 for the April exam and July 1 for the October exam). The CGFNS address is 3624 Market St., Philadelphia, PA 19104.

After obtaining a CGFNS certificate, the employing hospital will file for an H1 visa on behalf of the foreign nurse. The Bureau of Immigration and Naturalization Service returns the visa to the hospital, which will send it to the nearest U.S. embassy for delivery to the nurse. Because this visa restricts the holder to working at only one hospital in the United States, a new H1 visa must be obtained if the nurse wishes to work in another hospital or health care facility. Before coming to the United States, the nurse should write to the appropriate State Board for information about obtaining a license and for an application to take the NCLEX at the next available opportunity. The foreign nurse graduate may then move to the United States and practice nursing, usually with some restrictions, until the next NCLEX examination is given. Although the NCLEX examination is identical throughout the states, each state grants a license (that is, the designation "Registered Nurse") based on the individual's score.

The NCLEX is a 2-day-long, multiple-choice examination that evaluates a nurse's ability to systematically analyze and conceptualize nursing care using the scientific method of problem solving commonly called the "nursing process." Successfully obtaining a minimum score on the examination enables the recipient to obtain a license to practice nursing in that state. Generally, once a license is obtained in one state, other states will recognize that license and grant their state license by endorsement. A nurse who wishes to relocate or move to another state (remember that a new H1 visa is required) should contact the State Board of Nursing of the prospective employer's state before the anticipated move to inquire about obtaining a license by endorsement. Requirements for licensure by endorsement vary and may change periodically, so it is important to obtain the most current information from the individual State Board of Nursing.

The H1 visa may be extended annually for a total of 5 years. A resident alien who wishes to remain in the United States beyond this period must apply for permanent residency.

A WORD FOR CANADIAN NURSES

Like the United States, each Canadian province has its own nurse practice act and laws that vary slightly from province to province. All provinces, except Prince Edward Island and Ontario, require nurses to join the provincial nursing association to obtain a license. The provincial nursing association requires successful completion of the CNATS. Several U.S. states also accept the CNATS, thus exempting those Canadians who wish to practice in those states from taking the NCLEX. Those states include:

Alabama	Mississippi
Alaska	Missouri
Arizona	New Mexico
Arkansas	North Dakota
California	Ohio
Delaware	Pennsylvania
Georgia	Rhode Island
Idaho	Tennessee
Kentucky	Utah
Maine	Wisconsin

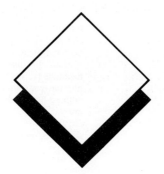

Appendix E
Commonly Used Abbreviations

NOTE: Abbreviations in common use can vary widely from place to place. Each institution's list of acceptable abbreviations is the best authority for its records.

° C	degrees Centigrade
° F	degrees Fahrenheit
μg	microgram
μm	micrometer
ʒ	dram
@	at
aa	of each
ABG	arterial blood gas
ac	before meals
ad lib	freely as desired
ADL	activities of daily living
Ag	silver, antigen
AIDS	acquired immunodeficiency syndrome
ALS	amyotrophic lateral sclerosis
AM	morning
ama	against medical advice
AMI	acute myocardial infarction
amp	ampule
ARC	AIDS-related complex
ARDS	adult respiratory distress syndrome
AS	aortic stenosis
ASD	atrial septal defect
Ba	barium
BE	barium enema
bid	two times a day
BM, bm	bowel movement
BMR	basal metabolic rate
BP	blood pressure
BPH	benign prostatic hypertrophy
BRP	bathroom privileges
BSA	body surface area
BUN	blood urea nitrogen
c̄	with
c/o	complains of
Ca	calcium, cancer, carcinoma
CAD	coronary artery disease
cap	capsule
CAT	computed axial tomography
cath.	catheter, catheterize
CBC	complete blood count
CBR	complete bed rest
CC	chief complaint
cc	cubic centimeter
CCU	coronary care unit, critical care unit
CDC	Centers for Disease Control
CEA	carcinoembryonic antigen
CFT	complement-fixation test
cg	centigram
CHF	congestive heart failure
CHO	carbohydrate

Cl	chlorine
cm	centimeter
cm³	cubic centimeter
CNS	central nervous system
CO	carbon monoxide
CO₂	carbon dioxide
COPD	chronic obstructive pulmonary disease
CPK	creatine phosphokinase
CPR	cardiopulmonary resuscitation
CSF	cerebrospinal fluid
CT	computed tomography
CVA	cerebrovascular accident, costovertebral angle
CVP	central venous pressure
D&C	dilatation and curettage
D5W	5% dextrose in water
db, dB	decibels
dc	discontinue
DIC	disseminated intravascular coagulation
diff	differential blood count
dil	dilute
DJD	degenerative joint disease
dl	deciliter
DM	diastolic murmur
DNR	do not resuscitate
DOE	dyspnea on exertion
dx, Dx	diagnosis
EBV	Epstein-Barr virus
ECF	extracellular fluid
ECG	electrocardiogram
ECT	electroconvulsive therapy
EDC	estimated date of confinement
EDD	estimated date of delivery
EEG	electroencephalogram
EKG	electrocardiogram
elix	elixer
EMG	electromyogram
ENG	electronystagmography
ER	emergency room
ERG	electroretinogram
ESR	erythrocyte sedimentation rate
ESRD	end-stage renal disease
EST	electroshock therapy
fʒ	fluid ounce
FANA	fluorescent antinuclear antibody test
Fe	iron
FEV	forced expiratory volume
FHR	fetal heart rate
FRC	functional residual capacity
FUO	fever of unknown origin
Fx, fx	fracture, fractional urine test

g, gm, Gm	gram
Gc, GC	gonococcus
GI	gastrointestinal
gr	grain
grav I, II, III, etc	pregnancy one, two, three, etc
gtt, gt	drop, drops
GTT	glucose tolerance test
GU	genitourinary
GYN, Gyn	gynecological
H₂O	water
h	hour
H⁺	hydrogen ion
h/o	history of
H&P	history and physical examination
HAV	hepatitis A virus
Hb	hemoglobin
HBAg	hepatitis B antigen
HBV	hepatitis B virus
Hct, HCT	hematocrit
Hg	mercury
Hgb	hemoglobin
HIV	human immunodeficiency (AIDS) virus
HLA	human lymphocyte antigen
hs	at bedtime
HSV	herpes simplex virus
I&O	intake and output
IC	inspiratory capacity
ICP	intracranial pressure
ICU	intensive care unit
IDDM	insulin-dependent diabetes mellitus
IE	immunoelectrophoresis
Ig	immunoglobulin
IgA, etc	immunoglobulin A, etc
IM	intramuscular
IOP	intraocular pressure
IPPB	intermittent positive pressure breathing
IV	intravenous
IVP	intravenous push; intravenous pyelogram
IVU	intravenous urogram
JRA	juvenile rheumatoid arthritis
K	potassium
kg	kilogram
KUB	kidney, ureters, and bladder (radiograph)
KVO	keep vein open
L	liter
L&A	light and accommodation
LBBB	left bundle branch block
LE	lupus erythematosus
LGV	lymphogranuloma venereum
LLL	left lower lobe
LLQ	left lower quadrant
LMP	last menstrual period
LNMP	last normal menstrual period
LP	lumbar puncture
LUL	left upper lobe
LUQ	left upper quadrant
LVH	left ventricular hypertrophy
m	meter
m, min, ♏	minim
MAP	mean arterial pressure
mgc	microgram
MCH	mean corpuscular hemoglobin
MCHC	mean corpuscular hemoglobin concentration
MCV	mean cell volume, mean corpuscular volume
mg	milligram
Mg	magnesium
MG	myasthenia gravis
MI	myocardial infarction
MICU	medical intensive care unit
ml	milliliter
mm	millimeter
mm³	cubic millimeter
mm Hg	millimeters of mercury
MRI	magnetic resonance imaging
MS	multiple sclerosis

MW	molecular weight
N	nitrogen
Na	sodium
NICU	neonatal intensive care unit
NIH	National Institutes of Health
nm	nanometer
NMR	nuclear magnetic resonance
NPO	nothing by mouth
NS	normal saline
O₂	oxygen
OD	right eye; optical density; overdose
OL	left eye
OOB	out of bed
ORIF	open reduction and internal fixation
OS	left eye
OT	occupational therapy
OTC	over-the-counter
oz, ℥	ounce
P&A	percussion and auscultation
Paco₂	partial pressure of carbon dioxide (arterial blood)
Pao₂	partial pressure of oxygen (arterial blood)
para I, II, etc	unipara, bipara, etc
PAT	paroxysmal atrial tachycardia
pc	after meals
PCG	phonocardiogram
Pco₂	partial pressure of carbon dioxide
PCP	pulmonary capillary pressure, phencyclidine
PCV	packed cell volume
PCWP	pulmonary capillary wedge pressure
PD	interpupillary distance; postural drainage
PE	pulmonary embolism, physical examination
PEEP	positive end expiratory pressure
PEG	pneumoencephalography
per	through, by way of
PERRLA	pupils equal, round, and reactive to light and accommodation
PET	positron emission tomography
PG	prostaglandin
pH	hydrogen ion concentration (acidity and alkalinity)
PID	pelvic inflammatory disease
PKU	phenylketonuria
PM	postmortem
PM	evening
PMS	premenstrual syndrome
PND	paroxysmal nocturnal dyspnea, postnasal drip
Po₂	partial pressure of oxygen
PO, po	orally
PPD	purified protein derivative
ppm	parts per million
prn	when required, as often as necessary
PT	physical therapy; prothrombin time
PTT	partial thromboplastin time
PUO	pyrexia of unknown origin
PVC	premature ventricular contraction
q	every
q2h	every 2 hours
q3h	every 3 hours
q4h	every 4 hours
qd	every day
qh	every hour
qid	four times a day
qn	every night
qod	every other day
qns	quantity not sufficient
R/O	rule out
RA	rheumatoid arthritis
RBBB	right bundle branch block
RBC	red blood cell; red blood count
RDA	recommended daily (dietary) allowance
RDS	respiratory distress syndrome
Rh +	positive Rh factor
Rh −	negative Rh factor
RHD	rheumatic heart disease
RLL	right lower lobe
RLQ	right lower quadrant

RML	right middle lobe		TAH	total abdominal hysterectomy
ROM	range of motion		TAT	tetanus antitoxin; thematic apperception test
ROS	review of systems		TB, TBC	tuberculosis
RS	Reiter's syndrome		TBG	thyroxin-binding globulin
RSV	Rous sarcoma virus		TG	triglyceride
RUL	right upper lobe		TIA	transient ischemic attack
RUQ	right upper quadrant		TIBC	total iron-binding capacity
Rx	take; treatment		tid	three times a day
s̄	without		TKO	to keep open
SB	sternal border		TLC	total lung capacity; thin-layer chromatography
SC	subcutaneous		TPN	total parenteral nutrition
sib.	sibling		TPR	temperature, pulse, and respirations
SICU	surgical intensive care unit		tr, tinct	tincture
SIDS	sudden infant death syndrome		TST	triple sugar iron test
Sig	write on label		UIBC	unsaturated iron-binding capacity
SLE	systemic lupus erythematosus		URI	upper respiratory infection
sol	solution, dissolved		UTI	urinary tract infection
sos	if necessary		V&T	volume and tension
sp. gr., SG, s.g.,	specific gravity		VC	vital capacity
SQ, subq	subcutaneous		VD	venereal disease
SR	sedimentation rate		VDA	visual discriminatory acuity
ss	half		VDH	valvular disease of the heart
SSS	sick sinus syndrome, specific soluble substance, short-stay surgery		VDRL	Venereal Disease Research Laboratory (test for syphilis)
stat	immediately		VS	vital signs
STD	sexually transmitted disease		VSD	ventricular septal defect
STS	serological test for syphilis		V_T	tidal volume
susp	suspension		W/V	weight/volume
T_3	triiodothyronine		WBC	white blood cell; white blood count
T_4	tetraiodothyronine		WNL	within normal limits
T&A	tonsillectomy and adenoidectomy		WR	Wasserman reaction
TAB	typhoid and paratyphoid A and B			

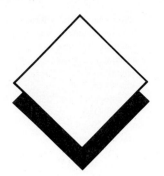

Index